P. E. S. PALMER · M. M. REEDER · The Imaging of Tropical Diseases

VOLUME 1

Springer

Berlin
Heidelberg
New York
Barcelona
Hong Kong
London
Milan
Paris
Singapore
Tokyo

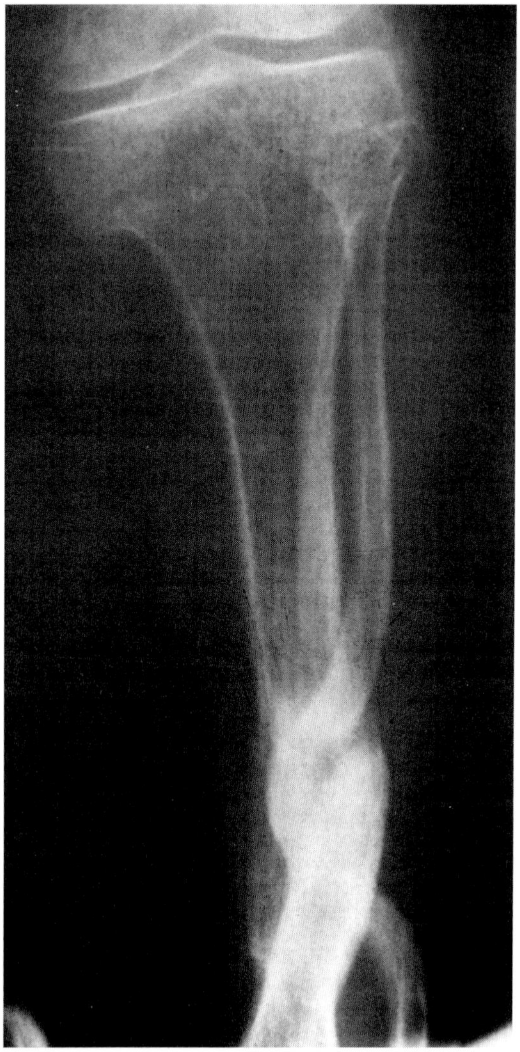

Ex Africa semper aliquid nova.
(Ascribed, perhaps incorrectly, to Pliny)

PHILIP E.S. PALMER · MAURICE M. REEDER

The Imaging of Tropical Diseases

With Epidemiological, Pathological and Clinical Correlation

VOLUME 1

Consulting Pathologist DANIEL H. CONNOR
Consulting Parasitologist IAN J. DUNN

Contributors
S.P. Bohrer · K.-H. Chang · D.H. Connor · I.J. Dunn · E.H.L. Gaensler
Y. Hiramatsu · J.-G. Im · B. Imalingat · J. Kendall · K. Kimura · D.B. Lewall · L.F. Mattoso
S. Mindel · R. Moncada · J.U.V. Monu · E.M. Moore · E. Palacios · P.E.S. Palmer
M.M. Reeder · P. Reeve · W. von Sinner · M. Stoopen · M.W. Wachira · S.J. Wambani

Springer

PHILIP E.S. PALMER, MD, FRCP, FRCR
Em. Professor of Radiology, University of California, Davis
Home address: 821 Miller Drive, Davis, CA 95616, USA

MAURICE M. REEDER, MD
Em. Professor of Radiology, University of Hawaii
Currently Adjunct Professor of Radiology
Uniformed Services University of the Health Sciences, Bethesda, MD 20814, USA
Home address: 12646 Travilah Road, Potomac, MD 20854, USA

2nd Edition (revised) of 'Radiology of Tropical Diseases', Maurice M. Reeder, Philip E.S. Palmer, published by
The Williams & Wilkins Company, Baltimore/London in 1981.

With 678 Figures in 2267 Separate Illustrations

ISBN 3-540-56028-9 Springer-Verlag Berlin Heidelberg New York

Library of Congress Cataloging-in-Publication Data
Palmer, Philip E.S. The Imaging of tropical diseases: with epidemiological, pathological, and clinical correlation/P.E.S. Palmer, M.M. Reeder. – 2nd, rev. ed. p. cm. Rev. ed. of: Radiology of tropical diseases/Maurice M. Reeder, Philip E.S. Palmer. © 1981. Includes bibliographical references and index.
ISBN 3-540-56028-9 (v. 1: alk. paper). – ISBN 3-540-62471-6 (v. 2: alk. paper)
1. Tropical medicine. 2. Diagnostic imaging. I. Reeder, Maurice M. (Maurice Merrick), 1933–. II. Reeder, Maurice M. (Maurice Merrick), 1933–. Radiology of tropical diseases. III. Title. [DNLM: 1. Tropical Medicine. 2. Diagnostic Imaging. 3. Radiography. WC 680 P1751 2001] RC961.5.P35 2001 616.9'883-DC21 DNLM/DLC
99-39417

Springer-Verlag Berlin Heidelberg New York
a member of BertelsmannSpringer Science+Business Media GmbH

Cover-Design: Erich Kirchner, Springer-Verlag, Heidelberg
Typesetting: K+V Fotosatz GmbH, Beerfelden
Printing and bookbinding: Stürtz AG, Würzburg

Printed on acid-free paper. SPIN 10039140 21/3130 ih – 5 4 3 2 1 0

Dedication

To our wives, Miep, Barbara, Norma, and Celina, without whose help, understanding, ... and patience, this book would never have been finished.

Foreword to the First Edition (1981)

Tropical radiology has been a stepchild of our specialty. It encompasses some of the most common diseases in the world, yet we seldom find them discussed in our literature. One reason for this paradox is that the affluent society of the temperate zones seldom suffers from tropical diseases, whereas the underprivileged tropical society has not had the luxury of adequate radiology or of a sufficiency of radiologists.

But the political and economic worlds are changing and with them the medical world. The underprivileged are demanding – and receiving – privileges, among which is the privilege of reasonable health care. Health organizations in the United States and United Nations, among others, are striving to control and prevent diseases in the Third World with some measure of success. A big and a little country, China and Israel, have managed to largely control their own parasitic diseases, setting an example for other nations to emulate. At the same time, certain tropical countries, specifically those in the Middle East, have prospered and can now afford, and hopefully will provide, better medical care. For these reasons, the incidence of tropical diseases in some parts of the tropics may be on the wane. Modern preventive medicine has come a long way, but there is still a long, arduous journey ahead.

Meanwhile, countless Arabs, Orientals, Caucasians and Blacks are traveling, and their microorganisms are traveling with them. As an example, I recently saw, in Cincinnati, a Vietnamese suffering from chronic smallpox osteomyelitis. (Incidentally, the roentgenograms were diagnostic.) At the same time, poverty, crowding, disease and drug addiction have made segments of our own privileged nontropical domain less privileged and ripe for attack by opportunistic foreign organisms that are lurking about looking for new bodies to inhabit. There is indication that the incidence of tropical disease is on the rise in the United States and Europe, as yet only slightly.

Great advances in the diagnosis, treatment, and prevention of tropical diseases have been made in recent years. These measures are now so effective that it is a needless tragedy for a child to be ravaged by chronic malnutrition from an unrecognized helminthic infestation, or for a patient to die of undiagnosed amebic liver abscess. It is essential today that every physician knows something about the tropical diseases that he or she may occasionally encounter, and where to quickly find appropriate detailed information.

Apart from all this, the roentgenology of tropical diseases is stimulating from an intellectual standpoint; it offers fascinating visual images of advanced disease, and an exciting challenge to decipher unfamiliar shadows and reconstruct their pathogenesis. It is (and should be) a matter of great satisfaction to the radiologist to be the first to recognize the presence of a serious tropical disease, such as amebiasis, and then to have the diagnosis verified and the patient cured.

My own tenuous role in the production of this book has been that of a catalyst. More than 15 years ago I heard a most fascinating lecture on African tropical diseases by a British colonial radiologist named Philip Palmer. A few years later, I was planning an issue of the journal *Seminars in Roentgenology* on diffuse diseases of the colon. In scouting about for authors of the various sections, I encountered a problem: Who would do "Tropical Diseases"? Palmer was still in Africa and, since communication and deadlines would be too difficult, I couldn't enlist him. So I looked about for an American expert on the subject, to no avail. It occurred to me that the Armed Forces Institute of Pathology (AFIP) must have considerable material on parasitic diseases. So, on my next consultant visit to the Radiology Section there, I recruited Maurice Reeder, a staff member, who knew only a little more about the subject than I, to write the article. Overriding his protests, I predicted that much of the material he would need was in the AFIP files.

Reeder did his homework and found my prediction false. He then went on a collector's hunt, scrounging for material and begging for cases from colleagues all over the world. He also reviewed the literature, perusing many exotic journals and books. Eventually he came up with a first class article on tropical intestinal diseases. I used him again for an article on tropical diseases of bone with similar results. In this gathering process, much more material came in than he needed, so, perforce, Reeder became a specialist in tropical radiology.

One of Reeder's many donors was Palmer, who subsequently moved to the United States. The two men finally met and continued their work together. This book is a culmination of that collaboration, and incorporates Palmer's 15-year experience in Africa and subsequent return visits, together with Reeder's experience in the U.S. Army, including 5 years in the Far East and Hawaii and 13 years at the Walter Reed Hospital and the Armed Forces Institute of Pathology in Washington, D.C., seeing patients and their diseases from around the world. Joining them in this endeavor are Herman Zaiman, a renowned parasitologist recently turned radiologist, and A.C. Johnson, once Chairman of Radiology at Christian Medical College in Vellore, India, and now residing in the United States. "Johnny" Johnson is not only an expert on tropical diseases, but also on snake swallowers. He has a spectacular roentgen movie of snakes swimming about in the stomach of a Hindu fakir that will make us both wealthy if he will only let me be the distributing agent.

The Radiology of Tropical Diseases contains carefully selected material culled from the extensive personal collections amassed by its authors, and from the literature. The book caps a long, arduous, and, I might add, successful effort to create an inclusive treatise on the subject. It will serve as a quick, reliable, unobtrusive consultant, not only for the radiologist, but also for other physicians. It is a veritable encyclopedia of parasitology and the clinical, roentgenologic, and pathologic aspects of tropical diseases. It is extremely well illustrated. If "a picture says a thousand words," this book speaks millions.

BENJAMIN FELSON, MD

Professor of Radiology
University of Cincinnati
School of Medicine
Cincinnati, Ohio

Preface

It was the late Professor Benjamin Felson who was the catalyst for the first edition of this book. We have not changed or added to the Foreword which he was kind enough to write when, after about ten years of work, the book came to publication. It was Ben Felson's great friend and colleague, Professor Harold Jacobson, who enthusiastically persuaded us that we should update the book and incorporate all the advances which have occurred since 1981. He freely gave to us his unparalleled experience and advice in the early stages. We assured our new publisher, Springer-Verlag, that this time it would only take a few years before we would be ready ... that was ten years ago.

We have learned a lot in that time: while much is unchanged, tropical medicine has in some ways become quite different. We had been fascinated as we wrote the first edition and reviewed a vast amount of material, to find how much diseases vary in different parts of the world. We learned then that there are many diseases that affect untold millions of men, women, and children and yet are often poorly understood. We found it difficult to reconcile the differing opinions of "tropical pathologists" and other experts and tried to take the middle view when differences seemed insoluble. None of that has changed. A few, but very few diseases are lessening. Smallpox has, we hope, disappeared entirely. Onchocerciasis, poliomyelitis, and perhaps guinea worm (dracunculiasis), filariasis, and even leprosy may soon be under control. There are successful vaccines for measles, typhoid, and pneumococcal and other infections, and if these vaccines can be delivered worldwide then these diseases, too, will become less important. Many infectious and parasitic diseases can now be successfully treated with new drugs. But at the other end of the scale, tuberculosis and malaria have spread and become more resistant to treatment. Malaria kills more than 2.7 million people every year, 1 million in Africa alone. And, as another example, the various forms of schistosomiasis infect the same number of people as the whole population of the United States. AIDS has become a major worldwide scourge and is changing the lifestyle, longevity, and population statistics of many countries. With it have come infections which previously were seldom seen in the tropics and even less often in the rest of the world. Another major source of injury and death is trauma, especially from motor vehicles; this is increasing rather than lessening. Malnourishment has brought with it a toll of infectious and chronic disease: worldwide, pneumonia is the cause of death of about one-third of the many thousands of children who do not live to be five years old.

Tropical diseases are spreading into the subtropics and temperate climates. Tourism and military intervention or rescue have rapidly increased, and many people visiting or returning by air or sea bring with them diseases previously known only in the tropics. Millions have been forced to migrate and whole families of refugees have spread infections into different climates: the climates themselves may be warming, allowing these tropical infections and parasites to survive in previously hostile surroundings. And, in the tropics, the many recent diagnostic and therapeutic advances are only too often unavailable to those who need them most.

Images from ultrasonography and computed tomography were just appearing when we wrote the first edition. Now both, particularly ultrasonography, are readily available over much of the world, and magnetic resonance imaging is adding further information. Although applied less widely, various radionuclides are providing helpful images of some tropical diseases. One of the main reasons for this 2nd edition has been the need to bring all these images together. Much that we knew only from autopsy and histopathological studies can now be seen with imaging. In many patients this has improved the accuracy of diagnosis. It is not really that tropical diseases have changed intrinsically, but that we can see and understand them so much better, particularly those which attack the central nervous system, abdominal and pelvic organs, and soft tissues, which could not be imaged successfully before.

But the growth of knowledge has not only been in imaging. Enormous strides have been made in unravelling the natural history of many tropical diseases: new laboratory techniques are available for the differential diagnosis of many of the infectious diseases, and there is a better understanding of genetic variations and of the effect of the environment, including nutrition, on patients with these diseases. The information gained from "geographic pathology" (now often known as geomedicine) has increased and includes far more than the incidence of cancer, which had provided the original impetus. Learning of all these advances and concentrating on those of importance to diagnostic imaging has meant that the completion of the second edition has taken much longer than we had anticipated.

We have again been extremely fortunate to have very experienced colleagues to guide us. Dr. Daniel Connor has for decades been an acknowledged expert on the pathology and indeed the clinical aspects and geography of tropical diseases. His own contributions to this field are unique and based on many years of personal experience in tropical Africa as well as at the AFIP and elsewhere. We were fortunate to be joined by Dr. Ian Dunn, from the University of British Columbia, who originally trained and had wide experience in parasitology but later became a radiologist. Virtually all that is written in this book has been reviewed by both Dan Connor and Ian Dunn and they have shared their knowledge with us. In the field of ultrasonography, we have had the advice and help of two experienced tropical sonologists, Dr. Sam Mindel, who for years was on the faculty of the University in Harare, Zimbabwe and Dr. M. Wachira, former Chairman of Radiology at the University of Nairobi, Kenya. As is shown by the list of contributors, we have worked with many other colleagues on different chapters: they all provided us with information and illustrations based on their own wide personal experiences, and added immensely to our knowledge.

The format of the book remains as it was in the first edition, combining the epidemiology, pathology, laboratory and clinical information to provide the background without which diagnostic images cannot be fully understood. We have tried to simplify and record the pathophysiology of these tropical diseases because many radiologists and other physicians do not have ready or immediate access to all this information. As in the first edition, we have seldom attempted to offer advice on treatment because it is changing and improving rapidly and is usually well beyond our personal expertise. But once the diagnosis has been established, it should not be difficult to learn of up-to-date treatment: imaging then can often record progress … or failure.

We still owe a considerable debt to those who helped us with the first edition and we have built on the work of Dr. Herman Zaiman and Dr. A.C. Johnson. While most of the chapters have been rewritten, they incorporate much of what we wrote before, because the underlying basics of tropical diseases have not changed.

Credit has been given throughout the text for numerous illustrations of gross specimens and photomicrographs from the collection of the AFIP. Many parasitology illustrations from the first edition were provided by Dr. Zaiman. Others for this second edition have come from Drs. Connor and Dunn; this has allowed us to present excellent radiological, pathological, and parasitology correlations, making it much easier to understand and then interpret the images.

Because their contribution was and is so valuable, it is a pleasure to repeat our acknowledgment to those who gave us helpful material and advice for the first edition; many have generously helped us again. We have attempted to list all those who assisted with this new edition and gave us pathological, clinical, and radiographic illustrations, but we suspect that we may not have succeeded completely because we have received so much help from so many throughout the world that some will inevitably have been overlooked. For this we must apologize: we have at times been overwhelmed with information and images, and it is misplaced records, not ingratitude, which must be blamed if we have failed to acknowledge help.

Bearing patiently and cheerfully with the vicissitudes of production, as well as the delays and problems which we gave them, have been our friends and colleagues at Springer-Verlag, who have taken all the information, illustrations, and bibliography and welded it into a whole. Inevitably we have added late paragraphs, new images, or new references well after claiming to have "finished" a particular chapter or section. We have again received skilled help from the Department of Medical Illustration of the University of California at Davis, and have benefitted from the ability of Springer-Verlag to take a vast number of images in different formats, including prints, negatives, scans, slides, and original radiographs, and from them produce high-quality illustrations. Their team has been led by Dr. Ute Heilmann, who has been responsible for the project from the very beginning. The medical desk editor, Ms. Ursula Davis, has provided immense support, not only by her knowledge but also through her willing understanding of the difficulties and constraints which we faced.

Mr. Rick mills has been our superb copy editor and Ms. Ingrid Haas had the arduous task of designing and laying out the book. Both have added the wisdom of their years in the publication business and have worked closely with us to obtain the best end result.

Mrs. Roberta Howering in California has typed about half the chapters in the book and retyped them many times until we were all satisfied: they often then had to be retyped again when some new information became available. Her willing help has been much appreciated.

And in the end, we find it difficult to improve on the final paragraph of the Preface we wrote for the first edition: "We have, of course, learned much in the process of putting this book together and, perhaps even more obviously, we have discovered how little we actually know and how much more there is to be learned concerning the radiology (*imaging*) of tropical diseases. Hopefully this book will be a stimulus to others to correct or amplify our thoughts and thus add to our knowledge. Radiology (*imaging*) has much to offer everyone, not least in tropical and developing countries. It does not have to be sophisticated and complex to bring benefit to millions of patients. More important is its contribution to the understanding of diseases, the clinical syndromes that result and the radiographic (*imaging*) changes which they cause. We hope that in the immense field of tropical medicine this book will play some small part: there is still so much more to do and, so far, so little done".

PHILIP E.S. PALMER

While wholeheartedly endorsing this Preface, which my friend and long time colleague, Philip Palmer, wrote for us both, I would like to add some personal remarks.

From the earliest days of man's habitation of the earth he has been forced to adapt to an ever-changing and often hostile environment. Paramount among these adaptations has been his struggle through the ages with the countless parasites and infectious organisms passed down by his animal ancestors. The fact that he has survived and even prospered in the face of such adversities is a tribute to his tenacity and adaptability. Even so, after 6000 years of recorded history, and considering the enormous strides mankind has made in the past century in the areas of medicine and public health, one's complacency must be staggered by the immense toll of human life and suffering still inflicted today by these same ageless organisms, particularly in the tropical regions of the world.

The astute physician in the modern era must recognize not only diseases endemic to his locale, but also those that can be imported from faraway places. Extensive civilian travel and military deployment, as well as increasing immigration, have brought millions of North Americans and Europeans into potential contact with parasitic and other tropical diseases. Most of these ailments require special alertness on the part of the clinician and the radiologist since they are often initially misdiagnosed, simulating other more common indigenous illnesses. In many of these diseases an unfortunate delay in institution of appropriate treatment prolongs illness and may prevent a complete cure or even contribute to a fatal outcome. Sadly, the vast majority of Tropical Medicine and Tropical Pathology textbooks and articles fail to mention the important role that conventional radiology and the modern imaging modalities of computed tomography, magnetic resonance imaging, and ultrasonography play in the diagnosis and, in some diseases like cystic echinococcosis, even the treatment of these maladies. Hopefully, this book will serve as a "wake up call" to all those who write about, and more importantly, treat tropical and parasitic diseases that modern radiology has a pivotal role to play in the diagnosis of over 60 of these diseases that affect more than two-fifths of the world's population.

I want to express my sincere appreciation to our contributing authors for their superb contributions now and in the past to the understanding of the myriad of parasitic diseases which continue to ravage over two billion of the world's populace even as we begin a new millennium in the history of mankind. To them and to my esteemed colleague, Dr. Philip Palmer, and the other great British radiologists of a prior era, Professor Sir Howard Middlemiss and Professor Peter Cockshott, who elaborated so brilliantly the radiological aspects of so many tropical diseases found on the continent of Africa and elsewhere, we all owe a great debt of gratitude which will only be repaid as we continue to make significant advances in the eradication of these timeless illnesses in the next century.

MAURICE M. REEDER

About the Authors

Dr. Philip E.S. Palmer was educated in England and gained his medical and radiological training at London University. He practiced diagnostic radiology in England for 8 years and then spent the next 15 years in Africa, first as a government radiologist in Matebeleland, in the then Federation of Rhodesia and Nyasaland, and then for 4 years as Professor and Chairman of Radiology at the University of Capetown, South Africa. During those years he traveled widely, especially in Africa, visiting, lecturing, and studying at almost all of the universities south of the Sahara. He also lectured in Cairo and Alexandria in Egypt, in Ethiopia and at many of the other major African medical centers.

He was an invited speaker at conferences in Jamaica and many major American universities, usually choosing tropical diseases as his subject. He was then appointed Professor of Radiology at the University of Pennsylvania and after 2 years became the first Professor and Director of Diagnostic Radiology at the University of California, Davis. He later became Chairman. He has been an invited speaker at many American universities and radiological societies, the American Society of Tropical Medicine, the AFIP, and many universities and international and national meetings in different parts of the world.

Dr. Palmer was appointed more than 20 years ago as an Advisor and Consultant to the World Health Organization Headquarters in Geneva, Switzerland. Since then he has often been asked to advise and teach in small and large hospitals and medical centers in the Pacific and Southeast Asian, European, African, Eastern Mediterranean (Middle East), and American Regions of the WHO. He has chaired or been a member of numerous WHO Expert committees and is editor, senior author, or co-author of the popular WHO Manuals of Ultrasound, Radiological Interpretation, Darkroom Technique and Radiographic Technique. These are available world-wide in more than 11 languages. He was for many years a member of the International Education Committees of both the International Society of Radiology and the Radiological Society of North America. He spent sabbatical years working and teaching in East and Southern Africa. He has been an examiner for the specialist degrees in Radiology for universities and colleges in West, East, and South Africa, as well as being an editor, guest editor, or reviewer for several journals. His publications include more than 220 articles in peer-reviewed journals, numerous textbook chapters, including contributions to textbooks of tropical diseases and parasitology. Dr. Palmer is an elected Honorary Fellow of the Romanian Society of Radiology and Nuclear Medicine, and of the West African and East African Radiological Societies. In 1993 he received the German International Roentgen Award (Roentgen Plakette) and in 1996 was the first Antoine Beclere Lecturer of the International Society of Radiology, at their meeting in Beijing, China.

Dr. Palmer is currently Emeritus Professor of Radiology at the University of California, Davis, and continues to be an Advisor to the World Health Organization.

In 2000 the President of the Radiological Society of North America honored him with a Special Presidential Award, for his 'Significant Contributions to the field of Radiology and the Radiological Sciences'.

Dr. Maurice M. Reeder was educated at Loyola College and the University of Maryland School of Medicine in Baltimore, and then spent 20 years as a career officer (Colonel) in the U.S. Army Medical Corps. He has worked as a radiologist in East Asia for 3 years, and for 3 years was a staff radiologist at the Registry of Radiologic Pathology at the Armed Forces Institute of Pathology in Washington, D.C. There he began to assemble what has become a vast collection of radiological and pathological material on tropical diseases, contributed by military and civilian radiologists from all over the world. There are currently over 4000 images of tropical diseases covering more than 50 diseases in this collection. He has lectured and written extensively on this subject, and has become well known as an expert in all aspects of tropical imaging. He has visited and taught in South America, Mexico, Canada, the Caribbean,

Europe and Asia and has had continuing experience in tropical diseases as Chief of the Department of Radiology at the Walter Reed Army Medical Center and Radiology Consultant to the Army Surgeon General from 1972 to 1977 and as Chairman of the Department of Radiology at the University of Hawaii School of Medicine and Radiology Consultant at Tripler Army Medical Center in Honolulu from 1978 to 1997. He is presently Adjunct Professor of Radiology at the Uniformed Services University of the Health Sciences in Bethesda, Maryland and is developing a permanent collection of Tropical Imaging for the U.S. Military with the 8000 image Reeder and Palmer collection as its core, as well as initiating a proposed International Registry of Tropical Imaging housed at USUHS.

Dr. Reeder is a Fellow of the American College of Radiology and a member of seven other Radiological and Tropical Disease Societies. He is the author of Reeder and Felson's "Gamuts in Radiology" (4 editions and CD-Rom) and of over 60 journal articles and book-chapters. He has lectured at over 200 universities, meetings, and conferences in different parts of the world.

Born in Canada, where he spent his early years, *Dr. Daniel H. Connor* graduated from Queen's University, receiving his M. D., C. M. in 1953. He trained at Emergency Hospital (now Washington Hospital Center) and did residency training in pathology at Emergency Hospital and George Washington University. He served in the US Army as Chief, Laboratory Service, Irwin Army Hospital and as Chief, Laboratory Service, 47th Field Evacuation Hospital. On leaving the Army he joined the permanent civilian staff of the Armed Forces Institute of Pathology, becoming Chairman, Department of Infectious and Parasitic Diseases and Registrar, Registry of Geographic Pathology in 1970. He continued in these positions until his retirement from Federal Service in 1987. Beginning January 1988 he has been visiting Professor, Department of Pathology at Georgetown University.

Dr. Connor's research interests have focused on infectious, parasitic, and tropical diseases. In pursuing these interests he has lived in tropical Africa for 5 years while studying onchocerciasis, buruli ulcer, endomyocardial fibrosis, and other diseases of the African hinterland. He has authored and co-authored 180 published papers and a variety of chapters for textbooks, and he co-authored and co-edited two definitive texts – *Pathology of Tropical and Extraordinary Diseases* (American Registry of Pathology, 1976) and *Pathology of Infectious Diseases* (Appleton & Lange 1997). He has served the World Health Organization as a consultant, temporary advisor, and as a member of various expert committees and scientific working groups. He served also the American Board of Pathology from 1972 through 1981, first as a consultant and then as a member of the test committee on medical microbiology, and he continues to serve the board as consultant. Other services include Chairman, U.S. National Committee, International Council of Societies of Pathology and the editorial boards of two peer-reviewed internationally orientated scientific journals.

Teaching has played a prominent role in his career. He has trained research fellows supported by the World Health Organization and the Pan American Health Organization as well as civilian consultants and scientists on sabbatical leave. These include Deans, Chairmen and distinguished scientists in Western countries, Asia, and Africa. At Georgetown University he received the best teaching award three times.

Ian J. Dunn became interested in tropical diseases while he was an undergraduate studying zoology at the University of British Columbia. In 1979 he went to graduate school at the University of Toronto, at first in the Masters course, then to complete his PhD in Parasitology in 1984.

Stimulated by his lecturers, he became interested in teaching and, while studying Diagnostic Parasitology, worked in the Tropical Disease Unit of the Toronto General Hospital. There he joined clinical teaching rounds in tropical medicine and gave laboratory courses at the University of Toronto.

He gained his medical degree from the University of Calgary and at the same time took a postdoctoral fellowship in intestinal physiology in the Intestinal Disease Research Unit. In 1986/1987 he was awarded a Health-Exchange Scholarship, which allowed him to study tropical diseases at the internationally recognized Christian Medical College in Vellore, India. He also spent time at Tribhuvan University in Kathmandu, Nepal and was able to visit a rural hospital in Pokhara. His scholarship travels ended at the Hospital for Tropical Diseases in Bangkok.

His radiology training was at the Dalhousie University in Halifax, Nova Scotia, and was followed by a Fellowship in abdominal imaging and intervention at the University of British Columbia, with additional training in angiography and cardiac imaging at the University of Toronto.

He is currently a Clinical Assistant Professor in the Radiology Department of the University of British Columbia and a consultant radiologist in Vancouver. He continues to write on parasitology and imaging. In July 2000 he moves to appointments in Calgary, Alberta.

List of Contributors (Volume 1 and 2)

STANLEY P. BOHRER, MD
Department of Radiology
Bowman Gray School of Medicine
of Wake Forest University
Medical Center Boulevard
Winston-Salem, NC 27157-1088, USA
Formerly: University College Hospital
Ibadan, Nigeria

KEE-HYUN CHANG, MD
Professor of Radiology, Director of Neuroradiology
Seoul National University Hospital
28 Yongon-dong, Chongro-gu
Seoul 110-744, Korea

DANIEL H. CONNOR, MD
Department of Pathology
Georgetown University, School of Medicine
Washington, DC 20007, USA
Home address: 11351 Morning Gate Drive
Rockville, MD 20852, USA

IAN J. DUNN, PhD, MD, FRCP(C)
Clinical Assistant Professor
University of British Columbia
Burnaby General Hospital
3935 Kincaid Street
Burnaby, BC, Canada V5G 2X6

ERIK H. L. GAENSLER, MD
Clinical Associate Professor
Department of Radiology
University of California
San Francisco, CA 94143, USA

YOSHIHIRO HIRAMATSU, MD
Professor and Chairman
Department of Radiology, Ohashi Hospital
Toho University School of Medicine
2-17-6 Ohashi, Meguro-ku
Tokyo 153, Japan

JUNG-GI IM, MD
Professor of Radiology
Director of Thoracic Radiology
Department of Radiology
Seoul National University Hospital
28 Yongon-Dong, Chongro-gu
Seoul 110-744, Korea

BENJAMIN IMALINGAT, MB, M. Med. (R)
Department of Radiology
The Kenyatta National Hospital, University of Nairobi
P.O. Box 19676
Nairobi, Kenya

JOAN KENDALL, MD
Department of Radiology
Queen's Medical Center
1301 Punchbowl Street
Honolulu, HI 96813, USA

KENJI KIMURA, MD
Director of Imaging
Hospital Los Angeles
Mexico, D. F., Mexico

DAVID B. LEWALL, MD
Comes de Rull, Casa C
Sispony, Andorra
Formerly: Chairman
Department of Medical Imaging KFSH and RC
Riyadh, Saudi Arabia

LUIZ FELIPPE MATTOSO, MD
Chief, Clinica Radiologica Luiz Felippe Mattoso Ltda.
Rua Bambina, 56
Rio de Janeiro, Brazil

SAM MINDEL, MB, BCh
2 Blandford Avenue
Oxford OX2 8DY, United Kingdom
Formerly: The University Hospital
Harare, Zimbabwe

ROGELIO MONCADA, MD, FACR
Professor of Radiology
Loyola University Medical Center
2160 S. First Avenue
Maywood, IL 60153-5500, USA

JOHNNY U.V. MONU, MD
Associate Professor of Radiology
Co-Head, Muskuloskeletal Imaging
University of Rochester School of Medicine
601 Elmwood Avenue
Rochester, NY 14642, USA

ELIZABETH M. MOORE, MD
Professor of Radiology
University of California Medical Center
Stockton Boulevard
Sacramento, CA 95817, USA

ENRIQUE PALACIOS, MD, FACR
Professor of Clinical Radiology
Louisiana State University, Health Center
1542 Tulane Avenue
New Orleans, LA 70112, USA

PHILIP E.S. PALMER, MD, FRCP, FRCR
Em. Professor of Radiology
University of California, Davis
Home address: 821 Miller Drive
Davis, CA 95616, USA

MAURICE M. REEDER, MD, FACR
Em. Professor of Radiology, University of Hawaii
Adjunct Professor of Radiology USUHS
Bethesda, MD 20814, USA
Home address: 12646 Travilah Road
Potomac, MD 20854, USA

PAUL REEVE, MB, MRCP (U.K.)
Specialist Physician
Health Waikato Ltd., Taumarunui Hospital
Private Bag 1002
Taumarunui, New Zealand
Formerly: Malwai and Vanuatu

WALTHER VON SINNER, PhD, MD
The Georgian Condo, Apt. 903
Collins Avenue 1621
Miami Beach, FL 33193, USA
Formerly: Head, Thoracic Radiology
KFSH and RC, MBC #28
Riyadh, Saudi Arabia

MIGUEL STOOPEN, MD
Editor-in-Chief, Mexican Journal of Radiology
Mexico, D.F., Mexico

M.W. WACHIRA, MB, M. Med. (R)
Department of Diagnostic Radiology
College of Health Sciences, Faculty of Medicine
Kenyatta National Hospital, University of Nairobi
P.O. Box 19676
Nairobi, Kenya

S.J. WAMBANI, MB, M. Med. (R)
Department of Diagnostic Radiology
College of Health Sciences, Faculty of Medicine
Kenyatta National Hospital, University of Nairobi
P.O. Box 19676
Nairobi, Kenya

Contributors to the First Edition

HERMAN ZAIMAN, MD
Radiologist and Parasitologist
Valley City, ND, USA
Formerly: Assistant Professor of Parasitology
Albert Einstein College of Medicine
New York, NY, USA

A. CHANDRAHASAN JOHNSON, MB, PHD, FRCR
Tulsa, OK, USA
Formerly: Chairman of Radiology
Christian Medical College
Vellore, Madras, India

With special thanks to

HAROLD G. JACOBSON, MD, FACR
Em. Professor of Radiology
Montefiore Medical Center
Bronx, NY 10463, USA

Contents (Volume 1 and 2)

Differential Diagnosis Index of Tropical Diseases

These lists refer only to the *major* diseases affecting each organ or system and are not meant to be exhaustive. When searching for the differential diagnosis of an abnormal finding on an image, use also Chapter 43, describing the variations in malignant neoplastic diseases in the tropics, or the similar Chapter 44, describing the variations in nonmalignant diseases. Both these chapters follow an anatomical format. The numbers after the individual diseases refer to the appropriate chapters. AIDS (8) has not been included in the lists.
The lists are in random order and do not in any way suggest the relative risks or frequencies of the various diseases. This is described in the specific chapters.

Abnormalities of the Alimentary Tract

A. Esophagus
Schistosomiasis (2)
Chagas' disease (4)
Tuberculosis (5)
Fungus diseases, especially candidiasis (6)
Malignant disease (43)
Corrosive strictures, hiatus hernia, achalasia (44)

B. Stomach
Schistosomiasis (2)
Tuberculosis (5)
Fungus diseases, especially candidiasis (6)
Ascariasis (10)
Anisakiasis (11)
Strongyloidiasis (13)
Malignant disease (43)
Burkitt's lymphoma (41)
Peptic ulcer disease; gastric outlet obstruction; hiatus hernia (44)

C. Duodenum and small bowel
Amebiasis (1)
Schistosomiasis (2)
Chagas' disease (4)
Tuberculosis (5)
Fungus diseases, especially candidiasis/histoplasmosis capsulatum (6)
Taeniasis (tapeworm) (7)
Giardiasis (9)
Ascariasis (10)
Anisakiasis (11)
Hookworm disease (12)
Strongyloidiasis (13)
Angiostrongyliasis costaricensis (13)
Intestinal capillariasis (14)
Tropical sprue; kwashiorkor (16)
Typhoid and paratyphoid fever (15)
Salmonella infections (15)
Malignant disease (43)
Burkitt's lymphoma (41)
Kaposi's sarcoma (42)
Crohn's disease (44)
Intestinal obstruction, intussusception, small bowel volvulus, hernia, obstructed hernia (44)

D. Colon
Amebiasis (1)
Schistosomiasis (2)
Chagas' disease (4)
Tuberculosis (5)
Fungus diseases, especially actinomycosis (6)
Ascariasis (10)
Strongyloidiasis (13)
Angiostrongyliasis costaricensis (13)
Salmonella infections (15)
Trichuriasis (17)
Bacillary dysentery (19)
Lymphogranuloma venereum (20)
Helminthoma (18)
Malignant disease (43)
Crohn's disease (44)
Ulcerative colitis (44)
Diverticulosis and diverticulitis (44)
Intestinal obstruction, intussusception, sigmoid volvulus, hernia, obstructed hernia (44)
Polyps (2/42/44)

E. Rectum and anus
Amebiasis (1)
Schistosomiasis (2)
Chagas' disease (4)
Tuberculosis (5)

Trichuriasis (17)
Bacillary dysentery (19)
Lymphogranuloma venereum (20)
Malignant disease (43)
Hemorrhoids, fissures, strictures (44)
Rectovaginal fistulae (1/6/20/44)
Ulcerative colitis (44)

F. Liver
Amebiasis (1)
Schistosomiasis (2)
Hydatid disease (3)
Tuberculosis (5)
Fungus diseases, especially histoplasmosis, actinomycosis (6)
Ascariasis (10)
Clonorchiasis, opisthorchiasis, and other liver fluke diseases (21)
Oriental cholangiohepatitis (21)
Malignant disease - hepatoma (43)
Burkitt's lymphoma (41)
Pentastomiasis (28)
Toxoplasmosis (45)
Kala-azar (46)
Kwashiorkor (16)
Portal hypertension/cirrhosis (2/44)

G. Gallbladder and biliary tract
Ascariasis (10)
Clonorchiasis, opisthorchiasis, and other liver fluke diseases (21)
Oriental cholangiohepatitis (21)
Biliary calculi (especially in the hemoglobinopathies) (31/44)

H. Jaundice (Unusual causes)
Hydatid disease (3)
Ascariasis (10)
Clonorchiasis (21)
Oriental cholangiohepatitis (21)
Calculi (44)

I. Spleen
Schistosomiasis (2)
Hydatid disease (3)
Tuberculosis (5)
Typhoid and paratyphoid fever (15)
Melioidosis (23)
Hemoglobinopathies (31)
Malignant disease (lymphoma) (41/43)
Pentastomiasis (28)
Kala-azar (46)
Tropical splenomegaly syndrome (44/46)
Tropical splenic abscess (44/46)
Malaria (46)

J. Pancreas
Carcinoma (43)
Pancreatitis (44)
Pancreatic lithiasis (44)

Respiratory Tract

A. Nasopharynx, mouth, hypopharynx and trachea
Fungus diseases, especially mucormycosis, phycomycosis, rhinosporidiosis, rhinoentomophthoromycosis (6)
Yaws and syphilis (35)
Rhinoscleroma (38)
Cancrum oris (noma) (39)
Malignant disease/postnasal carcinoma (43)
Burkitt's lymphoma (41)

B. Lungs
Amebiasis (1)
Schistosomiasis (2)
Hydatid disease (3)
Tuberculosis (5)
Fungus diseases (6)
Ascariasis (10)
Hookworm disease (12)
Capillariasis philippinensis (14)
Strongyloidiasis (13)
Paragonimiasis (22)
Melioidosis (23)
Plague (24)
Tropical eosinophilia (26)
Malignant disease, primary or metastatic (43)
Pentastomiasis (28)
Gnathostomiasis (46)
Malaria (pulmonary edema and shock lung) (46)
Unusual pneumonias (measles, whooping cough, blackfat lipid pneumonia) (44)
Bronchiectasis (44)

C. Mediastinum, pleura and chest wall
Amebiasis (1)
Hydatid disease (3)
Tuberculosis (5)
Fungus diseases, especially actinomycosis/nocardiosis (6)
Cysticercosis (7)
Paragonimiasis (22)
Melioidosis (23)
Plague (24)
Dracunculiasis (guinea worm) (27)
Pentastomiasis (28)
Malignant disease (41/42/43)
Rib and pleural lesions (43/44/46)

Cardiovascular System

A. Heart (25)
Amebiasis (1)
Hydatid disease (3)
Chagas' disease (4)
Tuberculosis (5)
Endomyocardial fibrosis (25)
Aneurysms (subvalvular or idiopathic aortic) (25)
Cardiomegaly, idiopathic/puerperal (25)
Idiopathic aortitis (25)
Hemoglobinopathies (31)
Burkitt's lymphoma (41)
Cysticercosis (7)
Kwashiorkor and malnutrition (16)
Hypertension (idiopathic) (25/44);
see also Schistosomiasis (2)

B. Pericardial effusions
Amebiasis (1)
Hydatid disease (3)
Tuberculosis (5)
Endomyocardial fibrosis (25)
Hemoglobinopathies (31)
Kaposi's sarcoma (42)
Rheumatic/viral (25/44)

C. Aorta, pulmonary arteries and peripheral arteries and veins
Schistosomiasis (2)
Idiopathic arteritis, aneurysms (25)
Pulmonary embolus and infarction (44)
Pulmonary hypertension (2/25/44)
Peripheral vascular disease, idiopathic gangrene, varicose veins (25/44)

Genitourinary Tract

A. Kidneys
Schistosomiasis (2)
Hydatid disease (3)
Tuberculosis (5)
Fungus diseases (especially candidiasis) (6)
Idiopathic arteritis (25)
Filariasis (with chyluria) (26)
Hemoglobinopathies (papillary necrosis) (31)
Malignant disease (43)
Burkitt's lymphoma (41)
Malaria (46)
Calculi (44)

B. Ureters and bladder
Schistosomiasis (2)
Hydatid disease (3)
Tuberculosis (5)
Fungus diseases (especially candidiasis) (6)
Malignant disease (43)
Calculi (44)
Calcification (2/5/44)

C. Urethra, vagina, penis, seminal vesicles, prostate
Amebiasis (1)
Schistosomiasis (2)
Tuberculosis (5)
Lymphogranuloma venereum (20)
Filariasis (26)
Elephantiasis (26)
Malignant disease (43)
Urethral strictures (44)
Rectovaginal and vesicovaginal fistulae (1/6/20/44)
Genital mutilation (44)

Central Nervous System

A. Brain and meninges
Amebiasis (1)
Schistosomiasis (2)
Hydatid disease (3)
Tuberculosis (5)
Fungus diseases (especially cryptococcosis) (6)
Cysticercosis (7)
Sparganosis (7)
Angiostrongyliasis cantonensis (13)
Neurotrichinosis (14)
Paragonimiasis (22)
Neoplasms (43/44)
African trypanosomiasis (44)
Toxoplasmosis (45)
Malaria (46)

B. Spine, including paraplegia
Schistosomiasis (2)
Hydatid disease (3)
Tuberculosis (5)
Fungus diseases (6)
Cysticercosis (7)
Spondylitis, including typhoid and pyogenic (15)
Dracunculiasis (guinea worm infection) (27)
Hemoglobinopathies (31)
Brucellosis (32)
Tetanus (33)
Syphilis (35)
Burkitt's lymphoma (41)
Malignant disease (43)

C. Peripheral nerves
Leprosy (34)

Soft Tissues

A. Soft tissue nodules without obvious calcification
Hydatid disease (3)
Tuberculosis (including breast) (5)
Fungus diseases (6)
Sparganosis (7)
Filariasis, especially onchocerciasis (26)
Guinea worm (Dracunculiasis) (27)
Tumoral calcinosis (29)
Yaws (35)
Leprosy (34)
Tropical ulcer (36)
Malignant disease (43)
Burkitt's lymphoma (41)
Kaposi's sarcoma (42)
Kala-azar, gnathostomiasis (46)
Miscellaneous (44)

B. Calcifications in the soft tissues
Hydatid disease (3)
Tuberculosis (5)
Cysticercosis, sarcocystis (7)
Filariasis (26)
Loiasis (26)
Onchocerciasis (26)
Dracunculiasis (guinea worm infection) (27)
Tumoral calcinosis/Kikuyu bursa (29)
Pentastomiasis (28)
Medicinal injection sites (44)

C. Other soft tissue diseases (e.g., edema, inflammation, ulceration, malignancy)
Amebiasis (1)
Hydatid disease (3)
Fungus diseases (6)
Cysticercosis (7)
Lymphogranuloma venereum (20)
Melioidosis (23)
Filariasis, elephantiasis, loiasis (26)
Onchocerciasis (26)
Dracunculiasis (guinea worm) (27)
Tumoral calcinosis (29)
Yaws and endemic syphilis (35)
Smallpox, monkey pox (40)
Leprosy (34)
Tropical ulcer, Buruli ulcer (36)
Ainhum (37)
Rhinoscleroma (38)
Cancrum oris (noma) (39)
Malignant disease (43)
Kaposi's sarcoma (42)
Tropical pyomyositis (30)
Gnathostomiasis (46)
Trauma (44)

D. Lymphadenopathy: in addition to all the usual "nontropical" diseases consider the following
Tuberculosis (5)
Atypical myobacteria (5)
Fungus diseases (6)
Lymphogranuloma venereum (20)
Plague (24)
Filariasis (26)
Dracunculiasis (guinea worm infection) (27)
Yaws (Treponematoses) (35)
Brucellosis (32)
Leprosy (34)
Malignant disease (43)
Burkitt's lymphoma (41)
Kaposi's sarcoma (42)
Kala-azar (46)

Skeleton

A. Skull, facial bones and spine
Hydatid disease (3)
Tuberculosis (5)
Fungus diseases (6)
Cysticercosis (7)
Typhoid and paratyphoid fever (15)
Hemoglobinopathies (31)
Yaws and endemic syphilis (35)
Brucellosis (32)
Tetanus (33)
Leprosy (34)
Cancrum oris (39)
Rhinoscleroma (38)
Malignant disease (43)
Burkitt's lymphoma (41)
Fluorosis, Paget's disease (44)

B. Long bones, hands and feet
Hydatid disease (3)
Tuberculosis (5)
Fungus diseases, especially mycetoma (6)
Salmonella osteomyelitis (15/31)
Melioidosis (23)
Hemoglobinopathies (31)
Yaws and endemic syphilis (35)
Brucellosis (32)
Leprosy (34)
Tropical ulcer (36)
Ainhum (37)
Malignant neoplasm (43)
Burkitt's lymphoma (41)
Kaposi's sarcoma (42)
Anomalies, carpal fusions/congenital hip dislocation (44)
Tibia vara/Blount's disease (44)
Osteomyelitis, acute/chronic (44)

C. Arthritis and other joint diseases – acute, chronic, neuropathic

Geography of Infectious and Parasitic Diseases

These lists should be used together with the lists of differential diagnoses based on organ or system involvement, so that the possible causes of illness in the traveler or visitor from the tropics may be determined and the specific chapters consulted for detailed information. However, the lists are in random order and do not in any way suggest the relative risks or frequencies of the various diseases.

The relevant chapter is indicated by the number after each disease. Only infectious and parasitic diseases are listed. For other diseases, consult Chapter 43 "Geographic Variations of Malignant (Neoplastic) Diseases in the Tropics" or Chapter 44 "Geographic Variations of Nonmalignant Diseases in the Tropics."

I. Diseases Found in Most Tropical Countries
Amebiasis (1)
Schistosomiasis (2)
Hydatid disease (3)
Tuberculosis (5)
Fungus diseases (6)
Taeniasis (tapeworm), cysticercosis, sparganosis (7)
AIDS (8)
Giardiasis (9)
Ascariasis (10)
Hookworm disease (12)
Strongyloidiasis (13)
Trichinosis (14)
Typhoid fever (15)
Kwashiorkor (16)
Trichuriasis (17)
Bacillary dysentery (19)
Lymphogranuloma venereum (20)
Filarial diseases (26)
Pyomyositis (30)
Brucellosis (32)
Tetanus (33)
Yaws and endemic syphilis (35)
Toxoplasmosis (45)
Malaria (46)
Kala-azar (46)

II. Diseases Commonly Found in Specific Tropical Regions

West Indies/Caribbean
All diseases listed in I
Tropical sprue (16)
Guinea worm infection (rare) (27)
Angiostrongyliasis costaricensis (13)

Central America/Mexico/Panama
All diseases listed in I
Chagas' disease (4)
Angiostrongyliasis costaricensis (13)
Paragonimiasis (22)
Plague (rare) (24)
Leprosy (34)

South America
All diseases listed in I
Chagas' disease (4)
Sparganosis (7)
Angiostrongyliasis costaricensis (13)
Paragonimiasis (22)
Melioidosis (23)
Plague (24)
Guinea worm infection (27)
Leprosy (34)

East Africa, North Africa, Arabia and Middle East
All diseases listed in I
Sparganosis (7)
Helminthoma (18)
Plague (24)
Guinea worm infection (27)
Smallpox (residual effects only) (40)
Leprosy (34)
Pentastomiasis (28)
Gnathostomiasis (Israel) (46)

West Africa
All diseases listed in I
Helminthoma (18)
Paragonimiasis (22)
Plague (24)
Guinea worm infection (27)

Leprosy (34)
Pentastomiasis (28)

Central and Southern Africa
All diseases listed in I
Helminthoma (18)
Plague (24)
Guinea worm infection (27)
Leprosy (34)
Pentastomiasis (28)

India and Sri Lanka
All diseases listed in I
Tropical sprue (16)
Paragonimiasis (22)
Plague (24)
Guinea worm infection (27)
Leprosy (34)
Pentastomiasis (28)
Gnathostomiasis (46)

Asia (including Japan and the Pacific Islands)
All diseases listed in I
Sparganosis (7)
Anisakiasis (11)
Angiostrongyliasis cantonensis (13)
Intestinal capillariasis (14)
Clonorchiasis, opisthorchiasis, and other liver fluke diseases (21)
Oriental cholangiohepatitis (21)
Paragonimiasis (22)
Melioidosis (23)
Plague (24)
Leprosy (34)
Pentastomiasis (28)
Gnathostomiasis (46)

1 Amebiasis

With Kenji Kimura, Miguel Stoopen, and Rogelio Moncada

Amebiasis is a widespread parasitic disease caused by the protozoan *Entamoeba histolytica*. This harmless-appearing, fragile microorganism, measuring 10–40 μm, has as its principal biological characteristic the ability to invade and destroy nearly every tissue of the human body. According to multiple reports it is probably colonizing the large bowel in 10–20% of the world's population, with an average of 12% as reported by the World Health Organization (WHO); it is most common in the poor developing countries of the tropics where sanitation and a clean water supply are inadequate or nonexistent. Out of the total number of infested individuals, about 50 million become symptomatic annually as a result of invasive amebiasis, and 40 000–100 000 deaths are reported per year. Amebiasis is the third leading cause of death from parasitic disease, surpassed only by malaria and schistosomiasis.

"Amebic dysentery" has for centuries conjured up a picture of steaming tropical jungles and sufferers dying with all the unpleasantness of an acute bowel infection. In fact, the disease is not confined only to the tropics but is worldwide in distribution and may affect not only the gut but the liver, chest, and other parts of the body. The illness may be so free from "dysentery" that it is often first recognized by the radiologist in patients who are suspected clinically of having colon cancer, cirrhosis, or an abscess of the liver or lung.

During the past 25 years, considerable progress has been achieved in the development of laboratory techniques to diagnose amebiasis, specifically using antibody titers for identification of the aggressive infectious stage of the parasite. Computed tomography (CT) and ultrasonography have made major contributions to the diagnosis and management of amebic liver abscess. Currently, the ability to diagnose colitis, hepatic abscess, and other clinical manifestations of this parasitic disease has improved early decision making, enabling implementation of the most appropriate form of therapy. Drugs such as metronidazole have had limited success in some segments of the population and, in some endemic areas, the morbidity and mortality have diminished. Even with these advances, however, the overall incidence of amebiasis in endemic areas is similar to that 30 years ago. There are still many unanswered questions about amebiasis from the biological, epidemiological, and clinical standpoints, and much remains to be learned about this ubiquitous and often devastating disease.

Synonyms

Amebiasis. Amebic dysentery. Amebic enteritis. Amebic granulomatous colitis. Ricaldoni and Berta's amebic inflammatory disease. *Sp:* Amibiasis. *Fr:* Amibiase. *Ger:* Amöbenbefall, Amöbiasis.

The ameboma is referred to as "pseudotumor", pseudocancer, Kartuli's amebic tumor, typhlitic or nonspecific granulomatous tumor, ligneous tumor, pseudotuberculoma or neoplastiform amebiasis. *Sp:* Amiboma. *Fr:* Amibome. *Ger:* Amöbom.

Definition

Amebiasis is infection by the pathogenic protozoan, *Entamoeba histolytica.* Other strains and species of amebae infect man, but only rarely are these pathogenic. The clinical significance of the other strains would be negligible were it not for mistaken diagnoses; they resemble and are sometimes mistaken for *E. histolytica.*

Geographic Distribution

It is estimated that up to 20% of the world's population harbor amebae, although only a small number (probably 5% or 6%) of these hosts develop invasive (and thus clinical) amebiasis. The parasite is found throughout the world, but is considered endemic between parallels 40° North and 30° South. Areas with the highest (*E. histolytica*) endemic activity include Asia, India, East and South Africa, Mexico, and portions of Central and South America. Thus, in Colombia 45% of the population may be infected, in Mexico 20%, and in Venezuela 17%. In Egypt

(Cairo), estimates vary from 20% to 40% of the population, and in India from 10% to 15%. St. Petersburg, Russia has a surprisingly high rate of infection for a nontropical city.
Logically, the incidence of amebiasis in the industrialized countries of Europe and North America is low. In the United States, it is currently estimated that less than 1% of the population may harbor amebae; however, as recently as 1967, over 12% of stools from 149 U.S. Army medical officers who had never been out of the United States contained *E. histolytica.* Subsets of the population may show an unusually high incidence of amebiasis, particularly homosexual patients who attend sexually transmissible disease clinics. Pomerantz et al. reported 1875 amebiasis cases among the homosexual community in New York, a higher number even than for tuberculosis (1307 cases) or hepatitis (1260 cases). Other studies of New York City male homosexuals have found between 19.6% and 31.7% of these patients to be infected with *E. histolytica.*
The existence of amebiasis in a community can be considered representative of the pathology of poverty, which implies deficiencies in the elemental rules of hygiene, lack of proper sewer systems, and irrigation with black or untreated waters. Therefore, it occurs primarily in developing overpopulated countries, even though it is a cosmopolitan disease that can be found in any part of the world in which humans and the parasite coexist. Certainly amebiasis is a common disease, although some of the above estimates appear high (...we hope!).

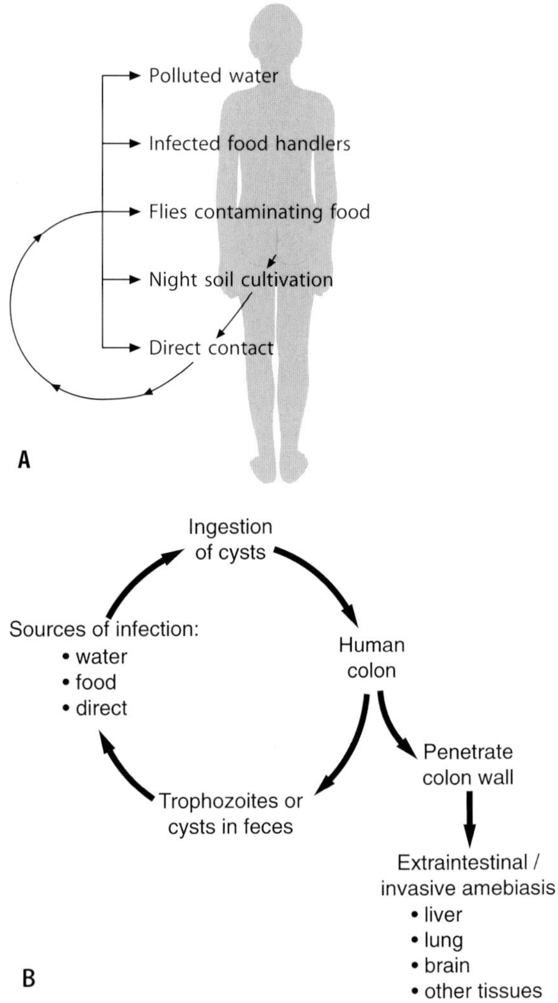

Fig. 1.1 A, B. Modes of transmission of amebiasis

Epidemiology

Humans usually acquire amebiasis by ingesting cysts of the protozoan *E. histolytica* in contaminated food or drinking water (Fig. 1.1). In most Western countries the infection is transmitted mainly by carriers who pass cysts and who work in restaurants or other public places. These human sources of infective parasites are either healthy hosts or convalescent patients with amebic disease; during the initial stage of the disease, they may discharge trophozoites in small numbers or up to millions a day. The quiescent stage of the disease may last from a few months to 2 years.
Throughout the tropics, water from polluted wells or broken plumbing and food contaminated by human "night soil" used for fertilization are significant sources of infection. Flies, cockroaches, and other insects may be vectors of the disease. Man is the principal host and reservoir of *E. histolytica*, even though amebic cysts can be found in the stools of various animals, including dogs, cats, pigs, rats, and some primates; however, these are not a frequent source of human infection. The parasite has also been experimentally inoculated in some mammals.
Amebiasis affects both sexes equally. Infections tend to be more common in adults than in children, but this certainly does not apply everywhere in the world. For instance, a study in Lagos (Nigeria) showed that 62% of all patients were under the age of 10 years and 75% of these were under 5 years. Infected infants under the age of 4 and 6 months have been reported in other series.
The amebic trophozoite is sensitive to minor temperature changes, cannot tolerate the low pH environment of the stomach, and can only survive out of its host for a brief period. Conversely, the infectious form of the parasite is the tetranucleated mature cyst, which is resistant to gastric secretions and other gastrointestinal enzymes and is known for its ability to survive adverse environmental conditions within or outside the host. Depending on temperature and degree of dehydration, the cysts re-

tain their infective capacity in soil and water for 8 days when the temperature ranges between 28° and 34 °C and for up to a month at 10 °C. The parasite is resistant to the conventional chlorine concentrations used to purify drinking water. The cysts are destroyed when exposed to 200 p.p.m. of iodine, to acetic acid, or to temperatures greater that 68 °C. They can also be removed by sand filtration.

Transmission of the disease occurs by ingestion of tetranucleated mature cysts which can be found in food and water contaminated by improper food processing, improper use of contaminated fertilizers, or faulty irrigation practices, and in unprocessed drinking water. Self-contamination can also occur due to poor habits of hygiene. However, it should be emphasized that only a small percentage of infested individuals become symptomatic from tissue penetration of the parasite. Clinical manifestations from intestinal or extraintestinal pathological lesions are designated as invasive amebiasis.

The natural history of amebiasis shows wide regional differences, with the percentage of infected patients and those with active disease varying from one area to another. In Mexico, it is estimated that one in every five infected patients will develop invasive amebiasis. However, in one sampling, 95% of 3000 infected Mexicans had ulcerative proctocolitis, a much higher percentage than in most endemic areas; there is a similar variation in the frequency of ameboma. These geographic variations are not fully understood. One possibility is that there is a synergistic action of the amebae with other elements in the flora of the bowel. Variations in host response and immunity, virulence and stage of the parasite, and possibly spontaneous mutations of avirulent into virulent strains of *E. histolytica*, are other factors that might influence the progress of infection. The clinical picture may also depend on the degree of exposure, and whether the infection is heavy, prolonged, or repetitive. Diet also influences the course of infection: malnutrition predisposes to more severe disease.

Pathophysiology

Intestinal amebiasis results from the ingestion of amebic cysts that contain a substance within their walls called quitina, which protects the parasites from adverse low pH and the enzyme-rich gastrointestinal environment. After passing through the unfavorable acid environment of the stomach, the cyst has its capsule dissolved in the alkaline content of the small intestine in preparation for colonization in the colon. Each cyst usually releases four active trophozoites which are carried along the small bowel (Fig. 1.2). Some are destroyed, but others produce strong proteolytic enzymes and hyaluronidases which can lyse the intestinal epithelium, making it possible for the trophozoites to burrow into the mucosa. This process occurs in association with bacteria (the exact mechanism is not understood) and produces ulcerations which, if they continue to progress, become the classical flask-shaped ulcers of invasive amebiasis. Specimens obtained from patients with invasive disease and from carriers reveal two genotypes of *E. histolytica* designated as "pathogen" and "nonpathogen," each generating phenotypic isoenzymes called zymodemes. According to Mirelman and other investigators, the existing bacterial flora may contribute to the pathogenic or invasive nature of the parasite. Experimental studies have demonstrated that bacterial-rich cultures increase certain aspects of the virulent functions in vitro. This controversial issue is yet to be resolved.

The majority of individuals infested with *E. histolytica* are asymptomatic. No symptoms will occur until there has been tissue invasion and ulceration, which marks the onset of clinical amebiasis. Until this happens, the individual is only an asymptomatic cyst passer or "carrier" because the parasite can and does live in the intestinal contents of many hosts without producing noticeable tissue reaction or symptoms.

There is, however, recent evidence that many asymptomatic "cyst passers" have tiny shallow amebic ulcers of the cecum (Connor). In tropical Africa postmortem examinations of indigenous peoples have revealed, on careful inspection of colonic mucosa, minute amebic ulcers. These are shallow, only a few millimeters across, usually in the cecum and frequently in the recesses between folds of plicae. Their detection requires close inspection. Clinically amebiasis is unsuspected in these patients and the ulcers would probably not be demonstrated by barium enema or colonoscopy. Patients harboring these small amebic ulcers may well be "asymptomatic carriers."

Many other amebae (*E. coli, E. moshkovskii, E. polecki, Iodamoeba bütschlii, Endolimax nana*, and others) may occasionally inhabit the human bowel without producing lesions or symptoms. Invasive amebiasis is confirmed by identifying hematophagous trophozoites in the stool (Fig. 1.2), or when biopsy specimens from involved bowel reveal trophozoites in the margins of ulcers and in the fibrin-rich exudate covering the base of the ulcers (Figs. 1.3–1.5).

Amebae within the lumen of the gut do not provoke significant antibodies, but those amebae which are invasive do, and this provides a useful serological test; once present, these antibodies persist long after invasion has ceased. Thus, they may indicate past rather than current infection but, if they are absent, clinical amebiasis can be excluded.

(Text continues on p. 6)

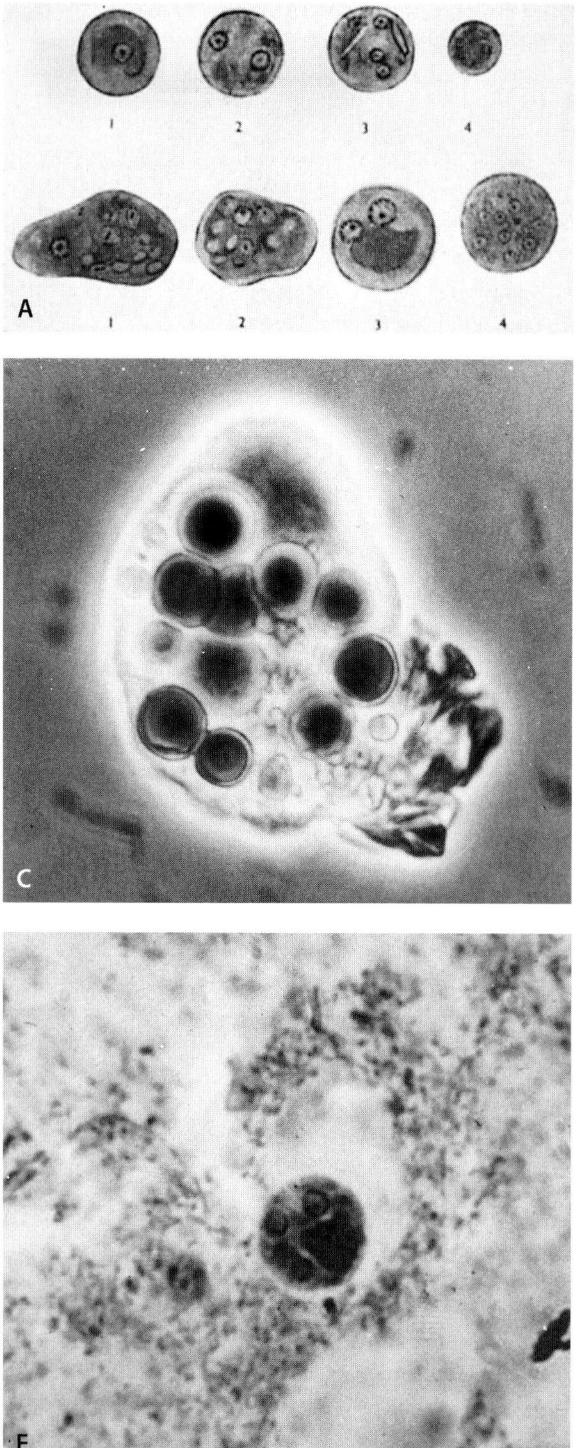

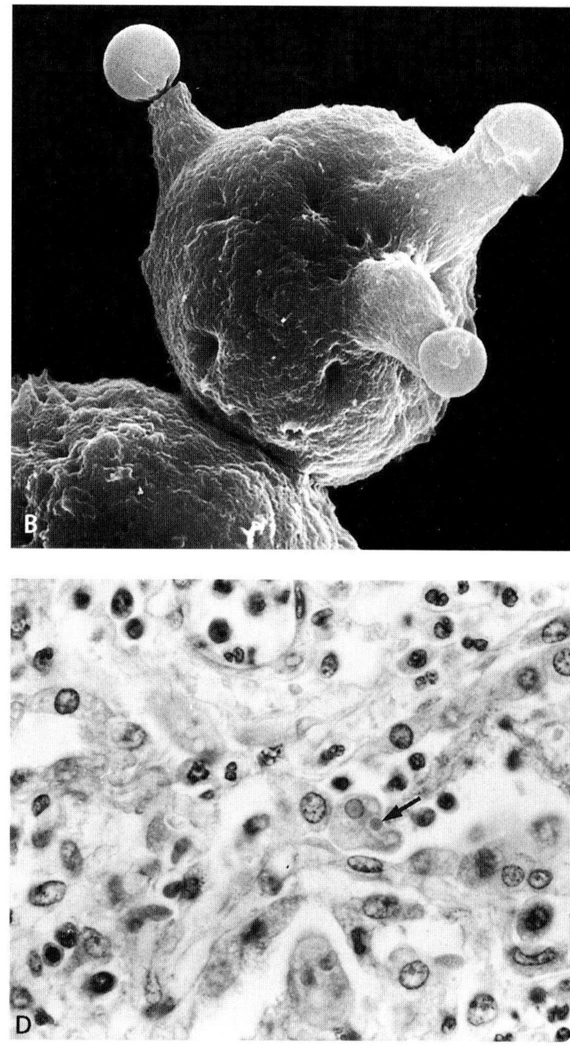

Fig. 1.2 A–E. *Entamoeba histolytica.* **A** Trophozoites (*1*), precysts (*2, 3*), and mature cysts (*4*) (*bottom row*). **B** Electron microscopy shows a trophozoite with three pseudopods simultaneously phagocytizing erythrocytes. ×2200. **C** Electron microscopy shows the presence of erythrocytes in phagolysosomes within an amoeba. ×2400. (**B, C** courtesy of Dr. Tsutsumi, Mexico City) **D** A single trophozoite of *E. histolytica* is in the *center* of the photograph. Note the slightly irregular ameboid outline and coarse cytoplasm, the spherical nucleus, and the tiny central karyosome. There is also an ingested erythrocyte in the cytoplasm (*arrow*). H&E, ×2000. (Courtesy of Dr. Daniel H. Connor) **E** *E. histolytica* cyst with four nuclei and chromatoidal bars

Fig. 1.4 A–D. *E. histolytica* trophozoites in tissue. **A** Numerous trophozoites are present in the submucosa of the colon. Those that enter lymphatics or venules may be carried to the liver or other organs and form the nidus of infection there. AFIP (Armed Forces Institute of Pathology) 625901. **B** Trophozoites surrounded by inflammatory cells in a submucosal abscess. ×440; AFIP 53-18759. **C, D** *E. histolytica* amid destroyed liver cells in hepatic abscesses. **C** ×240; AFIP 53-18758. **D** ×440; AFIP 53-3146 ▶

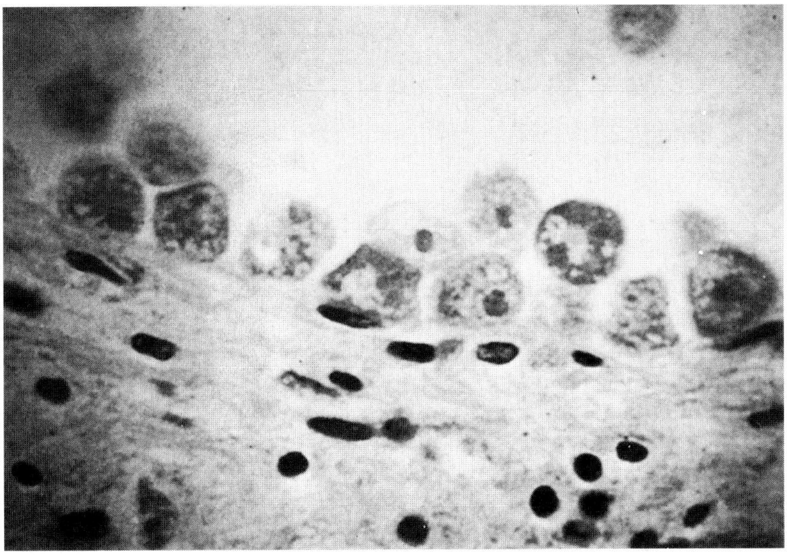

Fig. 1.3. Amebic infection begins when trophozoites attach to the epithelial cells of the colonic mucosa. Here trophozoites line the base of a shallow ulcer

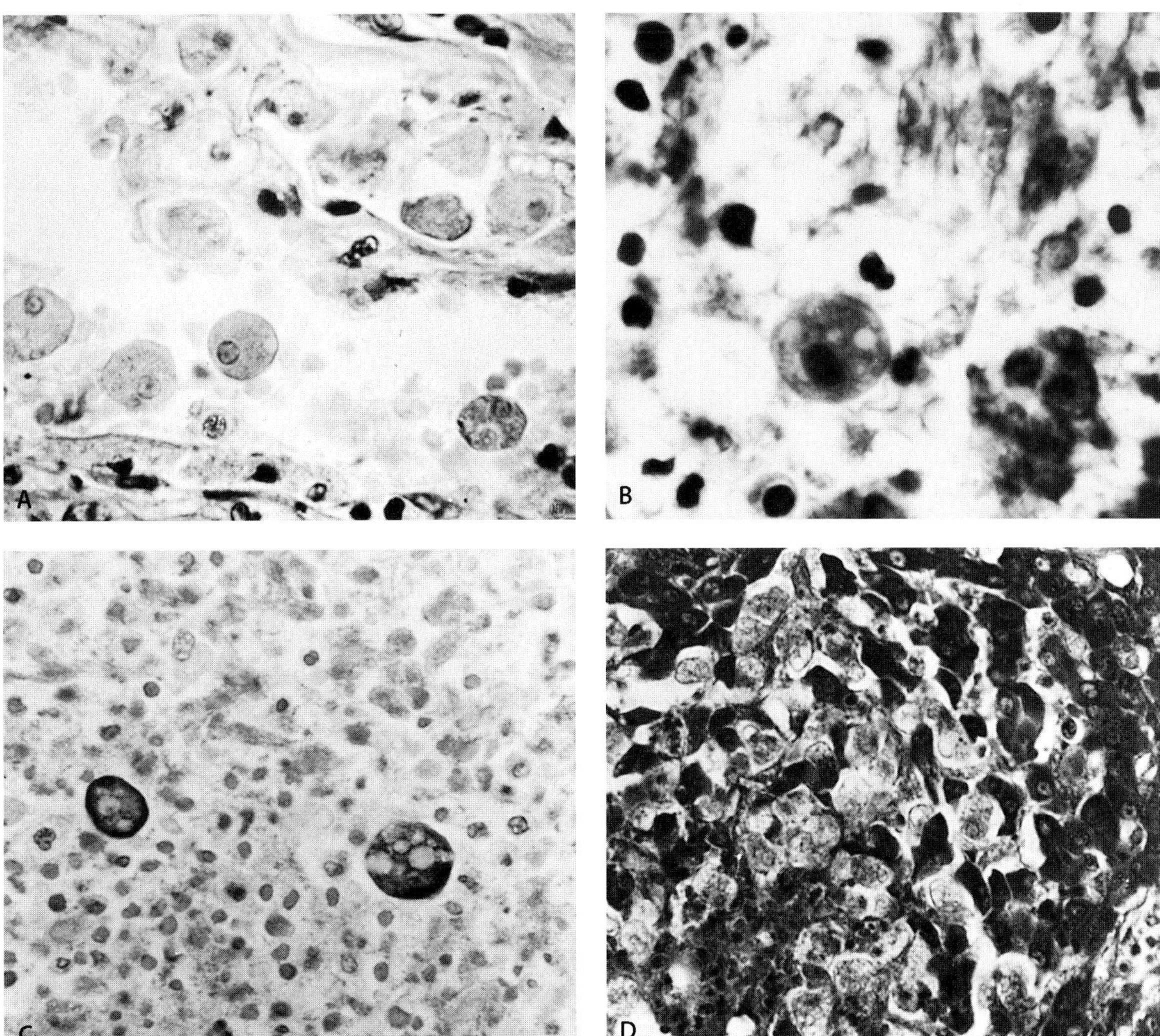

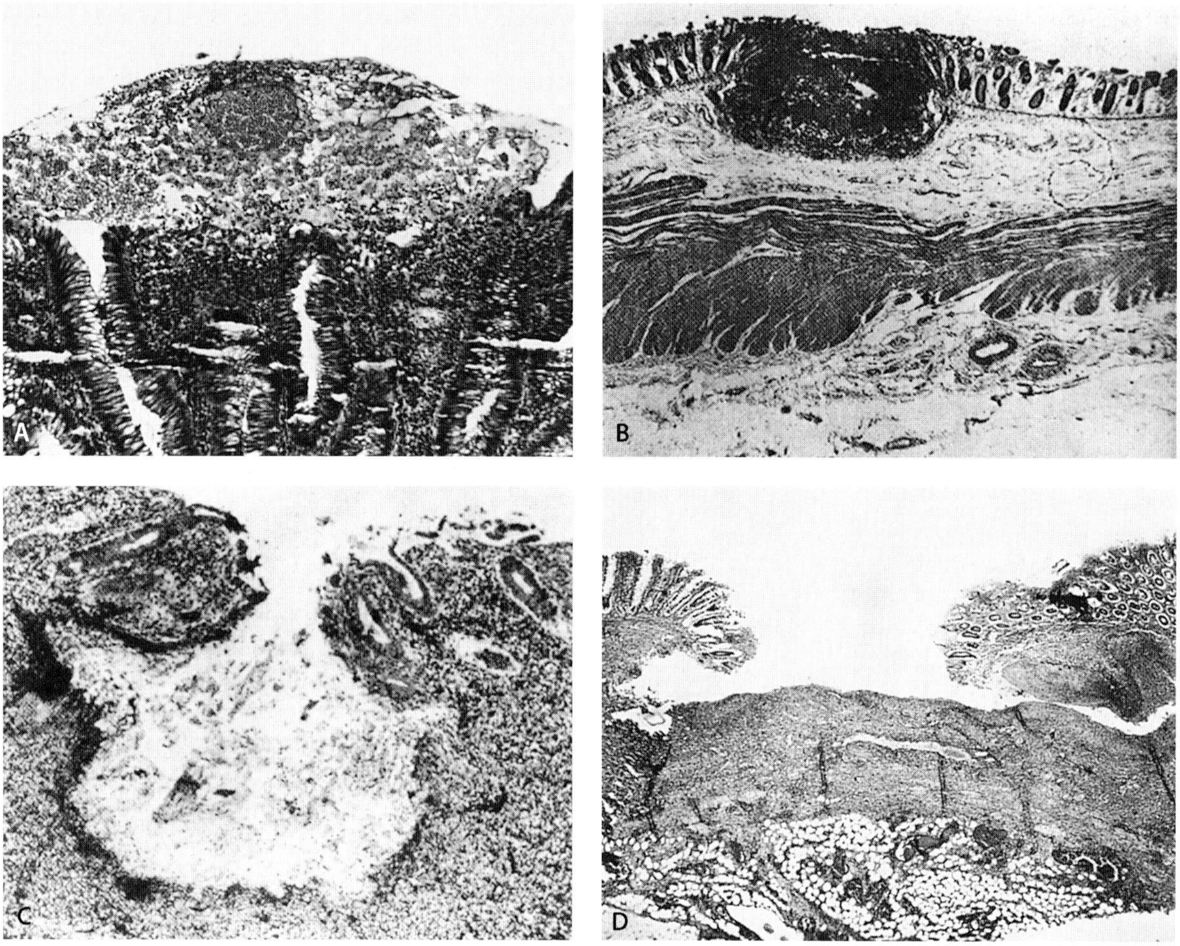

Fig. 1.5 A–D. Amebic ulcers - histological sections. **A** Early superficial erosion of the mucosa. The exudate contains numerous *E. histolytica* trophozoites. ×108; AFIP 69-7842. **B** Early amebic ulcer in the colon at low magnification. **C** Classical flask-shaped amebic ulcer of the colon extending through the mucosa into the submucosa with undermining. The extensive infiltrate of neutrophils surrounding the ulcer suggests secondary bacterial infection. **D** Section of an amebic ulcer of the colon showing characteristic undermining. The muscularis is partly eroded and the serosa is edematous and hyperemic. ×430; AFIP 58-15140

Pathology

Surgical or autopsy specimens highlight the two characteristic features of amebic lesions: (a) minimal inflammatory response and (b) extensive cellular destruction. Experimental animal studies at the molecular level have shown that organic tissue damage is not caused directly by the parasite, but actually by the liberated lysosomal enzymes from lysis of leukocytes and monocytes. Intracecal inoculation of *E. histolytica* trophozoites has produced a spectrum of superficial erosions, ulcers, and deep lesions giving origin to amebomas or perforations similar to those observed in human amebiasis.

Early Lesions: Adherence and Lysis

The keys to the pathogenesis and virulence of *E. histolytica* are the lectins and lytic substances produced by trophozoites. The lectins enable trophozoites to adhere to mammalian cells and then destroy them with lytic substances which include proteolytic enzymes, glycosidases, and pore-forming proteins. It is especially interesting that the pore-forming protein is essentially identical to a pore-forming protein of human T lymphocytes. Human defenses against amebiasis are most likely the antibodies and the enhanced cell-mediated immunity stimulated by exposure to these lectins and lytic substances. Without these lectins and lytic enzymes, *E. histolytica* would be just another commensal of the intestine, lacking the ability to adhere, erode, invade, produce ulcers or spread to the liver and other organs and cavities. The earliest lesions of man have not been studied but infections in experimental animals reveal early stages of increased mucin production by goblet cells, then adherence of trophozoites to surface epithelium, hyperplasia of crypts, edema of and hemorrhage into the lamina propria, and finally lysis and sloughing of epithelium. Thus, amebiasis begins when trophozoites adhere to surface epithelial cells. Next follows destruction of epithelial cells and then erosion and ulceration. Figure 1.3 is a dramatic illustration of the adherent and lytic effects of *E. histolytica.* A phalanx of trophozoites has eroded both the superficial epithelium and supporting lamina propria at every point of contact, and the line of destruction is as straight as the phalanx of trophozoites. This is one of the earliest and most dramatic lesions studied, because it demonstrates the two essential features of pathogenesis: adherence to, and lysis of, host cells.

Neutrophils and eosinophils are found in the superficial early lesions; eosinophils are no longer present in the chronic lesions. The destructive nature of the amebic parasite and its capacity to generate tissue lysis has justified the awarding of the *histolytica* appelation. Liberation of toxins, enzymes, avid phagocytic activity, and an efficient cytoplasm rapidly degrade the cellular and extracellular ingested material. It is generally accepted that the incipient lesions of invasive amebiasis demonstrate an intense inflammatory reaction, followed by extensive necrosis secondary to ischemia and the cytolytic action of the lysosomal enzymes liberated by the lysed leukocytes. An impressive feature of invasive amebiasis is the *restitutio ad integrum* of the affected organ. The regenerated tissues usually return to normal without the process of cicatrization. This is particularly evident in the colon, liver, and skin. This phenomenon is probably due to the lack of fibroblast activity, resulting in little inflammatory response, most likely due to the fibroblast-inhibiting factors generated by the parasite.

Intestinal Amebiasis

Invasive amebiasis can generate a variety of morphological alterations in the affected bowel with specific patterns, including: (a) ulcerative amebic rectocolitis, (b) toxic megacolon, (c) fulminant colitis, (d) ameboma, and (e) amebic appendicitis.

Ulcerative Amebic Proctocolitis. The earliest recognizable lesion in the ulcerative form of amebic colitis is one or more erosions of the colonic epithelium. These are followed by ulcers which usually occur at several closely linked sites; there is almost always healthy tissue between the areas of lytic necrosis. The ulcers are small, almost always multiple, and chiefly distributed in the cecum, sigmoid colon, and rectum (Figs. 1.5–1.7). They are elevated rounded lesions with a necrotic irregular center surrounded by an edematous ring. In the submucosa, small capillaries and venules become inflamed and sometimes thrombosed, which contributes to the mucosal necrosis. Amebae which are the progeny of the primary colonies may be squeezed out of, or overflow, the ulcers and be carried further down the bowel; the same process is repeated at multiple levels. At this stage, hitherto separate areas of pinhead ulceration spread below the mucosa and merge into large areas of lytic necrosis, causing the undermined flask-shaped ulcers characteristic of amebiasis (Fig. 1.5). Irregular and serpiginous ulcers of 1–5 cm length associated with edematous thickening of the colonic wall can also be observed. This process may be accompanied by bacterial invasion, and deeper penetration into the muscularis will occur (Fig. 1.6). Less commonly, deep penetration may be caused by the lytic action of the trophozoites.

Amebae migrate into the adjacent mucosa and submucosa, which becomes edematous. Perforation through the serosa is very uncommon, but can occur when tissue destruction is rapid and extensive (Fig. 1.7). Invasion of venules and lymphatics predisposes to thrombosis and septic embolization. Cysts form in the lumen of the gut, but not in tissue. Only cysts persist free in nature and can survive for long periods outside the body.

Toxic Megacolon. In acute, overwhelming infections, there may be massive distension and thickening of the colon with a great deal of destruction, edema, venous thrombosis, and perforation with an accompanying purulent peritonitis and very high mortality.

Ameboma. Ameboma is an uncommon pathological event of intestinal amebiasis, occurring most often in the cecum and ascending colon. A mass, often apple-core in appearance and resembling a carcinoma, originates from the colonic wall; it may measure 5–30 cm in diameter and may be multiple. How an ameboma develops is still a mystery; some authors believe that it is an amebic granuloma. Histologically, it shows abundant granulation tissue, edema, neovascularity, inflammatory cells, and live *E. histolytica.* The mucosa is generally ulcerated and there is marked thickening of the colonic wall with edema and hemorrhage.

Amebic Appendicitis. In Pakistan, Ahmed reported that 13 of 1400 histologically examined cases of appendicitis were of amebic origin. This is an uncom-

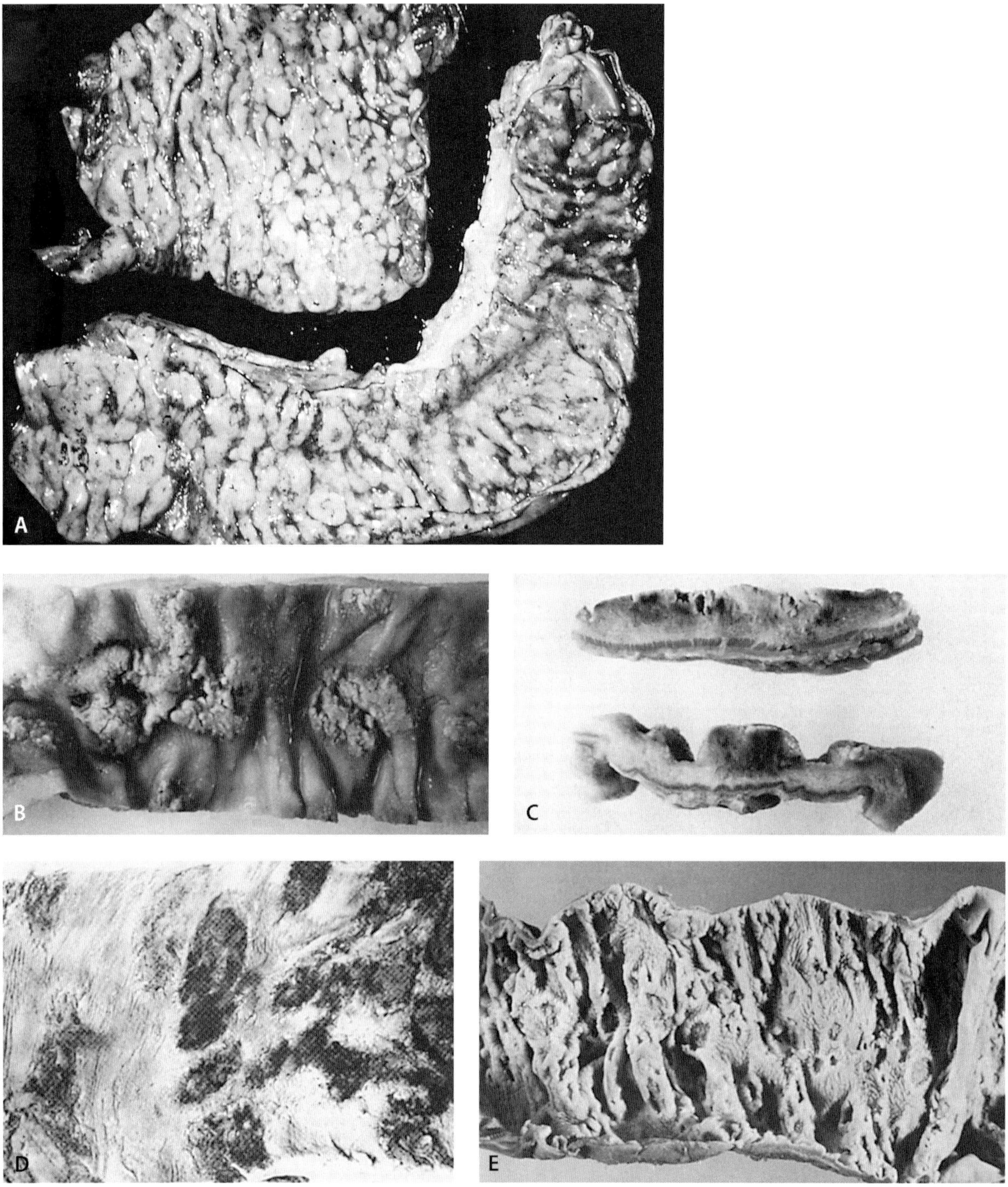

Fig. 1.6 A–E. Amebic ulcers of the colon-gross photographs. **A** Hyperemia and edema of the colonic mucosa with scattered superficial erosions and ulcers. **B** Amebic ulcers with ragged, heaped-up edges covered by an amorphous grey fibrinous exudate. ×75; AFIP 69-3234. **C** Vertical section of the same colon as **B**. Note the deep, ragged ulcers extending through the mucosa and submucosa but not through the muscularis. The colon is irregular, thickened, and rigid. AFIP 69-3550. **D** Deep, bleeding ulcers resulting from slough of necrotic tissue. These penetrating ulcers produce a "buffalo hide" appearance of the colon and may extend through the wall to the serosa. **E** Chronic amebic colitis with numerous well-defined, relatively small ulcers extending through the mucosa and submucosa to expose the muscularis. Many mucosal bridges are recognizable. AFIP 58-4840-3. (**B** from C.H. Binford, D.H. Connor, eds. *Pathology of tropical and extraordinary diseases.* Washington, DC, Armed Forces Institute of Pathology, 1976; **D** from J.E. Ash, S. Spitz: *Pathology of tropical diseases.* Philadelphia, Saunders, 1945)

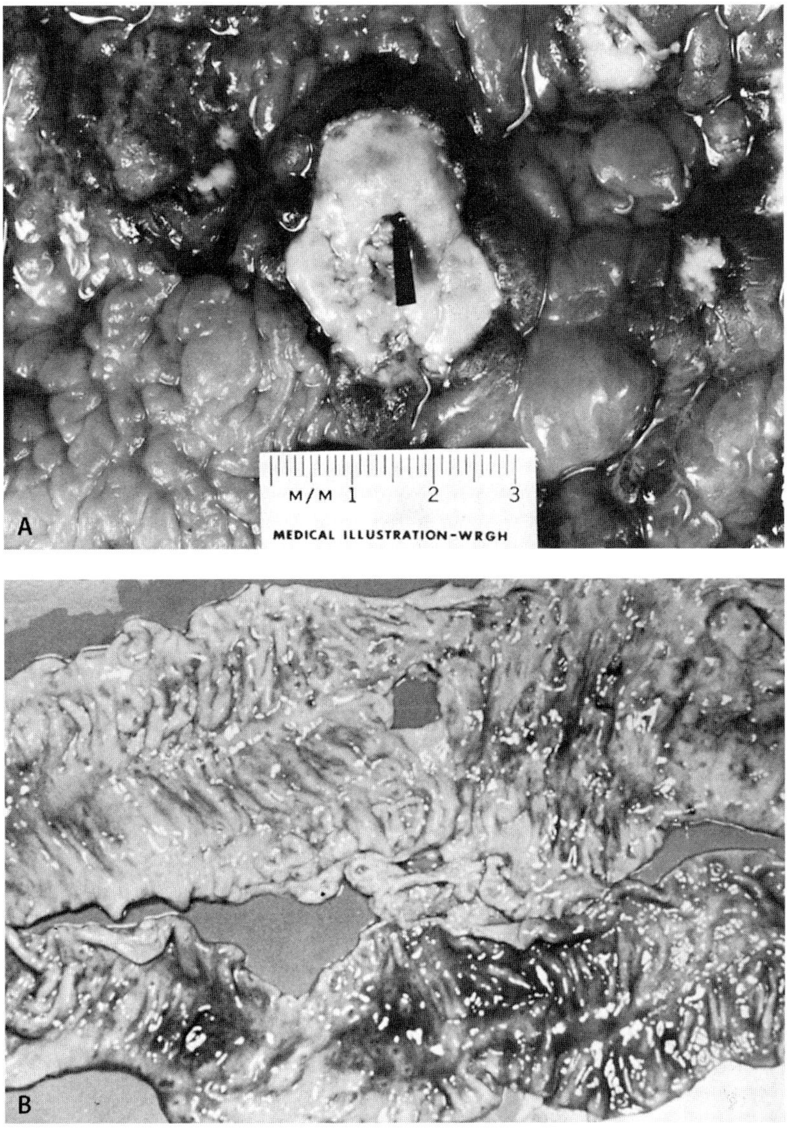

Fig. 1.7 A, B. Amebic colitis with perforation – autopsy specimens from two patients with colonic perforation leading to fatal amebic peritonitis. **A** Deep amebic ulcer which penetrated through the muscularis and serosa to cause a peritonitis. There were numerous other ulcers throughout the same colon. Note the markedly swollen mucosa around the ulcers caused by extensive mucosal and submucosal edema. AFIP 67 13734-A. **B** Diffuse ulceration of the colon with hemorrhage around many of the ulcers and perforation of the colon (*top center*)

mon entity, recognized postoperatively by the pathologist. The appendix shows suppurative inflammation with nodular mucosal ulcers. Once the etiology has been identified, conventional therapy for intestinal amebiasis must follow.

Extraintestinal Amebiasis

Spread of amebic infection to other parts of the body occurs by embolization or direct invasion. The colon and liver (Figs. 1.8, 1.9) are most frequently infected, but lung (Fig. 1.9), pleura, pericardium, brain (Fig. 1.10), genitalia, stomach, small bowel, spleen, and skin are other sites of infection; rare involvement of bone and aorta has been reported. Thoracic amebiasis is usually caused by direct spread from hepatic infection: over 75% of amebic infections in the chest develop from contiguous erosion of a liver abscess through the diaphragm (Fig. 1.9). Spread of amebae may take place by migration through the vertebral venous system to the brain and lungs without liver involvement, and direct spread from the gut to adjacent organs and tissues is common.

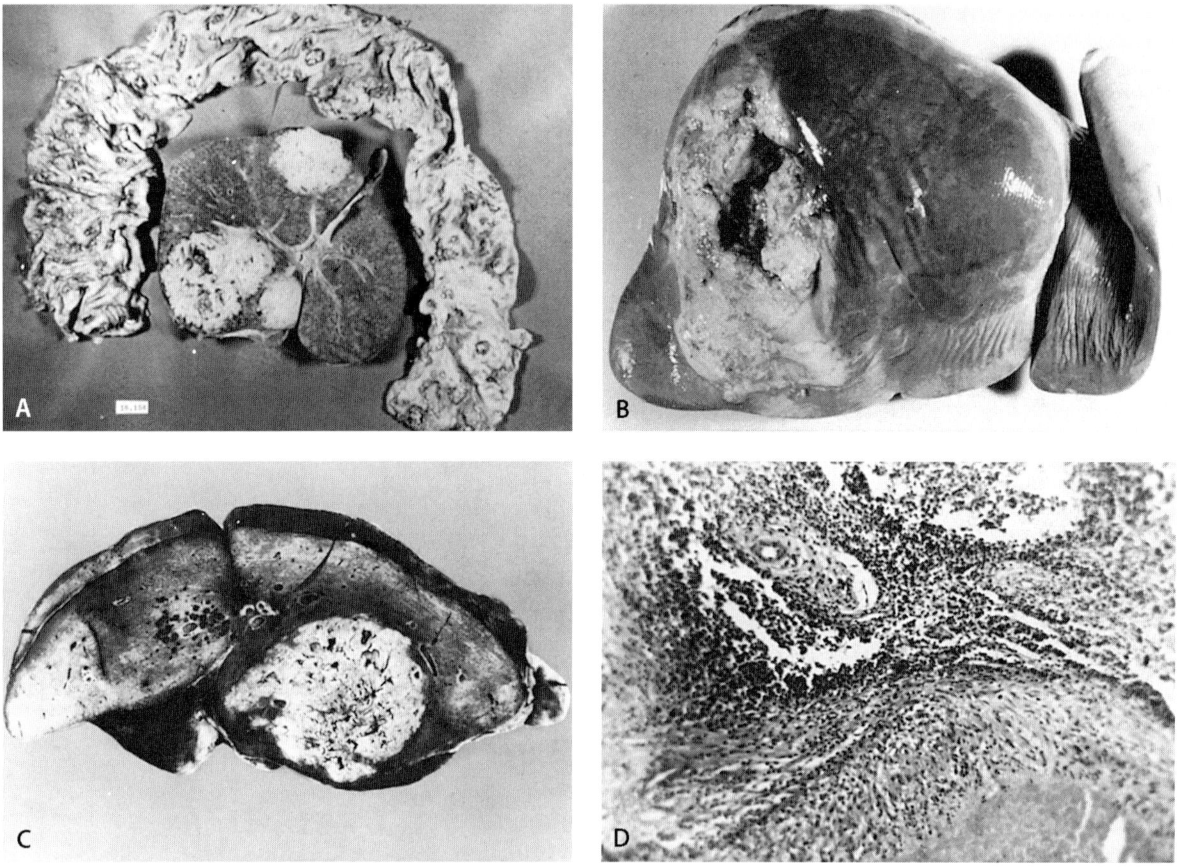

Fig. 1.8 A–D. Amebic abscesses of the liver. **A** Diffuse, well-defined amebic ulcers of the colon in a patient with fatal amebiasis. The cut surface of the liver contains multiple large amebic abscesses. (Courtesy of A.M. Fallis) **B** Huge abscess perforating through the surface of the right lobe of the liver. AFIP 1099409-1. **C** Large central hepatic abscess on cross-section. AFIP 53-4923. **D** Histological section of a hepatic amebic abscess with extensive inflammatory cell infiltrate, predominantly neutrophils. X112; AFIP 52-1160

Hepatic Abscess. Hepatic abscess is the most common extraintestinal lesion produced by *E. histolytica*, resulting from the embolization of pathogenic trophozoites into the portal venous system via the mesenteric-splanchnic circulation. The time lapse between the colonic mucosal-vascular penetration and damage to the liver parenchyma is unknown; however, experimental animal studies have demonstrated early hepatic alterations 3 hours after embolization of the trophozoites. The process begins with minimal dilatation of the sinusoids containing amebae, surrounded by varying amounts of polymorphonuclear leukocytes, some of which undergo lysis. Twenty-four to 48 hours later, the leukocytic lysis increases with proportional cellular necrosis of the adjacent liver tissue. By the fifth to seventh day, extensive necrosis with little inflammatory reaction can be observed. These experimental studies can be extrapolated to humans. Neutrophils tend to be sparse in amebic lesions generally, but especially so in amebic abscesses of the liver. The two essential features of any abscess are destruction of tissue and the accumulation of neutrophils and fibrin. The amebic "abscess" of liver therefore is considered somewhat of a misnomer because, although the "abscess" is characterized by necrosis, it contains few if any neutrophils after several days' development.

Macroscopically, the hepatic amebic abscess is identified as a well-delineated area where the liver parenchyma has been replaced by necrotic tissue of yellowish color and creamy consistency resembling anchovy paste. A rind of congested hepatic tissue surrounds the abscess. The necrotic center can be solid, soft, or semiliquid, sometimes containing mucus. The size of a hepatic abscess is variable, ranging from miliary spread to huge lesions that can replace 90% of the normal organ. At autopsy (Figs. 1.8, 1.9), the average size is 5–15 cm in diameter. Most abscesses occur in the right lobe, and they are more often single than multiple. A hepatic abscess may rupture into the peritoneal cavity followed rapidly by an acute peritonitis. Rupture can

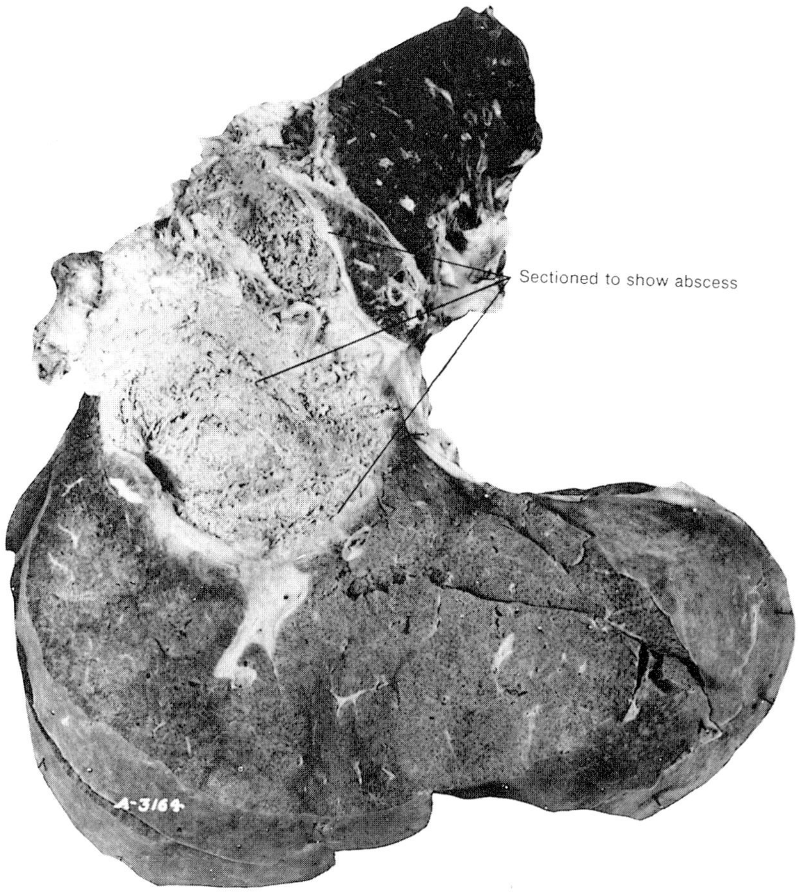

Fig. 1.9. Right lung and liver. Large hepatic amebic abscess in the dome of the right lobe of the liver, extending through the diaphragm and right pleura and causing an abscess in the right lower lobe. Thoracic amebiasis is almost always an extension of a hepatic abscess. The right hemithorax is involved by direct extension from an abscess in the right lobe of the liver, whereas a left lobe abscess may lead to empyema and lung abscess in the left hemithorax

also occur into the abdominal viscera, such as the stomach, duodenum, and colon, or into the biliary ducts, portal vein, or inferior vena cava, or toward the retroperitoneal space and, most frequently, the thoracic cavity (Fig. 1.9).

Cerebral Amebiasis. Spread of *E. histolytica* to the brain is thought to be hematogenous from the colon via hepatic, pulmonary, or vertebral veins. Lombardo et al., however, found intestinal symptomatology in little more than 50% of the cases of cerebral amebiasis which they reviewed. The reported incidence of amebic brain abscesses (Fig. 1.10) in patients with confirmed amebic liver abscesses varies from 0.6% to 8.1%; central nervous system infection without hepatic involvement is rare.

Cutaneous Amebiasis. Increasingly, cutaneous amebiasis is being recognized as complicating other forms of amebiasis. Surgical drainage from an amebic abscess in the liver or from the pericolic region after an appendectomy, or leakage from a perirectal or perianal abscess, allows implantation of amebae into small surface lesions, particularly around the drainage area. Perianal amebiasis can arise by direct spread from the rectum. Cutaneous ulcers, however they originate, are almost always tender, painful, and malodorous, but usually provoke little inflammation in adjacent tissue. Ulcers in the skin are generally shallow, and the edges are well defined: the floor of the ulcer is covered with a dirty gray slough (Fig. 1.11). Amebic ulcers of the trunk resemble those of the colon in that they are undermined and caused by extensive lytic necrosis. They contain few neutrophils and the trophozoites are concentrated in the exudate from the depths of the keratin pits, under the margin of the ulcer, and deep in the lesion along the line between necrotic and viable tissue. Only the trophozoite form of amebiasis is present in the skin, the cyst form never being found in man other than in the intestinal contents.

(Text continues on p. 14)

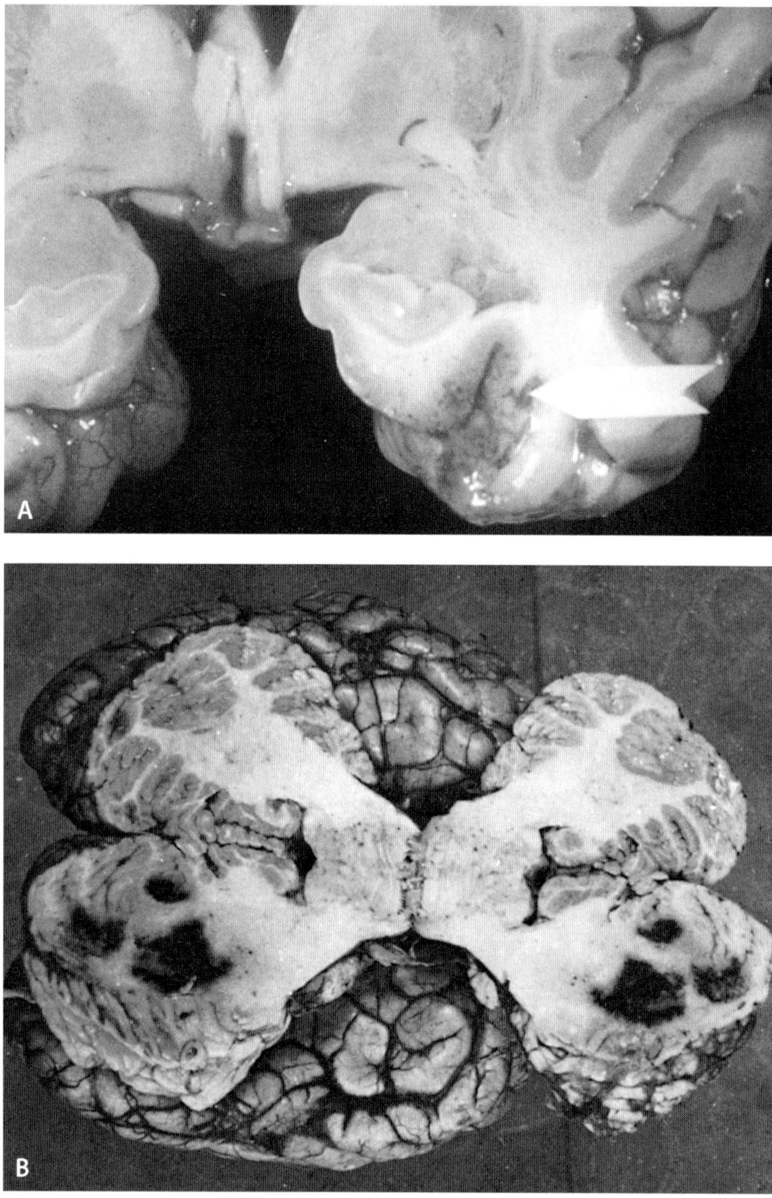

Fig. 1.10 A, B. Amebic abscesses of the brain in two patients. AFIP 203398-1

Fig. 1.11 A–D. Amebic ulcers of the skin in four different patients. **A** Large ulcer of the skin of the anterior abdominal wall which developed after drainage of an amebic abscess in the liver. Amebic skin ulcers are usually shallow, painful and malodorous, the edges are well defined, and the floor of the ulcer is covered with a dirty grey slough. The exudate near the margin of the ulcer may contain *E. histolytica* trophozoites. **B** Cutaneous ulcer which developed at the site of a midline surgical incision. Note a surgical drainage site nearby (*upper left*). **C** Extensive perianal and perineal bleeding from cutaneous ulcers caused by leakage from a perirectal amebic abscess. **D** Extension of colorectal amebiasis to anal skin in a 39-year-old man from the Democratic Republic of Congo. When trophozoites invade squamous epithelium, they cause epithelial hyperplasia, as shown here, which can be easily mistaken for squamous cell carcinoma. After trophozoites were identified in the biopsy specimen, the patient was treated with emetine hydrochloride and the lesion quickly healed. (**D** from D.H. Connor and F.W. Chandler, eds. *Pathology of infectious diseases*, Stamford, CT, Appleton & Lange, 1997) ▶

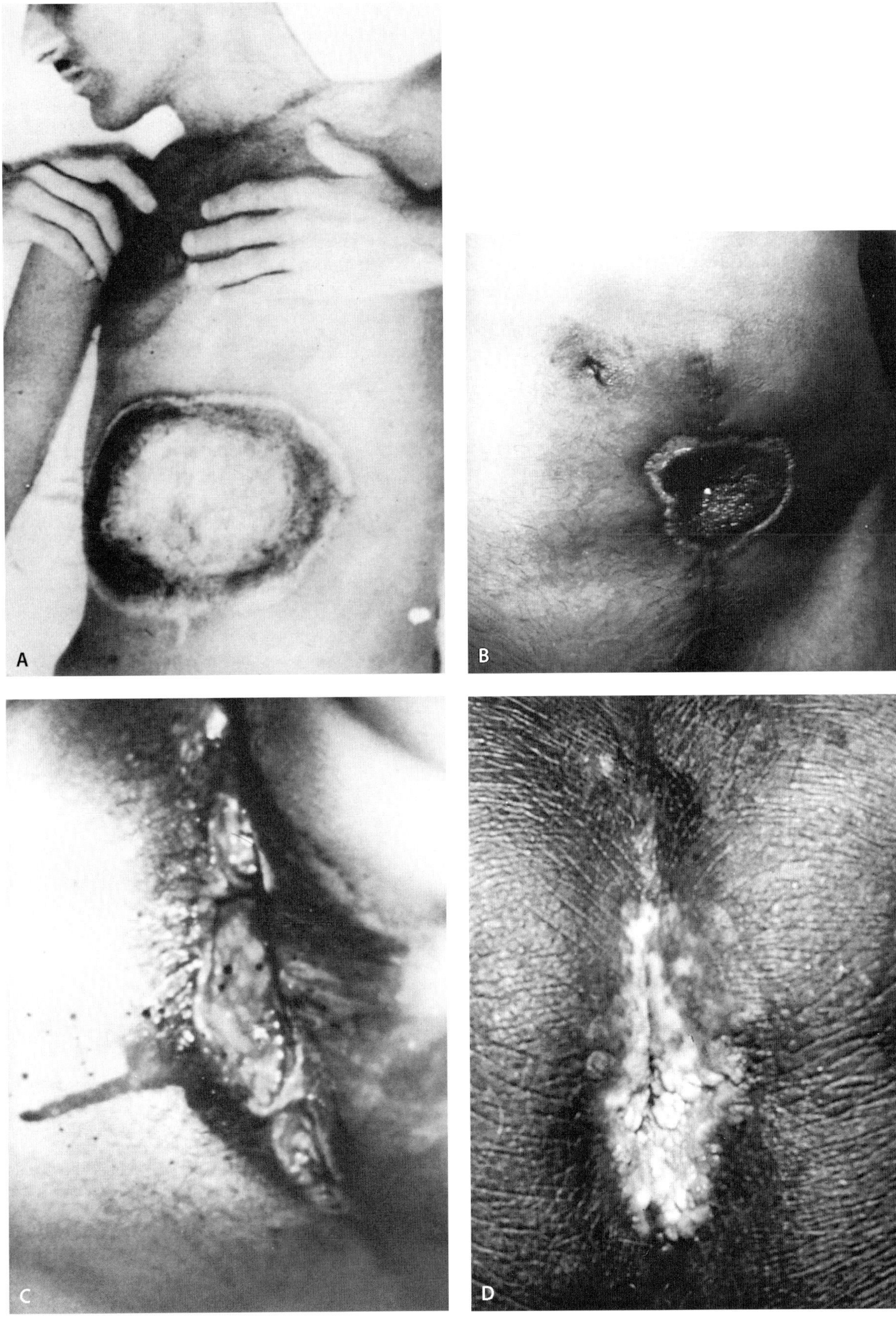
A
B
C
D

Amebiasis of anal skin (Fg. 1.11 C, D), genital skin, cervix, and penis causes hyperplasia of squamous epithelium punctuated by small shallow ulcers containing trophozoites. The hyperplastic epithelium raises the surface and gives it a "cauliflower-like" appearance resembling a squamous cell carcinoma; indeed, its gross appearance may cause the unwary clinician to misdiagnose perineal or genital amebiasis as a carcinoma or mycotic infection. Cutaneous infection is unlikely outside endemic areas unless the patient is already known to have severe amebiasis. Where the disease is common, cutaneous ulceration is not infrequent, but despite this the etiology is not always recognized immediately.

Laboratory Diagnosis

Identification of *E. histolytica* is essential to the laboratory diagnosis of amebiasis. Although this process may be as simple as a microscopic examination of a single stool specimen, difficulties often occur. The standard *ova and parasite investigation*, with three stool specimens, should be performed as a routine on all outpatients using direct and permanent stained smears in addition to concentration methods. The permanent stained smear remains the most valuable method in the detection and identification of amebae. Iron hematoxylin or trichromic acid stains yield characteristic cytoplasmic and nuclear features necessary in differentiating pathogenic from nonpathogenic organisms (see Fig. 1.2). Ninety percent of infected individuals can be confirmed with this technique. It is recommended that barium, laxatives, antibiotics, and soap enemas be avoided in order not to interfere with the test. Detection of amebae also depends on several factors ranging from appropriate collection and preservation of multiple fresh stool specimens (minimum of three over a 10-day interval), and concentration and staining methods, to training and experience of the microscopist. It is possible to cultivate trophozoites from fresh material and to hatch and cultivate trophozoite cysts in stools that are several days old.

Problems encountered at any step in the process may lead to false-negative reports. Likewise, inexperience in morphological recognition can lead to false-positive diagnoses with other nonpathogenic protozoa being mistaken for *E. histolytica*. In patients with diarrhea or dysentery, trophozoite identification should be emphasized whereas, with formed stool specimens, cysts will be more frequent and concentration methods become useful. The "steaming stool" examination or fresh biopsy material from a patient may provide a rapid inexpensive diagnosis. A warmed microscope stage and saline is ideal. The mobile trophozoites of *E. histolytica* can be diagnosed by two characteristic features: (1) presence of ingested red blood corpuscles (harmless amebae rarely contain red blood cells), and (2) rapidly protruding and slender pseudopodia (see Fig. 1.2). Amebic cysts can survive in contact with a little moisture for many years, but the vegetative forms of *E. histolytica*, which have pseudopodia, are not viable outside the body. (During the life cycle of this parasite in man, the trophozoite or "feeding stage" multiplies by simple binary fission in the large intestine. Eventually it rounds up and develops a wall protecting the infective form or cyst which is capable of surviving adverse environments in the host or externally when excreted with feces.) A dysenteric stool specimen with large numbers of white blood cells should alert the clinician to a superimposed bacterial colitis.

Sigmoidoscopy or colonoscopy biopsy specimens may also be helpful when several samples are obtained (five or more). The most rewarding specimens are obtained from the margins of small ulcers, but amebae in the process of migration may occasionally be found in the edematous areas between ulcers. If no ulcers are visible, biopsy should be performed where there is marked edema; even apparently normal mucosa may harbor the parasite. Despite repeated careful biopsies, there will be some patients from whom it is extremely difficult to obtain amebae, because they have few parasites. Rare false-negative biopsies can occur, even when the clinician and pathologist are experienced. *Histological diagnosis* is accomplished by identifying trophozoites in stained tissue sections (see Figs. 1.3–1.5). Hematoxylin and eosin staining demonstrates important cytological features within amebae and most often allows direct diagnosis. Periodic acid-Schiff staining is useful in locating organisms in multiple tissue sections. Genital and cutaneous lesions are examined similarly by smear and biopsy.

Amebic serology is useful where invasive or extraintestinal disease is suspected clinically. Over 60% of these patients with fever and right upper quadrant pain have no enteric symptoms and no history of dysentery. Stool examination for cysts and trophozoites will be positive in only a few of these individuals. Liver disease in particular can be confounding in situations where imaging is not available. Standard liver-function tests are of no value. Aspiration of amebic liver cysts is only likely to be needed if serology is not readily available, or occasionally for pain relief. Diagnostic aspiration often yields the characteristic "anchovy paste" fluid, which becomes thicker towards the end of drainage. This last thicker portion presumably contains debris from the wall of the cyst and with it live trophozoites. It is this smaller fraction that should be most carefully examined.

Serological tests that identify circulating ameba-specific antibodies are extremely valuable. The circulating antibodies were initially described in the early part of this century, through complement fixation and precipitation. Later, indirect hemagglutination and indirect fluorescent antibody tests (which are accurate and positive at low titers when tissue invasion occurs), as well as latex agglutination and other technological advances, heralded the progress in laboratory diagnosis of this parasitic disease. Currently, the enzyme-linked immunosorbent assay (ELISA) test for detection of the galactose-inhibitable adherence protein of *E. histolytica* (necessary for amebic adherence) in serum and feces appears to be the most reliable and sensitive serology test, with a virtual absence of false-negative results and a low 3.6% of false-positives. The ELISA and counterimmunoelectrophoresis (CIET) tests are highly sensitive and rapid; the CIET can be completed in 3 h and the ELISA titers in 1 day. If used together there are virtually no false-positives. The titers of ELISA are lower in intestinal amebiasis than in asymptomatic carriers; both tests are accurate for extraintestinal amebiasis. Such tests may remain positive for up to 2 years after the disease is eradicated, and can therefore be used to establish the diagnosis, but are less reliable as a therapeutic index.

Low serology titers may be unhelpful, requiring confirmation of invasion by microscopy. Also, serological testing is limited in the asymptomatic individual or as a screening procedure where antibody titers are negative or weak. Patients with high titers and positive imaging tests or other clinical evidence of extraintestinal disease should undergo therapy with both a luminal and a tissue amebicide.

Circulating *E. histolytica*-specific antibodies appear approximately 7 days after the initiation of symptoms of invasive amebiasis. Thus, the absence of serum antibodies 7 or more days after the onset of symptoms virtually eliminates amebiasis as a diagnostic consideration. A recombinant technology made of *E. histolytica* proteins (SREHP/MBP) has enhanced the serodiagnostic ability to detect invasive amebiasis, with a sensitivity of 79% and a specificity of 87%. Use of specific monoclonal antibodies against *E. histolytica* via immunofluorescence permits differentiation between the invasive and noninvasive abilities of the parasite. This technique requires samples of fresh feces. Reliability of this immunofluorescence test of 100% has been recently reported. The genotypes of invasive and noninvasive infestations correlate with the 1:10 ratio of symptomatic versus nonsymptomatic patients.

Immunoblot methods utilizing immunoglobulin A (IgA) antibodies of serum from patients with hepatic and intestinal amebiasis have shown that patients with hepatic abscess reacted to proteins greater than 200 kDa, while those with intestinal amebiasis reacted to proteins in the range of 145 kDa. IgG does not appear to increase in intestinal amebiasis and carriers, while a significant increase takes place in patients with active hepatic disease.

Finally, there is a latex agglutination test that can be performed anywhere for patients with intestinal invasive amebiasis. This test has an excellent correlation with the serology tests. Culture of *E. histolytica* can also be achieved with special media, but morphology and serology are more practical for identification of cysts and trophozoites and thus for confirmation of diagnosis.

Clinical Characteristics

The clinical spectrum of amebiasis is very wide: some patients have no symptoms while others may be desperately ill. Amebiasis can remain clinically silent and, in endemic areas, may be found incidentally at autopsy. Patients may be totally unaware of the invasive stage, and thus the history may be quite unreliable. There may have been no episode of dysentery, or it may have been so mild or occurred so long ago that it is overlooked. However, with invasive amebiasis, symptoms usually develop; they may occur as early as 8–11 days after infection, but more commonly the interval is much longer and the patient may even remain symptom free for months or years.

Similarly, the course of the disease is variable: there may be mild abdominal discomfort or acute dysentery with gripping abdominal pain, tenderness, and fever. Some patients have alternating constipation and diarrhea, whereas others have no clinical features of colonic infection. The initial attack may subside spontaneously after several days or may persist for weeks. Alternating periods of remission and exacerbation may continue for years in chronic amebic colitis. An unsuspected liver abscess may be discovered when there has been minor trauma to the rib cage, causing the abscess to rupture into the chest or abdomen and presenting as an acute emergency. In other patients, a lung abscess, pneumonia, or pleurisy may first bring the patient to medical attention.

Gastrointestinal invasion is more common among children, while hepatic amebiasis is more frequently seen in adults, with a 3 or 4:1 male to female ratio. There is less incidence of invasive amebiasis during pregnancy; however, it becomes more serious during the postpartum stage. It is more common among the malnourished and immunosuppressed, usually with grave consequences. The mortality is less than 1% in children with intestinal dysenteric amebiasis, but increases to 21.3%–40.2% when the course is complicated by intestinal perforation and peritonitis. Mortality from treated hepatic amebic abscess has gradually diminished from 2.0% to 0.2%, although it remains at 10.3% in some rural areas of Mexico.

Colon

Recurrent dysentery, with loose, mucoid, blood-stained stools, headache, and nausea are common symptoms in amebic colitis. Pain is most common in the right lower abdomen, but can occur with tenderness to palpation over any portion of the colon. Almost any variety of large bowel complaint can be caused by amebiasis, which must therefore be considered in differential diagnosis and evaluated by serological testing, repeated adequate examinations of fresh stool specimens, and/or sigmoidoscopy coupled with biopsy (repeated if necessary). If serological tests are negative, stool samples and biopsy may be unnecessary, but if they are positive, then the activity of the disease must be assessed.

Ulcerative Amebic Proctocolitis. This diarrhea-dysentery syndrome is characterized by mucosanguinous watery bowel movements associated with colic and tenesmus. There are four to six episodes of bloody diarrhea per day without fever or systemic manifestations. This syndrome has been termed "ambulatory dysentery" and resolves promptly with appropriate medical therapy. Mortality is 0.5%, but increases to 20%–40% with bowel perforation and peritonitis, which predominantly occur in children.

Fulminant Colitis and Toxic Megacolon. This is a grave and rapidly evolving disease with 20 or more episodes of bloody diarrhea during a 24-hour period. It is accompanied by severe abdominal pain and intense and constant tenesmus. There is nausea, anorexia, fever, rapid pulse, and hypovolemic hypotension. The patient suffers dehydration and prostration and may present to the emergency room in a state of shock. Massive thrombosis of the colonic wall venules with intestinal ischemia, infarction, and ischemic tissue necrosis are some of the features encountered in patients with severe colonic distention and abdominal hyperesthesia from toxic megacolon. Intestinal perforation worsens the prognosis. There is a high mortality despite palliative or radical surgical procedures.

Ameboma. Amebomas are pseudotumoral amebic granulomas that exhibit necrosis, inflammation, and edema of the mucosa und submucosa of the colon. Clinically, there is a bloody dysentery with abdominal pain and associated palpable colonic mass.

Amebic Appendicitis. In most patients, there are no distinguishing features between amebic appendicitis and conventional acute appendicitis. However, a preceding episode of bloody diarrhea may herald an amebic etiology.

Chronic Amebic Colitis. The term "chronic amebic colitis" has been applied to patients with nonspecific symptoms such as spasmodic colonic pain and alternating periods of diarrhea and constipation, with occasional mucus and *E. histolytica* cysts in the stool. Such patients may simply have an irritable colon or may be carriers of amebiasis. A diagnosis of amebic disease should be based on the identification of an intestinal wall lesion, a demonstrable trophozoite, and positive serological tests.

Liver

Hepatic abscess has protean clinical manifestations and is the most frequent extracolonic complication of amebic infection, occurring in up to one-third of all patients with colonic amebiasis. It may present at any age, but is 10 times more common in adults aged 20–60 years. It is three to four times more frequent in men. It is important to emphasize that, although the colon is the portal of entry of amebae, liver abscesses are often found in patients who have no dysentery or other colonic symptoms; in 59% of patients, there is no preceding history of diarrhea. Moreover, repeated stool examinations, and even culture and biopsy, may not demonstrate either cysts or trophozoites in every patient. Liver function tests are unreliable, but serological tests can be very helpful. In as many as 80% of such patients, the radiological and sonographic findings are highly significant, although not necessarily diagnostic. An abscess may sometimes persist within the liver for months before becoming clinically apparent. It frequently manifests itself by involvement of the chest. The clinical manifestations vary according to the stage and extent of the disease; however, there are some characteristic features. The onset is abrupt, beginning with sudden pain in the hepatic region, radiating towards the shoulder or subscapular area. Pain is exacerbated with deep inspiration, cough, and adoption of the right lateral decubitus position. In the minority of cases, where the abscess is located in the left lobe, the pain may be perceived to be in the epigastrium, radiating to the retrosternal area and occasionally to the precordium. There is an associated febrile course, reaching 38°–40°C, which can be accompanied by chills and profuse sweating. Other systemic symptoms include anorexia, nausea, vomiting, diarrhea, and weight loss.

The cardinal physical sign is a tender hepatomegaly, painful on digital pressure or percussion. However, if the abscess is subdiaphragmatic and the diaphragm is elevated, abdominal palpation may not reveal hepatomegaly. The patients are often anemic and have an elevated white blood cell count. Jaundice is noticeable in 8% of patients, of whom 70% will exhibit hepatic abscesses, heralding a poor prognosis. In isolated cases, jaundice is caused by porta-hepatic compression by a hepatic abscess.

Chest

Pleuropericardial and pulmonary manifestations are more common in adults aged 20–60 years, and are three to four times more frequent in men. In approximately 60% of patients, there is no preceding history of diarrhea. Such manifestations are the result of a communication or extension of a hepatic abscess into the adjacent thoracic cavity, although isolated case reports suggest that the infection can be primary or by inhalation, with adverse bronchopulmonary manifestations. Typically, an abscess located high in the right lobe of the liver generates an inflammatory reaction in the lower thorax as a result of the subphrenic process.

Amebiasis within the chest may present as an acute condition when such an abscess ruptures through the diaphragm into the pleura, pericardium, lung, or a bronchus. There may be severe shock, dyspnea, cough, and tearing lower chest pain. Rupture into the pericardium can cause a fulminating pericarditis or acute tamponade and may resemble a myocardial infarction with sudden onset, dyspnea, shock, and cyanosis. In other patients, the initial clinical features suggest lower lobe pneumonia or pleural effusion. The pleural fluid may be either purulent or a transudate caused by reaction to the subdiaphragmatic abscess. Fistulization into a bronchus produces a creamy chocolate-colored expectoration.

The frequency of chest involvement depends to a certain extent on the location of the abscess within the liver: clearly, the closer it is to the diaphragm, the more likely there will be perforation, a pleural exudate, or even pneumonia. In children, and occasionally in adults, the clinical picture of amebiasis may be that of a lung abscess presenting with purulent sputum, cough, pyrexia, and general malaise. These abscesses may be multiple, and can occur in any part of the lung. The liver need not be involved. The diagnosis may only be suspected when an apparently pyogenic lung abscess fails to respond to antibiotics; it may be confirmed by the discovery of amebae in the sputum.

Central Nervous System

Amebic abscesses may rarely occur within the brain or spinal cord and even more rarely may be the first evidence of the infection (Fig. 1.10). The clinical (and radiological) findings cannot be differentiated from cerebral or spinal abscesses of any other etiology. There may be some confusion (particularly when referring to the literature) because meningoencephalitis can be caused by other amebae. These are the free-living amebae, *Naegleria fowleri* and *Acanthameba astronyxis*, which can be found in mud around fresh water ponds and swimming holes. Human infection with *E. polecki* (normally a parasite in pigs and monkeys) has rarely been reported, is difficult to distinguish from *E. histolytica*, and is almost never symptomatic.

Skin

Although of less concern to radiologists, cutaneous amebiasis presents diagnostic pitfalls for both the clinician and the pathologist. Cutaneous amebiasis may involve anus, genital skin, vagina, and cervix, as a consequence of contiguous spread from colon and rectum. Amebiasis of the penis may develop after rectal intercourse. Amebic ulcers of the trunk (Fig. 1.11 A, B) are usually complications of penetrating amebic lesions of the colon, liver, pleura, peritoneum, or pericardium and are painful, tender, and malodorous. That amebiasis can involve skin must be kept in mind especially by those practicing in regions where amebiasis is common. The hyperplastic, cauliflower-like appearance of perianal, perineal, and genital amebiasis can be easily confused clinically with squamous carcinoma or a mycosis (Fig. 1.11 C, D).

Amebiasis versus Carcinoma

Amebiasis may mimic carcinoma, not only in the colon and rectum, where "napkin ring " or "apple core" constrictions can be caused by amebomas, but especially in skin and mucous membranes. Amebiasis of the anus, perineum, penis, and vulva may mimic carcinomas so strikingly that radical excisions have been done on the basis of clinical appearance alone. Amebiasis of the uterine cervix, by causing induration, swelling, and ulceration, may also be mistaken for carcinoma. Thus, benign amebic lesions may be inadvertently excised when anti-amebic therapy alone is indicated. Further complicating this diagnostic hazard is the fact that carcinomas may be colonized by *E. histolytica*. A patient with an amebic lesion resembling a carcinoma must

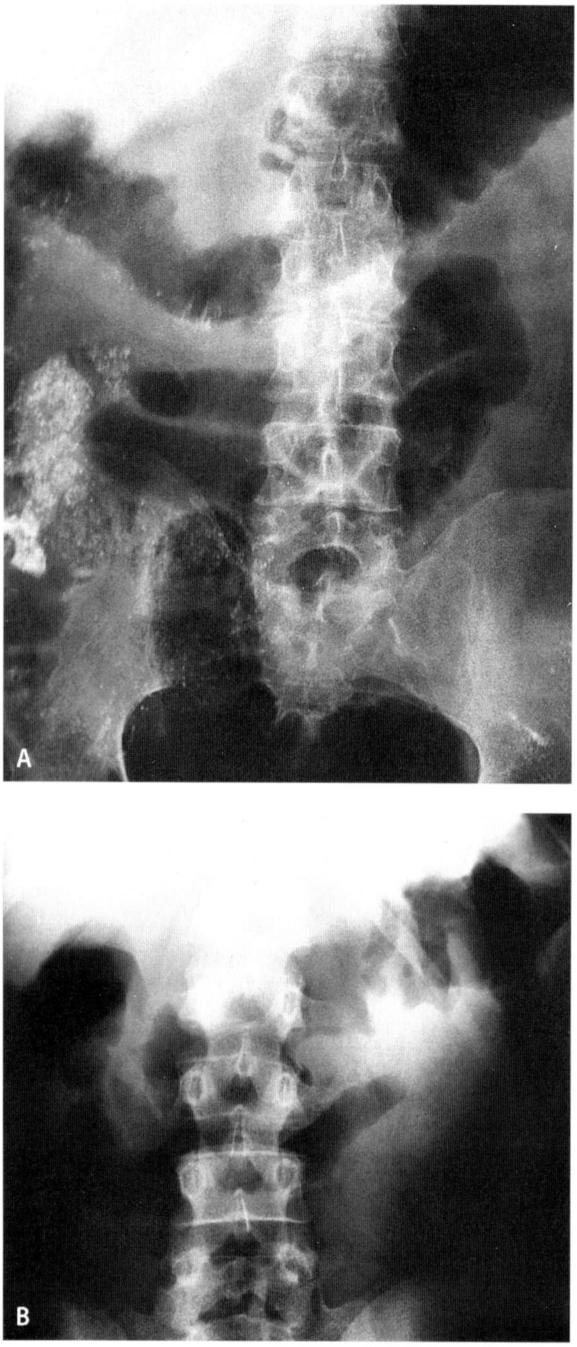

Fig. 1.12 A, B. Fulminant amebic colitis on plain film examination. **A** Note a diffuse antimesenteric ameboma narrowing the lumen of the proximal transverse colon. The distal transverse colon and several loops of small bowel in the mid-abdomen are distended, representing an ileus from peritoneal irritation. Opaque granular material represents ingested iodine-containing medication. **B** There is marked thumbprinting involving the transverse colon of another patient

therefore be rebiopsied if there is any suspicion of underlying malignancy.

Imaging Diagnosis

The radiological findings in amebiasis are many and varied. The radiologist, like the clinician, must have a high index of suspicion to suggest the correct diagnosis.

Intestinal Amebiasis

Plain Radiographs of the Abdomen

Abdominal films are of little value in the diagnosis of ulcerative amebic proctocolitis unless a perforation has occurred. They are of paramount importance in assessing the grave form of amebiasis, such as fulminant colitis, which co-exists frequently with an ameboma (25%) and hepatic abscess (30%) (Fig. 1.12 A). Gas in the colon serves as a natural contrast to outline alterations in the intestinal wall in patients with fulminant amebic colitis: (1) There may be a nonspecific pattern of right lower quadrant haziness with minimal colonic distension. (2) Thumbprinting may be present with deep indentations on the distended colon, segmental or generalized, predominantly in the transverse colon (Fig. 1.12 B). Thumbprinting represents areas of extensive edema and necrosis and is indistinguishable from the thumbprinting seen in ischemic colitis and other hemorrhagic or edematous processes.

Toxic Megacolon. This unfortunate, grave complication of amebiasis can appear during the course of a fulminant colitis. When the disease is fulminating, as it may be in children and younger adults, it resembles acute, rapidly progressive ulcerative colitis. The entire large bowel may be involved and occasionally the terminal ileum as well (even during the acute infection, an incompetent ileocecal valve is common). Only 0.5% of these patients develop this feared transmural disease with extensive muscle lysis damaging the myenteric plexus, resulting in loss of colonic muscle tone with massive dilatation of the large bowel (Fig.1.13). There is loss of the normal colon landmarks, including haustrations, as well as mucosal destruction and isolated islands of edematous mucosa projecting as pseudopolyps. In some patients, pneumatosis cystoides intestinalis can be appreciated, as well as all the findings of colonic wall destruction similar to ulcerative colitis. A toxic megacolon is a definite contraindication for barium enema examination because of the fragile nature of the severely ulcerated and often paper-thin bowel wall.

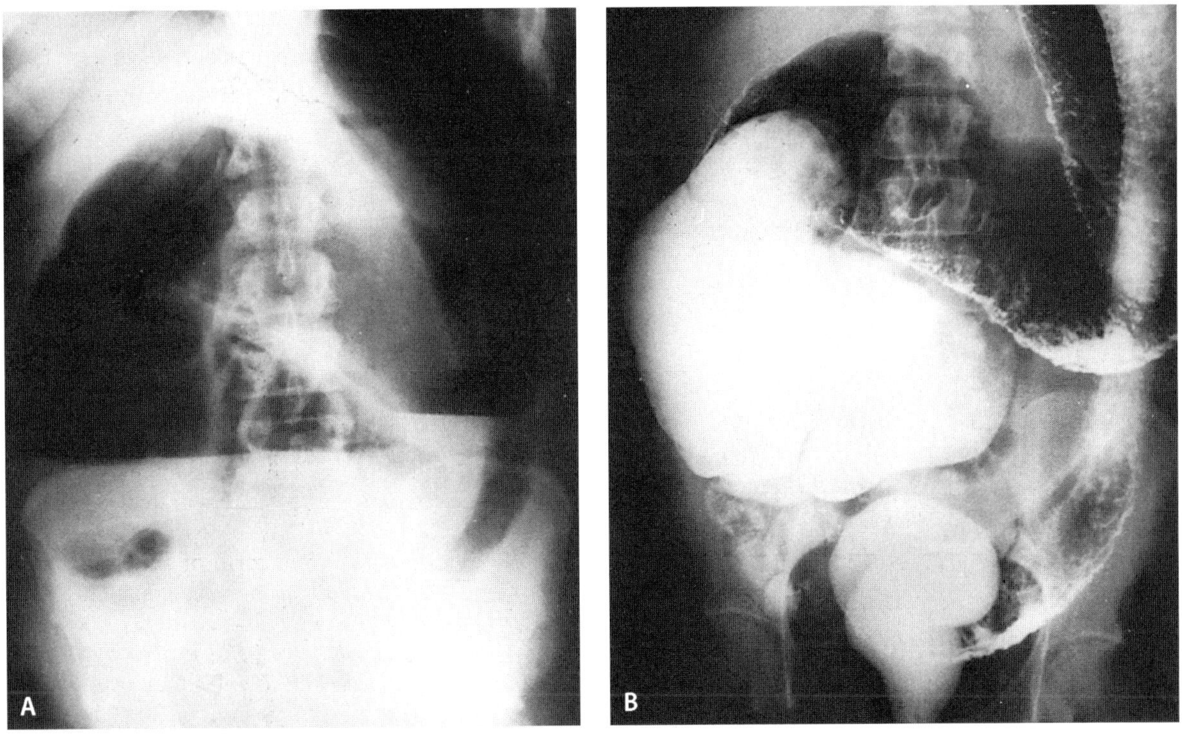

Fig. 1.13 A, B. Toxic megacolon in acute amebic colitis, similar radiographically to that seen in ulcerative colitis. In **A** there is marked distention of the colon with several air-fluid levels in the grossly dilated cecum and distal transverse colon on erect plain film of the abdomen. **B** A barium enema was performed in this case (sound judgment should prevail against such a potentially dangerous study) and shows innumerable small ulcers eroding the mucosa of the greatly distended colon. (Courtesy of Drs. Malcolm Hill and Henry Goldberg, San Francisco and *Am J Roentgenol*, 1967)

Unfortunately, multiple careful rectal biopsies and stool examinations may be negative, but the possibility of amebic colitis should be remembered because the results of surgery on the toxic megacolon of amebiasis are almost inevitably disastrous. Antiamebic therapy should always antecede surgery on all patients with colonic amebiasis (see Figs. 1.27 A and 1.33). Making the correct diagnosis is a greater problem in climates where both amebic and ulcerative colitis may occur than in the tropics, where ulcerative colitis is rare and toxic megacolon has a much higher probability of being amebic in origin.

Perforation. Sixty to eighty-seven percent of patients with fulminant amebic colitis progress to show single or multiple sites of perforation (see Fig. 1.7).

Amebic Typhloappendicitis. Three percent of invasive colonic amebiasis will be confined to the cecum and appendix. The appendix can be involved by direct extension from the colon; however, in 26% of cases, amebiasis is confined to the appendix. In Mexico, acute amebic appendicitis represents 1.6% of all cases. The traditional appendicolith or pneumoperitoneum is not a feature of this parasitic appendicitis.

Barium Enema

Single or double (air) contrast barium enema is a valuable method for diagnosing invasive amebiasis. It allows excellent evaluation of the mucosal abnormalities and provides information regarding alterations of the colon wall and caliber.

Ulcers. In the initial stages of the disease, the ulcers are small, confluent, and superficial, resulting in a fine granular appearance of the mucosa and discrete spiculation of its margin (Figs. 1.14–1.16). These findings are best demonstrated in the cecum, ascending colon, and rectosigmoid area. Alternating areas of spasm are common. Aphthous and linear ulcers are easily detected on double-contrast examinations (Fig. 1.16 A). Deep ulcers may penetrate the submucosa, giving origin to flask-shaped "collar button" ulcers (Figs. 1.17–1.20) similar to those observed in other ulcerative diseases of the colon. The large bowel wall is generally thickened.

Thumbprinting. A large number of digitiform areas of edema with segmental distribution deforming the colonic lumen is the rule. Edema, hemorrhage, and superimposed infection are found in these areas (Figs. 1.17–1.20).

(Text continues on p. 28)

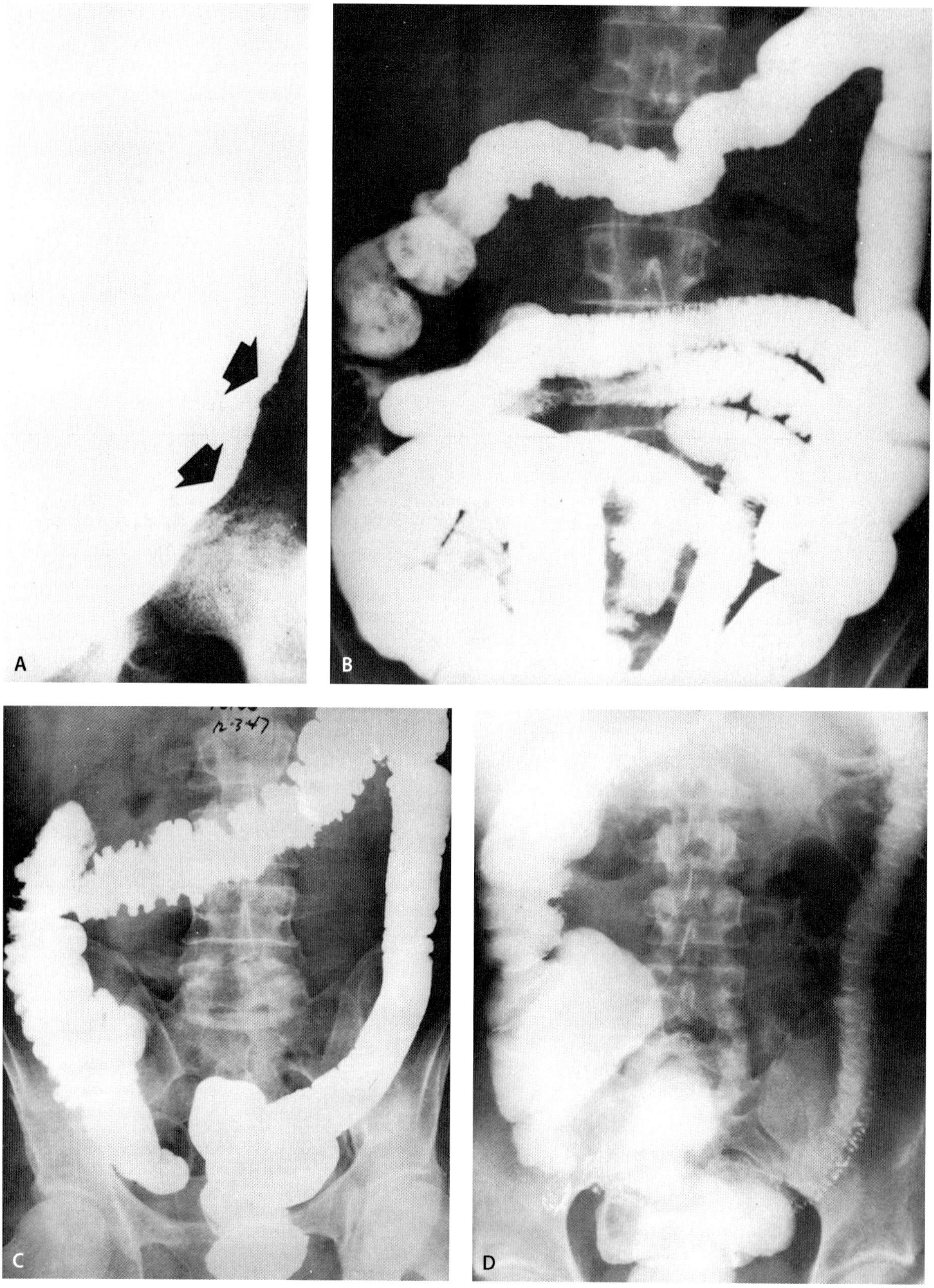
A
B
C
D

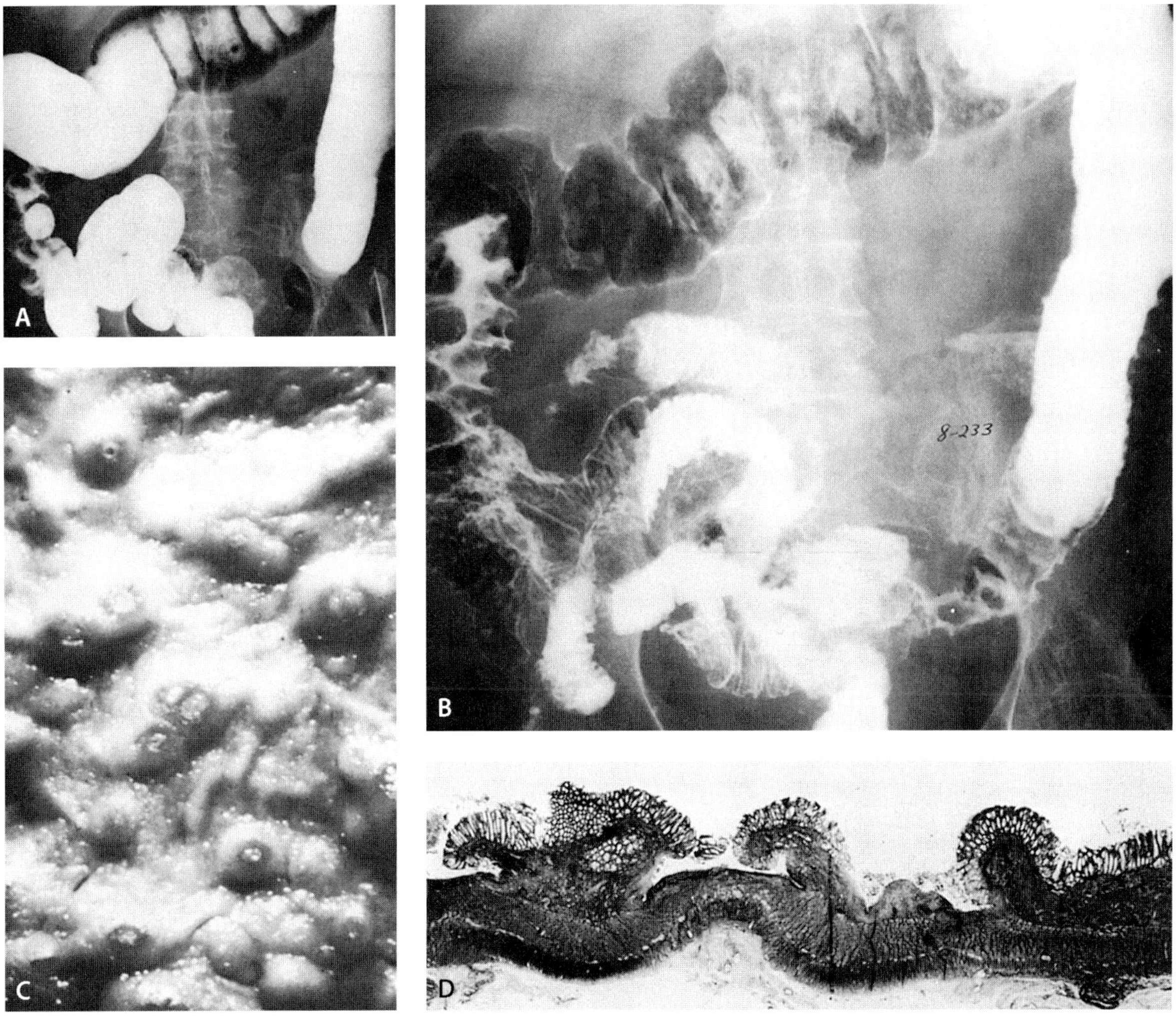

Fig. 1.15 A–D. Amebic colitis with ulceration and spasm in a San Salvador adult. **A, B** Note the spasm in the cecum and ascending and proximal sigmoid colon. There are mural spiculations and fine ulcerations along the ascending colon, and the cecum is slightly conical in shape. There are deeper ulcers extending into the submucosa of the descending and sigmoid colon. (Courtesy of Dr. Julio Astacio, San Salvador) **C** Multiple discrete, hemorrhagic ulcers atop mounds of heaped-up, edematous mucosa in the colon of another patient. **D** Such ulcers have characteristic undermining with extension deep into the submucosa, and at times into the muscularis. ×4.75; AFIP 54-10227

◄ **Fig. 1.14 A–D.** Amebic ulcers of the colon. **A** Fine marginal serrations (*arrows*) representing tiny mucosal spiculations in the distal colon in early, mildly symptomatic amebic colitis in a Korean child. (Courtesy of Dr. William Harshaw) **B** Fine mucosal spiculations and shallow ulcerations in the transverse colon of another patient with acute amebic colitis. Notice the marked spasm in the cecum, which was also involved and ulcerated. **C** Irregular haustral pattern and multiple superficial and slightly deeper mucosal ulcers in the transverse colon and hepatic flexure in another patient with amebic colitis. **D** Numerous well-defined, deep ulcers extending through the mucosa into the submucosa along the ascending, transverse, descending, and sigmoid colon. These are the flask-shaped ulcers seen histologically, which may resemble the collar button ulcers of ulcerative colitis radiologically. (Courtesy of Dr. Douglas Sheft, San Francisco)

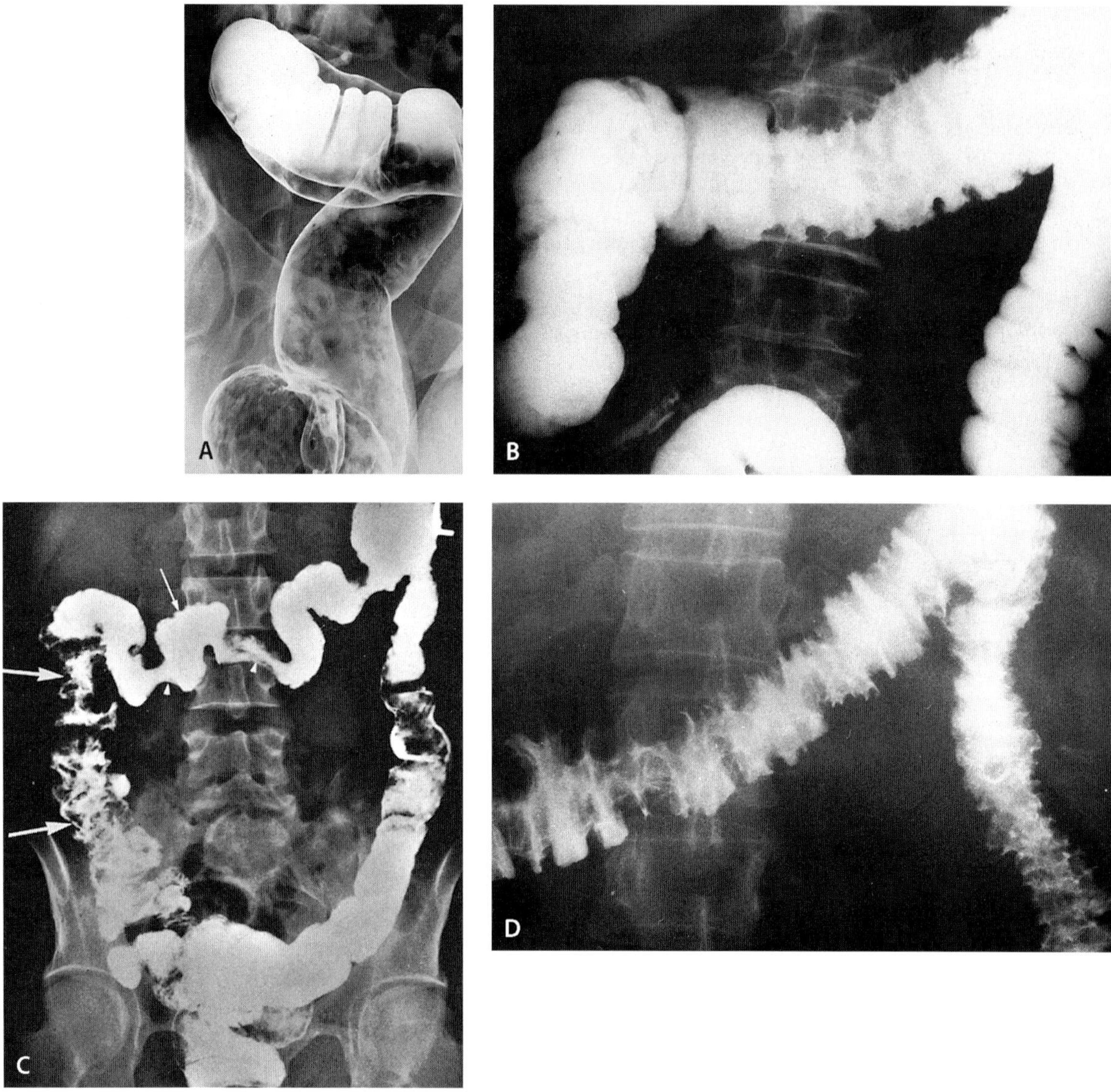

Fig. 1.16 A–D. Amebic ulcers in four different patients. **A** Air-contrast barium enema in a 22-year-old African patient shows numerous aphthous amebic ulcers in the rectosigmoid colon. (Courtesy of Dr. Peter Cockshott) **B** Barium enema in a Mexican patient demonstrates multiple ulcers in the mid-transverse colon and thumbprinting edema in the transverse and ascending colon. **C** Tiny spiculated mural ulcerations (*small arrow*) and multiple spastic areas (*arrowheads*) are seen in the transverse colon of another patient with amebic colitis. There is considerable mucosal edema, thickening, irregularity, and spasm in the ascending colon (*large arrows*). **D** Generalized ulceration of the transverse and descending colon with associated thumbprinting in a Mexican with colonic amebiasis. (**B, D** courtesy of Drs. Kenji Kimura and Miguel Stoopen)

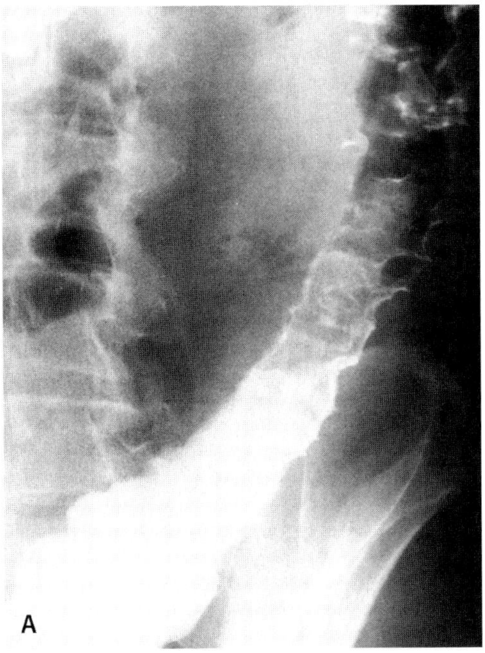

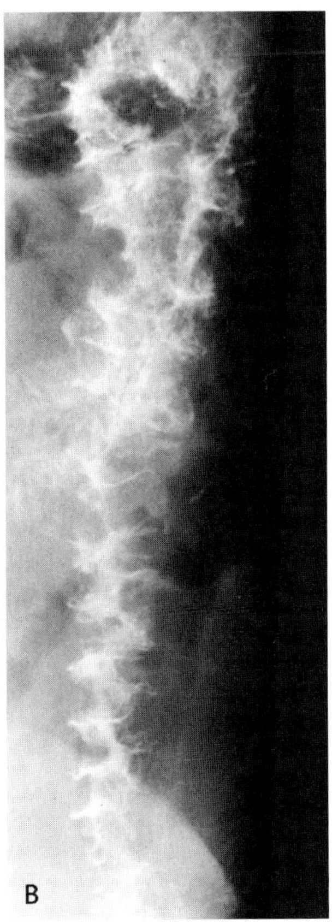

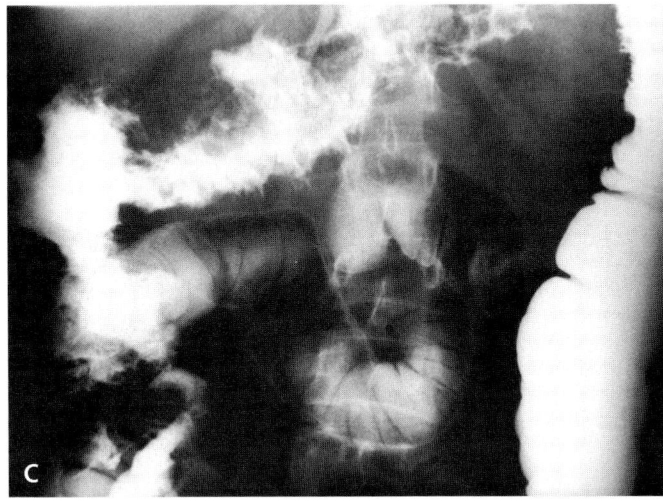

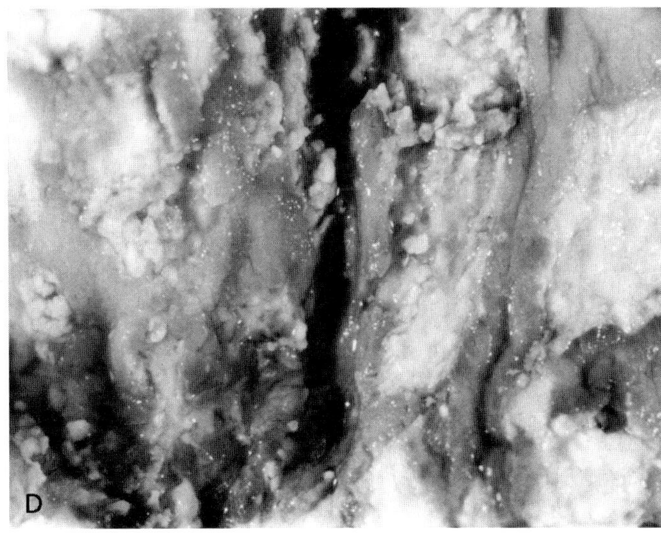

Fig. 1.17 A–D. Fulminant amebic colitis. **A, B** Effacement of the normal mucosa with multiple shallow and deep ulcers combined with thumbprinting secondary to necrosis and edematous thickening of the descending colon in two patients from Mexico and Africa. **C** Combination of multiple deep ulcers and amebomas involving the cecum and ascending, transverse and proximal descending colon in a Mexican with fulminant amebic colitis. (**A, C** courtesy of Drs. Kenji Kimura and Miguel Stoopen) **D** Confluent colonic ulcers in a 38-year-old woman with severe colonic amebiasis. A fibrin-rich exudate fills the ulcer craters on this surgical specimen; a colectomy was performed because her colitis became life-threatening. (Courtesy of Dr. Daniel H. Connor)

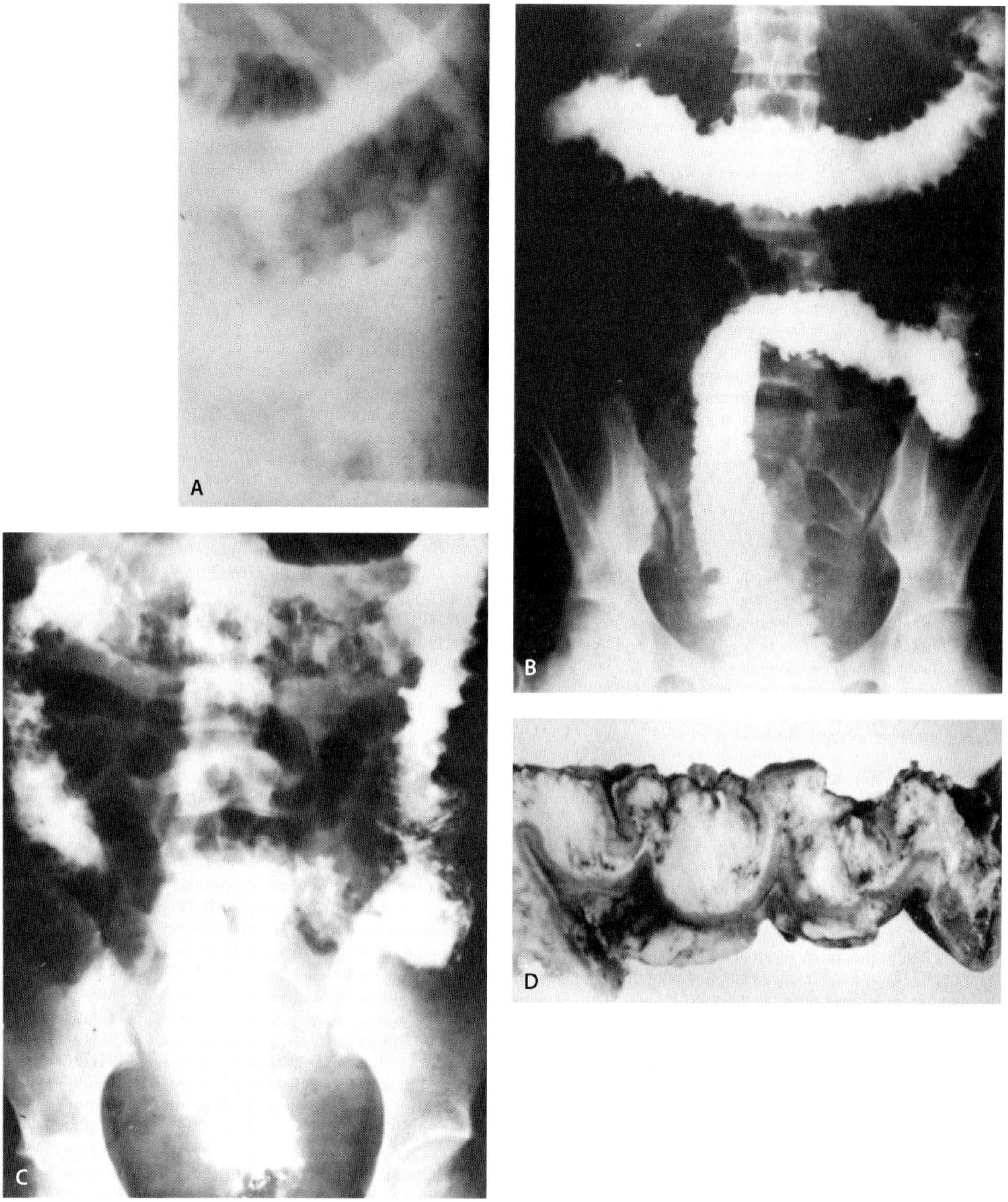

Fig. 1.18 A, B. Advanced amebic colitis in an 18-year-old woman from Sacramento, California. **A** Plain anteroposterior film of the abdomen shows a nodular mucosal pattern and thickening of the wall of the transverse colon. **B** Deep ulcers are seen throughout the colon together with multiple areas of thumbprinting from mucosal edema. There is intense spasm of the ascending and descending colon. The edematous mucosa and ragged outline of the thickened, ulcerated transverse colon correlate well with the plain film findings seen in **A**. **C** In a different patient from Canada there is partial filling of an irregular, ulcerated, thickened and spastic colon. The cecum never filled well on this examination. The rectum and sigmoid colon are straightened and lifted vertically out of the pelvis by a large perirectal abscess which has developed from extension of deep amebic ulcers of the rectum into the perirectal tissues. (Courtesy of Dr. Jack Tischler, Winnipeg) Similar findings are also seen in **B**. **D** Vertical section of a specimen of colon showing deep ragged ulcers extending through mucosa and submucosa and in some areas through muscularis. The bowel wall is markedly thickened, irregular, and distorted. ×6.5; AFIP 69-3640. (Courtesy of Dr. Daniel H. Connor)

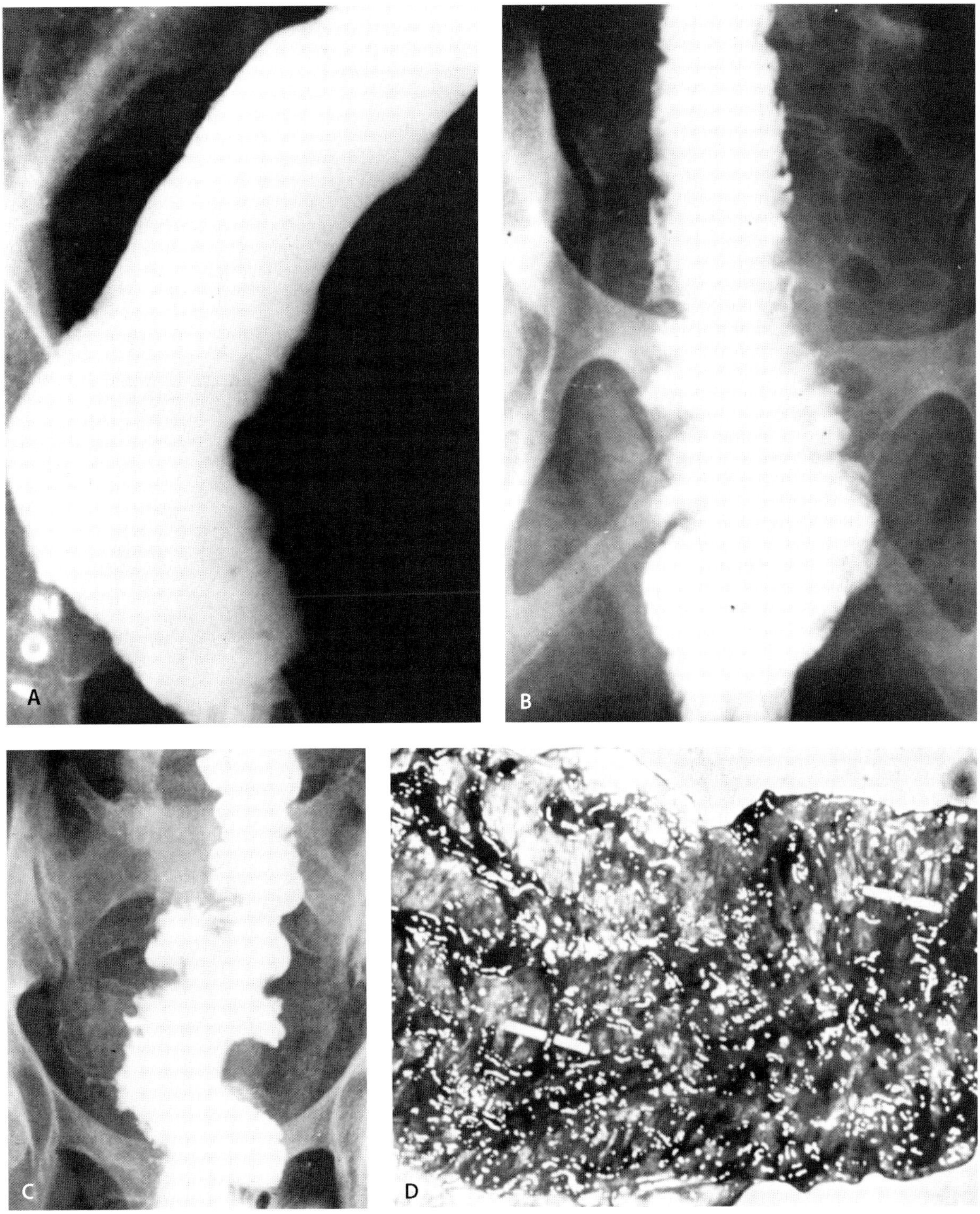

Fig. 1.19 A–D. Amebic proctitis in three patients. **A** Slight irregularity of contour of the rectum with shallow ulcers. **B** Extensive deep ulcers of the rectal mucosa extending through the submucosa and muscularis at right angles into the perirectal tissues with a large perirectal abscess straightening and elevating the rectosigmoid colon out of the pelvis in a patient from Sacramento. **C** Similar findings of markedly irregular rectal contour with deep ulcers and short right angle sinuses extending into the perirectal tissues in an African woman. A calcified uterine leiomyoma is seen in the right side of the pelvis. **D** Gross specimen of the rectum in fatal amebiasis showing red, hemorrhagic and ulcerated mucosa. Several mucosal bridges have markers placed beneath them

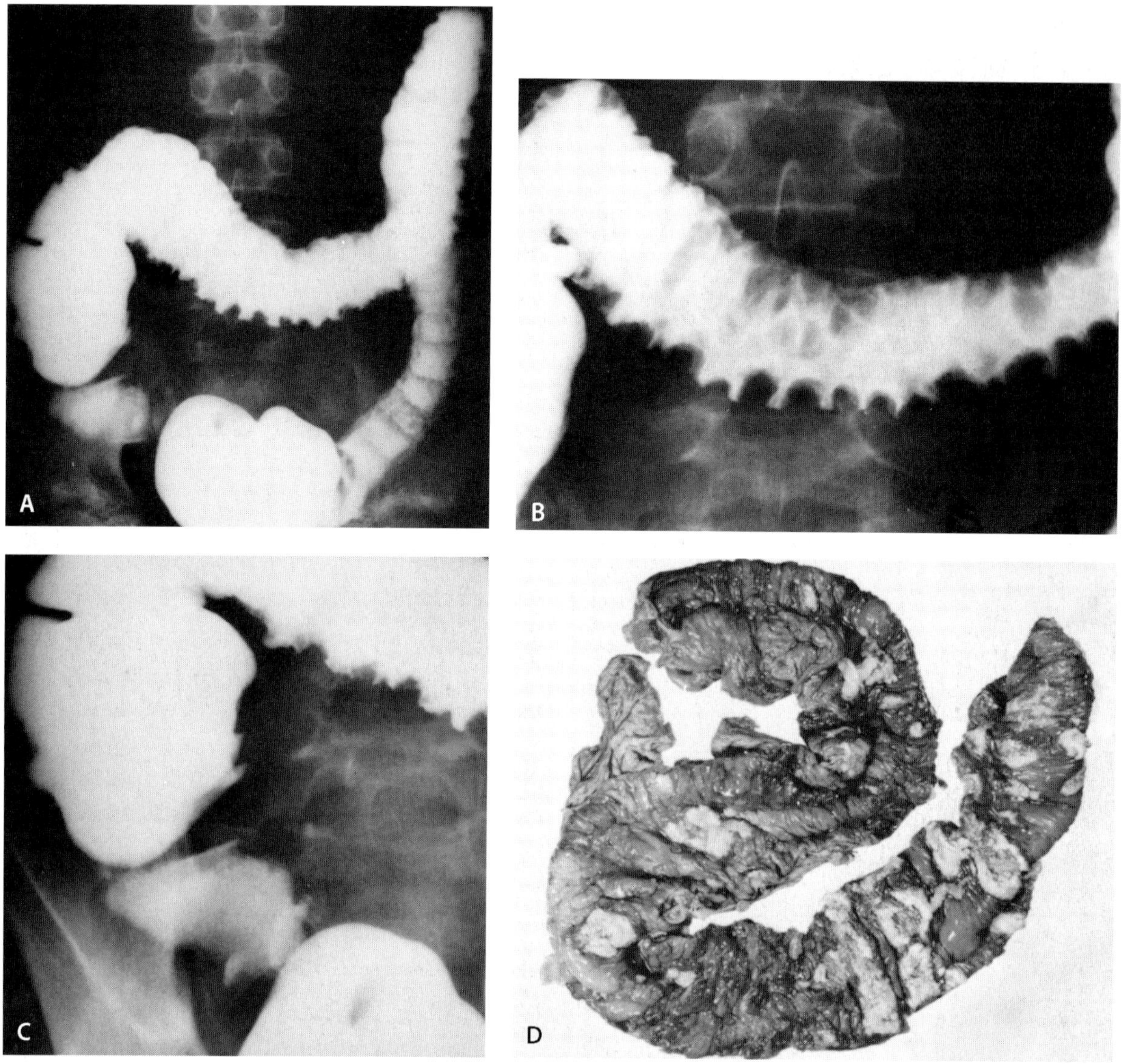

Fig. 1.20 A–D. Amebic colitis with cecal deformity, ulcers, and prominent thumbprinting of the mucosal pattern from extensive submucosal and mucosal edema. The thumbprinting is most intense in the transverse colon (**A–C**), whereas deep ulcers and irregularity of the ascending colon and cecum are best seen in **A** and **C**. The patient was a young American recently returned from Southeast Asia. **D** Gross specimen of the colon in fatal amebic colitis showing numerous large, ragged ulcers surrounded by heaped-up mounds of edematous mucosa. AFIP 67-13734-A. Extensive edema in the mucosa and submucosa occasionally produces prominent thumbprinting defects of the bowel contour in some patients with amebiasis. Thumbprinting is a nonspecific finding which may be caused by edema, hemorrhage, lymphoma, and other nonamebic forms of colitis

Fig. 1.21 A–D. Marked spasm of the involved section of colon is usually a prominent feature of acute amebic colitis. **A–C** Intense spasm of the right colon and cecum in three different patients preventing adequate visualization of the colonic mucosal pattern. In **B** there is also slight spasm and mucosal edema and spiculations giving a serrated appearance to the descending colon. Prolonged, intense spasm of the right colon and cecum should suggest the possibility of amebiasis, although tuberculosis, Crohn's disease, and other inflammatory conditions of the right colon may produce a similar appearance. If reflux is obtained into a normal-appearing terminal ileum, the probability of amebiasis is even more likely. In **A** the ileum appears normal, in **B** it appears thickened, ulcerated, and indurated in its distal portion, and in **C** it is not adequately filled. In **D** there is spasm of the entire descending colon, which shows superficial and some deep ulcerations. There is also an irregular wall contour of the transverse colon from edema and ulcers. The right colon, cecum, and rectum appear normal ▶

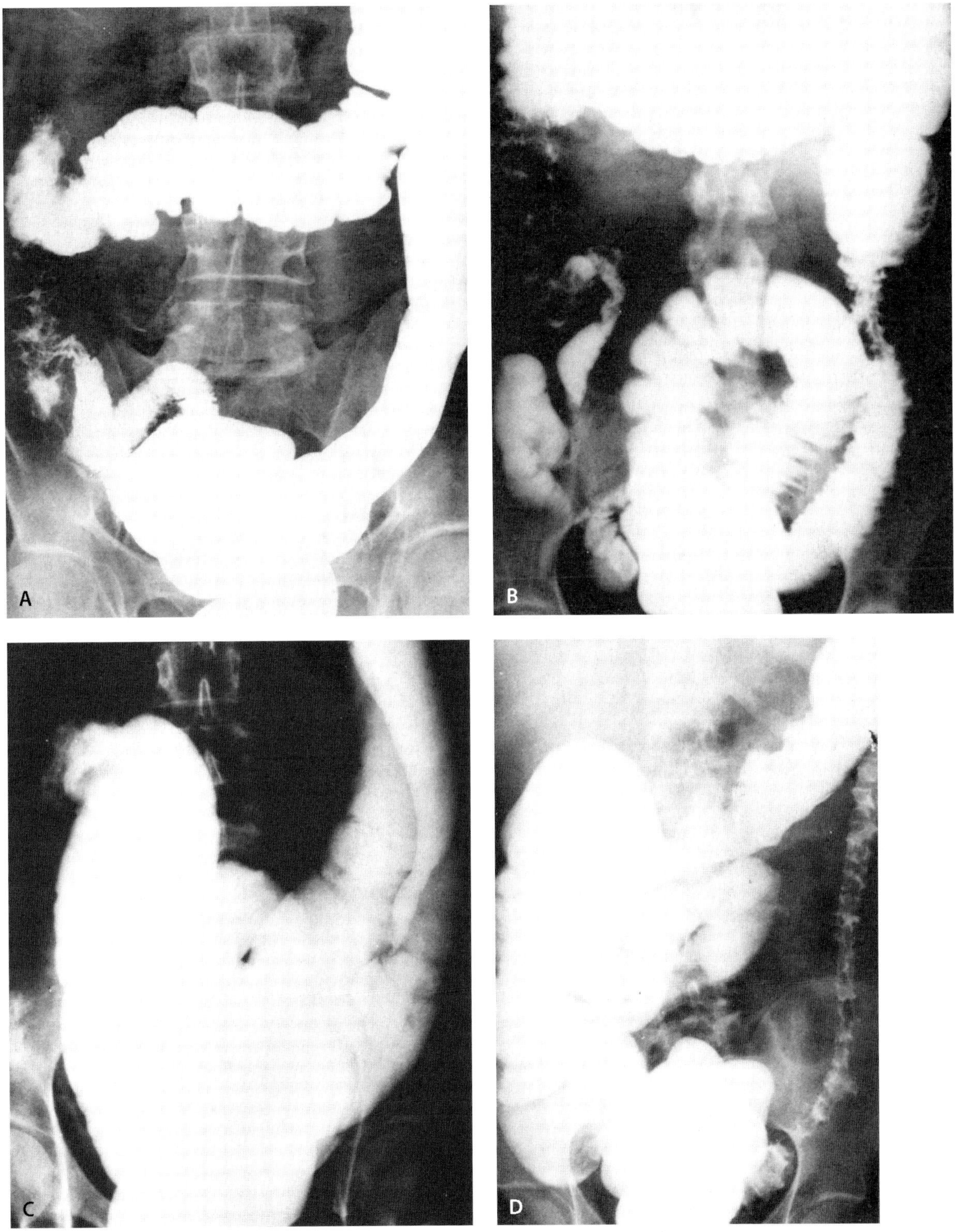
A
B
C
D

Cecum and Colon

The pathological findings of edema and ulceration are reflected by the radiological changes of a thickened, rigid bowel wall, swollen irregular mucosa, and multiple tiny ulcers with skip areas anywhere throughout the length of the large bowel.

The cecum is the primary site of involvement radiologically in 90% of patients with colonic amebiasis. Scattered areas of involvement may occur elsewhere in the large bowel, especially in the rectosigmoid colon, in up to 60% of such patients. In severe infections, the entire bowel may be involved.

In acute amebic colitis, the earliest roentgen sign is a granular mucosal pattern, often with tiny spiculations, which may occasionally extend throughout the bowel. This pattern is nonspecific and is the result of edema and multiple small ulcers in the mucosa. The bowel is often irritable and empties rapidly. It is difficult to distend any part of the involved bowel because of edema and spasm (Figs. 1.21, p. 27; 1.22). The ulcers may burrow deeper into the submucosa and have overhanging edges caused by undermining of the mucosa (these are the flask-shaped ulcers seen histologically - they may resemble the collar button ulcers of ulcerative colitis). They can be demonstrated more clearly radiologically at this stage and are often associated with muscle spasm and a thickened bowel wall (Figs. 1.14–1.22).

In the early stages of amebiasis, the outline of the cecum becomes hazy, indistinct, and irregular, and lacks its normal smooth, clear silhouette. It may appear that the bowel preparation has been inadequate, even when the cecum is actually empty. As the disease progresses, the wall becomes thickened, edematous and ulcerated, and the cecum becomes less mobile and relatively rigid, either in part or in whole: distension is possible with pressure, whereas in malignant disease the cecum is indistensible. A further difference is that in amebiasis there is a gradual transition from diseased to normal bowel without an abrupt change. These findings in the cecum should prompt a careful search throughout the rest of the bowel for similar areas, which occur most commonly in the rectosigmoid or transverse colon, although no part of the bowel escapes.

In the later stages, the cecum characteristically loses its normal sac-like appearance and gradually narrows until it becomes cone-shaped or pyramidal in outline (Figs. 1.23–1.26). The ileocecal valve often moves downward and may appear to lie close to the tip of the cecum. The valve is invariably thickened, rigid, and fixed in an open position, allowing reflux to occur in virtually all barium enema examinations, unlike in tuberculosis, in which reflux is uncommon. The combination of a conical cecum with a normal-appearing terminal ileum helps to rule out other entities, such as tuberculosis and Crohn's disease, in most patients, although the terminal 6 inches of ileum may be involved in 10% or more of patients with severe cecal amebiasis.

The sequence of changes throughout the colon is similar to that in the cecum. The earliest abnormality in the colonic mucosa is an exaggeration of the normal findings. The mucosal folds become enlarged, edematous, and more complex. Later, the mucosa is flattened and may appear smooth or granular and tiny ulcers can be visualized. There is alteration in motility caused by edema of the wall and often associated spasm (Figs. 1.21, 1.22); when spasm is present, cine or videotape studies are valuable. Even though mobility is decreased, the colon is not usually fixed.

Another less common radiological presentation of acute amebiasis, which may cause difficulty in diagnosis, is marked "thumbprinting" similar to that seen in ischemic bowel. There is marked mucosal edema, rigidity and narrowing extending over either short or long lengths of the colon (Figs. 1.17–1.20). In most patients it is possible to distinguish this appearance from ischemic lesions, because ulcers and skip areas more typical of amebic colitis may be recognized, or the cecum may have a characteristic amebic outline. However, there will be occasional patients in whom accurate diagnosis is not possible and rectal biopsy may show no trophozoites. Again, antiamebic therapy may be both life-saving and suggest the correct diagnosis.

As the disease becomes chronic, the bowel outline may become "pipe stemmed" and indistinguishable from end-stage ulcerative colitis. The normal haustral pattern is missing, and the bowel becomes smooth in outline and shortened.

Fig. 1.22 A–F. Disappearance of spasm, mucosal edema, and ulceration with reversion of the bowel towards a more normal appearance after antiamebic therapy in three different patients. **A, B** There is intense spasm and mucosal edema of the sigmoid colon on initial barium enema. Two months later, the colon appears normal after successful treatment for amebiasis. **C, D** Mucosal edema and spasm are seen in the proximal and distal sigmoid colon, preventing adequate distention of these segments on initial barium study. The midsigmoid colon between the spastic segments is dilated. Two weeks after a course of antiamebic therapy, the distal and midsigmoid colon fill normally. There is a residual short area of stenosis in the proximal sigmoid colon. **E, F** Initial barium study reveals prominent ulcers and a granular mucosal pattern involving the sigmoid colon, which is somewhat tubular and rigid. Five months later, after antiamebic treatment, no ulcers are identified and the colon has a more normal appearance, although it remains smooth and tubular with residual loss of haustrations. (**E, F** courtesy of Dr. Jack Farman, Great Neck) ▶

(Text continues on p. 33)

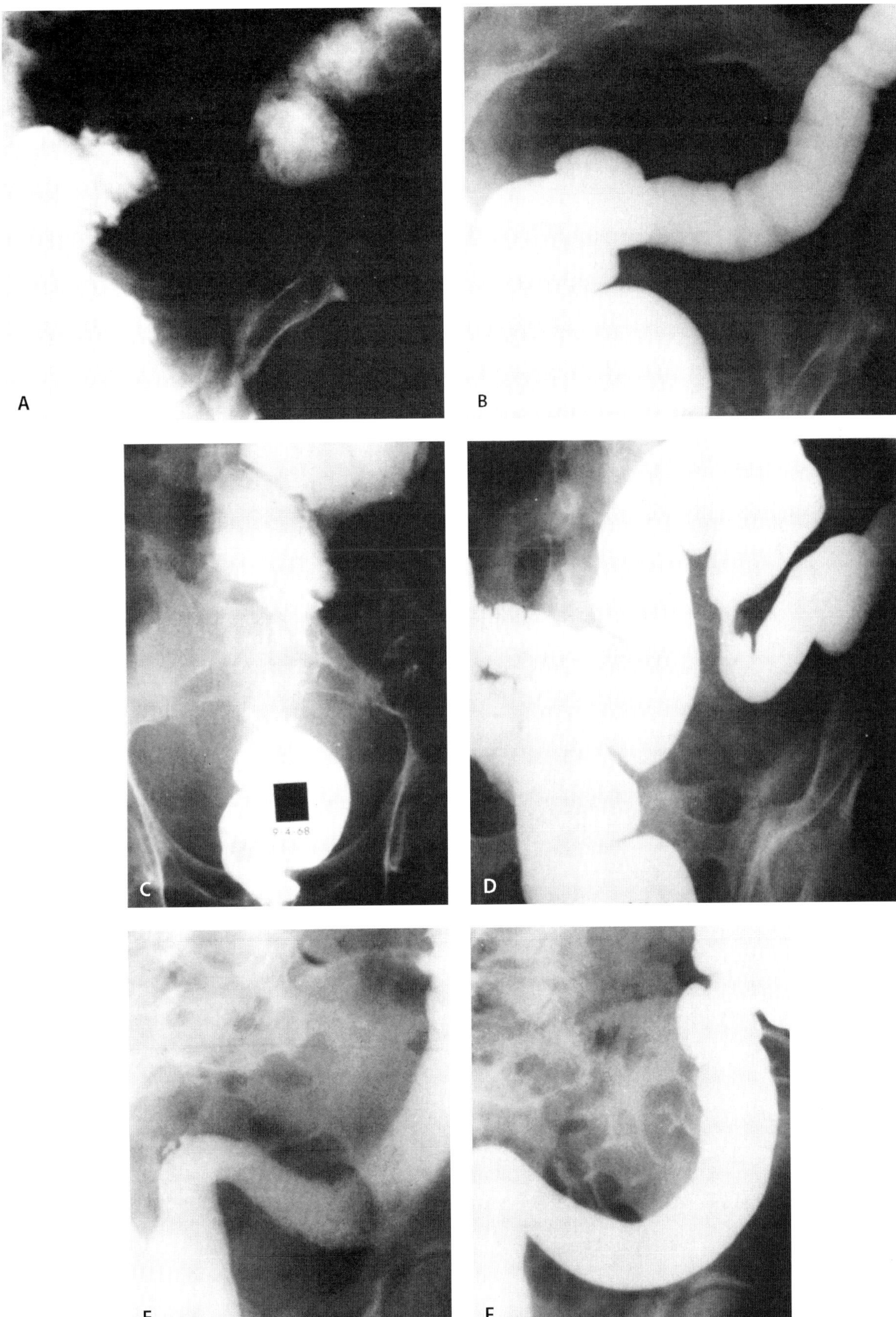
A
B
C
9-4-68
D
E
F

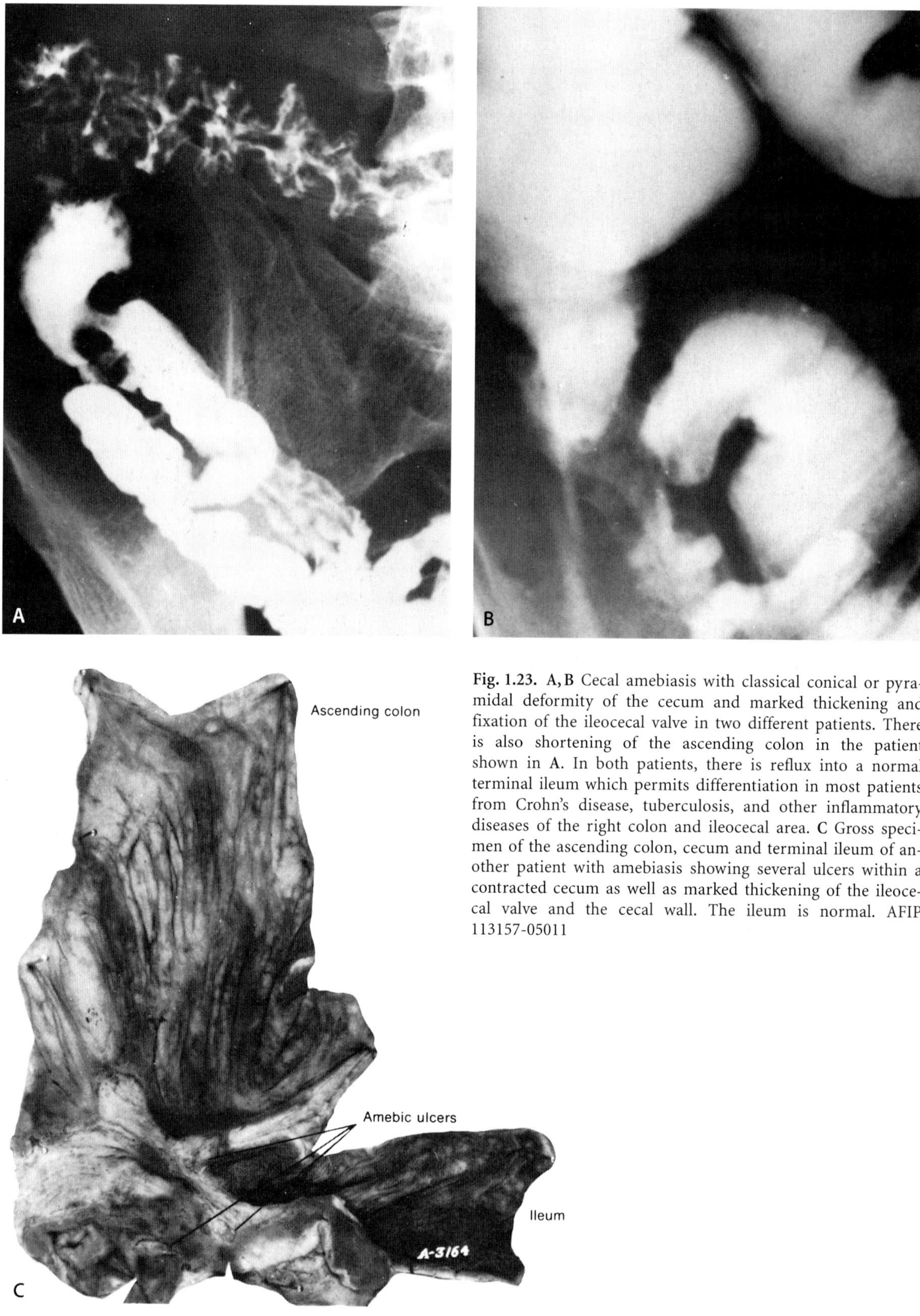

Fig. 1.23. **A, B** Cecal amebiasis with classical conical or pyramidal deformity of the cecum and marked thickening and fixation of the ileocecal valve in two different patients. There is also shortening of the ascending colon in the patient shown in **A**. In both patients, there is reflux into a normal terminal ileum which permits differentiation in most patients from Crohn's disease, tuberculosis, and other inflammatory diseases of the right colon and ileocecal area. **C** Gross specimen of the ascending colon, cecum and terminal ileum of another patient with amebiasis showing several ulcers within a contracted cecum as well as marked thickening of the ileocecal valve and the cecal wall. The ileum is normal. AFIP 113157-05011

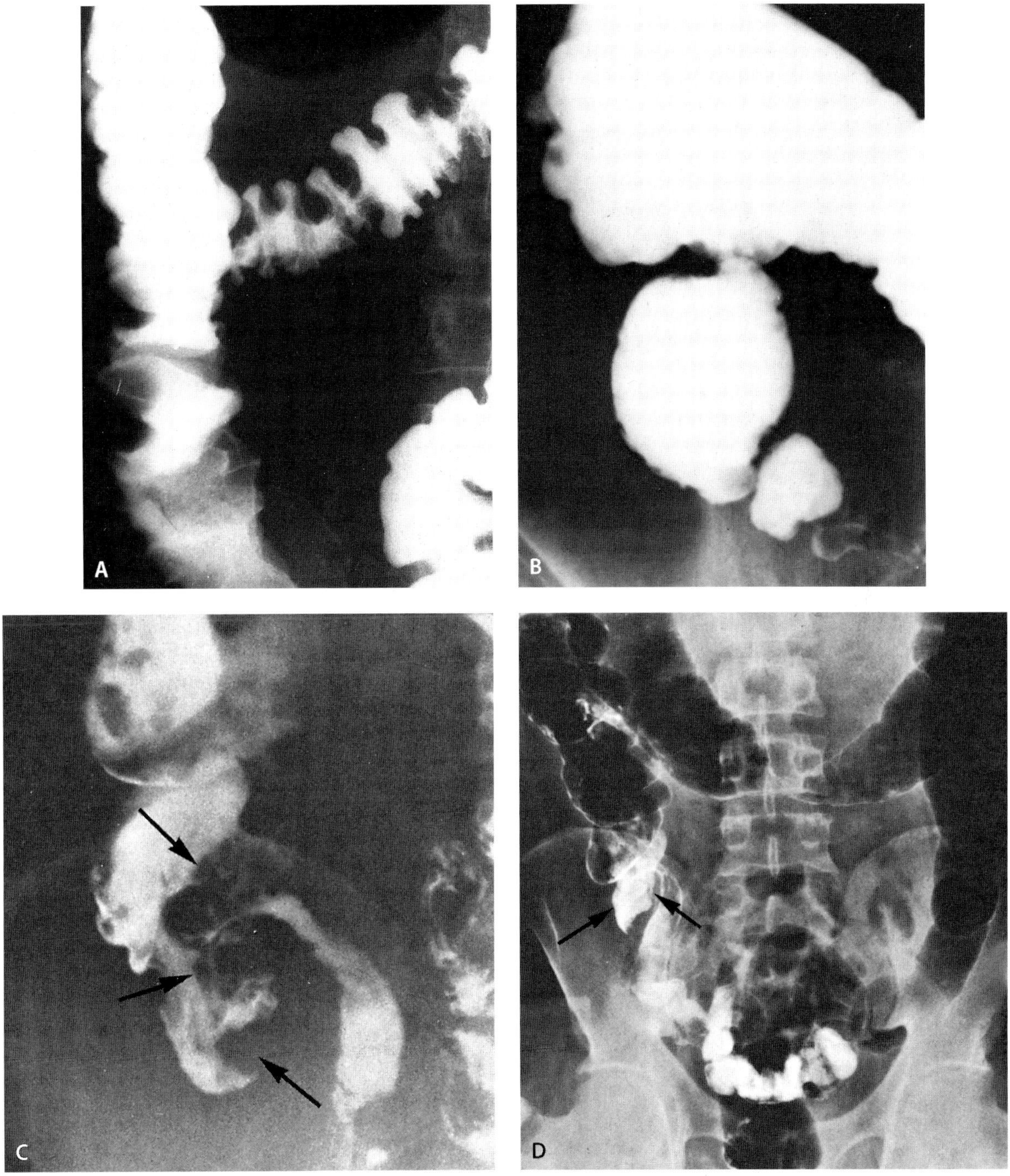

Fig. 1.24 A–D. Amebiasis of the cecum and ascending colon in four patients. **A** Multiple edematous, confluent wall masses resulting in a conical shaped cecum. There are milder segmental lesions in the transverse colon. (Courtesy of Drs. Kenji Kimura and Miguel Stoopen) **B** The cecum is markedly shrunken and deformed, and there are two separate skip areas of inflammatory stenoses involving the midascending colon and cecum. There are also ulcers in the cecum and lateral wall of the hepatic flexure. The cecal wall is thickened in the region of the ileocecal valve, but there is no significant reflux into the distal ileum. **C** Multiple amebomas (*arrows*) have produced filling defects in the cecal tip and ileocecal valve area. There is reflux into the slightly involved distal ileum because of the indurated, fixed ileocecal valve. **D** The cecum is short, narrow, and conical (*arrows*) with no visible haustra. The ileocecal valve is patulous and reflux has occurred into a normal-appearing terminal ileum. Skip areas of involvement are present in the ascending and midtransverse colon. Skip areas, stenoses, deep ulcers, and involvement of the cecum and right colon are also typical of two granulomatous diseases of bowel, namely Crohn's disease and tuberculosis. In both of these diseases, the distal ileum is commonly involved, which is unusual in amebiasis

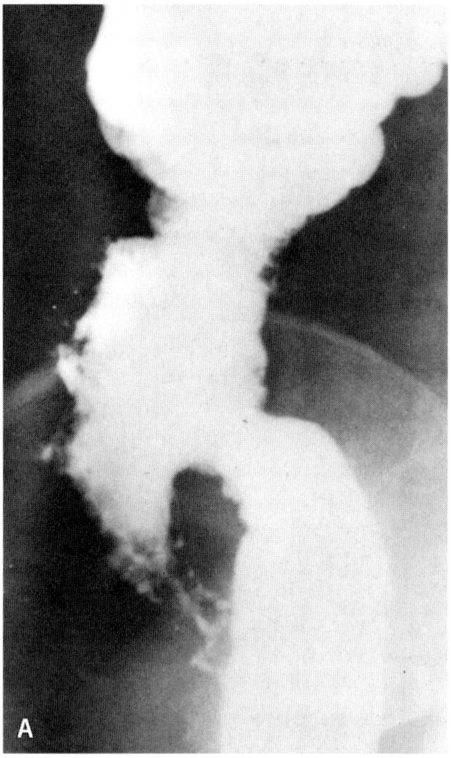

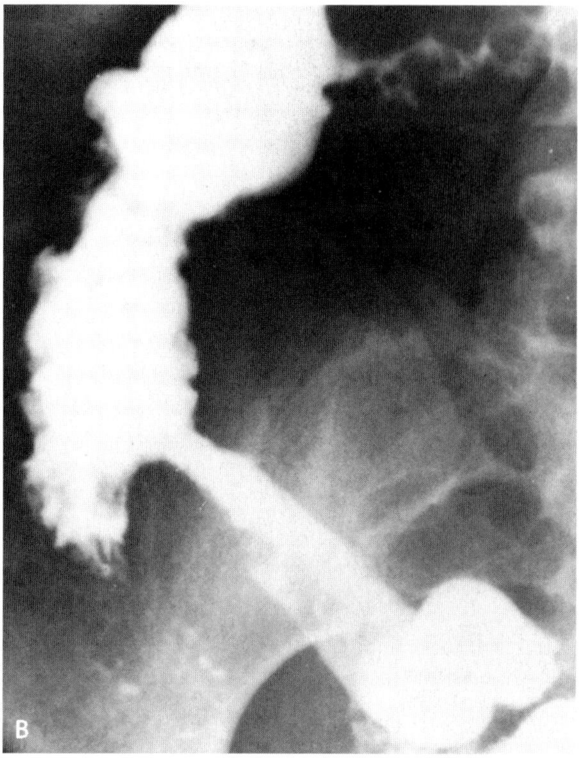

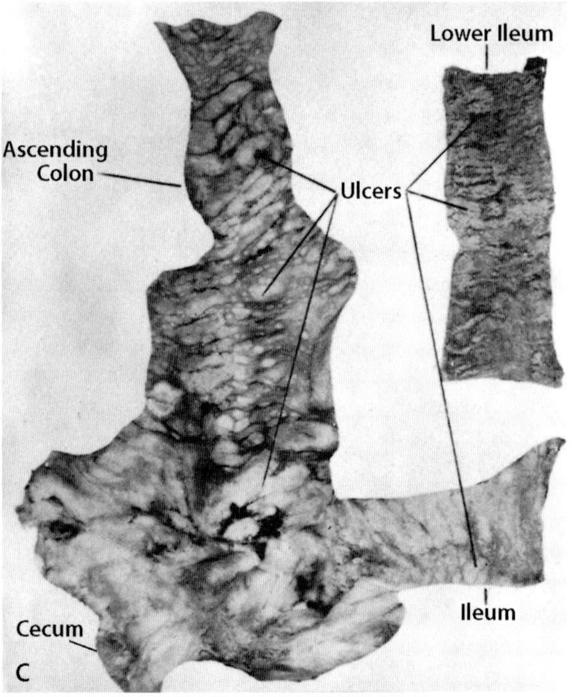

Fig. 1.25 A–C. Chronic amebiasis with acute exacerbation showing severe involvement of the cecum, ascending colon, and terminal ileum. **A, B** Numerous deep ulcers have undermined the mucosa and extended deep into the submucosa and muscularis. Several fistulas extend from the tip of the cecum, which is deformed in a typical conical or pyramidal shape. The ileocecal valve is fixed and incompetent as it is in most patients with amebiasis. In **B** there is also fixation, rigidity, ulceration, and a tubular appearance of the terminal foot of ileum. In addition there is marked spasm of the transverse colon. Such pronounced involvement of the ileum is unusual in amebiasis, occurring in about 10% of patients with colonic amebiasis. (Courtesy of Dr. Julio Astacio, San Salvador) **C** Gross specimen from fatal amebiasis showing numerous large, ragged, deep ulcers in the ascending colon and cecum with marked thickening and deformity of the cecal wall. Note the severe thickening around the ileocecal valve and ulceration and denudation of mucosa in the distal ileum, an uncommon finding in amebiasis. AFIP 196764-1

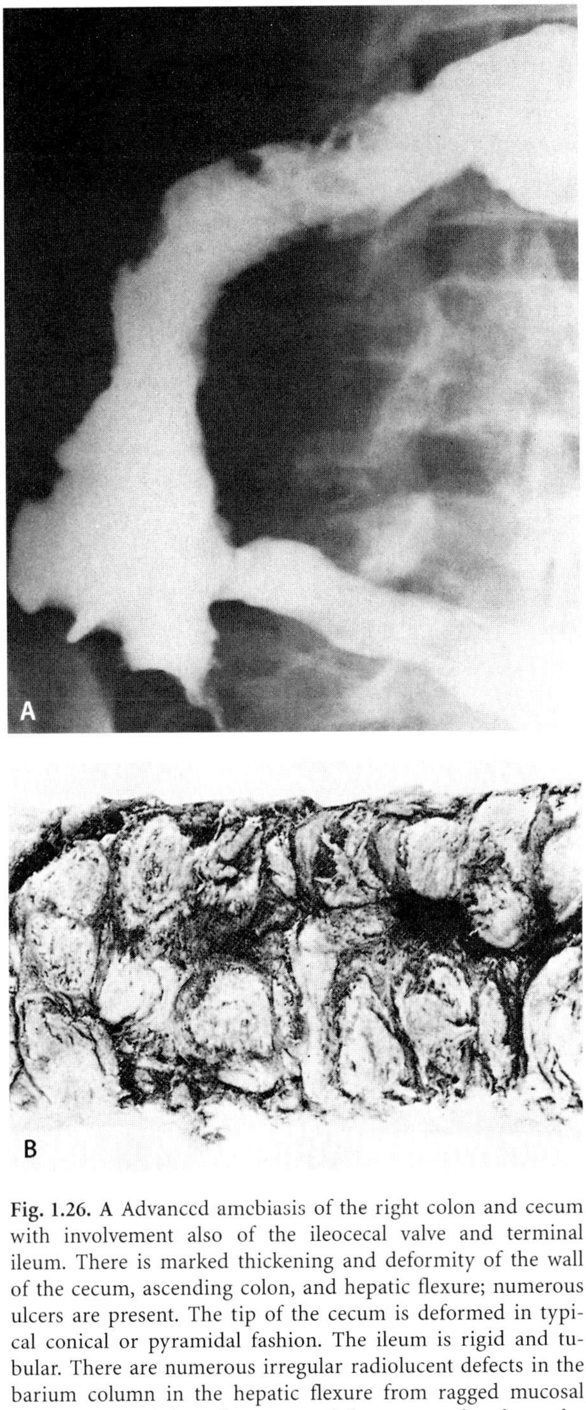

Fig. 1.26. **A** Advanced amebiasis of the right colon and cecum with involvement also of the ileocecal valve and terminal ileum. There is marked thickening and deformity of the wall of the cecum, ascending colon, and hepatic flexure; numerous ulcers are present. The tip of the cecum is deformed in typical conical or pyramidal fashion. The ileum is rigid and tubular. There are numerous irregular radiolucent defects in the barium column in the hepatic flexure from ragged mucosal remnants remaining after most of the mucosa has been denuded through severe ulceration. This appearance in some patients with chronic amebiasis can mimic pseudopolyp formation from mucosal tag remnants seen in chronic ulcerative colitis. **B** "Sea anemone" type of ulcerated mucosa in chronic amebic colitis. A shaggy yellow-white slough fills the large ulcers. Removal of this slough exposes the involved muscularis. There are ragged mucosal remnants which may project into the bowel lumen to cause irregularly shaped filling defects, such as those seen in **A**. AFIP 68-2723-3. (From *Hunter's tropical medicine*, 5th edn. Philadelphia, Saunders, 1976)

Alternatively, areas of colitis with ulcerations and narrowing from spasm, edema, or fibrosis may persist and superficially resemble Crohn's disease or diverticulitis (Figs. 1.27–1.29); fortunately these diseases are uncommon in many parts of the world, particularly in the tropics, but they may coexist with amebiasis in occasional patients.

In the final stages of chronic amebic colitis, strictures associated with shortening of the bowel occur and may resemble the end results of chronic ulcerative or granulomatous colitis (Figs. 1.30, 1.31); distinction may be impossible even histologically, unless trophozoites are recognized in the tissues.

Ameboma

Ameboma is a hyperplastic granuloma of the large bowel caused by bacterial invasion of an amebic abscess in the bowel wall (Figs. 1.32–1.39). It is characterized by marked thickening of the bowel, with dense fibrosis at the periphery and a core of acute and chronic inflammation and necrosis in the center. The resulting mass is firm and usually large and relatively fixed and tender to palpation. It may present as an eccentric filling defect in the bowel lumen (Fig. 1.36 D, E), but more commonly it causes a long, tapered area of stenosis or completely encircles the bowel to produce an apple-core lesion associated with a palpable mass and mimicking a carcinoma (Figs. 1.32–1.36). Barium enema can successfully diagnose 80% of the cases. The segment of large bowel that is affected shows an asymmetric or symmetric narrowing of the lumen, irregular edematous mucosa and poor distensibility.

These hypertrophic lesions are most frequent in the cecum and ascending and rectosigmoid colon, but an ameboma can occur anywhere in the large bowel. (An ameboma affecting the ileum has been reported, showing undermined ulcers with fibrosis and central debris.) An ameboma is usually associated with evidence of colitis elsewhere. The incidence of ameboma varies geographically, and, as with other changes of amebiasis, probably reflects the standard of hygiene and nutrition, recurrent infection, and general health of the patient.

Carcinoma of the colon, non-Hodgkin's lymphoma, and tuberculosis are the primary considerations in differential diagnosis. The ameboma is generally longer, with a transitional area that is gradual. Multiple concentric lesions are common (Figs. 1.28, 1.36), with rapidly detected morphological changes following the initiation of appropriate therapy (Figs. 1.37–1.39). The typical short "apple core" lesion of a colon carcinoma occurring on a background of normal colon is the norm. Occasionally a scirrhous linitis plastica lesion may extend for long segments.

(Text continues on p. 40)

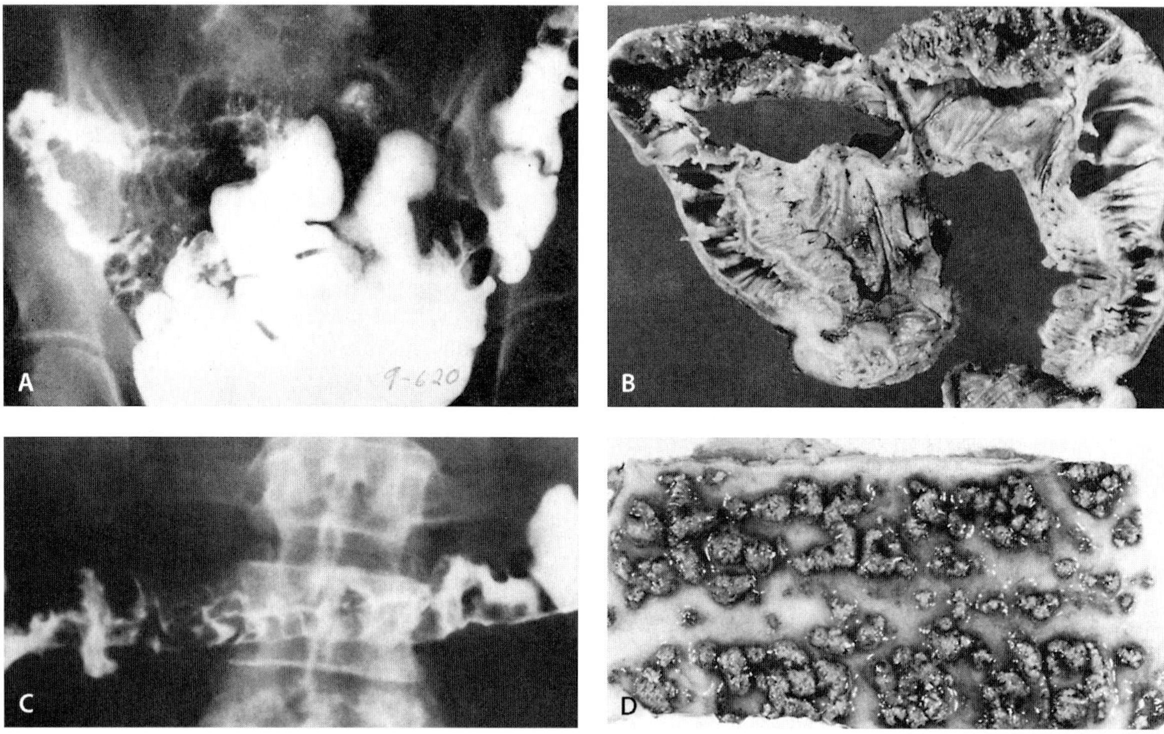

Fig. 1.27 A–D. Amebic colitis simulating Crohn's disease. **A** In this patient from New York City there is extensive involvement of the entire right colon, hepatic flexure, and proximal transverse colon with diffuse narrowing of the bowel lumen, deep ulcers leading to short, right angle sinus tracts and fistulas, and marked thickening of the bowel wall. The entire right colon is markedly shortened and there is a sharp cutoff between abnormal and normal bowel at the level of the mid-transverse colon. A cobblestone mucosal pattern is present in the transverse colon. There is a second skip area in the descending colon. These findings are identical to those of Crohn's disease, but at the time of surgery the patient was found to have amebic colitis. It is most unfortunate to establish such a diagnosis during or after surgery, since spread of the amebic infection often causes increased morbidity and mortality in such untreated patients. (Courtesy of Dr. William Seaman, New York City) **B** Specimen of the right colon, hepatic flexure, and terminal ileum of another patient with amebiasis. The specimen has been cut in half and opened to show the markedly thickened bowel wall and shaggy, severely ulcerated mucosa. In the region of the hepatic flexure, the bowel lumen is severely narrowed and the disease has extended through the submucosa and muscularis to the serosa and beyond. There is a hyperplastic granuloma about the cecum and ileocecal valve (lower part of specimen). AFIP 98-0787-2. **C** Cobblestone mucosal pattern caused by ulceration and heaped-up isolated mounds of mucosa involving a lengthy segment of the transverse colon in a patient from Colombia with amebic colitis. The appearance closely resembles granulomatous colitis. (Courtesy of Drs. Gonzalo Angel and Rodrigo Caro, Cali) **D** A segment of colon from fatal amebiasis in a Ugandan man. The colon is studded with numerous ulcers, some small, some confluent and covered with heaped-up gray exudate. These mounds of hyperplastic mucosa and fibrin appear as islands amid severely ulcerated and denuded mucosa and can occasionally present a cobblestone mucosal pattern radiographically similar to that seen in Crohn's disease. AFIP 69-3248. (Courtesy of Dr. Daniel H. Connor)

Fig. 1.28. Amebic colitis simulating Crohn's disease. There are multiple skip areas of narrowing and ameboma formation throughout the mid-ascending colon, transverse colon, proximal descending colon and mid-sigmoid colon, and thickening of the ileocecal valve, in a patient from the Marshall Islands of the mid-Pacific who was air evacuated to a U.S. military hospital in Hawaii where the initial diagnosis by a radiologist and clinician was probable Crohn's disease. Fortunately, the hospital's radiology consultant pointed out that Crohn's disease is virtually unknown in almost all Pacific Islands, as well as most of the tropics, whereas amebiasis is quite common. Further workup showed numerous amebae in the patient's stools and appropriate antiamebic therapy was begun ▶

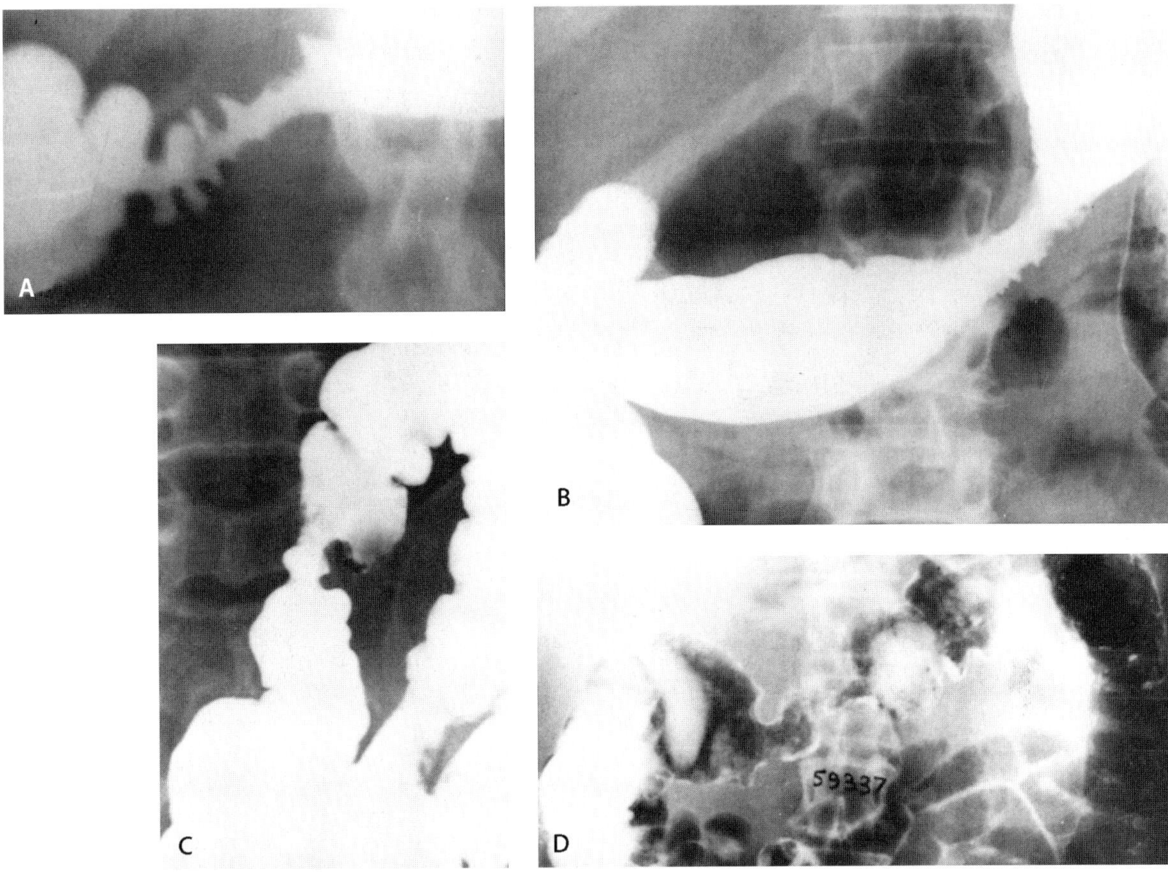

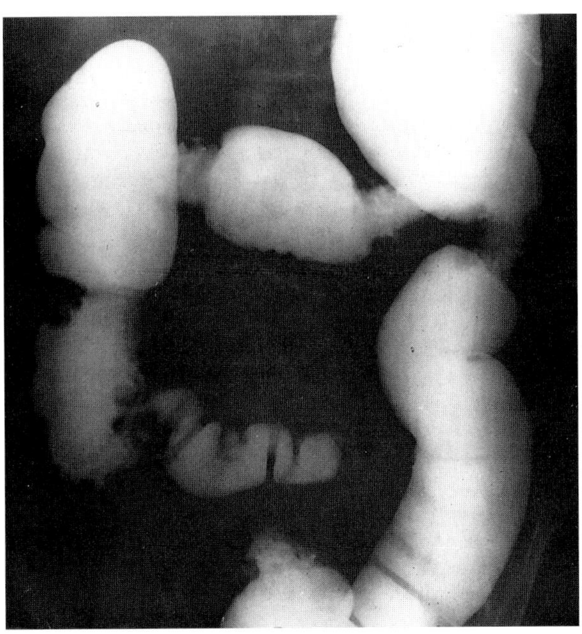

▲

Fig. 1.29 A–D. Amebic colitis simulating Crohn's disease. **A** Segmental narrowing and ulceration in the transverse colon. Notice the tapering distal edge and the relative preservation of mucosa, which, together with the length of the lesion, are more suggestive of a granulomatous process, such as amebiasis or Crohn's disease, than carcinoma. **B** Somewhat similar findings in the transverse colon of another patient with segmental amebic colitis. Note the deep ulcers throughout the narrowed segment of colon. There is considerable thickening of the bowel wall and tapering of both the proximal and distal edges, allowing differentiation from carcinoma but not from Crohn's disease. **C** There are short, stenotic, slightly ulcerated skip lesions involving the proximal and distal sigmoid colon with an intervening long normal segment of midsigmoid colon between these localized amebic granulomas (again, Crohn's disease and tuberculosis may cause similar findings). **D** Skip areas of stenosis from amebic granulomatous inflammation of the mid- and distal transverse colon in a patient from India. Notice the less involved segment of transverse colon between the two areas of stenosis. Fortunately, Crohn's disease is unusual in India and other tropical countries, where most patients with these patterns will have amebiasis or occasionally tuberculosis of the colon. (**D** courtesy of Dr. A. Chandrahasan Johnson)

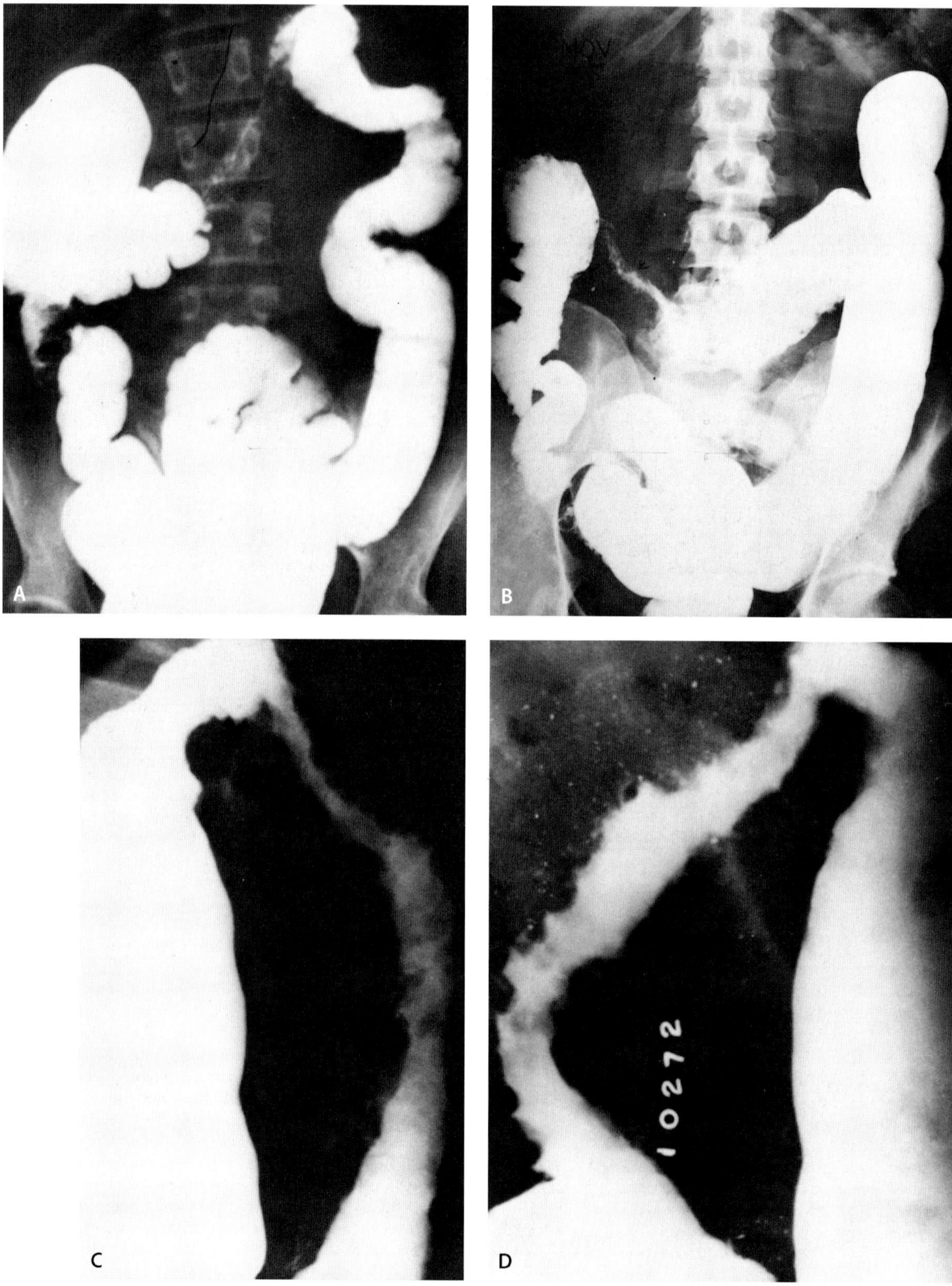
A
B
C
D
10272

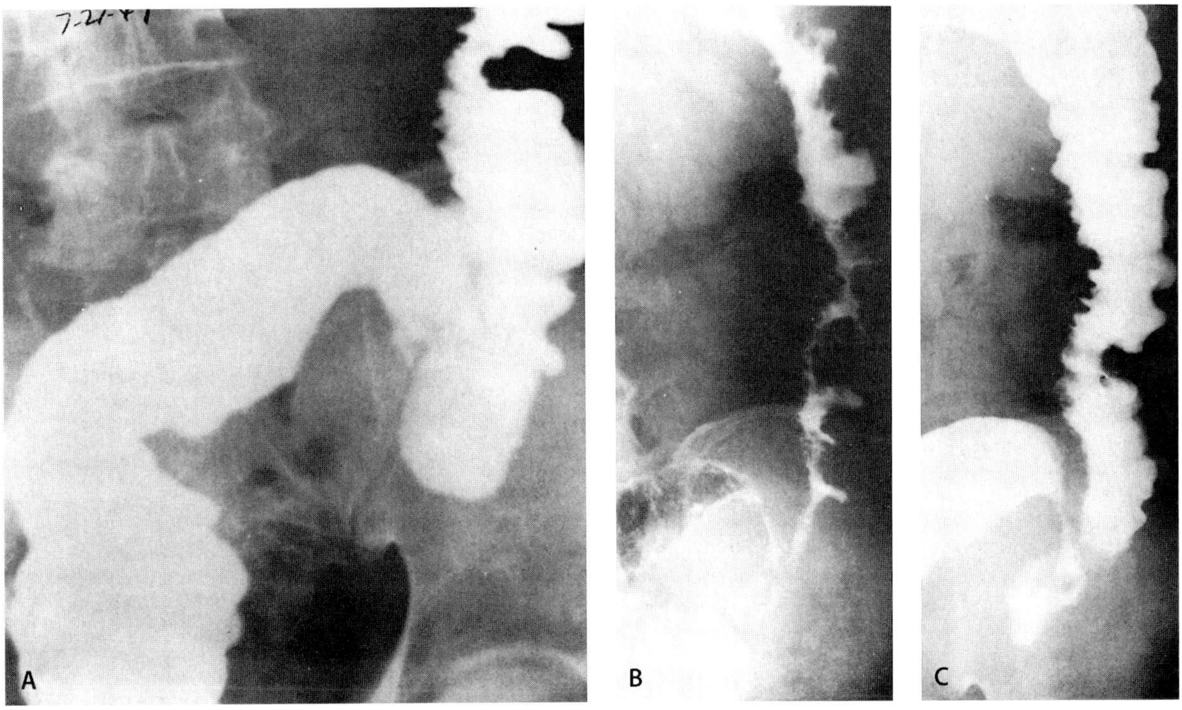

Fig. 1.31 A–C. Development of an amebic stricture of the sigmoid colon. **A** Initial barium enema shows irregular, distorted haustral markings and bowel contour of the rectosigmoid and descending colon. **B** Barium enema 6 months later shows a well-defined short stricture of the proximal sigmoid colon and intense spasm throughout the sigmoid and descending colon. **C** A film obtained several minutes later during the same study shows the spasm has relaxed and the descending colon is now well filled, outlining numerous ulcers and an irregular and distorted contour with exaggerated haustral markings. The short stricture, with a bowel lumen of less than 5 mm, is again identified in the sigmoid colon. The tapered distal edge of the stenosis, together with the obvious inflammatory changes in the descending colon, suggest a granulomatous colitis or amebiasis, rather than neoplasm

◀ **Fig. 1.30 A–D.** Amebic strictures of the colon. **A** A long stricture of the mid-transverse colon with associated ulcers in the splenic flexure and proximal descending colon and a markedly contracted and irregular cecum. The ileocecal valve is thickened but the terminal ileum is normal. Such skip areas of involvement in the colon are typical of a granulomatous colitis such as amebiasis. The contracted cecum and normal terminal ileum are highly suggestive of this diagnosis. **B** A long stricture of the proximal transverse colon associated with an irregular, ulcerated ascending colon and cecum. Note the conical deformity of the cecum with a normal terminal ileum, suggesting amebiasis. **C, D** Long areas of stenosis involving the splenic flexure and descending colon in a patient with advanced amebiasis. Note the deep ulcers and the marked thumbprinting caused by mucosal and submucosal edema. The bowel wall is markedly thickened, irregular, and stenotic, and there is a gradual transition from abnormal to normal bowel typical of an inflammatory rather than a neoplastic stricture

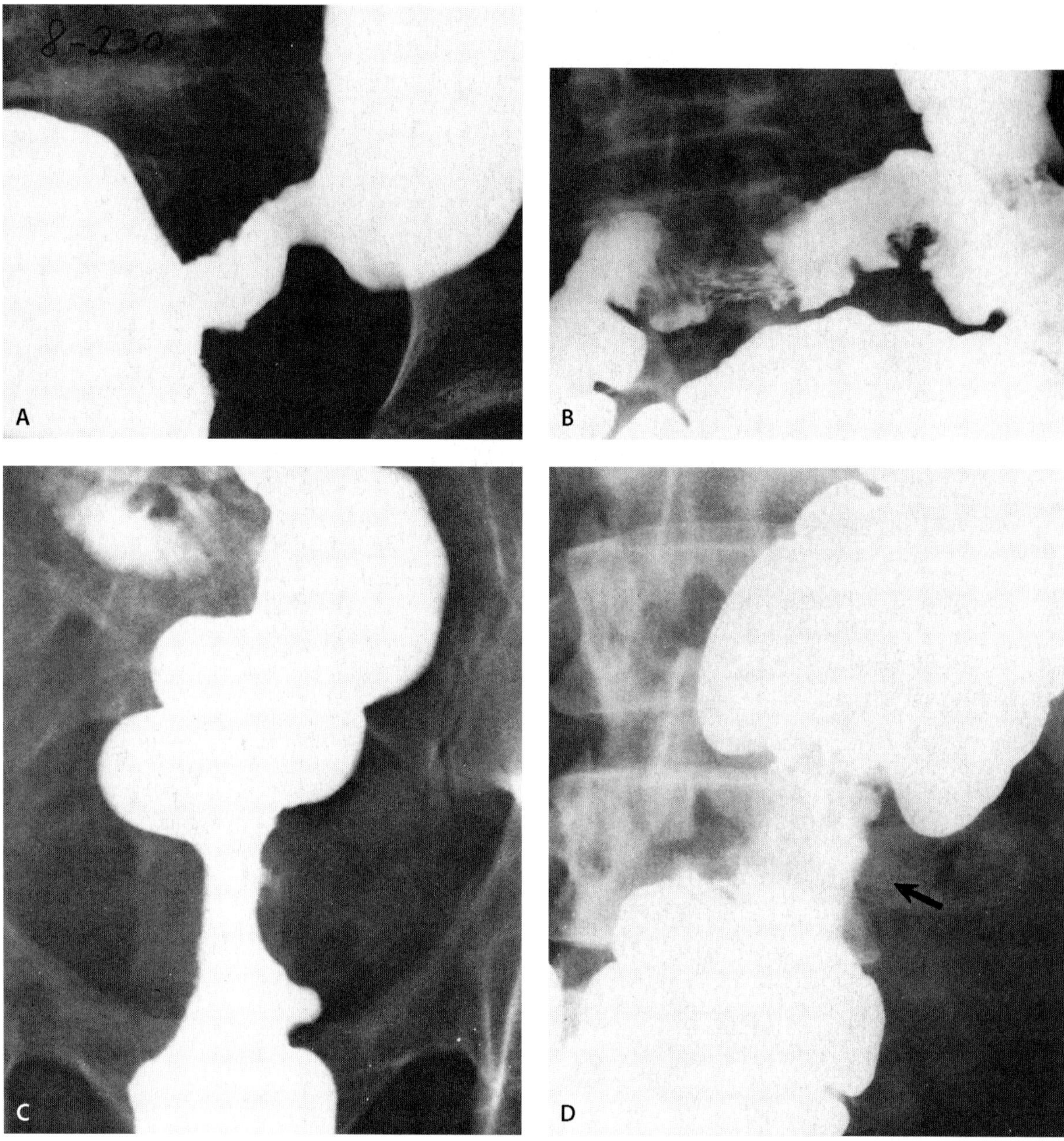

Fig. 1.32 A–D. Amebomas of the colon simulating the apple-core deformity of carcinoma. **A** Ameboma of the sigmoid colon. Note the tapered proximal edge and the tiny ulcerations within and adjacent to the annular constricting lesion, allowing possible differentiation from carcinoma. **B** Ameboma of the proximal transverse colon. Note that, despite the shelf-like edges of this lesion, there appears to be intact mucosa through the lesion. **C** Apple-core lesion of the rectum with deep ulcers along its left lateral aspect. There is also slight ulceration and an amorphous, somewhat tubular appearance of the dilated distal sigmoid colon. **D** Short apple-core lesion of the transverse colon (*arrow*) indistinguishable from carcinoma. The patient was a 25-year-old American soldier recently returned from Vietnam, which suggested the correct diagnosis of ameboma

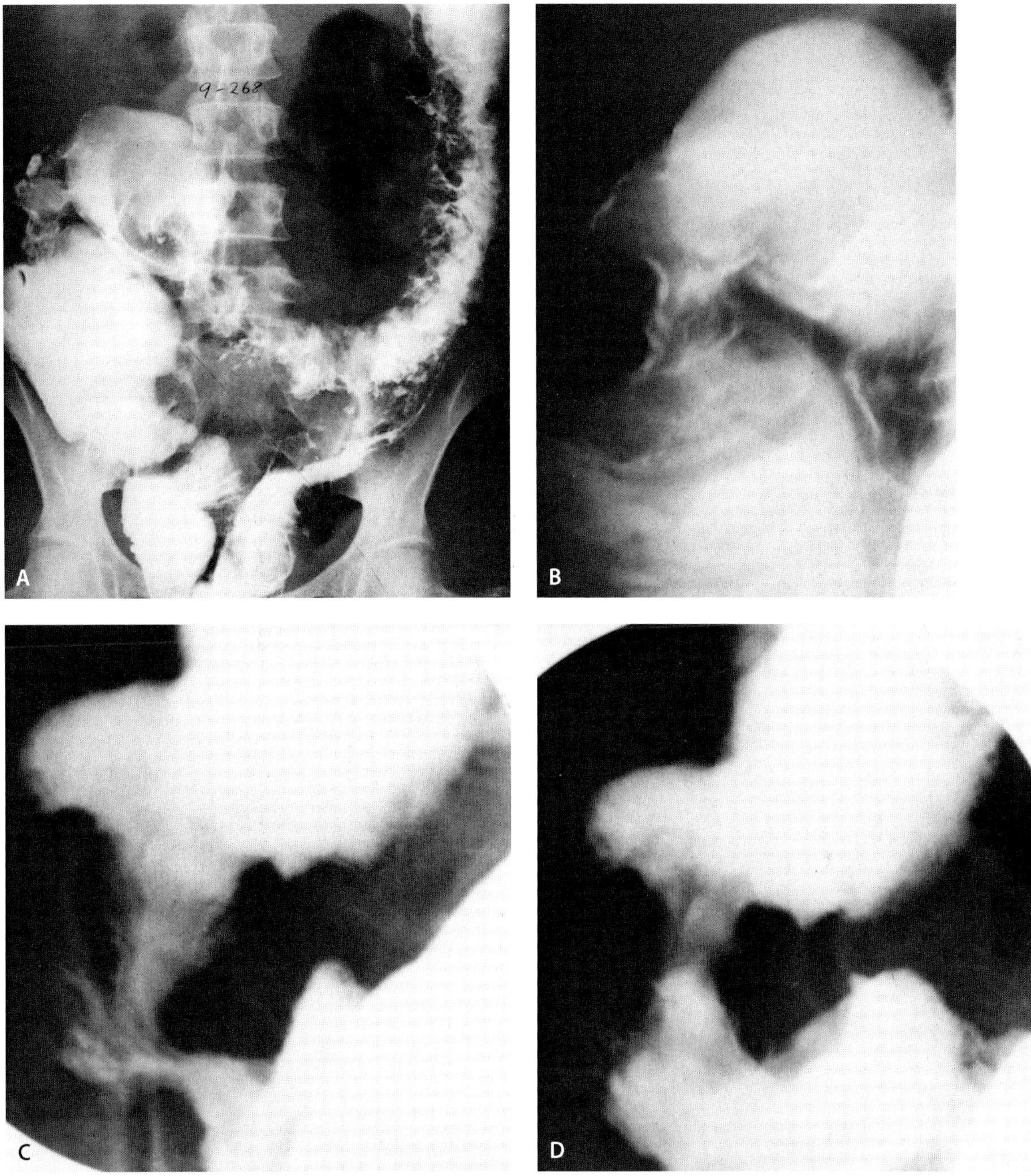

Fig. 1.33 A–D. Amebomas of the colon simulating carcinoma. **A** Apple-core lesion of the proximal ascending colon indistinguishable from carcinoma. However, there is extensive, deep ulceration and fistulous tract formation throughout the transverse and left colon and deformity of the cecum, which are the radiographic clues to the diagnosis of amebiasis. With many colonic amebomas, there will be radiographic evidence elsewhere of a colitis which may suggest to the astute observer that what resembles an annular carcinoma is in fact a granuloma caused by amebiasis or tuberculosis. **B** Close-up view of the hepatic flexure showing the classic apple-core deformity typical of carcinoma, but seen also in ameboma or tuberculoma. This patient, a young Puerto Rican adult, had the lesion resected because it was thought to be a carcinoma; he died postoperatively from generalized spread of his amebic infection, a tragic but common sequel to surgery on untreated colonic amebiasis. (**A**, **B** courtesy of Dr. Ehrlich, San Juan) **C**, **D** Annular cecal ameboma simulating carcinoma. Note that, although there is a persistent shelf-like edge distally, there is some pliability and distention and change in shape of the lesion along its proximal aspect, and there are deep ulcers within the lesion. These features should suggest ameboma in a young American housewife just returned from extensive travel in the tropics. Antiamebic therapy should be instituted before surgery in such a patient

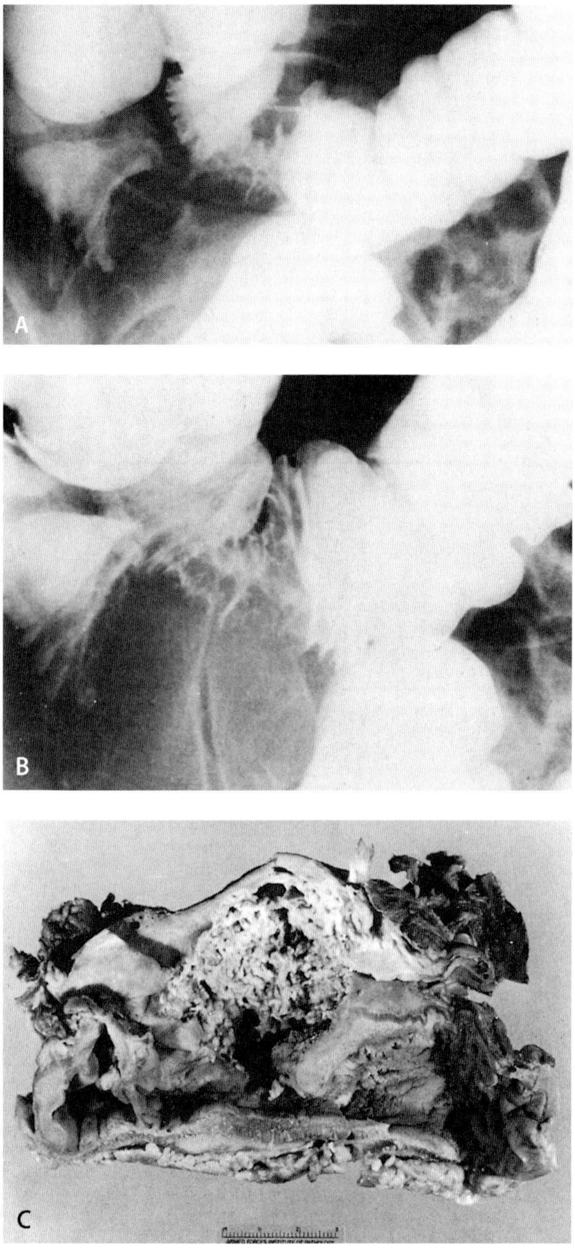

Fig. 1.34. A, B Large cecal ameboma with abscess formation and extension to involve the adjacent transverse colon. Note the large filling defect involving the tip of the cecum with the mass extending to involve the midtransverse colon with spiking of the mucosal pattern and narrowing of the bowel lumen caused by the abscess. **C** Gross specimen from another patient showing a large ameboma of the colon with extensive, eccentric abscess extending through the colonic wall into the pericolonic tissues. Note the markedly thickened colon wall at the site of the ameboma, the narrowed lumen, and the shelf-like edges of the lesion projecting into the lumen. This may appear radiographically as an annular, apple-core lesion with eccentric, extrinsic mass from the associated abscess. Barium may leak into such an abscess during a barium enema examination. AFIP 53-7738

Multiple lesions may occur in lymphoma, metastases, tuberculomas, fungal infections, and AIDS-associated lymphoma or Kaposi sarcoma of the bowel.

In countries where carcinoma of the colon is common, the distinction between ameboma and malignancy depends upon the awareness that such a granulomatous lesion can occur.

Characteristically, there is a smooth tapered narrowing from normal bowel into the ameboma, and the mucosa appears to be intact, although edema and tiny ulcers may be present in or adjacent to the lesion. The length of the lesion is variable and, in up to 50% of cases, the amebomas are multiple. The narrowed bowel is often longer than the constriction caused by malignancy (other than lymphoma or scirrhous carcinoma) and seldom causes obstruction, although there may be some dilatation proximal to the ameboma. Some amebomas mimic the typical apple-core appearance of carcinoma, and it is helpful to remember that cancer of the colon is uncommon in young people, and is rare in many parts of the tropics at any age.

The major differences between malignancy and ameboma can be summarized:

1. There is often inflammation and ulceration adjacent to an ameboma.
2. Evidence of amebiasis may be found elsewhere in the colon, especially in the cecum. There may be multiple amebomas, whereas primary malignancy of the colon is usually solitary.
3. There is a gradual transition from normal bowel to the area of stenosis in an ameboma. The edges of the lesion are often tapered rather than shelf-like. Colonic carcinoma usually causes an abrupt, localized narrowing.
4. The stenosis caused by ameboma is relatively incomplete, and obstruction is unusual. Malignant constriction is usually definite and obstructive. Obstruction in ameboma is usually the result of complications, such as rupture.
5. The bowel wall is not completely rigid and varies with pressure in amebiasis. Infilration by colonic carcinoma produces rigidity and the involved area can seldom be distended.
6. The mucosa may be intact throughout the area of stenosis in an ameboma. Carcinoma usually ulcerates and destroys the mucosa.
7. A barium enema seldom causes pain with an ameboma, but can be painful in obstructive malignancy.
8. Treatment for amebiasis may cause rapid regression over a 3- or 4-week period with eventual dilatation of the previously stenosed area, but antiamebic therapy produces no change in malignancy.

(Text continues on p. 44)

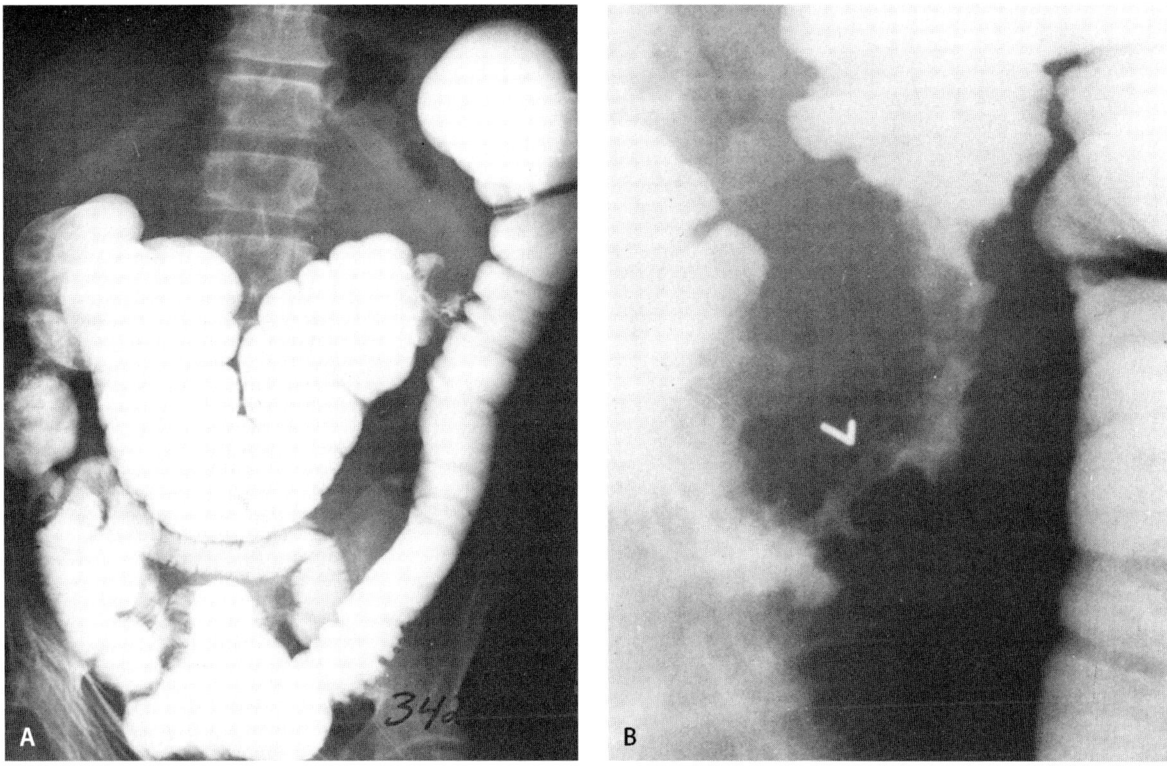

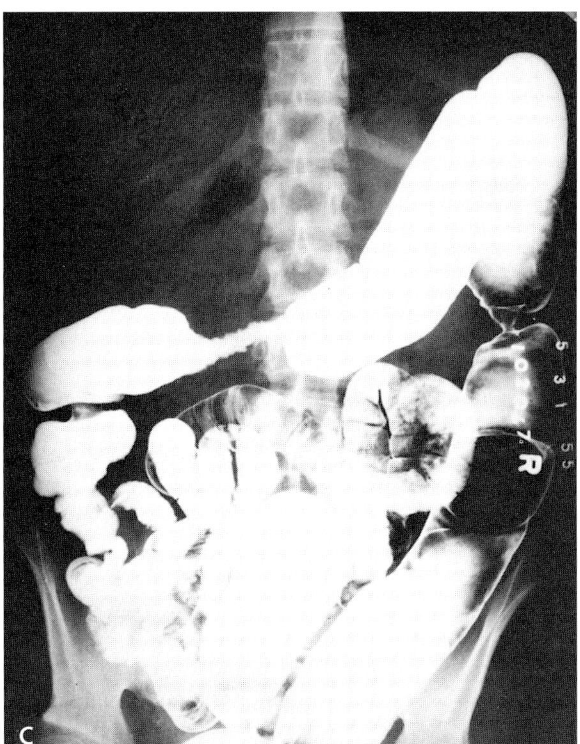

Fig. 1.35 A–C. Long tapering amebomas with associated evidence of amebic colitis in the right colon and cecum. **A** Lengthy lesion of the distal transverse colon with ragged ulcerated mucosa and tapered proximal and distal edges seen best on close-up view (**B**). Note the irregular, shortened right colon with contracted cecal tip and normal distal ileum typical of amebiasis in **A**. In **C** an ameboma of the midtransverse colon has multiple ulcers within the lesion and tapered edges, allowing possible differentiation from carcinoma. In addition, there is a contracted cecum and thickened ileocecal valve with normal distal ileum. There is also a localized short area of contraction in the proximal descending colon. The combination of cecal involvement, multiple skip areas, and a normal ileum strongly suggests amebiasis

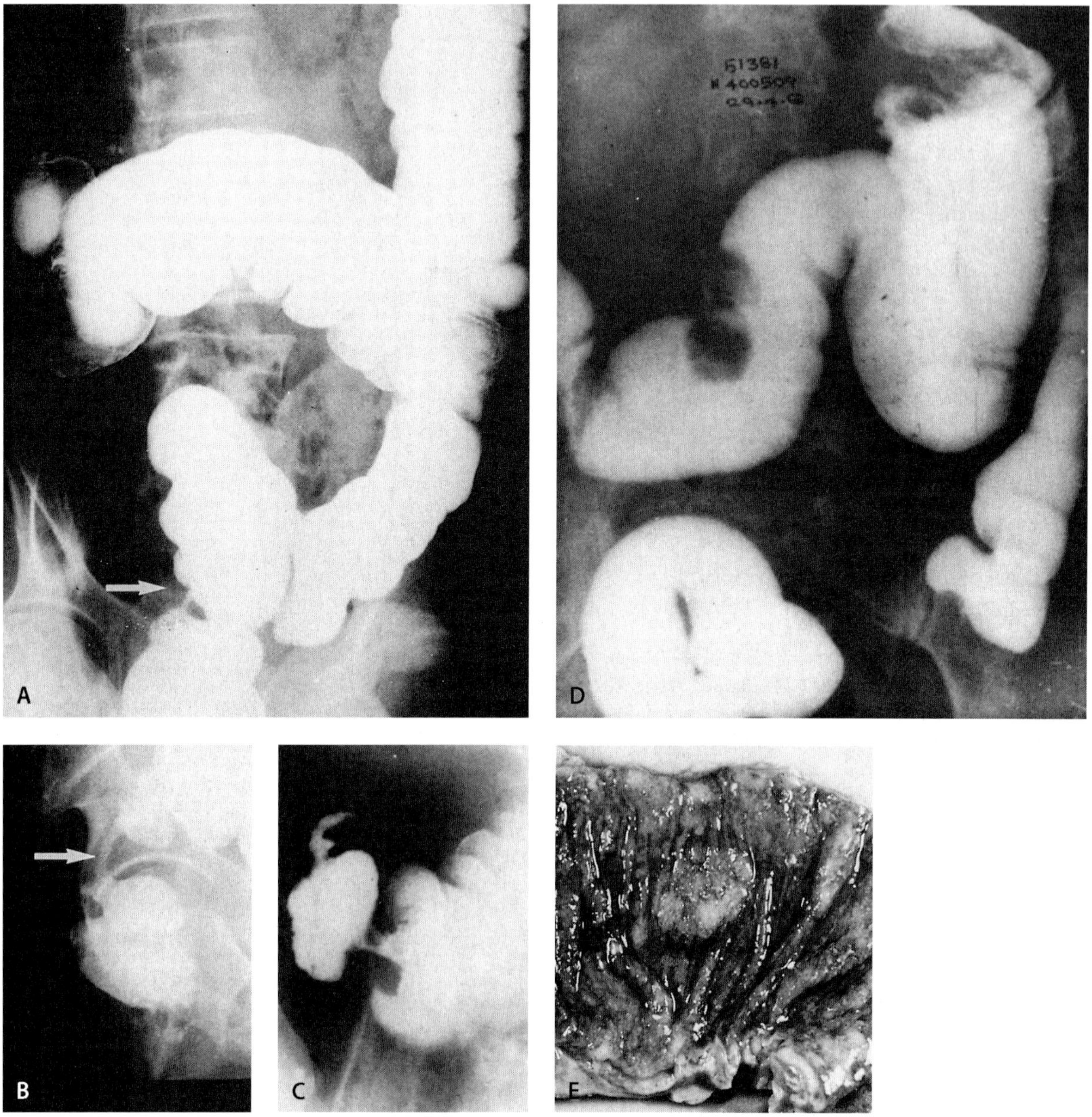

Fig. 1.36 A–E. Multiple amebomas of the colon. **A** Oblique view from a barium enema showing a short annular ameboma in the rectum (*arrow*) and two other short amebomas in the hepatic flexure. **B** Lateral spot film of the rectal ameboma (*arrow*). **C** Spot film of the hepatic flexure showing the two apple-core amebomas there. The presence of multiple such lesions in the colon favors a diagnosis of inflammatory disease, such as amebiasis, rather than carcinoma, which is rarely multiple. **D** Eccentric ameboma presenting as a filling defect along the superior aspect of the mid-transverse colon. There are other lesions in the splenic flexure and sigmoid colon in this patient from India. (Courtesy of Dr. A. Chandrahasan Johnson) **E** Gross specimen from another patient showing a localized amebic mass protruding into the bowel lumen. On barium enema, such a lesion would cause an eccentric filling defect as seen in **D**. There are also multiple ulcers of the adjacent mucosa

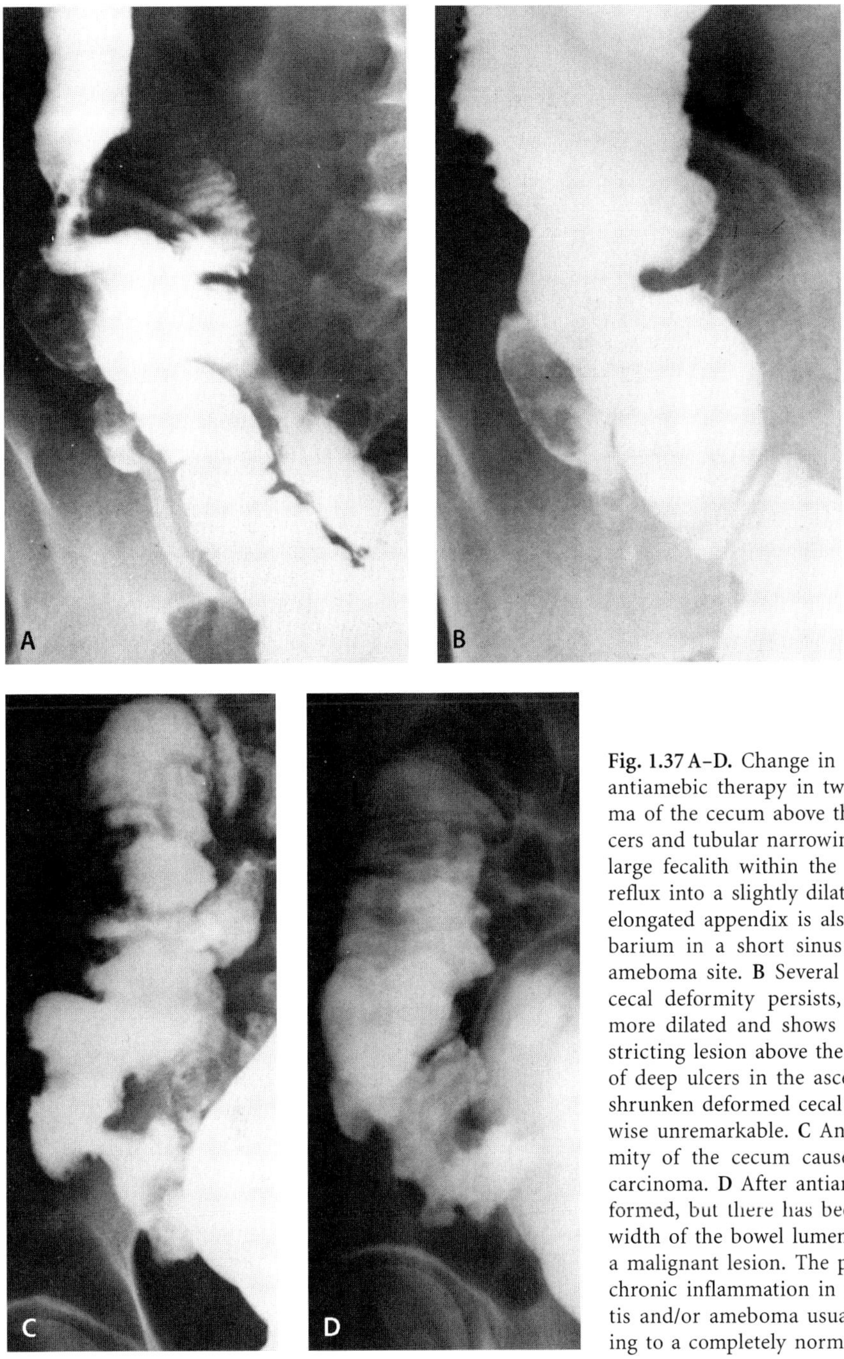

Fig. 1.37 A–D. Change in appearance of cecal amebomas after antiamebic therapy in two patients. A Large annular ameboma of the cecum above the ileocecal valve associated with ulcers and tubular narrowing of the ascending colon. There is a large fecalith within the contracted cecum and considerable reflux into a slightly dilated, but otherwise normal ileum. An elongated appendix is also filled. There is a small amount of barium in a short sinus tract extending medially from the ameboma site. B Several weeks after antiamebic therapy, the cecal deformity persists, but the right colon is now much more dilated and shows little evidence of the previous constricting lesion above the ileocecal valve. Note the persistence of deep ulcers in the ascending colon and the fecalith in the shrunken deformed cecal tip. The ileum is dilated, but otherwise unremarkable. C Another patient with apple-core deformity of the cecum caused by a large ameboma simulating carcinoma. D After antiamebic therapy the cecum is still deformed, but there has been a marked change in contour and width of the bowel lumen, which would not be anticipated in a malignant lesion. The presence of considerable fibrosis and chronic inflammation in patients with advanced amebic colitis and/or ameboma usually prevents the bowel from returning to a completely normal appearance after therapy

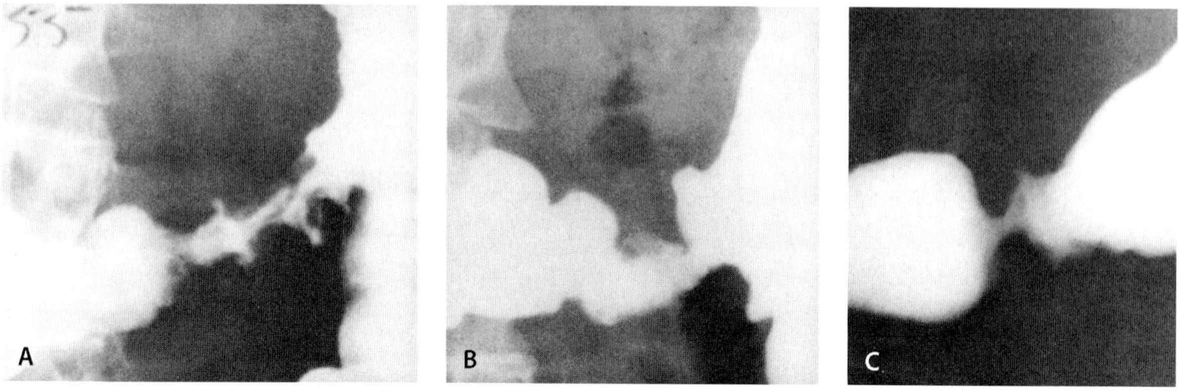

Fig. 1.38 A–C. Localized ameboma of the distal transverse colon and its response to antiamebic therapy over a 5-week period. In **A** the relatively long segment involved, together with slightly tapered edges and distortion but not destruction of the mucosal pattern in a relatively young adult, suggests amebic colitis with ameboma or Crohn's disease rather than carcinoma. A diagnosis of amebiasis was establisehd and antiamebic therapy begun. Follow-up barium enema 3 weeks later shows change in appearance of the involved segment with more localized stenosis now present (**B**). A further follow-up barium enema 2 weeks later (**C**) shows a tight stenosis over a very short segment. The bowel lumen is only 1 cm through the area of constriction. Note the tapering distal edge of the lesion suggesting a granuloma of the colon, such as ameboma or tuberculoma, insead of carcinoma. The patient was subsequently operated upon to avoid the possibility of future obstruction, and he did well postoperatively because his extensive antiamebic therapy precluded possible spread of the infection at the time of surgery

Distinguishing between amebiasis and carcinoma is important because there is a 17% mortality associated with surgery for amebomas (over 50% in one series). The typical clinical picture of an acute dysenteric syndrome, septic course, and abdominal distention is rarely, if ever, seen among the other potential diagnostic considerations. In most cases, endoscopic sampling or serological tests confirm the diagnosis. Unfortunately, even finding amebae in the stool or on rectal biopsy does not exclude malignancy, because the two conditions may coexist. In view of the risk of surgery in amebiasis, it is justifiable to treat the patient and assess the results radiologically after 3 weeks. In most patients, the area of stenosis will dilate, but in many the contour may remain irregular and distorted (Figs. 1.37, 1.38). After several months, some patients will have residual fibrotic stenosis (Fig. 1.38); in others the bowel returns to normal diameter (Fig. 1.39), and a few will have dilatation at the site of the prior ameboma.

Complications (Fig. 1.40)

There are several major complications of colonic amebiasis, some of which are specific circumstances that demand a laparotomy, e.g., suspected obstruction, perforation or appendicitis leading to peritonitis.

Intussusception. Children with amebic colitis may present to the radiologist with intussusception, and the diagnosis may not be realized until the barium enema is under way (Figs. 1.41, 1.42). Although the bowel wall in such cases is ulcerated, perforation is uncommon and reduction of the intussusception by enema should be preferable to surgical treatment, because the bowel will be extensively inflamed far beyond the intussusception. Amebomas are uncommon in children, but they can form a mass which may become the origin of an intussusception.

Perforation. The major complication of amebiasis in the alimentary tract is penetration of one or more ulcers through the serosa, causing a thoracic, subphrenic, or pericolic abscess, or peritonitis with or without internal or external fistula (Figs. 1.43–1.46). The radiologist must remember that a pericolic abscess may manifest itself only as rigidity and distortion of the bowel wall; it should be suspected when there is a palpable mass clinically but none can be demonstrated radiologically. The appendix may be involved, and an appendiceal abscess may occasionally be amebic in origin. Ischiorectal or perineal amebic abscesses are not unusual and often have associated perianal and perineal cutaneous ulceration.

Appendicitis – Amebic Typhloappendicitis. In the overwhelming majority of the cases, the coexistent involvement of other segments of the colon by amebic colitiis allows the observer to suspect the parasitic etiology.

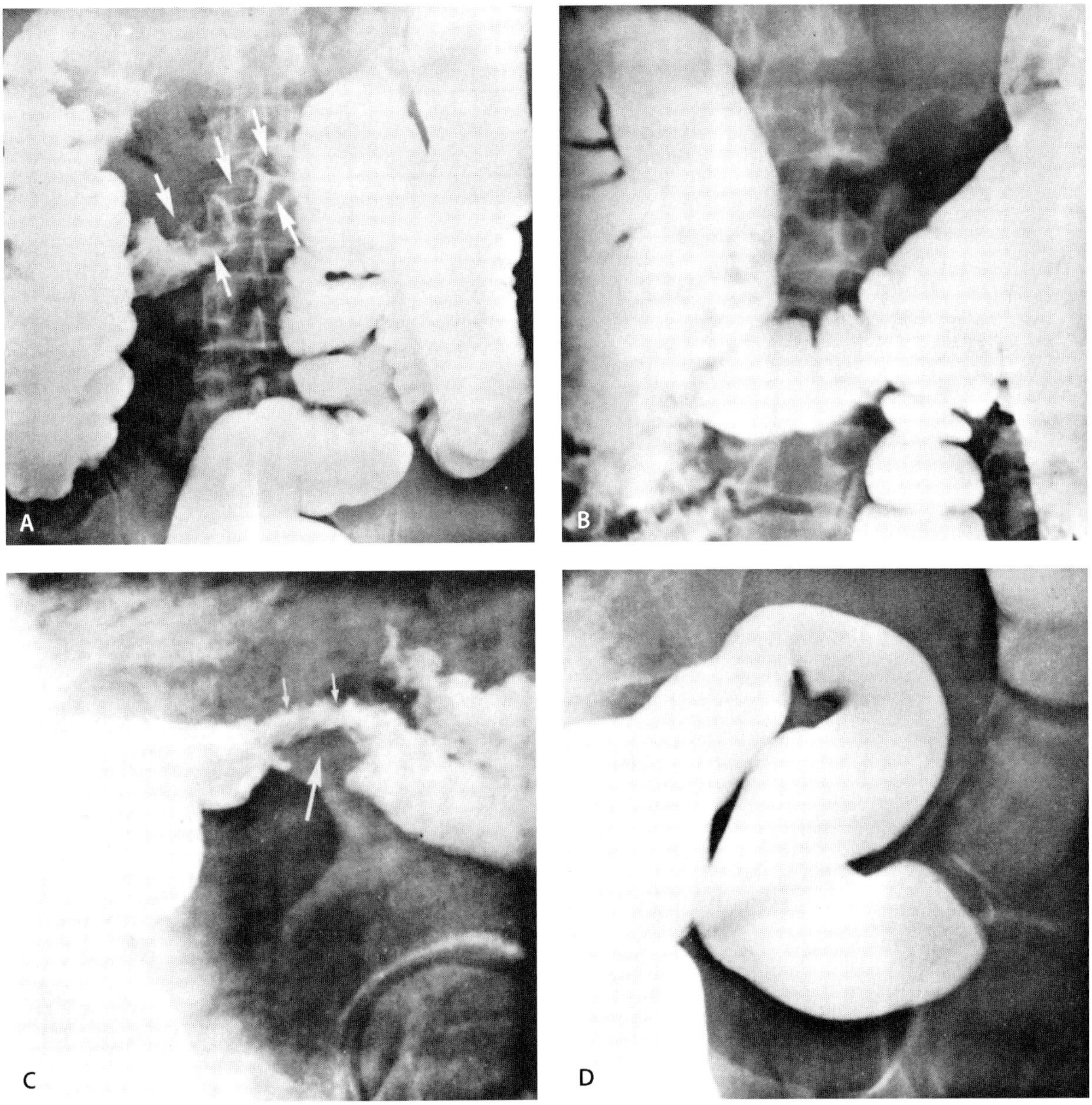

Fig. 1.39 A–D. Resolution of amebic colitis and amebomas following antiamebic therapy with return of the colon to a normal appearance (*restitutio ad integrum*) occurs in many patients. **A** There is a long narrow segment of the transverse colon which shows multiple contiguous filling defects (*arrows*) caused by amebomas in a patient whose stools were loaded with amebae. **B** Six weeks later, after intensive antiamebic therapy, the transverse colon has returned to a normal appearance and the patient had a complete recovery clinically. **C** In another patient, an asymmetric filling defect (*large arrow*) in the sigmoid colon simulates a carcinoma, but the presence of multiple tiny ulcerations (*small arrows*) on the opposite wall suggests the possibility of a localized inflammatory lesion such as ameboma. The diagnosis of amebiasis was established by stool examination. **D** Several months later, following complete recovery with antiamebic treatment, the sigmoid colon appears normal

Colonic Stenosis Following Amebiasis. Following amebicidal medical treatment, the colonic morphology undergoes *restitutio ad integrum* even in the most extensive and severe cases: some say only 0.1% of these patients present a sequela of stenosis. However, Martinez et al. found a persistent focal stenosis in 29% of metronidazole-treated patients who were examined several months following successful therapy. Retrospectively, a deep necrotic ulcerated area was the most common finding during the acute phase of the disease. Prado et al. reported stenosis in two out of eight patients. It is therefore recommended that a barium enema be performed after completion of treatment to assess for possible sequelae.

(Text continues on p. 51)

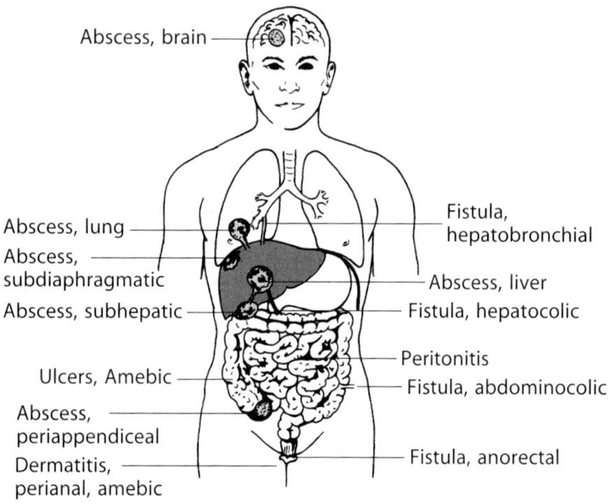

Fig. 1.40. Complications of amebiasis. (From J.E. Ash and S. Spitz: *Pathology of tropical diseases*. Philadelphia, Saunders, 1945)

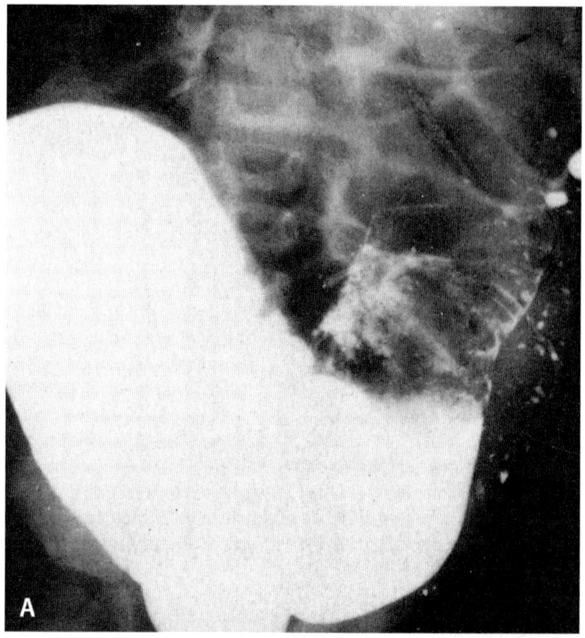

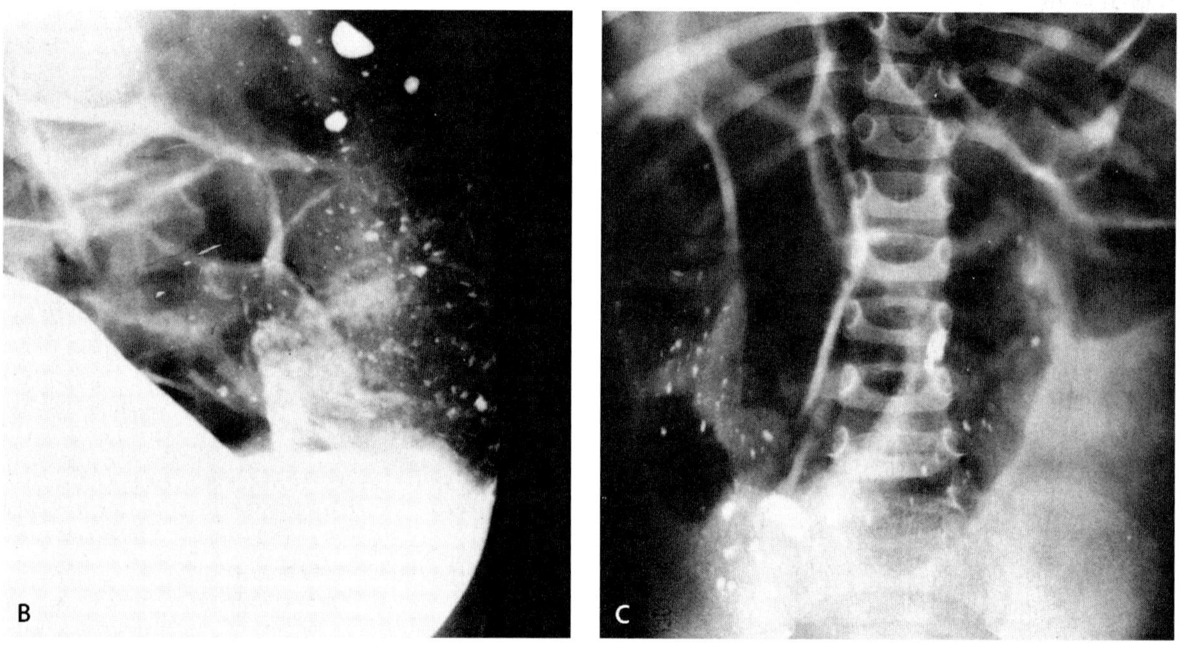

Fig. 1.41 A–C. Amebiasis with intussusception of an ameboma in a child from San Salvador. **A, B** Note the typical "coiled spring" appearance of the colon from an intussusception in the distal descending colon. There are globules of barium outside the colon secondary to an associated perforation causing a transmural peritonitis. **C** A plain film of the abdomen taken 2 days later, shortly before the child died, shows the mass in the left lower quadrant representing the unreduced intussusception, as well as scattered flecks of barium throughout the peritoneal cavity from the perforation. The proximal colon and multiple loops of small bowel are markedly distended as a result of the obstructing intussusception and transmural peritonitis. (Courtesy of Dr. Julio Astacio, San Salvador)

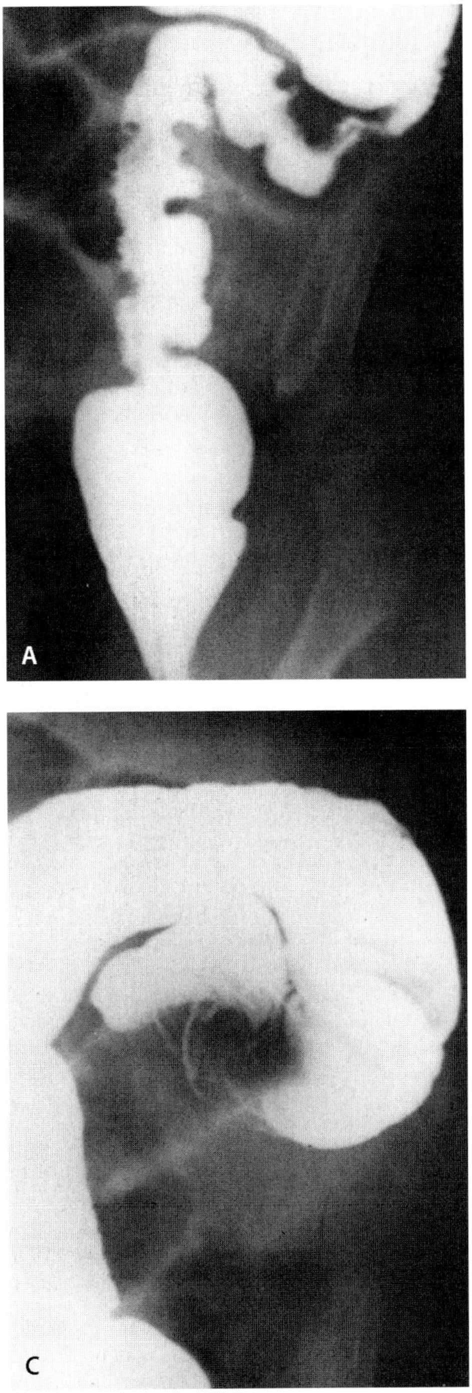

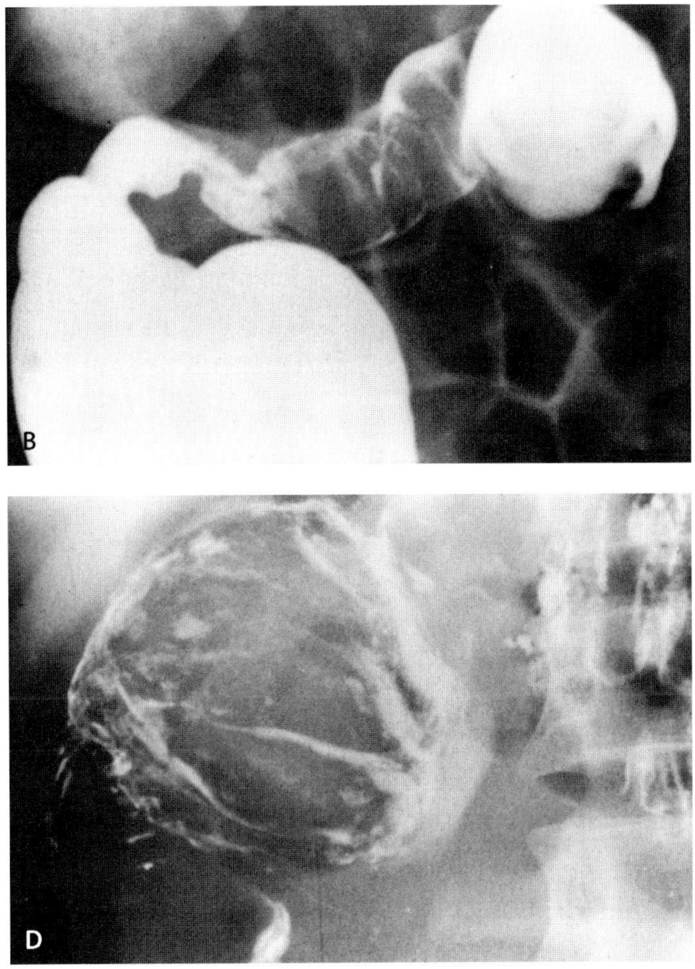

Fig. 1.42. **A–C** Intussusception in amebic colitis in a 4-year-old African girl. She had acute abdominal pain, vomiting, pyrexia, and blood in the stools. There was a palpable mass in the left lower quadrant, and a clinical diagnosis of intussusception was made. Barium enema (**A**) revealed ulceration and narrowing of the rectosigmoid colon. Further progress of the barium column revealed a prominent, long filling defect with the coiled spring appearance typical of intussusception (**B, C**). This colocolic intussusception was reduced to the cecum. Radiological reduction of an amebic intussusception is somewhat dangerous because of the risk of perforation of the bowel, but surgery can be even more hazardous because of the risk of spread of the amebic infection in the presence of the existing untreated amebic colitis. **D** Intussusception at the level of the hepatic flexure caused by an ameboma in a man from Zimbabwe

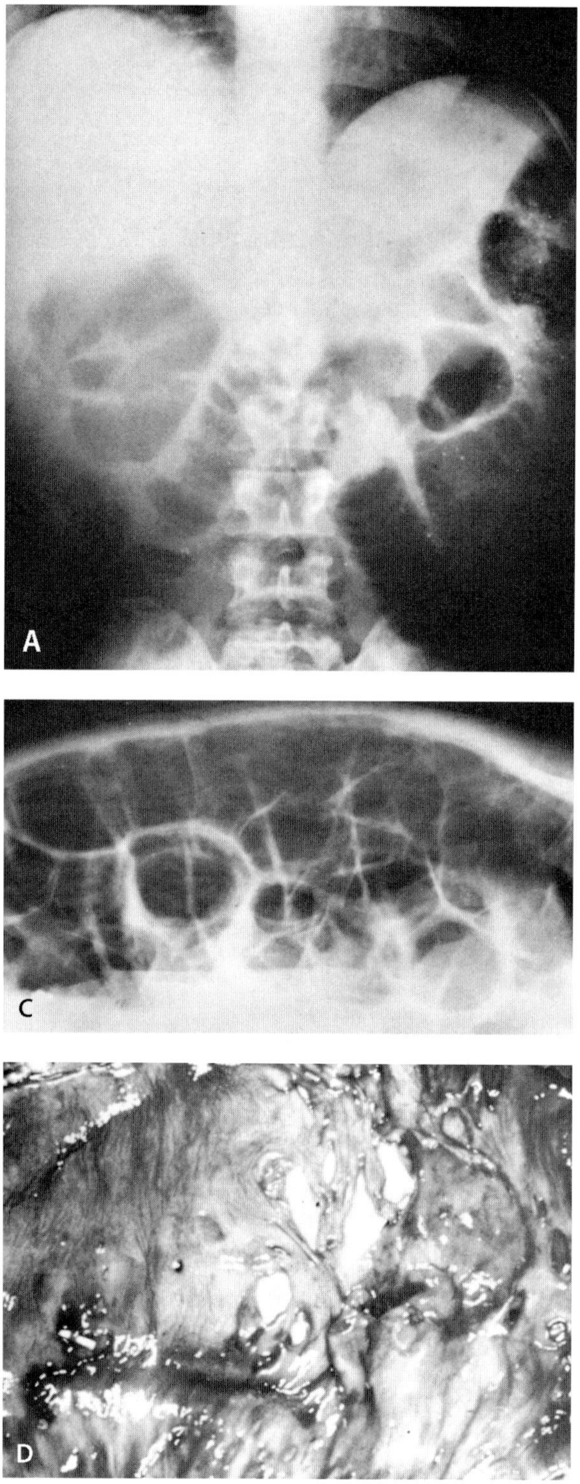

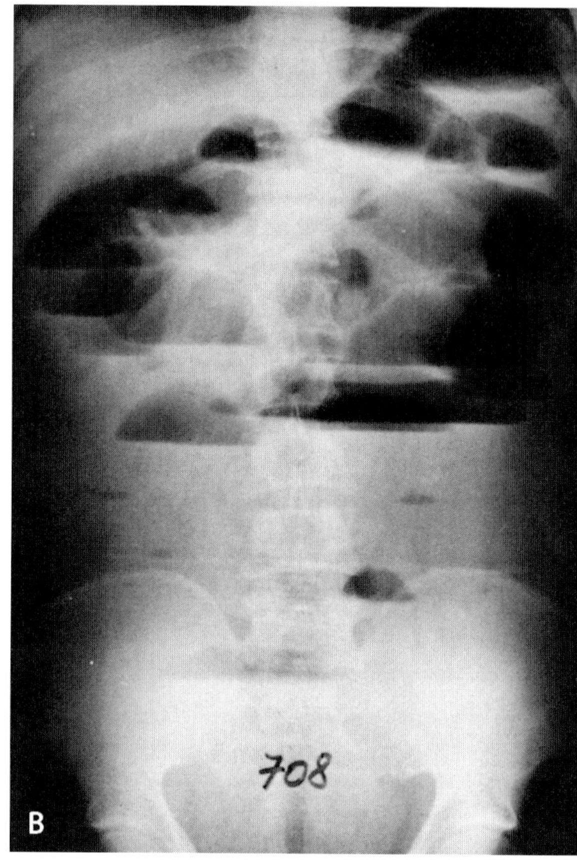

Fig. 1.43. A–C Peritonitis secondary to perforation of amebic ulcers through the serosa of the bowel in a Mexican adult. **A** AP supine view of the abdomen reveals multiple dilated loops of small and large bowel primarily in the midabdomen. Note the separation of the bowel loops caused by thickening of the intestinal wall and mesentery and the irregular thumb-printed contour of several loops from mucosal edema. Note also the slightly elevated right hemidiaphragm and large liver in this patient with hepatic amebic abscess as well as amebic colitis. **B** Upright view of the abdomen showing numerous air-fluid levels within both small and large bowel from severe paralytic ileus. There is also moderate ascites. **C** Lateral decubitus view showing marked distention of the colon and small bowel beneath the peritoneal surface. Fluid levels are seen in the more dependent loops. (A–C courtesy of Dr. Jorge Ceballos-Labat, Mexico City) **D** Gross specimen of a severely ulcerated, fragile colon with numerous large perforations (*white areas in center*) in another patient with fulminating amebic colitis and fatal peritonitis

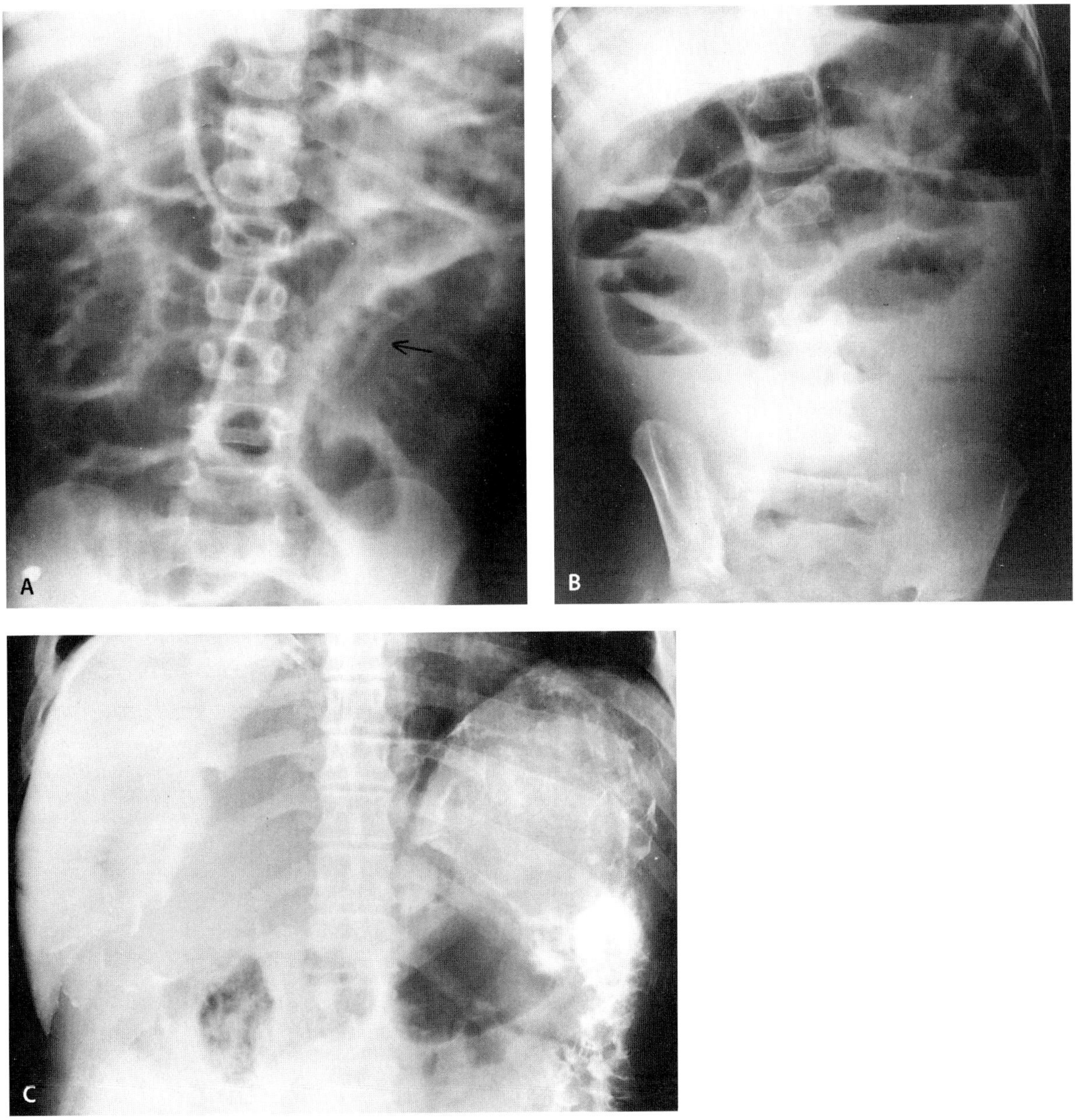

Fig. 1.44. **A, B** Amebic peritonitis in a child from San Salvador. Perforation of amebic ulcers through the colonic serosa led to fatal peritonitis manifest by generalized dilatation of small and large intestine and bowel wall thickening in several areas on AP supine (**A**) and erect (**B**) radiographs of the abdomen. Multiple fluid levels are present, primarily in the small bowel, on the erect view. The child also had ascariasis, with suggestion of at least one ascaris (*arrow*) seen in a dilated small bowel loop on the supine view (**A**). **C** In an African patient, marked leakage of barium from perforated amebic ulcers in the colon has led to huge collections of barium in both subphrenic spaces, especially on the right. This explains how subphrenic abscesses can develop following colonic perforation in patients with fulminant ulcerative amebic colitis. Multiple deep ulcers and areas of thumbprinting are seen in the partially filled descending colon on this ill-advised barium enema study

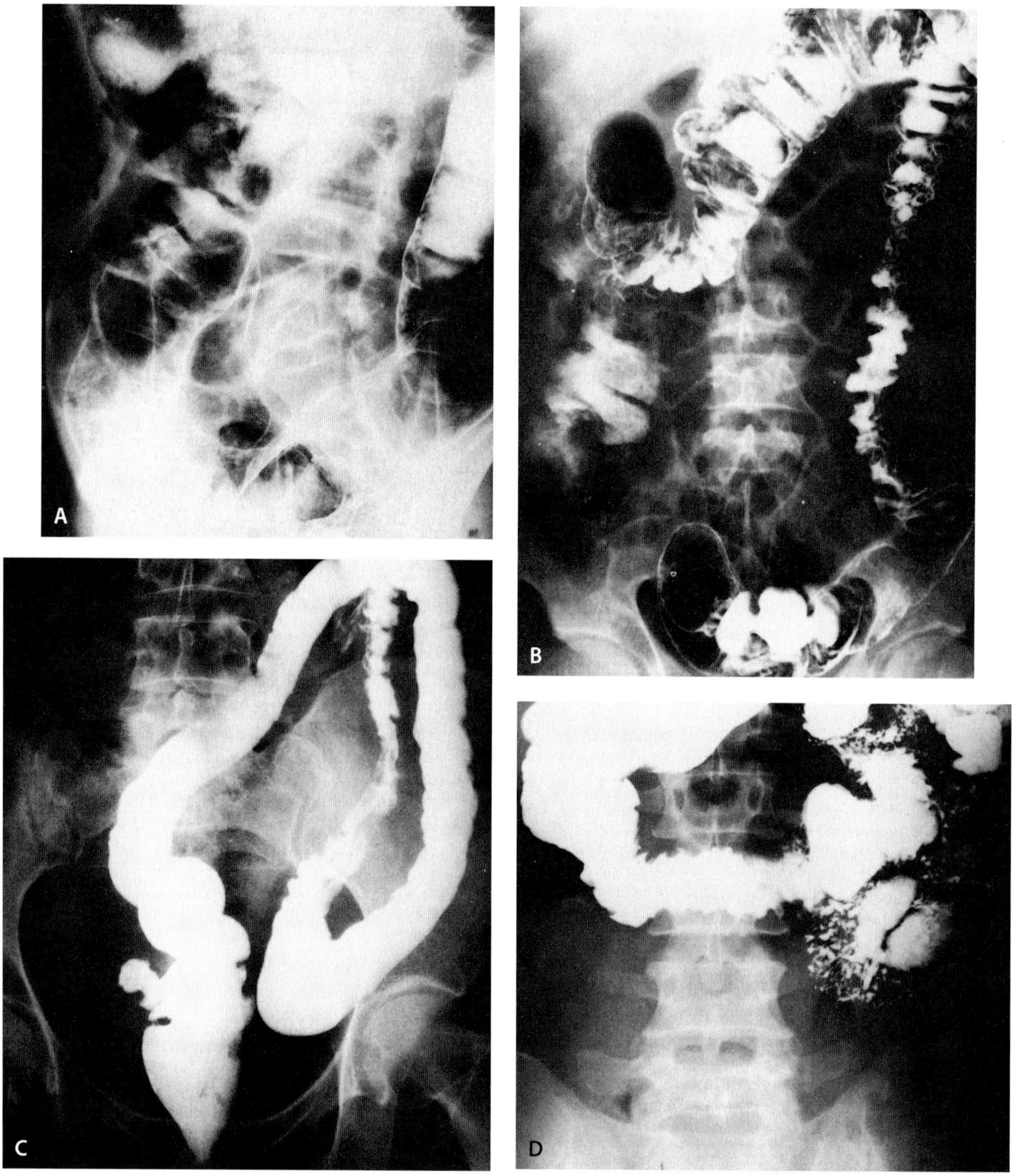

Fig. 1.45 A–D. Amebic pericolic abscesses. **A** There is an abscess in the right flank lateral to the ascending colon and outlined by gas within the abscess cavity. **B** Barium enema shows extensive extravasation of barium into the large abscess in the right flank and subhepatic area; the abscess displaces the ascending colon and hepatic flexure medially. **C** Perirectal abscess extending from the right lateral wall of the rectum deep into the pelvic soft tissues in another patient. The large pelvic abscess has caused straightening and lifting of the rectosigmoid colon out of the pelvis. Note the smooth, somewhat tubular contour of the sigmoid colon with loss of haustrations. **D** There is an irregular contour and marked mucosal edema of the third portion of the duodenum, caused by a large pericolic amebic abscess originating from the transverse colon, and identified on a barium enema performed 2 days after this upper gastrointestinal series in a patient from Colombia

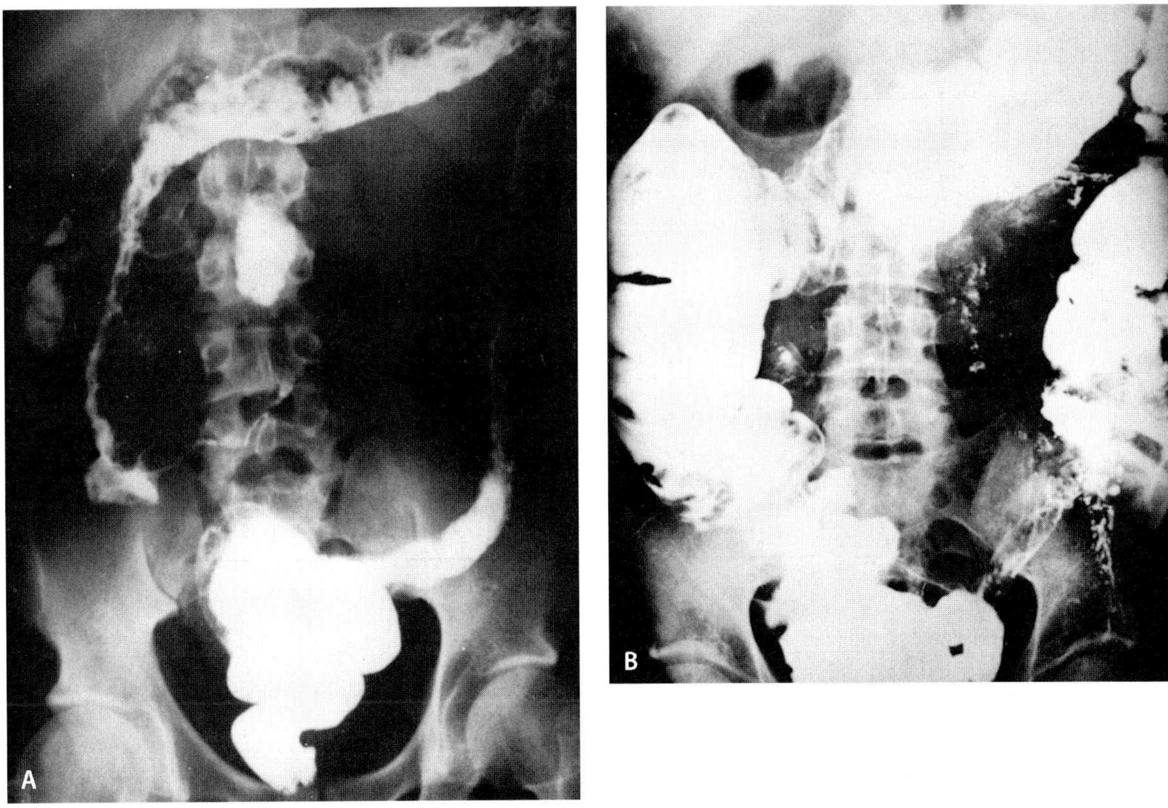

Fig. 1.46 A, B. Multiple fistulas and abscesses in two patients with advanced chronic amebic colitis. **A** There is diffuse stenosis and shortening of the colon from the cecum to the mid-sigmoid colon. The mucosa is severely ulcerated, especially in the ascending colon, and there are numerous long fistulous tracts extending from the ascending colon and cecum into the right flank, right upper quadrant, and midabdomen with large abscesses outlined by barium in the right flank and midabdomen. The ascending colon is displaced medially by the large flank abscess lateral to it. This appearance of a stenotic, shortened, ulcerated colon with multiple fistulous tracts and abscesses is indistinguishable from advanced Crohn's disease. **B** Multiple sinus tracts and fistulas extending into the left midabdomen and to the surface of the skin overlying the left lower quadrant, where a large, long ameboma is noted in the proximal sigmoid colon. There is also an area of stenosis in the proximal descending colon and considerable deformity of the cecum in this patient from San Salvador with chronic amebiasis. (Courtesy of Dr. Julio Astacio, San Salvador)

The Role of Ultrasonography in Intestinal Amebiasis

Ultrasound has an ever expanding role in the evaluation of the gastrointestinal tract. Knowledge of the normal and abnormal patterns have made it possible to recognize intestinal pathology. The "target," "donut," or "pseudokidney" signs produced by bowel wall thickening are not specific because they can be seen in neoplasms, chronic inflammatory disease, ischemic colitis, intussusception, and parasitic colitis (Fig. 1.47).

The typical clinical syndrome combines thickening of the colon wall of 8–17 mm with a hepatic abscess. Crohn's disease is the primary differential consideration for right-sided lesions, while alterations in the left colon may suggest ulcerative colitis.

The Role of Computed Tomography in Intestinal Amebiasis

Computed tomography is the best way to assess the presence and complications of amebic colitis and solid organ involvement. Subtle manifestations of grave complications such as perforation can be readily demonstrated. The intestine has limited response to adverse stimuli from infectious agents, ischemia, toxic events, or auto-immune diseases. Typically it responds with edema, hemorrhage, or ulcerations. This pathological morphology is grossly represented as generalized or focal wall thickening, sometimes with pericolic inflammation, which can be well demonstrated on CT (Fig. 1.48).

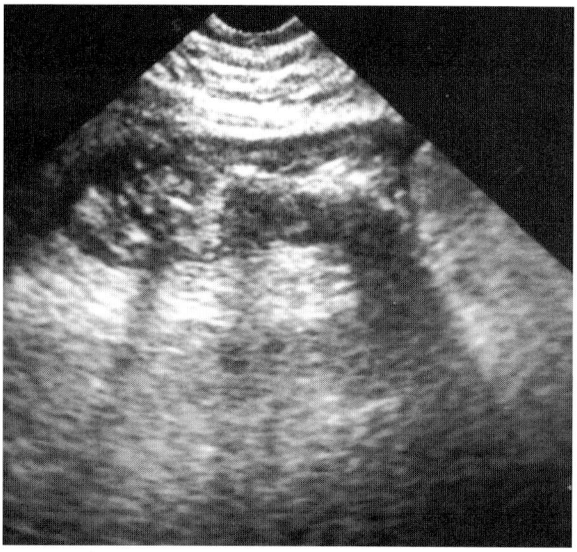

Fig. 1.47. Ultrasound study of amebic colitis, showing the typical image of a "pseudokidney" caused by thickening of the colon wall in amebiasis

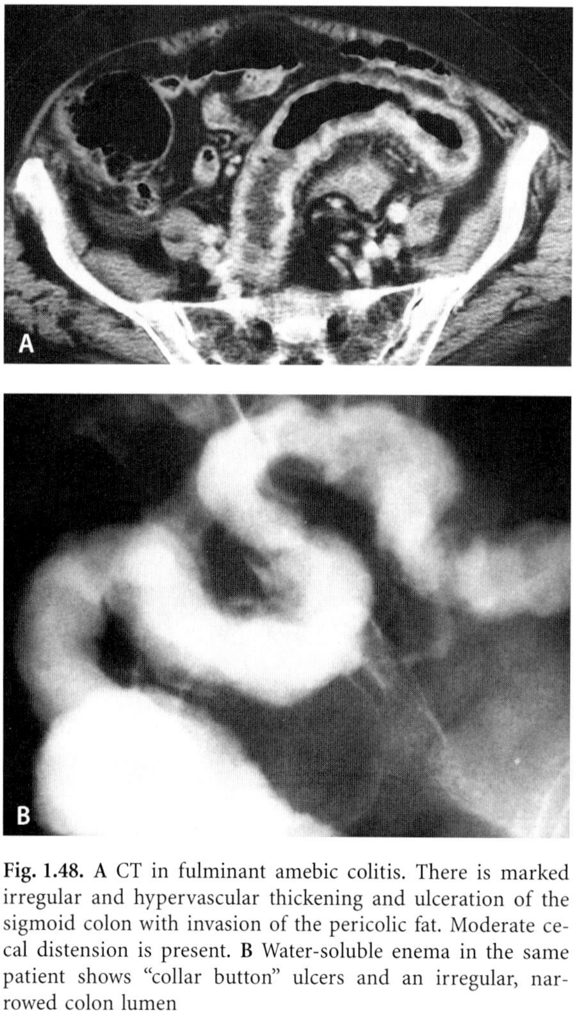

Fig. 1.48. A CT in fulminant amebic colitis. There is marked irregular and hypervascular thickening and ulceration of the sigmoid colon with invasion of the pericolic fat. Moderate cecal distension is present. B Water-soluble enema in the same patient shows "collar button" ulcers and an irregular, narrowed colon lumen

Differential Diagnosis of Amebic Colitis

The differential diagnosis of amebiasis of the colon includes the following disorders:

1. *Ulcerative Colitis.* Differentiation of amebic colitis from ulcerative colitis, granulomatous colitis, and tuberculosis may often be impossible radiologically. However, ulcerative colitis always involves the bowel in continuity and symmetrically and usually begins in the rectum and progresses proximally towards the cecum. In the late stage of the disease, the presacral space is increased and there is uniform diminution of the lumen and shortening of the colon with fewer flexures and convolutions, resulting in a distinct migration of the splenic and hepatic flexures. The ulcerations may be superficial; aphthous ulcers and, occasionally, "collar button" ulcers may be seen. By contrast, there may be skip areas of involvement in amebiasis, with intervening normal bowel, and the disease is more common in the cecum and right colon than in the distal colon. Deep ulcers, fistulous tracts, skip areas of stenosis, and pericolic abscesses are uncommon in ulcerative colitis but frequent in amebiasis.
2. *Granulomatous Colitis (Crohn's Disease).* In granulomatous colitis (and also tuberculosis), the ileum is involved in a high percentage of patients in whom there is cecal and right colon involvement, whereas in amebiasis the ileum is only occasionally abnormal even when there is extensive cecal disease. The asymmetry of bowel wall involvement and a somewhat greater tendency toward skip areas, aphthous ulcers, and a cobblestone mucosal pattern, as well as terminal ileitis, allow the differentiation of Crohn's disease from amebic colitis in many, but certainly not all, patients. Fortunately, Crohn's disease is rare or nonexistent in most of the tropical world whereas amebiasis is universal.
   The finding of *E. histolytica* cysts in the stool or trophozoites in biopsy specimens of the bowel may help in diagnosis, but the parasite can be found coincidentally in patients with granulomatous or other colitis. A therapeutic test may establish the correct diagnosis. In doubtful cases where treatment with amebicidal drugs has been instituted, there is no short-term improvement in patients suffering from Crohn's disease or tuberculosis.
3. *Tuberculosis.* Tuberculosis may mimic amebiasis with a conical, irregularly contracted cecum, but there is often intense spasm of the ileocecal valve in tuberculosis which prevents reflux into the ileum. If reflux does occur, the ileum is usually abnormal, with areas of ulceration, stenosis, and

fistulas; other more proximal portions of the small bowel are also often involved with tuberculosis. Skip lesions or granulomas within the bowel of tuberculous origin cannot be distinguished radiologically from amebiasis or Crohn's disease.

4. *Malignancy.* An ameboma may simulate and be indistinguishable from carcinoma (see pp. 33, 38–44), and a thickened bowel wall may resemble lymphoma.
5. *Ischemic Lesions of the Colon.* A history of bowel infarction is usually typical and the classical "thumbprinting" which changes rapidly even without therapy, permits the diagnosis with more confidence. Ischemic colitis is uncommon in most tropical areas, except when it is a complication of sickle cell disease. Unfortunately, the acute amebic colon may have "thumbprints" indistinguishable from ischemic colitis. Age and geographical location of the patient, response to treatment, and progress of the disease may be distinguishing features. Contrast-enhanced CT studies may at times pinpoint the ischemic nature of the colitis by clearly identifying thrombosis of the superior mesenteric artery or the splanchnic venous circulation.
6. *Pseudomembranous Colitis.* Antibiotic-induced alterations of the intestinal flora allow the growth and potentiation of *Clostridium difficile* via production of potent endotoxins that induce a severe inflammatory reaction with multiple whitish-yellowish pseudomembranes, representing mucus and inflammatory detritus covering the colonic mucosa. Abdominal pain, diarrhea, fever, and leukocytosis following antibiotic administration during the prior 6 weeks constitute the clinical picture and are the clues to search for *C. difficile* in feces or perform the more reliable toxin detection test.
7. *Actinomycosis.* Actinomycosis is rare and usually involves the appendix as well as the right colon. Seldom are there lesions elsewhere in the bowel. When sinuses erupt through skin, they are multiple and unlike those seen in cutaneous amebiasis. The mycotic grains and the pathological changes in biopsy or surgically excised specimens clearly distinguish the two diseases.
8. *Schistosomiasis.* Schistosomiasis involves the rectum and left colon in particular and can cause marked inflammatory polyposis. The cecum is rarely involved. Coincidental infections of schistosomiasis and amebiasis may be seen together in some geographical areas of the tropics.

The frequency of each disease on this list and therefore its weight in differential diagnosis varies throughout the world.

Amebiasis Elsewhere in the Gastrointestinal Tract

Esophagus. Direct involvement of the esophagus is extremely rare, but has occurred as a result of spread from a periesophageal abscess; clinically the patient may have dysphagia and pain. More important, obstruction and displacement of the esophagus from enlargement of the liver are recorded, presenting as dysphagia. In such patients, the hemidiaphragm (usually the left) is raised and fluoroscopy, or preferably ultrasound where available, shows reduced movement; a pleural effusion, with or without a pericardial effusion, is likely. Barium swallow shows that the esophagus is compressed and usually displaced posteriorly by the mass under the diaphragm. There is also lateral displacement, the direction depending on the location of the amebic abscess, whether in the left or right lobe of the liver. Typically, the lower end of the esophagus is rotated around the enlarged liver and the stomach is also displaced.
The differential diagnosis includes achalasia and esophageal carcinoma. The esophagus does not dilate to the same extent as in achalasia and restricted diaphragmatic movement suggests a subphrenic lesion. There should be no intrinsic mass within the esophagus in these amebic patients.

Stomach. Primary amebiasis of the stomach has not been recorded. An enlarged liver, however, can displace the stomach. Occasionally, an abscess in the left lobe of the liver can rupture into the stomach and, if the abscess also involves the diaphragm and pericardium, a pneumothorax or pneumopericardium may result (see Figs. 1.85 B, 1.101).

Duodenum. Edema of the duodenal loop can be demonstrated in some patients with amebiasis. The duodenum may become atonic and mildly dilated, and the mucosa is swollen and edematous, with spiking of the folds. Similar changes are found in other parasitic infections of the small bowel (e.g., giardiasis and strongyloidiasis) and there may be no distinguishing features. Such findings, associated with vague dyspeptic symptoms without demonstration of an ulcer, should suggest the possibility of parasitic infection, including amebiasis. The duodenal C-loop can be involved with inflammatory changes secondary to a pericolic abscess originating from amebic colitis in the adjacent transverse colon.

Small Bowel. Amebiasis does not affect the terminal ileum as an isolated finding, but will do so in 10% or more of patients where there is cecal involvement. Mucosal thickening, pseudopolyps, rigidity, and ulceration may be found. An ameboma of the ileum is recorded. An important distinguishing feature among amebiasis, Crohn's disease and tubercu-

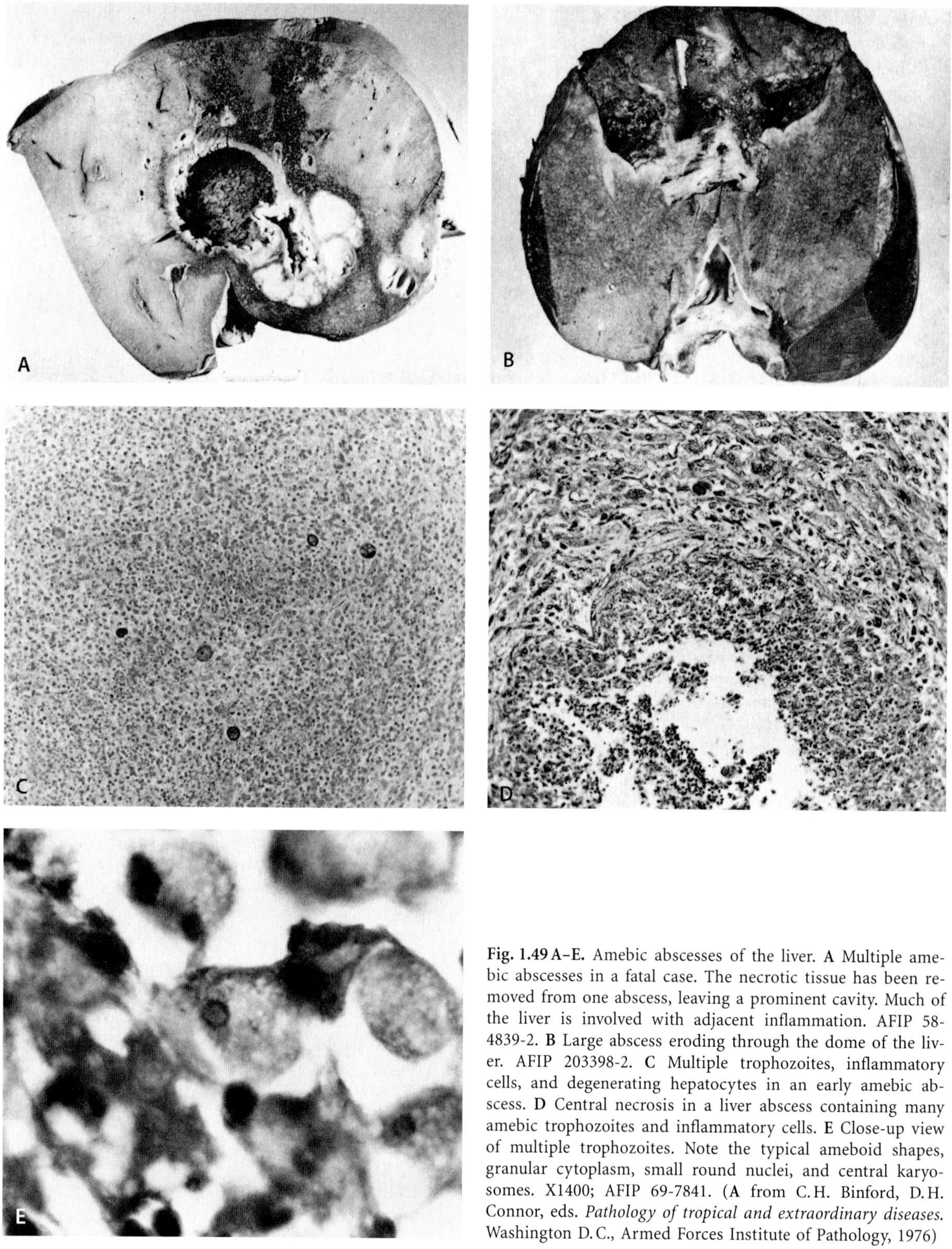

Fig. 1.49 A–E. Amebic abscesses of the liver. **A** Multiple amebic abscesses in a fatal case. The necrotic tissue has been removed from one abscess, leaving a prominent cavity. Much of the liver is involved with adjacent inflammation. AFIP 58-4839-2. **B** Large abscess eroding through the dome of the liver. AFIP 203398-2. **C** Multiple trophozoites, inflammatory cells, and degenerating hepatocytes in an early amebic abscess. **D** Central necrosis in a liver abscess containing many amebic trophozoites and inflammatory cells. **E** Close-up view of multiple trophozoites. Note the typical ameboid shapes, granular cytoplasm, small round nuclei, and central karyosomes. X1400; AFIP 69-7841. (**A** from C.H. Binford, D.H. Connor, eds. *Pathology of tropical and extraordinary diseases.* Washington D.C., Armed Forces Institute of Pathology, 1976)

losis in the ileocecal area is the high incidence of involvement of the ileum in the latter two diseases when the right colon is affected.

Gallbladder. Primary involvement of the gallbladder is not recognized, but an amebic liver abscess may cause oral cholecystography to be unsuccessful.

Amebic Liver Abscess

Plain Film Radiography

On plain film radiography, an amebic abscess of the liver (Fig. 1.49) is characterized by hepatomegaly and obscuration of the hepatic angle in both supine and erect views; ileus may be present, especially in the 30% of patients with hepatic abscess who show signs of invasive colonic amebiasis (Fig. 1.50). The gallbladder may be dense and distended. This combination is not usually seen in a subphrenic abscess or hepatoma, but can occur occasionally in acute cholecystitis.

If the abscess is in the center or lower part of the liver, it will enlarge in the anteroposterior diameter. When the abscess is closer to the diaphragm, it may restrict diaphragmatic movement, elevate the hemidiaphragm, or produce a localized bulge (Figs. 1.51–1.56). There may be an associated small pleural effusion and edema or pneumonitis in the lung above the diaphragm (Fig. 1.56). Attempts to differentiate the various causes of a "bulge" in a hemidiaphragm have been unsuccessful. Whether the bulge is medial or lateral depends entirely on the location of the underlying abscess and cannot be used to differentiate an amebic abscess from metastases, primary liver tumor, or any other cause of localized hepatic enlargement. Gas within a hepatic abscess is an indicator of a fistula to a hollow viscus, secondary infection by a gas-forming bacteria, or iatrogenic air from a previous percutaneous drainage or intervention (see Figs. 1.67, 1.83). Peritoneal signs may be indicative of perforation or rupture of a hepatic abscess into the peritoneal space.

Ultrasonography, CT and MRI (see pp. 68–82)

Nuclear Medicine Scan

Technetium-99m (^{99m}Tc) and dimethylaminodiacetic imaging can confirm the presence of a hepatic amebic abscess and often establish differentiation from other hepatobiliary pathology. A halo of radioactivity surrounding a photopenic defect are the typical findings which correlate well with ultrasound, CT

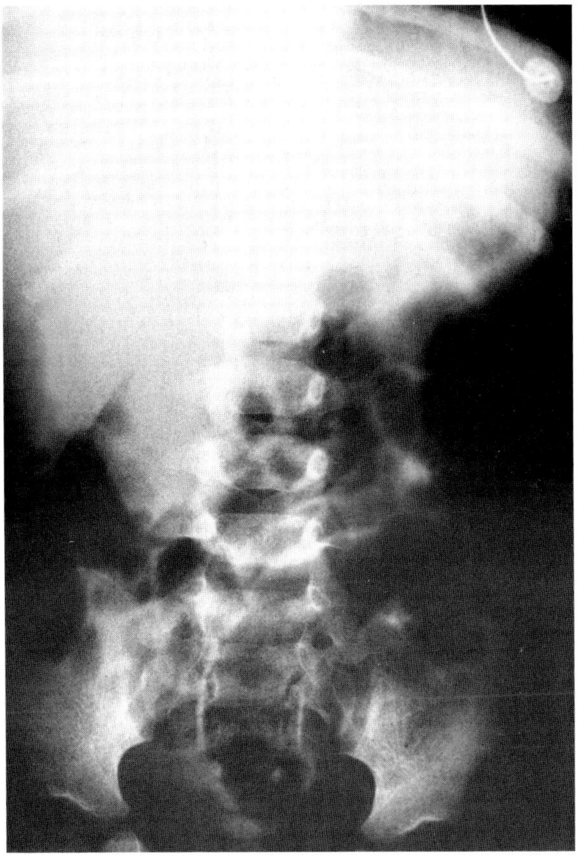

Fig. 1.50. Hepatomegaly and ileus, a common combination of findings in hepatic and intestinal amebiasis

and magnetic resonance imaging (MRI) (Figs. 1,56, 1.57–1.60). One or more filling defects or cold areas will be seen except where there are multiple very small abscesses or when the abscess is small and peripheral. Multiple scans should be made, including anteroposterior (AP), posteroanterior (PA), and right lateral views. If ultrasonography is unavailable, serial isotope scanning can also be used to assess the progress of antiamebic therapy, remembering that clinical and laboratory findings often lag behind improvement in the scan (Fig. 1.60).

The radioactive colloids of ^{99m}Tc and indium-113 (^{113}In) are phagocytosed by the reticuloendothelial cells in the liver. Ionic carrier-free ^{113}In (used previously) or gallium-67 (^{67}Ga) citrate accumulates at the perimeter of the abscess cavity in the region of hyperemia seen histologically and arteriographically. Liver scanning using ^{67}Ga citrate may be more accurate than the others in determining inflammatory activity and the size of an acute abscess. The gallium study will turn from hot to cold within days of antiamebic therapy. Assessment of resolution of the abscess and therapeutic effect should be accomplished with ^{99m}Tc sulfur colloid, usually at 3- to 4-

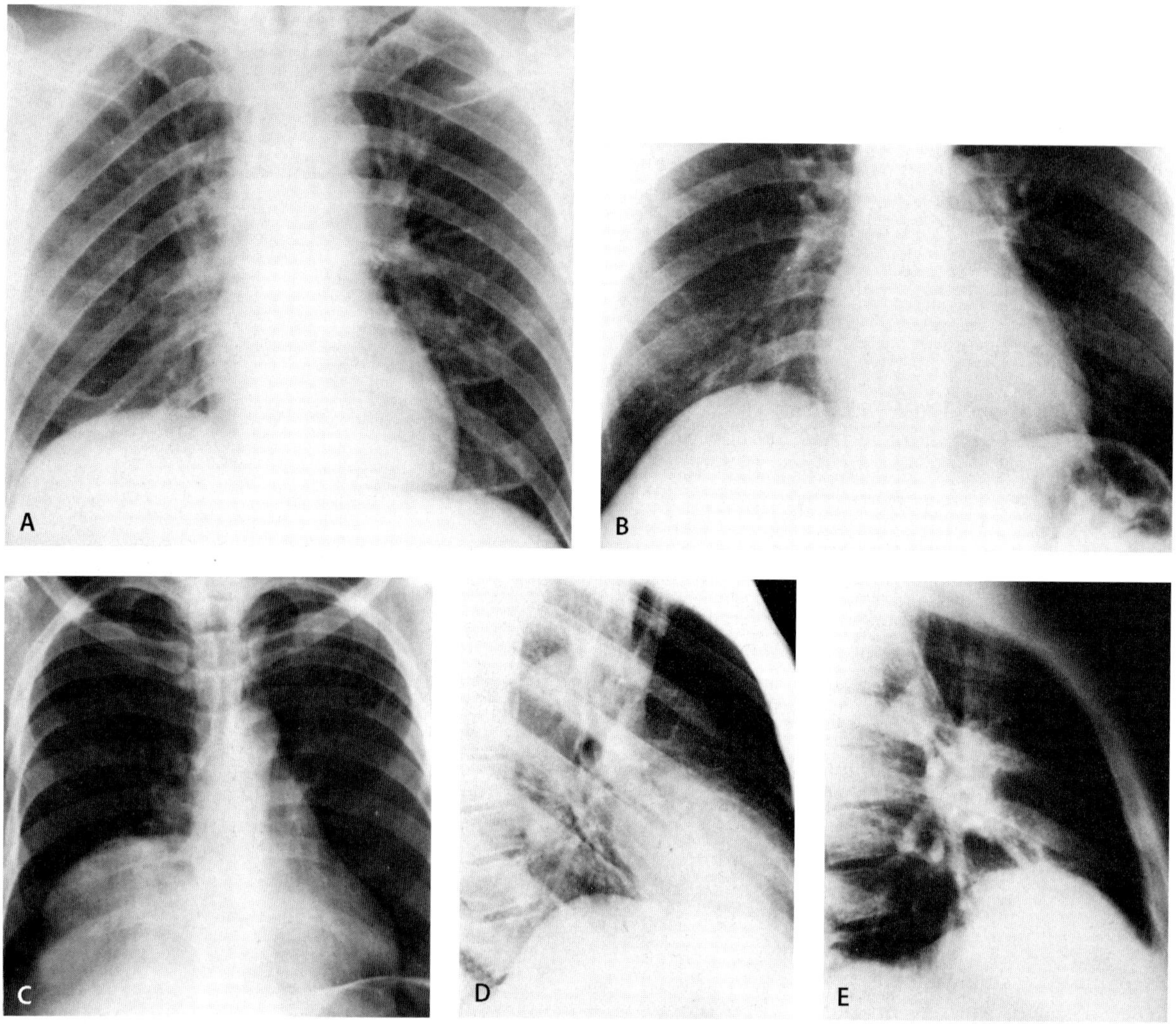

Fig. 1.51 A–E. Elevation of a hemidiaphragm is usually the earliest roentgen sign of an amebic liver abscess. The position of the bulge has little diagnostic significance. **A** Smooth generalized elevation of the right hemidiaphragm, whose movement was restricted on fluoroscopy when compared with the normal left side. **B** Elevation of the medial aspect of the right hemidiaphragm. **C** A prominent bulge in the midportion of the right hemidiaphragm affecting the medial but not the lateral aspect. In none of the above patients is there any reaction in the lung base or pleura. **D** Elevation of the diaphragm may be more clearly visible in the lateral view, where a small posterior bulge of the right hemidiaphragm is seen. **E** There is a large bulge in the midportion of the diaphragm on lateral view; the posterior portion is normal

week intervals. Nuclear tomography helps determine the extent of amebic involvement of the liver.

Isotope, CT and ultrasound scanning suggest that about 50% of amebic abscesses are solitary lesions in the right lobe of the liver only. Solitary abscesses in the left lobe are much less frequent, occurring in about 15% of cases. The remainder are multiple abscesses, some of which may coalesce into a large liver abscess. While the liver may become diffusely swollen, edematous, and tender in occasional patients, a true "amebic hepatitis" is not defined pathologically.

(Text continues on p. 63)

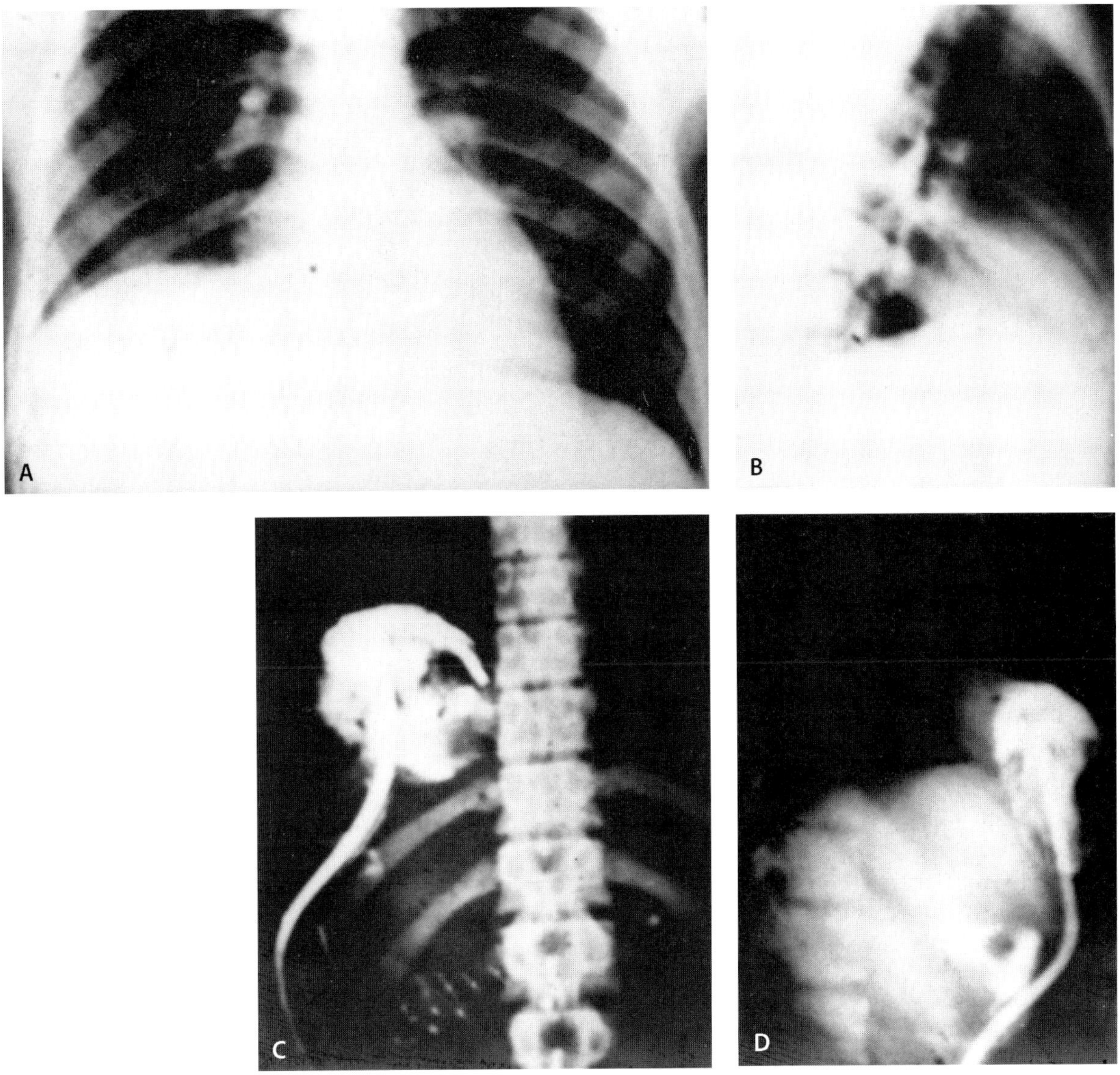

Fig. 1.52 A–D. Elevation of the right hemidiaphragm caused by an amebic liver abscess. **A** Posteroanterior and **B** lateral views of the chest reveal moderate elevation of a smooth right hemidiaphragm which showed restricted motion on fluoroscopy. There was no reaction in the lung or pleura above the diaphragm. **C, D** AP and lateral views of the lower thorax and upper abdomen after partial drainage of a large amebic abscess and injection of contrast media through the drainage tube to outline the extent of the abscess. The patient was a young American soldier serving in the Vietnam conflict

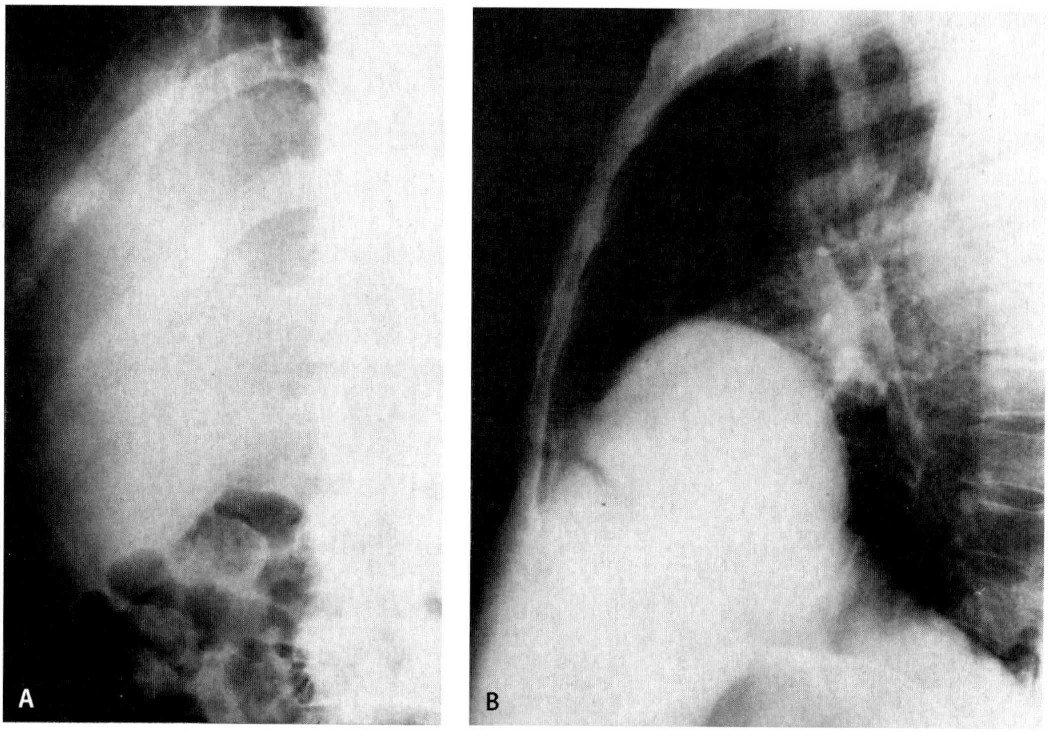

Fig. 1.53 A, B. The size of the liver involved with amebic abscess may be quite misleading when palpated through the abdominal wall. **A** The liver edge palpated below the right costal margin would suggest clinically that the liver is normal or only slightly enlarged; it is in fact enlarged considerably upwards with elevation of the right hemidiaphragm. **B** Lateral view of the same patient shows the marked bulge in the anterior portion of the right hemidiaphragm

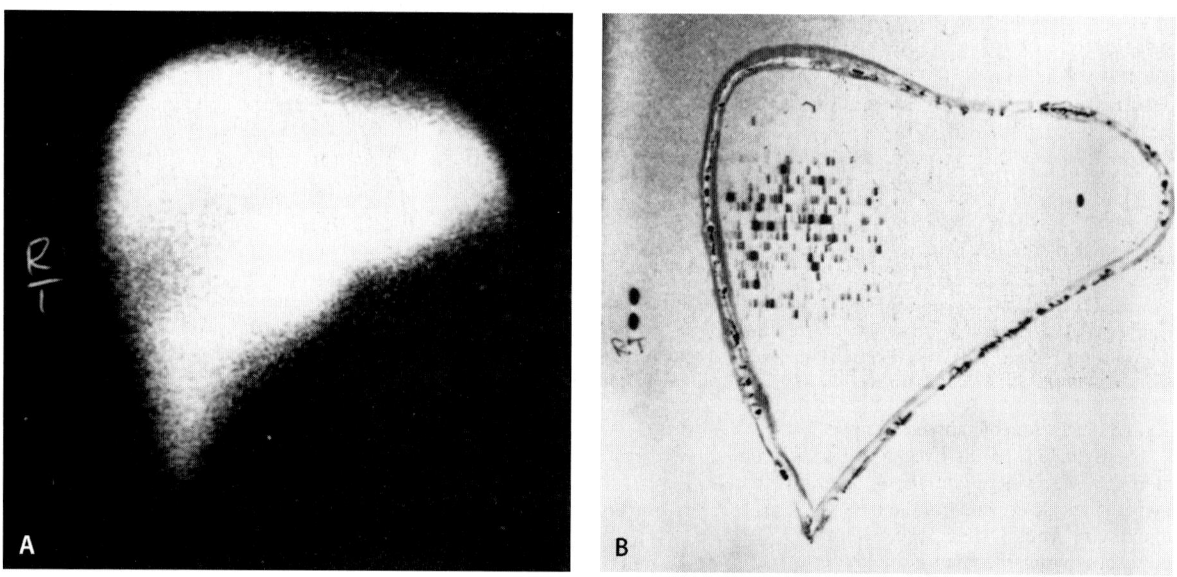

Fig. 1.54 A, B. Large amebic abscess identified by nuclear scanning. **A** The anterior projection of a ^{99m}Tc-sulfur colloid liver scan reveals a cold or photopenic lesion in the right lobe of the liver centrally and peripherally. **B** A follow-up study 24 hours later using ^{67}Ga citrate and image processing shows that the prior focal defect concentrates the nuclide. This is due to the inflammatory cells surrounding the amebic abscess. Technetium-99m sulfur colloid is a preferred radionuclide for imaging the liver. Gallium-67 citrate is used to determine inflammatory activity. The gallium study will turn from hot to cold within days of antiamebic therapy. Follow-up to demonstrate resolution and therapeutic effect is accomplished with ^{99m}Tc-sulfur colloid, usually at 3- to 4-week intervals. Occasionally nuclear tomography may aid in determining the extent of an abscess. (Courtesy of Dr. Bruce Mazat, Columbia)

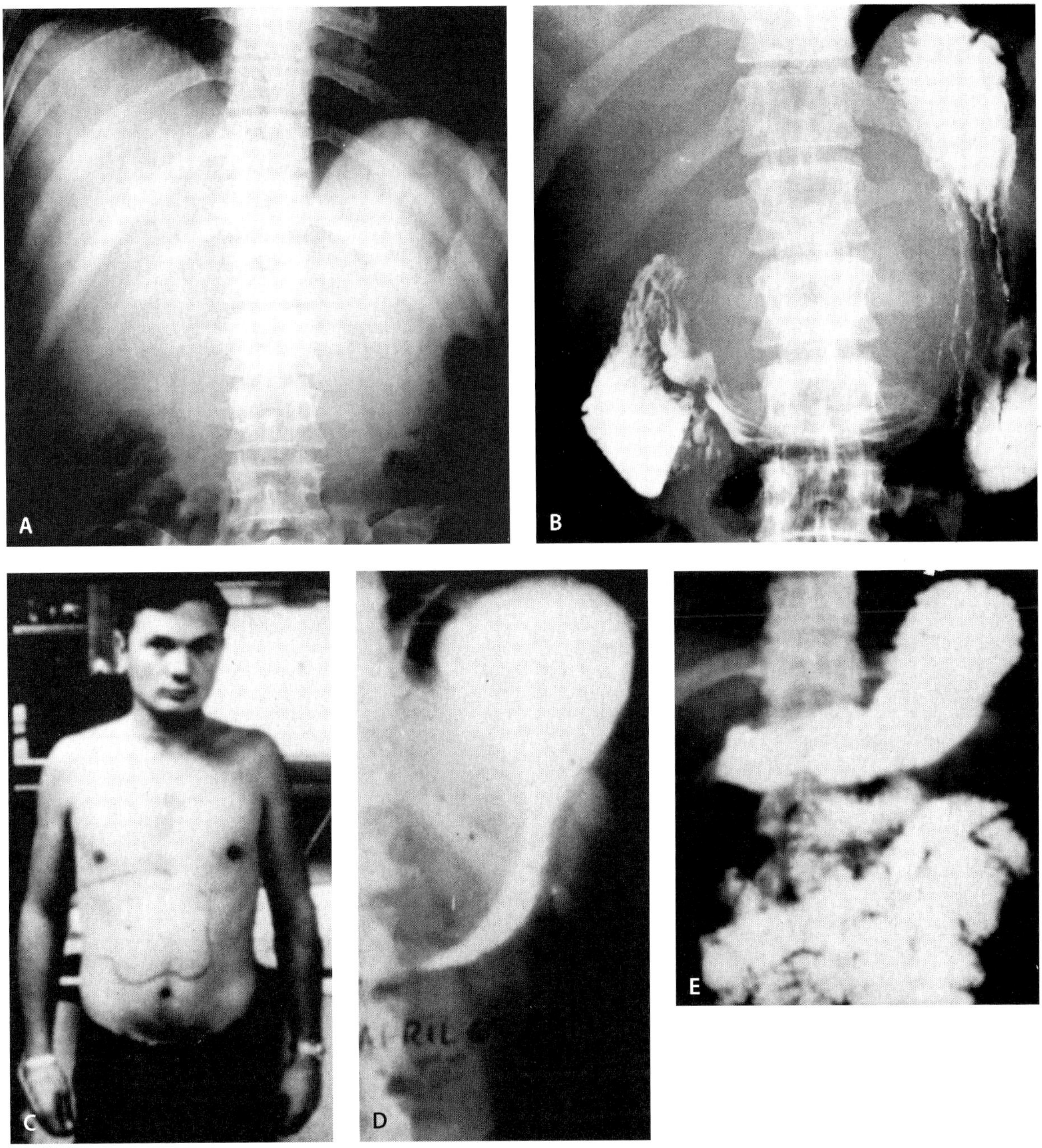

Fig. 1.55 A–E. Amebic abscesses involving the left lobe as well as the right lobe of the liver. **A** AP supine view of the abdomen of a Mexican patient shows massive generalized enlargement of the liver with marked elevation of the right hemidiaphragm from a right lobe liver abscess. There is a large mass occupying the midline of the abdomen and displacing the gas-filled stomach to the left as the result of a large left lobe abscess. **B** Barium-filled stomach of the same patient shows extrinsic pressure on the lesser curvature by the large abscess in the left lobe of the liver. (Courtesy of Dr. Jorge Ceballos-Labat, Mexico City) **C–E** Young American soldier who acquired amebiasis during the Vietnam conflict. **C** The liver was found to be markedly enlarged upon palpation; its outline is drawn over the anterior abdominal wall. **D** Initial upper GI series showed marked extrinsic compression and narrowing of the body and antrum of the stomach due to the large abscess in the left liver lobe. **E** An upper GI series several months later, after antiamebic therapy, shows the liver has returned to normal size; the barium-filled stomach also appears normal, with no extrinsic compression or displacement

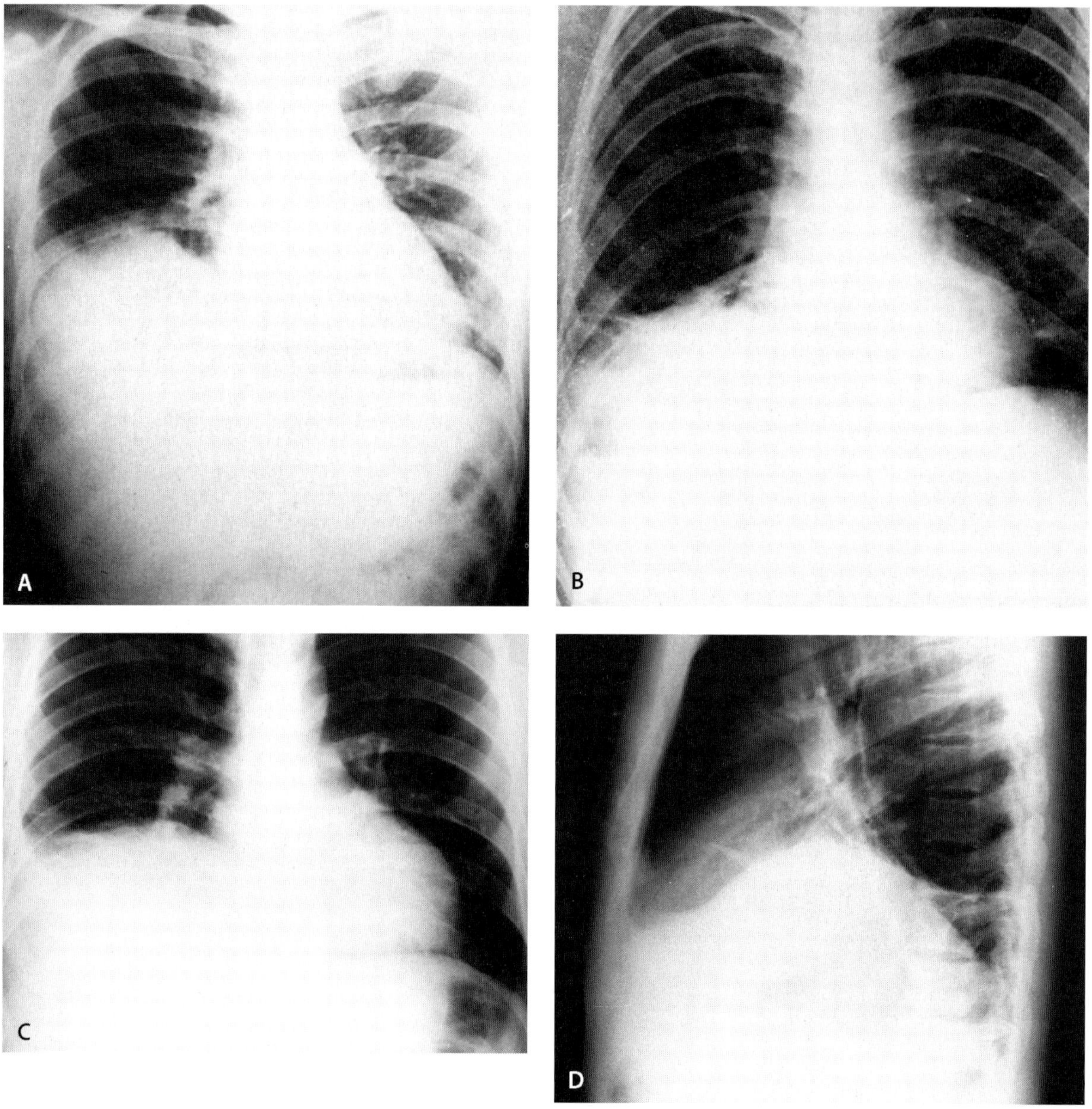

Fig. 1.56 A–D. Reaction in the lung and pleura above an elevated right hemidiaphragm in three patients with hepatic amebic abscess. **A** A Laotian youth with marked elevation of the right hemidiaphragm and massive liver enlargement. There is a patch of edema or pneumonitis at the right lung base above the indistinct outline of the raised diaphragm. **B** There is slight pleural effusion at the right base and costophrenic angle with minimal discoid atelectasis and hypoaerated, edematous lung above an elevated right hemidiaphragm in another patient with hepatic abscess. **C, D** Hepatic amebic abscess in a Mexican patient with focal elevation of the midportion of the right hemidiaphragm and associated pleuropulmonary findings of discoid atelectasis at the right lung base and a small empyema. (Courtesy of Drs. Kenji Kimura and Miguel Stoopen) These findings of localized edema, pneumonitis, discoid atelectasis, and pleural fluid or empyema are a common sequel to liver abscess and indicate spread of the amebic infection across the diaphragm to involve the pleural cavity and lung. At times, the radiographic appearance of an elevated hemidiaphragm may, in fact, be simulated by a subpleural effusion; this can best be demonstrated by ultrasonography or by a lateral decubitus film, which will show the pleural fluid layered along the lateral chest wall

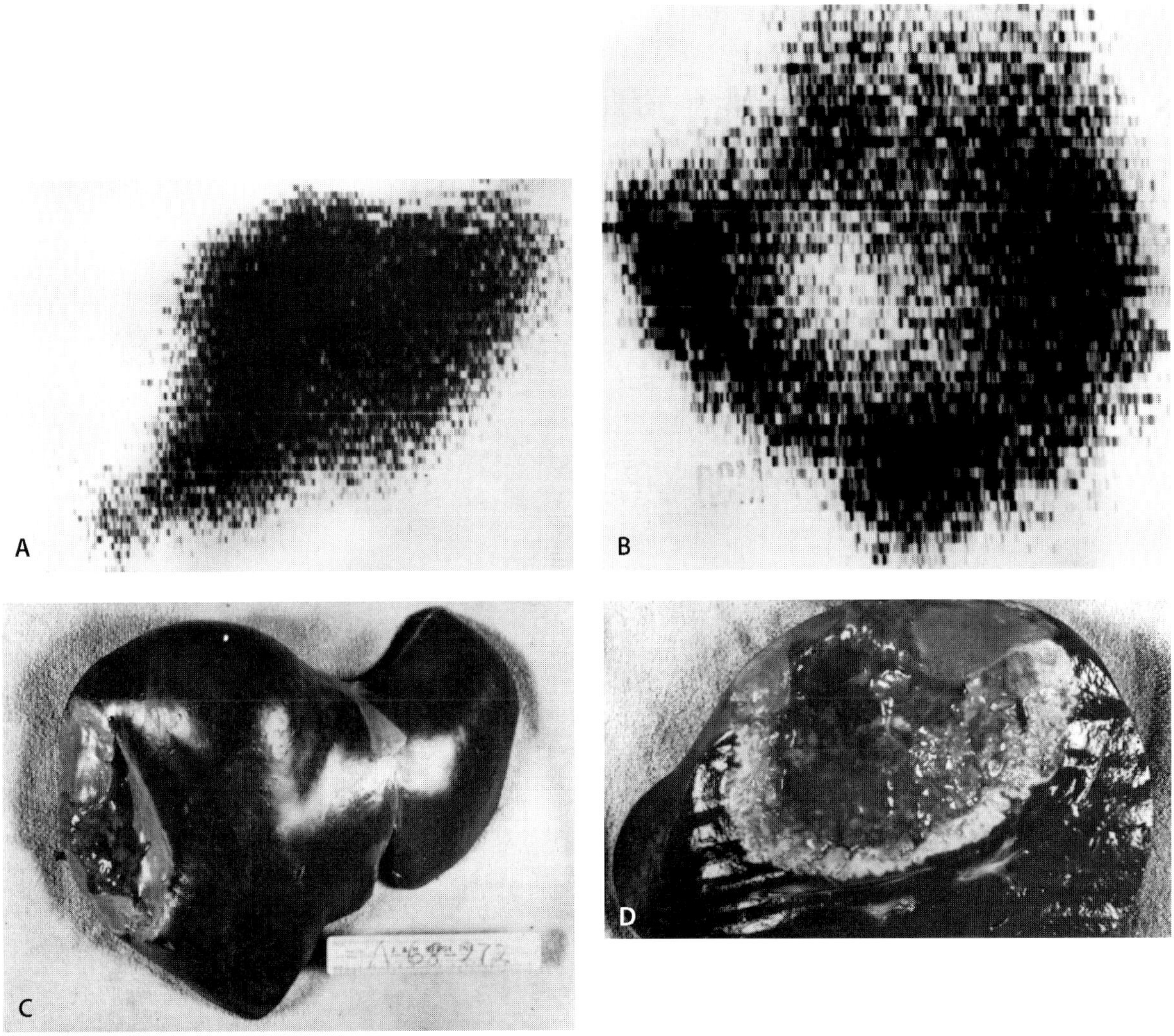

Fig. 1.57 A–D. Large amebic abscess in the periphery of the right lobe of the liver. Anteroposterior (**A**) and right lateral (**B**) views of a liver radioisotope scan show a large cold or photopenic defect occupying the lateral border of the right lobe (*RCM* right costal margin). On the lateral view this appears as a central defect because the abscess is seen "en face" rather than in profile as in **A**. **C, D** A large abscess of the lateral margin of the right lobe of the liver in another patient who died as the result of this serious complication of amebiasis. The abscess has perforated through the liver capsule. Extensive necrosis within the abscess is seen in profile (**C**) and "en face" (**D**) views of the autopsy specimen. Thick viscid debris resembling anchovy paste is often present in these ab scesses. AFIP 68-15508-1 and 2

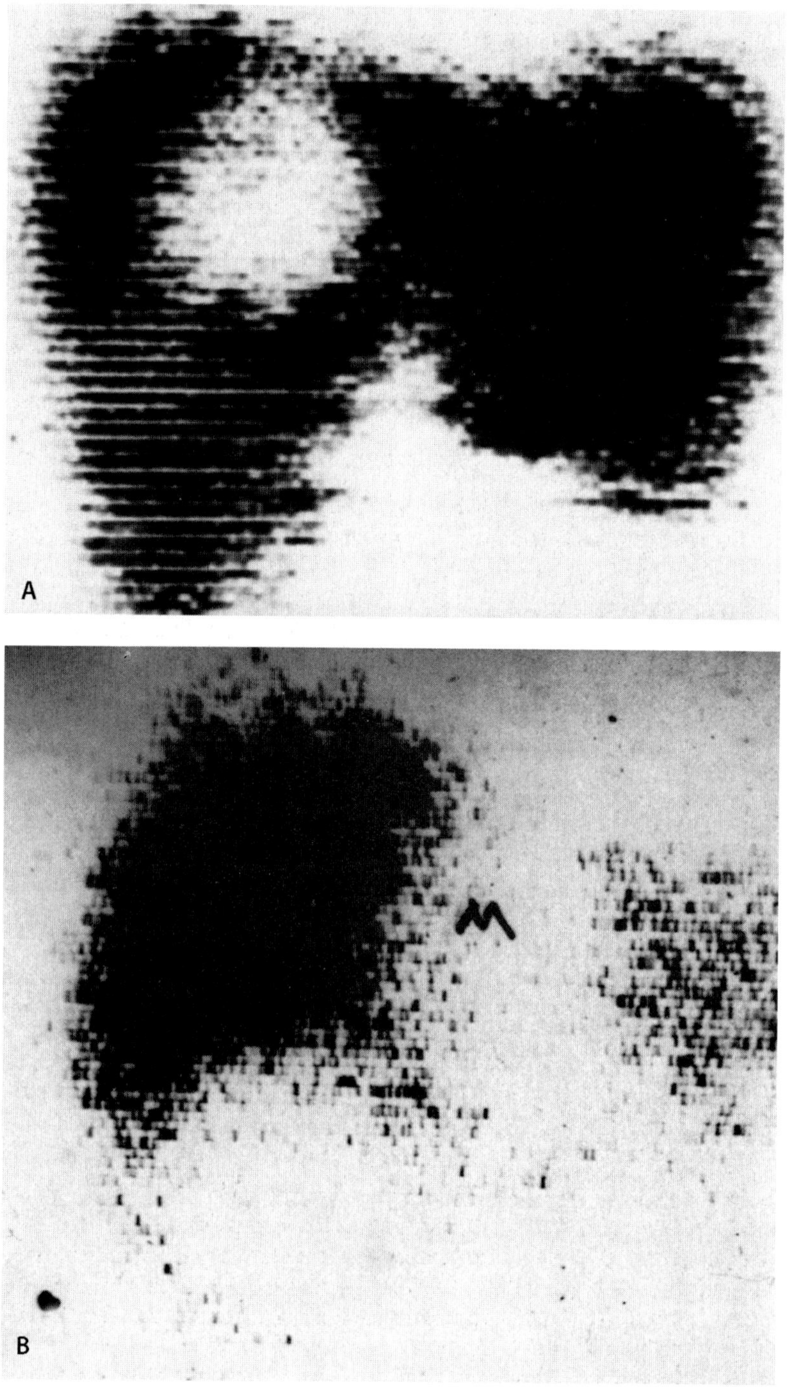

Fig. 1.58 A, B. Nuclear scans of large central amebic abscesses penetrating through the dome of the liver to involve the diaphragm in two patients. **A** A large central abscess of the right lobe with extension to the superior aspect of the liver presents as a large cold or photopenic lesion on nuclear scan. **B** Multiple large abscesses identified on ^{99m}Tc-sulfur colloid scan of the liver. There is a large central abscess extending into and replacing much of the left lobe of the liver. There is also a large abscess involving the inferior aspect of the right lobe. This second patient was a young American soldier who contracted amebiasis during the Vietnam conflict. Although desperately ill and almost succumbing from massive amebic involvement of the liver, he recovered after intensive antiamebic therapy. Central abscesses lying beneath the dome of the liver, as in these two patients, have a tendency to penetrate the diaphragm and involve the thorax with empyema or lung abscess, or even rupture into the pericardium

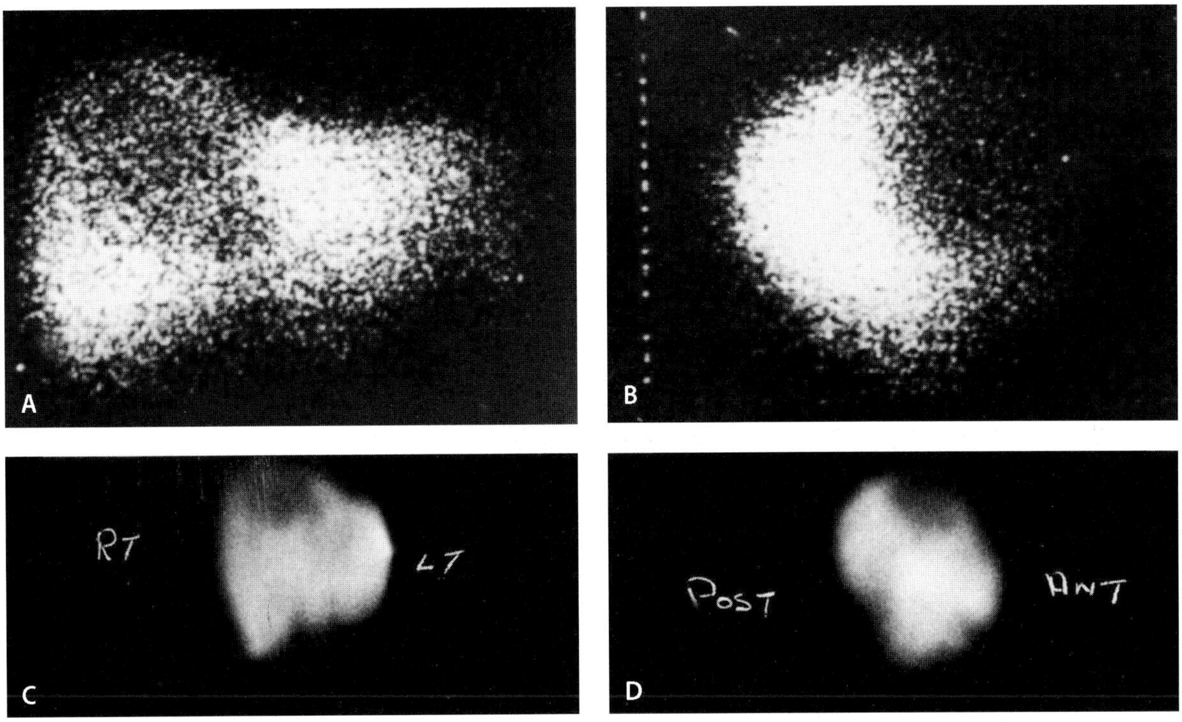

Fig. 1.59 A–D. Gamma camera studies of amebic liver abscesses. **A** Anteroposterior and **B** right lateral views of a huge central abscess in the right lobe of the liver which has extended to the anterior surface and dome with a prominent localized bulge. **C** Anteroposterior and **D** right lateral views of a gamma camera study show multiple amebic abscesses, the largest of which is penetrating through the dome of the right lobe of the liver, causing a prominent bulge there. Other abscesses are present along the anterior and posterior aspects of the inferior surface of the liver, seen best on the lateral view (**D**)

Arteriography

Selective celiac or hepatic arteriography may help demonstrate the location, size, and number of liver abscesses, but this technique is seldom used today. The abscesses displace and stretch the hepatic artery branches and cause one or more avascular filling defects during the capillary phase (Figs. 1.61, 1.62). There is usually a "rim" or blush of increased vascularity around the perimeter of the abscess, depending on the intensity of the inflammatory reaction (Fig. 1.61); a chronic abscess has less hypervascularity and a thinner blush surrounding the lesion. Arteriography is more sensitive than isotope scanning but less sensitive than ultrasound or CT scanning in detecting multiple small abscesses. Venous studies are rarely necessary, but with a large hepatic abscess there may be impaired drainage, compression, or occlusion of the portal or hepatic veins or even the inferior vena cava (Fig. 1.63).

Since the trophozoites are present in the hypervascular perimeter of the abscess, Mexican investigators previously experimented with giving high doses of amebicides (210–320 mg of dehydroemetine in 24–72 hours) by slow constant infusion through a catheter placed selectively in the hepatic artery. Results in gravely ill patients with extensive liver involvement were encouraging.

Pneumoperitoneography

In regions where the more sophisticated diagnostic modalities are unavailable, pneumoperitoneography may occasionally be a useful investigation in suspected cases of liver abscess. Adhesions between liver and diaphragm or the lateral thoracoabdominal wall are frequent, and local irregularity in the liver outline can be clearly demonstrated (Fig. 1.64). About 1000 ml of intraperitoneal gas (nitrous oxide or air) should be used, with the patient erect. Fluoroscopic control is helpful, but not essential.

(Text continues on p. 67)

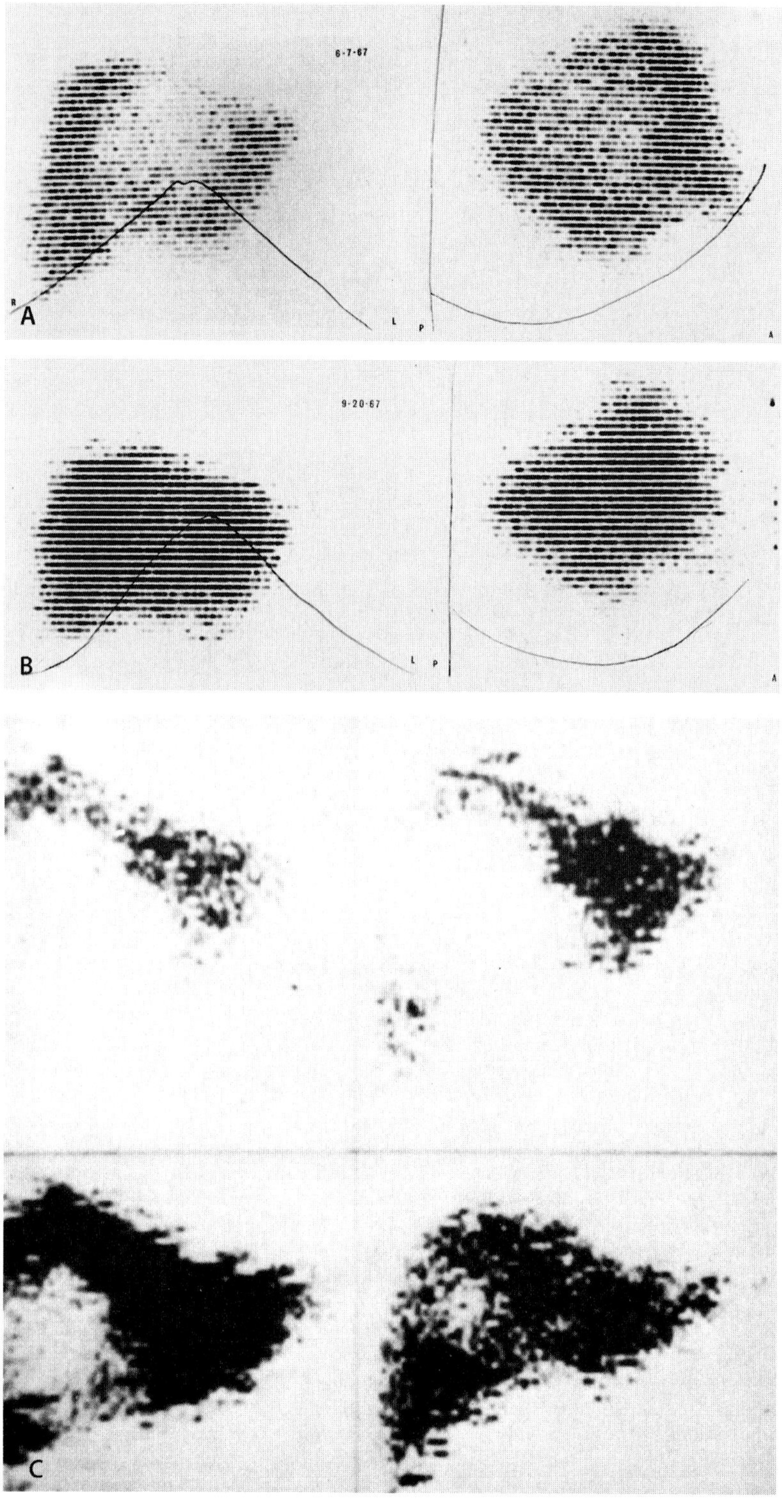

Fig. 1.60 A–C. Use of nuclear scanning to assess the size and number of amebic abscesses and their subsequent response to antiamebic therapy. **A** Anterior and right lateral liver scans, utilizing radioactive gold-198 colloid, demonstrate a large focal defect extending from the right lobe to the left lobe just below the dome of the liver in a young sailor. **B** After appropriate antiamebic therapy, a similar follow-up study 3 1/2 months later shows complete remission of this large amebic abscess and regeneration of normal liver tissue. **C** A series of four nuclear scans (anterior views) show a huge abscess replacing much of the right lobe of the liver with scattered involvement elsewhere in the liver parenchyma on the initial study. Subsequent studies show marked decrease in size of the huge right lobe abscess over a period of several months.

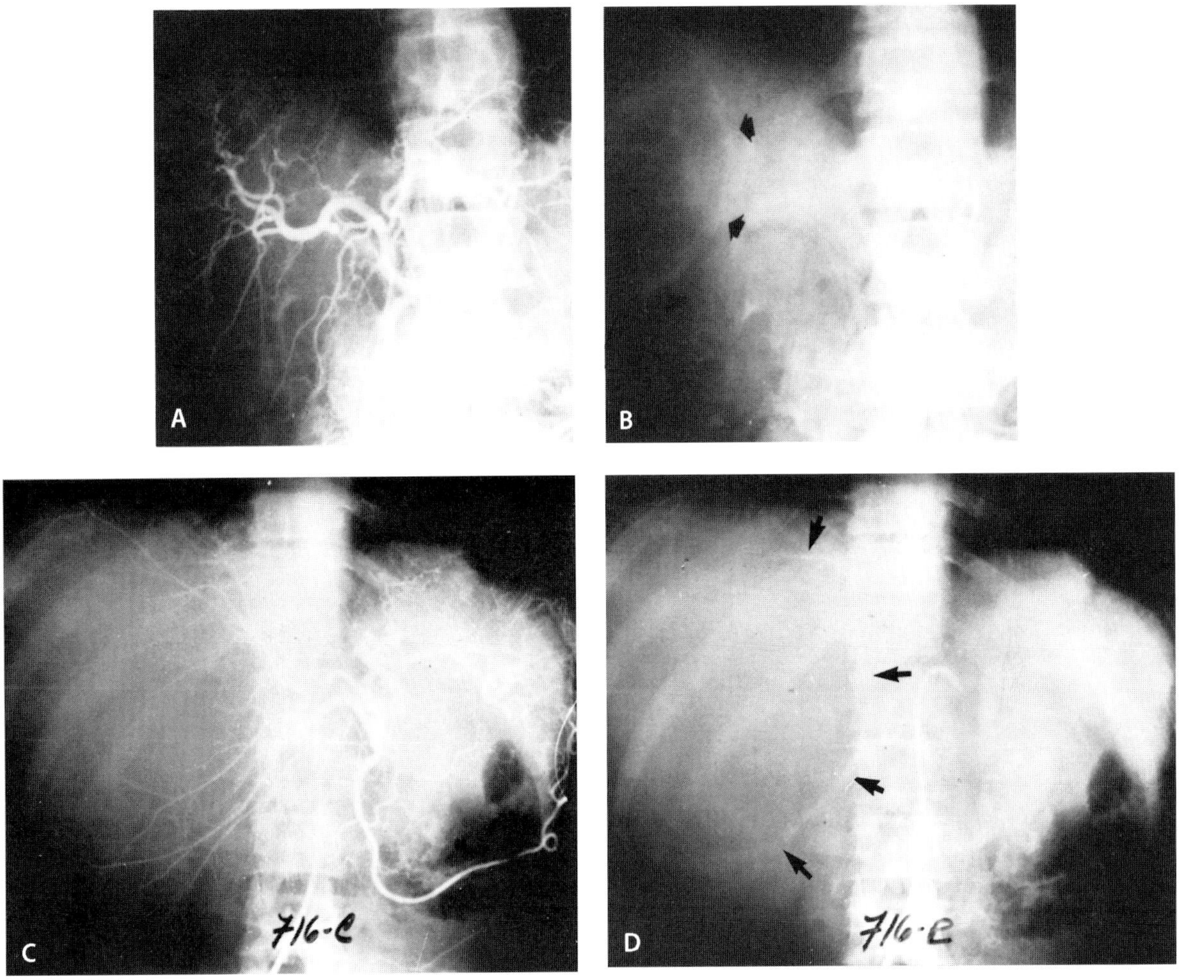

Fig. 1.61 A–D. Selective celiac arteriography in two patients with large amebic abscesses of the right lobe of the liver. **A** Arterial and **B** capillary phases of a celiac arteriogram in an American soldier. In the arterial phase, there is a large avascular area in the lateral aspect of the right lobe with some draping and stretching of peripheral arterial branches around this mass. The capillary phase (**B**) shows a large avascular filling defect and a rim or blush of increased vascularity around the margin of the abscess (*arrows*). This rim sign is caused by the inflammatory reaction and hypervascularity surrounding the abscess; the intensity of the blush depends on the extent and acuteness of the inflammation. **C** There is marked displacement and draping of hepatic artery branches around a huge amebic abscess in the right lobe, as seen on the arterial phase in a Mexican patient. **D** The capillary phase shows a large lucent area occupying much of the right lobe with some uptake of contrast medium in the surrounding compressed and inflamed wall of the abscess (*arrows*); this produces a rim sign around the abscess best seen here along its inferior margin. The only normal hepatogram is in the left lobe of the liver. There is also considerable uptake of contrast medium in the spleen. (**C**, **D** courtesy of Dr. Jorge Ceballos-Labat, Mexico City)

◀ **Fig. 1.60** (*continued*). There is still a small focal cold spot in the right lobe on the final study. Such serial hepatic nuclear scans offer a definitive method of assessing the success of antiamebic therapy in shrinking liver abscesses, although serial ultrasound or CT scans are much preferred in most countries

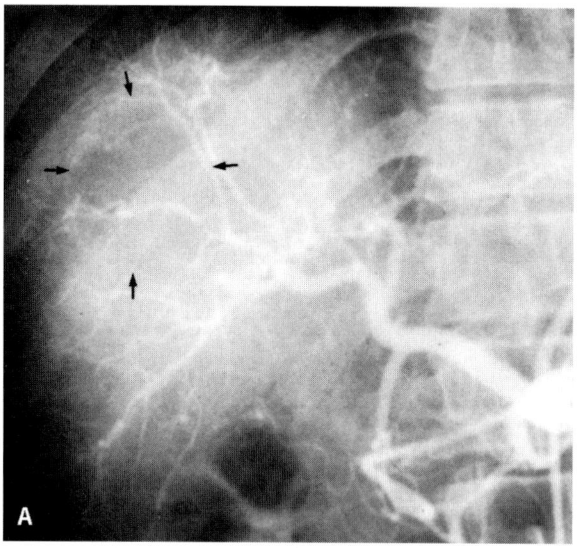

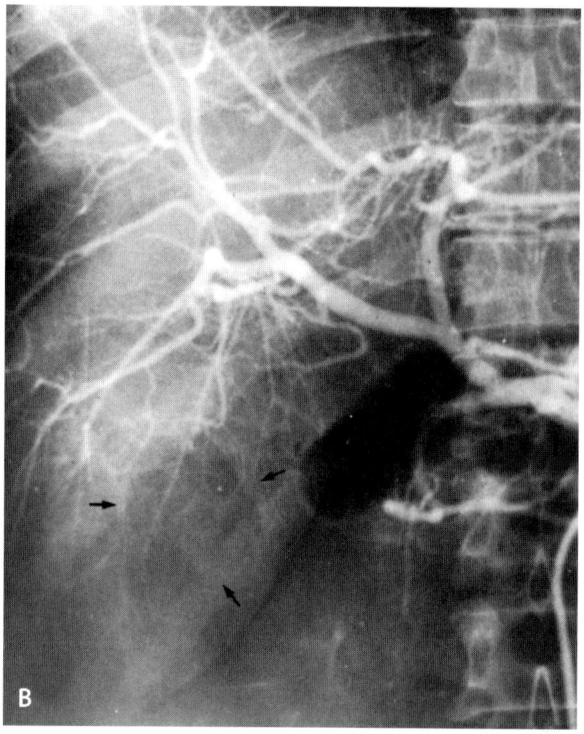

Fig. 1.62 A, B. Hepatic amebic abscesses in two patients showing large negative filling defects in the liver on celiac arteriography. **A** There is a radiolucent filling defect (*arrows*) in the right lobe of the liver with an otherwise normal hepatogram. Several major branches of the right hepatic artery are stretched and draped around this large abscess. **B** An abscess in the lower portion of the right lobe shows a prominent radiolucent filling defect (*arrows*) with surrounding stretched, very peripheral hepatic artery branches

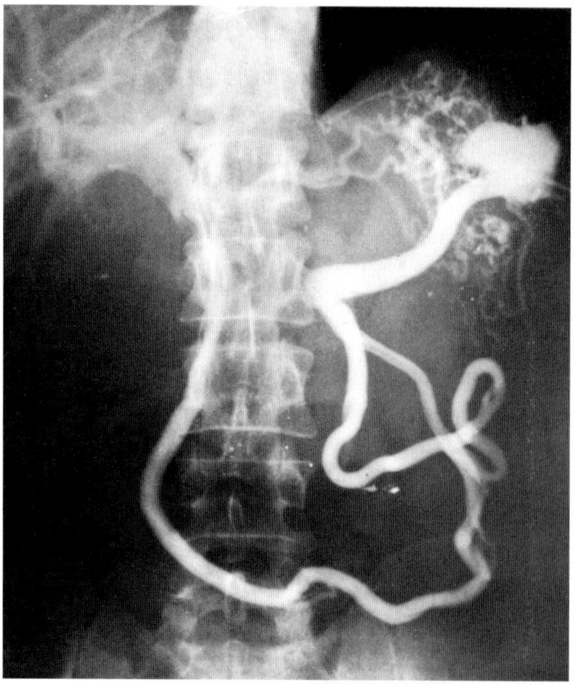

Fig. 1.63. Splenoportogram showing occlusion of the portal vein caused by large amebic abscesses in the right and left lobes of the liver. A collateral circulation has developed primarily via a patent umbilical vein bypassing the obstruction and eventually anastamosing with the splenic vein. This is the same patient as shown in Fig. 1.55 A, B. (Courtesy of Dr. Jorge Ceballos-Labat, Mexico City)

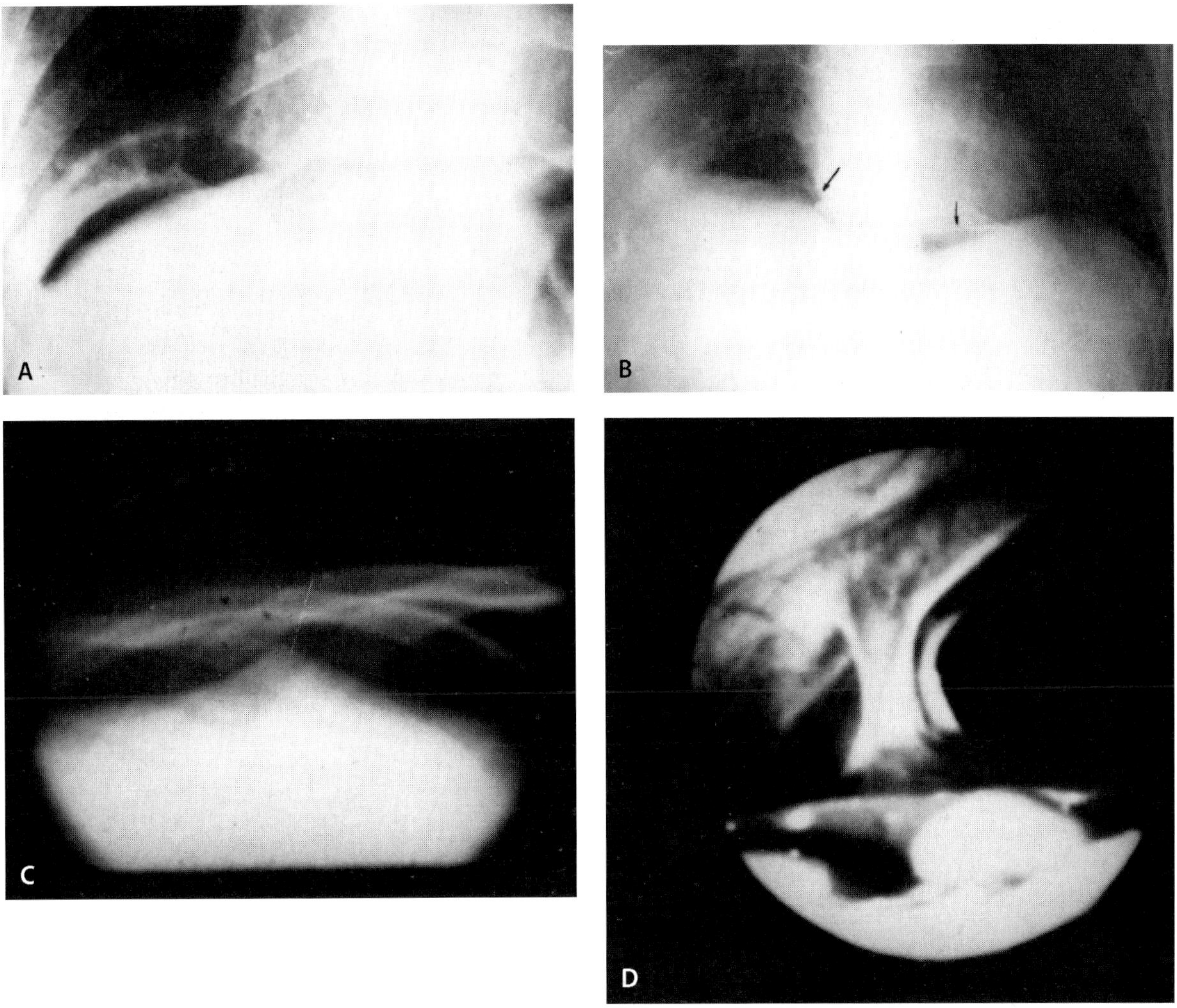

Fig. 1.64 A–D. Pneumoperitoneography in the diagnosis of hepatic amebic abscess, a procedure chiefly of historical interest and performed today only in areas where scanning equipment is unavailable. An abscess frequently causes adhesions between the liver and underside of the diaphragm; a pneumoperitoneum may demonstrate these as well as the outline of the liver when the diagnosis is in doubt. **A** Well-formed adhesions between the liver and the diaphragm suggest old disease rather than present activity in a patient with a diagnostic pneumoperitoneum. Note the lack of significant amebic activity in the adjacent lung and pleura. **B** In another patient, air from a pneumoperitoneum can be seen beneath the diaphragm in the midline over the uninvolved portion of the liver (*arrows*), but the liver is closely adherent to the diaphragm laterally as a result of perforation and adhesions. The amebic liver abscess has perforated into the thorax, causing an empyema at the costophrenic angle and a large abscess in the right lower lung. **C** Coned down view of the lateral thoracoabdominal wall of another patient in the left lateral decubitus position shows tenting of the lateral margin of the right lobe of the liver from a prominent adhesion between it and the thoracoabdominal wall. **D** Peritoneoscopy shows the thick adhesion between the liver (*bottom*) and thoracoabdominal wall (*top*) to good advantage

Direct Injection of Liver Abscess

Also, in areas lacking modern imaging equipment, direct injection of the liver abscess with a sterile suspension of a microfine barium sulfate using 3 ml of barium for each 500 cc of aspirated pus is a useful technique for sequential observation of the abscess (Fig. 1.65). The barium is taken up by the macrophages in the wall of the abscess and thus allows long-term visualization. This technique facilitates localization of the abscess, observation of increase or decrease in size, and early detection of rupture, and may even aid in differential diagnosis. Most abscesses have a round or oval cavity and a smooth outline, but some have irregular margins, probably due to debris within them. There is little risk to this procedure, and the end result is a small amount of barium included within the fibrotic nudule, persisting for many years (Fig. 1.66). It can be mistaken for calcification. Water-soluble contrast materials can be used, but are absorbed and thus not available for subsequent serial review (Figs. 1.67, 1.68).

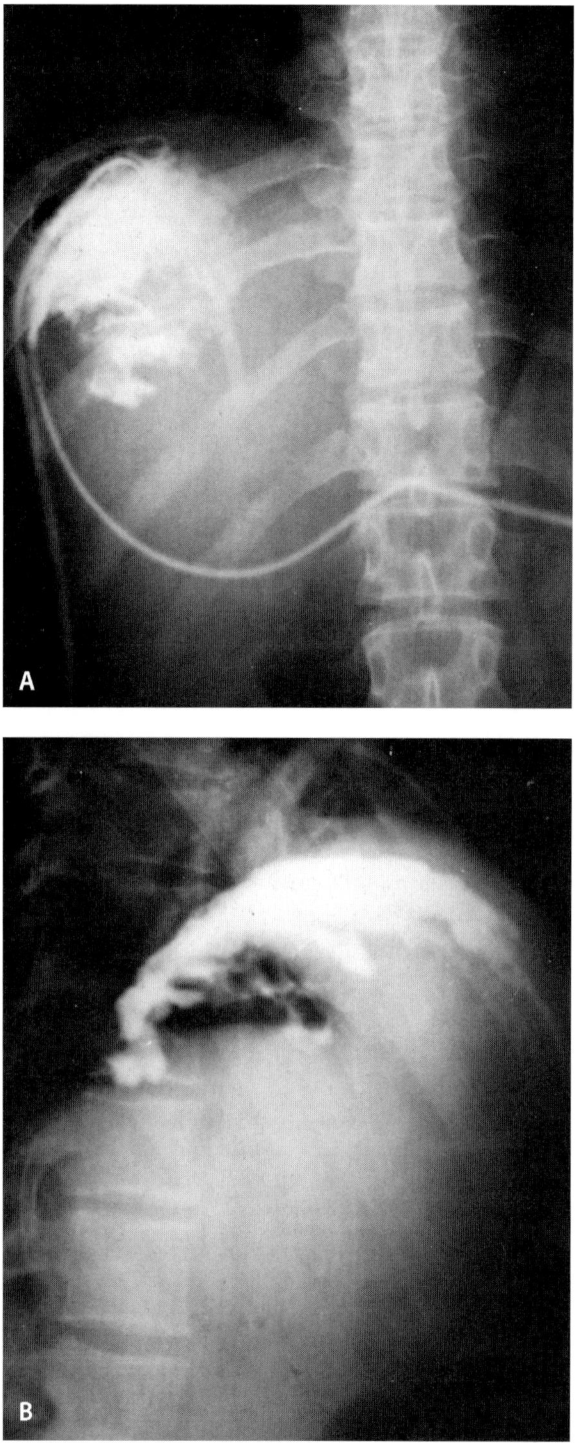

Fig. 1.65 A, B. Direct injection of barium through a drainage tube into a large amebic abscess in the right lobe of the liver. Note the marked elevation of the right hemidiaphragm on anteroposterior (A) and lateral (B) views taken after injection. In the lateral view, the full anteroposterior extent of the abscess can be appreciated as it lies below the thickened, irregular, fixed right hemidiaphragm. Note also in this view the air-containing abscess associated with the prominent localized bulge in the midportion of the raised diaphragm (*top of photo*)

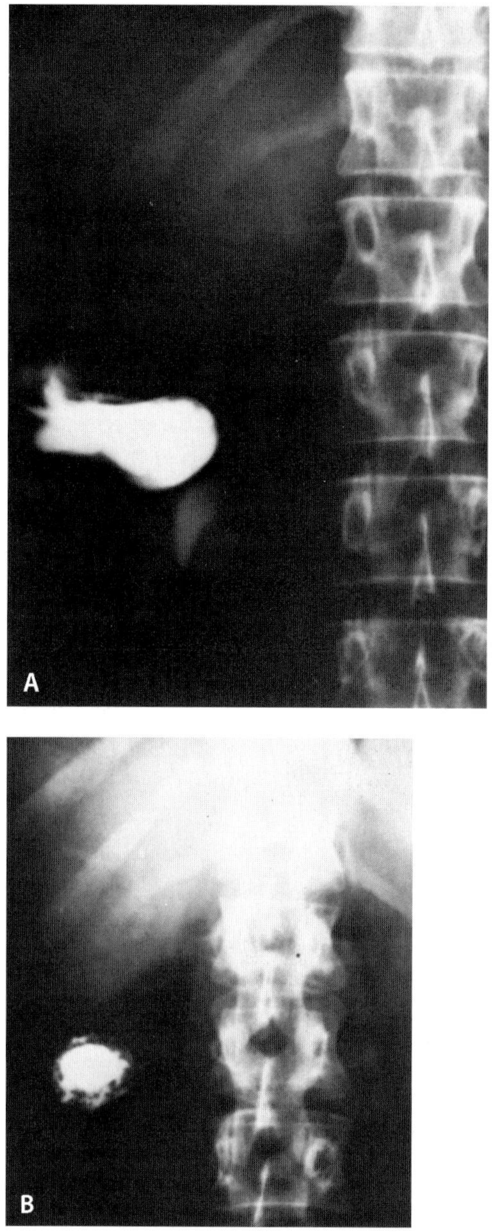

Fig. 1.66 A, B. Sequential evaluation of a hepatic amebic abscess after injection of the abscess cavity with barium. **A** Initial injection with barium after partial drainage shows rather smooth contours of a sizeable abscess in the lower portion of the liver. **B** Follow-up study many weeks later after antiamebic therapy shows over 65% reduction in the size of the abscess. Note that some barium has been engulfed by macrophages in the wall of the abscess, allowing accurate visualization of its size for many months or even years after treatment. Eventually there may remain only a small fibrotic nodule containing barium, which can be mistaken for a liver calcification years later

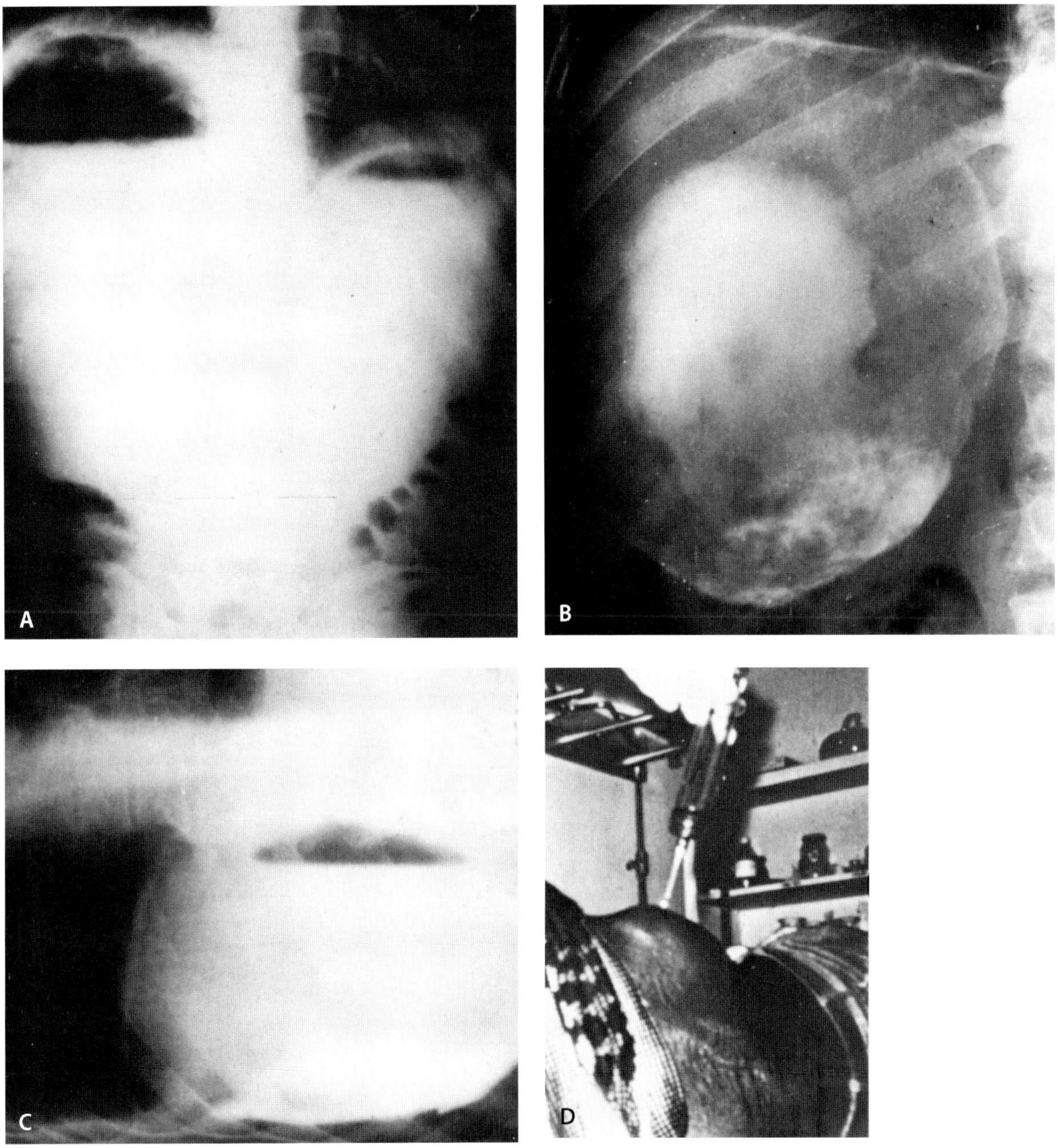

Fig. 1.67 A–D. Large gas-containing amebic abscess with bacterial infection, which has replaced most of the right lobe of the liver in a patient from India. Note the thickened, irregular, elevated right hemidiaphragm and the massive hepatomegaly which extends well across the midline into the left midabdomen. **A** Erect plain film of the abdomen shows a prominent air-fluid level within this huge abscess. There is a fluid level in the stomach as well. **B** Supine view after injection of contrast medium reveals the extent of this enormous abscess. **C** Right lateral decubitus radiograph shows a prominent air-fluid level. The injected contrast medium outlines the inferior and lateral margins of the abscess in this projection. (Courtesy of Dr. A. Chandrahasan Johnson) **D** Needling of a huge, bulging amebic abscess involving the liver and right flank of a different patient. After aspiration of a portion of the abscess contents, either barium or water-soluble, iodinated contrast medium may be injected to outline the cavity, a procedure utilized in some developing countries without access to modern scanning equipment. (Courtesy of E. Pike)

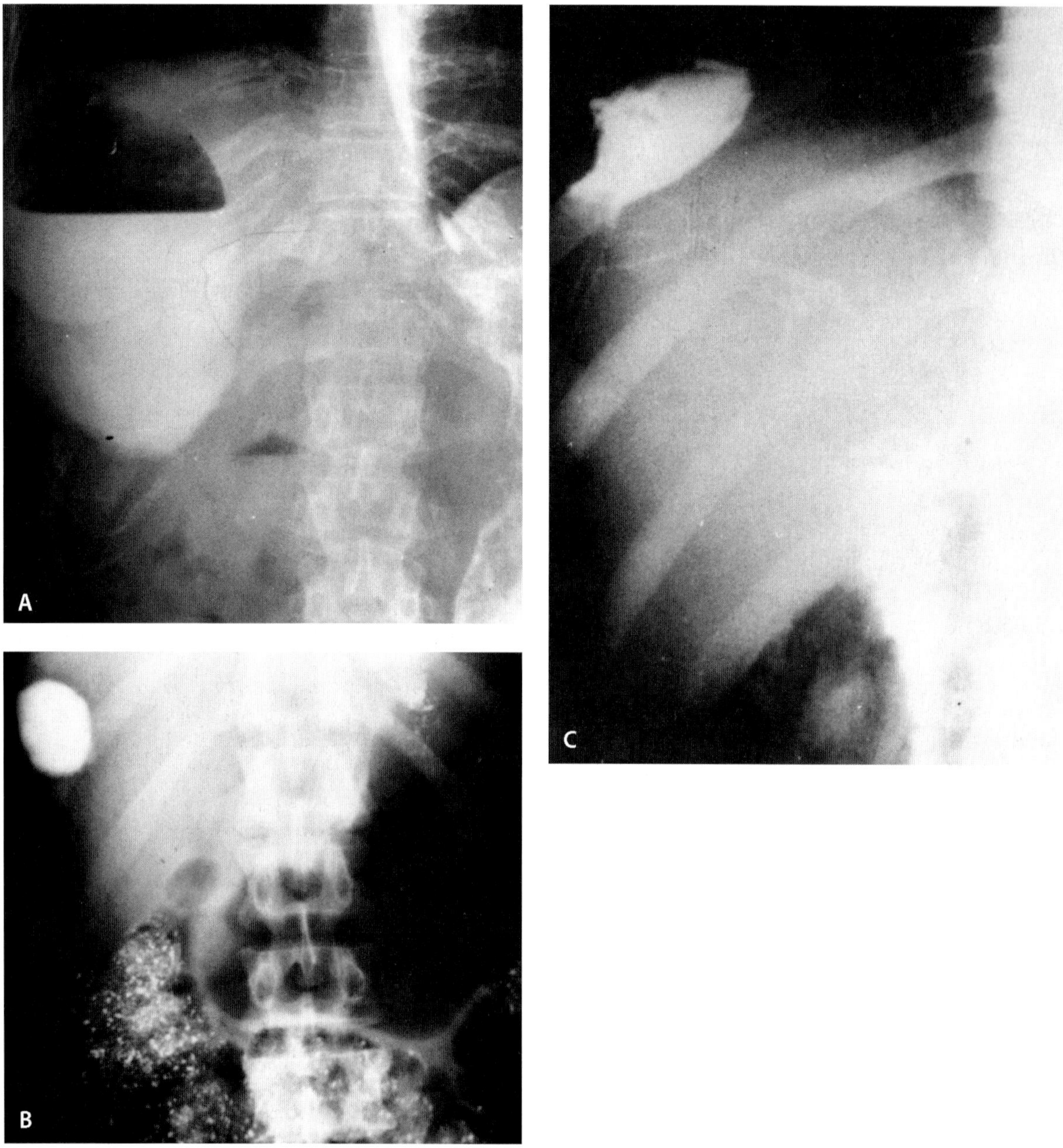

Fig. 1.68 A–C. Injection of amebic hepatic abscesses with water-soluble, iodinated contrast media in three patients. **A** Huge abscess in the right lobe of the liver in a Mexican patient. Note the prominent air-contrast level on erect film of the abdomen as well as the thickened, elevated, partially immobilized right hemidiaphragm. **B** A small abscess in the periphery of the right lobe injected with Hypaque. **C** Abscess involving the dome of the liver. The abscess has ruptured into peripheral bile ducts, outlining part of the biliary tree with contrast media

Current Imaging Techniques

Today, in developed countries where modern imaging techniques are available, amebic liver abscess is almost always evaluated by ultrasonography, CT or, less often, MRI. When there are multiple hepatic lesions of varying size, abscesses may be indistinguishable from metastases, unless it is possible to distinguish the inflammatory zone around them.

Ultrasonography. Ultrasonography is the ideal method for detection of hepatic abscesses, which may be rapidly and accurately localized (Figs. 1.69–1.73). Because this technology is readily accessible, noninvasive, relatively inexpensive, free from irradiation and painless, it should be recommended when an amebic abscess is suspected. The accuracy of ultrasonography in the diagnosis of hepatic abscess is estimated at greater than 90%, surpassing that of nuclear scanning and almost equal to the more complex and expensive CT and MRI. Ultrasonography should therefore be the first examination employed when the patient's clinical condition and chest and/or abdominal radiographs suggest a liver abscess. Sonography will not only show the abscess, but also any subphrenic or pleural effusions. While ultrasound will indicate if there is a pulmonary lesion when it is close to the pleura or diaphragm, a chest radiograph is always indicated to assess the exact extent of lung involvement. Whenever there are intrathoracic changes it is likely that the abscess is close to the diaphragm in the upper part of the liver, but it is essential that multiple planes of the liver are scanned, because more than one abscess may be present. Ultrasonography easily determines the intra- or extrahepatic location of the collection and also serves as a guide for needle puncture and placement of drainage catheters and monitoring until *restitutio ad integrum* can be confirmed (Fig. 1.72).

The ultrasound findings will vary, depending on the stage and evolution of the necrotic mass. Initially the lesion has greater echogenicity than the adjacent hepatic parenchyma when the necrotic center is solid, eventually converting to an echolucent area with posterior acoustic enhancement. The intervening stages show variable levels of internal echogenicity. In 5% of these patients, the solid echogenic central mass may resemble a solid hepatic mass of other etiology.

Not every amebic abscess will show a diagnostic ultrasonic appearance, but certain characteristics may suggest the diagnosis when hepatic abscess is clinically unsuspected.

1. Peripheral location within the liver
2. Predominantly fine low-level echoes at high gain
3. Slight posterior sonic enhancement
4. Well-defined border

A positive ultrasound scan will establish that there is an intrahepatic "tumor or abscess" and locate it accurately, but may not establish the precise diagnosis. A "negative" scan may be erroneous; small abscesses, single or multiple, may be better visualized by CT or MRI. An ultrasound scan may occasionally be falsely negative because, in its earlier stages, an abscess may be isodense with the liver or too tiny to visualize on initial scanning. If there is strong clinical indication of a liver abscess but the sonogram does not show one, it is important that the liver be rescanned after 12 or 24 hours. Alternatively, if the patient's condition warrants it, CT or MRI will probably show the abscess sooner.

In a 1990 report by Ahmed et al. from Cairo, 52 patients with amebic liver abscess underwent ultrasonography. Forty-two percent had an acute illness, usually with high fever, vomiting, sweating, right upper quadrant pain, and leukocytosis. The other 58% had a more chronic illness, usually with a dull ache in the right upper abdomen, weight loss, fatigue, moderate or low-grade fever, and anemia. Hepatomegaly and liver tenderness were present in all patients; fever occurred in 75%. The diagnosis was strongly suggested by amebic antibodies in high titer and hepatic abscesses were demonstrated by ultrasonography. Mean abscess diameter was 9.2 cm; 37% were larger than 10 cm. Most abscesses were solitary (81%), in the right lobe (73%), round or oval (78%), cystic (57%), and had a well-defined wall (53%). However, 43% were initially solid or heterogeneous. The latter lesions always developed a cystic pattern when ultrasonography was repeated. The diagnosis was confirmed by a good clinical response to metronidazole in 50 patients. Complications included right-sided pleural effusions or empyema (13%), ascites (13%), and jaundice (13%). Drainage of large abscesses was performed in four patients. All 52 patients survived and were cured.

Computed Tomography. The excellent contrast resolution of CT is capable of detecting small lesions, some even a few millimeters in diameter. This technique visualizes detailed margins of the lesion and clues in the arterial and venous parenchymal phases that allow differentiation from other pathology, such as a hepatic cyst, hemangioma, or solid neoplasm. *Helical CT* of the liver is now the diagnostic method with the greatest sensitivity, specificity, and anatomical resolution. In early amebic involvement of the liver, CT will show an ill-defined area of decreased attenuation compared with the surrounding normal parenchyma (Fig. 1.74 A). When there is actual abscess formation with central necrosis, the diagnosis

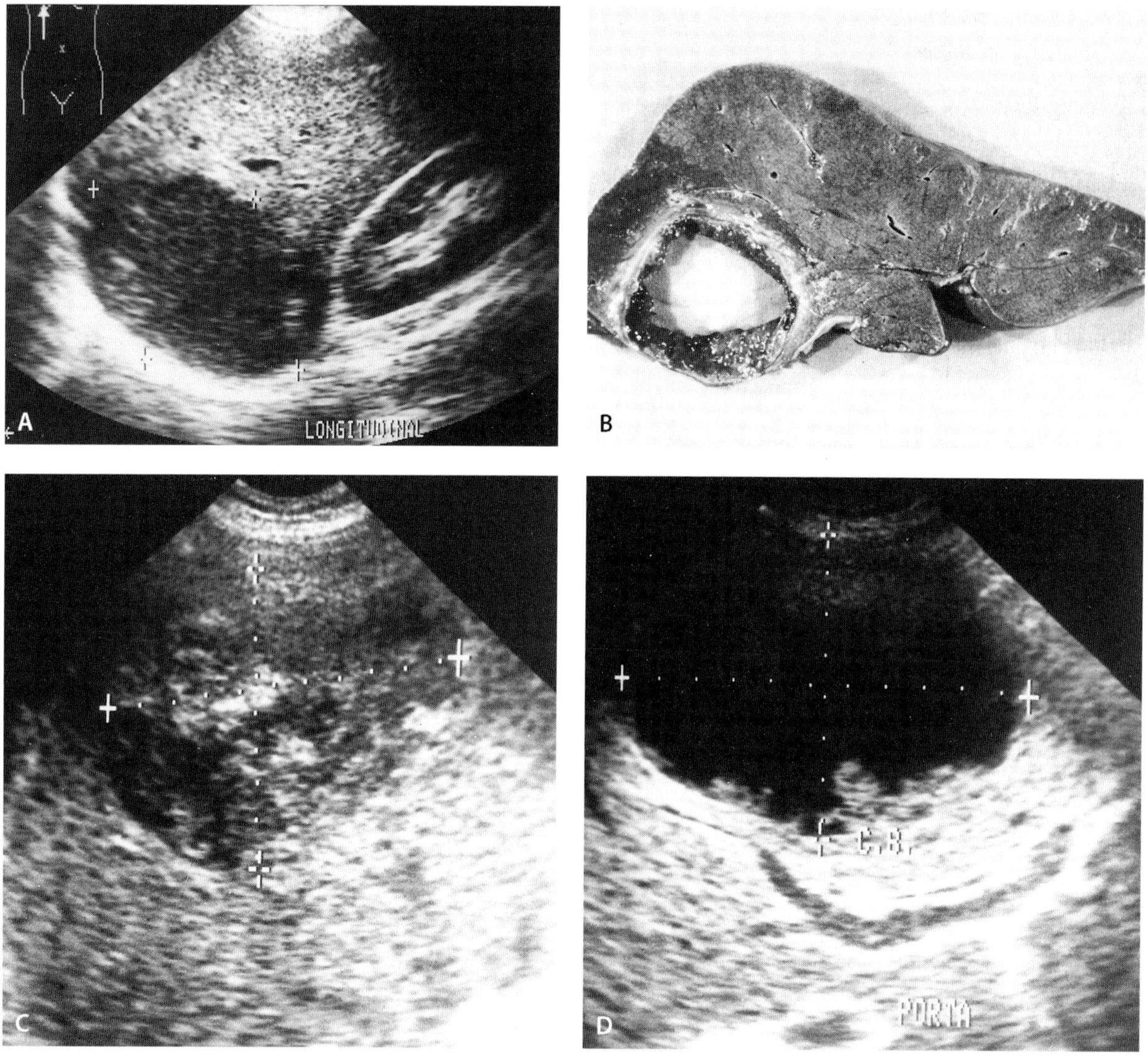

Fig. 1.69 A–D. Ultrasound diagnosis of hepatic amebic abscess in patients from Mexico. **A** Large abscess located posteriorly in the liver with some echogenicity of its contents. **B** Autopsy specimen of a large solitary hepatic amebic abscess. (Courtesy of Drs. M. Tanimoto and J. Aguirre, Mexico City) **C** Ultrasound examination during the acute phase of a hepatic amebic abscess in another Mexican. The necrotic solid component generates heterogeneous echogenicity. **D** Four weeks later, there is liquefaction of the contents with debris in the bottom of the abscess. (**A**, **C**, **D** courtesy of Drs. Kenji Kimura and Miguel Stoopen)

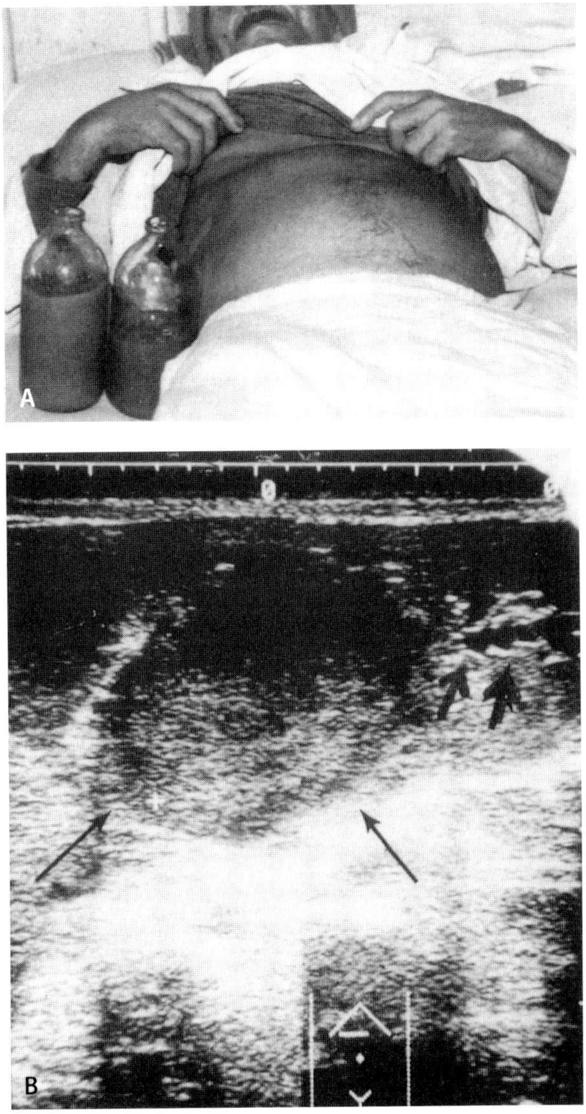

Fig. 1.70. A An Egyptian man with two amebic liver abscesses, a 15-cm cystic abscess in the left lobe and an 8×10 cm abscess in the right lobe causing obstructive jaundice. The bottles contain abscess fluid removed by percutaneous needle aspiration. There is a slight abdominal bulge beneath his index finger. B Ultrasonography of the liver shows the 8×10 cm abscess in the right lobe containing considerable echogenic debris (*small arrows*) and a dilated intrahepatic bile duct (*large arrows*). (Courtesy of Dr. L. Ahmed et al. and *Rev Infect Dis*, 1990)

is more easily established. A hypodense liver mass with attenuation values of 15–30 HU, which is avascular with well-defined margins and alternating hyper- and hypovascular peripheral halos following contrast media enhancement, can be demonstrated (Figs. 1.74–1.77); the central portion of the abscess shows no such enhancement. The abscess can be single or multiple and will usually produce a right pleural effusion and a small amount of perihepatic fluid; other abscesses may be present in the peritoneal cavity (Fig. 1.76), mesentery, spleen, or other abdominal organs. The extent of the disease and its response to therapy can be accurately assessed by follow-up CT scanning (Fig. 1.77).

(Text continues on p. 80)

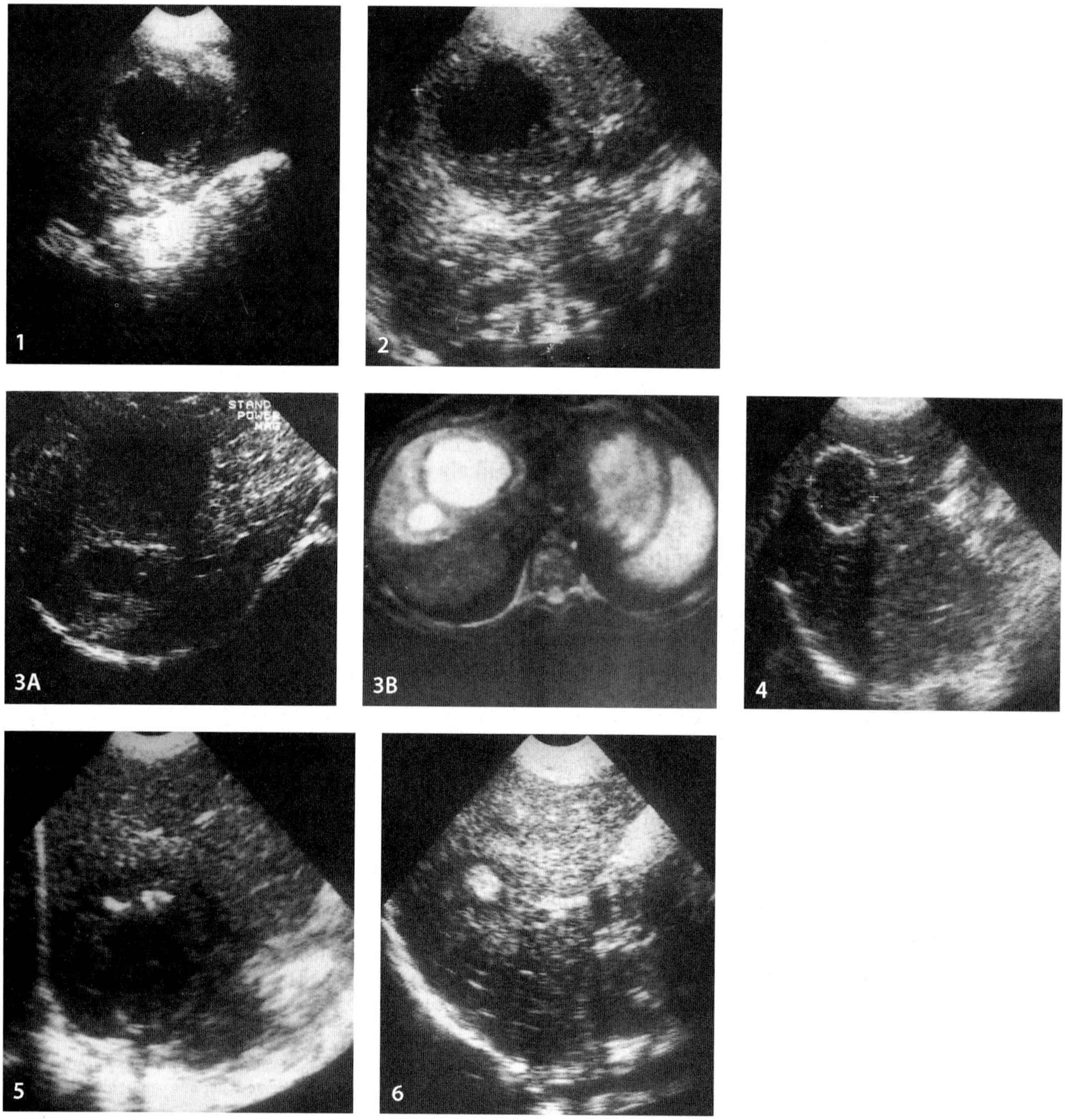

Fig. 1.71. Ultrasonographic findings in amebic liver abscesses in multiple patients from South Africa. **1** Sagittal scan showing large round lesion with central liquification and "halo" sign. **2** Transverse scan showing round lesion with central liquification and peripheral halo. **3A** Transverse scan showing two round well-defined hypoechoic lesions adjacent to one another. **3B** MRI of same patient shows the two lesions with high signal of the abscess contents and low signal of the abscess walls (halo sign) on T2-weighted image (TR1700, TE 100). **4** Sagittal scan showing a healing amebic abscess. An echogenic rim has developed around the residual lesion during the 18 months since initiation of antiamebic therapy. **5** Sagittal scan showing another healing abscess; echogenic deposits have developed at the lesion's periphery. **6** Sagittal scan of a healing amebic abscess; a small echogenic lesion developed from a previously hypoechoic abscess. (Courtesy of Dr. L. Oleszczuk-Raszke et al. and *Pediatr Radiol*, 1989)

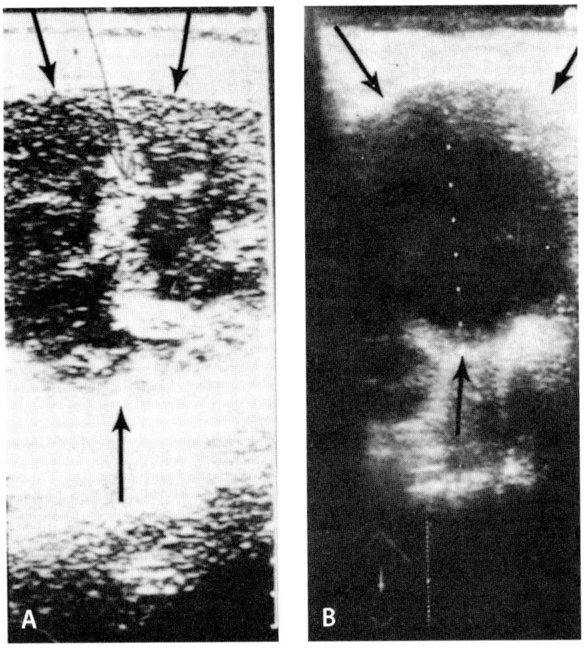

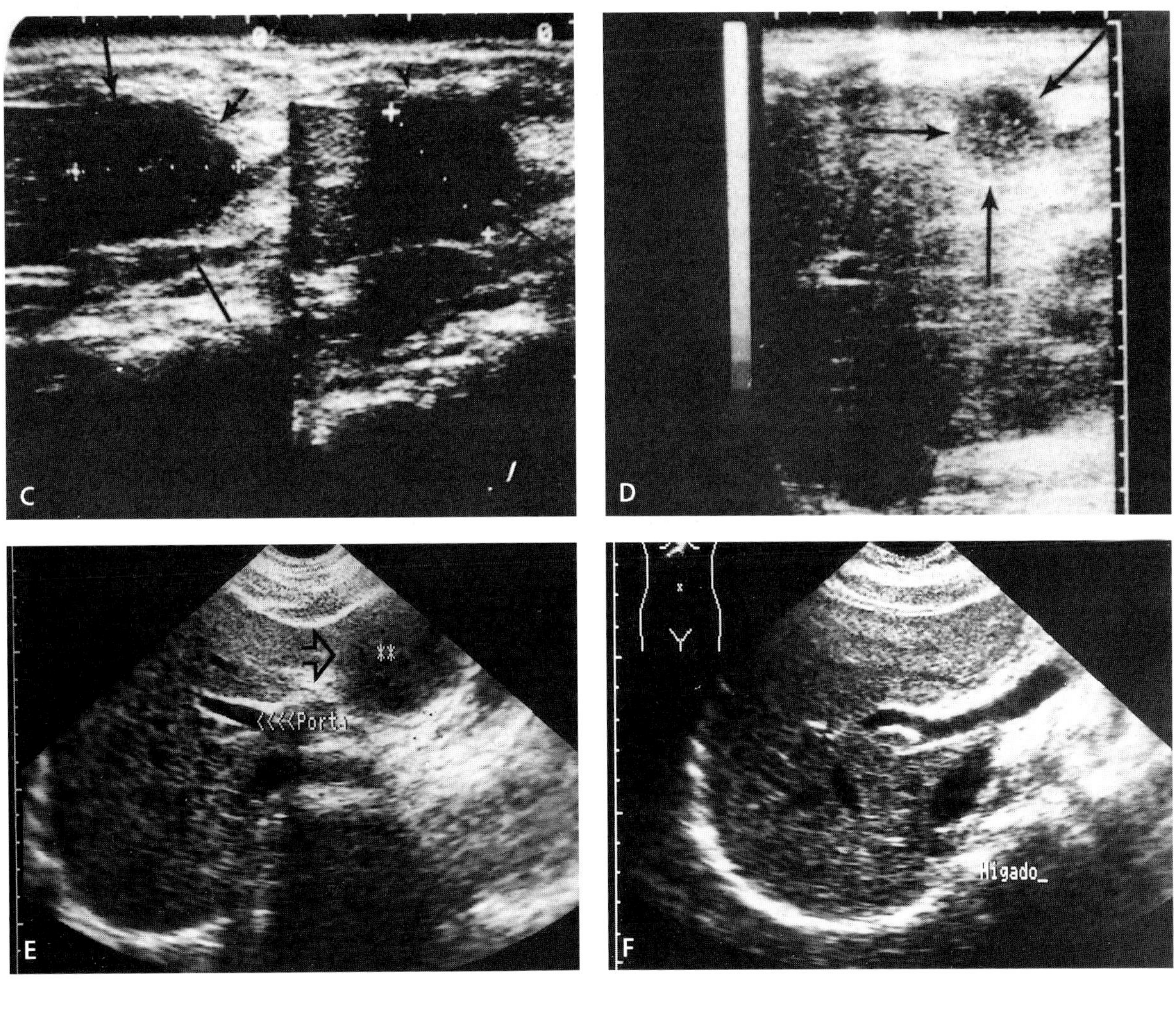

Fig. 1.72 A–F. Ultrasonographic resolution of hepatic amebic abscesses in three different patients. **A** Initial sonogram shows an 8-cm focal lesion (*arrows*) with a heterogeneous echo pattern in an Egyptian patient. **B** A follow-up scan 3 months later shows a well-defined abscess cavity (*arrows*) with liquification. **C** Hepatic sonogram in another Egyptian reveals a 5-cm amebic liver abscess (*arrows*) which underwent rapid resolution over a 2-week period with antiamebic therapy. **D** The abscess is much smaller (*arrows*) and shows increased echogenicity of its contents. A follow-up scan 4 months later showed complete resolution of the abscess. (**A–D** courtesy of Dr. L. Ahmed et al. and *Am J Trop Med Hyg*, 1989) **E** *Restitutio ad integrum* of a left lobe hepatic amebic abscess (*arrow*) in a Mexican patient, showing return to normal (**F**) following several weeks of medical treatment. (**E, F** courtesy of Drs. Kenji Kimura and Miguel Stoopen)

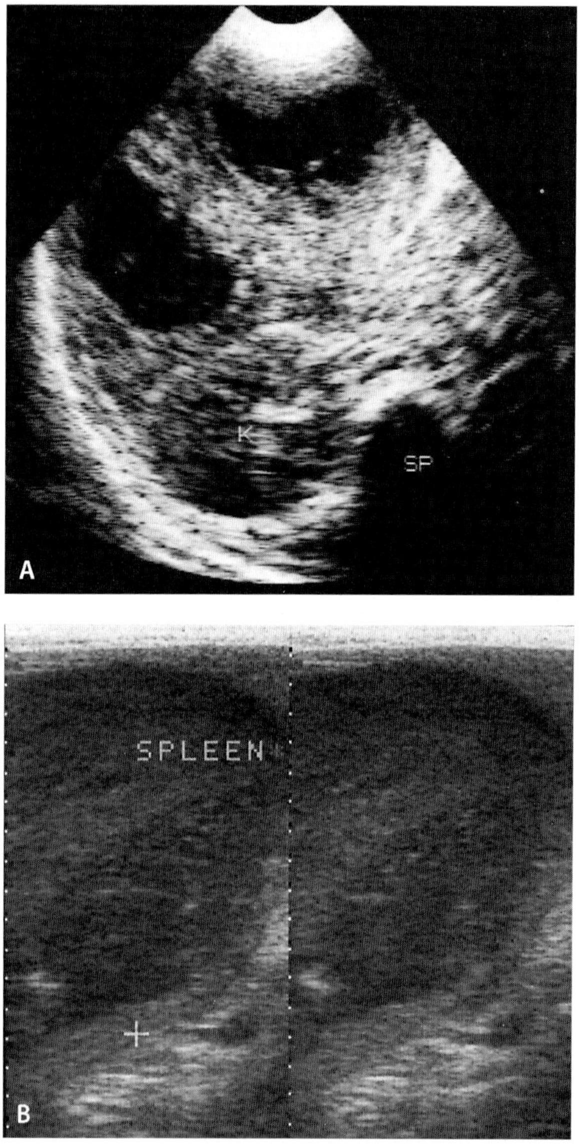

Fig. 1.73 A, B. Ultrasound studies of amebic abscesses of the liver and spleen in two South African patients. **A** Transverse scan of the liver showing two abscesses with irregular walls and "anchovy sauce" pus causing internal heterogeneous fluid/debris echoes. *K* Kidney; *SP* spine. **B** Large amebic abscess of the spleen in a second South African with heterogeneous internal echoes within the lesion. (Courtesy of Dr. Brian J. Cremin, Capetown)

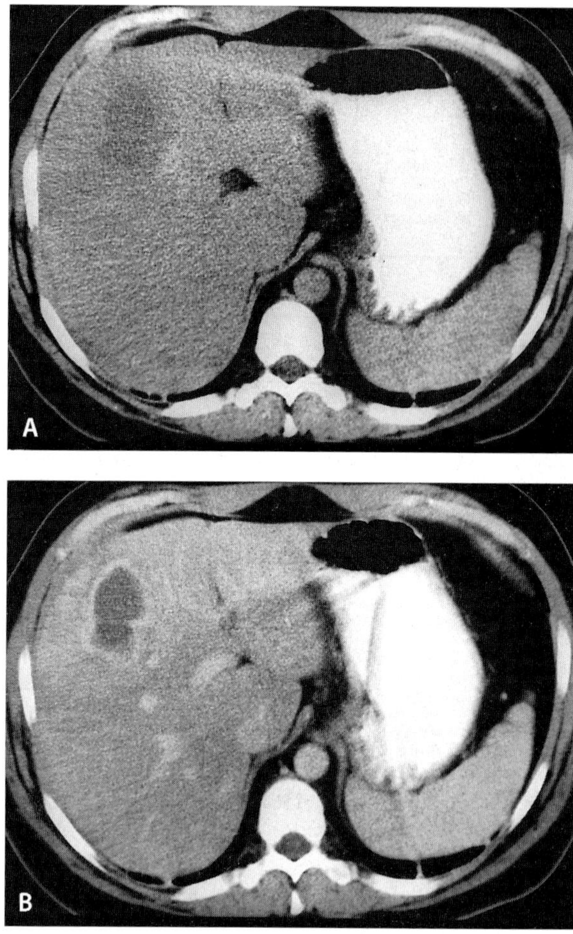

Fig. 1.74. **A** Unenhanced CT image of a right hepatic amebic abscess demonstrates a poorly defined low-density lesion with vague, irregular margins in a Mexican patient. **B** Contrast-enhanced CT image shows the abscess much better with a thick halo of hypervascular tissue in its wall. (Courtesy of Drs. Kenji Kimura and Miguel Stoopen)

Fig. 1.75 A–F. CT features of hepatic amebic abscess in six different patients, the first four (**A–D**) from Mexico. **A** Giant right hepatic abscess. **B** Giant left hepatic abscess with an irregular lobulated margin. The high density of its contents is caused by intracavitary bleeding from a prior diagnostic needle puncture. **C** Posterior hepatic abscess. Note the hypervascular halo immediately adjacent to the abscess cavity and a second hypodense halo corresponding to surrounding edema. **D** Hyperdense and hypodense halos surround another amebic abscess cavity. (**A–D** courtesy of Drs. Kenji Kimura and Miguel Stoopen) **E, F** Two other patients with large right lobe abscesses showing peripheral halos. The patient shown in **E** is from Kenya ▶

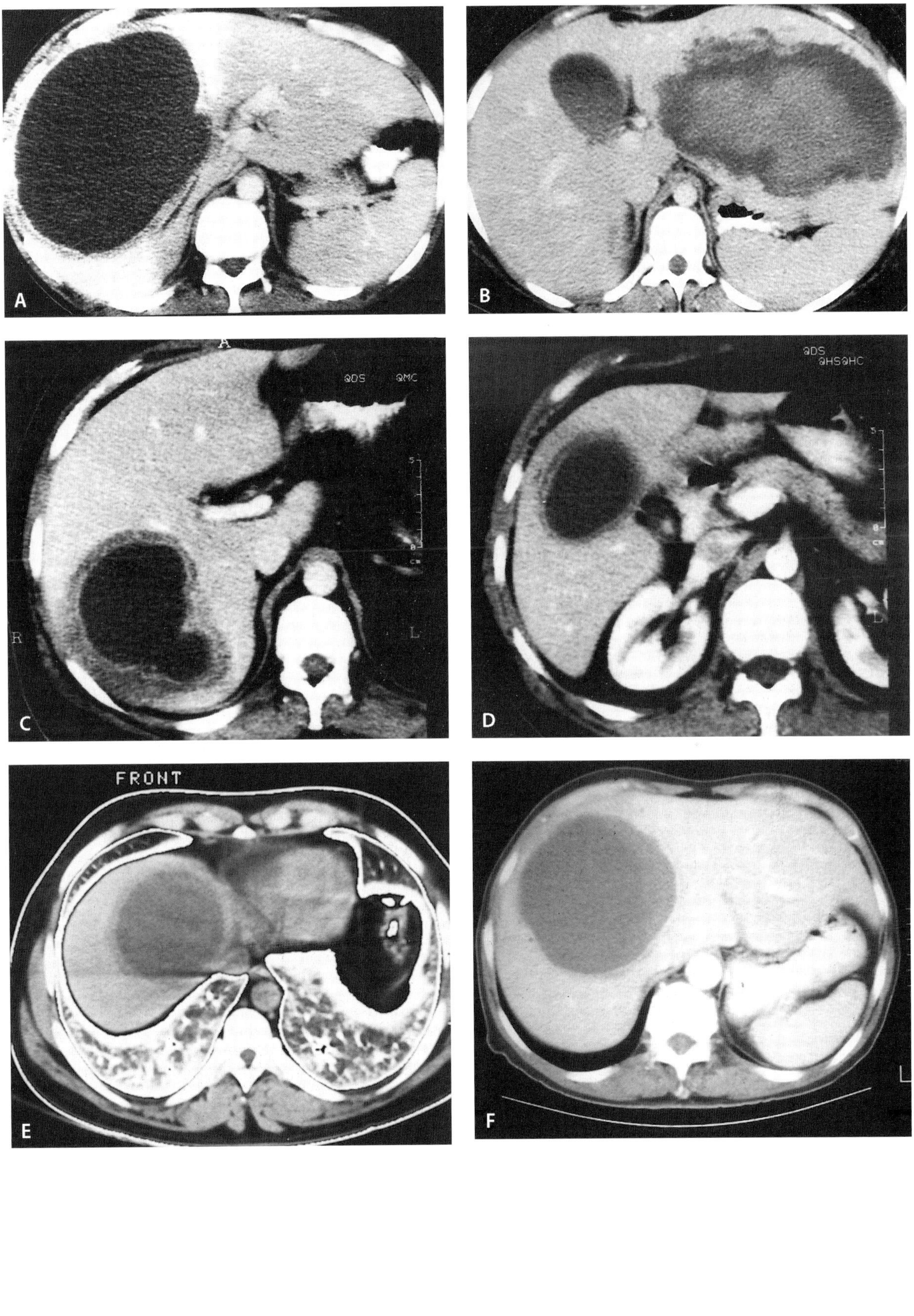
A
B
R
L
C
D
FRONT
E
F

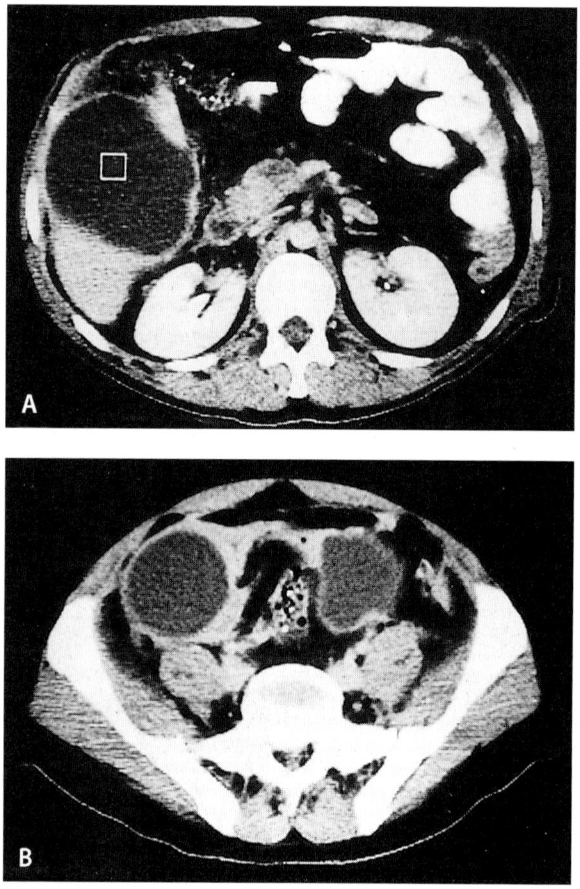

Fig. 1.76 A, B. Large amebic abscess in right lobe of liver (**A**) with two large abscesses in the peritoneal cavity (**B**) in the same patient

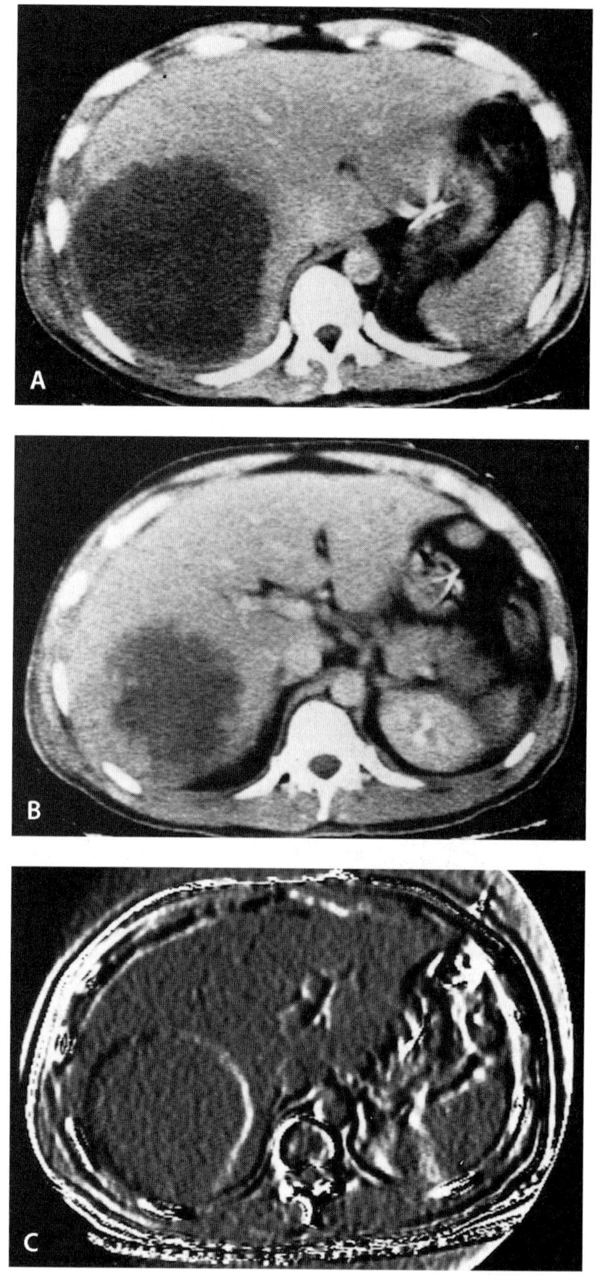

Fig. 1.77 A–C. CT scans obtained on a 16-year-old Sri Lankan man admitted to hospital in California. **A** Initial scan shows a huge low-density lesion in the right lobe of the liver, confirmed on further workup to be an amebic abscess. **B** After only 1 week of antiamebic therapy the abscess is significantly smaller with increasingly irregular borders and necrotic debris. **C** A filtered reconstructed negative image obtained at the same time shows the peripheral halo around the abscess to good advantage. (Courtesy of University of California Davis Medical Center)

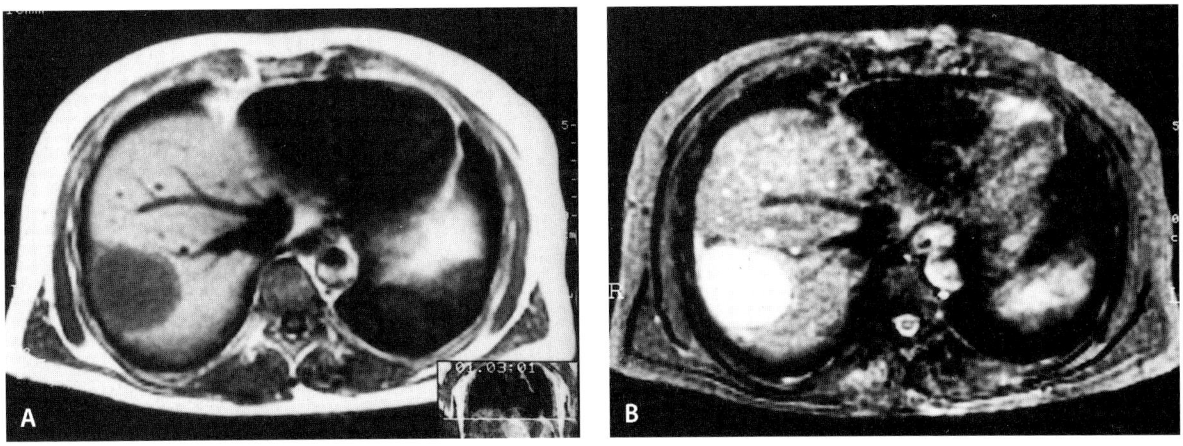

Fig. 1.78 A, B. MRI of hepatic amebic abscess. **A** T1-weighted image demonstrates hypointense contents and faint peripheral halos. **B** T2-weighted image shows high intensity of the contents and better outline of the surrounding halos

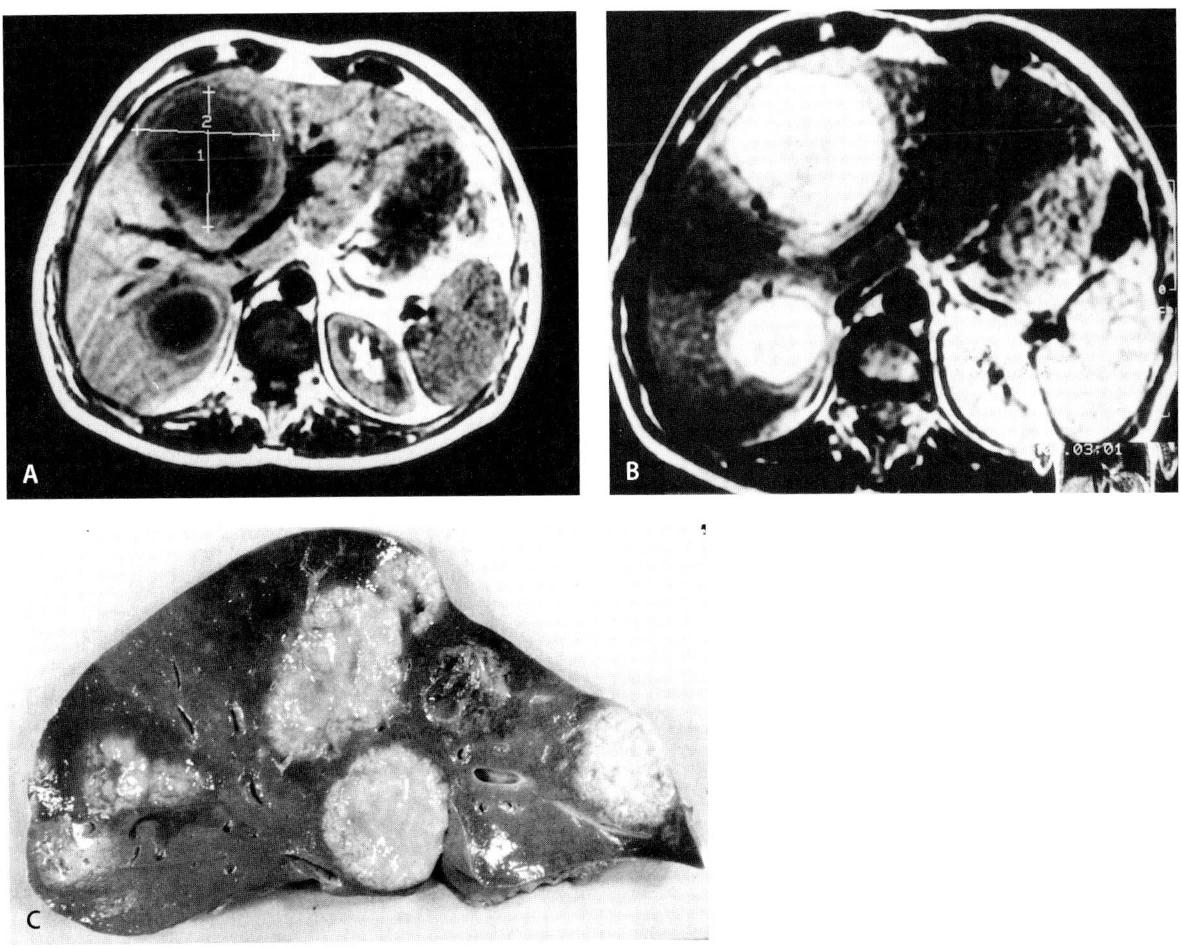

Fig. 1.79 A–C. MRI of multiple hepatic amebic abscesses in a Mexican patient. **A** T1-weighted image shows hypointense abscess contents and alternating peripheral halos around two right lobe abscesses. **B** T2-weighted image demonstrates hyperintensity in the abscess centers with some heterogenicity and alternating peripheral rings. (**A, B** courtesy of Drs. Kenji Kimura and Miguel Stoopen) **C** Autopsy specimen of the liver from another Mexican with multiple hepatic amebic abscesses. (Courtesy of Drs. M. Tanimoto and J. Aguirre, Mexico City)

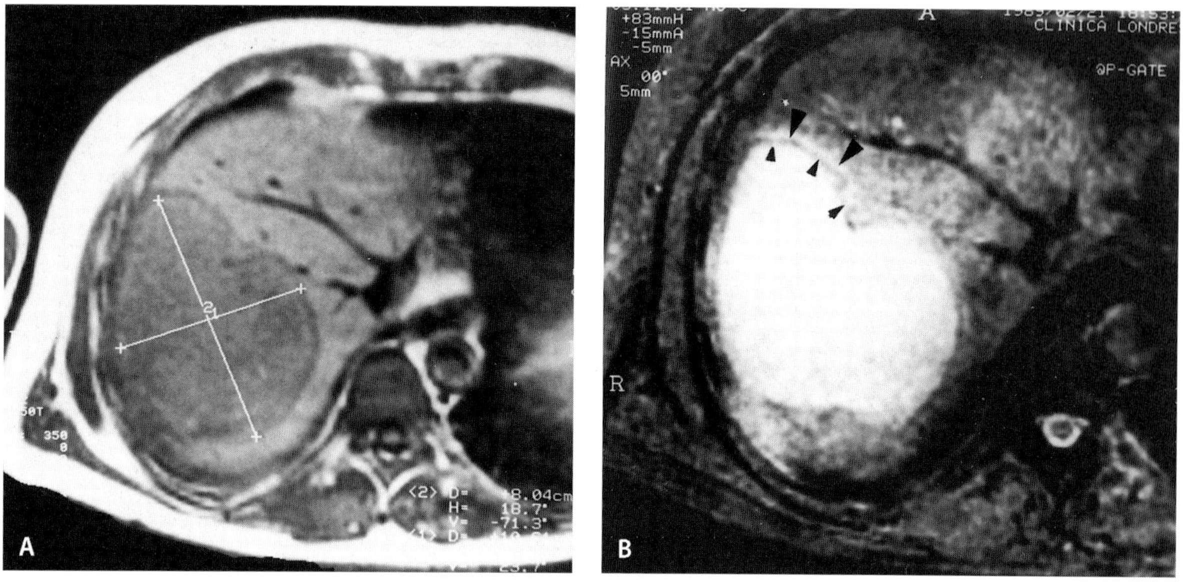

Fig. 1.80 A, B. MRI of giant hepatic amebic abscess in a Mexican patient. **A** T1-weighted image shows a peripheral ring of low intensity surrounding the 18-cm hypointense abscess. **B** T2-weighted image shows heterogeneous hyperintensity centrally and two well-defined low- and high-intensity peripheral rings (*arrowheads*). (Courtesy of Drs. Kenji Kimura and Miguel Stoopen)

Magnetic Resonance Imaging. Today, MRI of the liver is considered the most sensitive method for detection and characterization of focal hepatic lesions. MRI also provides a noninvasive type of imaging that can be an excellent monitoring guide during the evolution and regression of a hepatic abscess. In the initial stages, the hepatic abscess cavity is filled with thick necrotic material with small areas of cavitation. At this stage, MRI discloses, on a T1-weighted image, a homogeneous hypointense signal with clearly defined margins. On the T2-weighted image, the hypointense center becomes hyperintense, and heterogeneous in some, depending on the fluidity and debris of the necrotic exudate (Figs. 1.78–1.81).

During the evolution of the amebic abscess there may be signal variation and heterogenicity, generated by the changing contents of the cavity. In some cases, hemorrhage within the abscess may at times be responsible for its hyperintensity. The peripheral abscess wall and interface with the adjacent liver tissue may show an annular hypo- or hyperintense ring (Figs. 1.78–1.80).

The hypointensity of the ring on the T1-weighted image and its hyperintensity on the T2-weighted image probably correspond to the hypervascular area where vasculitis and thrombosis exist. This is the same phenomenon reported on isotope liver scanning, as well as in selective hepatic angiography, and represents the hyperperfused ring on the periphery of the abscess demonstrated by enhanced CT scanning. The above-described findings are not pathognomonic, as they can be seen in bacterial liver abscesses, hematomas, and necrotic neoplasms. Multiplanar demonstration of the abscess's relationship to the diaphragm, pericardium, and other vital neighboring structures can be readily demonstrated by MRI.

Fig. 1.81 A–F. MRI of large hepatic amebic abscess in a Brazilian patient. **A** T1- and **B** T2-weighted images show a huge right lobe lesion with low signal intensity on T1 and high signal of the abscess contents on T2. **C, D** T1- and T2-weighted images at a lower level in the liver on the same day. **E, F** Eight days later, after treatment with antiamebic drugs, chiefly Flagyl, and percutaneous catheter drainage, the abscess is markedly smaller and there is now largely localized edema remaining, which is dark or low signal intensity on T1 and bright or high signal intensity on T2. Compare these images with those taken 8 days earlier at the same level in the liver (**A, B**). (Courtesy of Dr. Felippe Mattoso) ▶

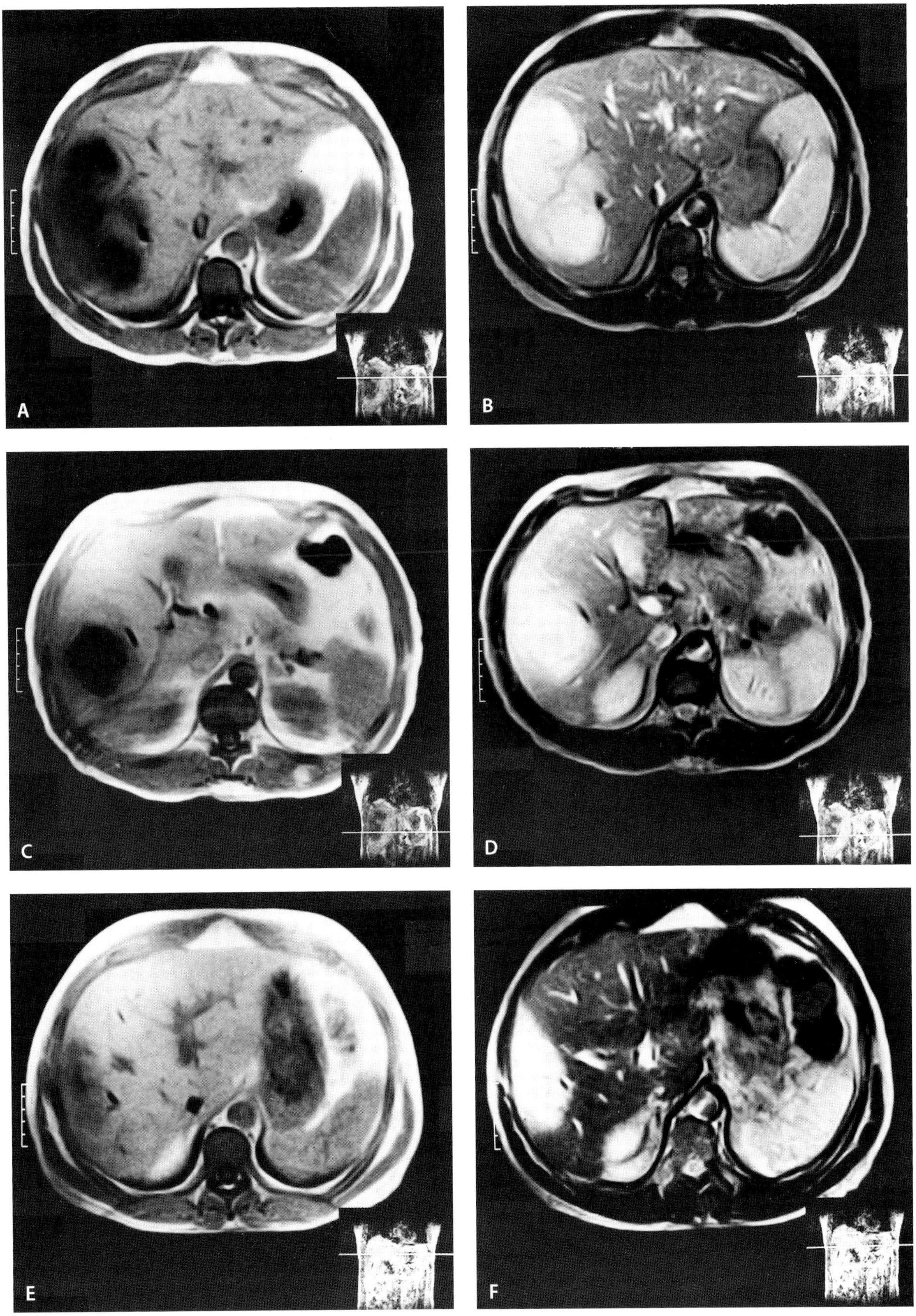
A
B
C
D
E
F

Complications

The complications of amebic abscess in the *right lobe* of the liver include rupture into the right subphrenic space, the pleural cavity, the lung, or through the lung into the bronchial tree (Fig. 1.82). Rupture into the peritoneal cavity may cause generalized peritonitis or localized abscess formation. Less commonly, the abscess may rupture into the bile ducts, duodenum, or colon and it has been known for the rupture to travel along the falciform ligament (Figs. 1.83–1.85 A). An abscess in the *left lobe* of the liver may rupture into the stomach (Fig. 1.85 B), peritoneum, retroperitoneal space, pleura, pericardium (see Fig. 1.101), lung or mediastinum.

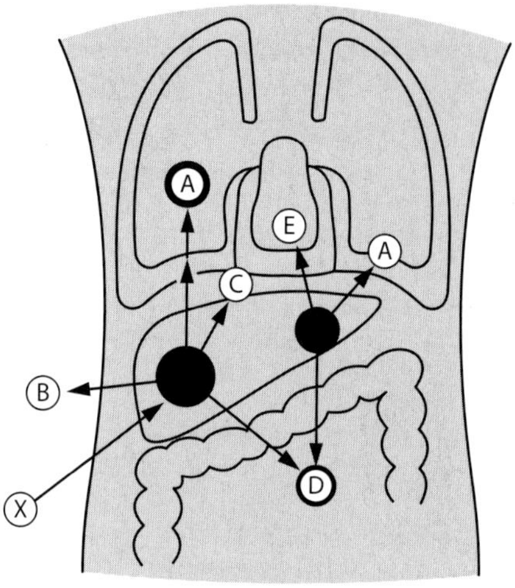

Fig. 1.82. The many directions in which an amebic liver abscess may rupture. The relative frequency of rupture is indicated by the thickness of the circles. *A* Rupture of an abscess in either the right or left lobe into the adjacent hemithorax with spread to the pleura and lung. *B* Penetration of a right lobe abscess to the surface with involvement of the chest or abdominal wall and rupture through the skin to cause amebiasis cutis. *C* Involvement of the subphrenic space as a localized abscess is rare since infiltration superiorly causes adherence to the diaphragm with subsequent penetration into the thorax. *D* Rupture of abscess of either lobe into the peritoneum, colon, or other adjacent viscera. From the right lobe, this may involve the hepatic flexure or duodenum, and, from the left lobe, the stomach or transverse colon. *E* Dangerous, often fatal, rupture of an abscess, usually from the left lobe, into the pericardial sac. *X* Introduction of external infection by aspiration. (From W.W. Davey: *Companion to surgery in Africa,* Edinburgh, E&S Livingstone, 1968; modified from Prof. D.S. Chapman, Durban)

Treatment

Prior to the introduction of metronidazole in the 1970s, the treatment of hepatic abscess required surgical drainage or aspiration, which was accompanied by a 25% mortality. Currently, conservative medical treatment has shown a favorable response in over 90% of patients and has reduced the mortality to 4%. The role of percutaneous catheter drainage is reserved for patients who do not respond to pharmacological treatment. Surgery is now indicated only for complicated abscesses or prevention of potential complications from strategically located large abscesses beneath the pericardial sac. Percutaneous catheter drainage can be beneficial by shortening the time of resolution and restitution of the liver parenchyma.

The sequence of events that highlight *restitutio ad integrum* under medical management generally takes between 5 and 23 weeks; isolated cases have persisted for longer than a year. A residual cyst at the site of a former hepatic abscess is a rare occurrence. Likewise, longstanding inactive amebic abscesses can rarely be manifest as solitary or multiple round calcifications in the liver (Fig. 1.86).

Intrathoracic Amebiasis

Thoracic amebiasis is nearly always secondary to hepatic abscess rupture across the diaphragm into three different thoracic compartments giving origin to (**a**) pleuropulmonary, (**b**) pericardial, and (**c**) mediastinal amebiasis. The high incidence of right hepatic lobe disease, particularly involving the bare area of the liver, shows a parallel high incidence of right pleuropulmonary disease. A left-sided abscess may rupture into the pericardium, while mediastinal amebiasis may occur from rupture of a subphrenic amebic abscess or pulmonary abscess, or both. The earliest radiological evidence of a hepatic abscess is restriction of movement and focal elevation of the diaphragm (Figs. 1.87–1.90), which occurs in 59% of patients with a range of 30–86%. Part or all of the affected hemidiaphragm may remain elevated for some months before any clinical features are noted. Next, a small pleural effusion may develop; a raised hemidiaphragm should suggest the need for an ultrasound scan, which will show not only the fluid but also the movement of the diaphragm, as well as the state of the liver. If sonography is unavailable, a lateral decubitus chest radiograph should be obtained to see if there is fluid present (Fig. 1.89 D), and fluoroscopy to assess diaphragmatic movement. The differential diagnosis includes phrenic nerve paralysis, subphrenic abscess, acute cholecystitis, and hepatic neoplasm.

(Text continues on p. 87)

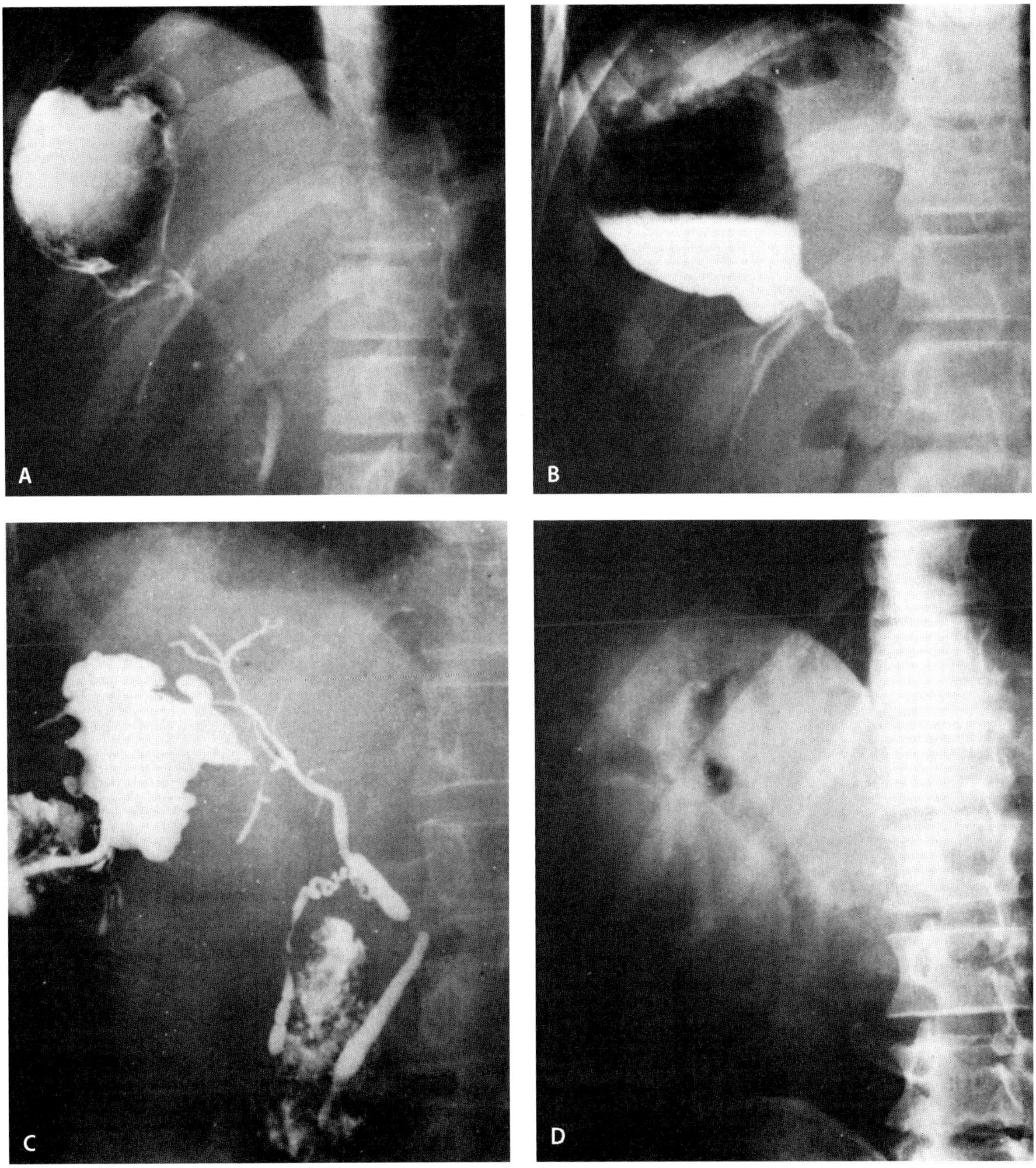

Fig. 1.83 A–D. Rupture of amebic liver abscesses into the bile ducts in three patients. **A** Supine and **B** erect views of the right upper quadrant reveal a large abscess in the right lobe of the liver after injection with Hypaque and air to outline its extent. Note communication of the abscess with the biliary tree, its ragged superior contour, and elevation of the right hemidiaphragm. **C** Contrast injected into a fistulous tract on the skin overlying the right upper quadrant of another patient fills a large irregular abscess in the right lobe of the liver. The abscess has ruptured into the biliary ducts and outlined the right hepatic, cystic, and common bile ducts. (Courtesy of Dr. Jorge Ceballos-Labat, Mexico City) **D** Air in a dilated common bile duct and biliary radicals after perforation of a right lobe abscess into the biliary system of a third patient

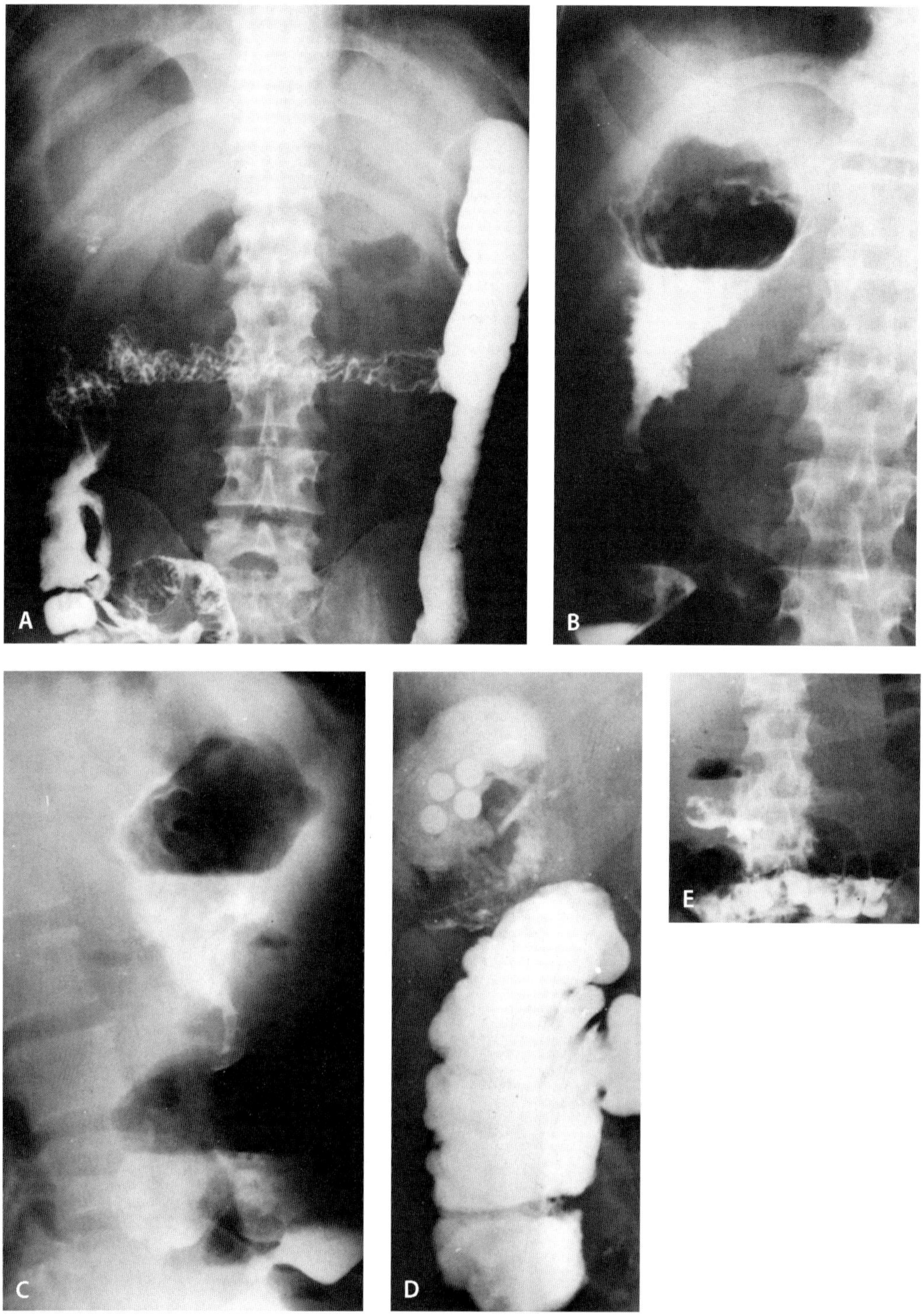
A
B
C
D
E

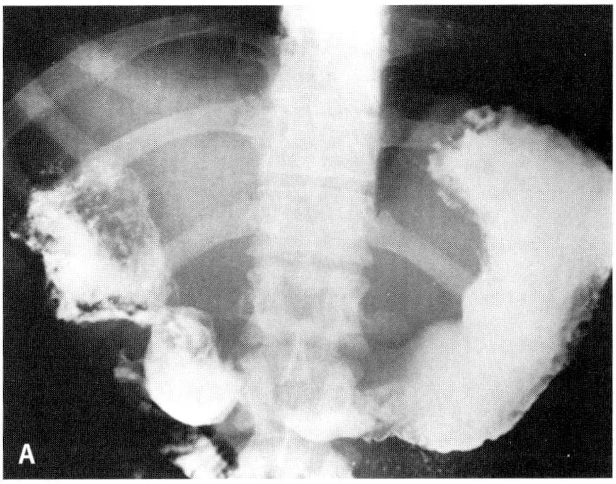

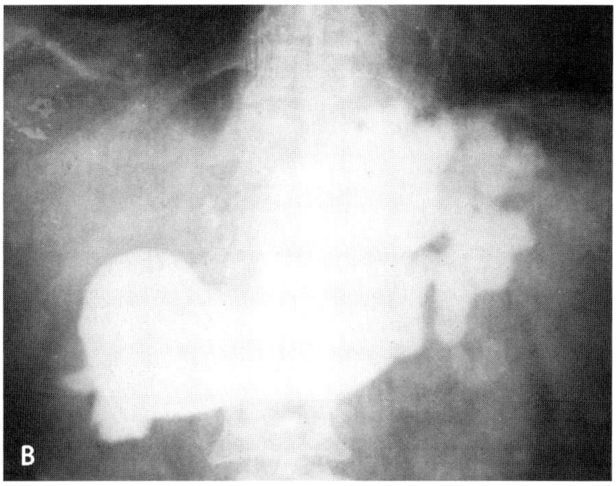

Fig. 1.85 A, B. Rupture of amebic liver abscesses into the duodenum and stomach. **A** A large right lobe abscess, which had ruptured into the first portion of the duodenal C-loop, is filled with barium during an upper gastrointestinal series on a Mexican. (Courtesy of Dr. Jorge Ceballos-Labat, Mexico City) **B** A large left lobe abscess which had perforated into the stomach is outlined with barium during a gastrointestinal series. The stomach is displaced towards the midline by the abscess. The wide communication between the stomach and abscess cavity is seen along the greater curvature of the stomach. There is also some elevation and irregularity of the right hemidiaphragm with pleural reaction above it, suggesting a penetrating abscess involving the dome of the right lobe of the liver as well. The patient was an Indian from a small village in Colombia

◀ **Fig. 1.84 A–E.** Rupture of right lobe amebic liver abscesses into the hepatic flexure and transverse colon in three Mexican patients. **A** Large gas-containing abscess in the right lobe with uncommon communication with the hepatic flexure of the colon via a narrow fistulous tract. The right hemidiaphragm is elevated. Note also the marked deformity, narrowing, and ulceration of the right colon and cecum with thickening and rigidity of the ileocecal valve and reflux into a narrow, rigid terminal ileum. These changes characteristic of chronic amebic colitis may be totally absent in many patients with amebic liver abscess; thus, a normal barium enema would by no means exclude amebiasis as the etiology of the abscess. **B** Anteroposterior and **C** right lateral views of the abdomen of the same patient after injection of contrast medium into the abscess. Note the prominent air-fluid level and irregular contour of the abscess on these erect views. The fistula extends to the gas-filled hepatic flexure, into which some of the contrast has spilled from the liver abscess. **D** In another patient, barium enema outlines a relatively normal hepatic flexure and right colon. However, some barium has spilled into a large abscess in the right lobe of the liver which had perforated into the hepatic flexure. Also noted are five treatment tablets within the abscess which had been given earlier by mouth and had passed into the abscess through the wide fistulous communication. **E** In still another Mexican, there is a fistula between a large abscess in the lower portion of the right liver lobe and the midtransverse colon. There is an air-fluid level within the liver abscess, with the air marking its superior extent on this erect film of the abdomen. The contrast medium outlines the irregular lower margin of the abscess, and the fistulous communication with the transverse colon is readily identified. (Courtesy of Dr. Jorge Ceballos-Labat, Mexico City

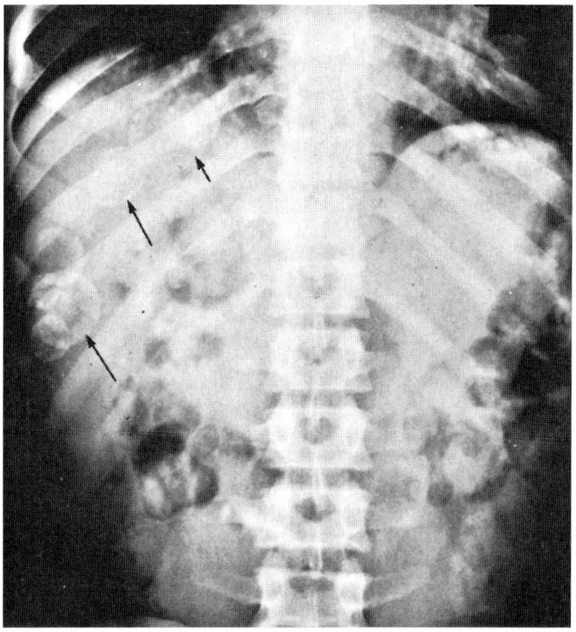

Fig. 1.86. Multiple old calcified hepatic amebic abscesses in a Kenyan adult. Multiple round calcific densities (*arrows*) are present in the liver from longstanding inactive amebic abscesses; such calcification is very uncommon in amebic abscesses anywhere in the body, and would much more likely be caused by old hydatid cysts where that parasitic disease is endemic. (Courtesy of Dr. L. Whittaker, Nairobi)

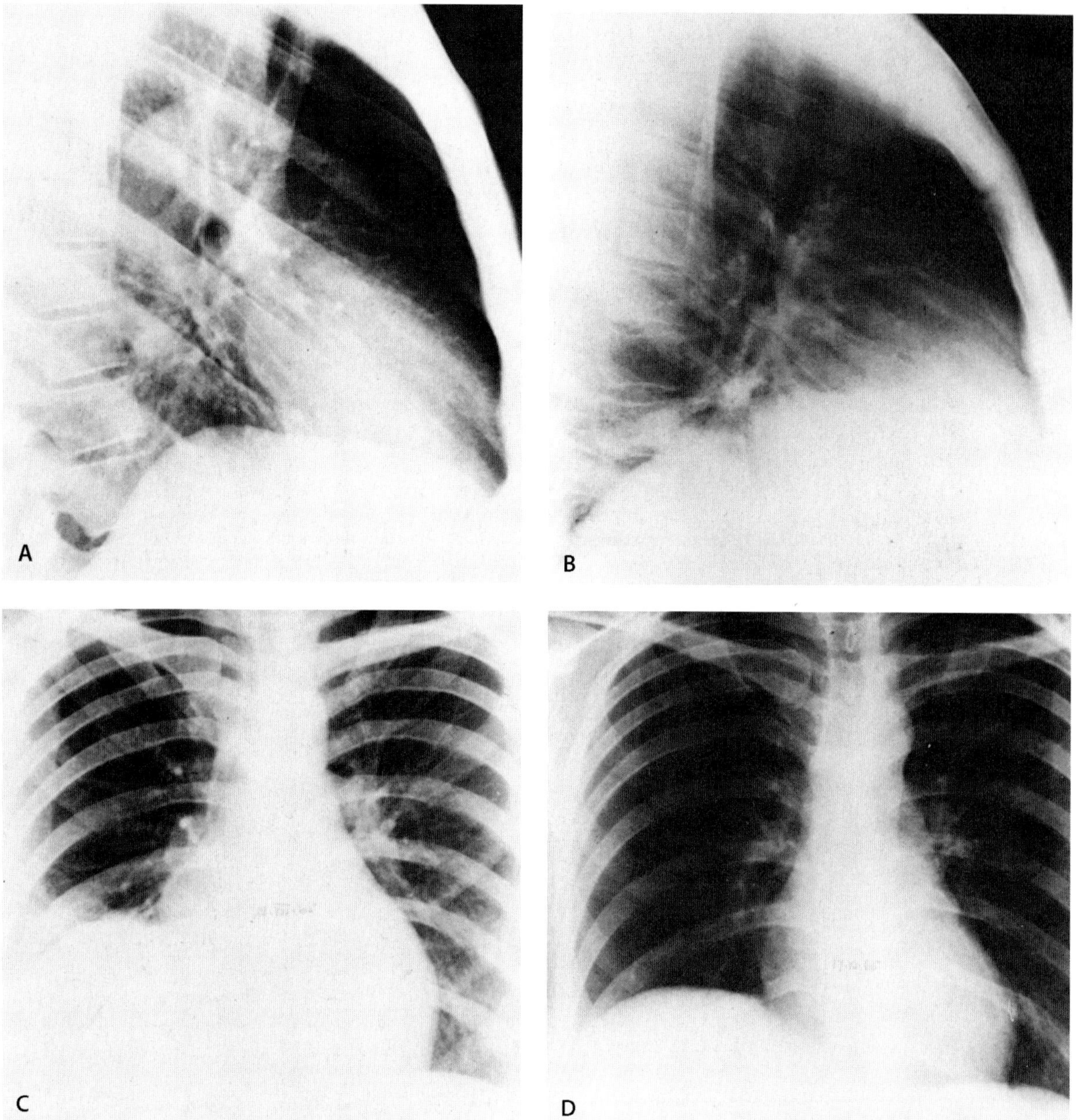

Fig. 1.87 A–D. Early roentgen changes in thoracic amebiasis. As the subphrenic liver abscess develops, the adjoining lung segment becomes edematous. **A** Lateral chest radiograph shows a bulge in the posterior portion of the right hemidiaphragm. **B** The same patient 10 days later. The outline of the diaphragm is indistinct and the posterior basilar segment of the right lower lobe shows patchy increased density. At this stage, adequate antiamebic treatment may return the lung to normal. **C** In a different patient, a PA chest film shows a markedly elevated right hemidiaphragm with a slightly indistinct outline and an amebic cloud in the lung above it. **D** Three months later, after treatment, the diaphragm has returned to a more normal position although still slightly elevated. Diaphragmatic motion is almost normal and the right lung base is now clear

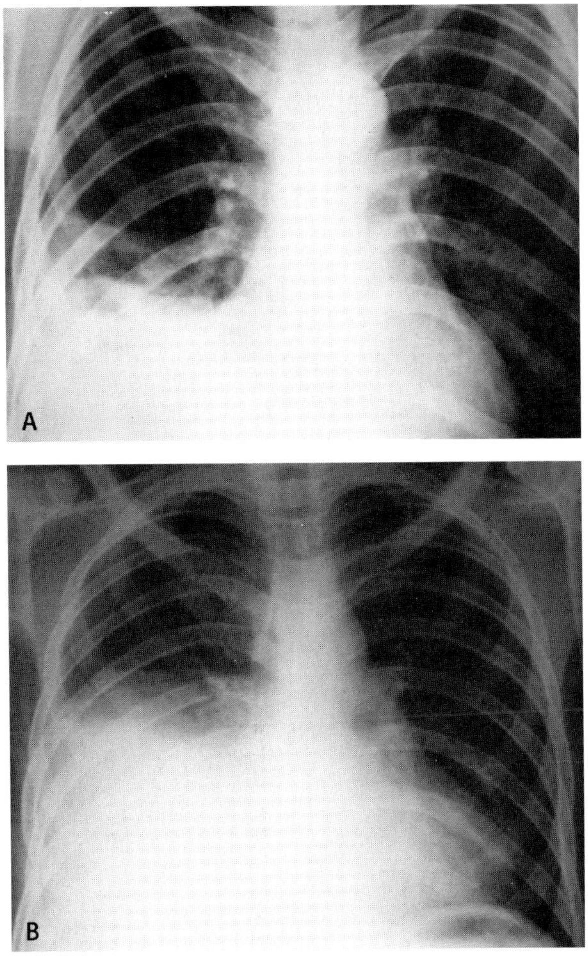

Fig. 1.88 A, B. Thoracic amebiasis in a Kenyan patient. A There is a hepatic amebic abscess containing air beneath an elevated right hemidiaphragm. Above the diaphragm can be seen an amebic haze and some volume loss in the right lung base as well as pleural fluid at the base and in the minor pleural fissure. B Follow-up chest radiograph shows increasing pleural effusion or empyema obscuring the right base and hemidiaphragm.

In most patients who develop intrathoracic amebiasis, there will be haziness and loss of definition of the outline of the elevated hemidiaphragm. Then a small triangular density, a "cloud," develops with the apex extending upwards and inwards toward the hilum and the base following the diaphragmatic outline (Figs. 1.87–1.90).

At this stage, the patient may complain of pain in the chest, with minimal physical signs. These early changes are probably the result of localized pulmonary edema above the stationary and inflamed hemidiaphragm.

By the time the patient has definite clinical complaints referable to the chest, the lung changes are radiologically more advanced, with pneumonitis or atelectasis of the lower lobe (Figs. 1.88–1.90). The original area of localized edema at the lung base will have spread to become a fluffy, irregular opacity overlying and obscuring the dome of the diaphragm, obliterating the costophrenic and cardiophrenic angles. Lateral views show that the right lower lobe is involved in most patients and the basal segments almost always. If pleural fluid is present, it may be a clear reactive exudate. As the infection progresses, the pneumonia in the lower lobe becomes more marked and more clearly defined. Necrosis with abscess formation follows (Fig. 1.90–1.95). At this stage, there is a large pleural effusion, no longer clear but with a high cell count. An amebic empyema may develop, usually quite rapidly within a few days (Figs. 1.94–1.98).

A small number of liver abscesses perforate directly through the diaphragm, following a "collar stud" or "dumbbell" track and presenting as a smooth round nodule above the diaphragm (Fig. 1.91). Free perforation into the pleural space does not always occur because pleural adhesions may be formed; when this happens, fluid extends along the major fissure and may only be seen in the lateral view of the chest. However, in most patients, there is an obvious pleural effusion as well as reaction in the lung above the liver abscess. Rupture of a hepatic or lung abscess (Fig. 1.95) will also generate an amebic empyema, completely filling the pleural space and producing compression atelectasis of the lung. Marked pleural thickening, especially at the lung base, is the usual end result of amebic empyema (Figs. 1.95, 1.98).

Isolated metastatic amebic lung abscesses may occur de novo without obvious infection of the liver and may involve any part of the lung, including the apices. These abscesses are not always associated with pleural fluid and the diaphragm may be entirely normal. They are clinically and radiologically indistinguishable from any other lung abscesses; they can have thick or thin walls, may contain fluid, or be relatively solid. They may be single or multiple. Only their response to treatment provides a clue to their origin, unless they rupture into the bronchus and amebae can be identified in the sputum. The prognosis is good if treatment is instituted early and maintained, but there may be considerable residual lung fibrosis with bronchial deformity and stenosis.

(Text continues on p. 93)

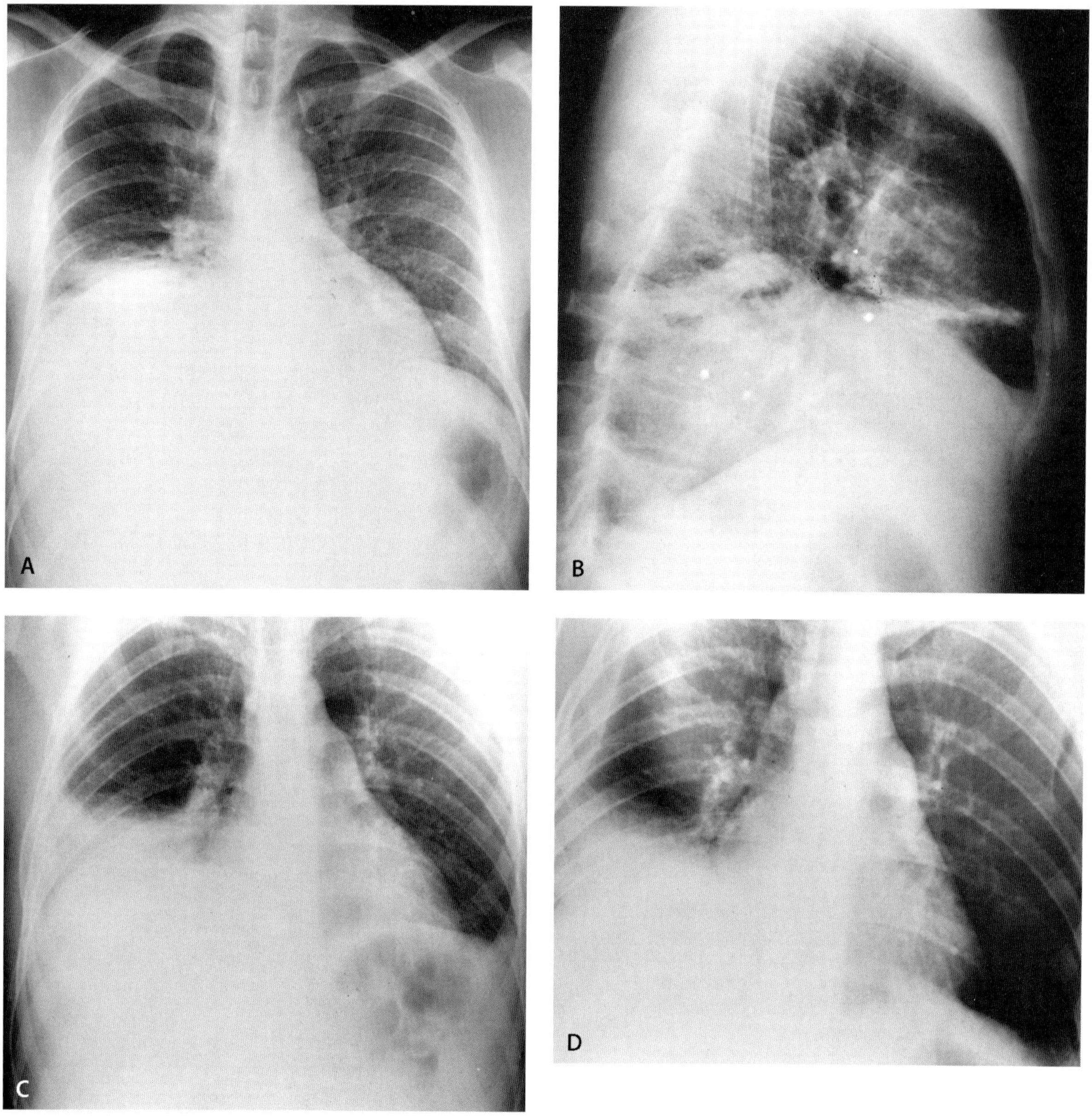

Fig. 1.89 A–D. Thoracic amebiasis in two patients. **A, B** In a Sri Lankan man, PA and lateral chest radiographs reveal hepatomegaly, elevation of the right hemidiaphragm with a localized hump in its midportion and some air in the underlying hepatic abscess, and an amebic haze and discoid atelectasis in the right middle and lower lobes, best seen on the lateral view (**B**). **C, D** In another patient with hepatothoracic amebiasis there is hepatomegaly, elevation of the right hemidiaphragm, volume loss and pneumonitis in the right lower lung, and a moderate pleural effusion or empyema of approximately 1000 ml at the right base, best seen on a lateral decubitus view (**D**). There is also slight pleural fluid obliterating the left costophrenic angle

Fig. 1.90 A–G. The development and progress of "amebic pneumonia." **A** The central portion of the right hemidiaphragm is elevated. The adjacent lung appears normal. **B** The liver infection has spread through the lymphatics. The diaphragm is partially immobilized and the segment of lung above the hepatic abscess becomes poorly expanded and edematous. **C** The amebic cloud of edema has increased in extent and there is now an area of consolidation in the right lung base overlying the diaphragm. **D** There is increasing pneumonia and beginning pleural effusion at the right base obliterating the outlines of the diaphragm and cardiophrenic and costophrenic angles. **E** There is now a definite lung abscess with thickened, irregular wall and central necrosis. At this stage, the pleural fluid may remain clear or, more commonly, become an empyema. The above changes in this patient's chest developed over a period of 10 days in spite of antiamebic therapy. The rate at which this process develops depends very much on the individual patient. **F, G** Autopsy specimens of a huge abscess in the right lobe of the liver (**F**) with a thickened diaphragm and pleura above it (**G**). There is pneumonitis in the right lung base

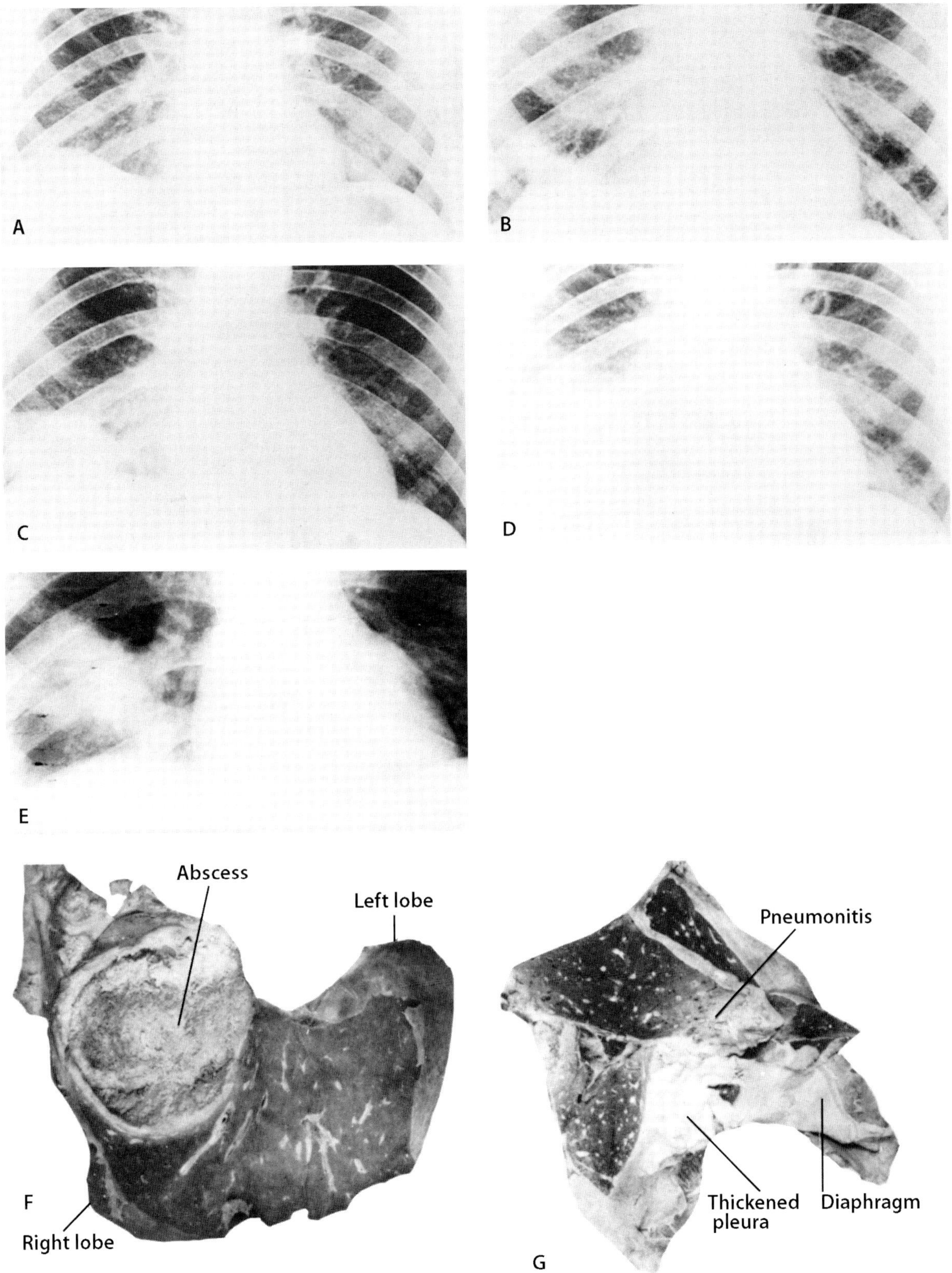
A
B
C
D
E
Abscess
Left lobe
F
Right lobe
Pneumonitis
Thickened pleura
Diaphragm
G

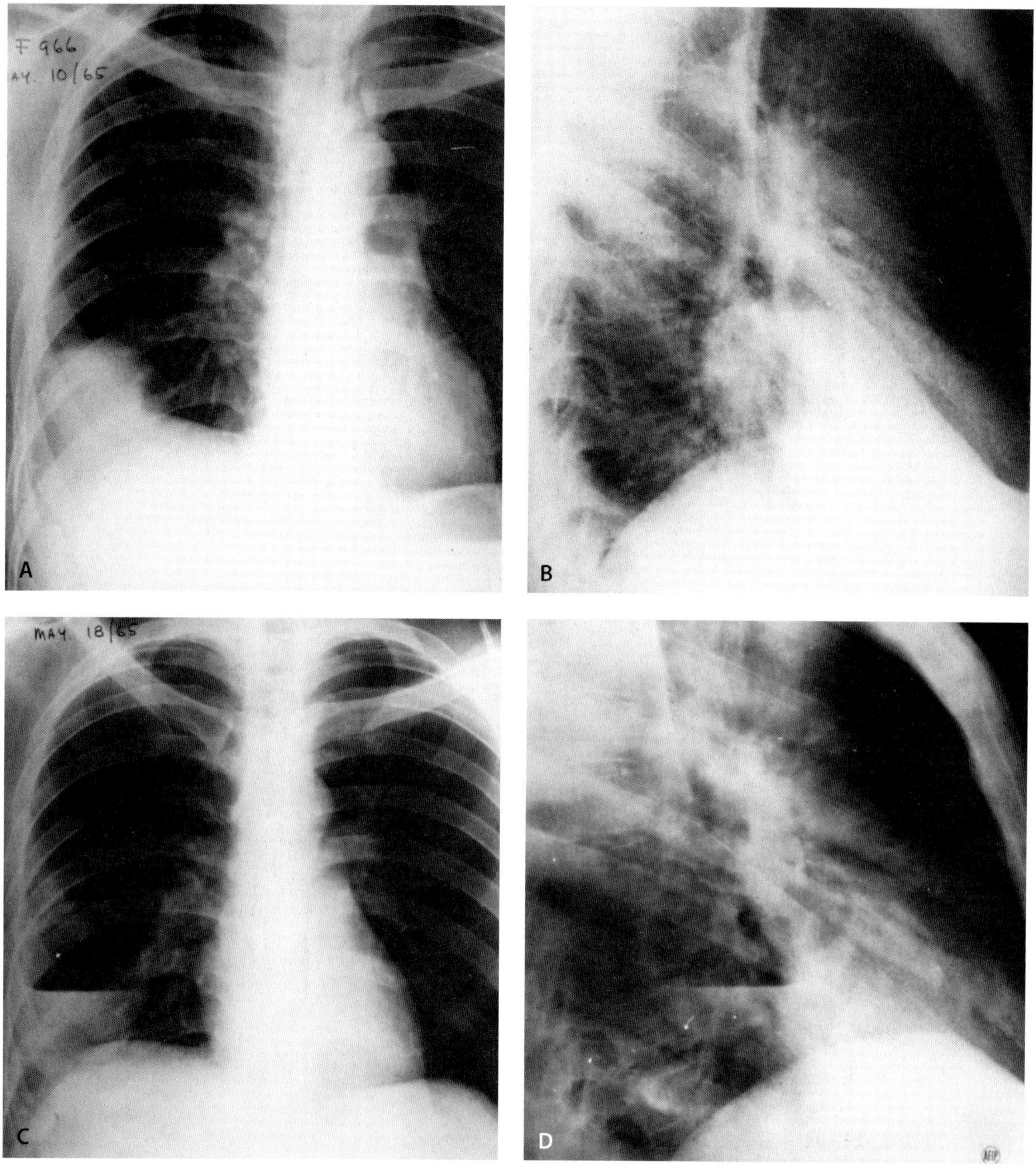

Fig. 1.91 A–H. Development of an amebic collar stud abscess. **A, B** May 10: PA and lateral views of the chest show a well-circumscribed mass in the lateral aspect of the right lower lobe immediately above the diaphragm. There is slight pleural reaction and fluid along the right lower lateral chest wall and costophrenic angle. **C, D** May 18: PA and lateral chest films show the abscess has ruptured into a bronchus with partial expectoration of its content. There is now a large air-filled cavity with a fluid level. **E** May 25: PA view shows a large thin-walled cavity in the same area previously occupied by the fluid-filled abscess (*upper arrow*). There is slight pleural reaction along the right lateral chest wall and base and a small air-fluid level below the right hemidiaphragm (*lower arrow*). **F** May 29: lateral view showing the patient has drained the abscess completely by coughing. The communication between the thin-walled lung abscess and the subphrenic liver abscess (*arrow*) is shown. There is a localized bulge in the midportion of the right hemidiaphragm caused by the liver abscess beneath it. This series of films shows the essential radiological findings when a liver abscess perforates directly through the diaphragm to produce a well-defined "dumbbell" abscess above it. **G** An autopsy specimen of a similar case. A large abscess in the right lobe of the liver has perforated through the dome of the liver and the diaphragm to produce a well-defined abscess in the right lower lobe of the lung. The *white marker* identifies the wide communication between the two abscesses. **H** Artist's rendition of a typical collar stud or hourglass amebic abscess as seen in the lateral projection. E–H see p. 91 ▶

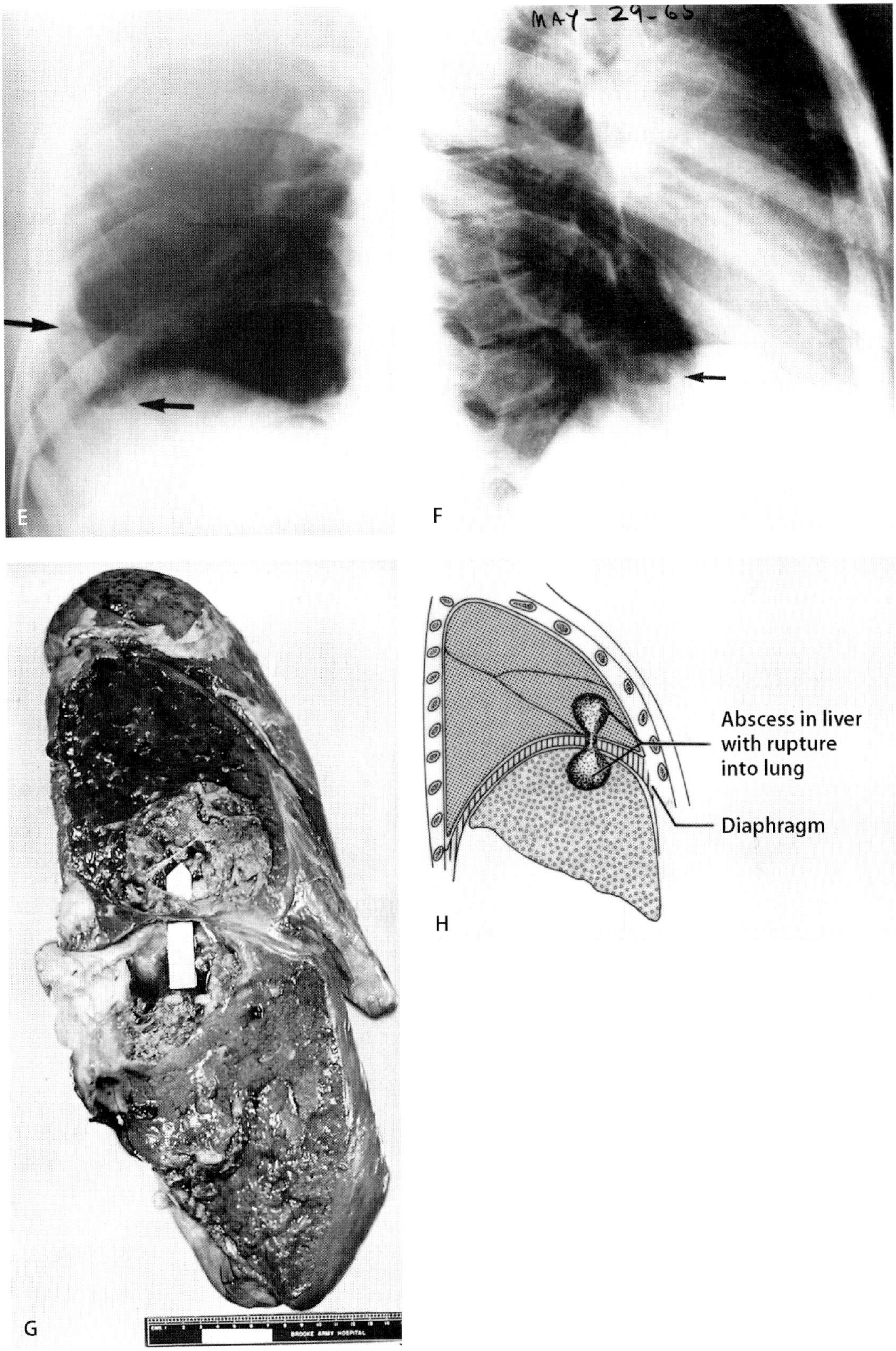
E
F
G
Abscess in liver with rupture into lung
Diaphragm
H

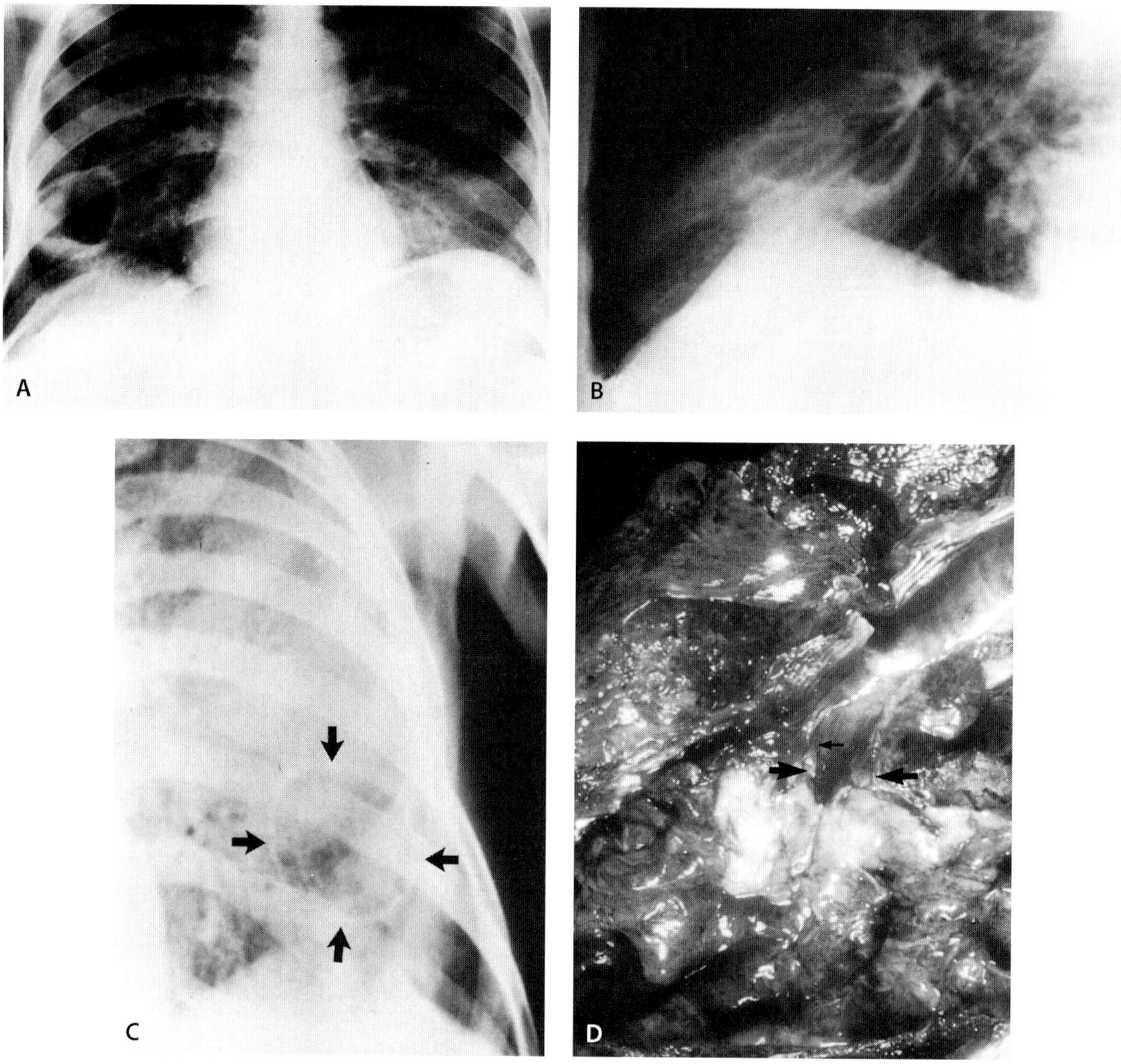

Fig. 1.92 A–D. This patient developed an amebic lung abscess above the right lobe of the liver and, at the same time, there was an amebic cloud of pneumonia above the left lobe of the liver, as seen on the PA view of the chest (A). The lateral view (B) shows the lung abscess above the midportion of the right hemidiaphragm, which shows a prominent upward bulge caused by the large hepatic abscess beneath it. The area of pneumonitis in the left lower lobe is in the posterior basilar segment. C The pneumonia persisted in spite of antiamebic therapy and eventually spread to involve the entire left lower lobe with development of an abscess in the original area of involvement. This abscess ruptured into a bronchus and an air-filled, thin-walled cavity resulted (*arrows*). The left hemidiaphragm shows a prominent bulge in its central portion, which is also indistinct because of the amebic abscess beneath it in the left lobe of the liver. The multiple abscesses in the lungs and liver eventually healed after prolonged therapy. D Gross specimen of a hepatopulmonary abscess (*lower*) communicating with a bronchus (*center*, see *arrows*)

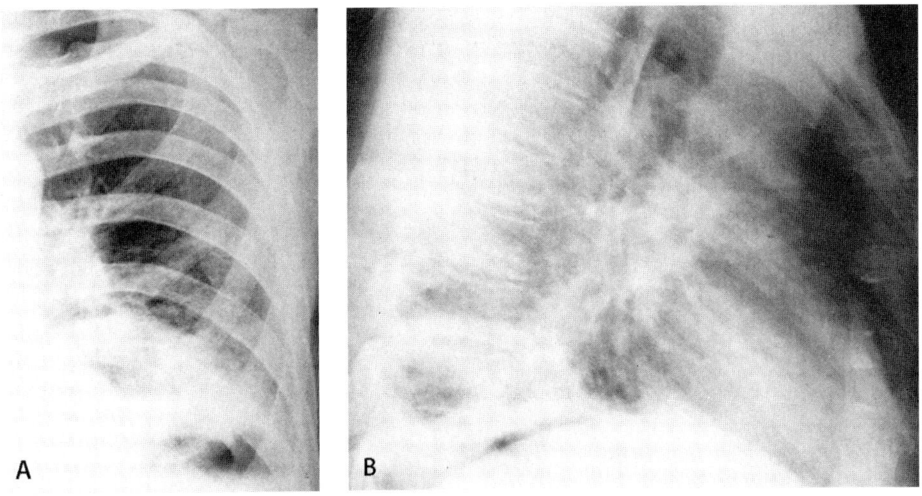

Fig. 1.93 A, B. Amebic abscess in the left lower lobe. **A** PA and **B** left lateral views of the chest show a thick-walled abscess in the posterior basilar segment of the left lower lobe. The left hemidiaphragm is slightly elevated and indistinct and there is slight surrounding infiltrate and minimal pleural effusion at the posterior costophrenic angle in association with the abscess. Left lung abscesses are decidedly less common than those in the right lung and usually develop from perforation of an amebic abscess in the left lobe of the liver through the diaphragm

A fistula to a bronchus occurs in 35% of all thoracic complications, basically communicating the hepatobiliary tract, or occasionally the pleura, chest wall, and skin, with the bronchial tree (Fig. 1.99 A, B). Bilioptysis is not an uncommon symptom. Other etiologies of bronchobiliary fistula include hydatid disease, trauma, biliary obstruction, and subphrenic abscess. Cutaneous fistulas can also develop outward to the skin through the pleura. Secondary involvement of the ribs from an amebic empyema can occur (Fig. 1.99 C).

Identical events may occur in either side of the chest, but are much less common on the left (Figs. 1.92 C, 1.93). There are no specific radiological features on the left side, other than the recognition of an enlarged left lobe of the liver and an associated pleural effusion in many patients. Perforation into the pericardium is an acute emergency, resembling a myocardial infarct and causing pericardial tamponade (Fig. 1.100). Pneumopericardium may complicate an abscess, which originated in the liver and has extended into the pericardium after first involving the lung or stomach (Fig. 1.101). An acute pericardial effusion in a patient with a fixed liver, but without a history suggesting a subphrenic abscess (such as from previous surgery), should lead to consideration of an amebic infection. The condition is so acute that it is unlikely to be a radiological problem. The end result may be constrictive pericarditis.

The diagnosis of thoracic amebiasis depends on the combination of a significantly elevated diaphragm on the affected side, hepatomegaly, and pleural effusion. Without these changes it is impossible to distinguish thoracic amebiasis from pulmonary infarction, pneumonia, pyogenic lung abscess, tuberculosis, or even malignancy.

(Text continues on p. 99)

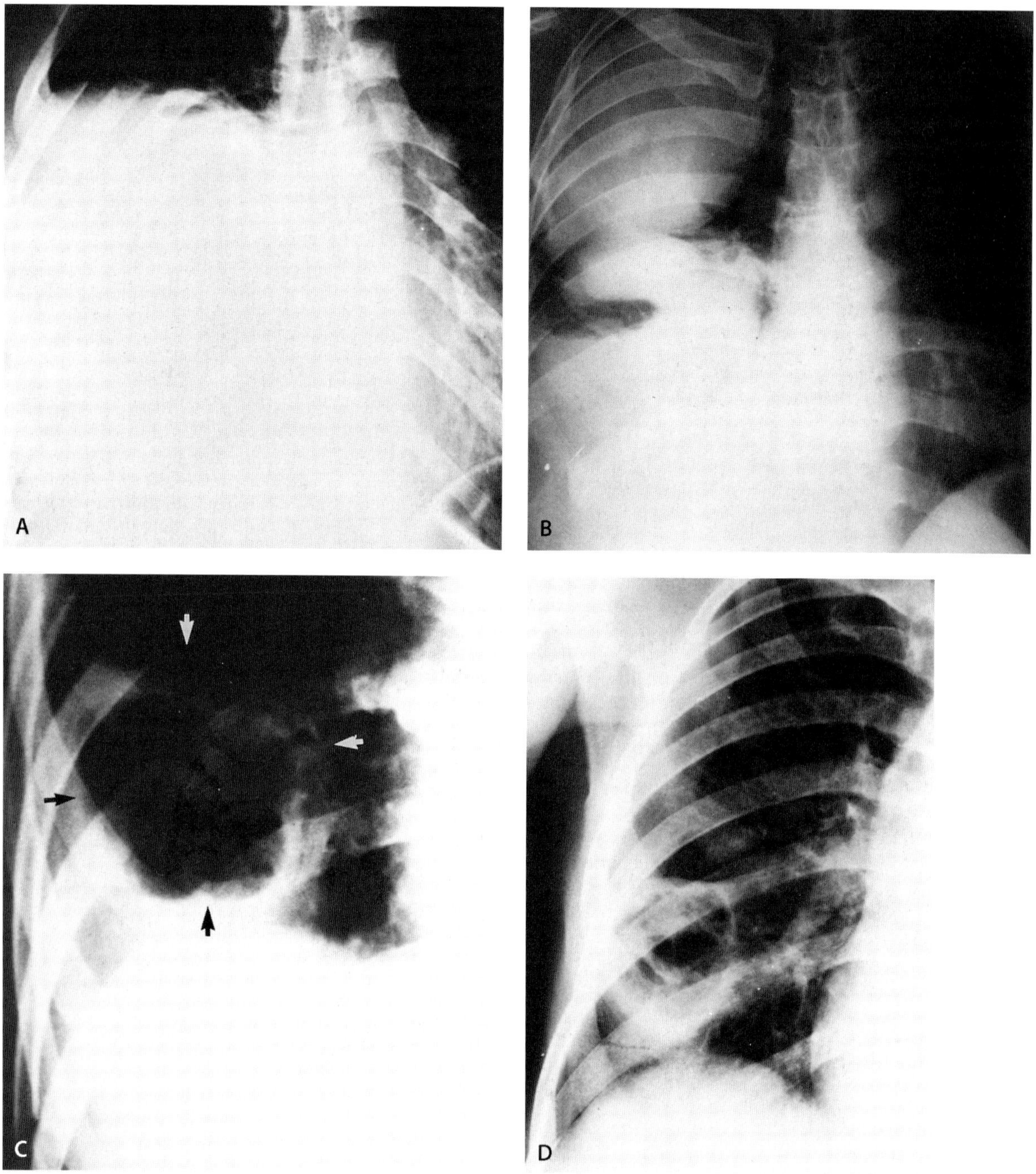

Fig. 1.94 A–D. Amebic lung abscesses vary considerably in size. **A** A huge amebic lung abscess filling most of the right hemithorax. There was an associated slight to moderate pleural effusion or empyema, but the diaphragm was only slightly elevated. Initial radiographic interpretation had suggested a massive empyema. **B** A large lower lobe lung abscess with a marked loculated empyema above it. There is also empyema below the lung abscess, obscuring the elevated right hemidiaphragm. **C** An amebic lung abscess with thick, irregular walls (*arrows*) in the right lower lobe. The lateral portion of the right hemidiaphragm and the costophrenic angle are obliterated by the abscess and associated small pleural effusion. **D** Another right lower lobe abscess with a thick wall, showing attachment to the midportion of the right hemidiaphragm

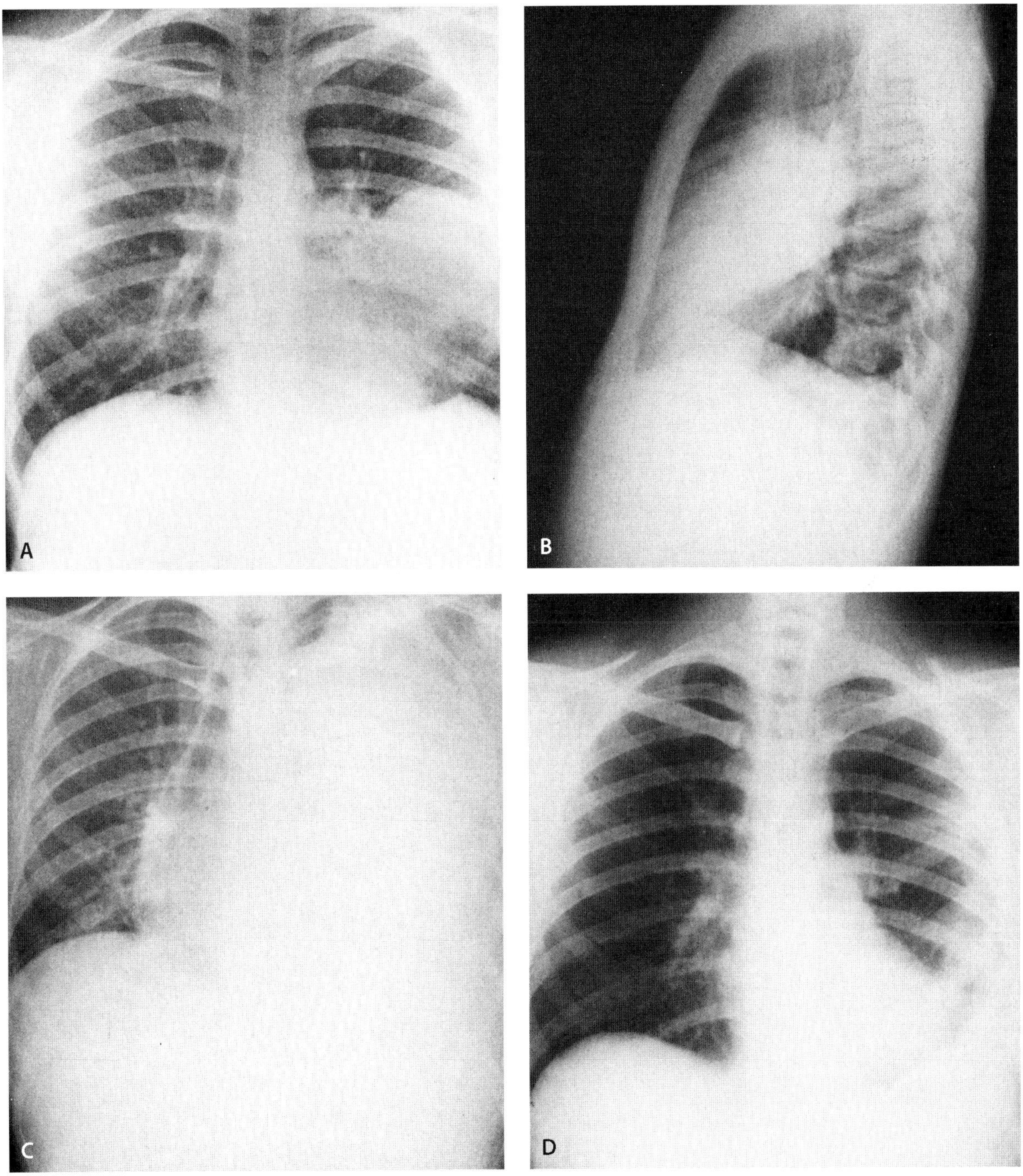

Fig. 1.95 A–D. Huge amebic lung abscess in the left lingula with rupture into the pleura, leading to massive empyema in young American soldier during the Vietnam conflict. **A, B** PA and lateral views of the chest, obtained on 20 and 22 June, 1963, show a large lobulated mass in the left lingula, obscuring the left heart border on the frontal view. There is slight tenting of the midportion of the left hemidiaphragm, and there was minimal fluid at the left costophrenic angle (not visible on the cropped PA illustration). The combination of a pulmonary mass and pleural and diaphragmatic changes should suggest an amebic lung abscess with subdiaphragmatic infection, especially in a febrile patient residing in or returning from an endemic area. **C** Chest film of June 24 shows the abscess has ruptured into the pleural cavity and caused a massive empyema, obscuring virtually the entire left hemithorax and displacing the mediastinum and heart to the right. **D** Four months later on October 18, there is residual pleural thickening along the left lateral chest wall, base, and costophrenic angle, but the patient was now clinically well after drainage of the empyema and successful antiamebic therapy. The pleural fibrosis will persist essentially unchanged in most patients as a reminder of their previous severe amebic empyema

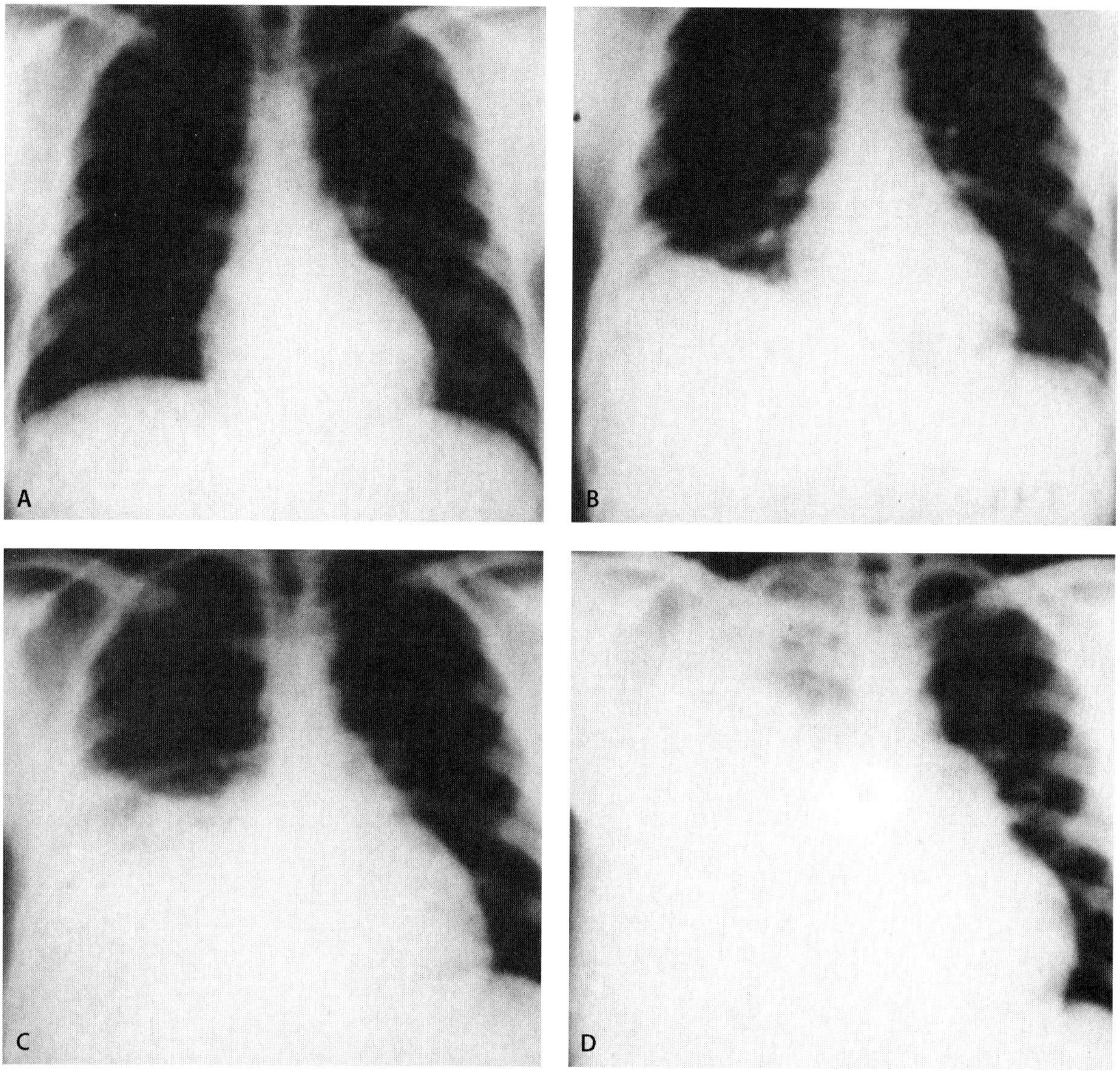

Fig. 1.96 A–D. Rapid development of amebic empyema over a 9-day period. **A** Initial PA radiograph shows a normal chest with sharp, nonelevated right hemidiaphragm and no evidence of pneumonitis or pleural effusion. **B** Three days later, the right hemidiaphragm is elevated and there is moderate pleural effusion at the right base and costophrenic angle. **C** Six days later, there is increasing fluid occupying the lower half of the right hemithorax. **D** After 9 days, there is massive empyema now filling almost the entire right hemithorax with purulent fluid. This case illustrates the dramatically swift development of empyema in many patients with thoracic amebiasis

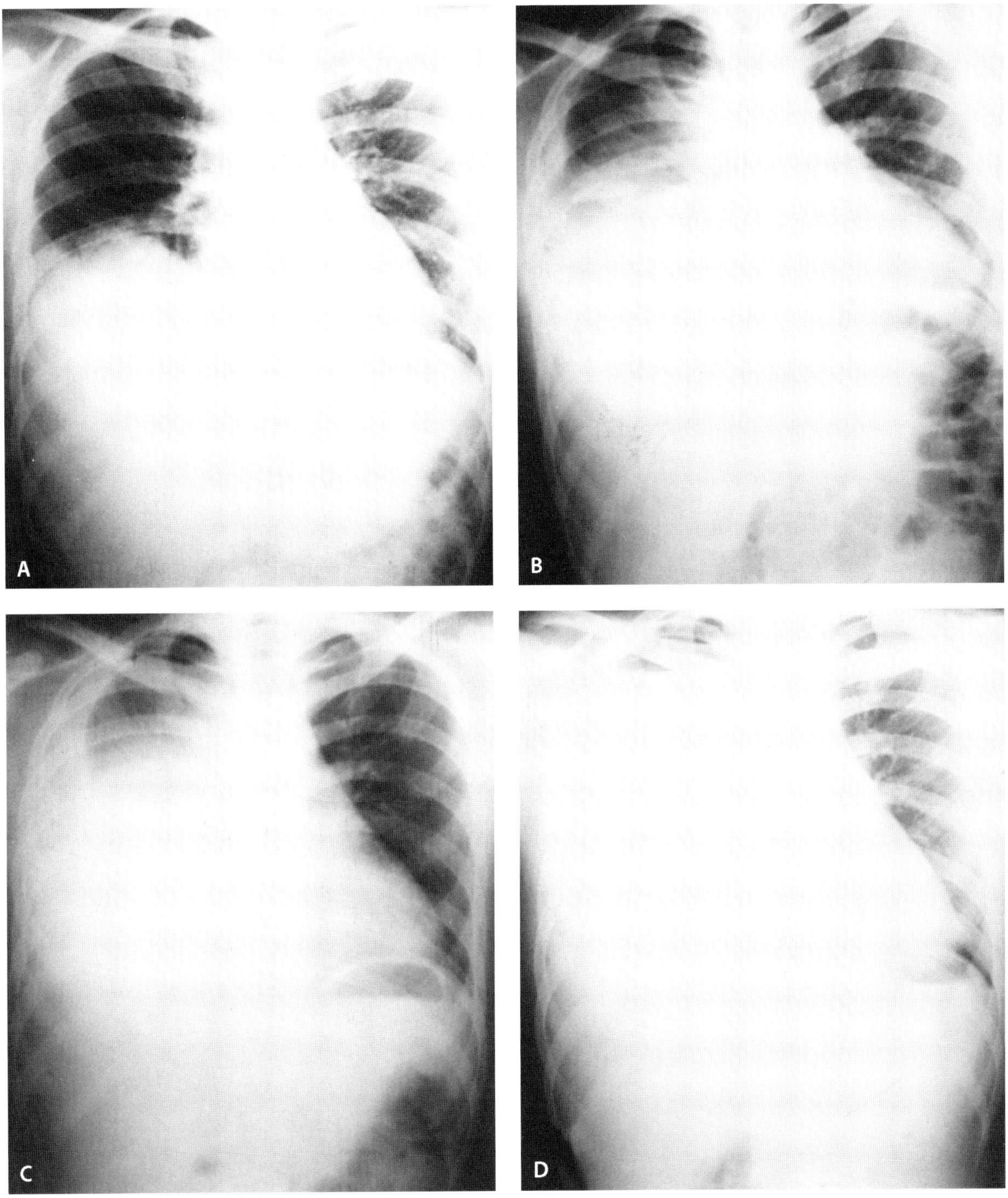

Fig. 1.97 A–D. Hepatothoracic amebiasis with massive empyema developing in a young Laotian man over a 2-week period. A Initial radiograph shows massive hepatomegaly. There is an amebic cloud of edema and pneumonitis in the right lower lung overlying the markedly elevated and indistinct right hemidiaphragm. B–D Serial films over the next 2 weeks again reveal marked hepatomegaly, elevation of the right hemidiaphragm and progressive development of amebic pneumonia in the right lung. There is an empyema initially at the lung base and lateral chest wall B, later progressing to fill virtually the entire hemithorax except for the apex (C, D). On the final film, there is a prominent air-fluid level overlying an otherwise opaque right chest which contained several thousand milliliters of purulent fluid. This was drained and, after vigorous antiamebic therapy, the patient recovered and was left with residual marked pleural thickening along the lower lateral chest wall and base similar to that seen in Fig. 1.95 D

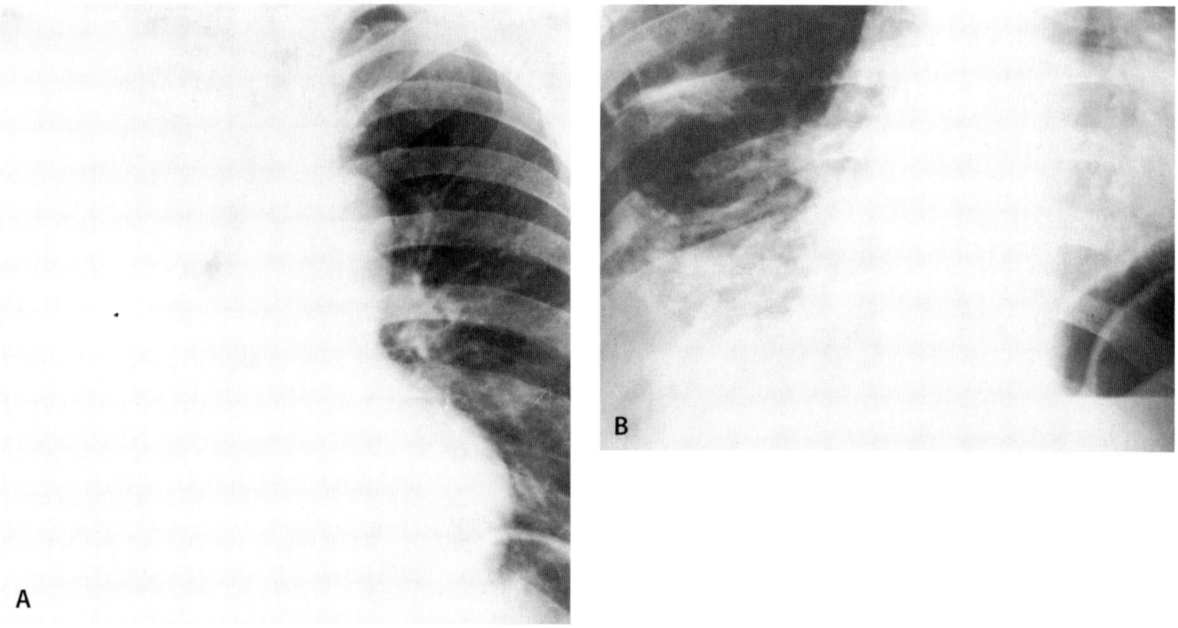

Fig. 1.98. Massive amebic empyema filling virtually the entire right hemithorax (**A**), with follow-up chest film 16 days later after drainage (**B**), showing residual inflammatory changes and subsegmental atelectasis in the right lower lung as well as slight residual pleural fluid and thickening. The right hemidiaphragm is totally obscured by the overlying pulmonary infiltrate and pleural reaction. Residual pleural thickening will persist throughout the patient's lifetime

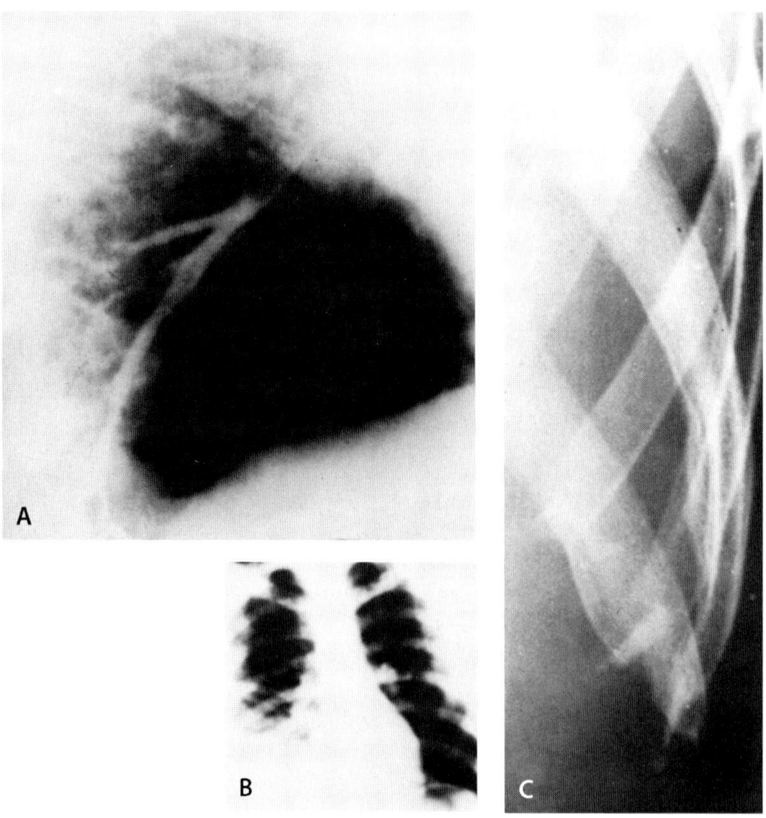

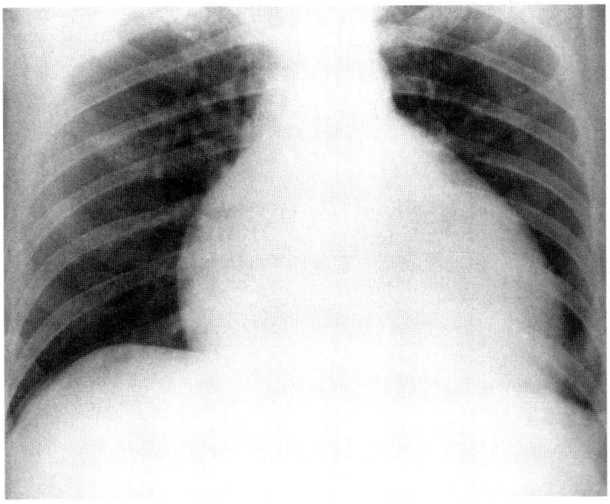

Fig. 1.100. Pericardial effusion with enlargement of the cardiac-pericardial silhouette, secondary to rupture of a left hepatic amebic abscess into the pericardium of a Mexican patient. (Courtesy of Drs. Kenji Kimura and Miguel Stoopen)

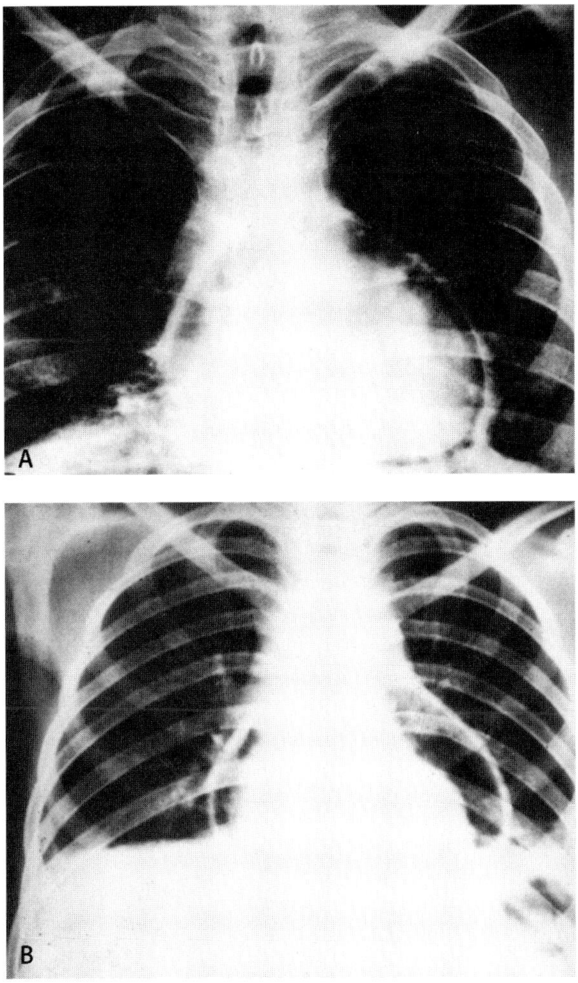

▶ **Fig. 1.101 A, B.** Pneumopericardium in two Mexican patients. An amebic abscess from either the right or left lobe of the liver, or even from the lung, may rupture into the pericardium and cause acute tamponade, usually resulting in death. Occasionally, pneumopericardium will be seen if a lung abscess has extended into the pericardium or if an abscess in the left hepatic lobe has perforated through the stomach into the pericardium. (Courtesy of Dr. Jorge Ceballos-Labat, Mexico City)

◀ **Fig. 1.99 A–C.** Other complications of intrathoracic amebiasis. **A** A bronchopleural-cutaneous fistula involving the bronchus to the posterior basilar segment of the right lower lobe is visualized by injection of the cutaneous fistulous tract with iodinated contrast media. **B** PA chest film of the same patient, showing elevation of the right hemidiaphragm and persistent chronic pleural and parenchymal inflammatory changes at the right base. **C** Periostitis involving the lateral aspects of several left lower ribs, which developed from drainage of pus through a fistula in a patient with amebic empyema

Amebiasis of the Brain

Amebiasis of the brain is a rare condition that occurs in less that 1% of patients with dysenteric amebiasis. However, it accounts for 4.2–8.5% of deaths due to amebiasis.

Pathology. The arrival of amebae to the central nervous system is by a hematogenous route, either secondary to intravascular rupture or through the systemic circulation combined with a paradoxical event across a patent foramen ovale or a pulmonary arteriovenous fistula. The systemic flow to the brain represents 20% of the cardiac output. Thus, once in the systemic circulation, the parasite can easily reach the central nervous system.

The lesions can be single or multiple, and range from microscopic to 5 cm in diameter. Grossly, they appear as a conglomerate of petechiae with softening of the brain and congestion. The larger lesions are necrotic with well-defined margins containing a yellowish-green exudate. The meninges may show a localized or generalized inflammatory response that may be indistinguishable from other types of acute purulent meningitis.

Clinical manifestations. Symptomatology includes convulsive disorder, hemiplegia, monoplegia, cranial nerve involvement, meningitis, and signs of increased intracranial pressure. The clinical behavior is basically that of an acute space-occupying lesion with spontaneous hemorrhage. Tumor and other parasitic infestations, such as cysticercosis, parago-

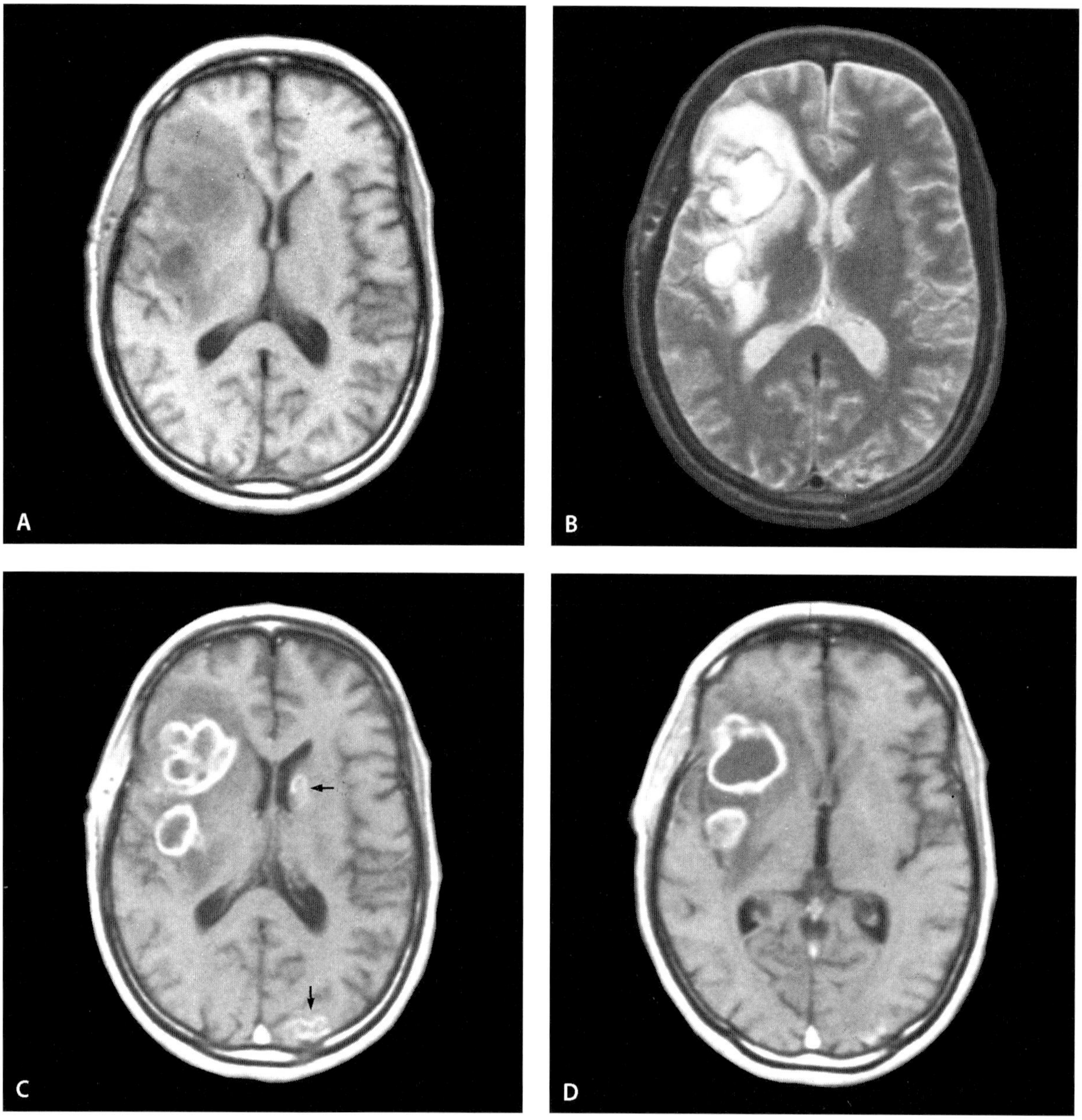

Fig. 1.102 A–D. MRI of multiple amebic brain abscesses in a 38-year-old South African man. **A** T1-weighted (SE 500/10) image shows multiple hypointense lesions in the right frontoparietal area. **B** On the T2-weighted (SE 260/90) image the lesions showed central hyperintensity of the abscess contents surrounded by low-intensity halos representing the abscess walls, which were in turn surrounded by hyperintense zones of edema. **C, D** Following intravenous gadolinium DTPA (0.1 mmol/kg), there was pronounced ring enhancement of all lesions, with demonstration of additional small lesions in the head of the left caudate nucleus and in the left occipital area (*small arrows* in **C**). (Courtesy of Drs. J.P. De Villiers and G. Durra and *Clin Radiol*, 1998) The patient, who was from a rural area, was admitted complaining of hemoptysis, dyspnea, and right upper quadrant pain. He appeared ill with a temperature of 38 °C, a tender liver, and signs of a right basal pleural effusion. He had slightly depressed consciousness, but no focal neurological signs. He was somewhat anemic but his white cell count was normal and he was HIV-negative. There was no change in the nature of his stools. A chest radiograph revealed an elevated right hemidiaphragm with a moderate right pleural effusion. Ultrasound of the abdomen demonstrated a 6-cm round hypoechoic lesion in the right lobe of the liver. Aspiration of the liver lesion under ultrasound guidance revealed pink pus. Microscopy revealed the presence of amebae and indirect hemagglutination for *E. histolytica* was positive at 1:4096, confirming systemic amebiasis. Stool microscopy was unremarkable. Oral metronidazole was initiated. On the same day, the patient developed a left hemiplegia with neck stiffness and a left upper motor neuron facial nerve palsy. A CT scan of the head revealed multiple low-density lesions in the right frontoparietal region of the brain and a single lesion in the head of the left caudate nucleus. Marked mass effect was present. The contrast-enhanced scan demonstrated ring enhancement of all lesions, with additional vague increased density noted in the occipital region.

nimiasis, and hydatid disease, are part of the differential diagnosis. Unfortunately, most cases go undiagnosed since cerebral amebiasis is rarely included in the list of potential etiologies. When an early diagnosis is made, a dramatic positive response to specific treatment is observed.

Imaging features. Amebic brain abscesses are hypodense on CT and hypointense on T1-weighted MRI with peripheral ring enhancement after intravenous contrast media; surrounding edema is present (Fig. 1.102). These abscesses, whether solitary or multiple, commonly involve cortical and deep grey matter. The frontal lobes and basal ganglia are the commonest sites of involvement; the left side is more common than the right by a ratio of 2.3:1. The CT appearance cannot be differentiated from other causes of brain abscess. The differential diagnosis also includes tuberculosis, nocardiosis, and metastases. The MR images do not differ significantly from those seen with pyogenic abscesses. T1-weighted images show central hypointensity with a surrounding thin rim of isointensity, presumably representing a capsule of granulation tissue (DeVilliers and Durra; also Dietz et al.). The T2-weighted images show central hyperintensity, presumably representing central necrosis and liquified brain. The presumed granulation tissue capsule is hypointense, and what is presumed to be surrounding edema is hyperintense, similar to that seen with pyogenic abscess. These findings are nonspecific for cerebral amebic abscess and, unfortunately, the premortem or presurgical diagnosis is only accomplished in a few patients. Because the condition is potentially lethal, it should be considered in differential diagnosis, especially in endemic areas, and metronidazole or other appropriate antiamebic therapy should be instituted after the diagnosis has been confirmed by serology or other laboratory tests. MRI is superior to CT in demonstrating small cerebral lesions, but neither modality is always available in most endemic regions, and thus the true incidence of brain involvement in amebiasis is probably underestimated.

◀ **Fig. 1.102** (*continued*). In this clinical setting these features were thought to be consistent with multiple brain abscesses. In view of the marked mass effect, the largest of the lesions was drained via craniotomy. Yellow-green pus was drained, but routine microscopic examination, bacterial stains, and culture revealed no organisms and cytological examination was normal. The patient's therapy was changed to intravenous metronidazole and ceftriaxone. A postoperative MRI demonstrated the findings enumerated in Fig. 1.102. The lesions in the left head of the caudate and occipital cortex had reduced in size since the initial CT scan prior to therapy. Postsurgical craniotomy changes were also present on all MR images. Clinically the patient had resolution of his neck stiffness and improved level of consciousness over 10 days

Other Sites of Amebiasis

Genital Amebiasis. Invasion of the genitalia is very rare and occurs mostly in women, with isolated reports in men. Amebic abscesses involving the genitourinary tract (including the fallopian tubes, vagina, and cervix) occur, but are not radiologically distinguishable from those caused by other organisms.

Vascular Involvement. Thrombosis, particularly of the mesenteric or portal vessels, may occur during acute amebiasis, as with any other infection. Usually it is a complication of the disease, but amebae have been recovered in large numbers from thrombi within the inferior vena cava. They become an important source of thromboemboli, giving rise to pulmonary or rare cerebral abscesses.

Commentary

Amebiasis remains an imposing public health challenge that affects millions of people with limited economic resources living in overpopulated developing countries. Despite the significant progress attained during the last few decades, including a diminishing mortality due to better understanding of the disease, availability of effective specific antiamebic medications, and generally improved patient care, it still remains a costly worldwide problem. The responsibility to eradicate this parasitic disease lies directly with the public health departments and political leaders of those countries who are charged with funding and building the necessary sewer infrastructures and modern water treatment plants to prevent further fecal contamination. Rural populations must be educated on the importance of avoiding contamination of water sources and how to protect and improve the quality of their drinking water. The following methods for water treatment are generally available and include simply teaching the "point-of use disinfection technique," either by traditional water boiling or by offering the new and relatively inexpensive household technology kit that includes a translucent high-density polyethylene plastic container with a wide single opening. Use of a nonrustable spigot and 5% calcium hypochlorite disinfectant solution is another method recommended by the World Health Organization with a modest cost of a few cents per year.

Bibliography

Abdel-Hakim M, Higazi AM: Broncho-pulmonary amoebiasis. *Dis Chest* 34:607–620, 1958

Abelouafi A, Ousehal A, Ouzidane L, Kadiri R: Ultrasonography in the diagnosis of liver abscesses apropos of 32 cases. [French]. *Ann Radiol* 36:286–292, 1993

Abuabara SF, Barrett JA, Hau T, Jonasson: Amebic liver abscess. *Arch Surg* 117:239–244, 1982

Adal KA, Kress K, Petri WA Jr: Determination of the pathogenicity of *Entamoeba histolytica*. *Clin Infect Dis* 16:340, 1993

Adams EB, Macleod IN: Invasive amebiasis I. Amebiasis liver abscess and its complications. *Medicine (Baltimore)* 56:315–323, 1977

Ahmed L, Salama ZA, El Rooby A, Strickland GT: Ultrasonographic resolution time for amebic liver abscess. *Am J Trop Med Hyg* 41:406–410, 1989

Ahmed L, El Rooby A, Kassem MI, Salama ZA, Strickland GT: Ultrasonography in the diagnosis and management of 52 patients with amebic liver abscess in Cairo. *Rev Infect Dis* 12:330–337, 1990

Ahmed M, McAdam KP, Sturm AW, Hussain P: Systemic manifestations of invasive amebiasis. *Clin Infect Dis* 15:974–982, 1992

Ahmed R, et al: Amebic appendicitis: a rare entity. *J Pak Med Assoc* 44:92–93, 1994

Albores-Saavedra J, Rosas-Uribe A, Altamirano-Dimas M, Brandt H: Cancer with superimposed amebiasis. *Am J Clin Pathol* 49:677, 1968

Alkan WJ, et al: The clinical syndrome of amebic abscess of the left lobe of the liver. *Ann Intern Med* 55:800–813, 1961

Allard JC, Lee VW, Foster J: Discordant uptake of technetium-99m DISIDA and technetium-99m sulfur colloid in an amebic abscess. *Clin Nucl Med* 13:114–116, 1988

Altemeier WA, Schowengerdt CG, Whiteley DH: Abscesses of the liver: surgical considerations. *Arch Surg* 101:258–265, 1970

Amoebiasis editorial. *Lancet* I:77–78, 1968

Anton AE, Cia MT, Celador AA, et al: Diagnostic and therapeutic criteria in amebic liver abscess. [Spanish]. *Rev Esp Enferm Aparato Dig* 70:461–464, 1986

Anzil AP, Rao C, Wrzolek MA, et al: Amebic meningoencephalitis in a patient with AIDS caused by a newly recognized opportunistic pathogen. Leptomyxid ameba. *Arch Pathol Lab Med* 115:21–25, 1991

Arroyo G, Elgueta R: Squamous cell carcinoma associated with amoebic cervicitis. *Acta Cytol* 33:301, 1989

Aucott JN, Ravdin JI: Amebiasis and "nonpathogenic" intestinal protozoa. *Infect Dis Clin North Am* 7:467–485, 1993

Badell Urdaneta A, et al: Intestinal amebiasis. *GEN* 29:125–151, 1975

Baker NM, Murray JA: Oesophageal obstruction due to an amoebic liver abscess. *Cent Afr J Med* 15:129–131, 1969

Balikian J, Uthman S, Khouri N: Intestinal amebiasis. A roentgen analysis of 19 cases, including 2 case reports. *AJR* 122:245–256, 1974

Balthazar EJ: Disorders of the appendix. In: Gore RM, Levine MC, Laufer I (eds) *Textbook of gastrointestinal radiology*. Saunders, Philadelphia, 1994, pp 1310–1341

Barnes PF, De Cock KM, Reynolds TN, Ralls PW: A comparison of amebic and pyogenic abscess of the liver. *Medicine* 66:472–483, 1987

Bautista O, Farril J, Guarner V, Baz-Diaz Lombardo G: Cirugia de la amibiasis invasora. *Arch Invest Med (Mex)* 2:437–444, 1971 (suppl 1)

Becker GL Jr, Knep S, Lance KP, Kaufman L: Amebic abscess of the brain. *Neurosurgery* 6:192–194, 1980

Berry M, Bazaz R, Bhargava S: Amebic liver abscess: sonographic diagnosis and management. *J Clin Ultrasound* 14:239–242, 1986

Bhargava S, Tandon PL, Sant MS, Gujral MS: Amoebic cervicitis masquerading as carcinoma cervix. *Indian J Pathol Microbiol* 29:382, 1986

Bhasin AS, Mittal KP, Shrivastava PN, et al: Resolution time of amoebic liver abscess by micro-opaque barium sulphate. *J Trop Med Hyg* 80:169–172, 1977

Bhoumik A: Amoebic infection of the female genital organs with a report of a case. *Indian Med Gaz* 86:355–357, 1951

Bia FJ, Barry M: Parasitic infections of the central nervous system. *Neurol Clin* 4:171–206, 1986

Blackett K: Amebic pericarditis. *Int J Cardiol* 21:183, 1988

Blumencranz H, Kasen L, Romeu J, Waye JD, LeLeiko NS: The role of endoscopy in suspected amebiasis. *Am J Gastroenterol* 78:15–18, 1983

Blyth DF, Pirie D: Haematogenous (amoebic) lung abscess. *S Afr Med J* 52:147–148, 1978

Bos HJ, et al: Serodiagnosis in amoebiasis [abstract]. *Trop Geogr Med* 29:204, 1977

Bruckner DA: Amebiasis. *Clin Microbiol Rev* 5:356–369, 1992

Bucco G: Localization of *Entamoeba histolytica* in the urinary tract. *Arch Ital Sci Med Trop Parasitol* 31:477–500, 1950

Bunnag TS, et al: Percutaneous splenic portography in amebic liver abscess. *Am J Roentgenol* 80:324–329, 1958

Caballero SA, Viveros RM, Salvatierra B, et al: Seroepidemiology of amebiasis in Mexico. *Am J Trop Med Hyg* 50:412–419, 1994

Cain GD, et al: Extensive stenosis of the colon and fistula formation following amoebic dysentery. *Gastroenterology* 61:898–900, 1971

Callicott JH, et al: Meningoencephalitis due to amebiasis. *JAMA* 206:579–582, 1968

Campbell S: Amebic brain abscess and meningoencephalitis. *Semin Neurol* 13:153–160, 1993

Cardoso JM, Kimura K, Stoopen M, et al: Radiology of invasive amebiasis of the colon. *AJR* 128:935–941, 1977

Cardoso M, et al: Detection of hepatic amebic abscesses by infusion tomography. *Gastrointest Radiol* 3:181–183, 1978

Caroline DF, Evers K: Colitis: Radiographic features and differentiation of idiopathic inflammatory bowel disease. *Radiol Clin North Am* 25:47–66, 1987

Carrillo N, Viloria A: Liver abscess. Diagnosis by the method of opacification. *GEN* 31:157–163, 1977

Carter B, Jones CP, Thomas WL: Invasion of squamous cell carcinoma of the cervix uteri by *Entamoeba histolytica*. *Am J Obstet Gynecol* 68:1607, 1954

Carter RF: Primary amoebic meningo-encephalitis: clinical, pathological and epidemiological features of six fatal cases. *J Pathol Bacteriol* 96:1–25, 1968

Carter RF: Primary amebic meningoencephalitis. An appraisal of present knowledge. *Trans R Soc Trop Med Hyg* 66:193–213, 1972

Cauron A, et al: Scanning of the hepatic blood pool in liver amebiasis. *Am J Roentgenol* 117:373–379, 1973

Cerva L, Novak K: Amoebic meningo-encephalitis. Sixteen fatalities. *Science* 160:92–96, 1968

Cervantes LF, Sanchez ME, Santillan JM: Tratamiento medico del ameboma del ciego y colon ascendente. *Arch Invest Med (Mex)* 2:427–436, 1971 (suppl 1)

Chadee K, Meerovitch E: *Entamoeba histolytica:* early progressive pathology in the cecum of the gerbil (*Merines unguiculatus*). *Am J Trop Med Hyg* 34:283, 1985

Chakravarti A: Pulmonary amoebiasis. *J Indian Med Assoc* 21:387–395, 1952

Chaves FJ, Cruz I, Gomes L, et al: Hepatic amebiasis-analysis of 56 cases. II. Laboratory and chest x-ray findings. *Am J Gastroenterol* 68:273–277, 1977

Chun D, Chandrosoma P, Kiyabu M: Fulminant amebic colitis: A morphologic study of four cases. *Dis Colon Rectum* 37:535–539, 1994

Citronberg RJ, Semel JD: Severe vaginal infection with *Entamoeba histolytica* in a woman who recently returned from Mexico: Case report and review. *Clin Infect Dis* 20:700–702, 1995

Cockshott WP, Braband H: Amebiasis. In: Rigler LG (ed) *Roentgen diagnosis,* 2nd edn. Grune & Stratton, New York, 1969, vol 3, pp 628–633

Cockshott P, Middlemiss H: *Clinical radiology in the tropics.* Churchill Livingstone, Edinburgh, 1979

Cohen C: Three cases of amoebiasis of the cervix uteri. *J Obstet Gynecol Br Commonwealth* 80:476, 1973

Connor DH, Neafie RC, Meyers WM: Amebiasis. In: Binford CH, Connor DH (eds) *Pathology of tropical and extraordinary diseases.* Armed Forces Institute of Pathology, Washington, DC, 1976, pp 308–316

Conter RL, Pitt HA, Tompkins RK, Longmire WP Jr: Differentiation of pyogenic from amebic hepatic abscesses. *Surg Gynecol Obstet* 162:114–120, 1986

Crawford AR: A case of amebiasis in early infancy. *J Pathol Bacteriol* 96:222–226, 1968

Cummins AS, Moody AH, Laloo K, et al: Rapid latex agglutination test for intraluminal amebiasis. *J Clin Pathol* 47:647–664, 1994

Dahnert W: *Radiology review manual, 3rd edn.* Williams & Wilkins, Baltimore, 1996, p 561

Dalrymple RB, Fataar S, Goodman A, et al: Hyperechoic amoebic liver abscesses: an unusual ultrasonic appearance. *Clin Radiol* 33:541–543, 1982

Daniels AC, Childress ME: Pleuropulmonary amebiasis. *Calif Med* 85:369–375, 1956

Das P, Pal S, Pal SC: Evaluation of the micro enzyme-linked immunosorbent assay, indirect hemagglutination and indirect fluorescence antibody techniques for serodiagnosis of amebiasis. *J Diar Dis Res* 2:238–242, 1984

Davey WW: *Companion to surgery in Africa.* E & S Livingstone, Edinburgh, 1968, pp 247–256

Davis A, Pawlowski ZS: Amoebiasis and its control. *Bull World Health Organ* 63:417–426, 1985

D'Cruz IA, Ramamoorthy K: Amoebic pericarditis. *J Indian Med Assoc* 49:342–343, 1967

De Silva PCC: Amoebiasis in infancy. *Br Med J* 2:1208, 1949

De Villiers JP, Durra G: Case report: amoebic abscess of the brain. *Clin Radiol* 53:307–309, 1998

Dietz R, Schanen G, Kramann B, Erpelding J: Intracranial amebic abscess: CT and MR findings. *J Comput Assist Tomogr* 15:168–170, 1991

Druckmann A, Schorr S: The roentgenological manifestation of amebiasis of the large intestine. *Am J Roentgenol* 54:145–148, 1945

Edington GM, Gilles HM: *Pathology in the tropics, 2nd edn.* Williams & Wilkins Co, Baltimore, 1976, pp 64–78

Elechi EN, Etawo US: Chest complications of amoebic liver abscess: a report of six cases from Nigeria. *East Afr Med J* 71:189–192, 1994

Elizondo G, Weissleder R, Stark DD, et al: Amebic liver abscess: diagnosis and treatment evaluation with MR imaging. *Radiology* 165:795–800, 1987

Escandon RC, Trevino N, Escobedo de la Pena J, et al: La amibiasis y el absceso hepatico amibiano en Mexico, un problema de salud publica de actualidad. *Rev Gastroenterol Mex* 61:378–386, 1996

Fadiran OA, Dare FO, Jeje EA, et al: Amoebic recto-vaginal fistula – a case report and review of literature [review]. *Cent Afr J Med* 39:172–175, 1993

Faegenburg D, Chiat H, Mandel PR, Ross ST: Toxic megacolon in amebic colitis: report of a case. *Am J Roentgenol* 99:74–76, 1967

Farid Z, Trabolsi B, Kilpatrick ME: Amoebic liver abscess presenting as fever of unknown origin (FUO). Serology, isotope scanning and metronidazole therapy in diagnosis and treatment. *J Trop Med Hyg* 85:255–258, 1982

Ferguson T, Burford T: Pleurobiliary and bronchobiliary fistulas. *Arch Surg* 95:380–386, 1967

Fishman EK, Kavuru M, Jones B, et al: Pseudomembranous colitis: CT evaluation of 26 cases. *Radiology* 180:57–60, 1991

Flores Barroeta F, Saavdra S, Velasco AF: Invasion de *Entamoeba histolytica* a diversos organos y tejidos en sujetos humanos. *Arch Invest Med (Mex)* 1:129–146, 1970 (supp 1)

Freeman O, Akamaguna A, Jarikre LN: Amoebic liver abscess: the effect of aspiration on the resolution or healing time. *Ann Trop Med Parasitol* 84:281–287, 1990

Ganayni GA, Attia RA, Naggar HM: Some immunological studies on amebiasis. *J Egypt Soc Parasitol* 24:357–362, 1994

Garcia Sainz M, Silva Arteaga R, Dela Huerta R: Amibiasis de organos genitales de ambos sexos. *Arch Invest Med (Mex)* 2:367–372, 1971 (suppl 1)

Gelfand M, Schnitzler MC: Amoebiasis in the African infant in Rhodesia. *J Trop Med Hyg* 69:144–146, 1966

Gendron Y, Talarmin FM, Simon P, et al: Hepatic amebiasis in French Polynesia. 16 cases in 2 years [French]. *Medecine Tropicale* 44:225–229, 1984

Geslien GE, Thrall JH, Johnson MC: Gallium scanning in acute hepatic amebic abscess. *J Nucl Med* 15:561–567, 1974

Ghosh P, Maneilla R, Ortiz L: Intestinal amebiasis: histopathologic features in experimentally infected mice. *Arch Med Res* 25:297–302, 1994

Gibney EJ: Amoebic liver abscess [review]. *Br J Surg* 77:843–844, 1990

Giorgio A, Amoroso P, Francica G, et al: Echo-guided percutaneous puncture: a safe and valuable therapeutic tool for amebic liver abscess. *GI Rad* 13:336–340, 1988

Godinez C, Quijano M, Jurado J, et al: Tratamiento quirurgico de la colitis amibiana fulminante. *Arch Invest Med (Mex)* 1:237–246, 1970 (suppl 1)

Goldman M: Evaluation of a fluorescent antibody test for amebiasis. *Am J Trop Med Hyg* 15:694–700, 1966

Gonzalez Montesinos F, Lee Ramos AF, Aguirre Garcia J: Influencia del sexo y la edad en la amibiasis invasora del higado. *Arch Invest Med (Mex)* 2:395–400, 1971 (suppl 1)

Gonzalez Ruiz A, Haque R, Rehman T, et al: Further diagnostic use of an invasive-specific monoclonal antibody against *Entamoeba histolytica. Arch Med Res* 23:281–283, 1992

Gordon F, Cuaron A, Munoz R, et al: Avances en la centelleografia hepatica. *Arch Invest Med (Mex)* 5:525–530, 1974 (suppl 2)

Guarner V, Jurado J, Baz-Diaz Lombardo G, et al: Tifloappendicitis amibiana. *Arch Invest Med (Mex)* 1:217, 1970 (suppl 1)

Guarner V: Tratamiento de la parasitosis producida por *Entamoeba histolytica*. In: Kretschmer RR (ed) *Amibiasis. Infeccion y Enfermedad por Entamoeba histolytica*. Editorial Trillas, Mexico, 1994, pp 261–281

Gupta RK, Pant CS, Prakash R, et al: Sonography in complicated hepatic amoebic abscess. *Clin Radiol* 38:123–126, 1987

Gutierrez G: Epidemiologia y control de la amibiasis en Mexico. *Arch Invest Med (Mex)* 17:375, 1986 (suppl 1)

Gutierrez G: Aspectos clinicos de la amibiasis invasora en los ninos. *Arch Invest Med (Mex)* 1:349, 1991 (suppl 2)

Gutierrez G, Munoz O: Epidemiologia de la amibiasis. In: Kretschmer RR (ed) Amibiasis. *Infeccion y Enfermedad por Entamoeba histolytica*. Editorial Trillas, Mexico, 1994, pp 207–225

Haque R, Kress K, Wood S, et al: Diagnosis of pathogenic *Entamoeba histolytica* infection using a stool ELISA based on monoclonal antibodies to the galactose-specific adhesin. *J Infect Dis* 167:247–249, 1993

Harding T, Lewis EA, Bohrer SP: Intra-cavitary barium sulphate in the assessment of amoebic liver abscess. *Clin Radiol* 22:68–73, 1970

Hardy R, Scullen DR: Thumbprinting in a case of amebiasis. *Radiology* 98:147–148, 1971

Hayden CK Jr, Toups M, Swischuk LE, Amparo EG: Sonographic features of hepatic amebiasis in childhood. *JCAR* 35:279–282, 1984

Healy GR: Serology. In: Ravdin JI (ed) *Amebiasis: human infection by Entamoeba histolytica*. Churchill Livingstone, New York, 1988, pp 650–653

Heinz KPW: Amoebic infection of the female genital tract-report of 3 cases. *S Afr Med J* 47:1795, 1973

Hernandez LF, Arredondo F, Prado J, et al: Absceso cerebral amibiano, informe de un paciente. *Rev Mex Radiol* 44:75–79, 1990

Hill MC, Goldberg HI: Roentgen diagnosis of intestinal amebiasis. *Am J Roentgenol* 99:77–83, 1967

Hingorani V, Mahapatra LH: Amebiasis of vagina and cervix. *J Int Coll Surg* 42:662–667, 1964

Hussain S, Dinshaw H: Ultrasonography in amebic colitis. *J Ultrasound Med* 9:385–388, 1990

Ibarra Perez C: Thoracic complications of amebic abscess of the liver. *Chest* 79:672–677, 1981

Ibrahim MS, et al: Detection of amoebic liver abscess by isotope scanning. *Br Med J* 1:1325–1328, 1963

Isaac F: Roentgen findings in amebic disease of the liver. *Radiology* 45:581–587, 1945

Islam N: A case of giant amoebic liver abscess. *J Trop Med Hyg* 70:68–73, 1967

Juimo AG, Gervez F, Angwafo FF: Extraintestinal amebiasis. *Radiology* 182:181–183, 1992

Juniper K Jr: Acute amebic colitis. *Am J Med* 33:377–386, 1962

Kasliwal RM, et al: Significance of the complement fixation text in diagnosis of amoebiasis in endemic area. *Br Med J* 1:837–838, 1966

Kean BH, Gilmore HR, Van Stone WW: Fatal amebiasis: report of 148 fatal cases from the Armed Forces Institute of Pathology. *Ann Intern Med* 44:831–843, 1956

Ken JG, van Sonnenberg E, Casola G, et al: Perforated amebic liver abscesses: successful percutaneous treatment. *Radiology* 170:195–197, 1989

Kessel JF, Lewis WP, Molina P, Turner JA: Indirect hemagglutination and complement fixation tests in amebiasis. *Am J Trop Med Hyg* 14:540–550, 1965

Kimura K, Stoopen M, Vazquez Saavedra J, et al: Estudio sobre los signos ultrasonograficos y la evolucion del absceso hepatico amibiano en 100 pacientes. *Rev Mex Radiol* 34:29–34, 1981

Kimura K, Stoopen M, Reeder MM, Moncada R: Amebiasis: modern diagnostic imaging with pathological and clinical correlation. *Semin Roentgenol* 32:250–275, 1997

Knigh TR: Survey for amebiasis: interpretation of data and their implications. *Ann Trop Med Parasitol* 69:35, 1975

Kolawole TM, Lewis EA: Radiologic observations on intestinal amebiasis. *Radiology* 122:257–265, 1974

Kretschmer RR, Lopez OM: Mecanismos efectores e immunidad amibiana. In: Kretschmer RR (ed) *Amibiasis. Infeccion y Enfermedad por Entamoeba histolytica*. Editorial Trillas, Mexico, 1994, pp 135–154

Krishnamoorthy P, Thomas K, Mathew O: Pulmonary amoebiasis. *Indian Pediatr* 4:195–197, 1967

Krogstad DJ, et al: Current concepts in parasitology. *N Engl J Med* 298:262, 1978

Krogstad DJ, Spencer H, Healy G, et al: Amebiasis: epidemiologic studies in the United States, 1971–1974. *Ann Intern Med* 88:89–97, 1978

Krogstad DJ: Isoenzyme patterns and pathogenicity in amoebic infection. *N Engl J Med* 315–390, 1986

Lam AH, de Silva M, Procopis P, Kan A: Primary amoebic (*Naegleria*) meningoencephalitis. *JCAT* 6:620–623, 1982

Landa L, Stoopen M, Aguirre Garcia J, et al: La ictericia en la amibiasis invasora del higado. *Arch Invest Med (Mex)* 5:531–540, 1974 (suppl 2)

Lawless, Knight V: Human infection with *Entamoeba polecki*. *Am J Trop Med Hyg* 15:701–704, 1966

Lecuna Torres V: Selective abdominal arteriography in the diagnosis of amebic liver abscess. *GEN* 29:153–167, 1975

Leder RA, Low VH: Tuberculosis of the abdomen. *Radiol Clin North Am* 33:691–705, 1995

Leonetti P, Moncany G, Soubeyrand J: Amebic abscess of the liver. Contribution of ultrasonics to developmental diagnosis apropos of 983 cases [French]. *J Radiol* 68:259–264, 1987

Le Roux BT: Pleuro-pulmonary amebiasis. *Thorax* 24:91–101, 1969

Levine SM, Stover JF, Warren JG, et al: Ameboma forgotten granuloma. *JAMA* 215:1461–1464, 1971

Lewis EA, Antia AU: Amoebic colitis: review of 295 cases. *Trans R Soc Trop Med Hyg* 63:633–638, 1969

Lewis EA, Antia AU: Amoebic liver abscess: a review of 113 cases. *West Afr Med J* 19:111–114, 1970

Limbos P, De Bergeyck E: Visualisation of the amoebic abscess of the liver with perfusion of diatrizoates (author's transl). *Acta Gastroenterol Belg* 40:159–166, 1977

Lombardo L, Alonso P, Saenz-Arroyo L, et al: Cerebral amebiasis-report of 17 cases. *J Neurosurg* 21:704–708, 1964

Lombardo L, Flores-Barroeta F: Amibiasis invasora cerebral. *Arch Invest Med (Mex)* 2:361–366, 1971 (suppl 1)

Luterman L, Alsumait AR, Daly DS, Goresky CA: Colonoscopic features of cecal amebomas. *Gastrointest Endosc* 31:204–206, 1985

Luvuno FM, Mitshali Z, Baker L: Toxic dilatation complicating fulminating amebic colitis. *Br J Surg* 69:56, 1982

Luvuno FM, Mitshali Z, Baker LW: Vascular occlusion in the pathogenesis of complicated amoebic colitis: evidence for an hypothesis. *Br J Surg* 72:123–127, 1985

Luvuno FM: Role of adhesive wraps in the pathogenesis of complicated amoebic colitis. *Br J Surg* 75:713–716, 1988

Lyche KD, Jensen WA, Kirsch CM, et al: Pleuropulmonary manifestations of hepatic amebiasis. *West J Med* 153:275–278, 1990

Ma P, Visvesvara GS, Martinez AJ: Naegleria and acanthamoeba infections: review. *Rev Infect Dis* 12:490–513, 1990

Majmudar B, Chaiken ML, Lee KU: Amebiasis of clitoris mimicking carcinoma. *JAMA* 236:1145, 1976

Martinez AJ, Sotelo-Avia C, Garcia-Tamayo J, et al: Meningoencephalitis due to *Acanthamoeba* sp: pathogenesis and clinico-pathological study. *Acta Neuropathol* 37:183–191, 1977

Martinez ER, Gilman R, Rabboni GH, et al: Amebic colitis: correlation of proctoscopy before treatment and barium enema after treatment. *AJR* 138:1089–1093, 1982

Martinez Baez M: Es la amibiasis una enfermedad tropical? *Arch Inv Med (Mex)* 2:161–164, 1971 (suppl 1)

Martinez Garcia M, Castro D, Armenta M, et al: Caracteristicas del absceso hepatico amibiano en un hospital rural del Altiplano Mexicano. *Arch Invest Med (Mex)* 17:351, 1986 (suppl 1)

Martinez Palomo A, Tsutsumi V, Anaya Velazquez F, et al: Ultrastructure of experimental intestinal invasive amebiasis. *Am J Trop Med Hyg* 41:273–279, 1989

Martinez Palomo A: Biologia de la *Entamoeba histolytica*. In: Martinez Palomo A (ed) *Amibiasis*. Ed Med Panamericana, Mexico, 1989, pp 17–410

Matsui T, Iida M, Tada S, et al: The value of double-contrast barium enema in amebic colitis. *Gastrointest Radiol* 14:73–78, 1989

McClatchie S, Sambhi JS: Amoebiasis of the cervix uteri. *Ann Trop Med Parasitol* 65:207, 1971

McKerrow JH: Pathogenesis in amebiasis: Is it genetic or acquired? *Infectious Agents and Disease* 1:11–14, 1992

Menon NK: Roentgenographic appearance of hepatopulmonary amebiasis. *Dis Chest* 46:219–222, 1964

Merten DF, Kirks DR: Amebic liver abscess in children: role of diagnostic imging. *AJR* 143:1325–1329, 1984

Messersmith RN, Chase GJ: Amebiasis presenting as multiple apple core lesions. *Am J Gastroenterology* 79:238–241, 1984

Middlemiss JH: Gastrointestinal parasites. In: Margulis AR, Burhenne HG (eds) *Alimentary tract roentgenology, 2nd edn*. Mosby, St. Louis, 1973, pp 1557–1574

Mills AE, Goldsmid JM: *Entamoeba histolytica*. In: Doerr W, Seifert G (eds) *Tropical Pathology, 2nd edn*. Springer, Berlin Heidelberg New York, 1995, pp 488–513

Mirelman D, Bralma R, Chayen A: *Entamoeba histolytica:* effect of growth conditions and bacterial associates on isoenzymes patterns and virulence. *Exp Parasitol* 62:142–148, 1986

Mirelman D: Ameba-bacterium relationship in amebiasis. *Microbiol Rev* 51:272–284, 1987

Moldwin RM: Sexually transmitted protozoal infections. *Trichomonas vaginalis, Entamoeba histolytica,* and *Giardia lamblia. Urol Clin North Am* 19:93–101, 1992

Morajkar RB, Menon PS, Wagh SS, et al: Left sided pleuropulmonary amebiasis, probably primary. *J Assoc Physicians India* 33:744, 1985

Munguia M, et al: Genital amebiasis. *Am J Obstet Gynecol* 94:181–183, 1966

Munoz O: Espectro clinico de la amibiasis en ninos. In: Kretschmer RR (ed) *Amibiasis. Infeccion y Enfermedad por Entamoeba histolytica*. Editorial Trillas, Mexico, 1994, pp 247–259

Myers HS, Cremin BJ: Clinical x-ray quiz. *Mod Med (South Africa)* 2:47–48, 1977

Myung K, Burch P, Jackson T, et al: Serodiagnosis of invasive amebiasis using a recombinant *E. histolytica* antigen-based ELISA. *Arch Med Res* 23:285–288, 1992

Nadler S, Cappell MS, Bhatt B, et al: Appendiceal infection by *Entamoeba histolytica* and *Strongyloides stercoralis* presenting like acute appendicitis. *Dig Dis Sci* 35:603–608, 1990

Nagar H: Surgical aspects of parasitic disease in childhood. *J Pediatr Surg* 22:325–331, 1987

Naidoo PM, Keeton G, Stein L, et al: Hepatic amoebiasis. A study of 32 cases in the Western Cape. *S Afr Med J* 48:1159–1160, 1974

Nanda R, Baveja B, Anand BS: *Entamoeba histolytica* cyst passers: clinical features and outcome in untreated patients. *Lancet* II:301, 1984

Nordestgaard AG, Stapleford L, Worthen N, et al: Contemporary management of amebic liver abscess. *Am Surg* 58:315–320, 1992

Nushan H, Miller B: Ameboma of the transverse colon. *Ann Intern Med* 37:372–379, 1952

Okuda K, Kanda Y, Fukuyama Y, et al: Spontaneous hepatobronchial communications preceding pyothorax in a patient with suspected liver abscess. *Gastroenterology* 65:124–126, 1973

Olatunbosun DA: Amoebiasis and its complications in Nigerian children: (a necropsy survey). *Trans R Soc Trop Med Hyg* 59:72–79, 1965

Oleszczuk-Raszke K, Cremin BJ, Fisher RM, et al: Ultrasonic features of pyogenic and amoebic hepatic abscesses. *Pediatr Radiol* 19:230–233, 1989

Orozco E: Pathogenesis in amebiasis (commentary). *Infectious Agents and Disease* 1:19–21, 1992

Pacheco CR: Complications toracicas del absceso hepatico amibiano. *Revista de la Facultad de Medicina (Mexico)* 13:25–37, 1970

Patra SB, Shukla GN, Giri DD, Mehta HS: Amoebic granuloma- an unusual cause of caeco-colic intussusception. *Postgrad Med J* 60:168–170, 1984

Perez Tamayo R, et al: Amoebiasis. In: Marcial-Rojas RA (ed) *Pathology of protozoal and helminthic diseases*. Williams & Wilkins, Baltimore, 1971, pp 145–188

Perez Tamayo R: Patologia de la amibiasis. In: Martinez-Palomo A (ed) *Amibiasis*. Ed Med Panamericana, Mexico, 1989, pp 42–78

Perez Tamayo R, Martinez RD, Montford I, et al: Pathogenesis of acute experimental amebic liver abscess in hamsters. *J Parasitol* 77:982–988, 1991

Perez Tamayo R: Fenomenos iniciales en la amibiasis hepatica experimental. *Rev Gastroenterol Mex* 59:62, 1994 (suppl 2)

Perez Tamayo R, Becker I, Montfort I, Perez Montfort R: Patobiologia de la amibiasis. In: Kretschmer RR (ed) *Amibiasis. Infeccion y Enfermedad por Entamoeba histolytica.* Editorial Trillas, Mexico, 1994, pp 155–187

Petri WA Jr, Clark CG, Diamond LS: Host-parasite relationships in amebiasis: conference report. *J Infect Dis* 169:483–484, 1994

Phillips SC, Mildvan D, William DC, et al: Sexual transmission of enteric protozoa and helminths in a venereal disease clinic population. *N Engl J Med* 305:603–606, 1981

Pittman FE, et al: Studies of human amebiasis. *Gastroenterology* 65:581, 1973

Pittman FE, Pittman JC, El-Hashimi WK: Studies of human amebiasis. III. Ameboma: a radiologic manifestation of amebic colitis. *Am J Digest Dis* 18:1025–1031, 1973

Pomerantz BM, Marr JS, Goldman WD: Amebiasis in New York City, 1958–1978: identification of the male homosexual high risk population. *Bull NY Acad Med* 56:232–244, 1980

Prado GA, Perez AN, Zavala B: Differential diagnosis of nonspecific and amebic ulcerative colitis. *Dis Colon Rectum* 15:147–149, 1972

Prado Vertiz A, Silva MC: Amibiasis en el nino. *Panorama Gac Med Mex* 103:287, 1972

Radin DR, Ralls PW, Colletti PM, Halls JM: CT of amebic liver abscess. *AJR* 150:1297–1301, 1988

Radke RA: Ameboma of the intestine: an analysis of 78 collected and 41 previously unreported cases. *Ann Intern Med* 43:1048–1066, 1955

Ralls PW, Henley DS, Colletti PM, et al: Amebic liver abscess: MR imaging. *Radiology* 165:801–804, 1987

Ralls PW, Barnes PF, Radin DR, et al: Sonographic features of amebic and pyogenic liver abscesses: a blinded comparison. *AJR* 149:499–501, 1987

Ralls PW, Barnes PF, Johnson M, et al: Medical treatment of hepatic amebic abscess: rare need of percutaneous drainage. *Radiology* 165:805–807, 1987

Ralls PW, Colletti P, Quinn M, et al: Sonographic findings in hepatic amebic abscess. *Radiology* 145:123–126, 1992

Ralls PW, Quinn MF, Boswell WD Jr, et al: Patterns of resolution in successfully treated hepatic amebic abscess: sonographic evaluation. *Radiology* 149:541–543, 1993

Ramachandran S, Goonatillake HD, Perera MV: Radiological surveillance in amoebic liver abscess. *J Trop Med Hyg* 78:133–134, 1975

Ramani A, Ramani R, Kumar MS, et al: Ultrasound-guided needle aspiration of amoebic liver abscess. *Postgrad Med J* 69:381–383, 1993

Ravdin JI: *Entamoeba histolytica* from adherence to enteropathy. *J Infect Dis* 159:420, 1989

Recio PM: Ameboma of the colon. *Dis Colon Rectum* 8:205–209, 1965

Reeder MM, Hamilton LC: Radiologic diagnosis of tropical diseases of the gastrointestinal tract. *Radiol Clin North Am* 7:57–81, 1969

Reeder MM: Tropical diseases of the liver and bile ducts. Semin Roentgenol 10:229–243, 1975

Reeder MM: *Gamuts in radiology, 3rd edn.* Springer, New York Berlin Heidelberg, 1994

Reeder MM, Palmer PES: Infections and infestations. In: Freeny PC, Stevens GW (eds) *Alimentary tract radiology, 5th edn.* Mosby, St. Louis, 1997, pp 888–951

Reeder MM, Glick S: Infectious colitis. In: Taveras J, Ferrucci J (eds) *Radiology.* Lippincott, Philadelphia, 1999

Remedios PA, Colletti PM, Ralls PW: Hepatic amebic abscess: cholescintigraphic rim enhancement. *Radiology* 160:395–398, 1986

Ridley DS, Warhurst DC: Misdiagnosis of amoebiasis. *Br Med J* 2:632, 1978

Roberts PP: Parasitic infections of the pleural space. *Semin Respir Infect* 3:362–382, 1988

Robinson AS, Levinson M: Amebic appendicitis associated with hepatic abscess. *Southern Med J* 77:1047–1048, 1984

Rojman JA, Korsten MA: Clinical spectrum of amebic colitis [Spanish]. *Acta Gastroenterol Latinoam* 13:733–739, 1983

Roudaut M, Tiendrebeogo H, Condat JM, et al: Pleuropulmonary manifestations in amebiasis. Sixty-one cases seen in Abidjan over a three-year period (author's transl) [French]. *Semaine des Hopitaux* 58:85–92, 1982

Roy DC, Ravindron P, Padmanabhan R: Bronchobiliary fistula secondary to amebic liver abscess. *Chest* 62:523–524, 1972

Ruiz-Moreno F: Amebic granuloma of the colon and the rectum. *Dis Colon Rectum* 6:201–205, 1963

Ruiz-Moreno F: Perianal skin amoebiasis. *Dis Colon Rectum* 10:65–69, 1967

Salako LA: Liver function tests in the diagnosis of hepatic amoebiasis. *J Trop Med Hyg* 70:19–22, 1967

Samuel E: Radiologic diagnosis of chronic amebic colitis. *Br J Radiol* 21:625–631, 1948

Saraswat VA, Agarwal DK, Baijal SS, et al: Percutaneous catheter drainage of amoebic liver abscess. *Clin Radiol* 45:187–189, 1992

Sargeant PG, Williams JE, Green JD: The differentiation of invasive and non invasive *E. histolytica* by isoenzyme electrophoresis. *Trans R Soc Trop Med Hyg* 72:519–521, 1978

Savitch I, Esser JD, Krige LP, et al: The use of technetium-99m-di-isopropyl - iminodiacetic acid imaging in the demonstration of a biliary-bronchial fistula. *S Afr Med J* 65:779–780, 1984

Schmidt AG: Plain film roentgen diagnosis of amebic hepatic abscess. *Am J Roentgenol* 107:47–50, 1969

Schumacher DJ, Tien RD, Lane K: Neuroimaging findings in rare amebic infections of the central nervous system [review]. *Am J Neuroradiol* 16 (suppl):930–935, 1995

Sepulveda B: La amibiasis invasora por *Entamoeba histolytica. Gac Med Mex* 100:201–254, 1970

Sepulveda B, Martinez Palomo A: Amebiasis. In: Warren KS (ed) *Tropical and geographical medicine.* McGraw Hill, New York, 1984, p 305

Shaff BL, Wolfowitz J: Enterocolic amoebic fistulae. *Br J Surg* 49:535–538, 1962

Sharma OP, Maheshwari A: Lung diseases in the tropics, Part 2. Common tropical lung diseases: diagnosis and management. *Tuber Lung Dis* 74:359–370, 1993

Sheehy TW, et al: Resolution time of an amebic liver abscess. *Gastroenterology* 55:26–34, 1968

Shih WJ, Reba RC, Tu YC, Yeh SH: Discordant ^{99m}Tc sulfur colloid and ^{113m}In chloride blood pool images in patients with acute amebic liver abscess. *Clin Nucl Med* 8:312–314, 1983

Sigler Morales, Mier y Diaz J, Melgoza Oritz C, et al: Amebiasis. Surgical treatment in 1989. *Rev Gastroenterol Mex* 54:185–189, 1989

Simjee AE, Patel A, Gathiram V, et al: Serial ultrasound in amoebic liver abscess. *Clin Radiol* 36:61–68, 1985

Smart MJ: Acute amebic dysentery - the radiological changes. *J Can Assoc Radiol* 13:95–99, 1962

Solan K: Amoebic pericarditis. Clinical meeting. *Proc Mine Med Off Assoc* 6:20, 1965

Stable GI, Irving HC, Simmons AB, et al: Case report: Hepatobronchial fistula complicating amoebiasis, treated by percutaneous catheter drainage. *Clin Radiol* 44:354–356, 1991

Stoopen M, Casal R, Elizondo L, et al: Las alteraciones angiograficas del abscesso hepatico amibiano estudio de 60 casos. *Rev Mex Radiol* 23:9–22, 1969

Stoopen M, et al: Utilidad de la angiografia en el diagnostico del absceso hepatico amibiano. *Arch Invest Med (Mex)* I (suppl):173–186, 1970

Stoopen M, Elizondo L, Landa L: Estado actual del diagnostico radiologico en la amibiasis. *Arch Invest Med (Mex)* 3:387–402, 1972 (suppl 2)

Stoopen M, Cervantes LF, Kawashima K, et al: Revision de la colitis amibiana cronica. *Arch Invest Med (Mex)* 4:211–216, 1973 (suppl 1)

Stoopen M, Hori S, Diaz Lopez A, et al: Evaluacion de la utilidad de la tomografia computada en el diagnostico del absceso hepatico (informe preliminar). *Rev Gastroenterol Mex* 44:239, 1979

Stoopen M, Kimura K: Le tecnologia de los ochentas: Ultrasonido, tomografia computada y resonancia magnetica han contribuido a mejorar el diagnostico del abscesso hepatico? *Rev Gastroenterol Mex* 54:167–175, 1989

Stoopen M, Kimura K, Cardoso M: Imagenologia del absceso hepatico amibiano: "Veinte anos despues". *Rev Mex Radiol* 45:165–171, 1991

Strang JI: Two-dimensional echocardiography in the diagnosis of amoebic pericarditis. A case report. *South Afr Med J* 71:328–329, 1987

Subramanyam BR, Balthazar EJ, Raghavendra BN, et al: Ultrasound analysis of solid-appearing abscesses. *Radiology* 146:487–491, 1983

Taneton K, et al: The study of hepatic amebiasis by radioactive rose bengal scanning of the liver. *Am J Trop Med Hyg* 15:16–21, 1966

Tannich E: Pathogenesis in Amebiasis. *Infectious Agents and Disease* 1:22–23, 1992

Tay J, Ruiz A, Schione H, et al: Frecuencia de la protozoosis intestinales en la Republica mexicana. *Bol Chil Parasitol* 49:9–15, 1944

Tchang S: Amebiasis in northern Saskatchewan: radiological aspects. *Can Med Assoc J* 99:688–695, 1968

Thomas JEP: Cutaneous amebiasis due to liver abscess. *Cent Afr J Med* 18:190–192, 1972

Thomas JA, Antony AJ: Amebiasis of the penis. *Br J Urol* 48:269, 1976

Tikly M, Denath FM, Hodkinson HJ, Saffer D: Computed tomographic findings in amoebic brain abscess. *S Afr Med J* 73:258–259, 1988

Trevino Garcia-Manzo N, Escandon RC, Escobedo de la Pena J, et al: Amebiasis in epidemiologic transition in Mexico: its morbidity and mortality trends in the Mexican Institute of Social Security. *Arch Med Res* 25:393–399, 1994

Trevino Garcia-Manzo N: Espectro clinico de la amibiasis en adultos. In: Kretschmer RR (ed) *Amibiasis. Infeccion y Enfermedad por Entamoeba histolytica.* Editorial Trillas, Mexico, 1994, pp 227–245

Tsutsumi V, Mena Lopez R, Anaya Velazquez F, et al: Cellular bases of experimental amebic liver abscess formation. *Am J Pathol* 117:8, 1984

Tsutsumi V, Martinez Palomo A: Inflammatory reaction in experimental hepatic amebiasis. An ultrastructural study. *Am J Pathol* 130:112–119, 1988

Ungar BLP, Yolken RH, Quin TC: Use of a monoclonal antibody in an enzyme immunoassay for the detection of *Entamoeba histolytica* in fecal specimens. *Am J Trop Med Hyg* 34:465–472, 1985

Varadarajan MG: Amoeboma of the large intestine. *Punjab Med J* 12:169–175, 1962

Veliath AJ, Bansal R, Sankaran V, et al: Genital amebiasis. *Int J Gynecol Obstet* 25:249–256, 1987

Venkataramaiah NR, Reinaerts HHM, Van Raalte JA, Shaba JK: Pseudomalignant cutaneous amoebiasis. *Tropical Doctor* 12:162, 1982

Verma RC, Ngo C, Yaghmai I: Patterns of gallium uptake in amebic liver abscesses. *Clin Nucl Med* 14:523–525, 1989

Villegas Gonzalez J, Naranjo Hernandez C, Aleman Velazquez P, et al: Amibiasis invasora cerebral en el nino. *Arch Invest Med (Mex)* 2:313–320, 1971 (suppl1)

Viranuvatti V, Chearanai O, Damrongsak C, et al: Selective coeliac angiography in amebic liver abscess. *J Med Assoc Thai* 60:35–38, 1977

Vogel H, Gonzales ER, Pekanan P, et al: Roentgen findings in amebiasis of the large intestine [German]. *Röntgenpraxis* 36:242–245, 1983

Wagner-Manslau C, Reiser M, Lukas P: Computertomographische Befunde bei der Amebiasis [German]. Radiologe 25:597–598, 1985

Walsh JA: Problems in recognition and diagnosis of amebiasis. Estimation of the global magnitude of morbility and mortality. *Rev Infect Dis* 8:228, 1986

Webster BH: Pleuropneumonic amebiasis. *Am Rev Respir Dis* 81:683–688, 1960

Weinfeld A: Roentgen appearance of intestinal amebiasis. *Am J Roentgenol* 96:311–322, 1966

Wruble LD, et al: Toxic dilatation of the colon in a case of amebiasis. *N Engl J Med* 75:926–928, 1966

2 Schistosomiasis

Schistosomiasis is one of the most protean diseases suffered by man. It was known to the Pharaohs over 5000 years ago. The presence of species of snails in Paleolithic sites in Africa, capable of carrying the immature stages of the parasite, raises the possibility of an even older history. The ancient Egyptians recognized the malady causing "the bloody urine and stools" and knew that it was caused by worms. It now infects about 200 million people throughout the tropical world and its literature is vast and complex describing many aspects of the disease in many languages. Bilharz first described the etiology in 1851, but it was not until 1913 that Myairi recognized the snail as the intermediate host. It was many years later, in 1957, that schistosomiasis was first described in Southeast Asia. The Mekongi subspecies was not accepted until 1978. It is truly a continuing modern plague, yet the life cycle of this blood fluke is such that the adoption of simple but strict hygiene would probably eradicate the disease within a generation. Surveying the subject, one must wonder both at man's failure to rid himself of this affliction and at his ability to live with it.

Synonyms

Schistosomiasis: Bilharzia. Bilharziasis. Katayama disease. Kin Kiang fever. Egyptian splenomegaly. Cercarial dermatitis. Swimmer's itch. Collector's itch. Dew itch. Sawah itch. Snail fever. Yangtze fever. Koganbyo. Clam digger's itch. Kichocho. Haemic distomiasis.
Schistosomiasis haematobium: *Sp:* Esquistosomiasis urinaria. Hematuria de Egypto. Hematuria de los paisos calidos. *Fr:* Schistosomiase urinaire. Bilharziose. Hematurie du Cap. *Ger:* Blasenbilharziose.
Schistosomiasis mansoni: *Sp:* Esquistosomiasis intestinal. *Fr:* Schistosomiase intestinale. *Ger:* Darmbilharziose.
Schistosomiasis japonica: *Sp:* Esquistosomiasis japonesa. *Fr:* Schistosomiase japonaise. *Ger:* Schistosomiasis japonica.

Definition

Schistosomiasis is an infection with parasitic blood flukes (worms) which are digenetic trematodes, schistosomatidae. Four species regularly affect man: *S. haematobium, S. mansoni, S. japonicum,* and *S. intercalatum.* Four more have limited geographic distribution: *S. mattheei, S. mekongi, S. incognitum,* and *S. rodhaini.* Within these species there are some strains, such as the Formosan strain of *S. japonicum,* which live for only a short period within man and may fail to reach maturity. There are other species, normally parasites of cattle or birds (zoonotic), which also occasionally infect man but do not usually cause significant symptoms or radiological changes. However, they can confuse laboratory tests. When they do rarely cause symptoms, the illness is less severe.

Geographic Distribution

The World Health Organization estimates that at least 200 million people are infected with schistosomiasis and 400 million more are at risk in at least 76 countries. It is second only to malaria as a cause of morbidity and mortality from parasites.
The importance of schistosomiasis is shown by a 1997 survey of an island on Lake Victoria, Tanzania. Eighty-six percent of 1695 villagers on the island were infected with *S. mansoni,* with children and adolescents being at highest risk. Forty-three percent of those infected had suffered from bloody diarrhea in the 2 weeks before the survey. The later stages of the infection, such as periportal fibrosis, were rare.
The disease is found naturally in other primates, such as baboons and chimpanzees in Africa and monkeys such as the capuchin, marmoset, and macaque in South America and the West Indies. *S. mansoni* parasitizes wild rodents in Africa and South America. *S. japonicum* parasitizes about 40 species of mammals, including water buffalo, cattle, horses, pigs, dogs, cats, rodents, and goats. It is generally agreed that the animal hosts of *S. japoni-*

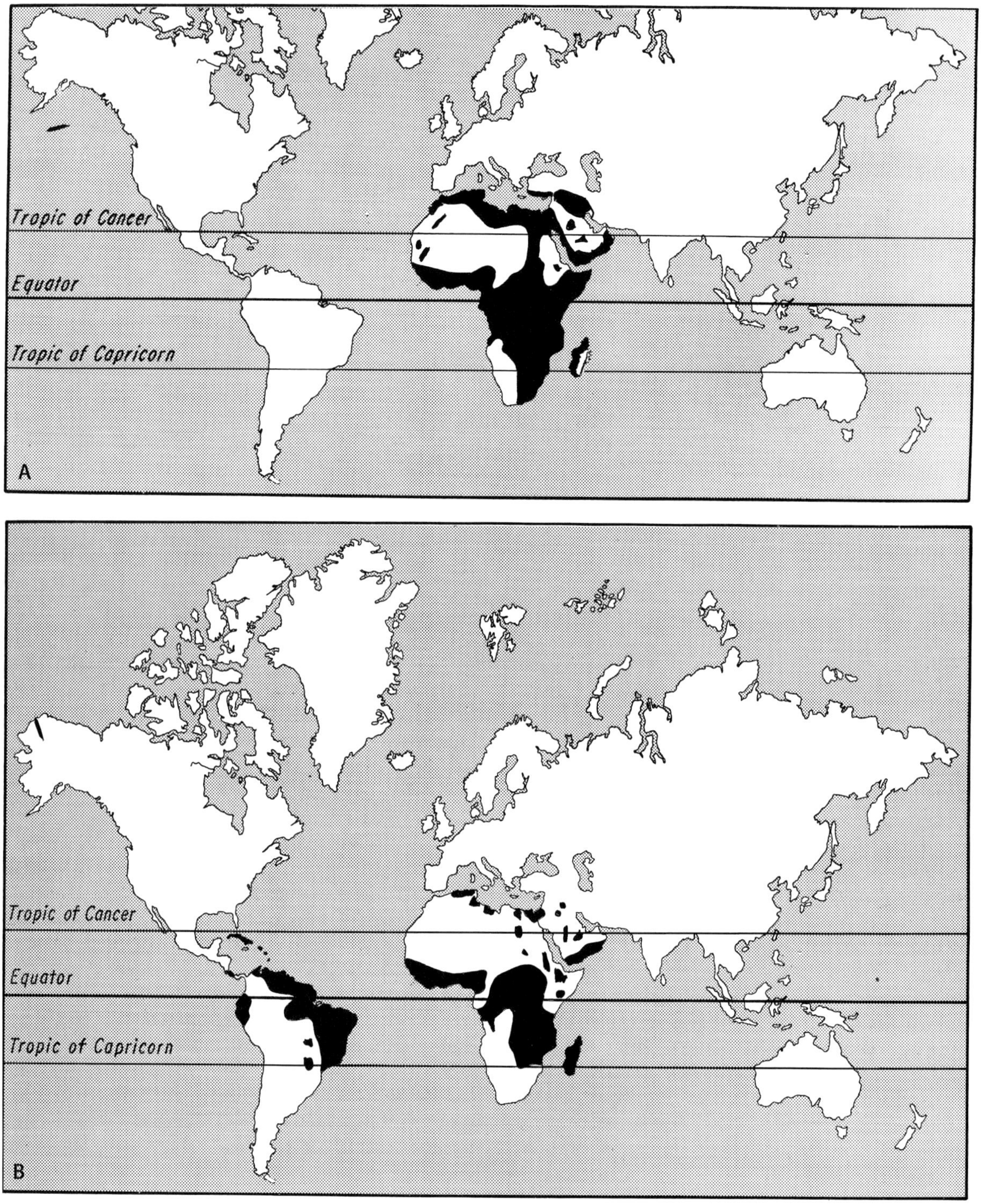

Fig. 2.1. **A** Geographic distribution of *S. haematobium*. **B** Geographic distribution of *S. mansoni*. **C** see p. 111

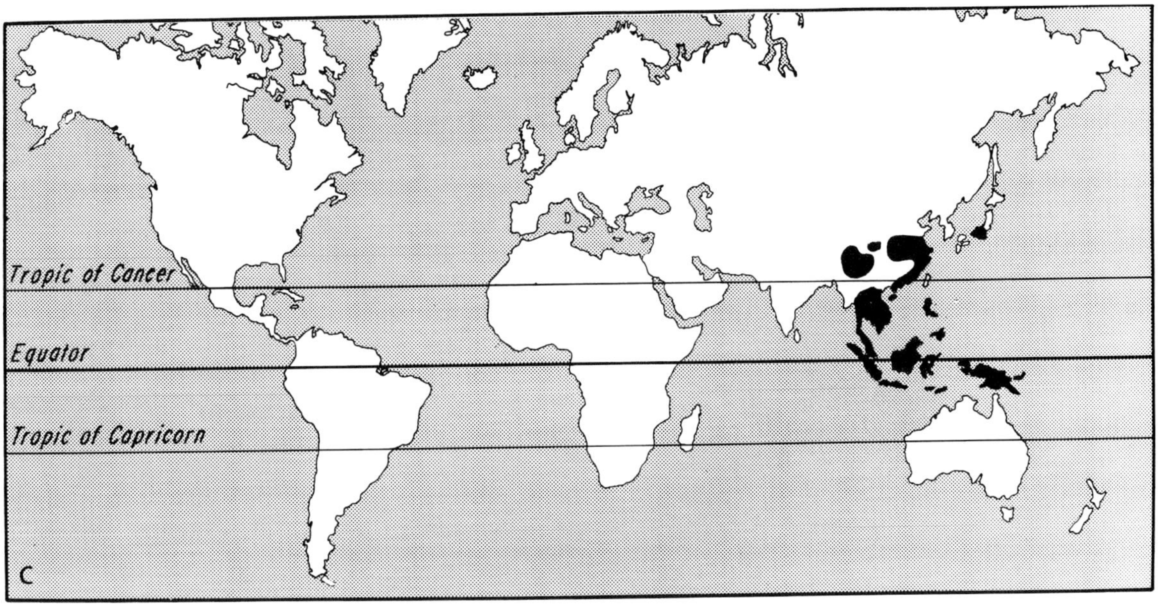

Fig. 2.1 (*continued*). C Geographic distribution of *S. japonicum*

cum have significance to humans as reservoirs of the disease, but their importance in containing the infection varies regionally.

S. haematobium occurs throughout Africa, on the islands of Madagascar and Mauritius, around the southern shores of the Mediterranean, and in the Middle East, including Turkey (Fig. 2.1 A). It primarily involves the urinary tract and the portal system, but can affect the colon and lungs as well.

S. mansoni is prevalent throughout Africa, especially in the north, and is also endemic in Arabia, the northern part of South America, Puerto Rico, and other islands of the Caribbean (Fig. 2.1 B). It was imported into the New World via the slave trade. It affects primarily the colon, portal system, and lungs.

S. japonicum occurs in the coastal and river areas of China, particularly the Yangtze Basin and the Shanghai River, Japan, Taiwan, the Philippines, Celebes, and other western Pacific islands; it is found in isolated areas of Cambodia, Thailand, Laos, and Myanmar (Burma) (Fig. 2.1 C). It primarily affects the colon, small bowel, portal system, and lungs, but it may be found in the urinary tract.

S. mekongi is found in the Mekong Delta, and in Laos, Cambodia, and Thailand.

S. intercalatum is found only in the Democratic Republic of Congo and equatorial Africa, including Gabon, Cameroon, Chad, Guinea, and the Central African Republic. It affects primarily the digestive tract and the portal system.

S. mattheei is found in southern Africa (South Africa and Zimbabwe). *S. incognitum* is found in India, and *S. rodhaini* in the Democratic Republic of Congo. Not all authorities agree that these are of significance for human infection.

There is considerable overlap in distribution and combined infections are common, especially with *S. haemotobium* and *S. mansoni.* Despite this, *S. japonicum* probably affects the largest number of people because of the density of population within its geographic area.

Owing to immigration, there are thousands of Puerto Ricans and other immigrants in New York and other American cities who harbor *S. mansoni* or other schistosomes. Similar immigrant pockets of schistosomal infection exist in many other nontropical countries, especially in major cities. Members of the Armed Forces, other travelers and members of organizations such as the Peace Corps and relief workers are all at risk.

In many parts of the world, schistosomiasis is almost a "normal" part of human existence, reinfection is usual, and many of the effects of the disease are not regarded as abnormal by the local populace.

Epidemiology and Pathology

Although there are variations between the species of worms which infect man, there is a common pattern. The adults do not multiply in man, are long lived (3–30 years), and produce large numbers of eggs. Because of repeated reinfection, the worm burden tends to increase, and the immunity given by the initial exposure is not complete. Many of the

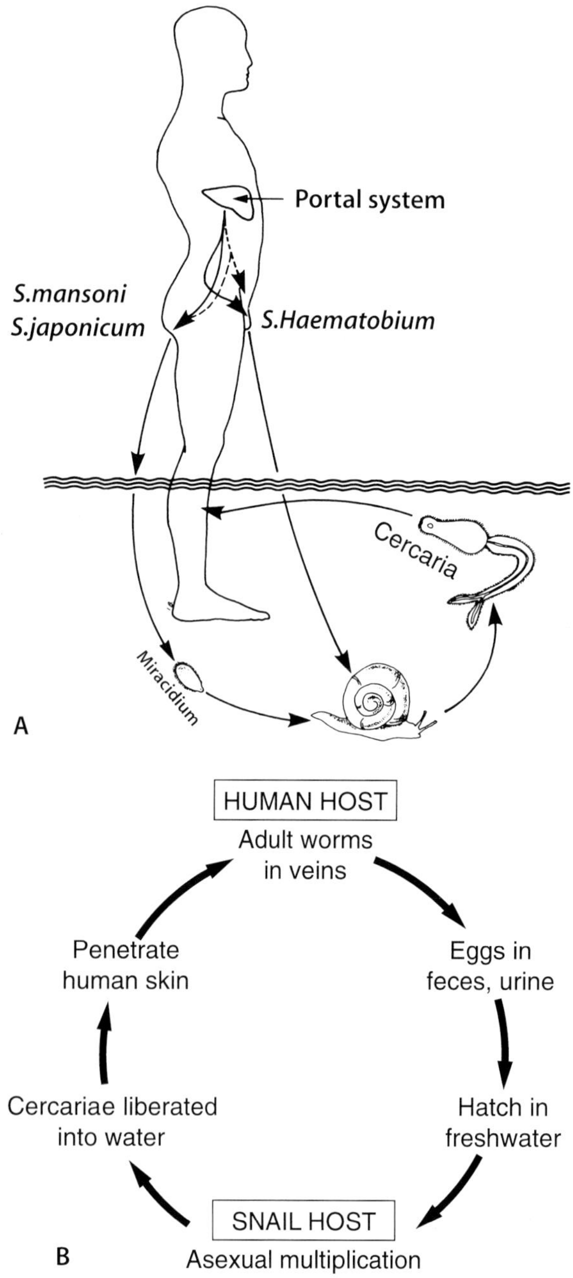

Fig. 2.2 A, B. The life cycle of the schistosomes (bilharzia)

eggs remain embedded in human tissues and organs and the ill health of infected persons represents the total combination of reactions to the parasites and the eggs (Fig. 2.2), varying with the anatomical site, the individual response of the host, and the intensity of the infection. The clinical disease in particular reflects the acuteness or chronicity of the infection and whether there are few or many worms.

Schistosomiasis is primarily an infection of the vascular system, from where it spreads to damage multiple organs. The worms (blood flukes) live and copulate in the portal vein and its mesenteric tributaries or, for *S. haematobium*, in the vesicle plexus of veins. The adult worms are strictly intravenous parasites, attached to the wall of the vein by two suckers (Fig. 2.3 C). The female spends much of her life in the male gynecophoral cleft and they migrate together along the vessel wall, against the bloodstream, with the aid of their suckers. Some worms, however, lose their hold and become emboli.

The male worm is shorter and wider than the female (Fig. 2.3 A, B). The species vary in size but are in the range of 16 mm×0.75 mm for the male and 25 mm×0.3 mm for the female. The female leaves the male after copulation and migrates further upstream (retrograde) to reach the smallest venule possible. There the eggs are deposited. The various species have different egg-laying capacities, which have been estimated to be as high as 3500 eggs per day in the case of *S. japonicum* and a mere 300 eggs per day in the case of *S. mansoni*. Within the individual species, the substrains vary also. For example, the South African and Tanzanian strains of *S. mansoni* produce far fewer eggs than similar species of the same schistosome in Egypt and Brazil.

Each species has a preferential site for depositing its eggs, although unexpected distribution can occur: The eggs of *S. haematobium* are usually deposited in the wall of the urinary bladder or ureters. The eggs of *S. mansoni* are usually deposited in the rectum or large intestine. The eggs of *S. japonicum* are usually deposited in the small intestine, the proximal large bowel, or the rectum. However, it is not unusual for the eggs of *S. haematobium* to be in the walls of the bowel, and the eggs of *S. mansoni* or *S. japonicum* are occasionally found in the bladder.

Eggs of all species are oval, and vary in size from 120 to 60 μm. All eggs have a spine by which they become fixed in the tissues (Fig. 2.4), although whether this is the function or purpose of the spine is unknown. *S. haematobium* has a narrow, finely tapered terminal spine, whereas *S. mansoni* has a thick lateral spine, about 20 μm long. The spine of *S. japonicum* is very small and may not be seen. The shells of *S. haematobium* eggs are not acid-fast, while those of *S. mansoni* are; this helps to distinguish the eggs in tissue sections. There are other

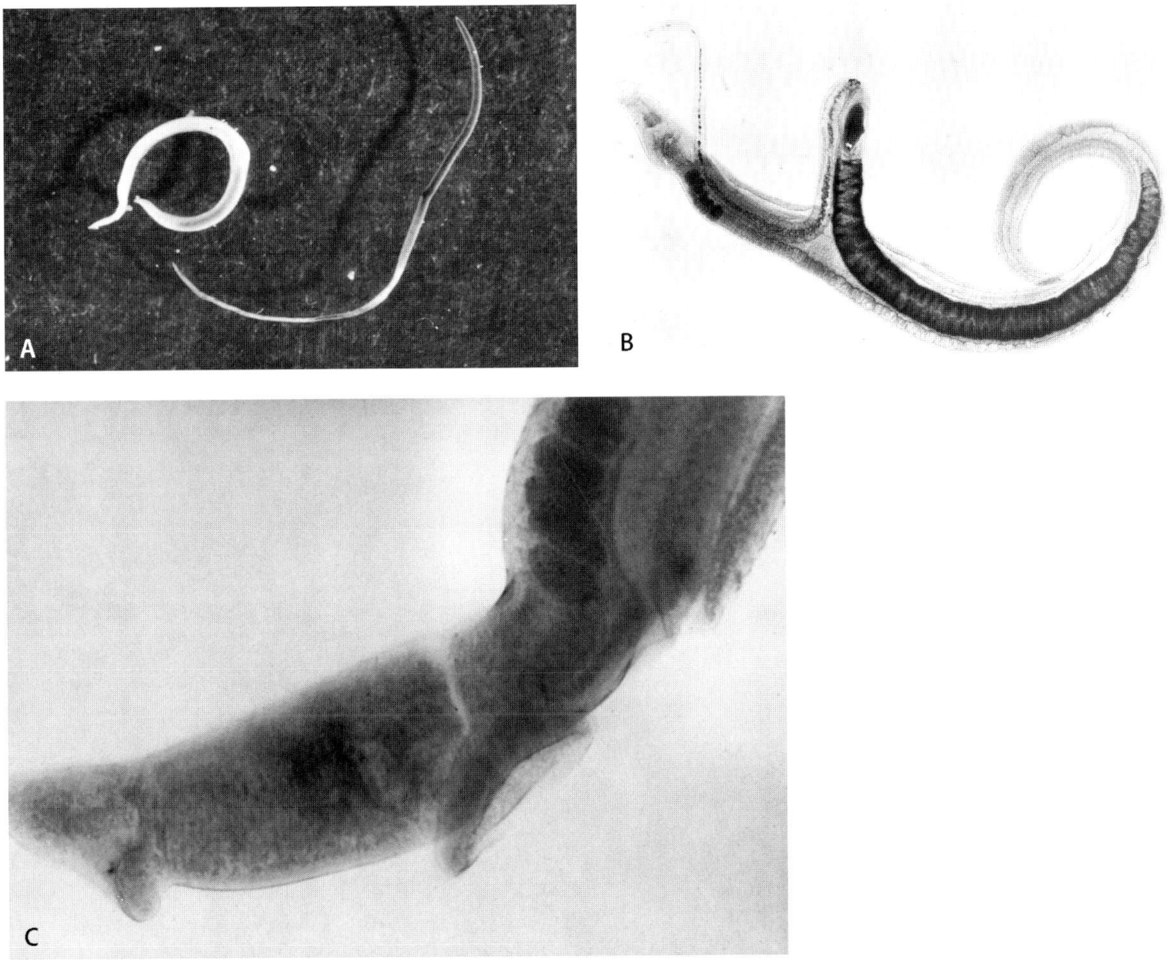

Fig. 2.3. A Adult *Schistosoma mansoni* flukes: the shorter, wider male is on the left with the longer, more slender female on the right. B Male and female *S. japonicum* worms copulating. The longer female lies in the gynecophoral canal of the male. C The sucker near the end of the male *S. mansoni* by which it attaches itself to the wall of the vein in the portal system. The dark testes can be seen above the beginning of the gynecophoral canal, on the right

schistosome eggs with terminal spines, e.g., *S. mattheei*, which are very common in cattle in the tropics (92% of cattle at slaughter in Zimbabwe). They may be recovered from both the stools and urine of man, and accurate identification is essential because they seldom cause clinical symptoms.

The shell of the schistosome egg consists of chitin and, when mature, each egg contains an embryo called a micracidium. Two possible fates await the eggs:

1. They may fail to attach to the wall of the capillaries and become emboli, traveling and lodging almost anywhere in the body. Many accumulate in the liver, but if there is already portal hypertension, with a collateral circulation, the eggs may be carried to the lungs, brain, and other organs. They provoke the production of discrete granulomas in which the eggs are trapped and incarcerated: eventually they disintegrate and phagocytes remove their contents. The granulomas heals, forming a nodular scar within which are the calcified remnants of the eggs and shells. Granuloma formation is initiated by the alpha tumor necrotizing factor, and the higher the alpha factor, the more granulomas are produced. Unencapsulated eggs do not stimulate granuloma formation, but secrete a toxin which causes severe liver damage. The acute syndrome (Katayama disease, pp. 122–124) is the result of the circulating immune complexes, not a reaction to mature worms or eggs.

The extent of the tissue reaction depends on many factors, including host genetics, allergy, load of infestation, and repetitive infections; but, whatever the reaction, the result is fibrosis. When this occurs in a vessel, especially in the lungs, there is blockage with damage, to both the intima and the wall. A

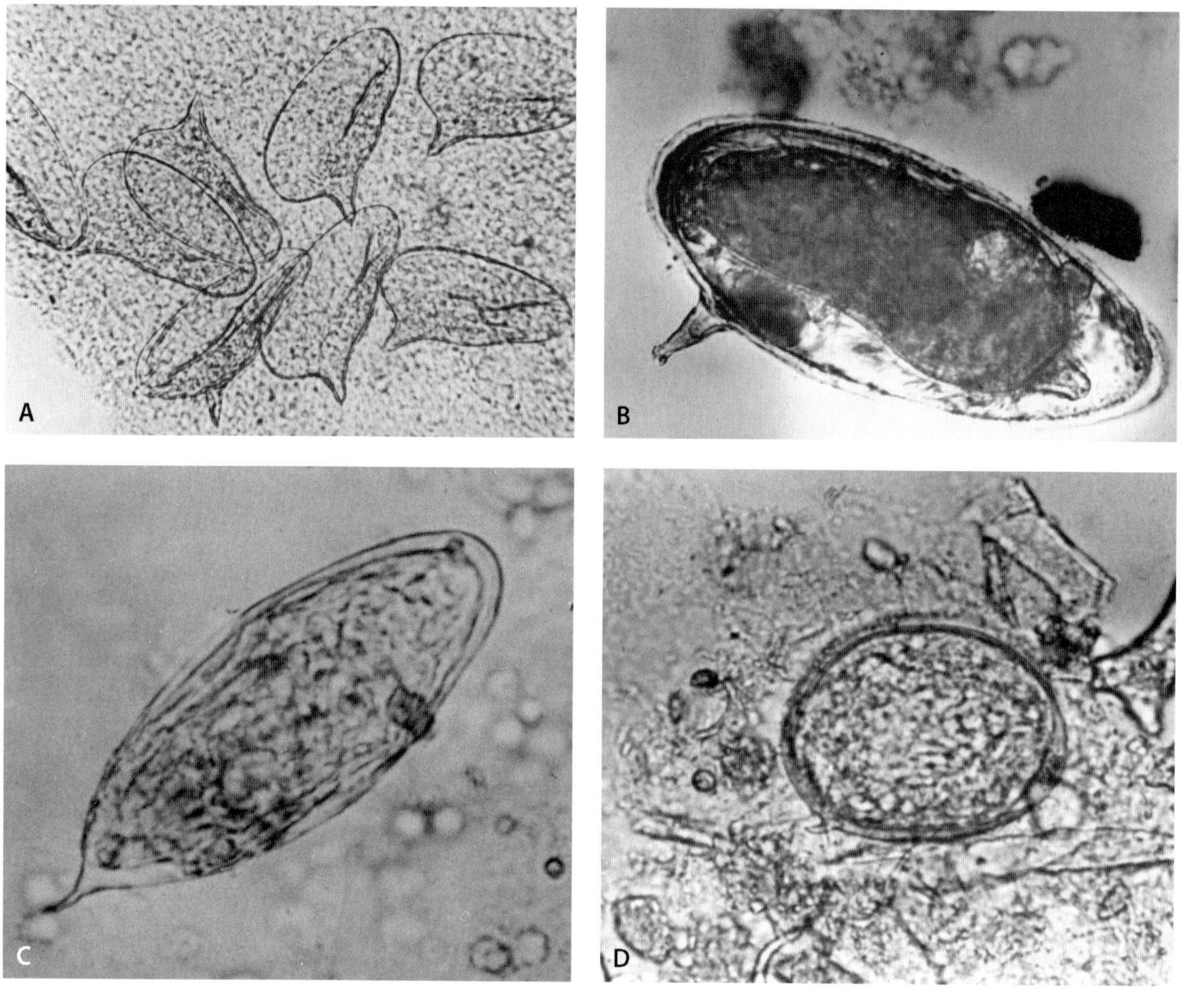

Fig. 2.4 A–D. The three main species of schistosomes. **A** Multiple eggs of *S. mansoni* (press preparation from a colon biopsy). **B** Single eggs of *S. mansoni* from a stool specimen, showing the prominent lateral spine. (Stained with iodine; courtesy of Barbara Drake, Hackensack) **C** An *S. haematobium* egg with a short terminal spine, seen in a urine specimen. **D** An *S. japonicum* egg in stool, showing a tiny lateral spine. (Courtesy of John Hall)

dumbbell-shaped granuloma develops which eventually recanalizes to form small arteriovenous fistulas and sometimes aneurysms. These are the angiomatoids which are characteristic of pulmonary schistosomiasis (see p. 118, Figs. 2.59–2.61). Elsewhere the progressive fibrosis, combined with obliterative endarteritis, causes the urinary, bowel, or hepatic changes of chronic schistosomiasis.

Dead worms embolizing to the liver and elsewhere, especially during treatment (or for other reasons), may also initiate inflammatory and fibrotic reactions; thus granulomas can be caused by dead worms, as well as by eggs.

Solitary granulomas may be large enough to produce symptoms, which will depend on the anatomical location. The granulomas in the spinal cord may lead to paraplegia, or in the colon, resemble an ameboma or carcinoma. Schistosome papillomas within mucosa represent a similar hyperplastic granulomatous reaction and can be found in the colon, bladder, and cervix or body of the uterus. No organ escapes, not even the heart.

Another type of reaction may form around a few eggs and is mainly allergic. There is infiltration by lymphocytes, plasma cells, and large numbers of eosinophils. The vessels become dilated and congested and the lymph nodes enlarged. The severity of such allergic reactions depends on the load of infection and on repeated infection: allergic reactions are responsible for the "acute phase" which is seen clinically.

The diffuse effects of schistosomiasis may also be caused in large part by allergy. Repeated infections also enhance the immune response, so that more eggs are trapped in the tissues and larger granulomas are formed around each egg. The diet of the in-

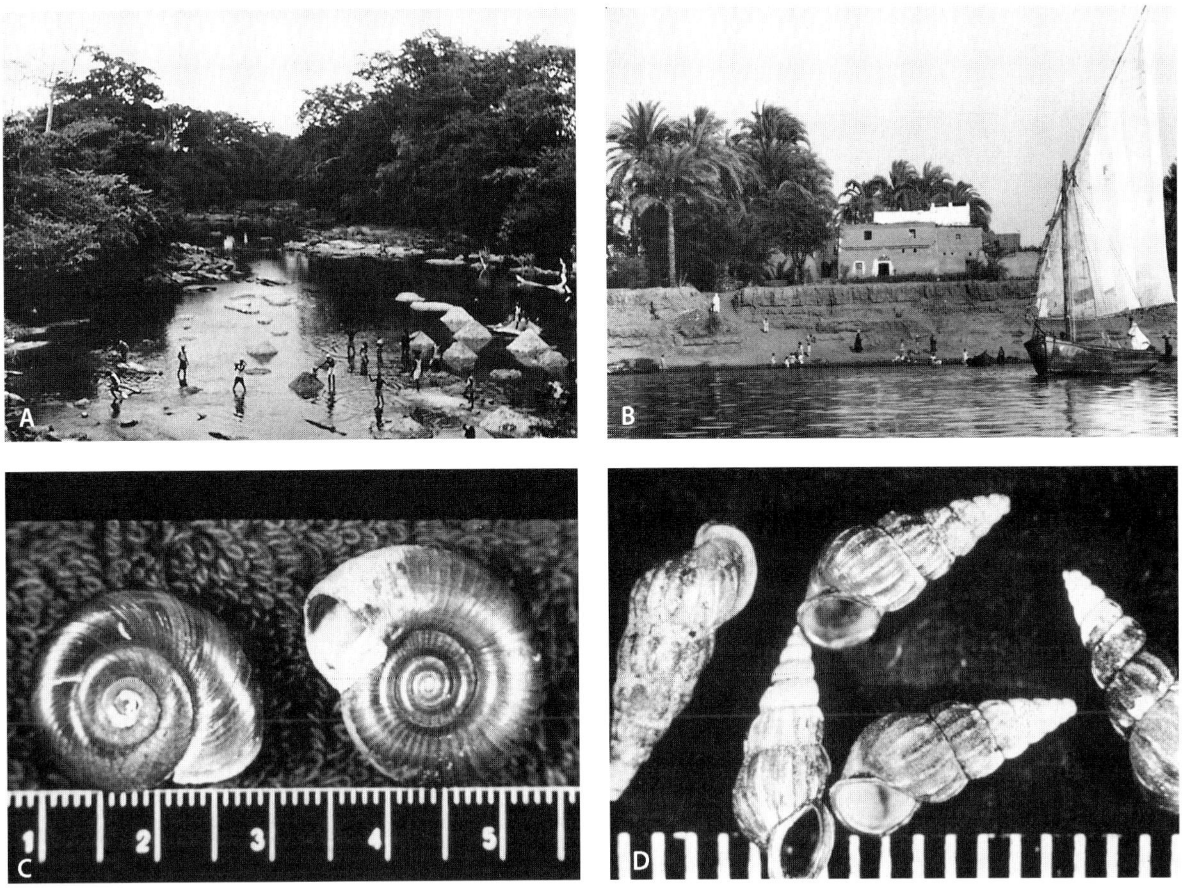

Fig. 2.5 A–D. Slowly moving fresh water in the tropics is the major source of schistosomiasis. **A** A West African river with villagers gathering sand, washing clothes and becoming infected. **B** The Egyptian Nile, source of life...and death. **C** The shells of *Australorbis glabratus* snails (*Biomphalaria* spp) from the island of Saint Lucia in the Caribbean. These snails are natural hosts for *S. mansoni*. **D** *Oncomelania* snails shells. These mollusks are intermediate hosts for *S. japonicum*

fected person influences the parasites, by affecting the defense mechanisms: low levels of vitamins D and C make the individual less resistant to schistosomal infection, but also make the ova abnormal.

2. The alternative is that the enclosed miracidium secretes an irritating lytic substance which produces an acute necrotizing arteriolitis. (There is a hypersensitivity element in this reaction.) In conjunction with mechanical forces related to peristaltic activity, the eggs then leave the host through the wall of the intestine or urinary tract by passing through the wall of a blood vessel. They escape into the lumen of the gut or urinary tract: if the miracidia lie deeper in the tissues, they produce tiny abscesses (sometimes referred to as "egg abscesses") which may rupture in the same way.

When the eggs have been released from the host and reach fresh water, they hatch and release the miracidia, which require a specific snail as their host (Fig. 2.5). The snails are found in slow-moving streams, especially in water which is used for irrigation, such as in paddy fields or sugar plantation, and (where endemic) in almost any open water, natural or artificial (Fig. 2.5). One of the difficulties in controlling schistosomiasis is that the snail eggs are transported in the feathers of water birds, and thus spread widely. The snails are sensitive to water temperature, altitude, and many other factors: for example, they are not infected by the miracidia if the water temperature is below 15 °C. The miracidia are attracted to the snails chemically and swim towards them at a rate of 7 m per minute. (The snail's pace is not recorded.) Each species requires a particular genus of snail (mollusk), usually one of the many species in the family Planorbidae, most commonly the genus *Biomphalaria* for *S. mansoni* and the genus *Bulinus* for *S. haematobium*. There are two other genera, *Planorbarius* and *Ferrissia*, which are of limited importance. In Asia the snails are species of *Oncomelania* and *Tricula*, the latter particularly acting as host for *S. mekongi*. Other freshwater snails serve as hosts for nonhuman schistosomes, contributing to schistosomal dermatitis (see p. 122). Each species need particular snails, but species have

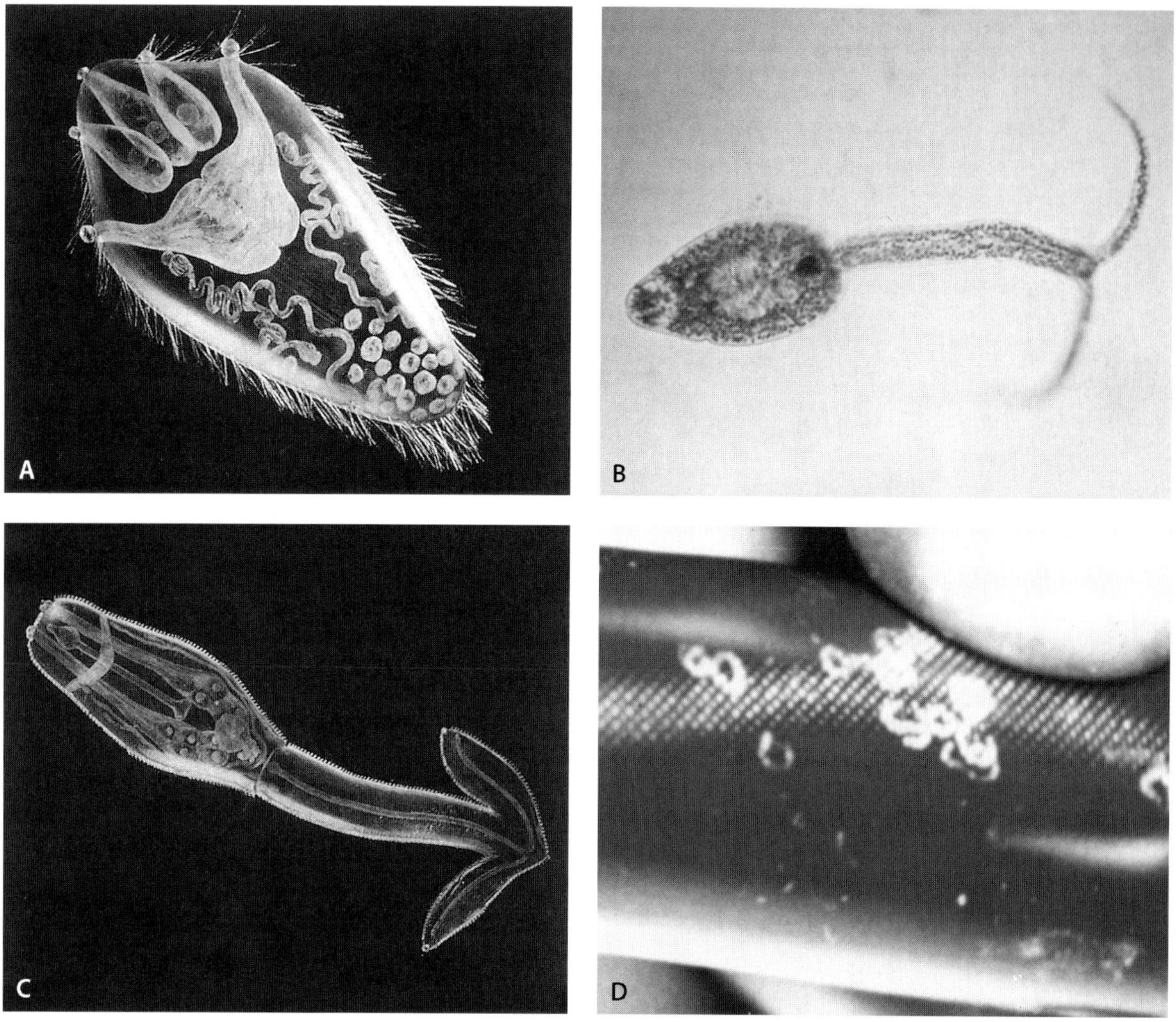

Fig. 2.6. **A** The recently hatched miracidium of a schistosome. ×1000; MIS 218934-42. **B** The fork-tailed cercaria which swims through water to penetrate the skin of man. **C** The fork-tailed cercaria of a schistosome. ×1000; MIS 218934-44. **D** Adult *S. japonicum* flukes trapped in a blood filter placed in the inferior vena cava of a patient with schistosomiasis. This is sometimes used as a way to reduce the adult worm population within the body. (**A**, **C** from Marty and Andersen 1995)

adapted to the local environment so that the host for *S. mansoni* in Africa is not the same as the snail which it inhabits in South America.

Some snails can survive out of water for weeks and, if infected, the sporocysts which develop from the miracidia can live with them. A maximum of 98 days has been recorded, but this will vary in different climates and conditions.

Within the snail, the miracidium develops into an adult sporocyst from which thousands of larval cercariae are released (Fig. 2.6). This release from the snail is stimulated and altered by many factors: for example, the snail releases *S. mansoni* as a response to light, usually about 2 hours after the stimulus. The total output is shed within 5 hours. Therefore, the risk of *S. mansoni* infection will be much less in the early morning and the late evening than between 10 a.m. and 2 p.m. *S. japonicum* is shed at night and different stimuli are involved for other species, as well as different time ratios.

The cercariae of *S. mansoni* and *S. haematobium* continually swim vertically upward in the water, then sink down to the bottom; those of *S. japonicum* remain just under the surface water film. Each cercaria has five pairs of glands and penetrates the skin of the host with a combination of lytic secretions and vibration, taking 3–5 minutes. This, too, may be affected by the environment of the cercaria, such as the quality and quantity of the water. In particular, a low concentration of heavy metal ions reduces the rate of penetration and the ability of the cercariae to mature. Penetration occurs through the

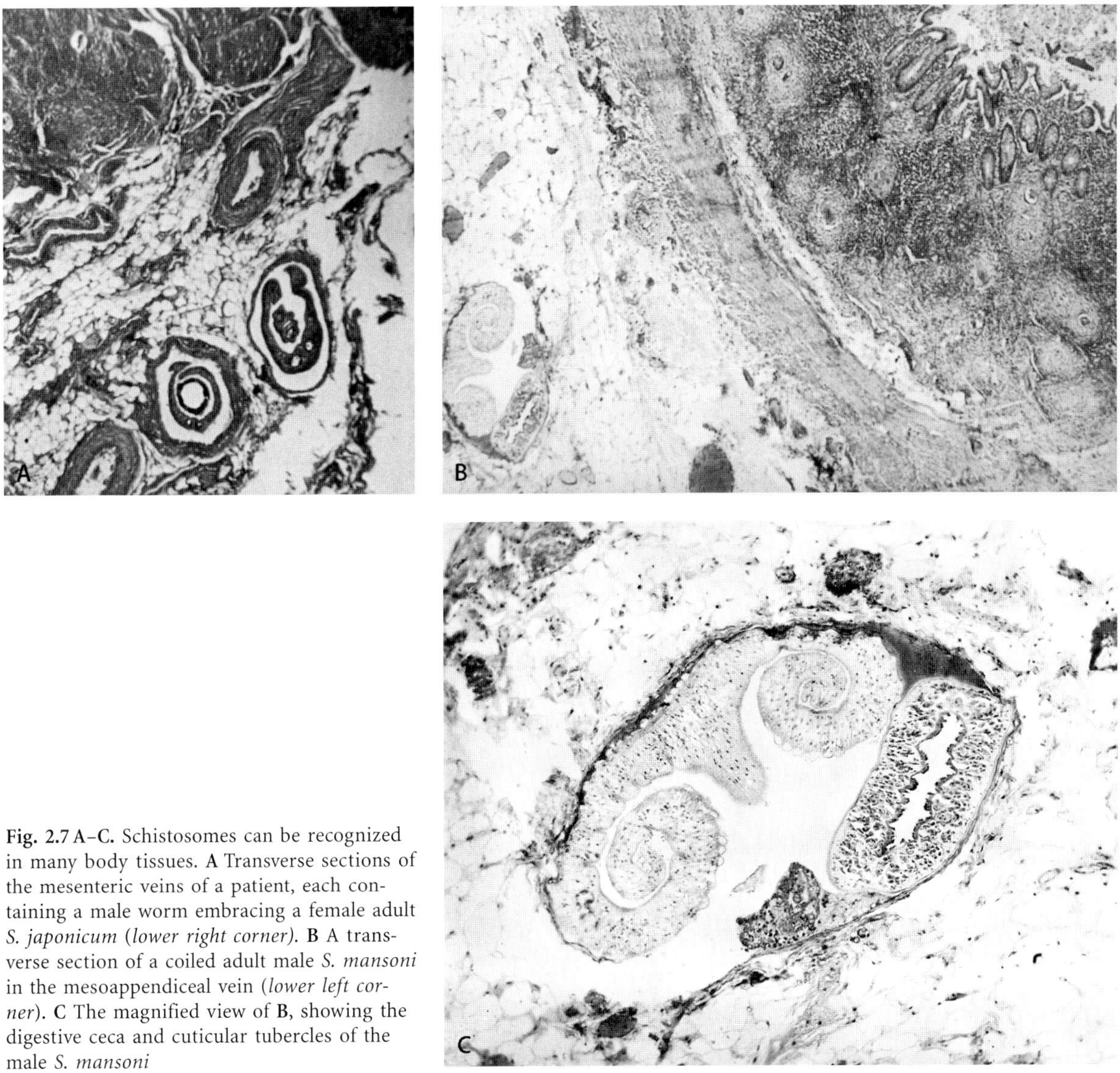

Fig. 2.7 A–C. Schistosomes can be recognized in many body tissues. **A** Transverse sections of the mesenteric veins of a patient, each containing a male worm embracing a female adult *S. japonicum* (*lower right corner*). **B** A transverse section of a coiled adult male *S. mansoni* in the mesoappendiceal vein (*lower left corner*). **C** The magnified view of **B**, showing the digestive ceca and cuticular tubercles of the male *S. mansoni*

skin or buccal mucous membrane, but cercaria which are swallowed are destroyed in the stomach.

After penetration, the larvae shed their tails and become schistosomula, then enter the lymphatics and pass through the thoracic duct into the right side of the heart; whether they also enter the veins after penetrating the skin is disputed. From the right heart they then travel through the lungs. If the capillary diameter is too small, the schistosomula can stretch the vessel to move through to the left side of the heart and via the mesenteric capillaries to the portal system and liver; this journey may take from 10 to 21 days. In the liver they mature and the "intestinal" species return in pairs to the portal system, where they may live for 30 years or more. Maturation can also occur in other organs, especially the lungs, but copulation is uncommon outside the liver. Vesicle plexus schistosomes apparently reach the vesicle veins by collateral circulation.

Adult schistosomes, while alive in the veins, do not cause any inflammation (Fig. 2.7). However, the continued presence of the adult schistosomes is associated with increased but not complete protection against reinfection by cercariae. In general, the dead eggs and dead worms cause more reaction than either do when living, but no stage in the life cycle is entirely harmless and there are minor differences between the individual species.

There are two common pathological processes in schistosomiasis: (1) the formation of granulomas (pseudotubercles) and (2) an obliterative endarteritis.

Superimposed on these pathological processes will be the nutritional state of the patient, which in many parts of the tropics will mean a low protein intake, anemia from other parasites, and general dietary deficiency. These variations are so important that a heavy infection with schistosomes may have few and minor sequelae in some countries and yet cause severe complications in others. All the factors involved in host reactions are not fully understood.

Schistosomiasis may depress the immune system, resulting in an increased risk and severity of hepatitis B infection, and increasingly severe consequent liver damage. All schistosomes, but especially *S. intercalatum*, can prolong *Salmonella* infections, or permit early recurrence even after effective treatment if the schistosomiasis has not also been treated.

There are specific pathological changes caused by the different strains of schistosomiasis.

1. *The alimentary tract. S. mansoni* and *S. japonicum* mainly affect the alimentary tract, primarily the large bowel. Following the discharge of hundreds of eggs through the mucosa, a fibrotic reaction develops, but at the same time other eggs may be deposited within the bowel wall and are no longer able to migrate because they have been trapped. Each egg causes an inflammatory reaction which heals with fibrosis and the contained embryo dies. Granulomas form in the submucosa (Fig. 2.8) and may become heaped up into a polyp. Strictures and ulceration are late manifestations.
2. *The genitourinary tract.* The majority of urological infections occur with *S. haematobium*. (If you have difficulty remembering which schistosome species invades the urinary tract, remember that "*haematobium* causes hematuria".) The resulting inflammatory changes will principally involve the ureters and bladder, but renal damage may also occur (see p. 121). Granulomas caused by *S. haematobium* have been identified in the testes and there are numerous reports of their occurrence in the female genitalia, cervix, ovary, and endometrium.

   In the bladder and ureter the changes may vary considerably between different populations. Thus obstruction of the bladder neck is frequently found in Egypt, but seldom seen in southern Africa (see p. 129).
3. *The lungs.* The earliest reports of schistosome ova in the lungs were in 1885 and since then the literature has grown considerably. Pathologists agree that *S. haematobium* is found about twice as frequently in the lungs as *S. mansoni*, although radiologists will find that *S. mansoni* and *S. japonicum* cause more marked radiological changes than *S. haematobium*. Some authors suggest that portal hypertension and collateral circulation are essential to shunt sufficient numbers of eggs to the lungs and that only then do pulmonary changes develop: this may be significant but is probably not the only explanation. It is possible that there is a difference between the various species of schistosomes.

S. haematobium causes few changes in the lungs. In some patients there may eventually be diffuse fibrosis, with numerous ova, particularly in the peribronchial regions. There may be mild emphysema and some endarteritis.

S. mansoni and *S. japonicum* cause more severe and widespread effects. These are of two types: (1) the effect on vessels, which may be either direct or remote; and (2) the formation of parenchymal granulomas, which may be solitary and relatively large or, more commonly, multiple and almost invisible radiologically.

Vascular damage occurs when the eggs become anchored in the small pulmonary vessels and do not reach the capillaries. Due to a lytic secretion the eggs become embedded and then covered in the intima, causing local damage to the wall of the vessel. This damage is both mechanical, due to the actual presence of the ova, and toxic. The resulting inflammatory reaction surrounds the eggs and extends both ways to form the "dumbbell" granuloma which eventually blocks the lumen of the vessel inwardly, and at the same time pushes outwards to cause a pseudoaneurysm (Figs. 2.59–2.61). This process provokes fibrosis and new blood vessels are formed, both intra-arterially and para-arterially. These vessels link up and may also connect with the pulmonary veins, which become involved in the granulomatous process. Eventually these new vessels dilate, partly because the normal channels are blocked and there is increased vascular flow through the new vessels, but also because of the arteriovenous connections. These "angiomatoids" are pathognomonic of the endarteritis of pulmonary schistosomiasis. They are a major cause of schistosomal pulmonary hypertension. As the pressure increases, the branches of the pulmonary artery become affected, as occurs with any longstanding increase in pulmonary pressure. The main pulmonary artery also dilates, sometimes reaching aneurysmal width, but this is due not only to pulmonary hypertension, but also to the direct effect on the main pulmonary artery wall by eggs which have traveled through the vasa vasorum. The ova thus deposited cause local fibrosis and weaken the pulmonary artery, causing the aneurysms of the major branches which may be a striking abnormality seen on the chest radiograph (Figs. 2.62, 2.63).

Within the pulmonary circulation the anastomotic vessels may become so numerous that they resemble small angiomas; this occurs in both *S. mansoni*

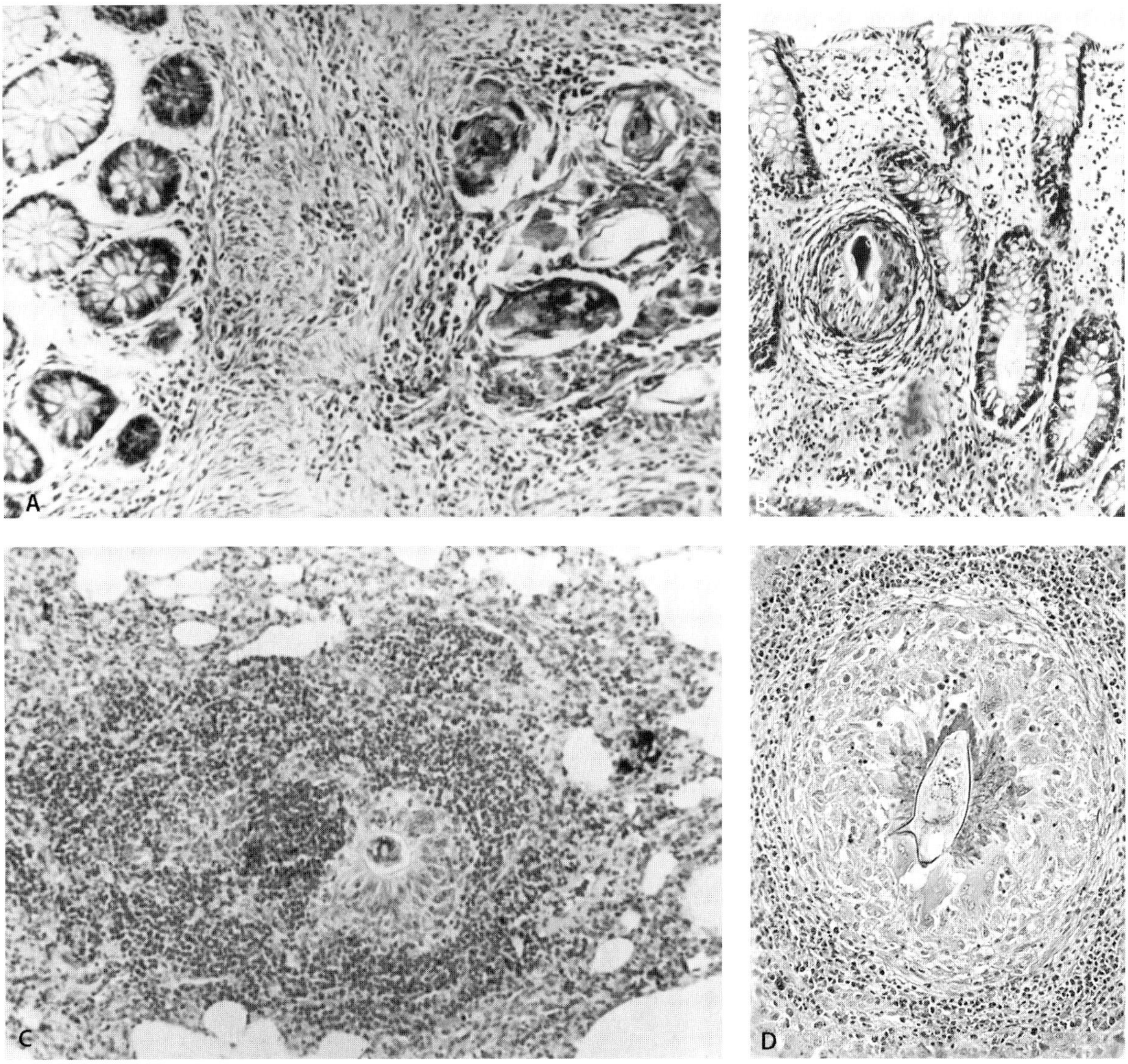

Fig. 2.8 A–D. The granulomas of schistosomiasis. **A** *S. mansoni* eggs in the bowel, stained with H & E. One of the eggs (*on the right*) clearly shows the lateral spine. **B** An *S. mansoni* egg in a granuloma of the large bowel. **C** An *S. japonicum* egg in the lung of a monkey. There is a marked eosinophilic infiltrate surrounding the granuloma. (Courtesy of E. Sadun, Washington) **D** An egg of *S. mansoni* surrounded by a marked foreign body reaction, cellular infiltrate, and early connective tissue proliferation: this is a pseudotubercle. ×170; AFIP 64-12055

and *S. japonicum* infections. Schistosomal cor pulmonale occurs fairly frequently in endemic areas but perhaps not as often as would be expected in view of the number of infected people. Where schistosomiasis is common, it must be considered as a possible cause in all patients presenting with cardiac failure. The associated aneurysmal dilatation of the pulmonary artery which occurs in some patients may be useful in excluding a rheumatic or arteriosclerotic origin.

There are other vascular changes in schistosomiasis, not directly related to the eggs and occurring without the granulomatous reaction which surrounds the egg. There are two varieties: arteritis and hyaline thrombi. The arteritis results from a fibroid necrosis of the vessel wall, with disruption of the elastic fibers, and is very similar to the arteritis of collagen disease. It is thought to be a local allergic reaction. The changes can be so severe that this form of arteritis can also disturb the pulmonary circulation and contribute to the pulmonary hypertension.

Hyaline thrombi may be found in many arteries, arterioles, and venules. Microscopically there are hyaline, polypoid masses beneath the vascular endothelium. These hyaline thrombi are multiple and found throughout the lungs and are yet another factor contributing to the pulmonary hypertension. It is possible that these hyaline masses are the result of embolization of eggs or even worms.

Much less common is the finding of a larger *Bilharzia* granuloma, the bilharzioma. This is a solitary lesion, which can occur anywhere in the lungs or heart, and may persist unchanged for some years or may shrink or increase in size. Pathologically it is a granuloma around an egg (or occasionally a worm), which has penetrated the vessel wall with minimal damage. Radiologically, it can be difficult to distinguish from any other granuloma, or even a small neoplasm.

The most common histological finding, the bilharzial "tubercle," 0.1–0.5 cm in size, is the least common radiological presentation and the most difficult to recognize (Figs. 2.58, 2.59). The tubercle is formed when the egg provokes a granuloma surrounded by histiocytes within the lung parenchyma and the inflammatory reaction becomes chronic, with the granuloma resolving to a focus of fibrosis and scarring. These small granulomas are always related to the bronchioles or alveoli. In some patients the alveoli fill with a serofibrinous exudate which may progress to become patchy consolidation characteristic of bronchopneumonia. The live adult schistosome in the lung is harmless; an exactly similar granulomatous lesion may develop around a dead worm, forming either a small tubercle or the much larger bilharzial granuloma. These "bilharziomas" do not contribute to the pulmonary hypertension.

The granulomatous-fibrotic changes must be differentiated from the acute reaction which occurs during treatment or the fleeting reaction during the stage of acute infection (the Katayama syndrome, see p. 122). Although it is difficult to obtain histopathological material at this phase, because it is transient and heals completely both clinically and radiologically, it is probable that there are no significant residual histological changes and no permanent damage. These reactions are probably allergic.

4. *The liver, spleen, and portal system.* Unfortunately, the story of schistosomiasis in the human body does not end with involvement of the gastrointestinal and genitourinary tracts or the lungs. Not all the eggs shed by the female worms in the mesenteric venules are trapped in the colon, small bowel, bladder, ureters, and/or lungs, or are passed to the outside in feces and urine to perpetuate the life cycle of the parasite. Many eggs and worms are forced back into the portal veins from mesenteric venules. Here they penetrate the walls of the small portal veins and lodge in the periportal connective tissue, where they incite an inflammatory cell reaction, eventually leading to multiple granulomas in the liver followed by fibrous tissue formation (Figs. 2.42–2.45). These lesions obstruct the small portal veins before they enter the hepatic sinusoids, causing a presinusoidal pattern of cirrhosis, known as Symmers' fibrosis. Initially, the fibrous tissue is confined to the portal tracts, with hepatic cells being uninvolved. Therefore, portal hypertension occurs long before there are measurable changes in liver function, in direct contrast to Laënnec's (postsinusoidal) cirrhosis.

There are three types of intrahepatic vascular lesions in schistosomiasis: (1) substitution by granulomas; (2) sclerosis and narrowing of portal venules; and (3) intrahepatic thrombophlebitis. Newly developed sleeve-like capillary networks surround the portal vein and probably form intrahepatic shunts between the portal and systemic circulations. There may also be extensive development of portal systemic collaterals outside the liver that help to lower the portal pressure with resultant esophageal, gastric, and mesenteric varices which can be quite dramatic in their size and number (Figs. 2.54–2.58). There is an increase in blood flow through the hepatic artery to compensate for the decreased portal flow. Late in the disease, hepatic fibrosis becomes more generalized, the liver decreases in size, and there is less destinction between presinusoidal and postsinusoidal cirrhosis.

Laboratory Diagnosis

The accurate diagnosis of schistosomiasis depends on the identification of the eggs and on the serological tests. Eggs can be recovered from urine or stools. The excretion of eggs occurs with a circadian rhythm and peaks about noon; urine should therefore be collected between 10:00 a.m. and 2:00 p.m. (1000–1400 hours). Quantitative urine filtration is the most reliable method. For stool, cellophane fecal thick smears (Kato) are best. If not readily identified by urine or stool tests, eggs can be reliably found by rectal biopsy; three or four specimens should be taken from the region of the first rectal valve, immediately pressed between two slides, and examined under the microscope. This method takes a few minutes, permits accurate identification of the schistosome species, and obviates the need for time-wasting stool or urine examinations. There is little or no risk attached to it. (Local bleeding may be prevented by direct pressure or, very occasionally, by the application of 10% silver nitrate to the bleeding area. Only very rarely is electrocauterization required.) There are no contraindications except possibly in very young children, very elderly patients, and those who are on anticoagulant therapy or have a bleeding tendency. It has been suggested that rectal biopsy should be avoided during an acute febrile state, but if there is a strong possibility of schistosomiasis, then the establishment of the diagnosis is of more importance than this theoretical contraindication.

Miracidial hatching is often successful, but takes time and experience.

Serological and Skin Tests

The serological diagnosis of schistosomiasis is generally accurate, but can be falsely negative, particularly in patients with longstanding infections. There are numerous tests from which to choose. The most reliable are indirect immunofluorescence (IIF) (a titer of 1:16 is diagnostic) and an enzyme-linked immunosorbent assay (ELISA) (a titer of 1:32 is diagnostic). A fast ELISA, using purified adult worm microsomal antigen, is excellent and may be the best test. Also available are the circumoral precipitin test (COPT), the cercaria-Hullen reaction (CHR), and total and fractionated soluble adult worm antigens (SWAP). While many of these tests are useful, they should not be used as the sole basis for treatment because avian schistosomes may produce confusing results. These tests are more important as an indication for further attempts to find the ova and this is where rectal biopsy may be particularly useful, because 20% of people infected with schistosomes will not pass ova, making positive identification in the stool very difficult in the early stages. Furthermore, confusion can be caused by finding nonviable eggs of *S. mattheei* or other nonhuman (avain or cattle) schistosomes, especially in North America and other temperate climates.

Of course, hematuria alone is a valid indication of infection in the right population. Microhematuria can be detected by reagent strips (dip sticks), which will recognize blood and protein. They are nonspecific but particularly useful in children. For more accuracy, a low-intensity infection may require a 24-hour urine collection. The great difficulty in many populations is to distinguish an active from previous infection, particularly after treatment, and for this situation, the circulating schistosome antigen is probably the most reliable test.

The skin tests are accurate at the time of the first exposure, but do not indicate which cercaria are present. This is a histamine release phenomenon, triggering mast cells. If there is a delayed reaction it usually indicates previous infection, because skin tests remain positive in about 50% of patients after treatment, even when the infection is eradicated. False-positive tests may indicate infection with a nonpathogenic species and false-negative results occur most frequently in children. There is a specific skin test for *S. mansoni*, but patients with trichinosis also react strongly to the *S. mansoni* antigen (the reverse does not happen).

Used together, the skin and serological tests are a very accurate index of either active or previous schistosomal infection. They do not indicate the extent, nor necessarily the activity, but if these tests are negative the likelihood of the current illness being due to schistosomiasis is slight.

Bladder calcification

There are only a few causes of bladder wall calcification (see p. 152), none of which resemble the eggshell calcification which is seen radiographically in *S. haematobium* infections. This calcification is due to large numbers of calcified eggs in the bladder wall. However, while indicating that the patient has had schistosomiasis, this does not show whether there is still active infection. The quantity of calcified or other dead eggs found in the urine is related to the number of accompanying embryonated eggs rather than the stage of the disease. But, unknown to the patient (or physician), calcified eggs are discharged in the urine and the number in the bladder wall slowly decreases over the years when there is no reinfection; thus, there may be less calcification in the bladders of elderly people than in their younger neighbors.

Bladder calcification, then, is a strong indication that the patient has, at some time, had schistosomiasis. It provides no further information.

Kidneys

Kidney damage, with marked hydronephrosis, may be the end result of urinary tract outflow obstruction, but the renal parenchyma may be damaged by schistosomiasis even if the lower urinary tract is relatively normal. This can occur in both *S. haematobium* and *S. mansoni* infections, and renal biopsy is useful to establish the cause. There is a high frequency of renal disease in hepatosplenic *S. mansoni* infections, particularly the nephrotic syndrome. An immuno-complex glomerulonephritis is a possible explanation because the many vascular collaterals allow the antigen-immune complexes to bypass the phagocytes in the liver and settle in the kidney or elsewhere. Electron-dense deposits in basement membranes of the glomeruli, together with laminated bodies near the mesangial cells, have been found in *S. mansoni* infections. The severity of renal damage can be correlated with the load of *S. mansoni*, but, as so often happens with schistosomiasis, there is geographic variation in both the severity and the rate of progress. A segmental but locally diffuse sclerosing glomerulonephritis occurs in severe cases; occasionally there may be glomerular capillary aneurysms.

Hematological Status

In some parts of the world, in Asia particularly, but also in Egypt and elsewhere, blood loss from hematuria and/or colonic disease can be sufficient to cause anemia. The fluke does not consume much blood but hematuria can cause blood loss equivalent to 37 mg of iron daily, and colonic-rectal loss can account for 26 mg. However, when a patient is anemic this may not be the sole reason and other causes should be sought. Eosinophilia may be high but is not invariable, especially during chronic infections. A routine check of the blood urea is advisable to exclude renal damage.

Equivocal Laboratory Tests

There are occasions when the positive identification of the parasite is not possible and yet immediate treatment may be indicated:

1. When there is a positive history of exposure, together with a strong clinical indication.
2. When more than one of the following are also present: eosinophilia or a history of hematuria, or of the Katayama syndrome, or of freshwater swimmer's itch (saltwater swimmer's itch, also known as seabather's eruption, is not related to schistosomiasis but to larvae of the species phylum Cnidaria). Equally important is a positive radiographic examination or ultrasound scan.
3. When a positive serology is found and yet parasites may not be identified, as in the invasive stage (the Katayama syndrome) or in the early stages of a light or subclinical infection. Rarely, this can also occur when there has been a predominantly unisexual infection or when infection occurs at an ectopic site.

Clinical Characteristics

As has already been noted, there are many factors which affect the complicated life cycle and behavior of the schistosome. This is also true of the clinical manifestations. At every stage in the cycle of invasion and maturation there is some clinical reaction: it varies with the individual, with the immune status, with the parasitic load, with the species of schistosome, and with many other factors, which include the patient's age and general state of nutrition and health, as well as the presence of other schistosomes or parasites. Previous infection only provides a limited protection. Chimpanzees can be successfully immunized, but so far (1999) there is no tested human vaccine. Reinfection may produce an illness differing from the primary infection, and the nature of that reaction may depend on whether or not the patient is currently infected.

Katayama Syndrome

The acute stage of infection with any of the schistosomes is known as the "Katayama syndrome." This name was originally given to an urticarial fever in China, which in about 1907 was recognized to be the result of early infection with *S. japonicum*. Later the syndrome was seen in early schistosomiasis caused by any schistosome. It follows exposure to infected water about 3–9 weeks previously. The majority of patients who exhibit this syndrome will not have been previously infected by schistosomes and the syndrome may therefore be seen in travelers returning from endemic areas. For example, six out of seven American tourists exposed to river water in west Africa were ill within 4 weeks and became seropositive for *S. mansoni*. The Katayama syndrome is similar to serum sickness, an antibody-antigen reaction with raised IgE and IgG. It can be life threatening. Eggs will eventually be found in the urine or feces between 40 and 50 days after the contact, but may take over 90 days to appear, by which time the "Katayama" stage may be long past.

At the stage of exposure to the cercaria, many patients will exhibit no clinical reaction and have no complaints. Indigenous populations in particular seldom develop cercarial dermatitis. In the nonsensitized, there may be burning and irritation of the skin (swimmer's itch) followed in some cases by urticaria within the first 24 or 48 hours. This may have no clinical significance, being due to avian or animal cercaria. In fact, some authorities distinguish the clinical appearance of a cercarial dermatitis, which is a maculopapular rash which can last about 2–3 weeks and is not due to human schistosomiasis, and restrict the term "schistosomal dermatitis" to the short-lived specific itchy, papular rash which results from contact with human schistosomes. In everyday practice, however, the history of an itchy rash or transient sunburn, with ill health after contact with fresh water in the tropics, is significant and important. About 25% of patients will feel tired and "off color." These complaints may have no clinical significance, being due to animal cercaria. If the infection has been massive, there may be very severe skin irritation and the condition may be mistaken for sunburn or other skin allergy.

This is followed by a latent period, which usually lasts from 3 to 9 weeks and then the patient may complain of headache, backache, chills, fever, night sweats, nonproductive cough, abdominal discomfort, and profound anorexia and distaste for food. The temperature will vary from 99° to 105°F (37.2°–40.6°C). Urticaria and/or diarrhea occurs in 25% of cases. This probably coincides with the stage of migration of the larvae through the blood vessels and can be associated with radiological changes in the chest and elsewhere. The most constant finding on examination of the blood is eosinophilia, which frequently may reach between 15% and 50%; in a few cases it can even reach 90% or 20000 eosinophils per mm^3. Again, individual variation is considerable and patients may be asymptomatic or moderately or extremely ill. When the acute infection is massive in a patient not previously exposed to any schistosomes, the resulting illness can be serious and life threatening. Headache and neck stiffness may be severe, tenderness can develop over the liver, and the cough can be extremely troublesome. The serological tests should be positive, but a negative test at this stage does not exclude schistosomiasis.

For all species of schistosomes, the acute abdominal symptoms probably represent the invasion of the hepatic and portal veins, the mesenteric vessels, and lymphatics. Thereafter, the symptoms are related more specifically to the eggs than to the worms. The passage of eggs through the intestinal wall will be accompanied by diarrhea, with mucus and extravasated blood. Other embolic ova lodge in the small intestine, appendix, heart (cardiac arrhythmia can develop), pancreas, kidneys, adrenals, ovaries, fallopian tubes, lymph nodes, retroperitoneal tissues and omentum. Especially in *S. japonicum* infections, the embolic eggs may become lodged in the brain and may cause an ecute encephalitis, with loss of consciousness and extensor plantar responses, the EEG may be abnormal. In some patients there have been transitory paralysis, visual impairment, incontinence, ataxia, and even seizures and coma. Wherever they lodge, all eggs may cause a local cellular or granulomatous reaction.

Chronic Schistosomiasis

When the illness becomes chronic it is different for each species. In *S. haematobium* infections urinary symptoms predominate, with hematuria and recurrent urinary infection. Some patients have experienced testicular tenderness and tingling. There may be changes in the ejaculate (presumably when the seminal vesicles or prostate are infected). Patients will notice a decrease in the volume of the ejaculates, which may be watery and yellow. Hematospermia does not always occur, but may be found on microscopy, which will also show schistosomal ova and an increase in the number of polymorphs. There is no decrease in spermatozoal motility. Female partners have been found to be infected, but it seems unlikely that this is transmitted from the male. A common clinical diagnosis is a nongonococcal urethritis. Renal schistosomiasis usually presents clinically because of the obstruction and infection which has affected the lower urinary tract, but an immune complex glomerular nephritis may occur, presenting clinically as albuminuria, hypertension, and a finding of glomerular changes on renal biopsy or autopsy. There is variation in the histopathological findings, which have been classified by the African Association of Nephrology (Barsoum). This type of renal schistosomiasis is the result of longstanding chronic infection, often over 10–15 years. Renal amyloidosis may be the eventual outcome of schistosomal glomerulopathy. All three major species of schistosome may affect the kidneys. In *S. haematobium* infection as well as urinary tract involvement, there may be granulomatous disease of the colon; the latter often occurs in conjunction with mucosal polyps and causes, diarrhea, though this varies in extent in different countries and in different people. In *S. japonicum* infection, the disease may affect the small bowel as well as the colon, liver, and lungs; cerebral infections may cause epilepsy. Infection with *S. mansoni, S. japonicum*, and *S. intercalatum* particularly may affect the liver, causing cirrhosis, portal hypertension, and splenomegaly. Esophageal varices develop, with resulting hemorrhage, and pulmonary hypertension may be an added complication. It is necessary to reemphasize that the worms cannot multiply within the body and that most of the clinical manifestations result from dead worms or eggs. Many, perhaps the majority of infected persons are asymptomatic, often for many years.

The clinical and laboratory investigations for each patient depend on the symptoms. When there is hematuria caused by *S. haematobium*, ultrasound and subsequently intravenous urography may be indicated. Cystoscopy may show multiple papillomas within the bladder. *S. mansoni* and *S. japonicum* infections require barium examination of the bowel and/or colonoscopy, which may be quite normal even during an active infection. Other patients will show clusters of small, yellow, nodular pseudotubercles or plaques beneath the normal mucosa of the rectum and biopsy will show that these contain eggs. The bowel wall may have only glistening granulation tissue or the reaction may be such that actual polyps are found; sometimes these are quite large and may resemble a neoplasm.

In endemic areas, children are usually exposed to schistosomiasis early in life. Very few children avoid the parasitic onslaught and in some areas infection is almost universal. For instance, in Niger (West

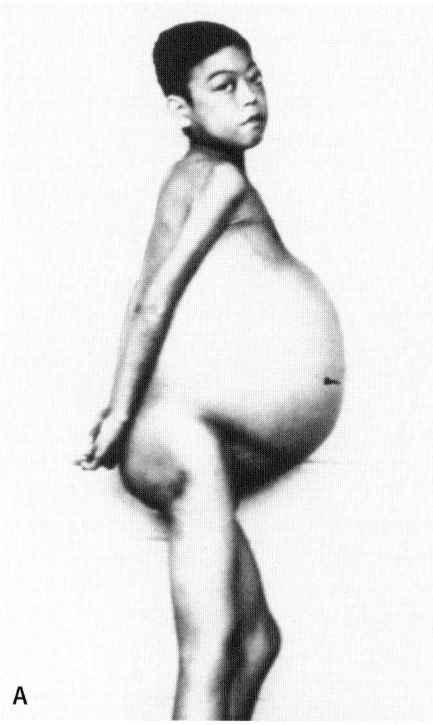

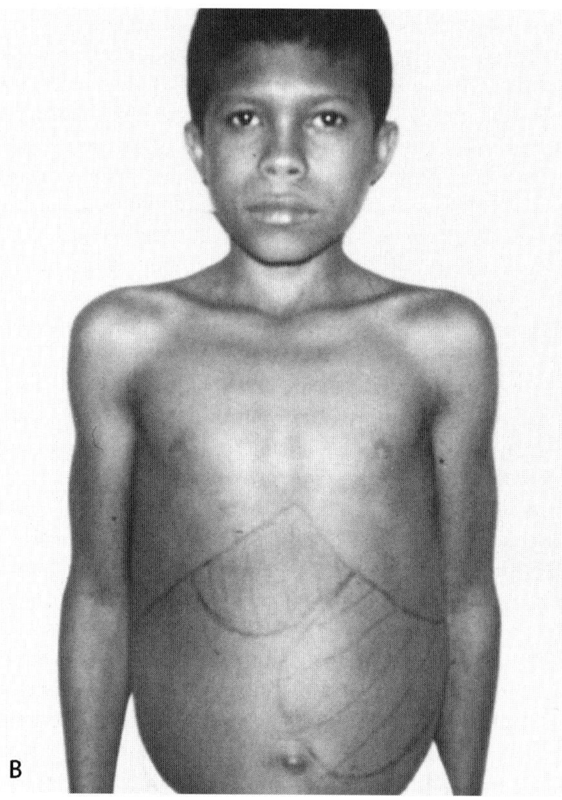

Fig. 2.9 A, B. The sad effect of advanced schistosomiasis in two different children in the tropics. There is hepatomegaly and massive splenomegaly from long-standing presinusoidal cirrhosis and portal hypertension: both children are anemic, malnourished, and suffer from ascites, which is especially marked in the child in A

Africa) over 80% of children are infected and in rural Zambia the rate is nearly 70%. However, wherever there is a piped water supply, the prevalence decreases considerably. Depending on the severity and constancy of the exposure, on general health, and on other factors, there may be a latent asymptomatic period of 2–25 years before the portal manifestation of *S. mansoni* or *S. japonicum* infections becomes apparent. An enlarging left upper quadrant mass, or gastrointestinal bleeding from esophageal and gastric varices, is frequently the initial complaint causing the patient to seek medical attention. Although the liver is enlarged initially, liver function studies may be nearly normal even at this stage, while hypersplenism and anemia will usually be present. The spleen is often massive; in fact, for centuries this disease was known as “Egyptian splenomegaly” (Fig. 2.9). There is often malnutrition and ascites. The development of esophageal varices is an indication of chronic irreversible liver disease. The first attack of schistosomiasis may present as a change in intellectual level, particularly in schoolchildren: they develop difficulty in concentration. Active schistosomiasis has been shown to affect spatial relationships and numerical ability. Chronic schistosomiasis does not affect growth, physical activity, or the general level of intelligence of children in endemic areas, until it has progressed to cause significant cirrhosis.

Clinical Summary

The clinical findings can be summarized as follows:

1. During the acute phase of infestation: urticaria, pruritus, cough, fever, and eosinophilia; abdominal pain and, less commonly, CNS symptoms.
2. After a few months, general debility, ill health and anemia, headaches.
3. At the stage of oviposition: hematuria or bloody stools with dysentery.
4. There may be side-effects, such as persistent and severe *Salmonella* infections or increased miscarriages and stillbirths. Hepatitis B infections may also be more frequent and severe.
5. Finally, portal cirrhosis, esophageal varices, hemorrhoids, pulmonary fibrosis and hypertension, urinary infection, carcinoma of the bladder, chronic rectal bleeding with rectal prolapse, anemia, and infections.

Many of these changes will be irreversible. During the acute phase the administration of steroids may reduce the permanent effects: even the hypersplenism may subside, but once the granulomas are established it is difficult to prevent their progress. Surgery may be required to reliever urinary obstruction, to manage portal hypertension, and to deal with the effects on the bowel. Urinary schistosomiasis is associated with an increased incidence of bladder carcinoma (a complex etiological relationship) and there is an increased incidence of bowel cancer in patients with *S. japonicum* infections. Whether *S. mansoni* or *S. haematobium* infections cause increased cancer of the colon is still controversial. There is no evidence linking schistosomiasis with cancer of the lung.

Imaging Diagnosis

The chest radiograph is either normal or shows increased vascular and interstitial markings and minimal enlargement of the hilar lymph nodes. Miliary tuberculosis in its early stages or a simple virus infection may be suspected. The changes are not specific but, in conjunction with a significant history and eosinophilia, they may help to confirm the diagnosis. Skin tests are variable; the complement fixation test is usually positive. The chest radiograph returns to normal with or without treatment.

In the abdomen there are three sonographic (and CT) findings which contribute to the diagnosis of the Katayama stage of acute schistosomiasis.

There may be a nonspecific hepatosplenomegaly and, particularly in series from Brazil, splenomegaly: the left lobe of the liver may be more enlarged than the right. The liver is sonographically homogeneous or, in a few cases, hyperechoic. Liver enzymes may be slightly abnormal. At the same time there may be periportal and juxta pancreatic lymphadenopathy, particularly in children. The lymph nodes are sharply outlined and round or oval, with a thin surrounding hypoechoic halo.

Ultrasonography may also show multiple small nodules throughout the liver parenchyma. In schistosomiasis mansoni they have been described as hypoechoic, but in schistosomiasis japonicum they are hyperechoic. There are not many reports of these findings and the different echogenicity is more likely to reflect a different clinical pattern than an intrinsic difference in the reaction to the two species. The histopathology has not been described (1999), and it is not known whether such findings are always present. Differences will not be surprising because there are many variations in response, even to the same species of schistosome. These nodules may persist in spite of adequate therapy: they may be 4–5 mm in diameter and are well shown on CT scanning, being hypodense with delayed contrast enhancement. Even with a second course of treatment, it may take 20 weeks before the liver in sonographically normal although the patients's clinical condition will have improved long before this. The natural history without treatment has not been described (1999).

In subacute schistosomiasis, echogenic lesions in the liver are thought to be due to portal vein branches (in cross-section). It probably takes from 3 to 5 years to develop stage one periportal (Symmers) fibrosis when patients have a high-intensity infection. With low infection rates, it may take much longer. There is no evidence of portal hypertension during the Katayama stage. It should be emphasized again that the diagnosis is only reliably made when correlated with the clinical findings, a raised eosinophilia, and, preferably, the finding of eggs in the feces or on biopsy.

The acute phase of *S. japonicum* infection results in CNS involvement in about 2% of patients, possibly because the eggs of *S. japonicum* are the smallest of the more common species. There is a focal pattern of egg distribution in the brain, resulting in a wide variety of symptoms, not only headache but speech impairment, disorientation, memory loss, visual disturbances, seizures, and coma; in a few patients there may be spasticity, cranial nerve findings, and various patterns of paralysis. CT scans of the brain may show edema around low-density inflammatory foci, which are often multiple and contrast enhancing with edema. In some cases there may be a mass effect, causing shift with pressure on any part of the ventricular system. The CSF pressure may be slightly raised, but all the findings will be very variable, depending on the distribution and the number of eggs. In most cases there has not been a clear correlation between the parasite load and the possibility of CNS involvement or its extent. The diagnosis will be made in the usual way, by serology or recognition of the ova in stool or urine. If treated appropriately, and with steroids, complete resolution can be expected within about 8 weeks, matched by an improvement of clinical symptoms and signs.

This pattern of CNS involvement must be distinguished from the mass effect which is found in chronic cerebral schistosomiasis affecting patients who have been previously and often repeatedly infected (p. 198).

Imaging changes other than in the acute state are different with each type of infection and will be discussed separately.

Schistosomiasis haematobium

There is no doubt that ultrasonography has added significantly to the understanding of urinary tract schistosomiasis, by permitting surveys of children and adults and providing accurate information on the results of treatment. However, there are conflicting results in various reports, which again shows how much individual variation there is between populations, even villages, seemingly infected with the same schistosome to the same extent. Anyone working in a particular country or locality must determine the effect of schistosomiais in their own patients, but it is possible to give a general review.

Many different studies have been made to assess the value of various imaging methods in suspected or proven schistosomiasis haematobium. Ultrasonography, which is noninvasive, radiation free, and inexpensive, is an excellent way to assess morbidity. It is the most widely available method for studying the liver and spleen size, and for detecting liver disease (periportal fibrosis and portal hypertension). In the early stages of liver disease there is some observer variation: as the disease progresses, the results become more consistent. Ultrasonography is also an excellent way of detecting hydronephrosis and thickening of the bladder wall; it can demonstrate early malignant change in the bladder and can assess residual urine. It is not so accurate in finding ureteric lesions (hydroureter, calcified ureteric granulomas) or bladder wall calcification and is less accurate with renal or bladder calculi. It is quite unreliable in the detection of mesenteric or other abdominal calcification, including calcification of the liver.

Intravenous urography is excellent in demonstrating the whole urinary tract, particularly ureteric lesions (stenosis, dilatation, poor peristalsis), bladder wall calcification, and bladder capacity.

Plain radiography of the abdomen is of little assistance unless there is bladder or ureteric calcification, when it becomes a very useful investigation. It can also show calcification in the seminal vesicles. Plain radiography can also detect moderate or advanced intestinal or nonvisceral calcification but, in the earlier stages, does not show calcification as clearly as computed tomography (CT), which is excellent for the demonstration of calcification in any site or organ, including pelvic tissue; it is also excellent for recognizing other lesions in the urinary tract. It can demonstrate CNS lesions, with or without contrast enhancement. Myelography is useful for spinal schistosomiasis, but not as accurate as CT or magnetic resonance imaging (MRI).

Magnetic resonance imaging is most important in the CNS, particularly for imaging the brain and spinal cord. While it can demonstrate urinary tract and other intra-abdominal schistosomiasis, it has little advantage over ultrasonography or CT. It is much less accurate in the demonstration of any calcification.

Wherever schistosomiasis haematobium is endemic, 60–70% of children aged 4–14 years will have bladder lesions; about 20% of boys and 2–5% of girls in this age group will have hydronephrosis. Ureteric lesions will usually be bilateral, but not symmetrical. Between 10% and 15% of these children will have ureteric lesions only, which may reflect the stage of the infection. The vast majority of ureteric lesions, over 90%, will be in the lower third of the ureters.

In adults in the same endemic areas, about 50–60% of men and 20–30% of women will have bladder lesions, but only about 15% of men and less than 10% of women will have hydronephrosis. This is less than among the children.

In some series there is a positive relationship between the severity of the bladder lesions and the egg count. In other series there is no correlation.

In areas where the infection occurs but is not known to be endemic, the prevalence is much less; surveys show that in supposedly schistosome-free areas, 10% of children and 16% of adult men and perhaps 5%–10% of adult women may have active infections. In these nonendemic areas, hydronephrosis is very uncommon at any age, unless there is bladder calcification. Once there is bladder calcification, visible on imaging, hydronephrosis becomes twice as common as it is in patients who have no visible calcification. Bladder calcification, even when quite heavy, makes little difference to bladder function because the ova are predominantly in the mucosa and submucosa, not in muscle. Difficulty in micturition in patients with schistosomiasis is likely to be evidence of cystitis or bladder neck thickening (see p. 129).

Ultrasonography

In the urinary tract, ultrasonography can detect hypertrophy of the bladder mucosa, thickening of the bladder wall (which is normally less than 5 mm when the bladder is distended), and bladder calcification. If the ureters are easily demonstrated by ultrasonography, they are probably thickened and abnormal; in some patients calcification will be seen, but ultrasonography is not a reliable way to demonstrate early ureteric changes. Dilatation of the renal collecting system can be detected very early, and represents the result of significant ureteric dysfunction. (Increased proteinuria, more than 1 g per liter in midday urine, strongly suggests that there is urinary tract stasis and may suggest the need for imaging.)

Because of the strong association between schistosomiasis haematobium and squamous cell carcinoma of the bladder, particular care should be taken during ultrasonography to accurately record bladder wall thickening. Repeat ultrasonography is advisable after treatment; about 70% of schistosomal bladder lesions will regress significantly in less than 12 months (after treatment with praziquantel). If a bladder lesion does not improve, long-term follow-up is required to exclude malignancy. Over 90% of patients who have schistosomal carcinoma of the bladder will have ureteric obstruction; of those with a nonschistosomal bladder carcinoma (transitional cell) less than 25% will have ureteric obstruction.

There are authorities who believe that the liver is not affected by *S. haematobium*; however, there are others, equally eminent, who state that all schistosomes cause similar liver pathology, some more commonly than others. An International Expert Committee, convened by the World Health Organization (together with UNDP and the World Bank), met in Cairo, Egypt in 1991 to draw up criteria for assessing the extent of schistosomal infections as demonstrated by ultrasonography (see pp. 166–168). This very experienced committee provided separate guidelines for *S. haematobium, S. mansoni*, and *S. japonicum*. Module 4 for *S. haematobium* (Annex B, p. 24 of the report) is "The record sheet for *S. haematobium* pathology-ultrasound findings: Liver Pathology," which leaves no doubt that this group is convinced that *S. haematobium* does indeed affect the liver.

There is, nevertheless, no question that liver pathology occurs more frequently and perhaps more severely with *S. mansoni* infections: the description of the ultrasonographic findings is therefore on pp. 166–170. The practicing radiologist will more often be concerned with the extent of the changes rather than the specific schistosome, and certainly will not be able to distinguish between the schistosomes by hepatic ultrasonography.

Radiography

Plain radiography of the abdomen is of no assistance until calcification has developed in the bladder and ureters, although in severe infections calcified eggs may also be seen in the soft tissues. (Early calcification is much more clearly seen by CT.) Intravenous (contrast) urography will provide very useful diagnostic information. All the early findings will be in the ureters and bladder; the kidneys remain normal until later in the disease.

Ureters

The earliest change in the ureters is persistent filling of the lower segment in all films of the urography series. At this stage the ureters are not dilated or otherwise abnormal in many patients, but dilatation of the filled distal, intrapelvic segment is the next change (Fig. 2.10). The widening may be slight or marked, but there may be no visible stenosis. The earliest ureteric constriction is within the bladder wall, and there will also be changes in ureteric peristalsis. This has been confirmed by fluoroscopic studies.

In the early stage of ureteric dilatation, before there is visible ureteric calcification, the lower ureter will have a ragged outline and a beaded internal appearance, with some irregular dilatation because of acute "pseudotubercles" in the submucosa. As they heal these may cause strictures. Over 80% of the earliest strictures in the ureter lie radiologically within the bladder wall and next in order of frequency are those 2–5 cm (1–2 inches) above the orifice (Fig. 2.11). Later there may be local stenosis with irregular dilatation both above and below the stenotic segment. In more advanced cases there are multiple strictures, and gross irregularity throughout the length of the ureter, almost always bilateral but seldom symmetrical. Eventually dilatation may affect the whole ureter because there is extensive involvement of the ureteric wall.

Even at an early stage fine calcification may be seen in the ureters, beginning with skip areas but eventually coalescing so that the ureters are calcified throughout their full length from bladder to kidney and visible on plain radiographs (Figs. 2.12, 2.13).

When the bladder is not calcified, the ureters may show normal peristalsis (even if there is some constriction within the bladder walls). However, as soon as the bladder shows calcification, the rate of lower ureteric peristalsis is halved compared with normal. When the lower third of the ureters become dilated and calcified also, the upper ureter may continue to show normal peristalsis. When there is no normal peristalsis at all in the lower ureters, there may even be reverse peristalsis. As the calcification spreads up the ureter, there will be a matching reduction in the rate of peristalsis. By the time there is hydronephrosis and hydroureter, peristalsis is negligible and in the end, when renal function is decreased, with marked dilatation of the whole system, there will usually be no peristaltic activity (Fig. 2.19c). The presence of added secondary infection will hasten these changes. Apart from research investigations, there is no clinical indication for ureteric fluoroscopy except when reflux is suspected but cannot be demonstrated on cystography.

Bladder

In the bladder the changes are similar; the bladder outline first becomes hazy and indistinct, due to submucosal edema and pseudotubercles (Fig. 2.14). There are some significant geographic variations in the bladder changes. In West African children there may be a marked bladder reaction, probably due to severe "urticarial" edema of the bladder wall (Fig. 2.20). The large circular filling defects are so marked that they may be mistaken for sarcoma botryoides. It is possible that this pattern occurs only when there is

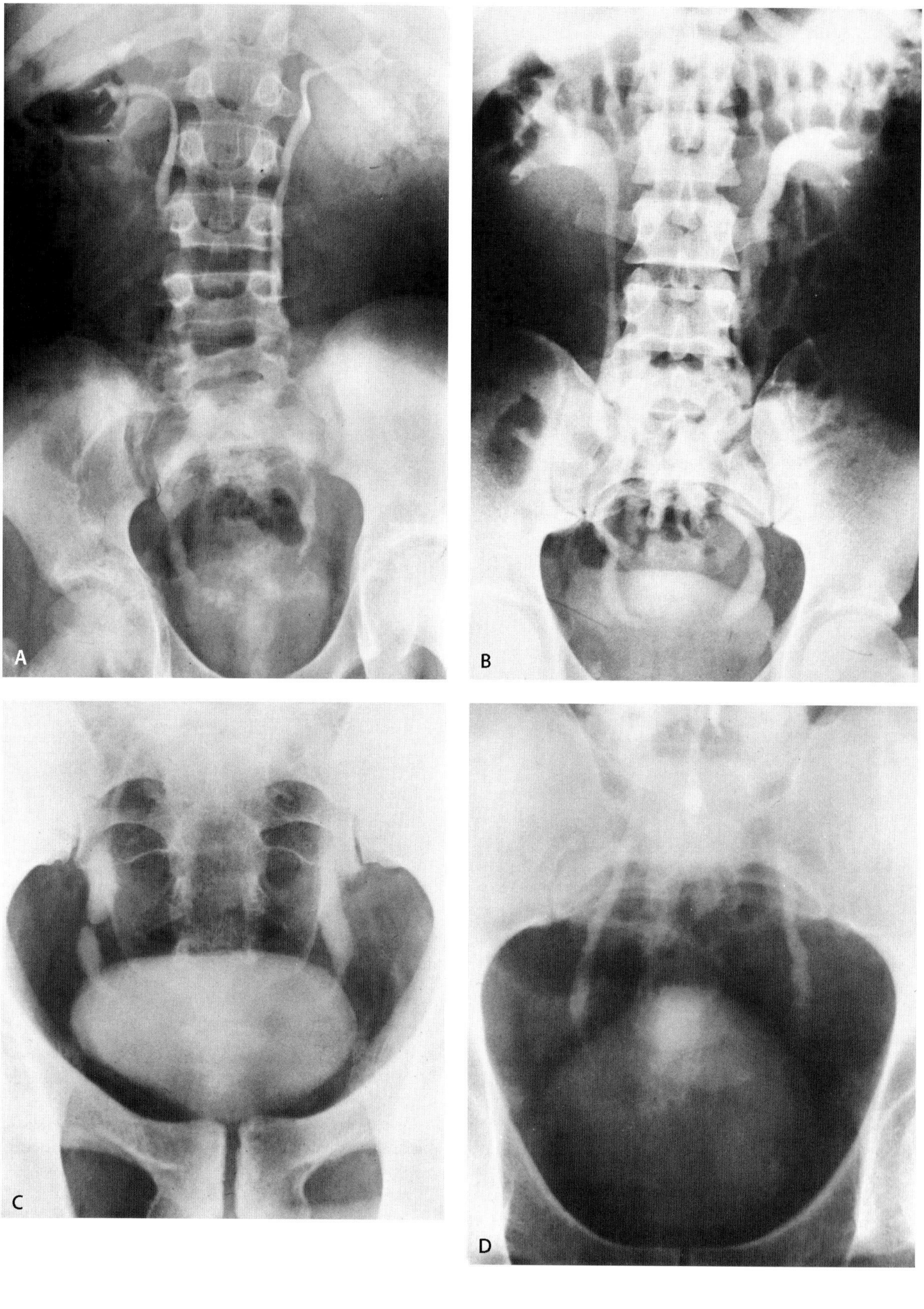
A
B
C
D

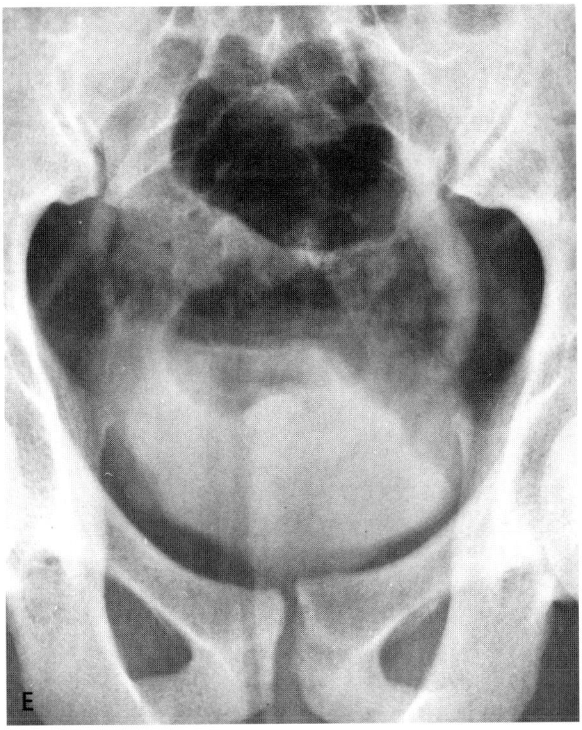
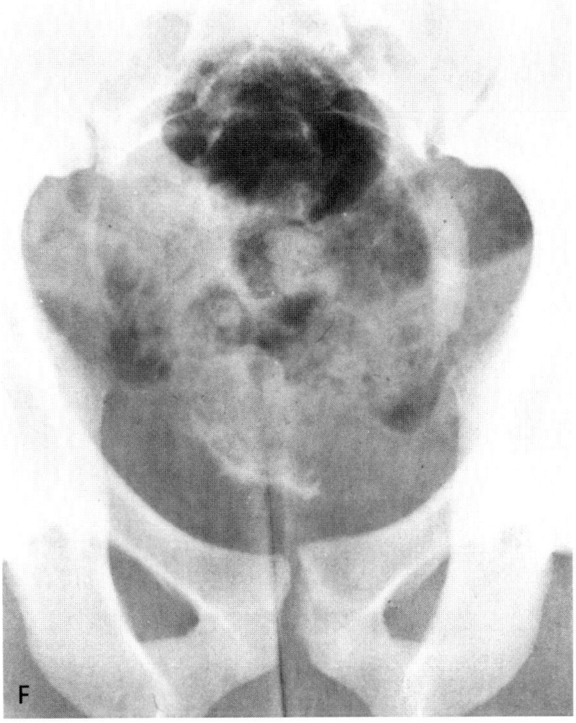

◄ **Fig. 2.10 A–F.** The early changes in schistosomiasis of the ureter. **A, B** Intravenous urograms of two African men. Kidneys are normal, but both ureters are filled throughout their length and the lower thirds are dilated, irregular, and with beading due to multiple intrinsic constrictions. Their bladders do not show any calcification. **C** In another patient there is narrowing of both ureters close to the bladder and in the right ureter there is a segment of dilatation between two areas of stenosis, with dilatation also above the upper narrowing. **D** Persistent filling in the lower half of both ureters, with a long constriction in the right ureter just above the bladder. Both show irregular areas of constriction and dilatation. **E** As this bladder fills, the lower ureters are irregular, with the left more dilated than the right. **F** After micturition (same patient as **E**) the bladder is empty, the right ureter is irregular but normal in diameter, whereas the left ureter is persistently filled and dilated, with a long constriction close to the bladder

recurrent infection after a period free from the disease; massive urticaria of this sort is not so common in Egypt or southern Africa, where the infection is endemic. In adults there are likely to be multiple small, rather flat papillomas, requiring cystoscopy or ultrasonography to distinguish them from malignancy (Figs. 2.20, 2.21). A therapeutic trial may provide the answer in an endemic area, but follow-up ultrasonography every 10–12 months is advisable. The bladder wall is often ulcerated and thickened, making the differential diagnosis extremely difficult in some patients, even on cystoscopy.

In Egypt a syndrome of "bladder neck obstruction" has been described and is relatively common, probably because of the eggs entering the muscles of the urinary bladder and provoking a partial hyperplasia which proceeds to fibrosis. The area of the trigone is the most affected and hypertrophies to form a prominence bulging into the vesicle lumen between the ureteric orifices. As this prominence undergoes fibrosis, it atrophies and shrinks, leaving the mucosa and muscularis as a mass which is pushed forward over the internal urethral orifice. Infiltration of the bladder neck by schistosomes produces inflammatory obstruction and then dilatation and atrophy of the detrusor muscle, so that a dilated bladder in these patients may occupy the greater part of the pelvis. Such marked bladder outlet changes are not reported outside Egypt.

As the granulomas become fibrotic, the bladder wall shows calcification, but the calcium is not within the fibrous tissue. Rather, it is entirely submucosal, in the eggs. It has been reckoned that "sandy" radiopaque areas contain between 500 000 and 1 00 000 per gram and that as few as 100 000 eggs per cm^3 can be detected on a radiograph. Whether the eggs are visible radiologically depends on how evenly they are dispersed through the tissues. The extent of calcification in the bladder in schistosomiasis is roughly correlated with the number of free calcified eggs present in the bladder lumen, but the excretion of eggs in the urine is related to the activity of any infection and is not affected by the presence or extent of bladder calcification.

(Text continues on p. 134)

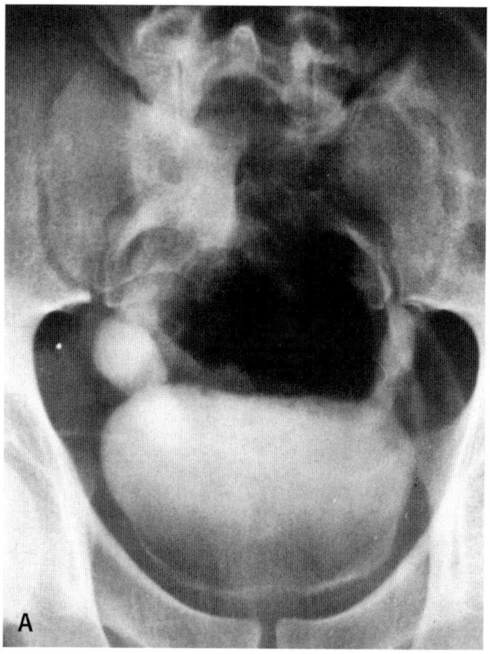

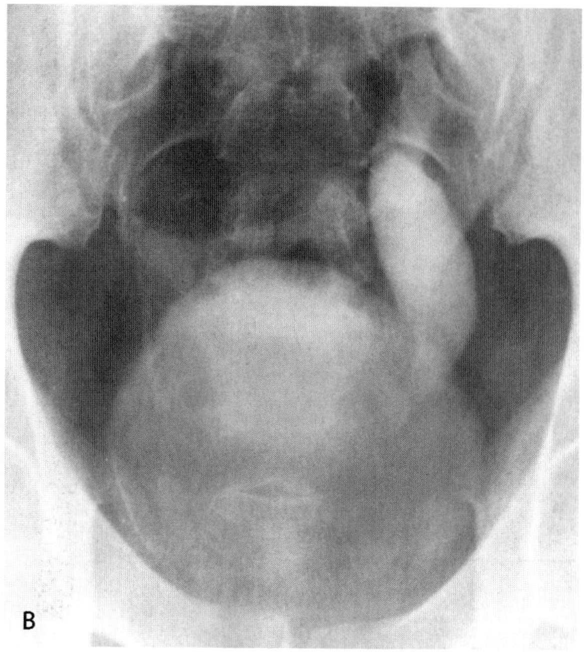

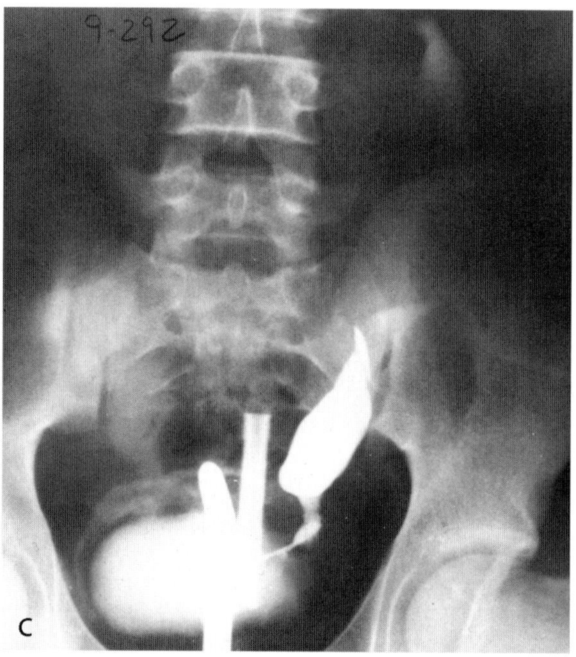

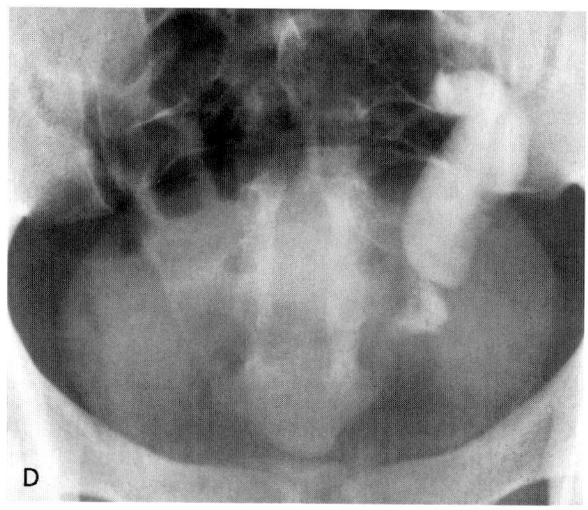

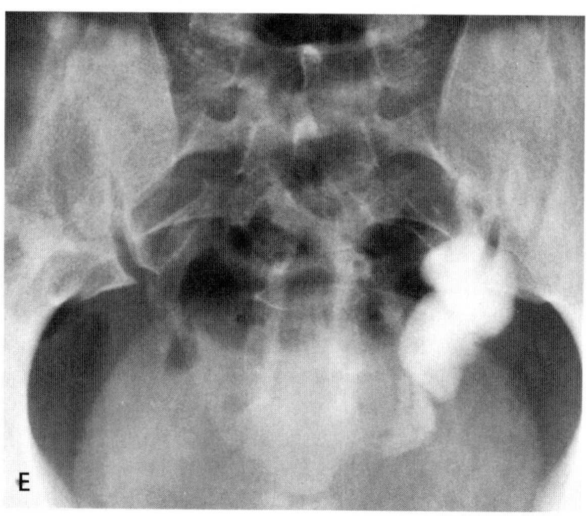

Fig. 2.11 A–E. Progressive stages of ureteral schistosomiasis. **A** Dilatation of both ureters, more marked on the right side with stenosis at the opening into the bladder. **B** Marked dilatation of the left ureter, showing the typical narrowing as the ureter enters the bladder wall. The right ureter is not distended or even filled, so it may be normal. **C** Ascending urography in another patient shows stenosis of the distal segment of the left ureter within the bladder wall and marked dilatation above it. A slight amount of constrast is visible in the hydronephrotic left kidney. AFIP 68-1093-2. **D, E** Two phases of peristalsis in the same dilated ureter. Again, the portion of the ureter within the bladder wall is much less dilated and there is marked stenosis at the ureterovesical junction. In all these patients there is bladder calcification, at different stages

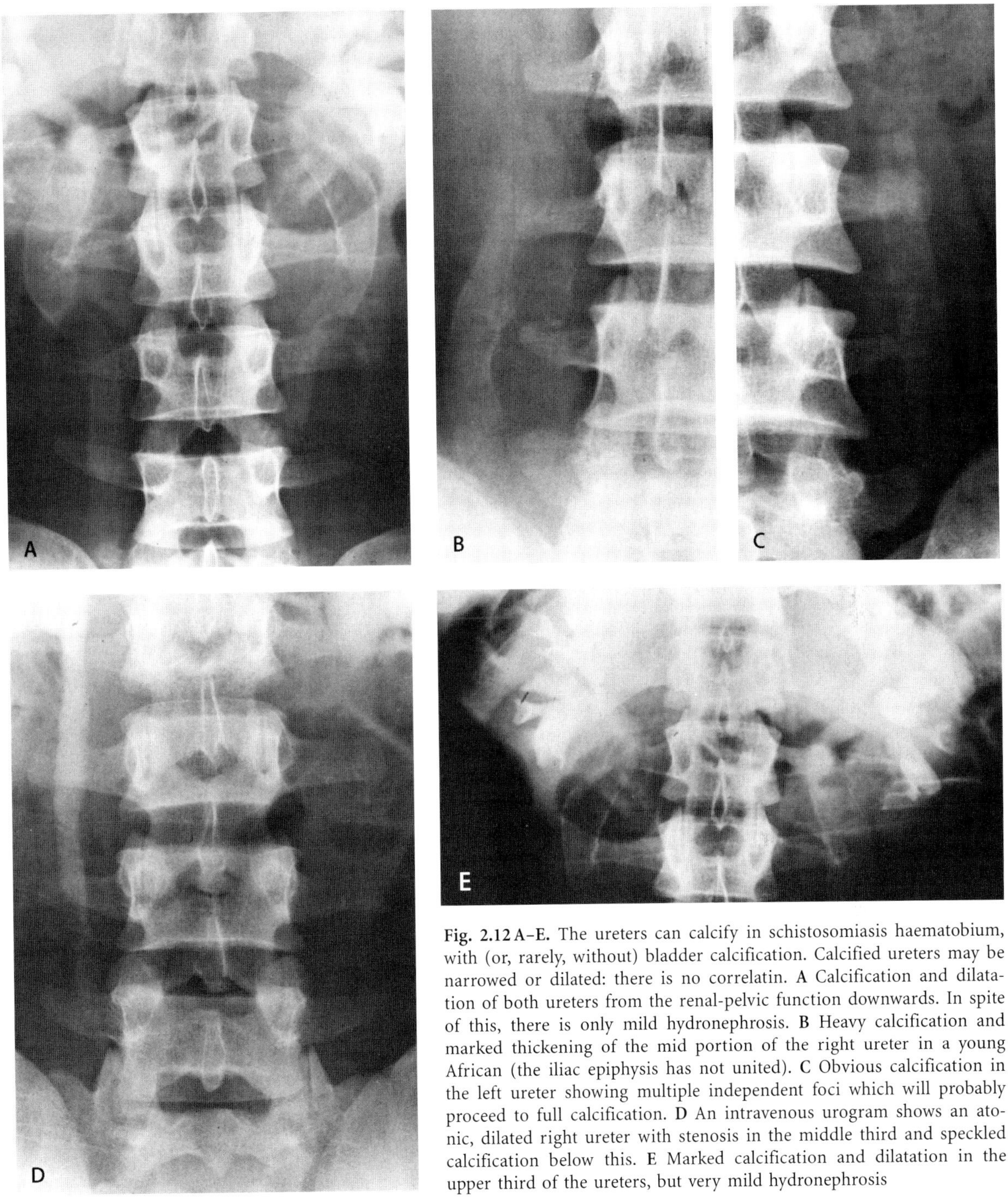

Fig. 2.12 A–E. The ureters can calcify in schistosomiasis haematobium, with (or, rarely, without) bladder calcification. Calcified ureters may be narrowed or dilated: there is no correlatin. A Calcification and dilatation of both ureters from the renal-pelvic function downwards. In spite of this, there is only mild hydronephrosis. B Heavy calcification and marked thickening of the mid portion of the right ureter in a young African (the iliac epiphysis has not united). C Obvious calcification in the left ureter showing multiple independent foci which will probably proceed to full calcification. D An intravenous urogram shows an atonic, dilated right ureter with stenosis in the middle third and speckled calcification below this. E Marked calcification and dilatation in the upper third of the ureters, but very mild hydronephrosis

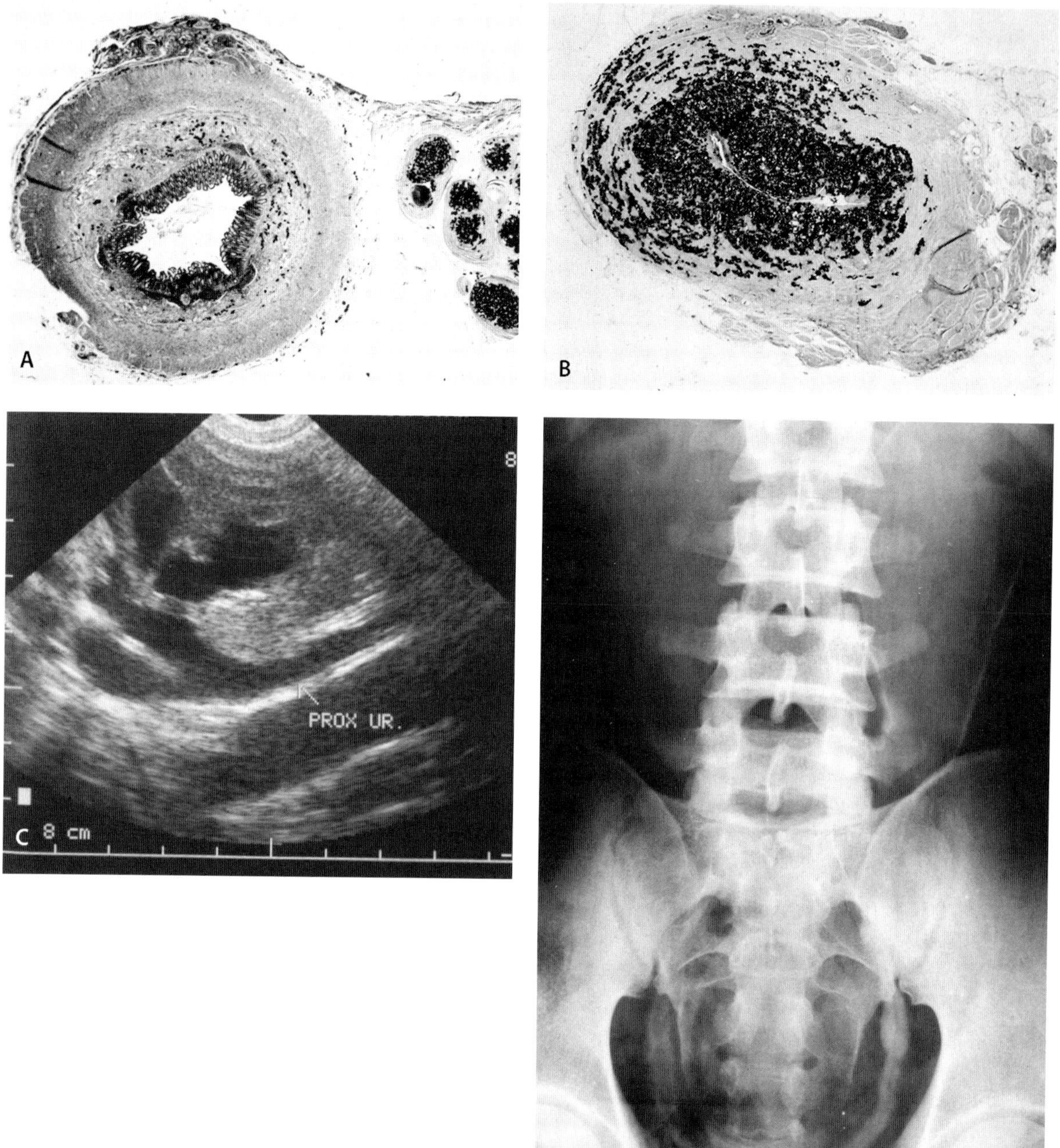

Fig. 2.13 A, B. Cross-sections of two different ureters in schistosomiasis: both show marked thickening and fibrosis of the ureteric walls and calcified *S. haematobium* eggs. **A** Multiple eggs in the wall of the ureter and in the periureteral tissues, but the lumen of the ureter is still patent. ×2 3/4; AFIP 66-3065-24. **B** A very large number of eggs causes massive periureteral calcification, with so much narrowing that the lumen of the ureter is almost obliterated. ×4 1/2; AFIP 66-3065-1. **C** A transverse ultrasound scan of the ureter of a 12-year-old South African boy showing marked hydronephrosis, a dilated extrarenal pelvis, and a dilated and thickened ureter (*PROX UR* proximal ureter) due to schistosomiasis. There is some debris in the renal pelvis as a result of an associated urinary tract infection. (Courtesy of WHO and Dr. Brian J. Cremin, Capetown) **D** Extensive ureteric calcification in a patient from Egypt. There is gross left hydronephrosis outlined with calcification. The lower end of the left ureter is very thick and the lumen has been virtually obliterated. The bladder also shows calcification. On intravenous urography the left kidney was not functioning; there was mild hydronephrosis of the right kidney, perhaps due to renal calculi which could be seen on the plain abdominal film but not in this contrast study. There is, however, calcification of the lower end of the right ureter but the lumen has not been obliterated. AFIP 68-8615-1

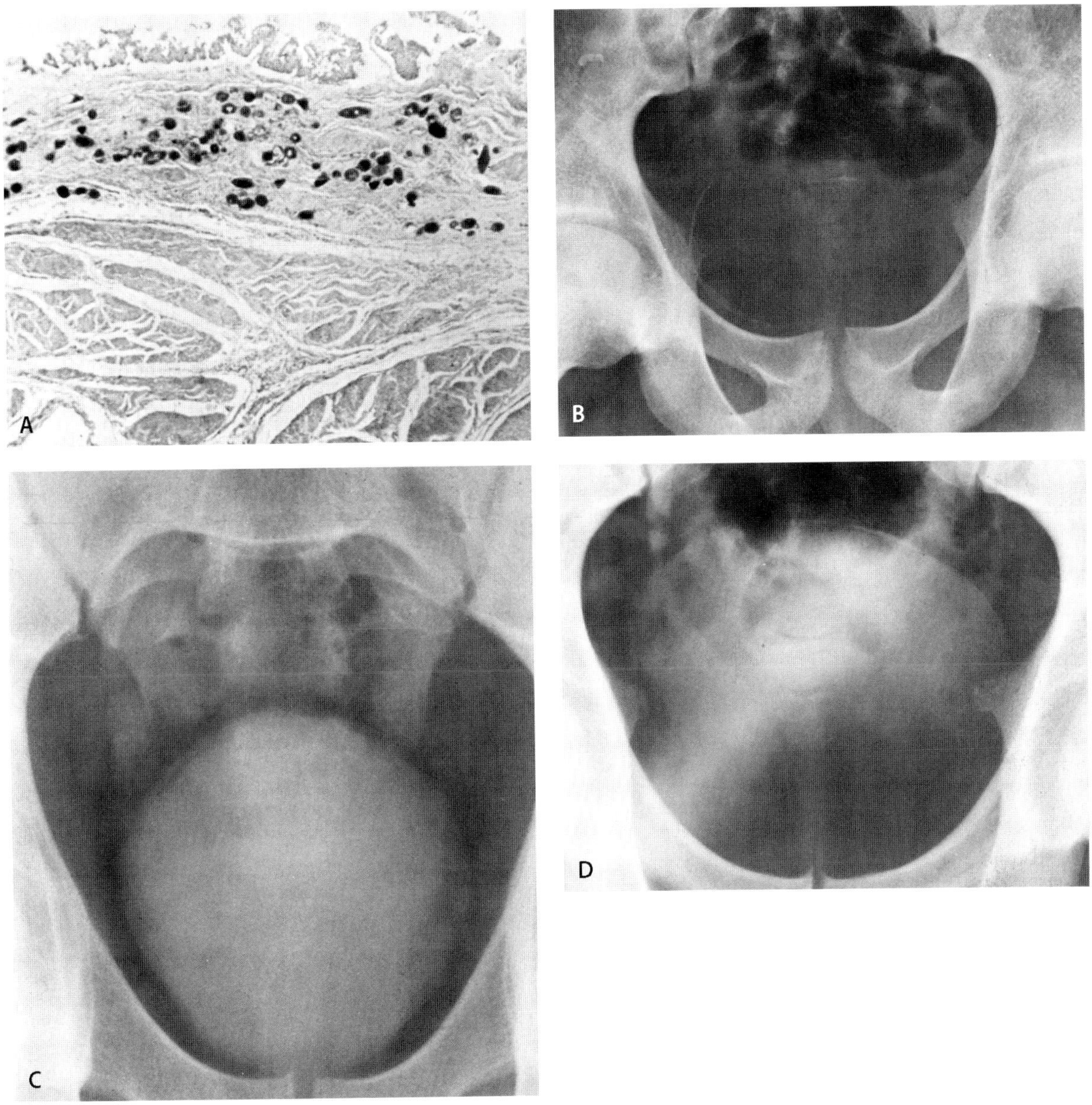

Fig. 2.14 A–F. Radiologically visible calcification in the bladder is due to schistosome eggs in the bladder wall, almost always in the submucosa. The pattern of calcification is very variable in both position and extent. **A** *S. haematobium* eggs in the bladder wall, lying between the mucosa and the muscle. This amount of calcification might be only just visible radiologically. There must be at least 100000 eggs per cm^2 for calcification to be visible on plain radiographs. In this patient, the normal urinary bladder epithelium has undergone squamous cell metaplasia. **B** Very early bladder calcification visible on the right side and across the base. There may be a short length of calcification also in the top of the bladder. **C** The outline of the bladder is hazy and there is edema of the wall. The contrast medium within the bladder is separated by the dark line of the mucosa from the calcification in the wall (best seen across the right half of the dome of the bladder). **D** The right side of the dome of the bladder is hazy and thickened: linear calcification is visible across the dome in the submucosa, with the mucosa showing as a negative linear shadow. (The right ureter is a little dilated and irregular.) **E, F** see p. 134

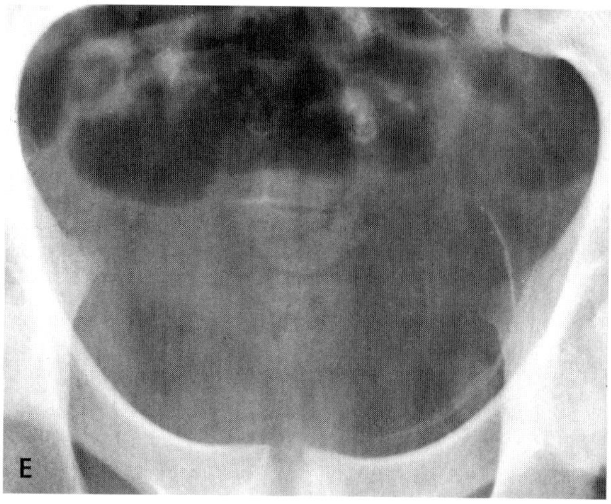

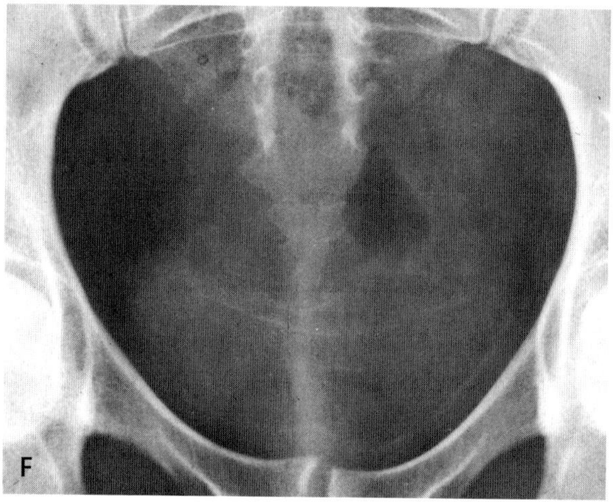

Fig. 2.14 (*continued*). **E** Calcification is visible only on the left side of the bladder, as a double arc. **F** Very faint calcification but almost around the whole bladder. (The dome of the bladder is inverted, due to external pressure)

In other words, a heavily calcified bladder does not shed more eggs than one which is lightly calcified. In both, the activity of the infection or the secondary infection is more significant than the quantity of eggs in the bladder wall.

Bladder calcification can resolve partially or completely, either from reabsorption of calcified eggs in situ or rupture of the eggs from the submucosa into the bladder and passage in the urine. An excretion rate of about 2 000 000 eggs per year is necessary to allow decalcification. If all the calcified eggs are discharged the bladder wall may return to relative normality. Calcified bladders are less common in old age, suggesting that this may be part of the natural history of the disease.

The pattern of calcification is variable. It may be fine and granular, fine and linear, thick and irregular, encircling the whole bladder or only segments, more marked on one side than the other, or at the base or the vault (Figs. 2.14–2.19). The shell-like rim of calcification has little or no effect on bladder capacity or emptying, because it does not indicate fibrosis but only the deposition of the eggs in the submucosa (Figs. 2.18, 2.19). Cystography, either intravenous or retrograde, will frequently show clearly that the calcification lies outside the translucent bladder mucosa (Figs. 2.18, 2.19). Later the bladder does become fibrosed, shrunken and contracted, and (as already noted) the degree of calcification may regress. At this stage the capacity of the bladder often becomes restricted, and there may be secondary infection; some surgical intervention will eventually be required.

Both the clinical and the radiological features may be changed by repeated schistosomal infections, with recurrent edema and congestion (Figs. 2.20–2.22). In addition to the almost inevitable secondary infection, ureteric and bladder calculi are relatively common (Fig. 2.23), although there is some geographic variation in incidence. In chronic schistosomiasis haematobium there is a higher incidence of malignant disease wherever patients have urinary schistosomiasis (Figs. 2.24–2.26). This is not a simple "cause and effect" association. Schistosomal bladder malignancy is predominately squamous cell in type. It is not entirely certain why it occurs, although the association is beyond question. The bladder mucosa becomes hyperplastic and undergoes squamous metaplasia, almost always with infection. This evolves into squamous carcinoma, which usually spreads laterally and from the mucosa into the bladder wall and surrounding tissues, with lymphatic spread to the para-aortic lymph nodes. Whether this carcinoma arises from prolonged irritation of the bladder epithelium from urinary stasis and sepsis, or from carcinogens in the urine of patients (a high level of tryptophan) is undecided but, in the early stages, the differential diagnosis of bladder wall thickening by either ultrasonography or cystography can be very difficult.

Fig. 2.15. **A** Faint calcification in the left lower quadrant of the bladder. **B** A rim of calcification around the whole bladder. **C** Calcification surrounding the bladder (with external pressure on the left side of the dome); the lower half of the left ureter is bifid and remains filled because of a constriction at the bladder wall. **D** A rim of bladder calcification of varying thickness, with calcification in the lower part of the left ureter. **E, F** The same African patient. When the bladder is filled, calcification is clearly visible around the lower half on both sides and across the base. After micturition (**F**) calcification can be seen around the whole of the bladder. The double-dome has no clinical significance ▶

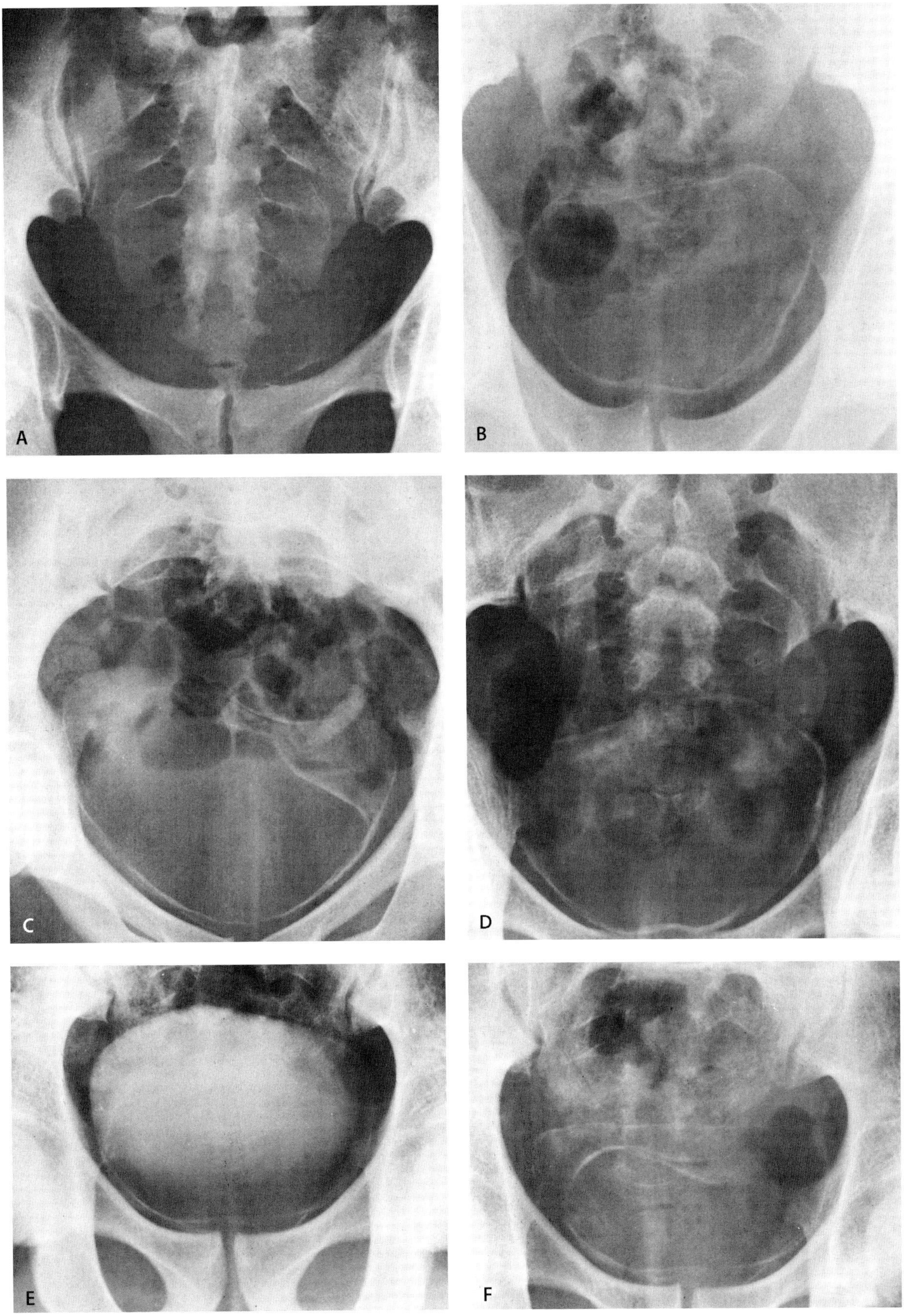
A
B
C
D
E
F

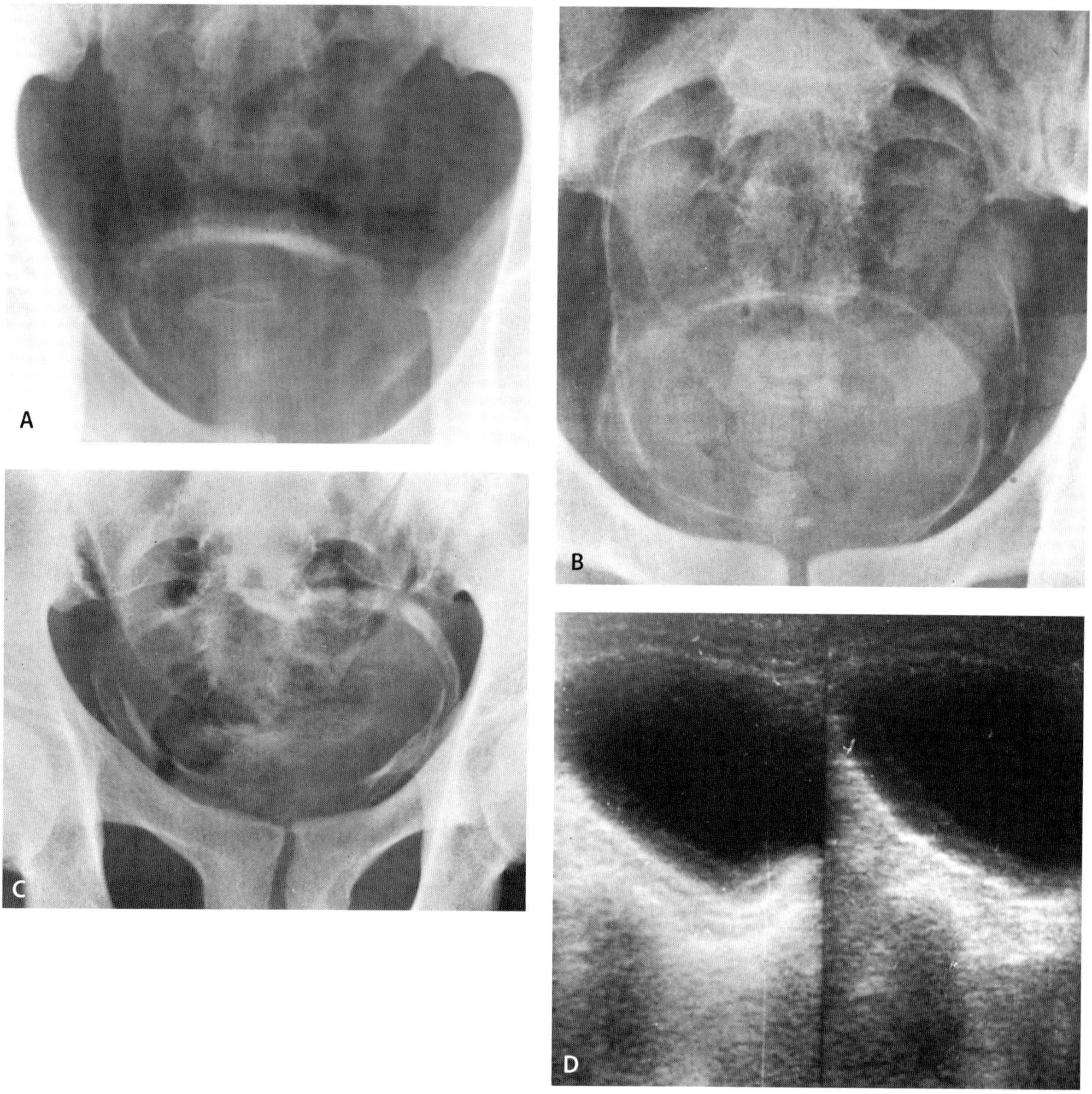

Fig. 2.16. **A** Thick calcification across the fundus of the bladder with less marked calcification of varying density on both sides. **B** In this bladder there are two quite distinct circles of calcification; this is all in the wall of the bladder and this double layer has no clinical significance. **C** Thicker, multi-layered calcification of the entire bladder wall; there is no explanation why there should be more eggs deposited on one side (in this bladder, *on the left*). There is no clinical correlation. **D** Two transverse ultrasound scans of a bladder, showing calcification and thickening of the bladder wall. (An Egyptian patient; courtesy of Prof. M.R. El Meligi, Cairo) **E, F** see p. 137

Reflux from the bladder up the ureters is a late complication of the ureteric and bladder abnormalities (Fig. 2.19). Reflux does not occur in the early stages because of the ureteric stenosis. As fibrous tissue replaces the granulomas, the ureters become aperistaltic and dilated. Vesicoureteric reflux eventually occurs in about 30% of patients who have a significantly calcified bladder. It is interesting and important to note that, despite reflux for many years, renal disease develops slowly, even when there is both hydronephrosis and hydroureter. Children, in particular, often respond well to treatment and the post-therapy urogram may be surprisingly normal. In chronic infections, when the bladder has become contracted, the ureters are calcified and the disease is longstanding, ascending urinary infection does occur, but the average patient manages to avoid this for longer than might be expected. There is no clinical evidence that such reflux contributes significantly to the development of hypertension in

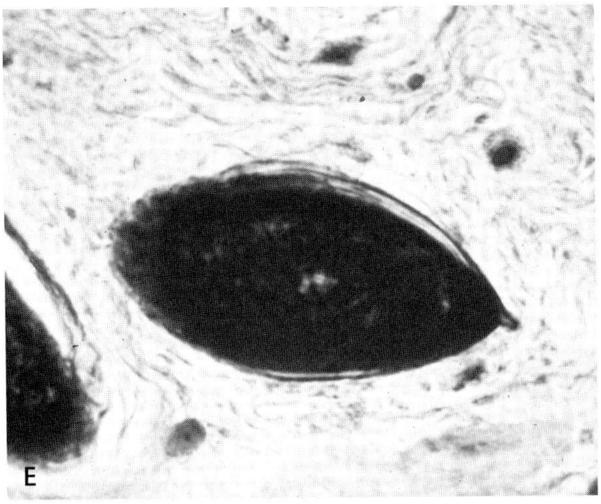

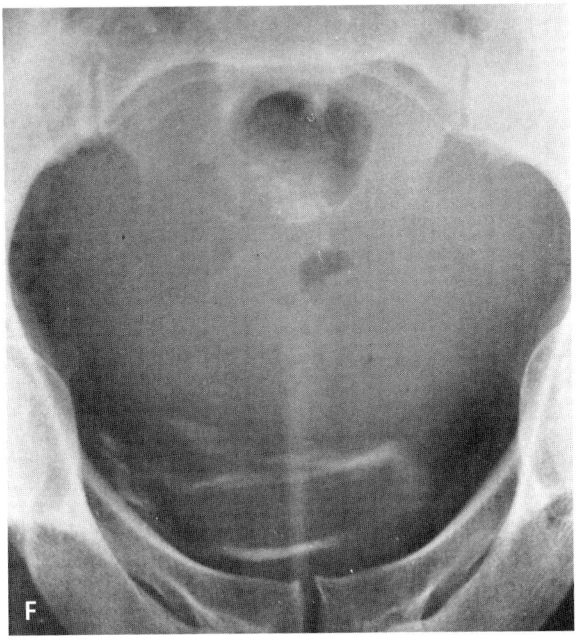

Fig. 2.16 (*continued*). **E** The eggs of *S. haematobium* in the wall of the bladder. AFIP 66-3065-53. **F** This bladder is empty and collapsed due to the pressure of an enlarged, pregnant, uterus. This was an incidental finding

patients with *S. haematobium* infection. However, in *S. mansoni* infection there is evidence of glomerular disease, almost certainly of immunological origin. Such renal disease has been invariably associated with hepatosplenic schistosomiasis (see p. 121).

Hydronephrosis is not always due to reflux: because the incidence of ureteric involvement in the presence of bladder disease may reach as high as 40%, hydronephrosis can be due either to the reduced bladder capacity and high intravesical pressure, or to stricture of the ureter or, in about one-third of the cases, to involvement of the ureter and subsequent dilatation and aperistalsis without obvious stricture or bladder shrinkage.

In the chronic stage if ultrasonography does not give enough information, the radiological examination must include a good plain radiograph: if ureteric calcification is suspected but has not been clearly demonstrated, oblique views may be added to the routine anteroposterior (AP) views of the abdomen. If necessary, an additional view angled 15° caudally towards the pelvis will demonstrate the bladder more accurately. It may be advisable not to use ureteric compression, but rather to use a high-dose urography technique, so that the exact state of the ureters may be demonstrated: applying pressure to an inflamed ureter may alter its tone and thus its appearance. The examination of the bladder should include a postmicturition film angled upwards (cranially) at 15° and centered over the symphysis pubis. This will demonstrate the base of the bladder without distortion, as well as confirming the bladder emptying.

Various methods have been described for assessing the ureters before surgery. Perfusion pressure flow studies and diuretic isotope renography, with wash-out, have been used to show the presence or absence of obstruction. Diuretic renography provides an accurate assessment in the majority of cases, but there can be false-positives and perfusion studies should follow before surgery. Technitium-99m diethylene triamine penta-acetic acid (DTPA) is used, followed by furosemide (20 mg) to produce diuresis. However, a reasonably accurate assessment of both renal function and the state of the ureters can be obtained from intravenous contrast urography, with laboratory tests if needed.

Urethral stenosis from schistosomiasis does occur, but gonorrhea is much more likely to be the commonest cause of such a stricture in most countries of the world.

Calcification may also be seen in the seminal vesicles (Fig. 2.27) and, rarely, in the spermatic cord. Schistosomiasis of the testes (bilharzial orchitis) causes edema and, in some patients, the testicular granuloma may simulate a mass. This can be detected by ultrasonography but could be mistaken for testicular malignancy, leading to unnecessary orchiectomy. As many of the patients will be young men, treatment for schistosomiasis and reassessment, and perhaps ultrasound-guided biopsy, are advisable. The fallopian tubes may be infected and blocked, causing a pelvic mass, but calcification has not been recorded. It may well be demonstrated in the future, as CT becomes more widely available. *S. haematobium* may be recovered from the cervix uteri, but has no significance for the diagnostic radiologist, except that the ultrasonographic appearance of the edematous schistosomal cervix may resemble carcinoma and even clinically it can be very difficult to differentiate.

(Text continues on p. 140)

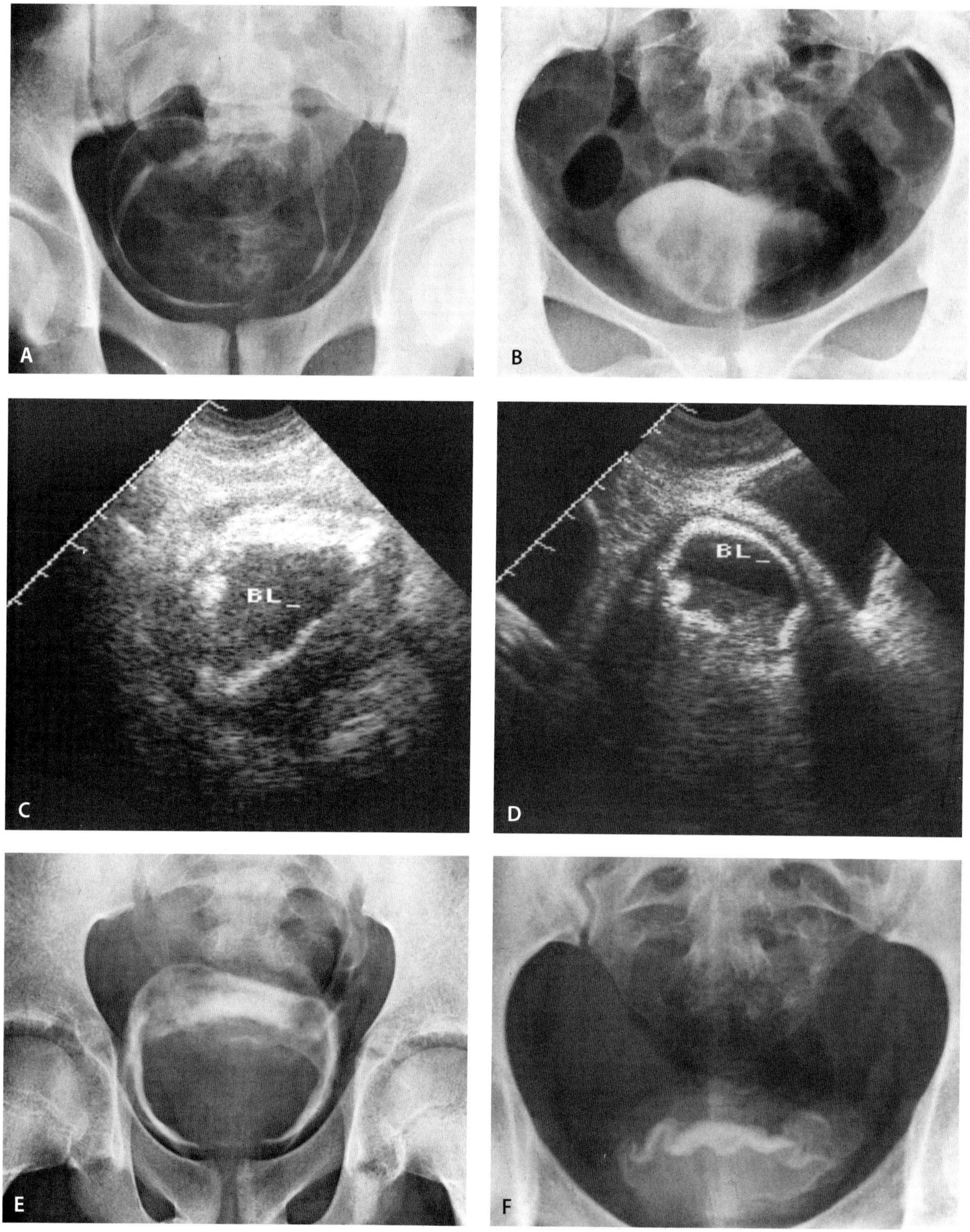

Fig. 2.17. **A** Thick and thin calcification in the same bladder. **B** Very heavy bladder calcification, distorted by the gas in the colon. The thin negative line of the mucosa shows very clearly over the right side of the fundus. **C, D** Ultrasound scans of two patients from Zimbabwe. Both have well-marked calcification, but are totally different. There is thickening of the bladder wall in each patient. *BL* Bladder. (Courtesy of Dr. Sam Mindel) **E** Heavy calcification almost completely surrounding the bladder. The lower part of the left ureter is also calcified. **F** Thick "serpiginous" calcification across the fundus of an empty bladder. It is probable that the calcification does not seem so thick and irregular when the bladder is full. As this figure illustrates, heavy calcification does not usually prevent the bladder from emptying

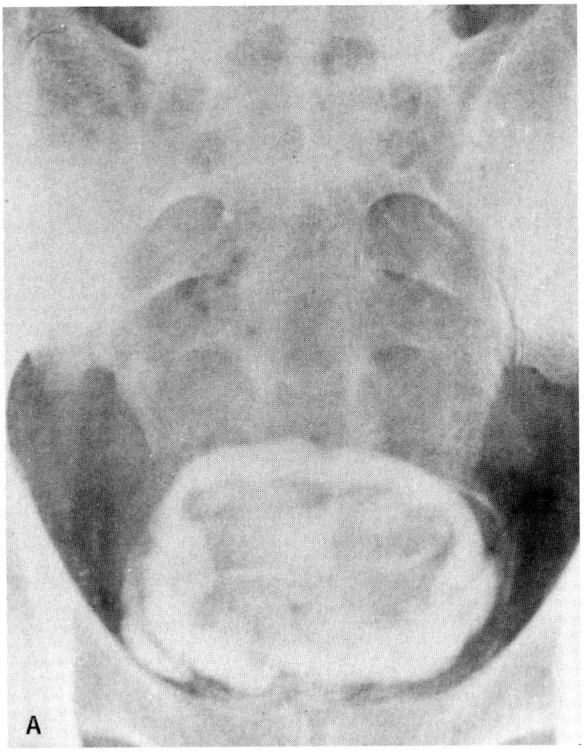

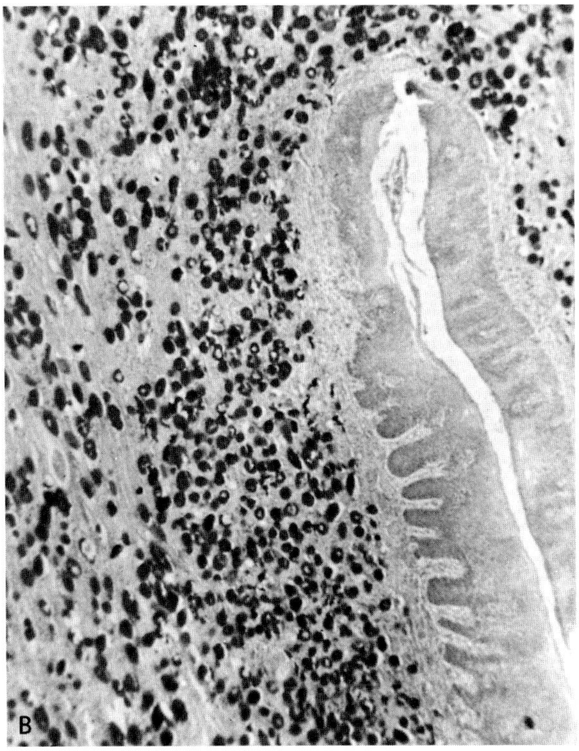

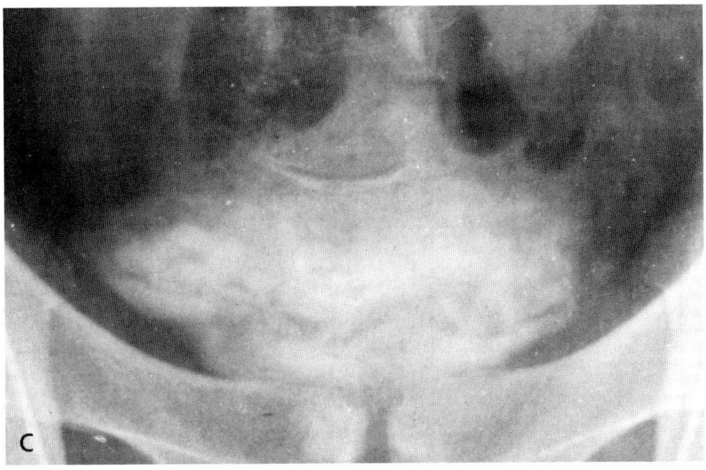

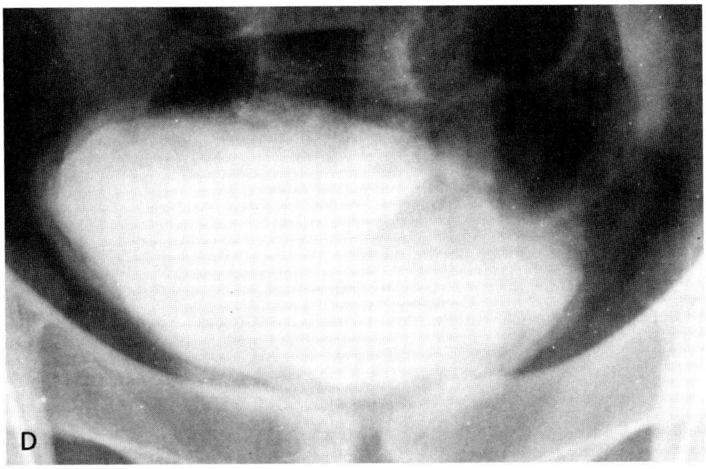

Fig. 2.18 A–F. Extremely heavy bladder calcification in schistosomiasis haematobium. **A** Dense, with the calcification in the submucosa and bladder wall of an African patient. **B** Histological section showing countless calcified *S. haematobium* eggs within the bladder wall and marked squamous metaplasia of the bladder mucosa. **C** The heavily calcified (empty) bladder of an Egyptian male patient. **D** The bladder of the same patient when filled on intravenous urography. In spite of the very heavy calcification, the bladder still has the capacity to expand, and contracts quite well during micturition. The wall of the bladder does not become fibrotic and lose its capacity to expand until quite late in the disease, unless there is severe superimposed cystitis. Although this bladder is heavily calcified, it is still possible to see the radiolucent shadow of the mucosa between the central contrast and the bladder wall. There is dilatation of the lower end of the left ureter due to stenosis in the distal segment. **E, F** see p. 140

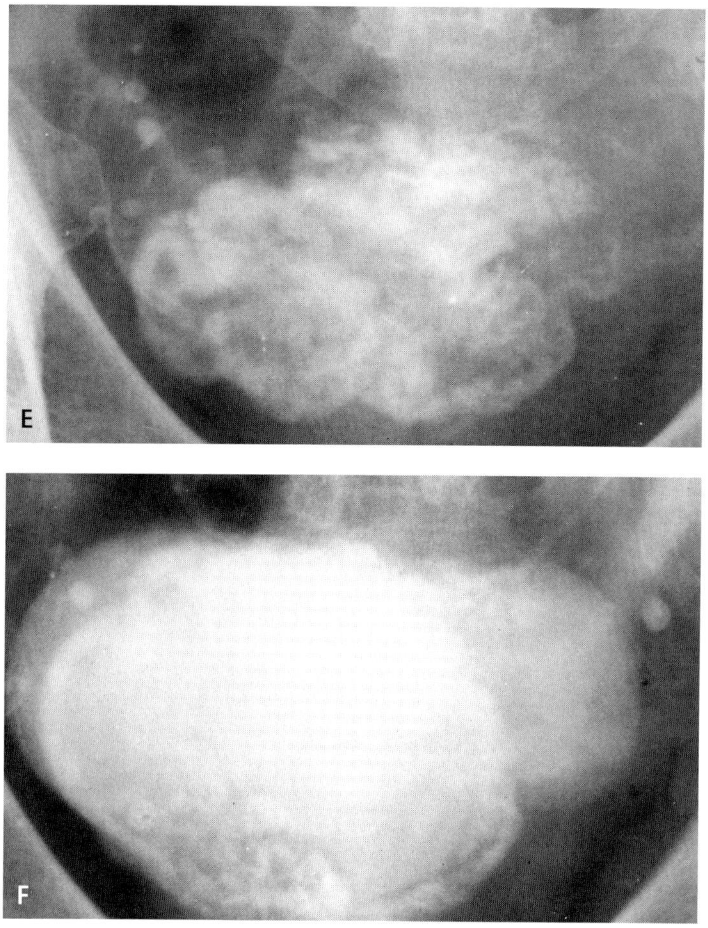

Fig. 2.18 (*continued*). E Another Egyptian patient with dense serpiginous calcification throughout the distorted wall of the bladder. However (F), this does not prevent distention of the bladder which fills well during intravenous urography. In F, the left ureter is dilated. (C–F AFIP 22-9499-532/283)

Unfortunately, both schistosomiasis and carcinoma of the cervix not infrequently coexist. Schistosomiasis has been implicated in the causation of vesicovaginal fistulae. However, it seems more likely that schistosomiasis is a complication rather than a cause of fistula, but it has been shown to delay healing because of the fibrosis which schistosomiasis causes.

Computed tomography of the urinary tract should not be the primary imaging procedure for schistosomiasis haematobium, although the scans can clearly demonstrate the calcified eggs in the bladder, in the ureters, and in the surrounding tissues. It may be most useful in the differential diagnosis of bladder wall thickening and the exclusion of carcinoma, or the staging of a tumor. Apart from this, because the ureteric and bladder functional changes are not dependent on the extent of calcification, CT is not usually necessary.

(Text continues on p. 150)

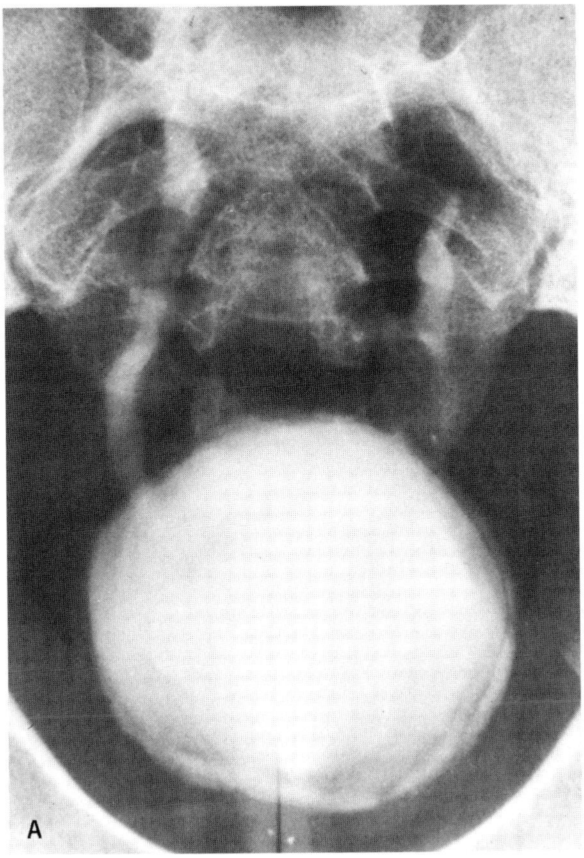

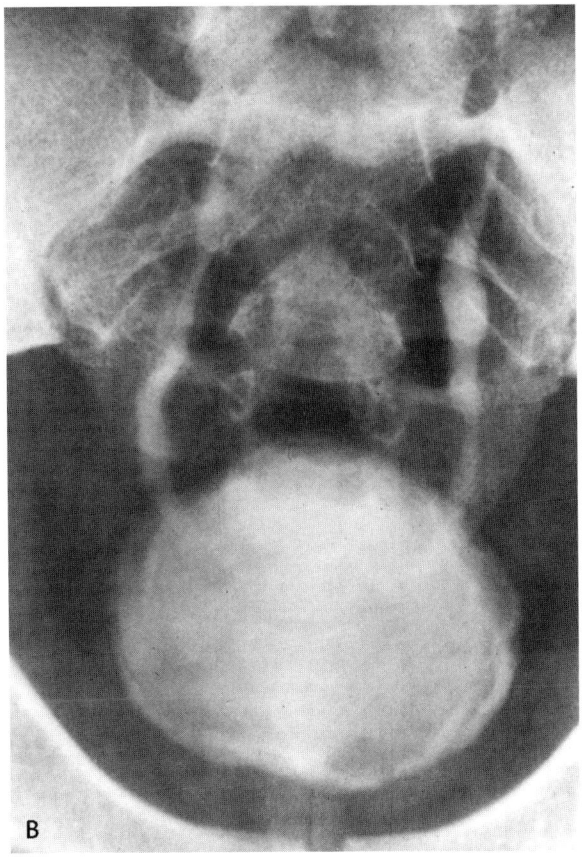

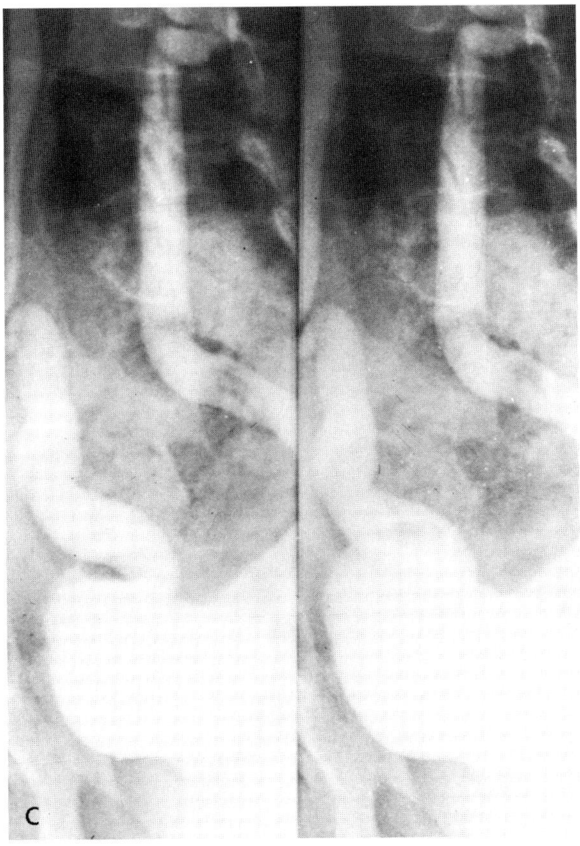

Fig. 2.19 A–G. Bladder calcification, even if quite heavy, does not usually cause problem in micturition. **A** The contrast-filled bladder of a young African male, with quite thick surrounding calcification. The bladder capacity and shape remain relatively normal. Both ureters are a little dilated, but this is probably due to ureteric infection. **B** At the start of micturition the bladder wall becomes irregular and starts to contract in the normal way. There is some reflux, particularly up the left ureter, which at a later stage may become clinically significant (see **C** below). On both **A** and **B** the negative line of mucosa can be seen, not only around the bladder, but on either side of the right ureter. **C** Marked reflux up both ureters during voiding cystourethrography in another patient with advanced schistosomiasis. The ureters are both dilated, smooth, and aperistaltic. The bladder is small and fibrotic and cannot expand to its normal capacity. The urethra was normal. **D–G** see p. 142

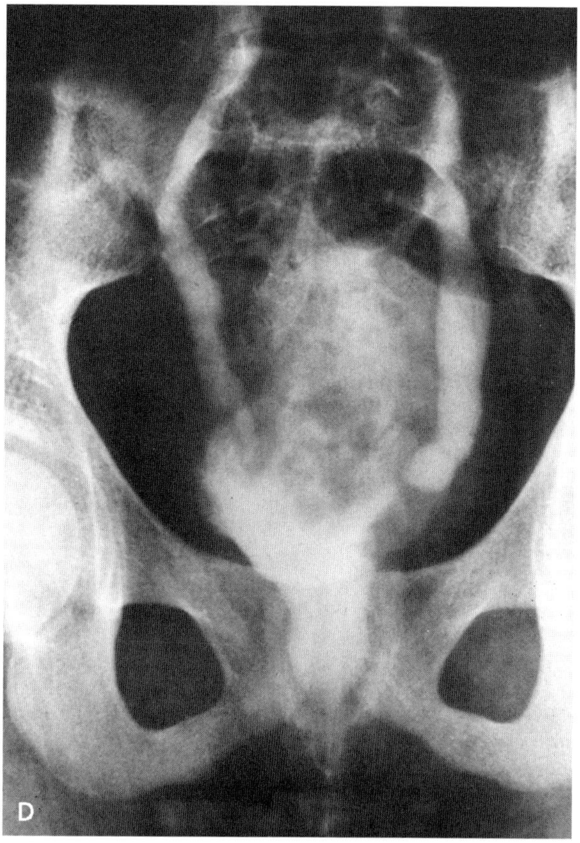

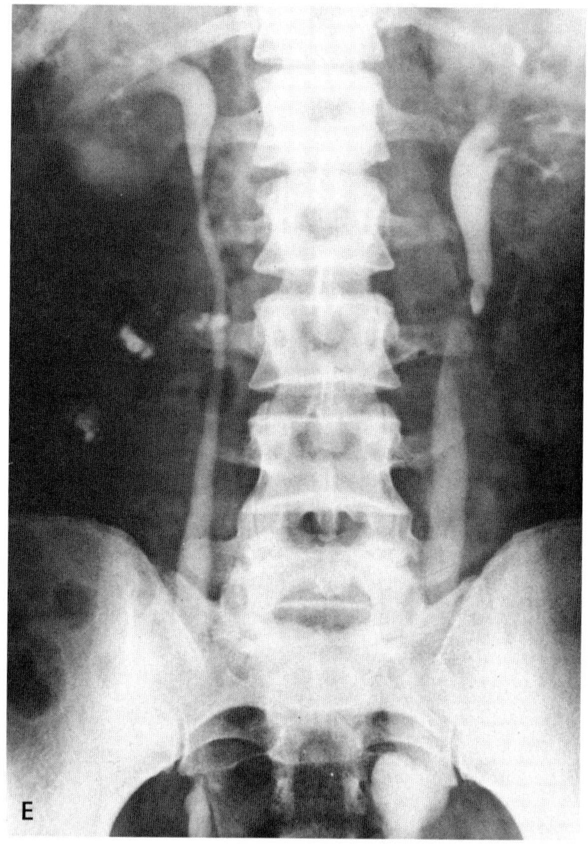

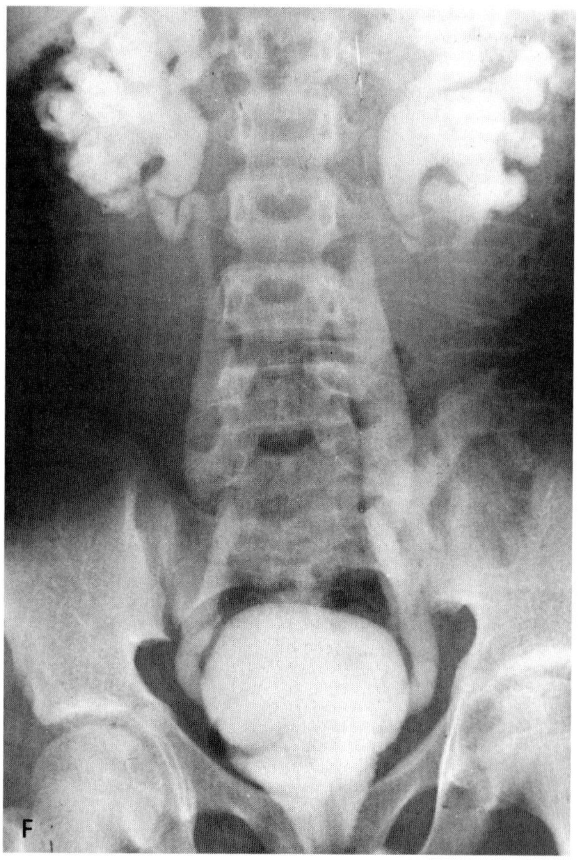

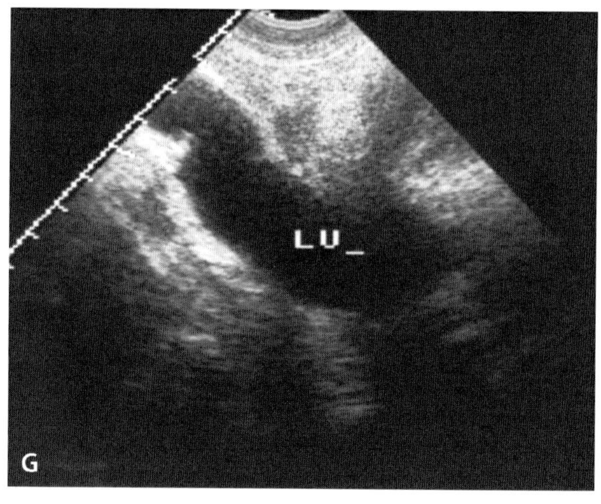

Fig. 2.19 (*continued*). **D** Reflux up both ureters from a contracted, nodular bladder. In this patient there is still beading and irregularity of both dilated ureters. **E** An intravenous urogram on a Caucasian patient showing several stenotic areas in the lower third of both ureters, with local and general dilatation. Despite this, the kidneys are within normal limits and do not yet show any caliceal dilatation. **F** Gross bilateral hydronephrosis and hydroureter demonstrated by reflux from a retrograde cystogram. The ureters are atonic and have lost the beaded appearance. As well as schistosomiasis, there is likely to be a urinary tract infection. **G** An ultrasound scan of an African from Zimbabwe showing a grossly dilated left ureter (*LU*). (Courtesy of Dr. Sam Mindel)

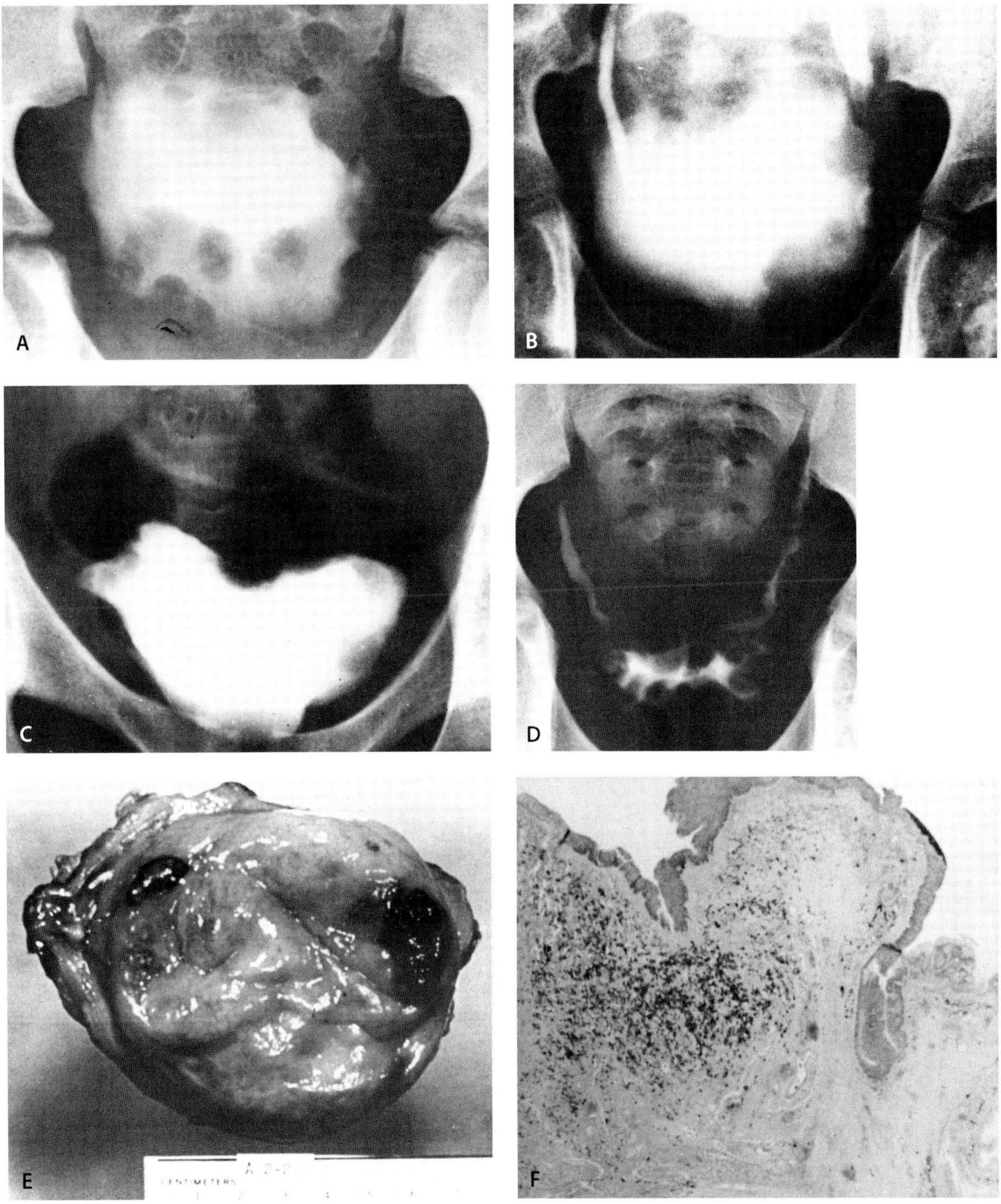

Fig. 2.20 A–F. Severe acute bladder reaction in three different Nigerian children, due to urticarial edema of the bladder wall and mucosa. It is probable that these changes occur when there has been reinfection with *S. haematobium* after a period free from the disease. There are large round filling defects within the bladder of each child. **D** is the same patient as **A**, with the bladder empty after micturition. These masses can be mistaken for sarcoma botryoides. The swelling disappears rapidly with appropriate treatment and the bladder usually returns to normal. In **B** and **D** the ureters are dilated and irregular, with areas of stenosis. **E** Polypoid-like lesions in the bladder of a 10-year-old Egyptian child. There were red elevated polyps at the apex of the bladder and along the right ureteric orifice. These sharply localized, active lesions are not uncommon in *S. haematobium* infection, suggesting that the adult flukes remain at one site for some time. There were eight pairs of adults in the bladder vasculature in this patient. **F** The cross-section of a similar polyp from another patient, showing large numbers of calcified schistosome ova in the lamina propria and submucosa. There is marked squamous cell metaplasia of the bladder mucosa. This type of polyp is not easily recognized on contrast cystography, but can be demonstrated with ultrasound and easily seen on cystoscopy. (**E** AFIP 229499-881; **A**, **D** courtesy of Dr. Stanley P. Bohrer)

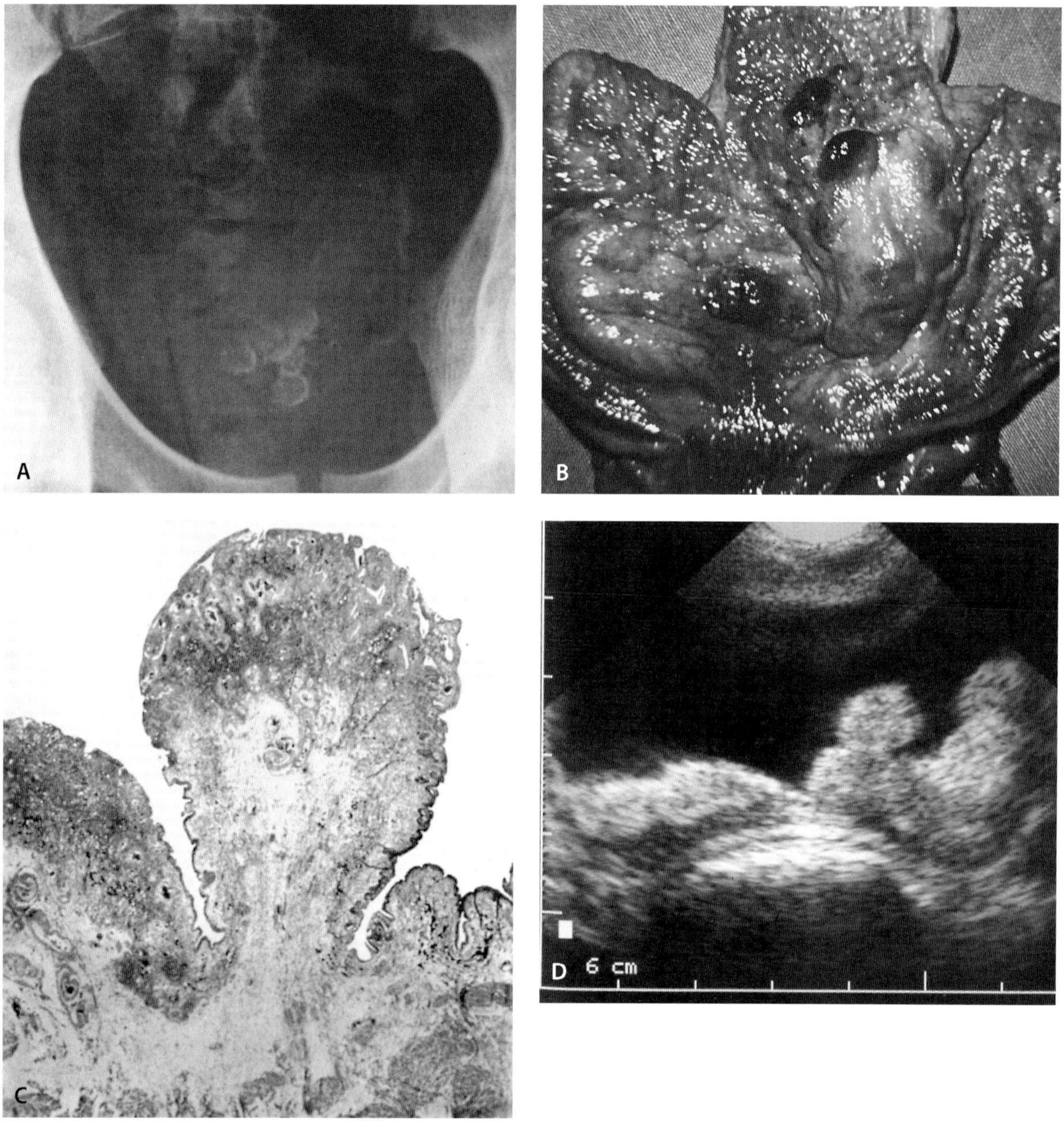

Fig. 2.21 A–D. Schistosomal bladder polyps. **A** Calcification along the base of several small polyps and in the wall of the left side of the bladder. This pattern is not very common. **B** The inside of a similar bladder with three schistosomal polyps and edematous, nodular, inflamed mucosa. **C** Histology of a similar polyp with adult *S. haematobium* schistosomes in the venules of the large polyp and in the veins of the lamina propria. There are also multiple calcified schistosome eggs in the submucosa and lamina propria. ×8; AFIP 68-2723-8. **D** The ultrasound scan of a similar polyp in a young African patient. (Courtesy of Dr. Brian J. Cremin, Capetown)

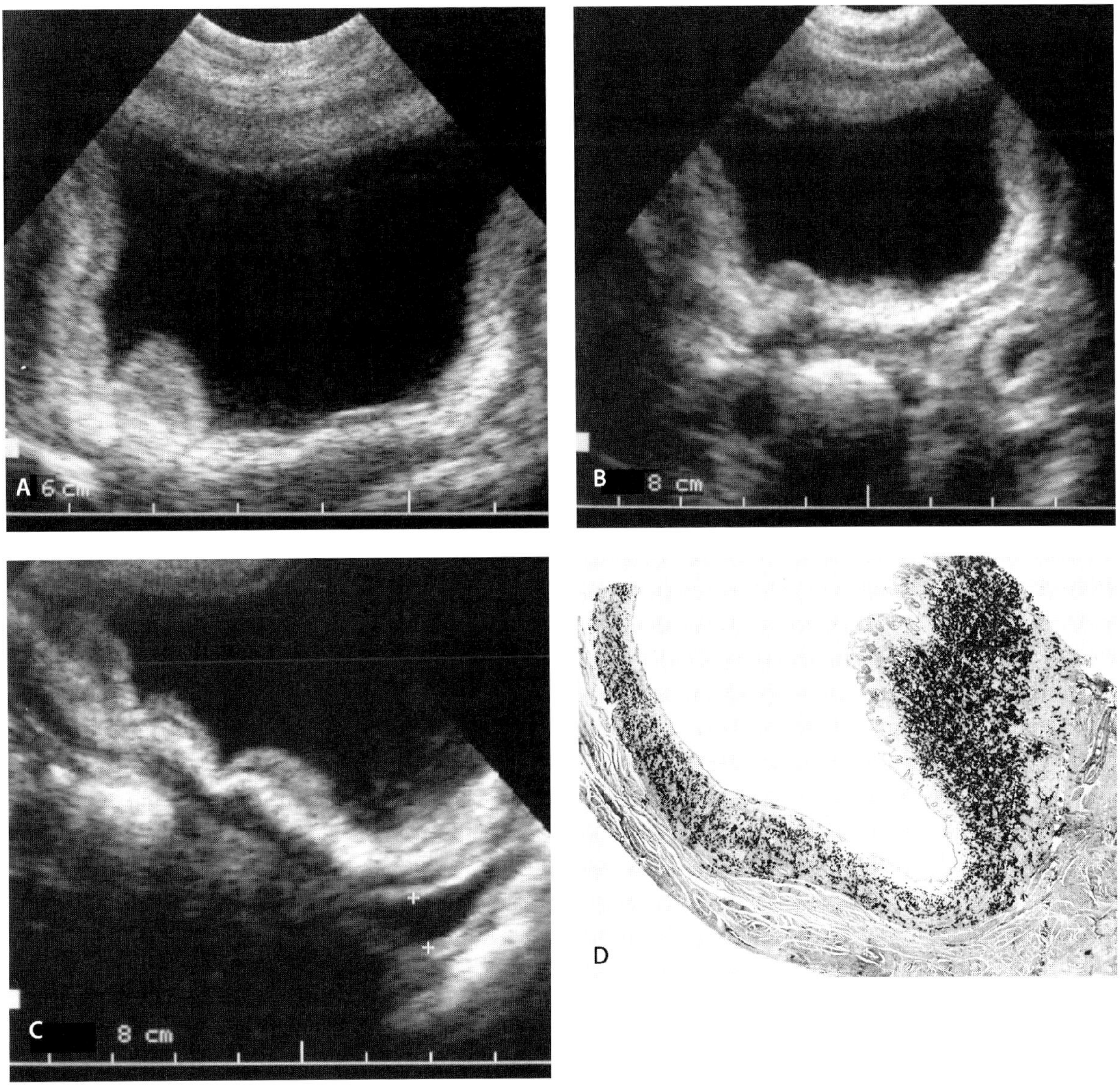

Fig. 2.22 A–C. Ultrasound scans showing gross thickening of the bladder wall and of the ureter (**B**) in a 12-year-old boy from South Africa. (Courtesy of Dr. Brian J. Cremin, Capetown and WHO) **D** The histology of a similar bladder, showing multiple calcified ova, marked mucosal swelling, and squamous metaplasia. AFIP 66-3065-54

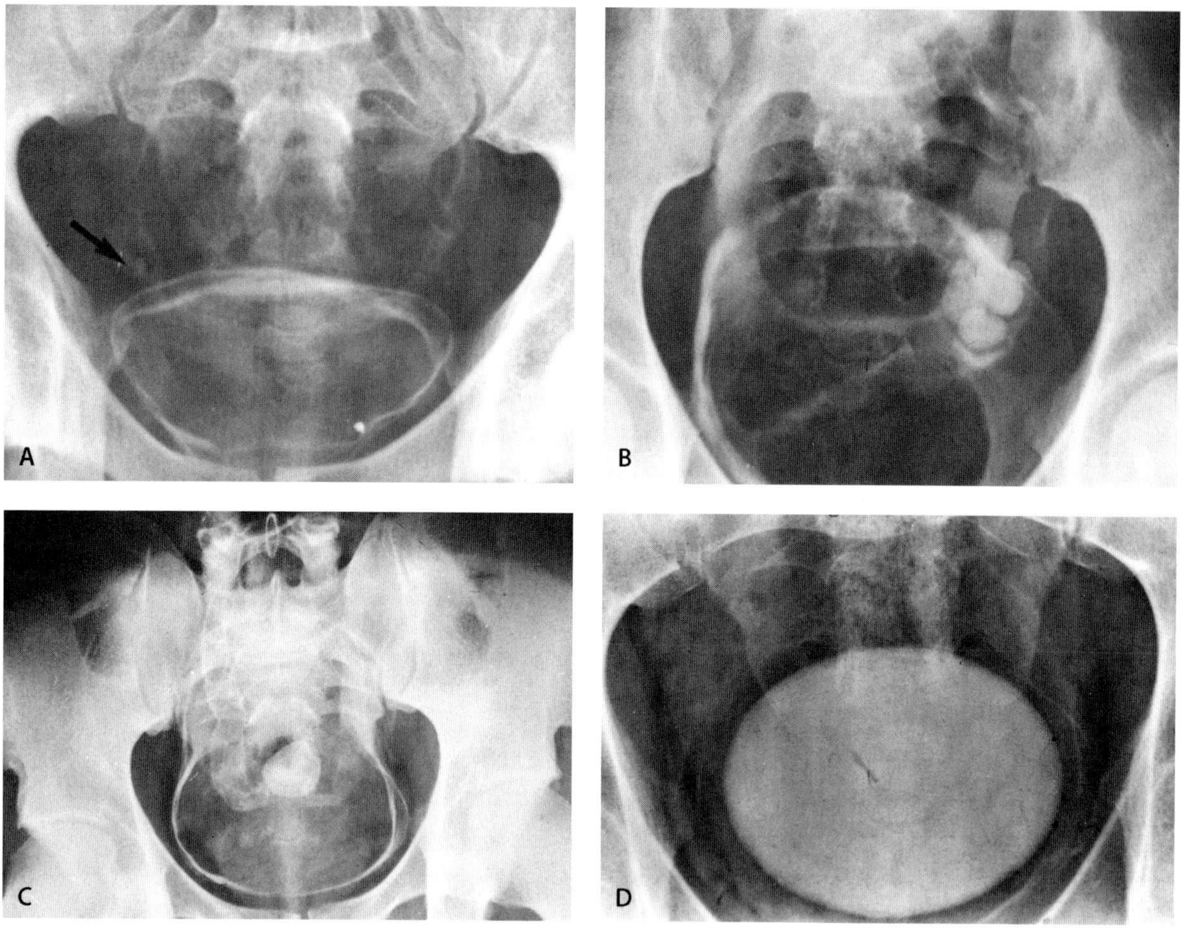

Fig. 2.23 A–D. The incidence of urinary calculi associated with schistosomiasis varies considerably throughout the tropics, although recurrent infection is common. Calculi are not related to the extent of ureteric or bladder calcification. **A** A small calculus (*arrow*) in the distal right ureter of a patient with a moderately calcified bladder. **B** Multiple calculi in the lower end of the left ureter. (Both ureters are dilated and the bladder wall is calcified.) These calculi were originally thought to be in the bladder diverticulum, but a repeat examination did not show any: it was unlikely that there were any pills in the colon, and there did not seem to be any rational explanation. It was then realized that the ureter was grossly dilated, so widely that the stones could pass easily upwards into the kidney and were, therefore, not always visible on a pelvic radiograph. Reexamining the patient erect restored the calculi and the reputation of the radiologist. **C** Another African patient with dilated, calcified ureters, a calcified bladder wall and a moderate sized bladder calculus. There is no correlation between the extent of the ureteric calcification and that in the bladder wall. **D** A very large calculus occupying the whole of the bladder, surrounded by thin calcification in the bladder wall. (This is a plain radiograph, not a contrast cystogram)

Fig. 2.24 A–F. Chronic schistosomiasis is associated with a significantly increased incidence of carcinoma of the urinary bladder. A malignant mass is probably most easily recognized by ultrasonography, which will also show thickening and infiltration of the bladder wall and demonstrate the extent of the tumor very accurately. These six ultrasound scans are all from different patients (all Africans from Zimbabwe) and clearly show tumors of different sizes in different parts of the bladder. *M*, mass; *P*, prostate; *R*, rectum; *Bl*, bladder. The patients were men (**A–C**) and women (**D–F**), age 40–70 years. (Courtesy of Dr. Sam Mindel) ▶

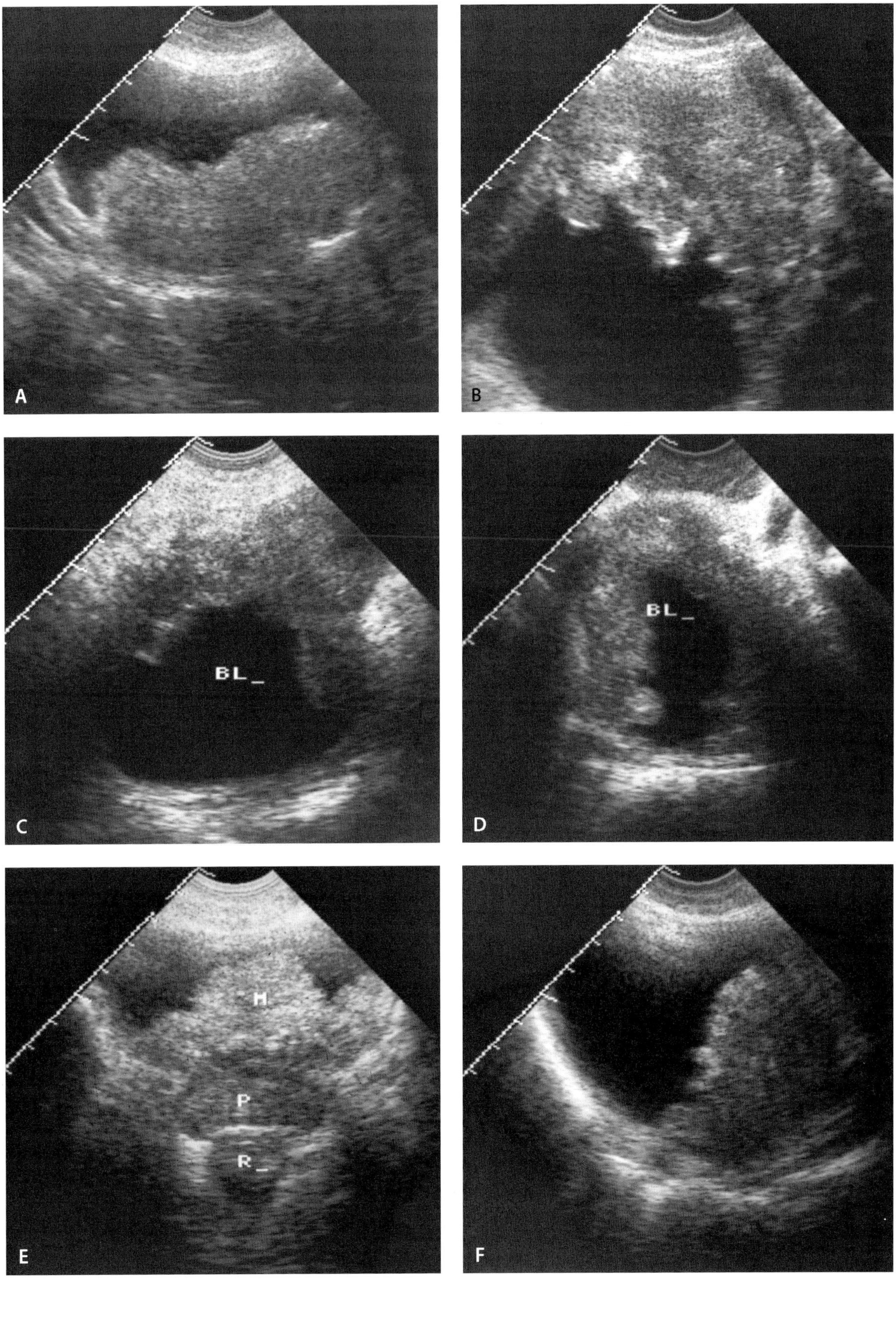
A
B
BL
C
BL
D
H
P
R
E
F

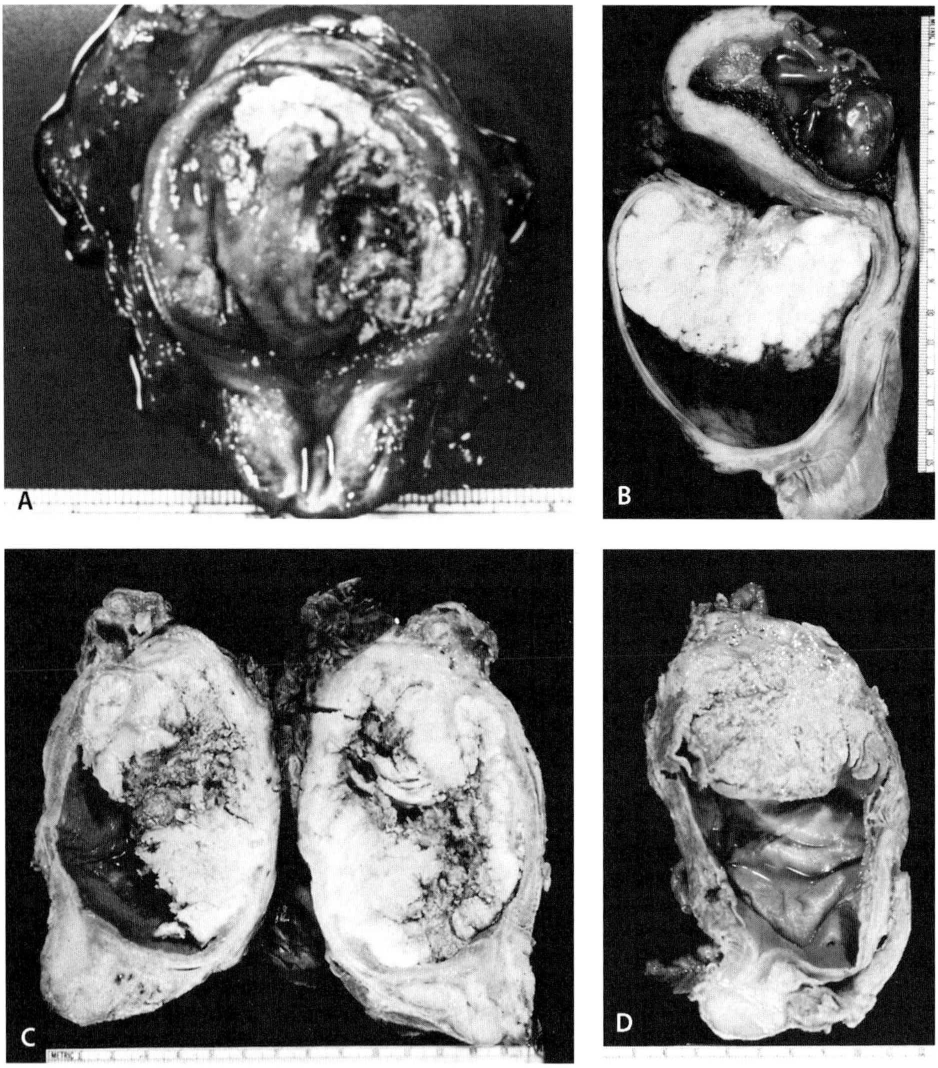

Fig. 2.25 A–D. The macroscopic appearance of schistosomal carcinoma of the bladder. **A** A large ulcerating squamous cell carcinoma of the left posterior wall of the bladder of a 26-year-old Egyptian male. The bladder contained 156000 eggs per gram of tissue, together with 18 pairs of adult worms. The very white area near the top of the bladder is due to squamous metaplasia and leukoplakia; scattered over the remainder of the bladder are: numerous confluent, sandy (granulomatous) patches. **B** A large carcinoma of the bladder in a pregnant woman. The fetus is seen in utero above the bladder. AFIP 66-3065-52. **C** A huge carcinoma virtually filling the bladder cavity. AFIP 63065-32. **D** A large carcinoma of the fundus of the bladder. AFIP 66-3065-50. It is unusual to see calcified eggs within the tumor, either on section or radiographically

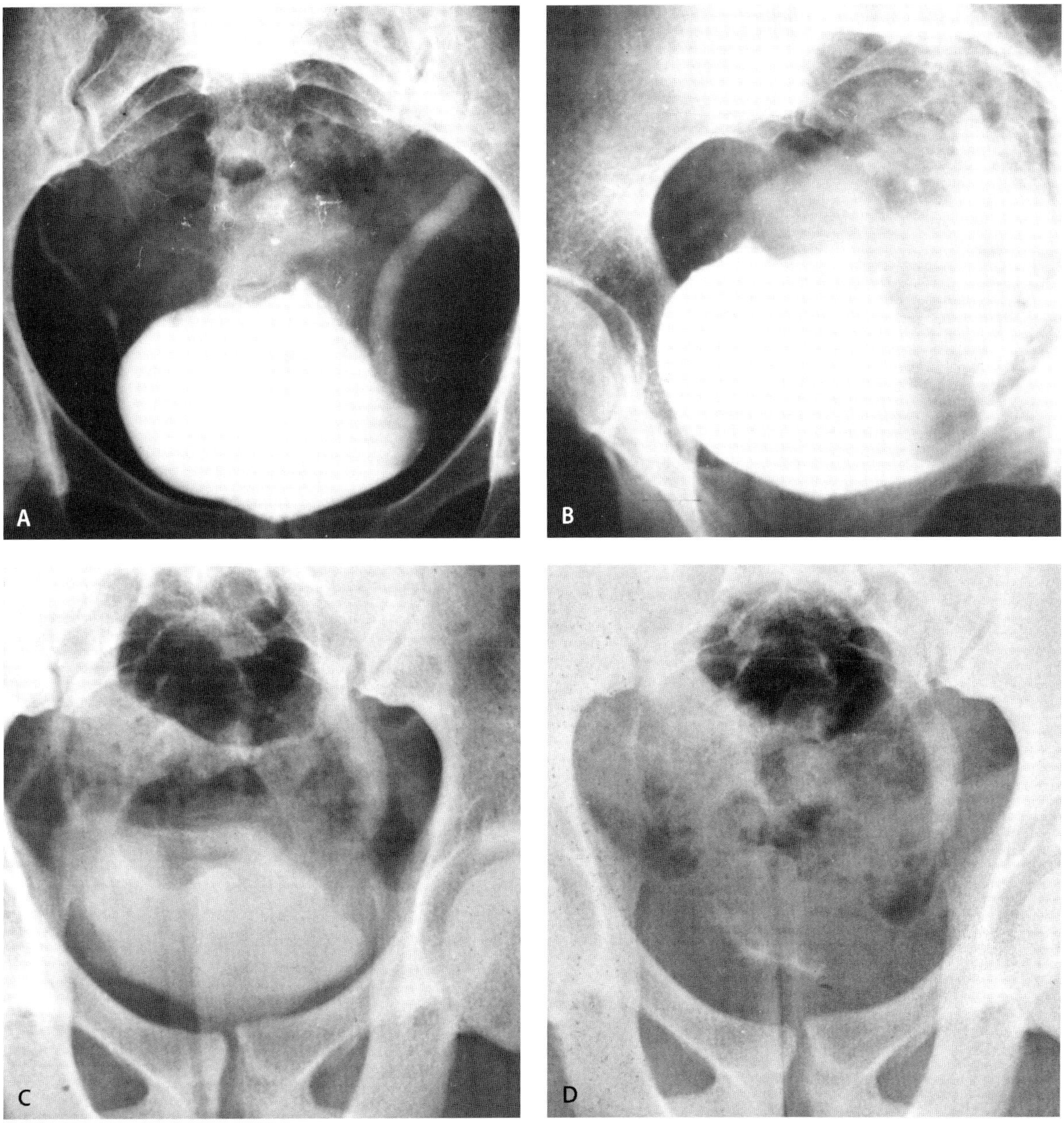

Fig. 2.26 A–D. The cystographic appearance of carcinoma of the bladder in three patients. **A, B** Patients from Egypt. **C** is an African with a similar carcinoma which is partially obstructing the left ureter; after micturition (**D**) the ureter remains filled, and although the bladder empties completely there is still a significant soft tissue shadow in the pelvis because the bladder wall is thickened by both the neoplasm and the schistosomal fibrosis

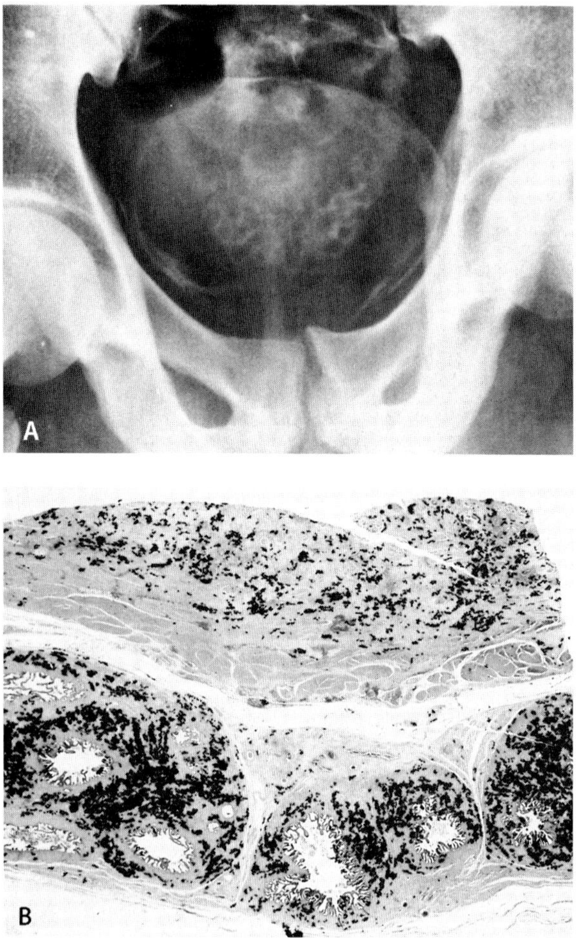

Fig. 2.27. A Schistosomiasis of the seminal vesicles. Eggs can be deposited in the seminal vesicles, which will then show as calcification behind the bladder and adjacent to the ureters. This bladder is also calcified. **B** Histological section showing innumerable calcified eggs of *S. haematobium* in the seminal vesicles. With this number of eggs there is almost always fibrosis and muscle hypertrophy. ×2; AFIP 66-3065-23

Lungs

Radiological abnormalities in the chest are uncommon in patients infected with *S. haematobium*, despite the fact that *S. haematobium* eggs are found about twice as frequently in the lungs as *S. mansoni* eggs. In a previously reported personal series of over 15000 patients of all ages, of whom at least 70% were known to be infected with *S. haematobium*, and all of whom had chest x-rays, there was not one patient in whom a diagnosis of pulmonary schistosomiasis was entertained. In a similar smaller series reported from Zambia (Northern Rhodesia) of 255 cases, all known to have bilharziasis and all under the age of 30 years, there were no abnormal pulmonary findings. And yet it should be emphasized that, pathologically, every second case will show ova in the lungs.

Radiologically there are three distinct patterns which, although rare in clinical practice, may be significant. The first, the Katayama syndrome (Fig. 2.28 A), has already been described on p. 125 and the radiological changes in *S. haematobium* at this stage are identical to those of *S. mansoni*.

The second pattern is the reaction around the larvae either when they embolize a small vessel or die during treatment. This is a local immune reaction similar to others in the Löffler syndrome. There is likely to be a peripheral blood eosinophilia. There will be scattered hazy foci of consolidation in both lungs, changing in both size and position at short intervals, and without any specific distribution. There is not likely to be any long-term result. There is no lymphadenopathy (Fig. 2.58).

The third pattern is often found by chance in the elderly patient when a routine chest radiograph shows a pattern of fine, generalized, interstitial fibrosis, distributed equally throughout both lungs (Fig. 2.28 B); it is nearly always symmetrical and not confined to the lung bases. There are no abnormal clinical findings and in most patients the degree of dyspnea is no more than would be expected from the patient's age. The cardiac outline is normal and there is no cor pulmonale or clinical cyanosis. The microscopic findings are those of diffuse fibrosis with numerous eggs in the peribronchial regions; emphysema is not a marked feature. Even in endemic areas this is uncommon, but when seen it is typical, as is the striking disparity between the obvious radiological findings and the lack of clinical disability. Eventually, pulmonary hypertension and cor pulmonale may develop but in *S. haematobium* this is a later change compared with the more rapid deterioration in *S. mansoni* infections.

Bilharziomas caused by *S. haematobium* do not appear to have been reported. It must be emphasized that the vast majority of patients with *S. haematobium* infections, even if lifelong, will have normal chest radiographs.

(The cardiovascular changes are similar to those of *S. mansoni*; see pp. 192–194).

Colon

The large bowel is not commonly affected by *S. haematobium* but this can occur, especially in combination with *S. mansoni* (see Fig. 2.32). The most common presentations are of a granulomatous type of colitis (often in the transverse colon) and proctitis (Fig. 2.29).

Rectal and colonic calcification may be seen, most commonly in the right side of the colon. It is always associated with bladder or ureteric calcification. The pattern varies with the state of distention of the

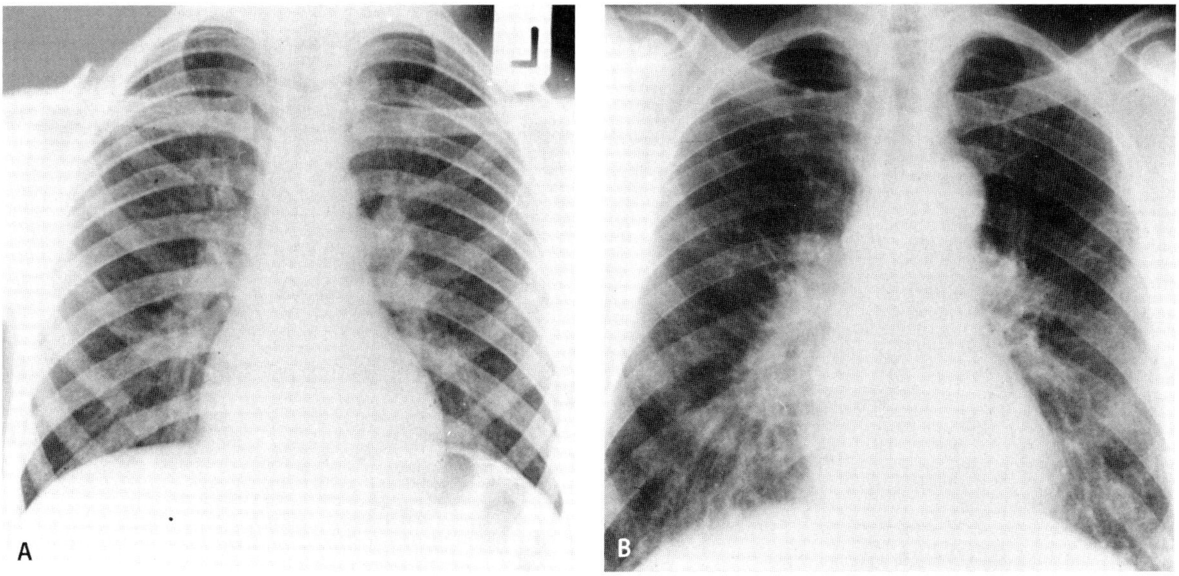

Fig. 2.28 A, B. *S. haematobium* does not prominently affect the lungs, but may be seen at quite different stages: **A** Katayama stage of an acute *S. haematobium* infection. This young adult had not previously been exposed to schistosomiasis when he bathed in a Central African lake 4 weeks before this radiograph. The day after swimming he noticed that his arms were "sun burnt" and 3 weeks later he developed an irritating cough and felt off color. He had a low fever and a poor appetite, blood showed a 20% eosinophilia. The chest radiograph shows an increase in vascular markings with a faint nodular pattern throughout both lungs; the hila are prominent. There were no focal lesions and the findings were transient. There was an immediate clinical response to antischistosomal therapy and his chest radiograph returned to normal. **B** In the late stage of schistosomiasis the appearances are quite different. This elderly Zimbabwe African was known to have had *S. haematobium* infection for most of his life. He came to hospital because he fractured his leg; he was a little short of breath. Both lungs show marked interstitial fibrosis and there is enlargement of the main pulmonary arteries. Pulmonary hypertension has many causes and there is no way to distinguish schistosomiasis, nor, at this stage, will specific therapy have any significant effect

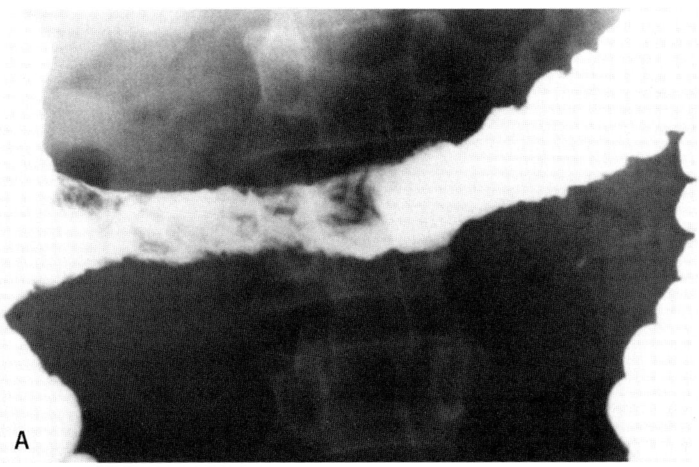

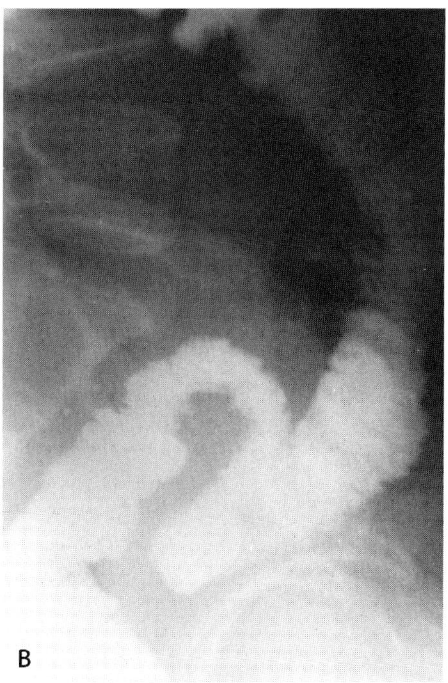

Fig. 2.29 A, B. *S. haematobium* can cause a granulomatous reaction in the large bowel. **A** Superficial ulceration and edema causing irregularity of the right half of the transverse colon in a 30-year-old African. The normal haustral pattern is lost and the lumen is slightly narrowed. **B** Extensive granulomatous proctocolitis of the rectosigmoid colon in another African patient. Normal haustration can be seen in the descending colon, just visible at the top of the radiograph

bowel and may therefore change frequently. The calcification may be laminar or amorphous or corrugated. If the bowel is distended, the laminar or linear pattern is likely, whereas the corrugated pattern is more common in the rectum, especially when empty. Calcified eggs may be recognized on CT and, rarely, as bright echoes on ultrasonography in the pericolonic or perirectal tissues. There is no clinical correlation between the extent of colitis or polyposis and the presence of bowel calcification.

Central Nervous System

It is very rare for *S. haematobium* to affect any part of the central nervous system, but it can happen. Paraplegia due to granulomatous arachnoiditis and to transverse myelitis are recorded (Fig. 2.65). (One patient with transverse myelitis was pregnant.) But the majority of CNS symptoms will be due to *S. mansoni* or *S. japonicum* (see p. 198).

Differential Diagnosis (S. haematobium)

The differential diagnosis of calcification of the bladder is not difficult in most patients because each cause has a very different appearance. Calcification can be due to amyloidosis, in which it is very spotty. Some chemicals and drugs, such as cyclophosphan, may cause quite heavy calcification, but the bladder will be small and does not expand. Tuberculosis can cause localized calcification in one, or perhaps, two areas of the bladder, usually a small flat area. Carcinoma which has been treated by radiotherapy may also calcify when it heals, associated with scarring and distortion of the bladder outline and localized to one area. There is nearly always residual local thickening. In schistosomiasis the bladder calcification follows the shape of the bladder, is seldom associated with distortion except in the final stages, and does not usually affect bladder distention or contraction. It is by far the commonest cause of bladder calcification and is very characteristic. It is the only cause of bladder calcification in which there is likely to be calcification of the ureters as well.

In those who have acquired the infection recently (such as travelers), as opposed to those who have lived with it for many years, it is important to recognize the early signs of prolonged ureteric filling during contrast urography. This may be the only evidence of the infection. Later the irregularity and beading of the ureter, the stenosis, and the dilatation can be recognized by ultrasonography or radiography at a time when the bladder may still be normal. Following treatment, particularly in those who have not been previously infected, follow-up ultrasonography and intravenous urography after 6 months will ensure that there has been no ureteric stenosis or dilatation.

The findings of calcified eggs in the gallbladder, in any part of the bowel, in the seminal vesicles, or in the female genital tract is also a strong indication of schistosomiasis.

If ultrasonography shows hepatic periportal fibrosis, this is a strong indication of schistosomiasis (see p. 166).

Schistosomiasis mansoni

The main imaging findings in *S. mansoni* infections reflect the pathological changes in the bowel, portal system, and lungs.

Large Bowel

The earliest radiographic changes in the colon include an edematous mucosal pattern with mural spiculations or tiny ulcers, often accompanied by spasm and incomplete distention of the involved segment (Fig. 2.30). Later, there is loss of haustration, chiefly in the descending and sigmoid colon (Figs. 2.31–2.34). Although any part of the bowel may be affected, in schistosomiasis mansoni the changes will be most marked in the distribution of the inferior mesenteric artery.

Where there has been a heavier infection and chronic exposure, there may be multiple granulomatous polyps, usually 1–2 cm in diameter, especially in the rectum, sigmoid, and descending colon (Figs. 2.31, 2.32). The polyps begin as submucosal granulomas which lift the overlying mucosa and acquire a short stalk. They are very friable and vascular and bleed easily. They can become quite extensive and coalesce into a large hemorrhagic granuloma from which all the normal mucosa has been lost (Figs. 2.33, 2.34). These masses may become so large that there is obstruction or intussusception. Rectal prolapse can occur. Such lesions simulate carcinoma.

Polyp formation varies in different countries; polyps are not uncommon in Egypt, Arabia and other parts of Africa where *S. mansoni* infections predominate and are particularly common where there are combined *S. mansoni* and *S. haematobium* infections, but less frequent in *S. mansoni* infections alone. In the Western hemisphere, colonic polyps are uncommon; in fact, radiologically detectable schistosomal colonic disease is rather uncommon except in severely infected individuals, in whom the most common finding is a stenosing granulomatous process with extensive pericolonic infiltration resembling granulomatous colitis.

(Text continues on p. 159)

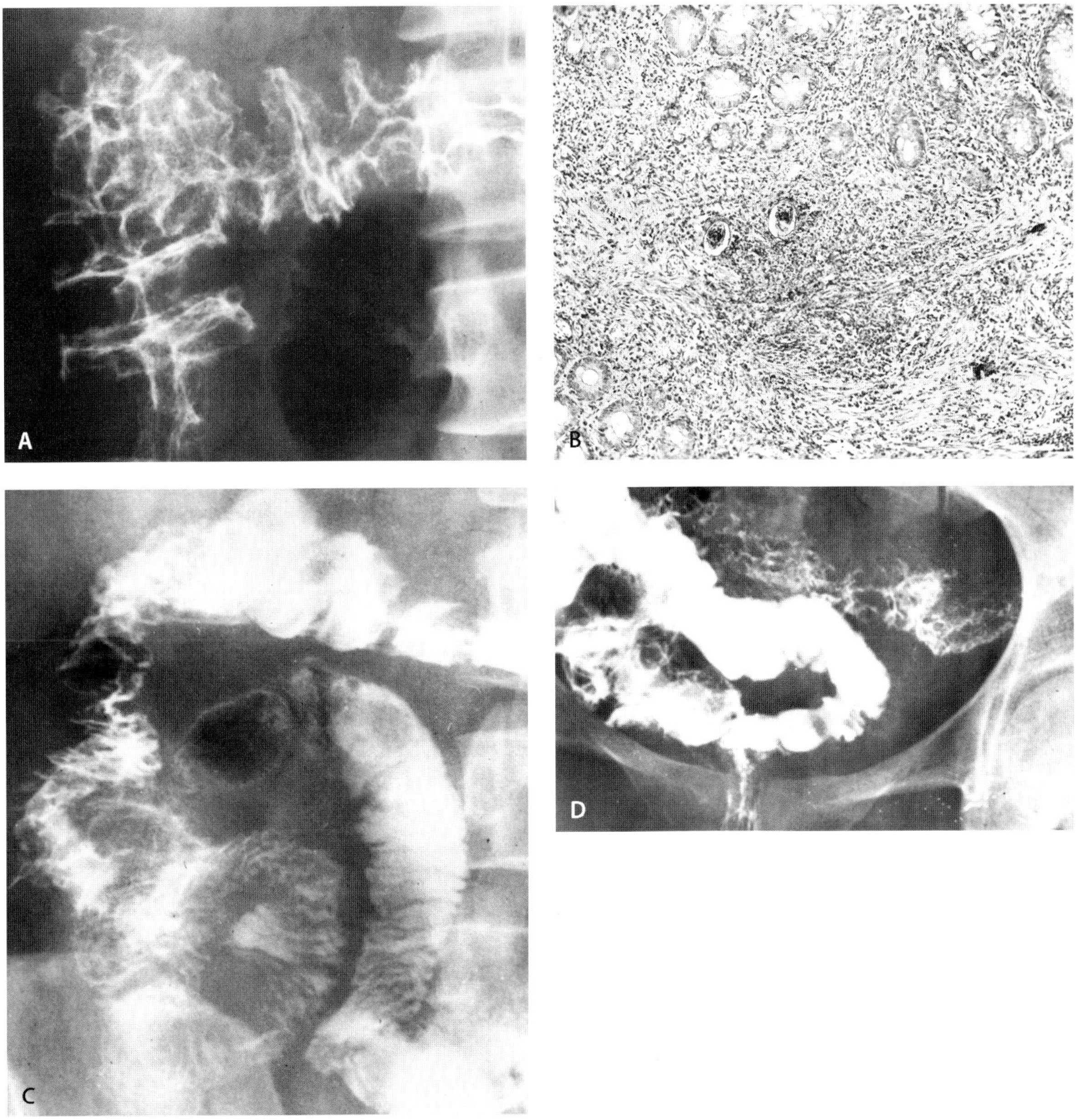

Fig. 2.30 A–D. The early changes of schistosomiasis mansoni of the colon. **A** Because there are many tiny punctate mucosal ulcerations, a barium double contrast enema will show a fine granular mucosa, as in this hepatic flexure. There is local spasm, making it difficult to distend the colon completely. **B** The marked inflammatory cell reaction surrounding eggs of *S. mansoni* in the submucosa of the rectum. ×100; AFIP 53-8656. **C** The terminal ileum and right hemicolon (after partial evacuation of a barium enema). The terminal ileum is normal, except for slight external pressure due to a granulomatous mass in the pericecal and appendiceal tissues. The cecum is irregular and spiculated and there is considerable spasm in the ascending colon. The clinical diagnosis was acute appendicitis, but the cecum was found to be encased in a 0.5-cm-thick fibrous wall, which extended to involve the ascending colon and around the appendix. Histologically there were multiple schistosome eggs and granulomas and an intense serosal eosinophilic granulomatous exudate in the pericecal fat, possible due to the recent death of the adult female schistosome outside the cecum. Rectal biopsy was also positive for *S. mansoni* eggs. **D** Edema of the mucosa, associated with irregularity and spasm. A previous rectal biopsy had show schistosome eggs. All these patients were Puerto Ricans living in New York. (**A** was a 19-year-old male, **C** a 42-year-old male, and **D** a 37-year-old female). All had a chronic history of abdominal pain, diarrhea, and weight loss

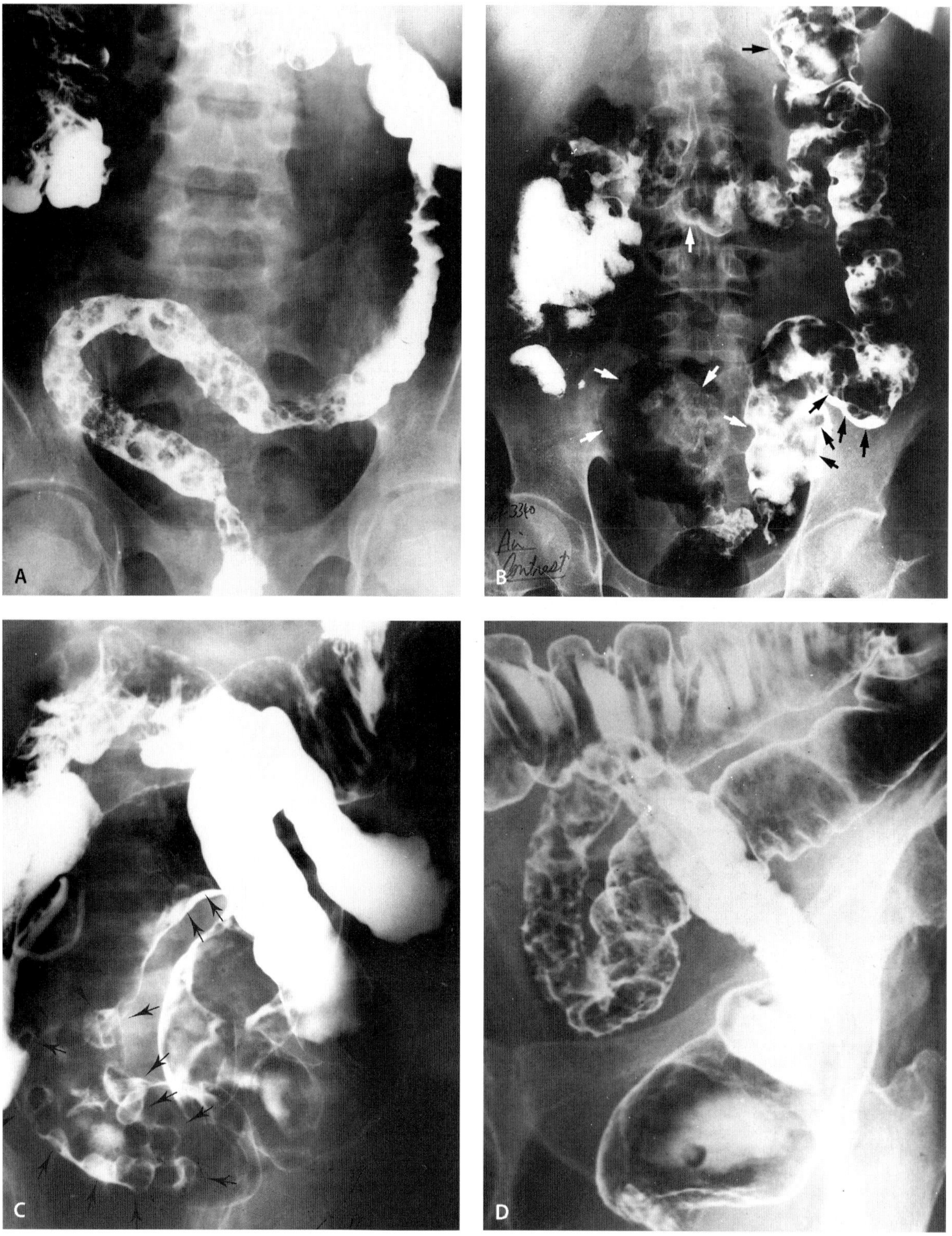
A
B
C
D

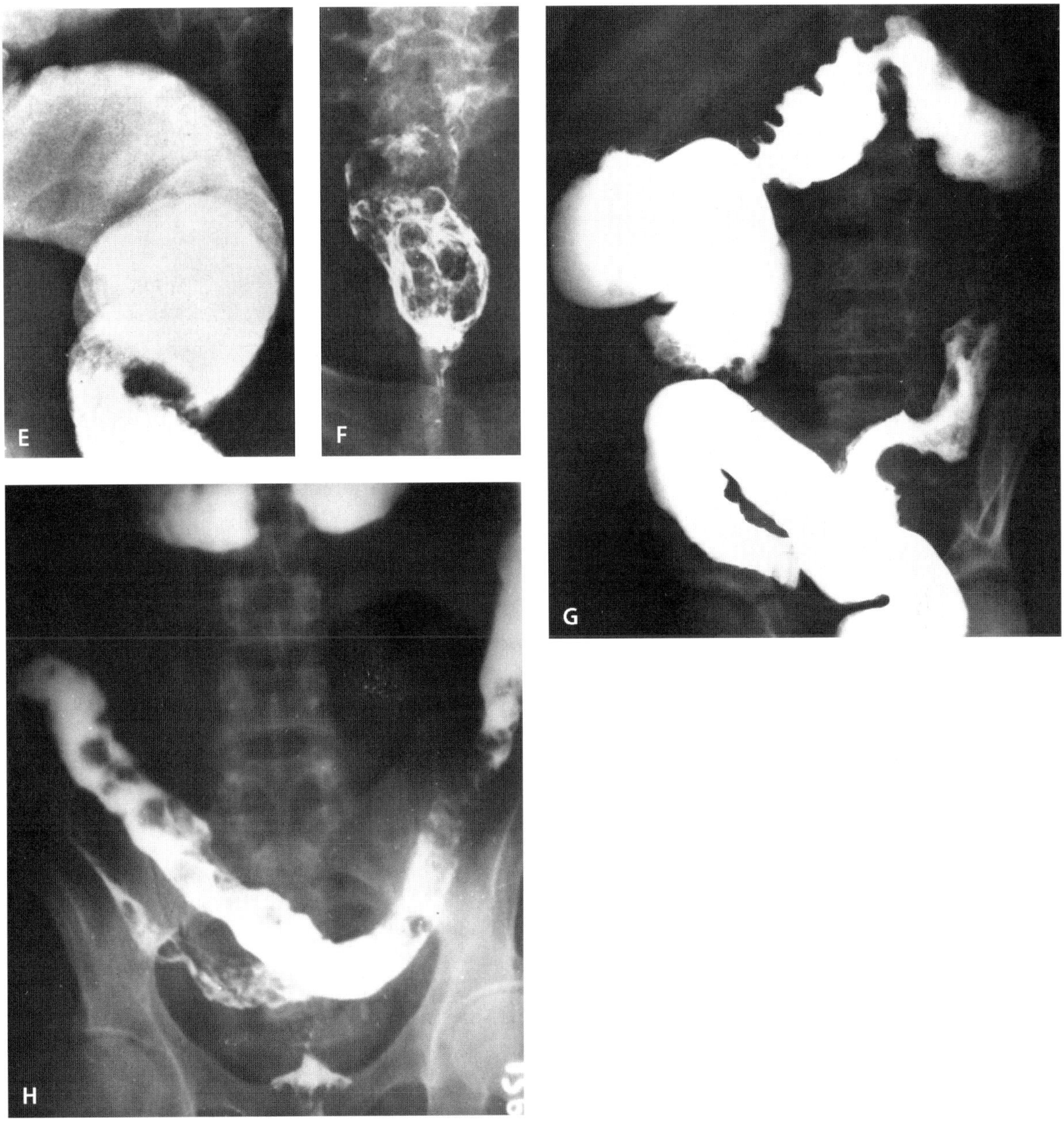

◀ **Fig. 2.31 A–H.** Schistosomal polyposis in the colon and rectum. **A** Multiple polyps throughout the rectosigmoid colon, which was displaced out of the pelvis by a large pericolic bilharzial (schistosomal) abscess. There is mural spiculation, loss of haustration and spasm in the descending colon, with scattered strictures. There were *S. mansoni* eggs, blood, and pus in the stools. The patient was a 20-year-old Egyptian male complaining of bloody diarrhea, fatigue, and abdominal swellings. He had hepatosplenomegaly and anemia. (Courtesy of Dr. Hafez Hassan, Cairo) **B** Schistosomal polyposis *arrows* extending from the rectum to the transverse colon in a 42-year-old Egyptian (air-barium enema). **C** A 22-year-old Egyptian patient with marked schistosomal polyposis, (*arrows*) in the rectum and sigmoid (air-barium contrast enema). (**C, D** Courtesy of Dr. N.A. El Masry, Cairo) **D** Extensive granulomas and polyposis of the sigmoid colon and rectum in a Brazilian patient with schistosomiasis mansoni. (Courtesy of Dr. J. Phillips et al. and *Radiology*, 1975) **E, F** A barium enema on a 16-year-old Puerto Rican girl who had a 6-year history of recurrent diarrhea and abdominal pain. There is a polypoid mass arising from the left lateral rectal wall in the frontal view (**E**), more clearly seen in the post evacuation film (**F**). (Courtesy of Dr. J. Medina et al. and *Radiology*, 1965) **G** Multiple areas of irregular narrowing, muscosal ulceration, spiculation, and granulomatous polyps, with a length of intense spasm in the mid-descending colon. The proximal colon is more normal. (Courtesy of Dr. John Ebersole, Lancaster) **H** Tubular narrowing of the entire rectum, sigmoid, and descending colon with numerous large (2 cm) polyps, with some areas of spasm, due to schistosomiasis mansoni in an Egyptian patient. (Courtesy of Prof. Kassem, Cairo)

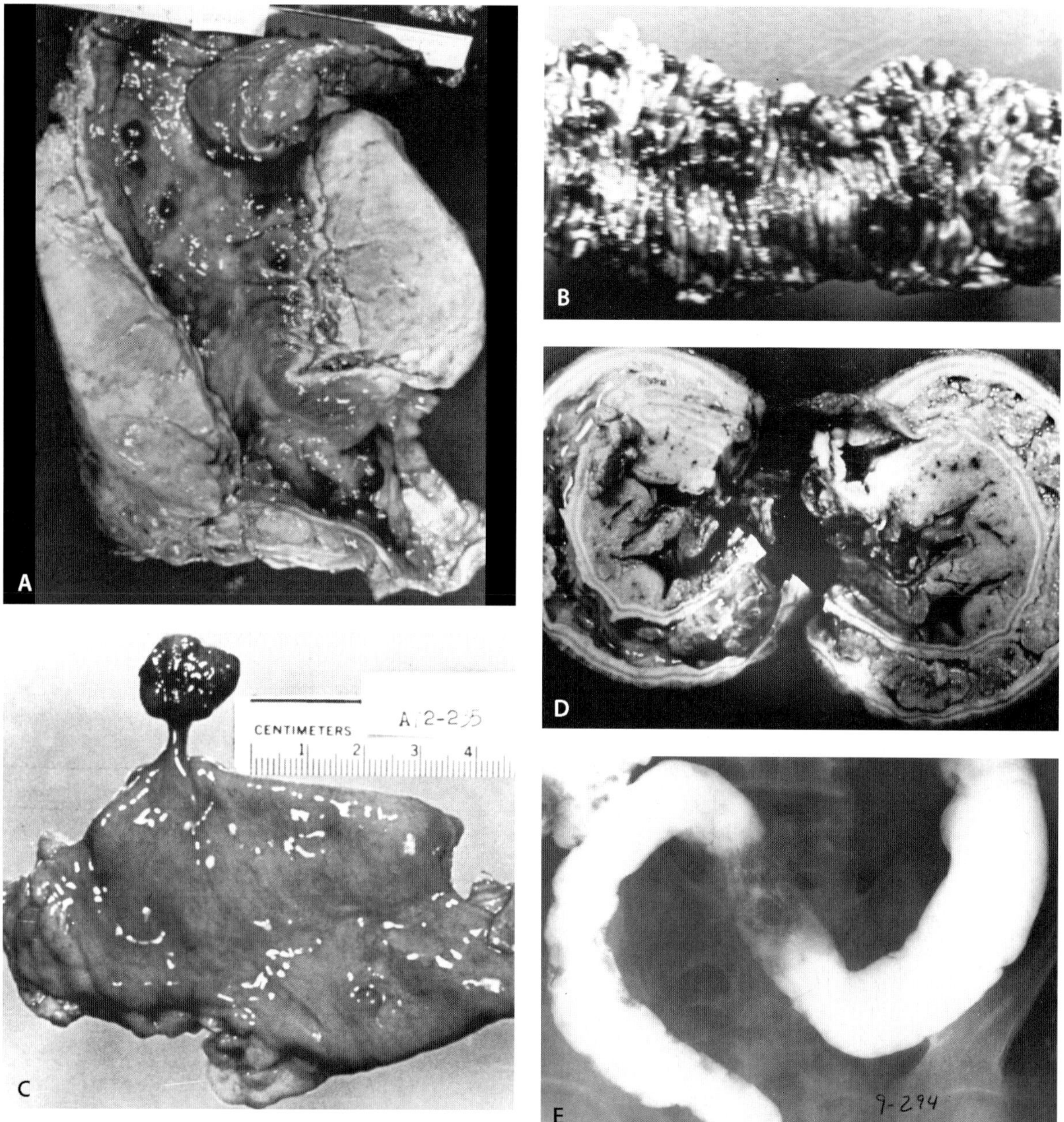

Fig. 2.32 A–E. Colonic and rectal polyps are usually multiple and associated with a marked inflammatory reaction. **A** The hemicolectomy from an Egyptian patient with combined *S. haematobium* and *S. mansoni* infections. A large bilharzioma is surrounding the rectosigmoid colon and displacing it arteriorly and upwards. There are several polyps. There were about 23 000 *S. mansoni* eggs and 1500 *S. haematobium* eggs per gram of tissue, with numerous *S. mansoni* adult schistosomes in the irregular fibrous masses in the colonic serosa and the bilharzioma. There were similar but less severe serosal changes throughout the remainder of the colon and small intestine. Clinically the mass was thought to be malignant. AFIP 76-2329. **B** Multiple polyps in the colon of a 20-year-old Egyptian male with schistosomiasis mansoni. (Surgically resected: courtesy of Dr. Jerome H. Smith, Tucson) **C** A large inflammatory polyp on a short stalk in the sigmoid colon of a 10-year-old Egyptian boy. The polyp contained numerous *S. haematobium* eggs and a few of *S. mansoni*. There is a much smaller sessile polyp (*lower right*). There is a geographic variation in the frequency of polyps: they are not uncommon in Egypt and elsewhere in Africa, particularly in combined infections. They are not so frequent in Brazilians with *S. mansoni* infection. Polyps are also found in Schistosomiasis japonica. **D** Transverse sections of the colon of an 18-year-old Egyptian male with combined *S. mansoni* and *S. haematobium* infections. There are multiple polyps almost filling the lumen and the colonic wall is very fibrotic and thickened. (Courtesy of A.W. Cheever) **E** Schistosomiasis mansoni causing thickening of the colonic wall, with narrowing and rigidity of the pelvic colon; the normal haustral pattern has been lost and there are multiple polypoid lesions in the rectum and sigmoid colon. There was also a large pericolic mass of fibrofatty granulation tissue displacing the bowel. AFIP 68-1095

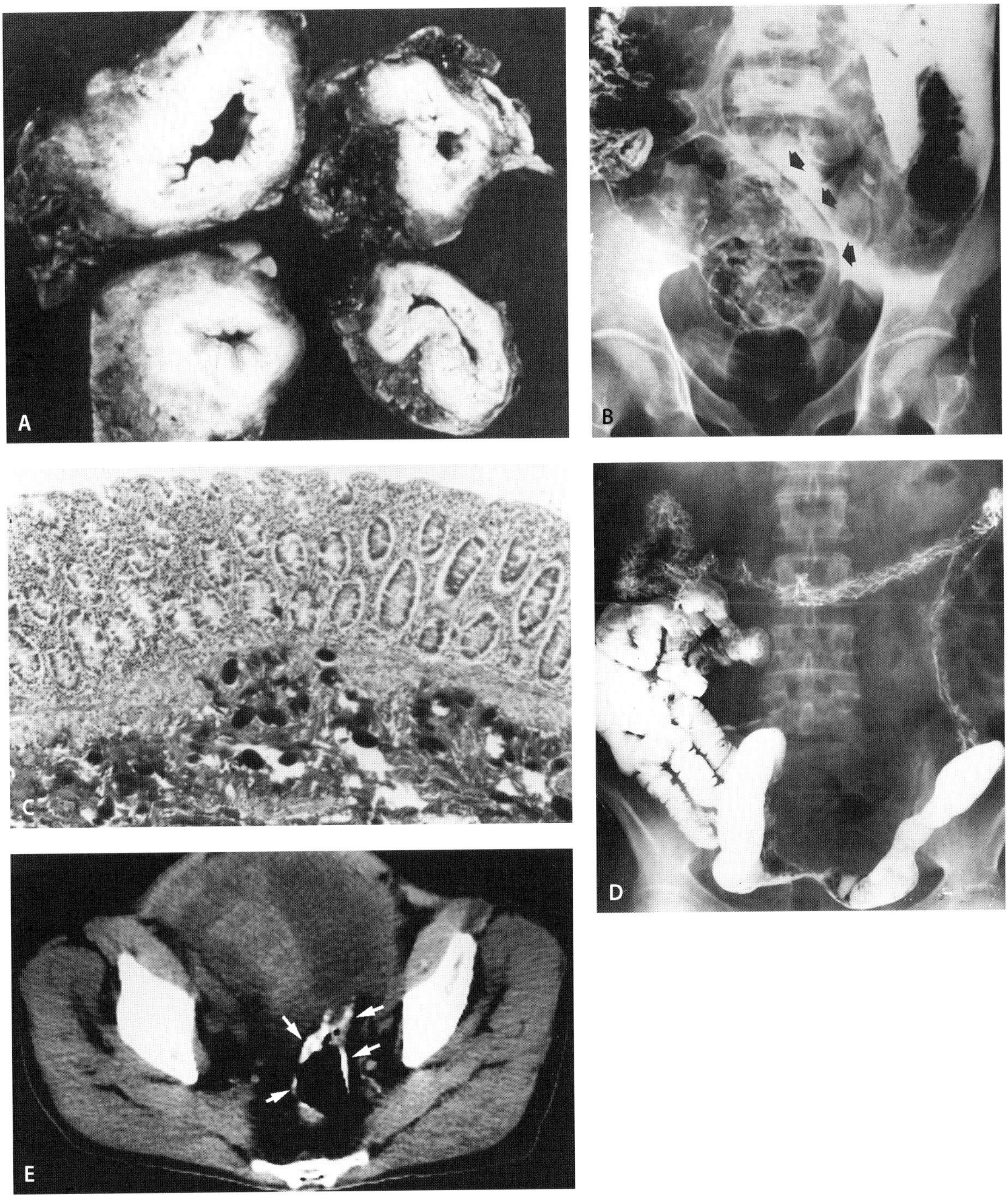

Fig. 2.33 A–E. Schistosomiasis mansoni can cause marked granulomatous thickening of the bowel wall and, eventually, strictures. **A** Transverse sections of a stenosed segment of bowel from an 18-year-old Egyptian male. Elsewhere in the colon there were multiple polyps. This tissue contained 111 000 *S. mansoni* and 1500 *S. haematobium* eggs per gram, and was almost entirely inactive when removed. **B** Peritoneography combined with a double barium-air contrast study of the colon shows marked thickening of the wall of the distal colon (*arrows*) in a patient with *S. mansoni*. (Courtesy of Dr. Morton Meyers, New York) **C** Histological section through the colon of a different patient with chronic schistosomiasis mansoni showing an inflammatory reaction in the mucosa and many calcified schistosome eggs in the submucosa: there is marked collagen and fibrous tissue formation, which results in narrowing of the bowel lumen and eventually stricture or stenosis. AFIP 68-4761. **D** This barium enema shows stenosis of the rectum and a stricture in the midsigmoid colon. Throughout the rectosigmoid there is loss of haustral markings and the bowel has become tubular and rigid. Proctoscopy confirmed the rectal stricture, which was thought to be malignant until the biopsy showed edema, granulomas, and multiple schistosome eggs. AFIP 68-9019-15. **E** CT scanning can show calcification in the wall of the colon. This is the nonenhanced CT scan of an 86-year-old Japanese man showing calcification in the wall of the colon (*arrows*). *S. japonica* were found in his stool

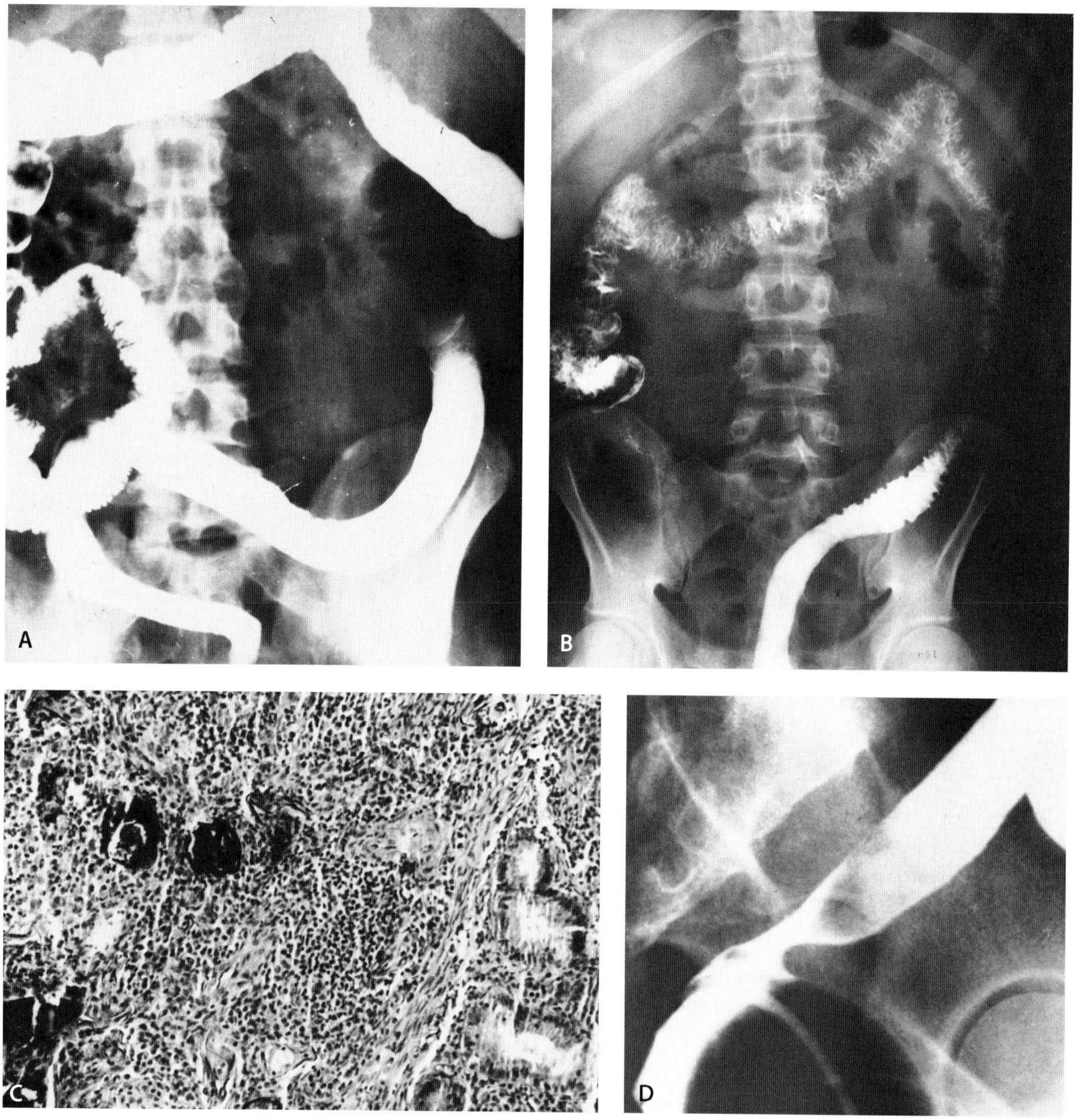

Fig. 2.34 A–I. The end results of schistosomiasis in the colon may be diffuse bowel thickening or local strictures. In these patients with diffuse loss of haustrations, there is narrowing and rigidity of the colon. In **A** this is evident from the mid transverse colon to the rectum. The patient was a 33-year-old Puerto Rican male and biopsy of the sigmoid showed multiple schistosome eggs. He had been treated 17 years previously. In **B** the sigmoid colon is shortened, narrowed, and rigid. A polyp found on sigmoidoscopy at 15 cm showed schistosome eggs. Biopsy of his rectum (**C**) showed multiple calcified eggs of *S. mansoni* in the submucosa with a marked eosinophilic inflammatory reaction. H & E, ×100; AFIP 68-9019-11, 68-9019-9, 68-9004-1. **D** The shortened, straightened, and narrowed sigmoid colon of the same patient as in **B** and **C**. AFIP 68-9018-2. **E–I** see p. 159

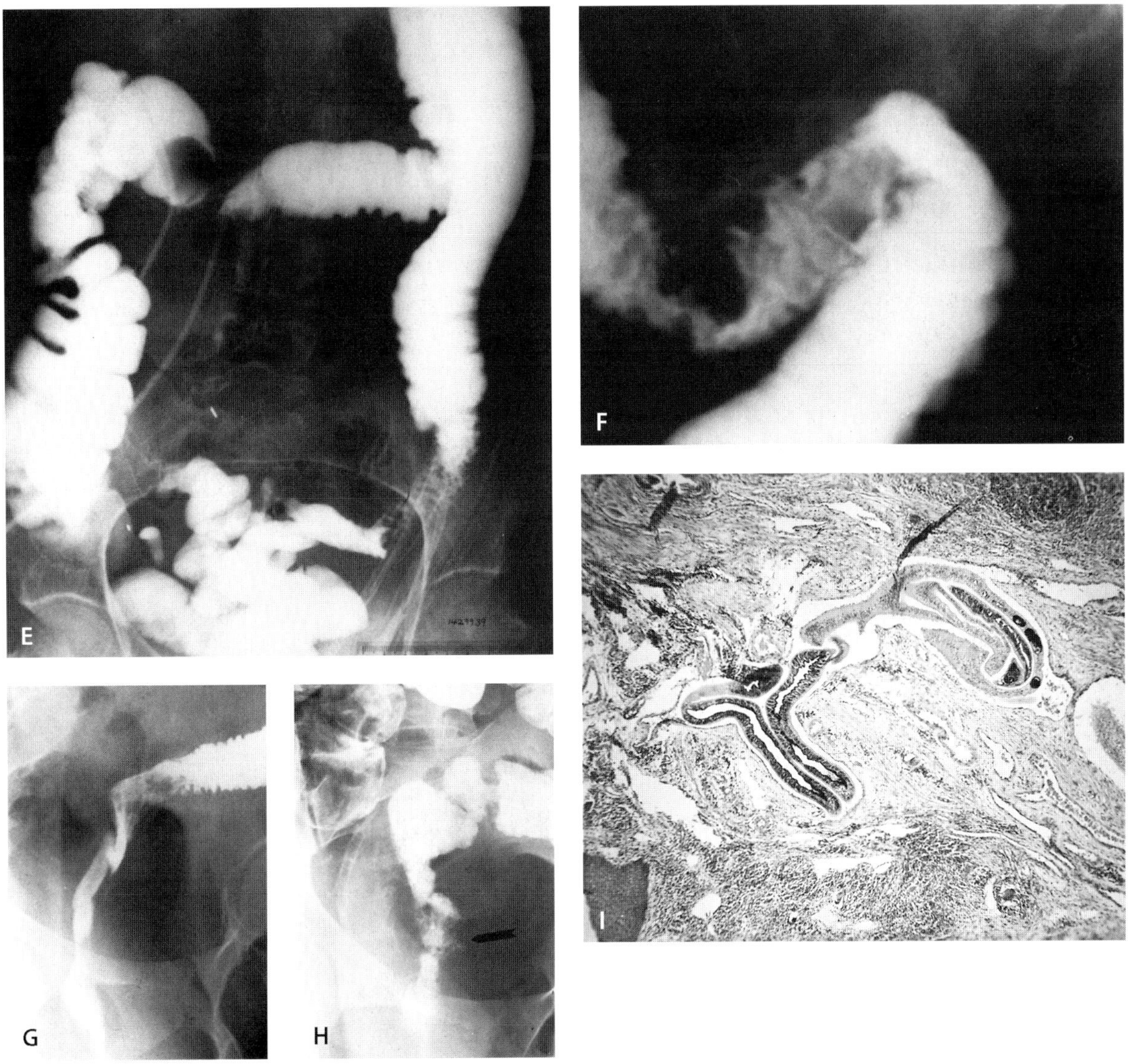

Fig. 2.34 (*continued*). **E** A barium enema through a midtransverse colon colostomy shows a long area of stenosis, with irregular thickened mucosal folds in the sigmoid colon. There was also (**F**) a second irregular stricture with tapered edges below this. The stool contained *S. mansoni* and histologically there were multiple schistosomal granulomas. (This 33-year-old Puerto Rican female had presented with mechanical large bowel obstruction at the level of the sigmoid colon.) **G, H** Similar narrowing and stricture in the rectum and rectosigmoid of a Nigerian patient, shown by a barium enema. He was positive for *S. mansoni*. (Courtesy of Dr. Stanley P. Bohrer) **I** The final insult: hemorrhoids *and* schistosomiasis

Strictures may develop (Figs. 2.33, 2.34) and can be mistaken for carcinoma or Crohn's disease. Calcification in the eggs may be seen in the bowel and surrounding tissues (Fig. 2.35). It is best demonstrated by CT, but often can be seen on plain radiography, usually in the left side of the abdomen. As described in *S. haematobium* (see pp. 150, 152) it will have a very variable appearance, depending on the distention of the bowel. It can be spotty, laminar, corrugated, or amorphous. Near the rectum, the inflamed hypertrophic rectal mucosa may show a converging pattern of calcification towards the anus. Although many patients with colonic schistosomiasis will have diarrhea and bleeding, there is no close correlation between the number of calcified eggs, and the number and size of the polyps or the extent of colitis. Unlike adenomatous polyps, those from schistosomiasis are inflammatory and the majority will resolve after proper treatment. Unfortunately, the pericolonic fibrosis does not improve significantly with any therapy.

There are some parts of the world where schistosomal colonic polyps are very uncommon, e.g., in South America, although the egg count does not dif-

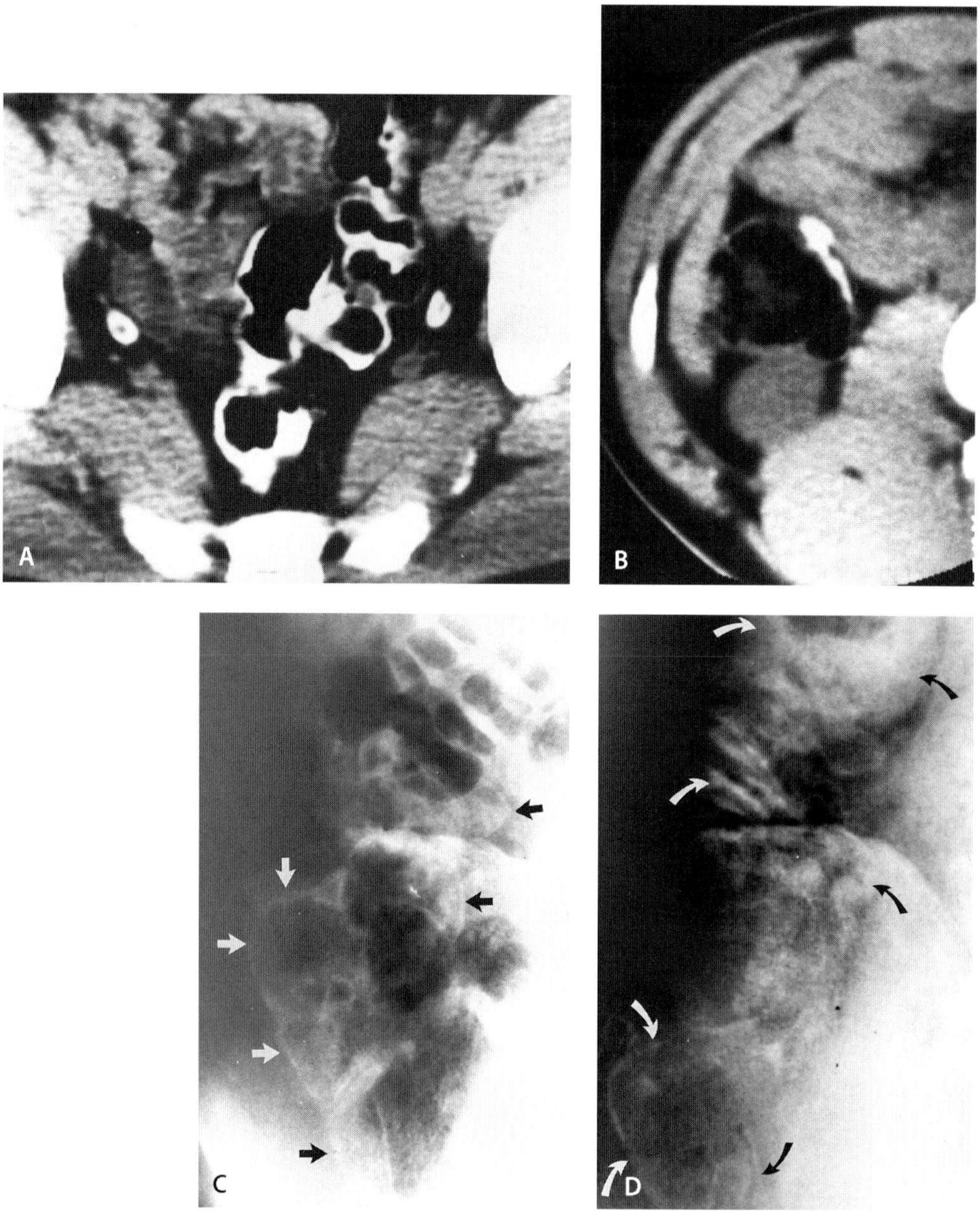

Fig. 2.35 A–G. Schistosomal calcification of the intestine. **A** A nonenhanced CT scan of a 46-years old Egyptian may showing dense calcification of the sigmoid colon. **B** The right colon of the same patient. A CT scan without contrast. He was known to have urinary schistosomiasis but had never had any bowel complaints. **C, D** Plain radiographs show the calcified eggs (*arrows*) in the bowel wall of a different Egyptian man: the pattern varies with the degree of bowel distension. In **C** there is a laminar calcification, and in **D** the pattern is more amorphous when the bowel is emptier. **E–G** see p. 161

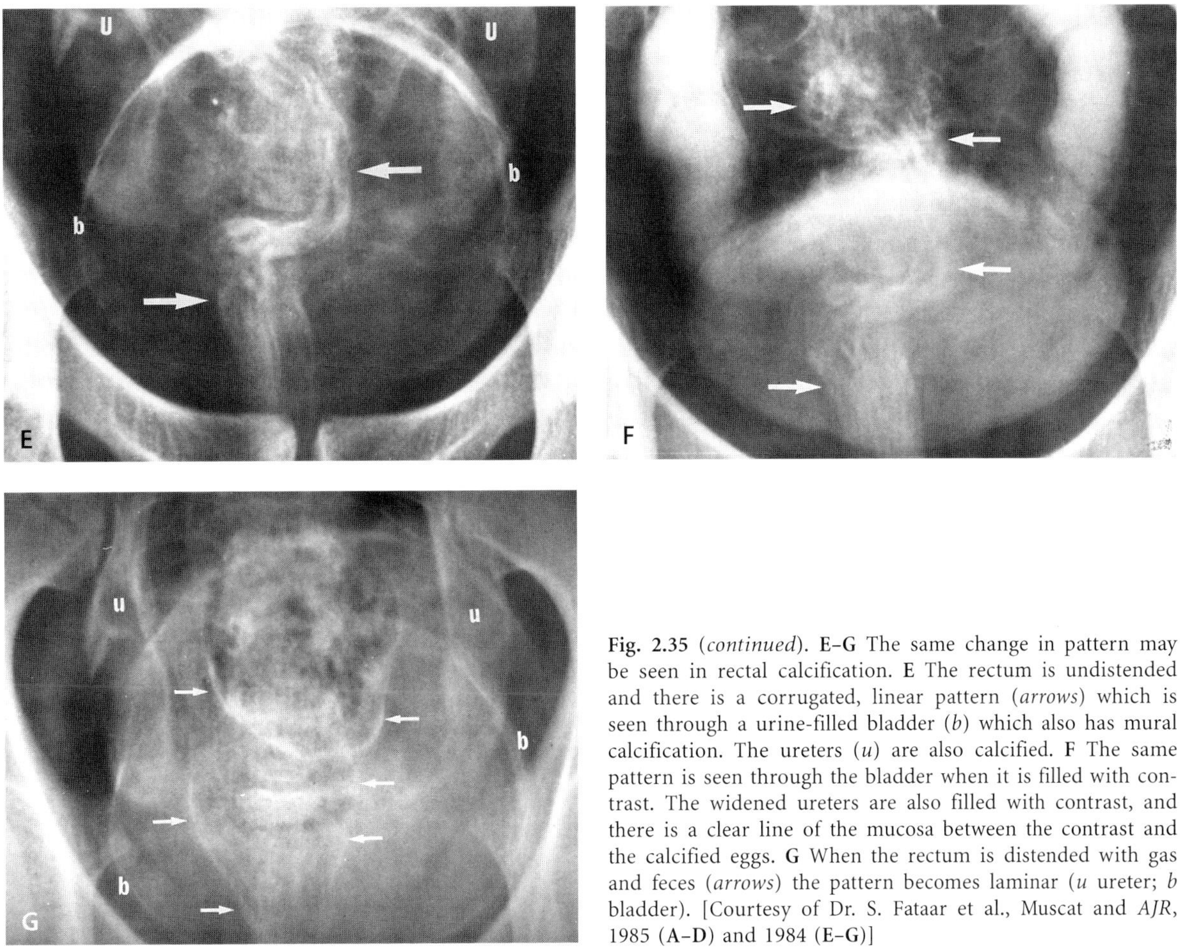

Fig. 2.35 (*continued*). **E–G** The same change in pattern may be seen in rectal calcification. **E** The rectum is undistended and there is a corrugated, linear pattern (*arrows*) which is seen through a urine-filled bladder (*b*) which also has mural calcification. The ureters (*u*) are also calcified. **F** The same pattern is seen through the bladder when it is filled with contrast. The widened ureters are also filled with contrast, and there is a clear line of the mucosa between the contrast and the calcified eggs. **G** When the rectum is distended with gas and feces (*arrows*) the pattern becomes laminar (*u* ureter; *b* bladder). [Courtesy of Dr. S. Fataar et al., Muscat and *AJR*, 1985 (**A–D**) and 1984 (**E–G**)]

fer significantly from those countries in which colonic polyps are found more frequently. The reason for this is not fully understood.

Pericolonic schistosomal abscesses or pelvic granulomas may be large enough to compress the pelvic colon and displace it laterally and anteriorly. Large, solitary bilharziomas may occur, either in the bowel wall or mesentery, and can be mistaken for carcinoma.

Small Bowel

S. mansoni does not commonly cause radiological changes in the small bowel although ova may be recovered from the duodenum, jejunum, and upper ileum (Figs. 2.36, 2.38). When the infection is severe, the radiological changes resemble other parasitic infections or regional enteritis, and it may be difficult to distinguish the etiology even on histological examination.

Acute mesenteric ischemia has been caused by *S. mansoni*, but in a patient who was dehydrated and who had previous splenectomy because of splenomegaly. There were many eggs in the thrombosis.

Patients with chronic schistosomal bowel infection become anemic and they have a protein-losing enteropathy. In one series from Egypt, well over half the patients had marked clubbing of the fingers and pain, swelling, and tenderness around the wrists, knees, and ankle joints. Radiographically there was periosteal reaction and new bone formation, particularly around the wrists. Treatment for the schistosomal polyposis improved the patient's swelling and tenderness but the clubbing persisted and the periosteal reaction did not improve. There was some correlation between the extent of the polyposis and the finger clubbing, but those who had hepatosplenomegaly had this only to a moderate degree. It is possible that clubbing may be more frequent than is reported, because many middle aged and older patients in the tropics have chronic lung disease from other causes, and clubbing is not unexpected.

(*Text continues on p. 164*)

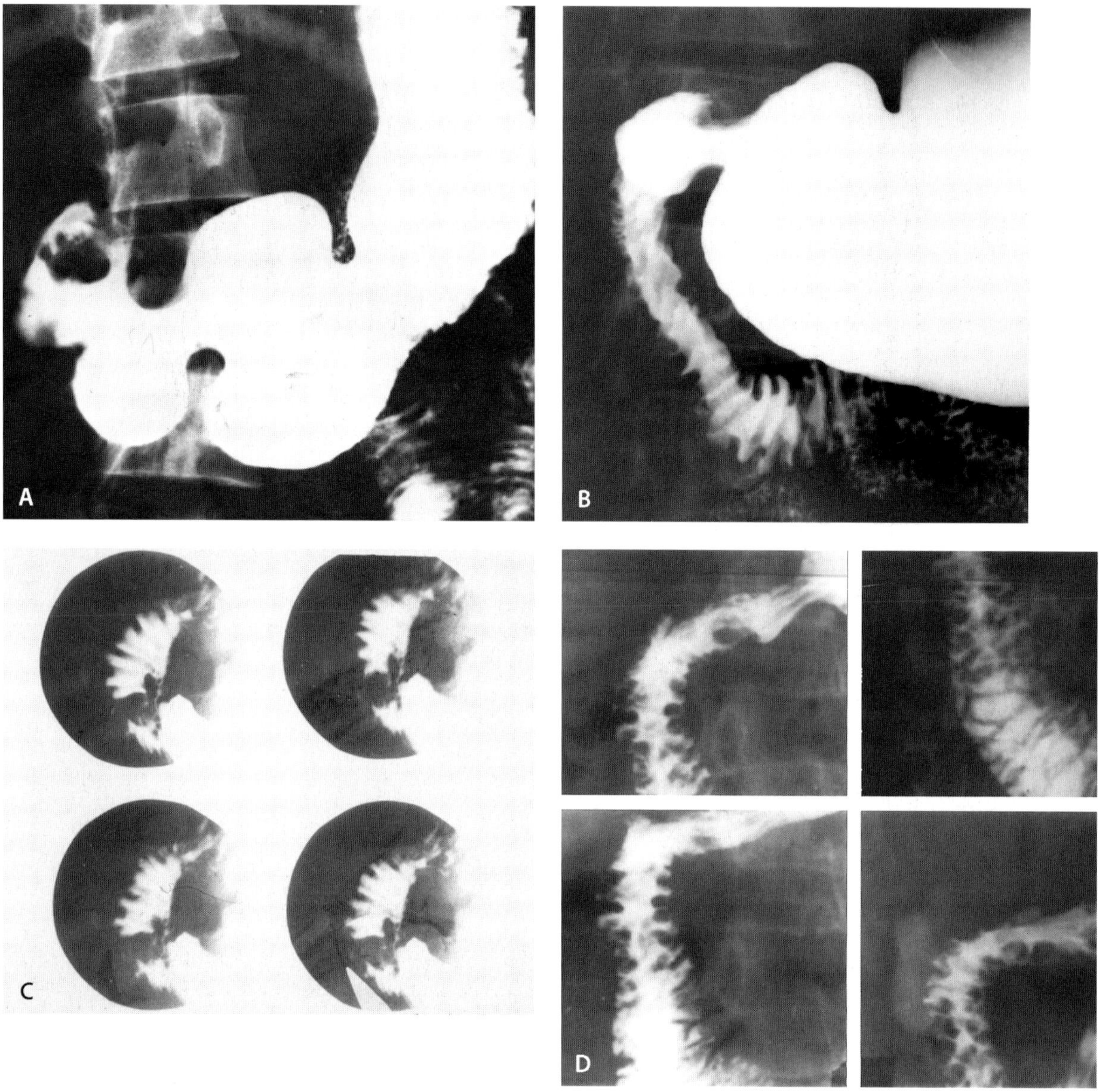

Fig. 2.36 A–D. All varieties of schistosomiasis can affect the duodenum; patients present clinically with vague symptoms suggesting peptic ulceration. **A** Marked deformity and narrowing of the pylorus and duodenum in a 22-year-old Puerto Rican male with a 4-year history of pain and vomiting, with weight loss in the fast few months. The stomach is dilated. At surgery the pylorus was involved in a 5×5 cm mass, adherent posteriorly to the pancreas, gallbladder, and first part of the duodenum. There was local lymphadenopathy. Histology showed chronic peptic duodenal ulceration, with schistosomal granulomas in the submucosa of the first part of the duodenum, and also in the lymph nodes, where there were multiple schistosome eggs. There were similar findings in the appendix and liver AFIP 68-9019-7. **B** The edematous second and third parts of the duodenum of an African from the Sudan. There was decreased peristalsis. He had portal hypertension and hepatomegaly due to *S. mansoni*. (From P. E. S. Palmer, in: Simpkins K. C. ed. *A textbook of radiological diagnosis, vol 4, 5th edn.* London, H. K. Lewis, 1988, pp 678–705) **C** Four views of the first and second part of the duodenum of a Chinese patient with schistosomiasis japonica. (Courtesy of Prof. Xing-Rong Chen, Shanghai) **D** The very edematous duodenum of a patient from Iran with schistosomiasis mansoni

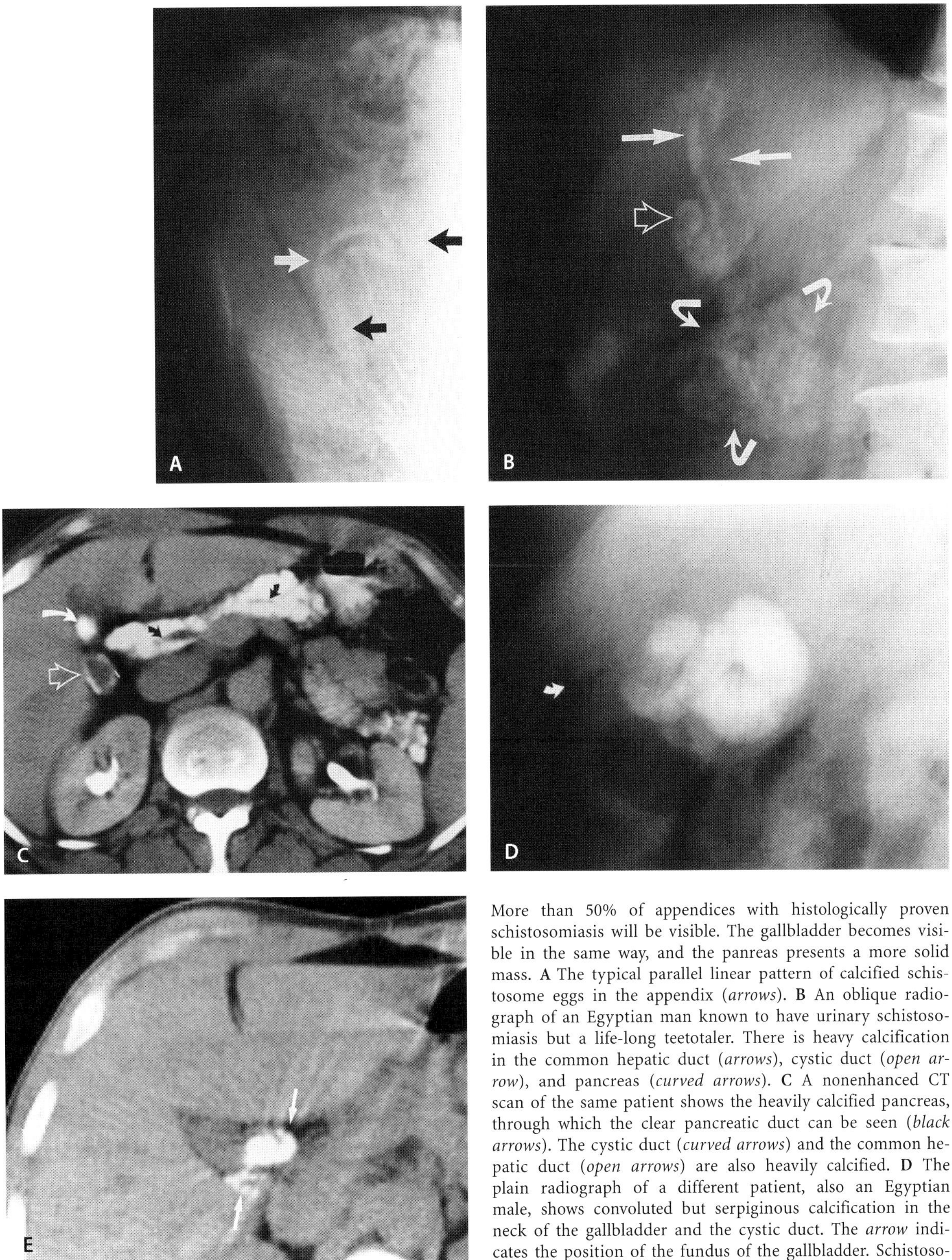

Fig. 2.37 A–E. Schistosomal calcification of the appendix, gallbladder and pancreas. The eggs of any schistosome can be deposited anywhere, calcified, and become clearly visible on imaging when present in sufficient numbers. Appendiceal calcification is not uncommon, especially with *S. haematobium*. More than 50% of appendices with histologically proven schistosomiasis will be visible. The gallbladder becomes visible in the same way, and the panreas presents a more solid mass. **A** The typical parallel linear pattern of calcified schistosome eggs in the appendix (*arrows*). **B** An oblique radiograph of an Egyptian man known to have urinary schistosomiasis but a life-long teetotaler. There is heavy calcification in the common hepatic duct (*arrows*), cystic duct (*open arrow*), and pancreas (*curved arrows*). **C** A nonenhanced CT scan of the same patient shows the heavily calcified pancreas, through which the clear pancreatic duct can be seen (*black arrows*). The cystic duct (*curved arrows*) and the common hepatic duct (*open arrows*) are also heavily calcified. **D** The plain radiograph of a different patient, also an Egyptian male, shows convoluted but serpiginous calcification in the neck of the gallbladder and the cystic duct. The *arrow* indicates the position of the fundus of the gallbladder. Schistosomal granulomas could be mistaken for calculi both on radiography and ultrasonography. **E** The CT scan of a different Egyptian patient showing dense calcification in the neck of the gallbladder (*arrows*). [Courtesy of Dr. S. Fataar, Muscat, and *Br J Radiol*, 1996 (**B, C**) and 1990 (**D, E**)]

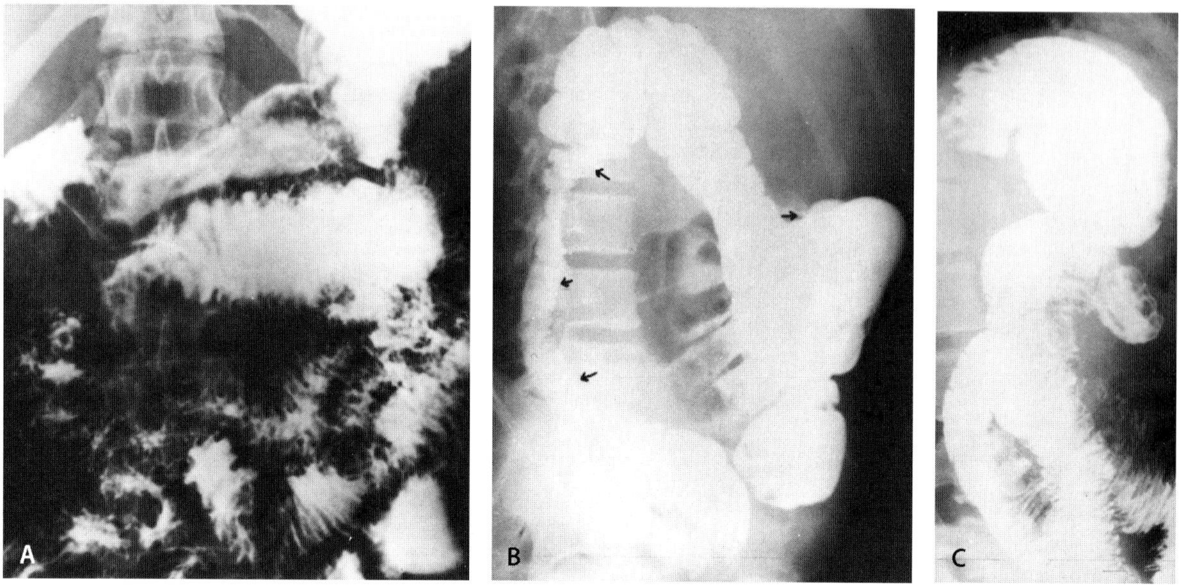

Fig. 2.38 A–C. Schistosomiasis can involve the small bowel, either directly or by adhesions. **A** Alternate dilatation and contraction of several loops of jejunum, with prominent valvulae conniventes due to mucosal edema, with flocculation and segmentation of the barium. This pattern is often seen in *schistosomiasis japonica*, resembling malabsorption, but this particular patient was a Puerto Rican with *S. mansoni* eggs in the stool and on rectal biopsy. (Courtesy of Dr. A. Chait and *AJR* 1963 and AFIP 68-9019.5) **B, C** *Schistosomiasis mansoni* causing a large pericolic bilharzioma and abscess in a 40-year-old Puerto Rican male. The mass is adherent to the descending colon (**B**, *arrows*) and to multiple loops of jejunum (**C**). It involved the mesentery and extended to the anterior abdominal wall. (Courtesy of Dr. Ehrlich, San Juan)

Biliary Tract and Pancreas

Calcification may be seen in the main hepatic ducts, the common hepatic, cystic, and common bile ducts, and also the pancreatic duct (Fig. 2.37). Such calcification is tubular and irregular and can be quite dense. There is seldom ductal obstruction, although this has been reported at least once. Biliary and pancreatic ductal calcification is probably a little more common in mixed infections with *S. haematobium* and *S. mansoni* and may persist after treatment. Pancreatic calcification (which may occur in *S. haematobium* infections alone as well as in mexed infections) is not associated with alcohol intake.

The tubular calcification may be seen on plain radiographs and the irregularity in the ducts can be demonstrated by cholangiography. It is well shown by CT as calcified ring densities or, depending on the section, parallel tubular lines.

Esophagus and Stomach

Esophageal and gastric varices (see Fig. 2.54) are commonly found in *S. mansoni* (and *S. japonicum*) infection because of portal cirrhosis but intrinsic changes in the esophagus and stomach due to direct schistosomal infection are very unusual. Eggs have been deposited in the wall of the stomach, causing a granulomatous mass resembling a carcinoma, but this is extremely uncommon. A schistosomal ulcer has been recorded on the greater curvature of the stomach; both radiologically and at surgery it was thought to be malignant. Antral narrowing due to schistosome-induced fibrosis occurs rarely (Fig. 2.39). There are no specific radiological characteristics of schistosomal involvement of the stomach, and because schistosomiais may coexist with other conditions, there is no way that any method of imaging can exclude either fibrosis or malignancy.

Fig. 2.39 A–E. Schistosomiasis seldom involves the stomach but occasionally granulomas involve the gastric antrum and eventually cause narrowing due to fibrosis, as in these four patients. **A** Multiple calcified eggs in the gastric mucosa. AFIP 60–1300. **B, C** The pyloric antrum is narrowed and the duodenal loop is edematous. In **D** stomach duodenum and jejunum all show edema and areas of narrowing. In **E** there is narrowing of the gastric antrum (*arrows*) due to fibrosis caused by schistosome granulomas (*S. mansoni*). There are also pressure defects on the fundus of the stomach due to gastric varices as a result of portal hypertension. This is most common cause of deformity of the stomach in patients with schistosomiasis ▶

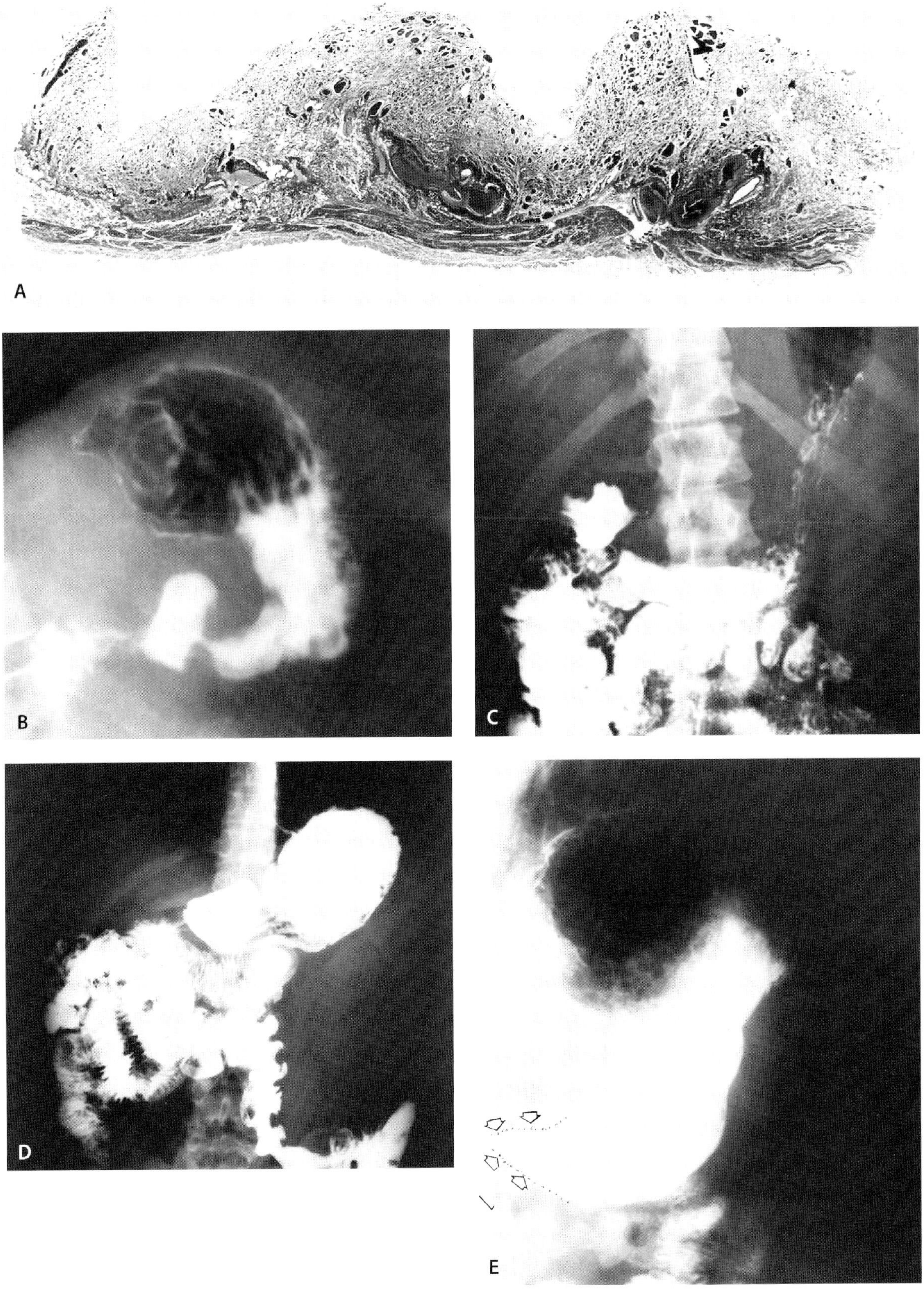
A
B
C
D
E

Portal System

In this section on the portal system, illustrations relating to both *S. mansoni* and *S. japonicum* (Figs. 2.40–2.57) are grouped in order to facilitate comparison of the radiological appearances of these infections (for S. Japonicum text, see p. 197).

Ultrasonography

Ultrasonography of the liver is very important in schistosomiasis, and especially in *S. mansoni*, given its particular association with liver pathology. The earliest evidence of infection is loss of the normal smooth liver outline. In the left lobe, the surface becomes wavy, the posterior margin convex or straight, and the caudal margin rounded instead of concave. At some stages the caudal margin will become sharp. Measurements of liver size must be established within each locality; there is too much geographical variation to provide reliable standards.

An early change in the liver is thickening around the portal vein and its main branches. This becomes highly echogenic, especially around the porta hepatis. There may be enlargement of the splenic veins and when portal hypertension develops, there is usually splenomegaly. As this increases, multiple varicosities and collateral veins will develop, including short gastric, paraumbilical, coronary, and esophageal veins. Visualization of any collateral veins is abnormal (see p. 169).

There are standard WHO criteria allowing the grading of the pathology due to *S. haematobium* (and for other schistosomes also). These are useful to permit accurate comparison in epidemiological surveys in different countries. In the liver, criteria are based on the width of the periportal echogenic bands. As with the bladder, there is considerable variation in the extent of the disease in different regions of the tropics.

When surgery is considered for severe liver disease, the diameters and blood flow velocity of the portal vein and hepatic artery can be measured using a Doppler duplex technique. Pre- and postsurgical studies allow accurate assessment for treatment. When successful, there should be a decrease in the venous portal blood flow to the liver and an increase in the arterial hepatic blood flow. Probably the best vein to use for the diagnosis of portal hypertension is the splenic vein, although some authorities prefer the portal vein.

A few patients with chronic persistent hepatitis will show early periportal fibrosis and this must be differentiated from early schistosomiasis. If there is no periportal fibrosis on ultrasonography, there is unlikely to be hepatosplenomegaly.

The direct detection of esophageal varices with ultrasonography can be very difficult. With careful scanning it may be possible to show some of the dilated vessels around the cardia. An alternative is to use an ultrasonographic scoring system, rating periportal fibrosis, portal vein diameter, spleen size, and portal-systemic anastomoses. With experience this can provide a fairly accurate, noninvasive means of screening for esophageal varices. It correlates strongly with prior gastrointestinal hemorrhage.

Apart from the liver changes, in 80% of patients who show periportal fibrosis there will be thickening of the wall of the gallbladder. There will usually be omental thickening also.

The findings on hepatic ultrasonography are so accurate and reliable that they should replace liver biopsy as a method of confirming the diagnosis of schistosomiasis.

The World Health Organization staging, to record the severity of hepatic disease in schistosomiasis by ultrasonography, is based on the following criteria. All measurements for hepatomegaly assume that there is no other reason, such as cardiac failure or leishmaniasis.

A. Liver outline: This is normally smooth (grade 0). Grade (1) is slightly irregular. Grade (2) is grossly irregular.

B. Measurements, taken in longitudinal cross-section with the transducer above the aorta, from the upper to the caudal margin of the left lobe, provide standards which must be reassessed locally in endemic countries, and with allowance for the height of the individual.

Left lobe in adults:
Normal (0) is 70 mm or less
Enlarged (1) is more than 70 mm

Right lobe in adults is measured in the right midaxillary view:
Normal (0) is more than 140 mm
Small, shrunken (1) 140 mm or less

Another sign of abnormality in adults (not in children) is the finding of echogenic "spots" in the liver parenchyma which are not part of the portal system.

C. Periportal veins: The inner diameter of the portal vein, measured midway between the porta hepatis and the bifurcation, is normally 12 mm or less. If over 12 mm, it is abnormal.

Periportal echogenicity is assessed by the average of three outer to outer measurements (maximum transverse outer diameter) of the increased width of echodensity around branches of the portal vein, measured between the first and third branches.

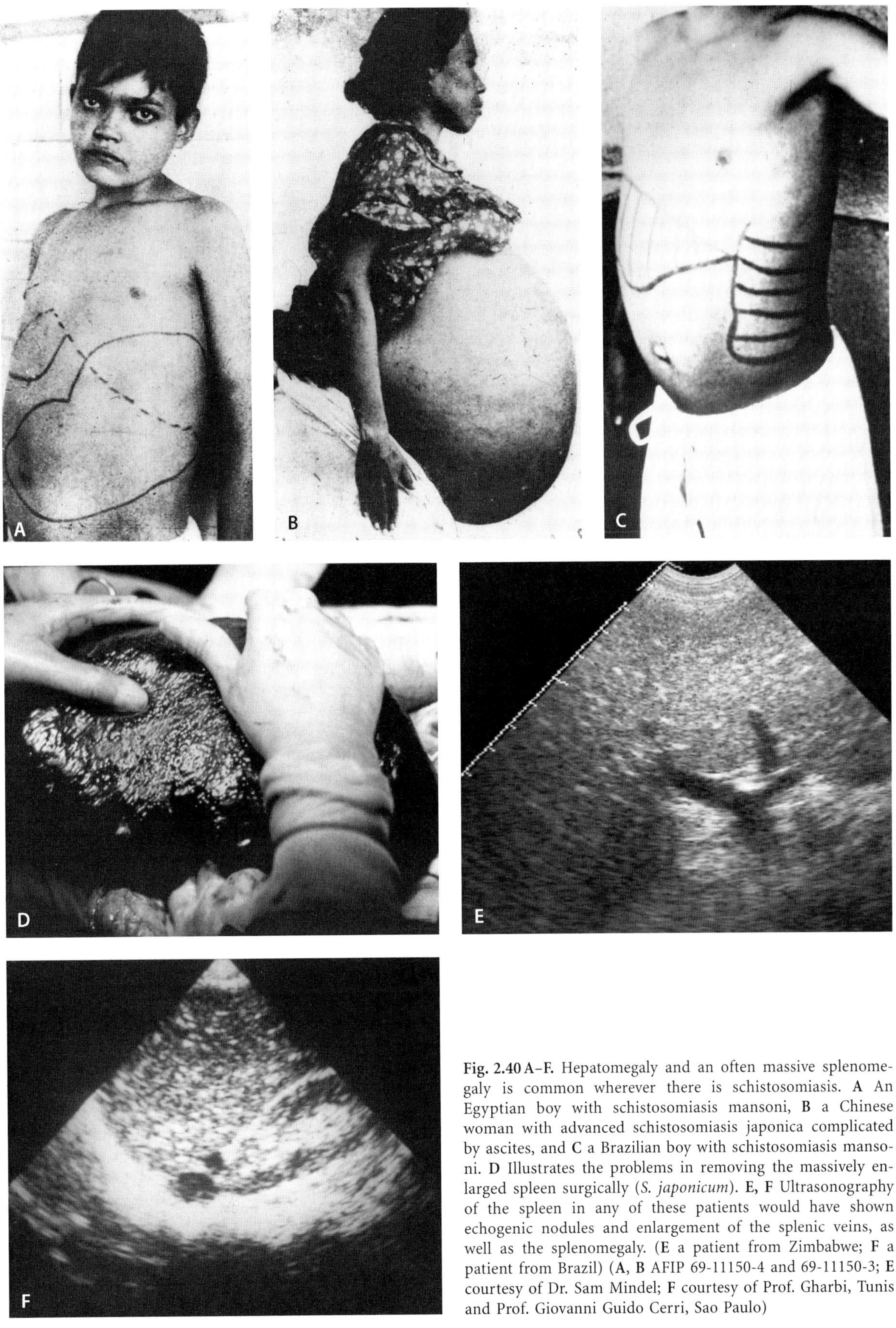

Fig. 2.40 A–F. Hepatomegaly and an often massive splenomegaly is common wherever there is schistosomiasis. **A** An Egyptian boy with schistosomiasis mansoni, **B** a Chinese woman with advanced schistosomiasis japonica complicated by ascites, and **C** a Brazilian boy with schistosomiasis mansoni. **D** Illustrates the problems in removing the massively enlarged spleen surgically (*S. japonicum*). **E, F** Ultrasonography of the spleen in any of these patients would have shown echogenic nodules and enlargement of the splenic veins, as well as the splenomegaly. (**E** a patient from Zimbabwe; **F** a patient from Brazil) (**A, B** AFIP 69-11150-4 and 69-11150-3; **E** courtesy of Dr. Sam Mindel; **F** courtesy of Prof. Gharbi, Tunis and Prof. Giovanni Guido Cerri, Sao Paulo)

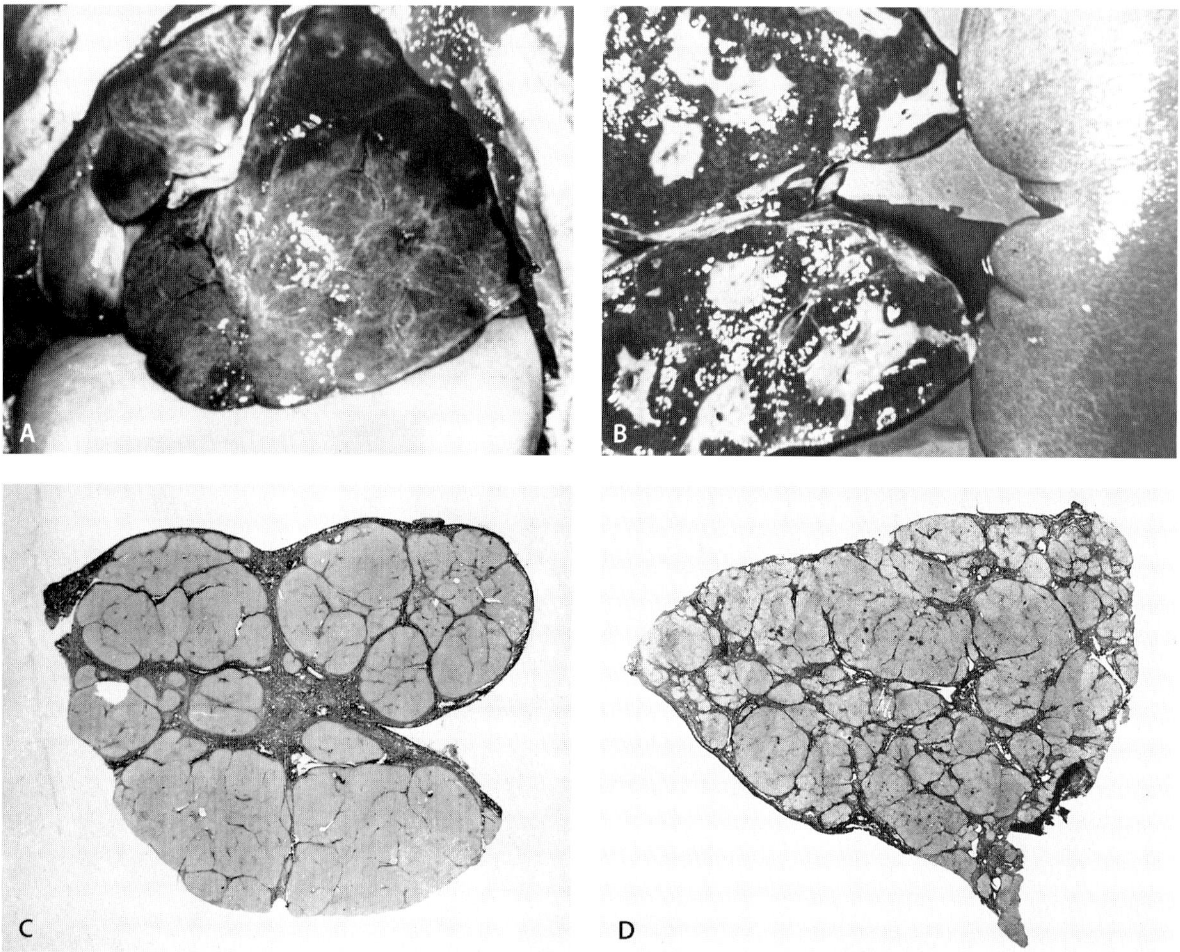

Fig. 2.41 A–D. The liver has a very characteristic appearance in schistosomiasis. **A** The autopsy specimen of a liver of a 27-year-old Brazilian male who died of hematemesis associated with hepatosplenomegaly secondary to schistosomiasis mansoni. There were a total of 183 active adult pairs of worms counted at autopsy. The external surface of the liver is bosselated, which is the typical appearance: sometimes the liver is smooth or finely nodular. **B** The cut surface of the same liver showing marked periportal fibrosis: the intervening liver parenchyma appears fairly normal. It is possible to have severe disease but show less portal fibrosis. Next to the liver is the edge of the enlarged spleen, which weighed 700 g. **C, D** Cross-sections of the livers of different patients showing the marked periportal fibrosis, septal thickening, and nodular cirrhosis seen in advanced schistosomiasis mansoni or japonica. (**C, D** AFIP 5426643 and 5427250)

Normal (0) equals less than 3 mm, Grade (1) 3–5 mm, Grade (2) greater than 5–7 mm, Grade (3) greater than 7 mm.

D. The gallbladder must be assessed when full, i.e., when the patient has been fasting (no food, only water to drink for 6 hours or more). If the gallbladder is not full, the wall will show on ultrasound scans as a double line. All measurements are of the anterior wall on the longitudinal view of the full gallbladder; the thickness of the wall should be less than 5 mm. When the wall thickness is 5 mm or more, this is abnormal (grade 1). (It must be noted that many ultrasonographers use 3 mm as the maximum thickness of a normal full gallbladder wall in the fasting patient. Less than 5 mm is therefore a safe margin to allow for variation between observers. The gallbladder wall may thicken for other reasons, such as cardiac failure or dengue fever.)

E. The spleen should not be more than 120 mm (12 cm) in length, measured in the midaxillary line. It may, of course, be larger due to causes other than schistosomiasis, such as malaria or leishmaniasis.

F. Collateral veins are almost always abnormal. If there are none, this is normal (0). If the observer is not certain, this is grade (1); if veins are definitely present, this is grade (2). If there are collateral veins, the record should include which veins have been seen, the coronary, paraumbilical, or short gastric.

G. Ascites is abnormal (excluding other causes); if there is none this is (0), if the observer is undecided this is grade (1), and if definitely present, this is grade (2). There are minimally different criteria for grading schistosomiasis japonica (see pp. 246–252).

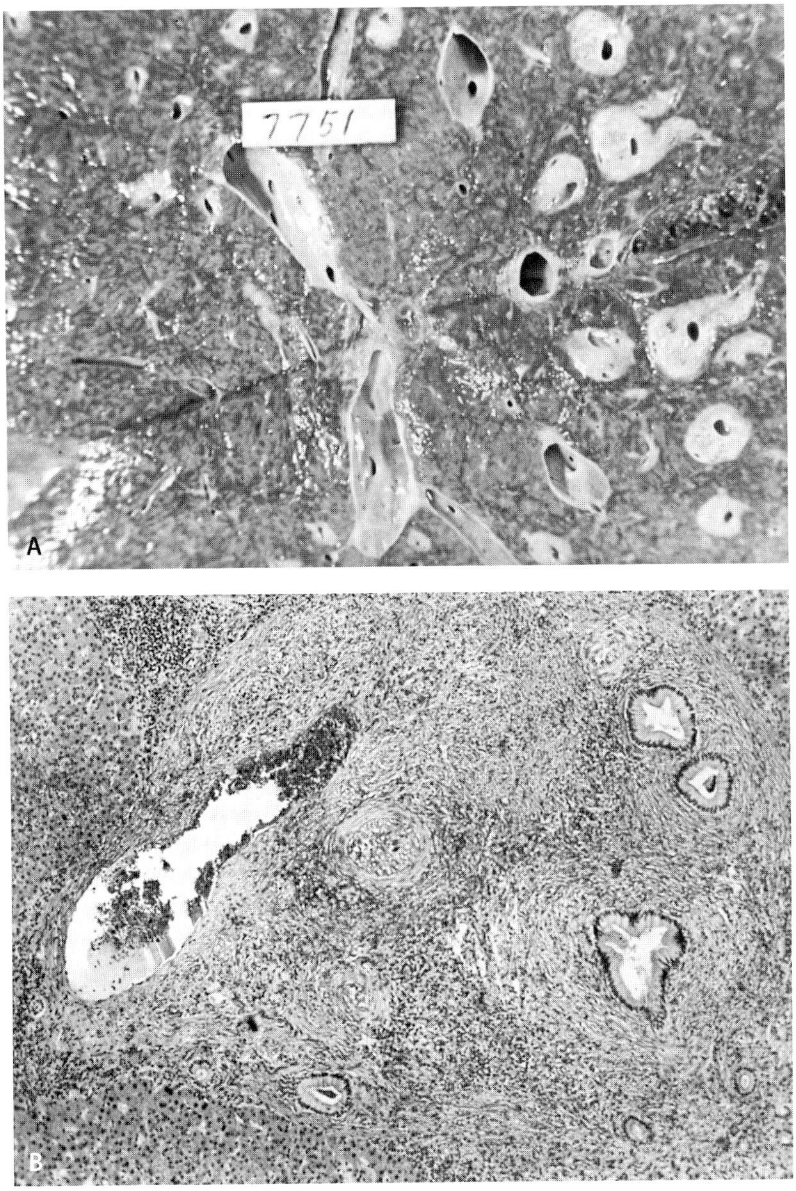

Fig. 2.42 A, B. Periportal fibrosis (or pipe stem fibrosis) is characteristic of hepatic schistosomiasis. **A** The cut surface of the liver of a patient who died from schistosomiasis mansoni. The periportal fibrosis is due to embolization of eggs from the mesenteric vessels. **B** The histology of the same liver showing extensive fibrosis involving a periportal triad. The portal vein is on the left and several bile ducts are on the right. (Courtesy of L. Millman, New York City) This periportal fibrosis can be demonstrated by ultrasonography

Portal Hypertension

For many years splenoportography and splenic manometry have been used to assess portal hypertension in schistosomiasis (see p. 186). Ultrasonography, with duplex Doppler, can effectively replace these invasive methods and is also an excellent method to assess postoperative improvement. Many studies from different countries confirm the close correlation between the ultrasound grading levels and the level of portal hypertension. The best index and correlation may be of the diameter of the splenic vein, measured at the hilus (normally less than 9 mm), but the size of the portal vein and superior mesenteric vein must also be measured. There is direct and accurate correlation between the diameter of the splenic vein and the intrasplenic pressure.
The mean velocity of the blood flow in the splenic vein may be normal, in spite of the increased diameter; it is likely to exceed that of the superior mesenteric vein.

(Text continues on p. 172)

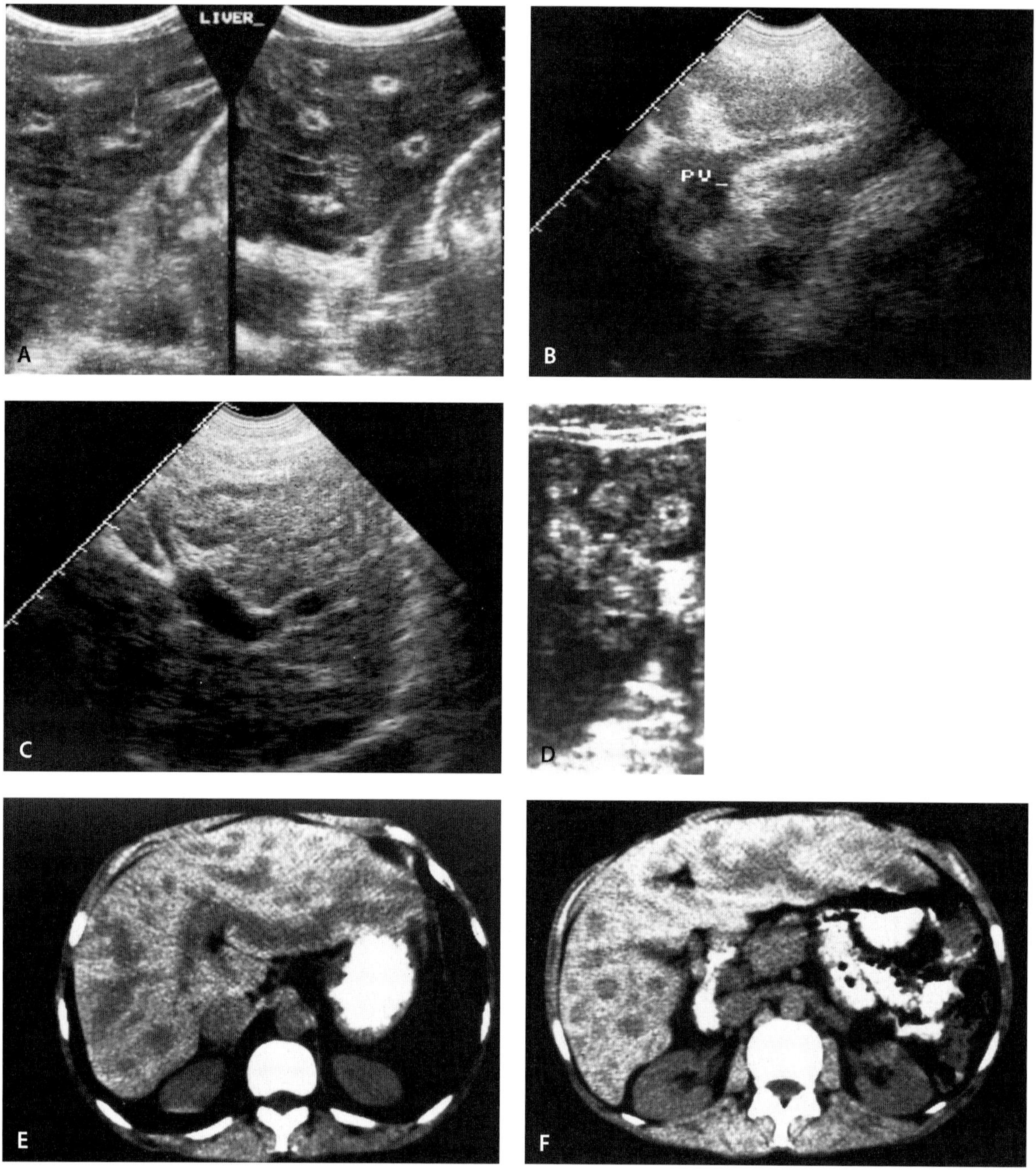

Fig. 2.43 A–L. The characteristic periportal fibrosis of hepatic cirrhosis due to *S. mansoni* infections can be demonstrated by both ultrasonography and CT scanning. Both will show the dense bands which show the portal vein branches into the periphery of the liver. On ultrasonography the bands are echogenic, while on CT they are of low density but enhance strongly with contrast, becoming either homogeneous or denser than the surrounding liver. Depending on the angle, the foci can be rounded or linear and the branching pattern allows differentiation from metastases. **A** Transverse ultrasound scans of the left lobe of the liver of an African from Kenya, showing well-marked periportal fibrosis due to *S. mansoni*. (Courtesy of WHO and Dr. M.W. Wachira) **B, C** Similar periportal fibrosis in an African from Zimbabwe. (Courtesy of S. Mindel) **D–H** A middle-aged Egyptial male who had splenectomy 2 years earlier for portal hyperension. **D** Transverse sonogram showing thick echogenic circles surrounding the portal vein branches. **E, F** Nonenhanced CT scans show both round and linear patterns of low density throughout the liver. **G–L** see p. 171

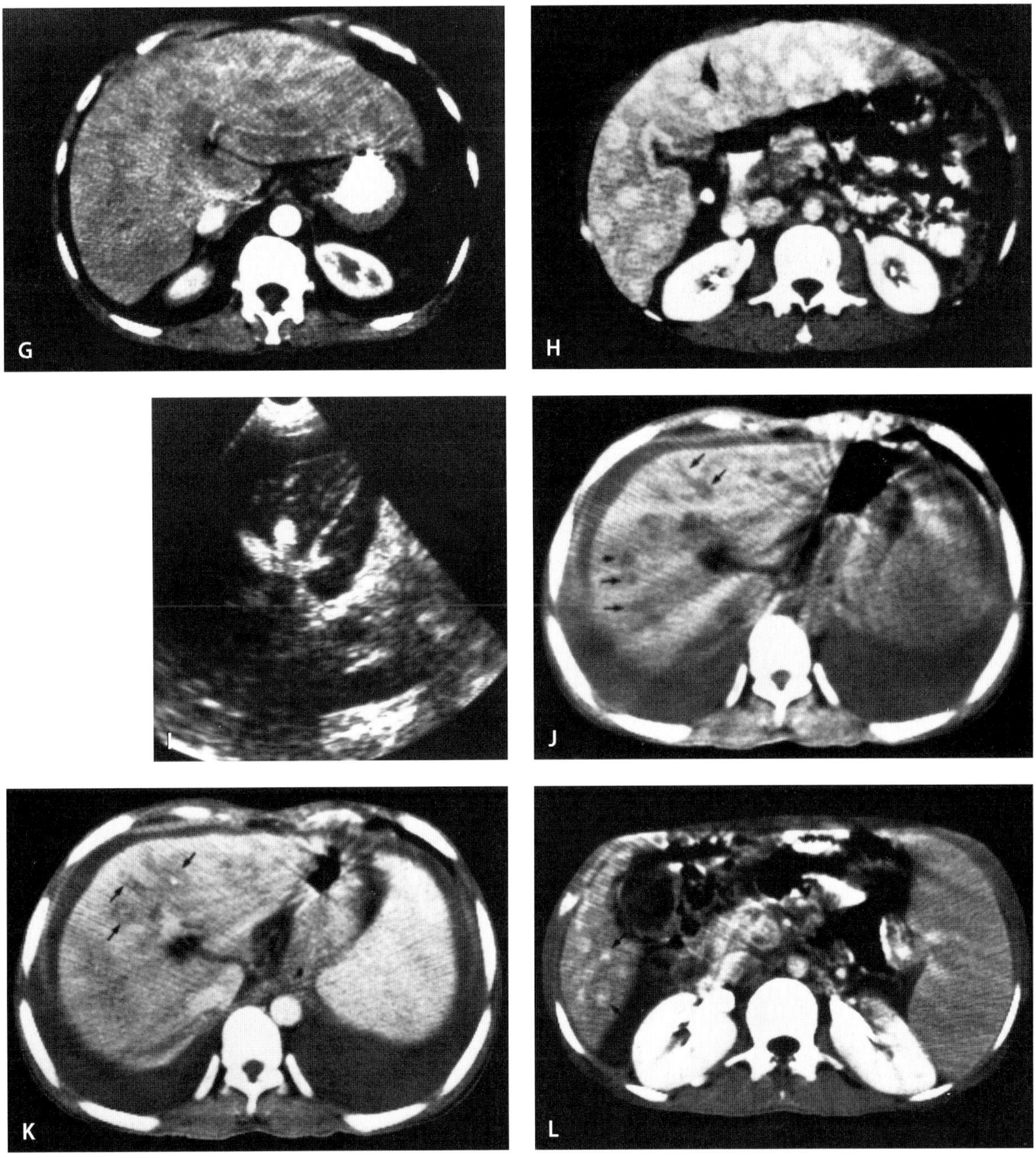

Fig. 2.43 (*continued*). **G** In the early phase of contrast scanning, the inferior vena cava has just filled, and there is compression of the left main portal vein. **H** One minute later there is contrast enhancement of both the linear and circular zones: this pattern persists for several minutes. **I–L** The same pattern in a younger Egyptian male who had severe hematemesis due to esophageal varices. There is the same typical appearance of periportal fibrosis on ultrasonography (**I**), nonenhanced CT scan (**J**), the early contrast phase (**K**), and four minutes later (**L**). The CT scans of **J** and **K** are at the same level. (**D–K** courtesy of Dr. S. Fataar, Muscat and *AJR*, 1985)

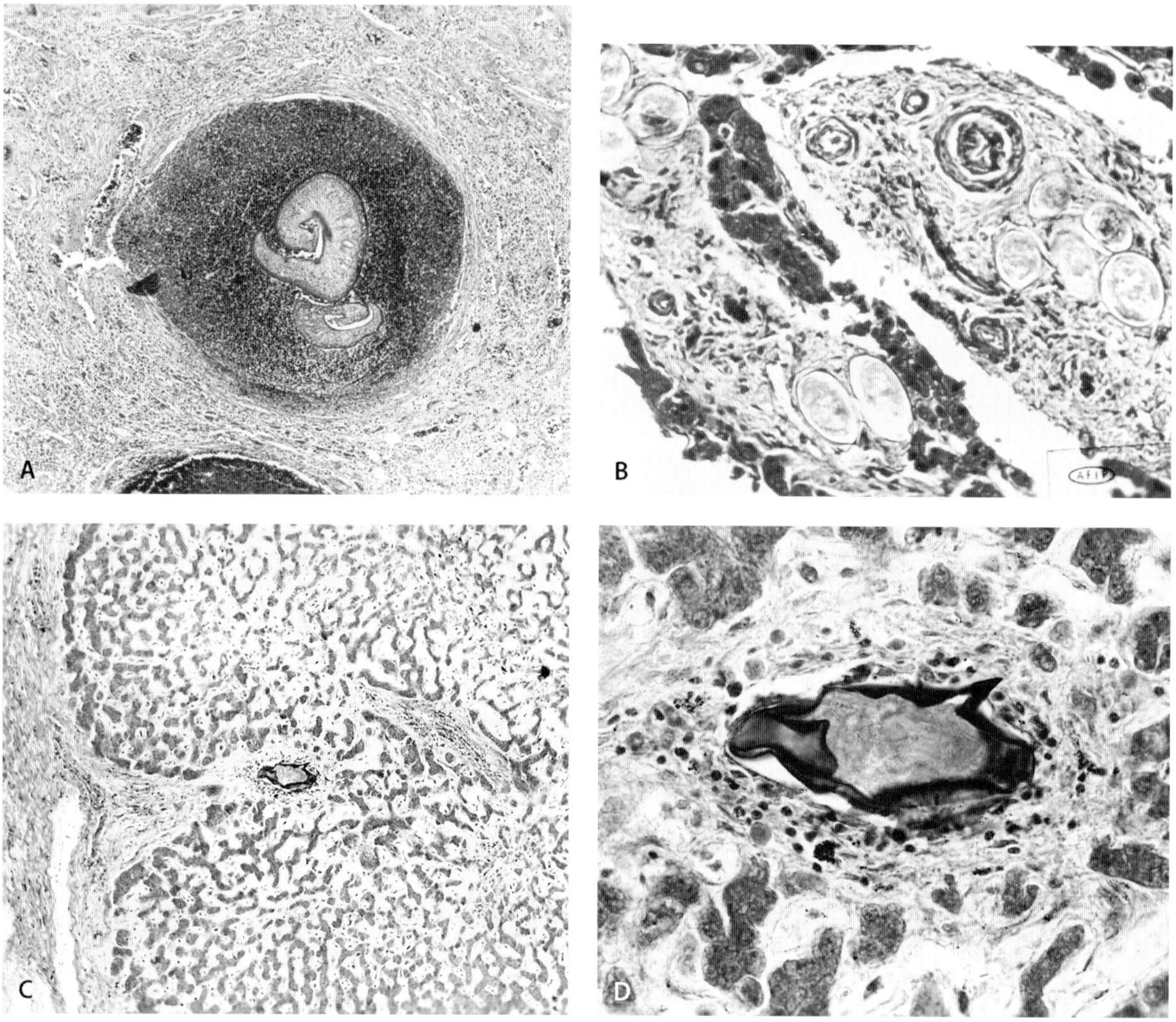

Fig. 2.44. A Cross-section of human liver showing adult male and female *S. mansoni* in a small liver abscess. ×50, AFIP 65-3024. **B** Multiple schistosome eggs in a different liver have caused an intense fibrosis and hepatic cell destruction. AFIP 68-4761-3. **C** A single *S. mansoni* egg in a liver sinusoid surrounted by minimal inflammatory reaction. ×54. **D** Magnification of the same *S. mansoni* egg, showing the lateral spine. ×270, AFIP 67-4754 and 67-4753

The blood flow in hepatic veins may not be increased. The grading of periportal fibrosis correlates well with the risk of bleeding. If worse than grade (1) and if the spleen is more than 11 cm in length, there is a significant risk of bleeding. A palpable liver and the portal vein diameter do not give a good correlation with the risk of hemorrhage.

Following successful surgery, there is usually a decrease in the size of the portal vein and an increase in the size of the hepatic artery. Mean blood velocity in the portal vein will be decreased but there will be no change in the blood flow velocity in the hepatic artery. It should be noted that preoperatively, splenic vein thrombosis is not uncommon, which will invalidate some of the usual measurements. As expected, there is a difference depending on the type of surgery, when devascularization is compared with a distal splenorenal shunt. After devascularization, the portal blood flow velocity is usually decreased, whereas it is increased following splenorenal shunt.

Radiography

Radiography, with or without angiography, is less important whenever ultrasonography is available. But it may be useful in some circumstances.

In advanced *S. mansoni* infections, plain radiographs of the abdomen may show moderate to marked splenomegaly without splenic calcification. The stomach may be displaced medially and the splenic flexure of the colon displaced downward by the enlarged spleen, which at times extends below

(Text continues on p. 181)

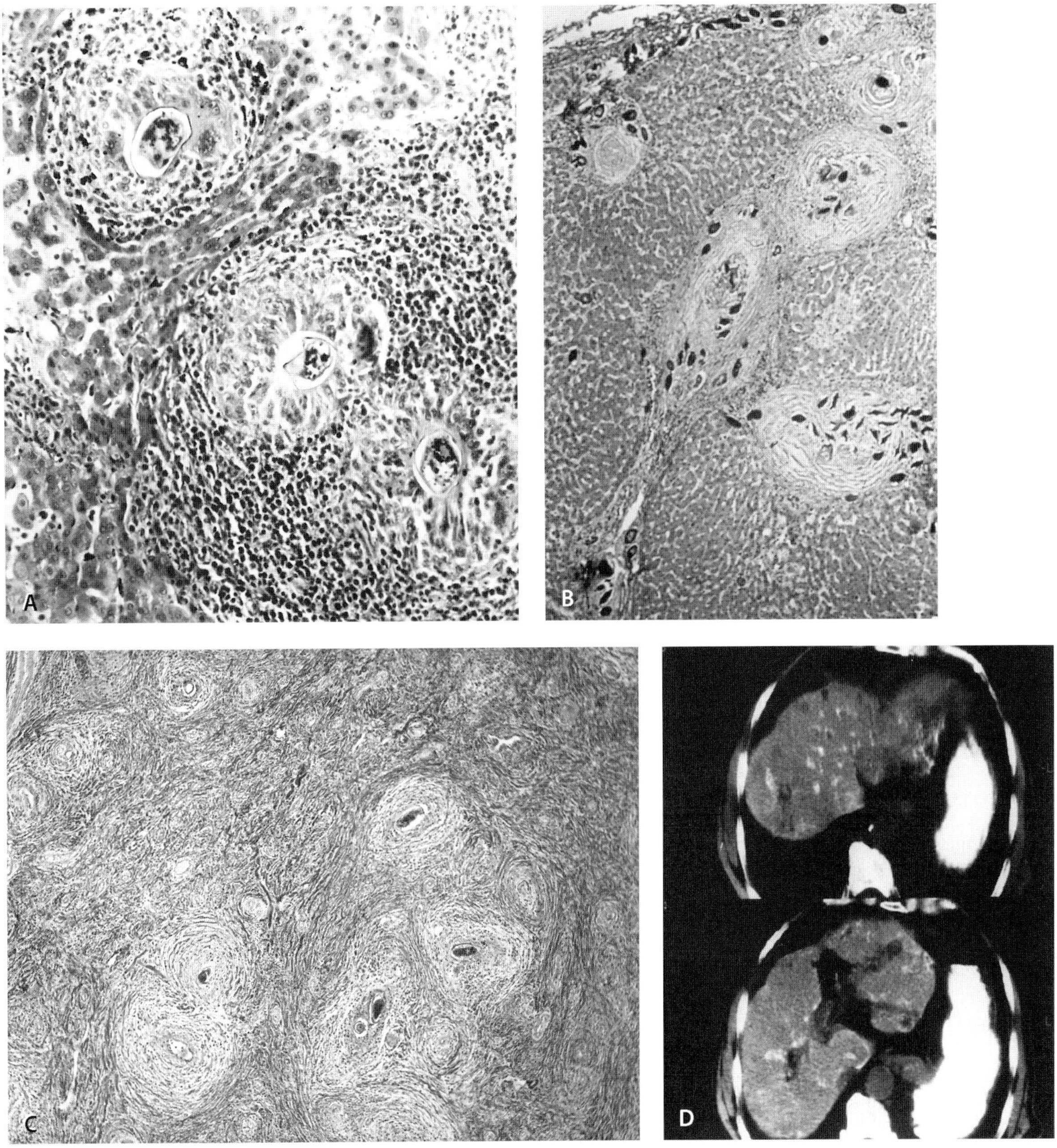

Fig. 2.45 A–D. Schistosome granulomas in the liver cause a marked inflammatory reaction and eventually fibrosis. **A** *S. mansoni* eggs within granulomas, surrounded by intense small cell inflammatory reaction. **B** *S. japonicum* eggs in several liver granulomas with intense surrounding fibrosis. **C** Intense hepatic fibrosis around several granulomas with virtually no recognizable liver cells remaining. **D** If there are sufficient eggs surrounding these granulomas, there may be a pattern of dense nodules (spots), as seen in this patient from Hong Kong with schistosomiasis japonica. There is also septal and capsular calcification (see Figs. 2.43–2.47). (**D** courtesy of Dr. H. Cheung, Hong Kong)

Update. It is reported (C. Frank et al., *Lancet* 355, pp. 887–891, 2000) that about 15–20% of Egyptians are seropositive for Hepatitis-C virus. This large reservoir of chronic hepatitis is probably linked to mass-treatment for schistosomiasis prior to the 1980's. This will affect the appearance of images of the liver.

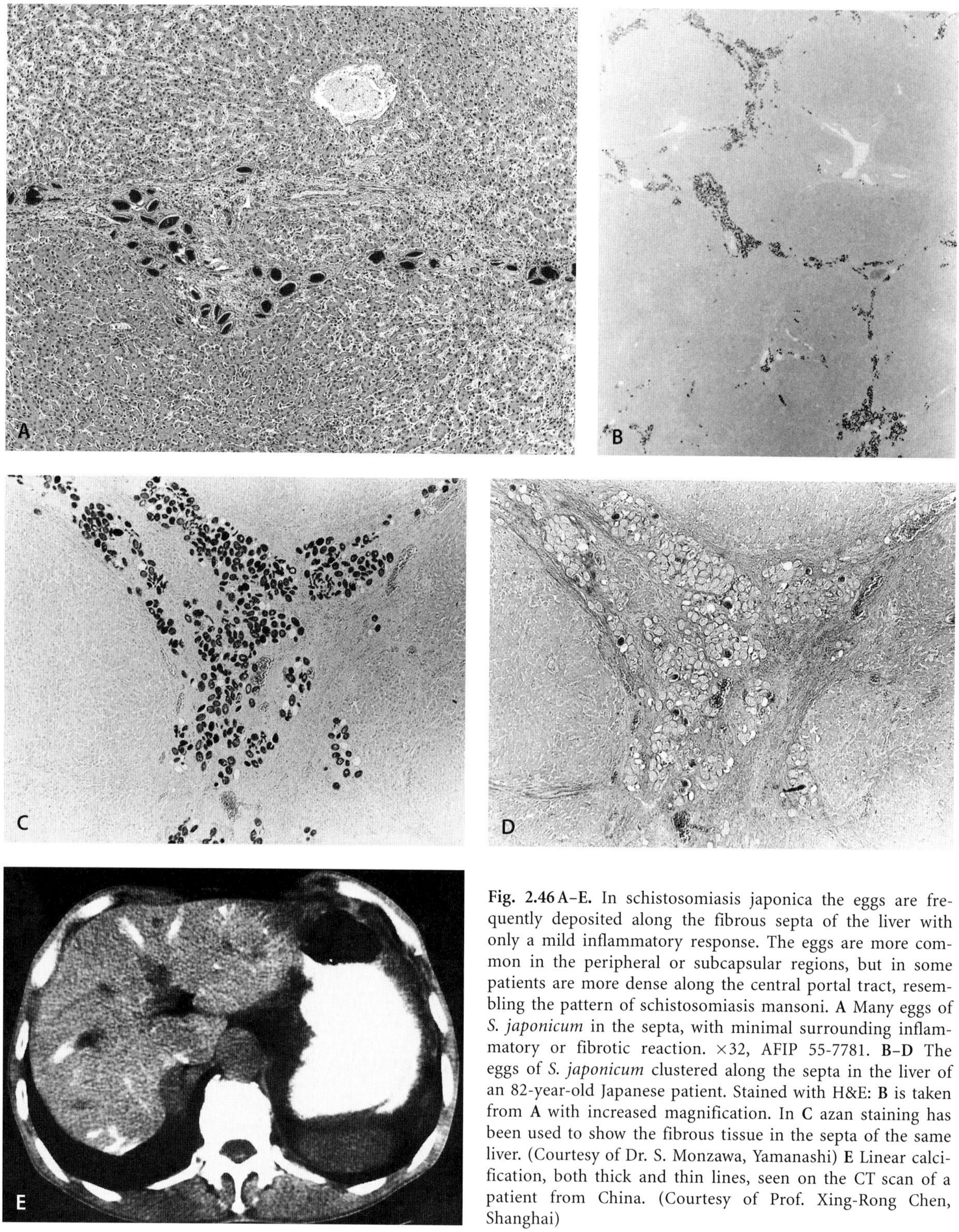

Fig. 2.46 A–E. In schistosomiasis japonica the eggs are frequently deposited along the fibrous septa of the liver with only a mild inflammatory response. The eggs are more common in the peripheral or subcapsular regions, but in some patients are more dense along the central portal tract, resembling the pattern of schistosomiasis mansoni. **A** Many eggs of *S. japonicum* in the septa, with minimal surrounding inflammatory or fibrotic reaction. ×32, AFIP 55-7781. **B–D** The eggs of *S. japonicum* clustered along the septa in the liver of an 82-year-old Japanese patient. Stained with H&E: **B** is taken from **A** with increased magnification. In **C** azan staining has been used to show the fibrous tissue in the septa of the same liver. (Courtesy of Dr. S. Monzawa, Yamanashi) **E** Linear calcification, both thick and thin lines, seen on the CT scan of a patient from China. (Courtesy of Prof. Xing-Rong Chen, Shanghai)

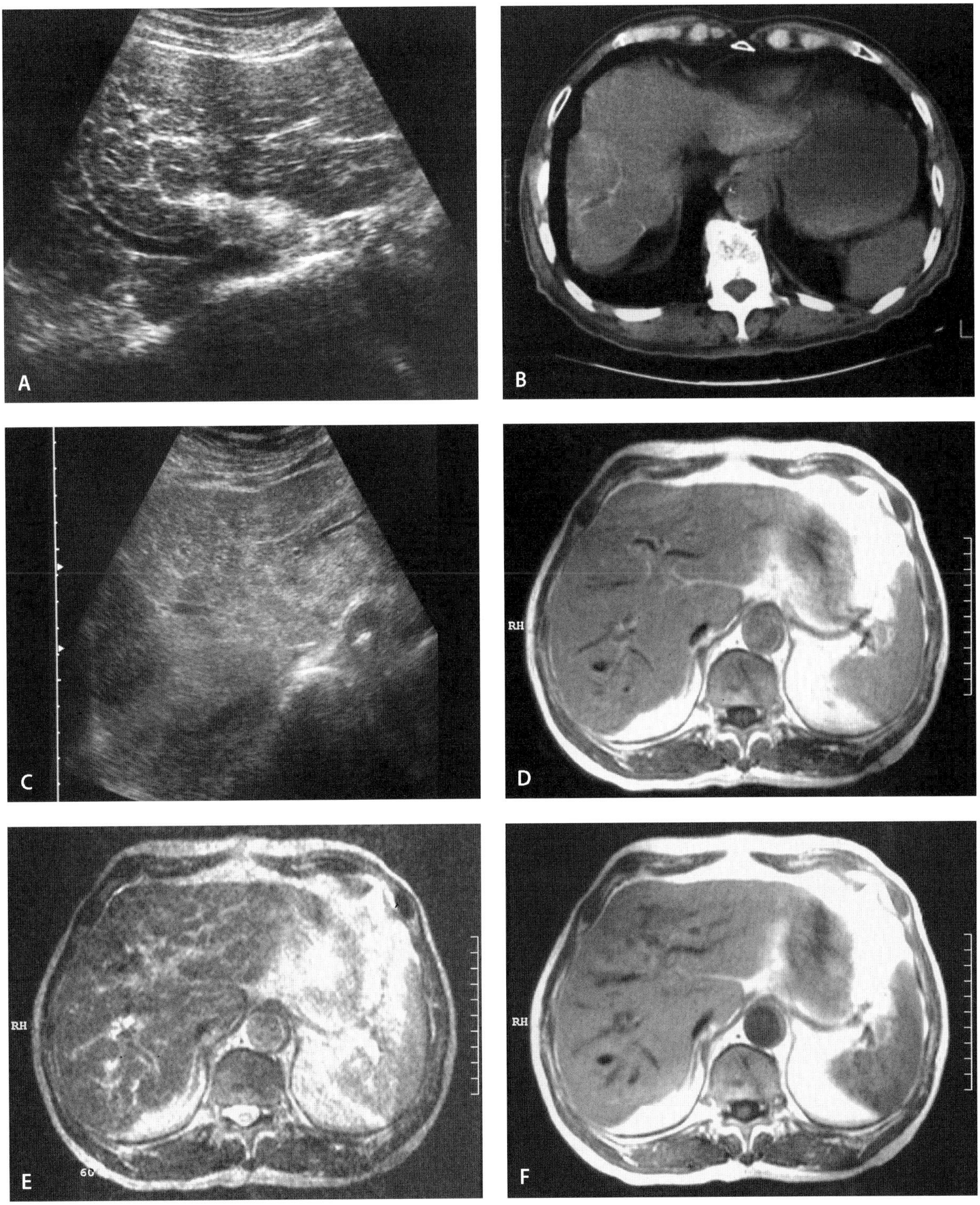

Fig. 2.47 A–F. Scans from Hong Kong, showing (**A**) echogenic lines on ultrasonography and (**B**) the same calcified septal lines on CT. MRI is not always as useful as CT or ultrasonography and the septa may be poorly demonstrated. The (**C**) ultrasound and (**D–F**) T1, T2, and postgadolinium MRI sequences at approximately the same level, in another Chinese patient from Hong Kong. (All courtesy of Dr. H. Cheung, Hong Kong)

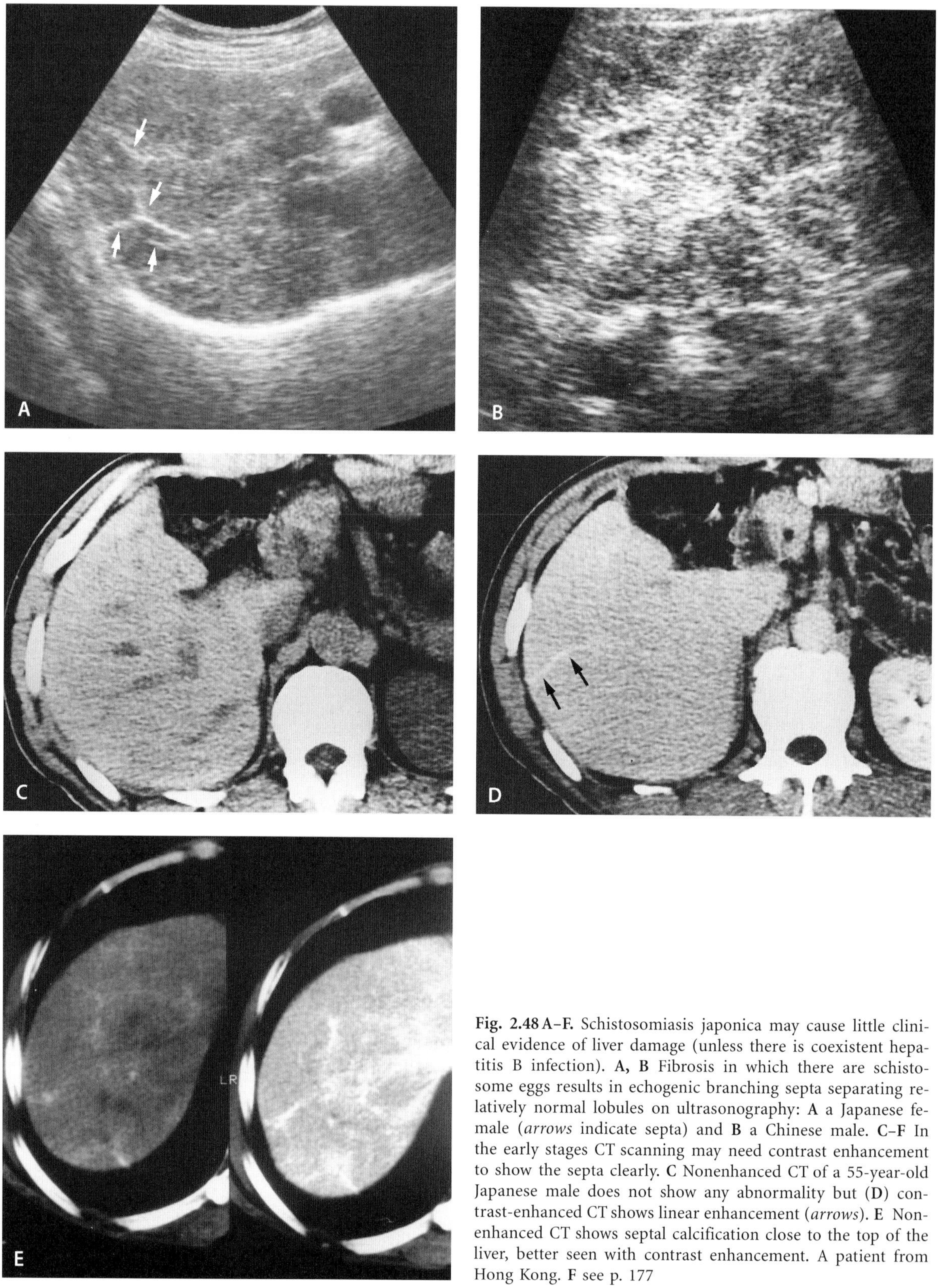

Fig. 2.48 A–F. Schistosomiasis japonica may cause little clinical evidence of liver damage (unless there is coexistent hepatitis B infection). **A, B** Fibrosis in which there are schistosome eggs results in echogenic branching septa separating relatively normal lobules on ultrasonography: **A** a Japanese female (*arrows* indicate septa) and **B** a Chinese male. **C–F** In the early stages CT scanning may need contrast enhancement to show the septa clearly. **C** Nonenhanced CT of a 55-year-old Japanese male does not show any abnormality but (**D**) contrast-enhanced CT shows linear enhancement (*arrows*). **E** Nonenhanced CT shows septal calcification close to the top of the liver, better seen with contrast enhancement. A patient from Hong Kong. **F** see p. 177

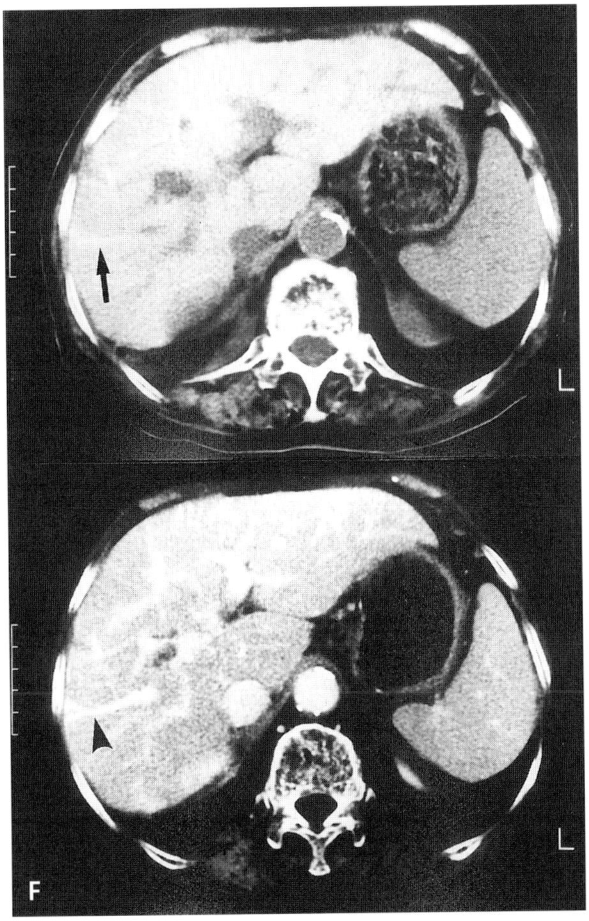

Fig. 2.48 (*continued*). **F** Similar pre- and postenhancement scans of a 77-year-old Japanese patient known to have had a positive stool examination for *S. japonicum* 54 years previously. The faint linear density seen on the nonenhanced CT (*arrow*) is much more clearly seen after enhancement (*arrowhead*). (**A, C, D, F** courtesy of Dr. S. Monzawa, Yamanashi; **B, E** courtesy of Dr. H. Cheung, Hong Kong)

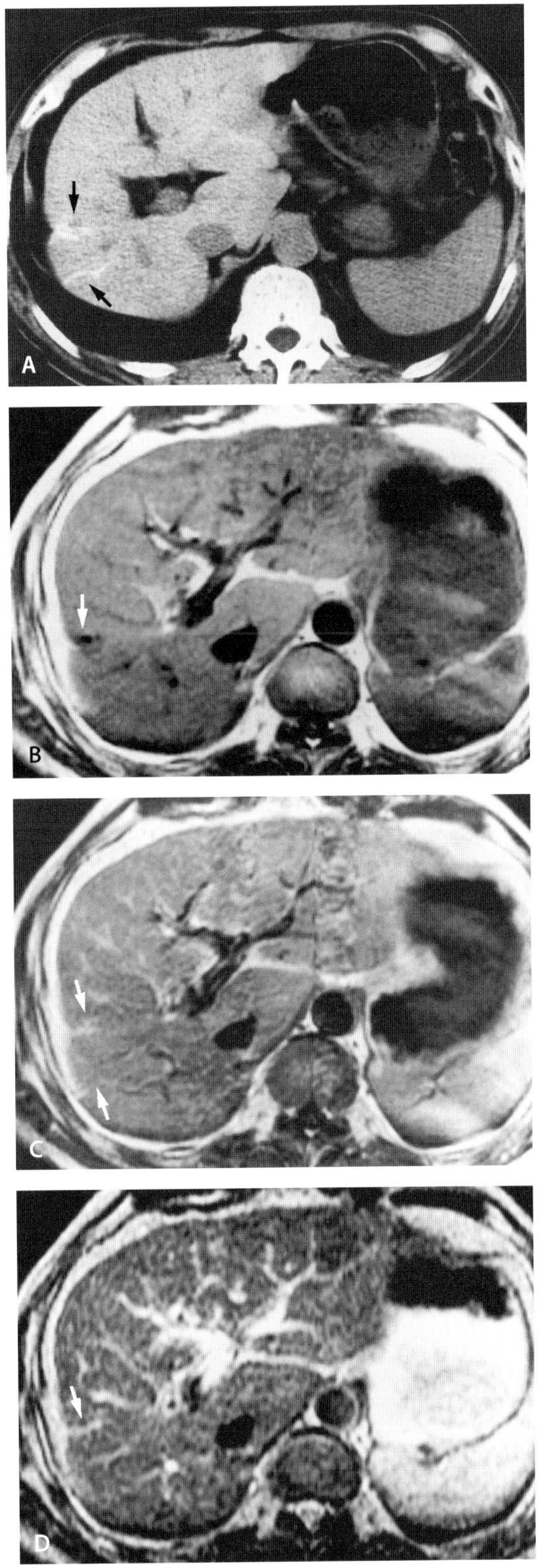

▶

Fig. 2.49 A–D. CT and MRI scans of a 61-year-old Japanse patient with histologically proven schistosomiasis japonica. **A** CT shows two linear, calcified septal lines (*arrows*). **B** On T1-weighted MRI, only the anterior line is seen (*arrow*), at low intensity. After gadolinium-DTPA (**C**) both lines are again seen (*arrows*) and are slightly enhanced. On T2-weighted MRI (**D**) the posterior line cannot be identified (*arrow* indicates anterior line). (Courtesy of Dr. S. Monzawa, Yamanashi)

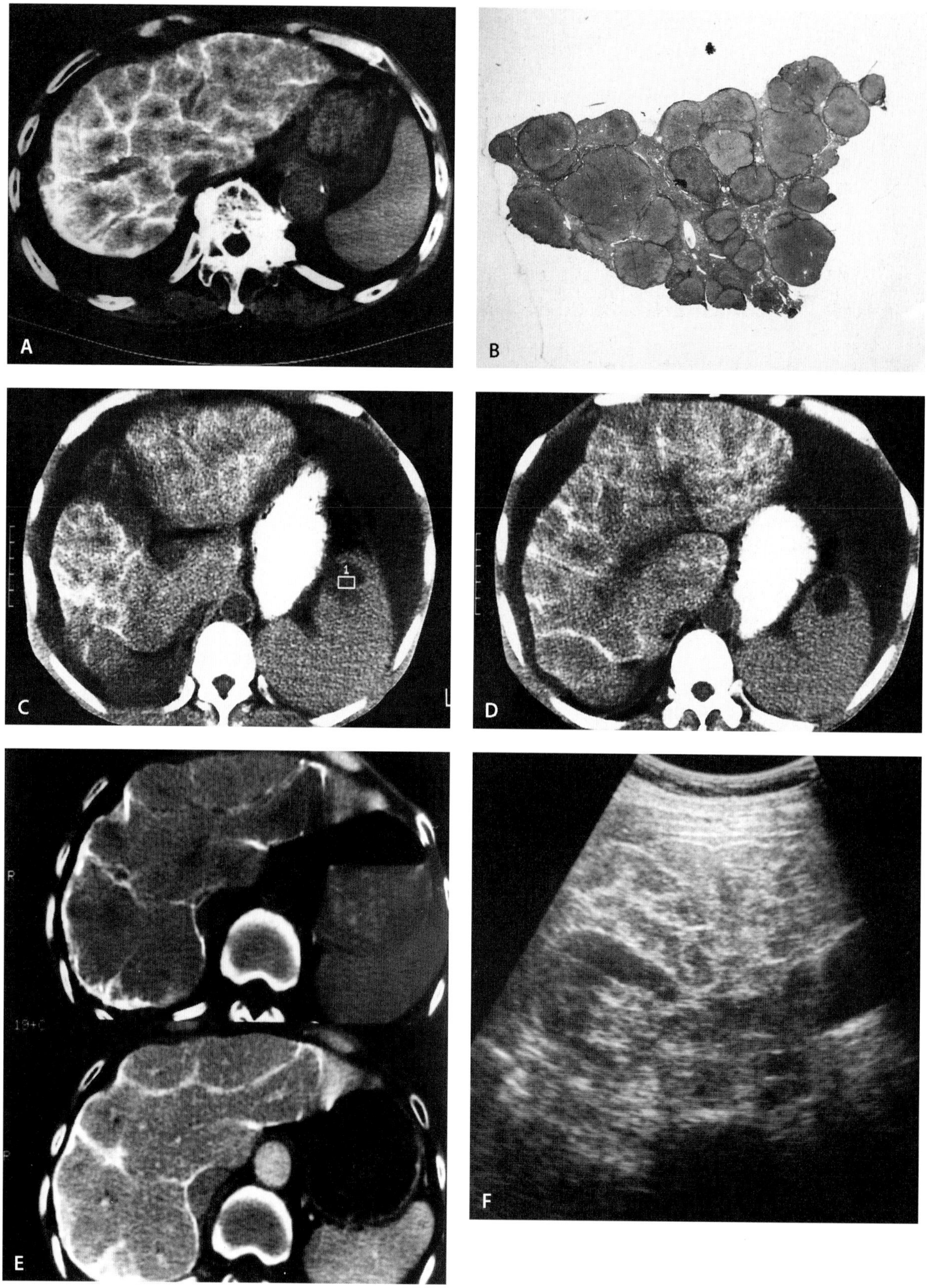
A
B
C
D
E
F

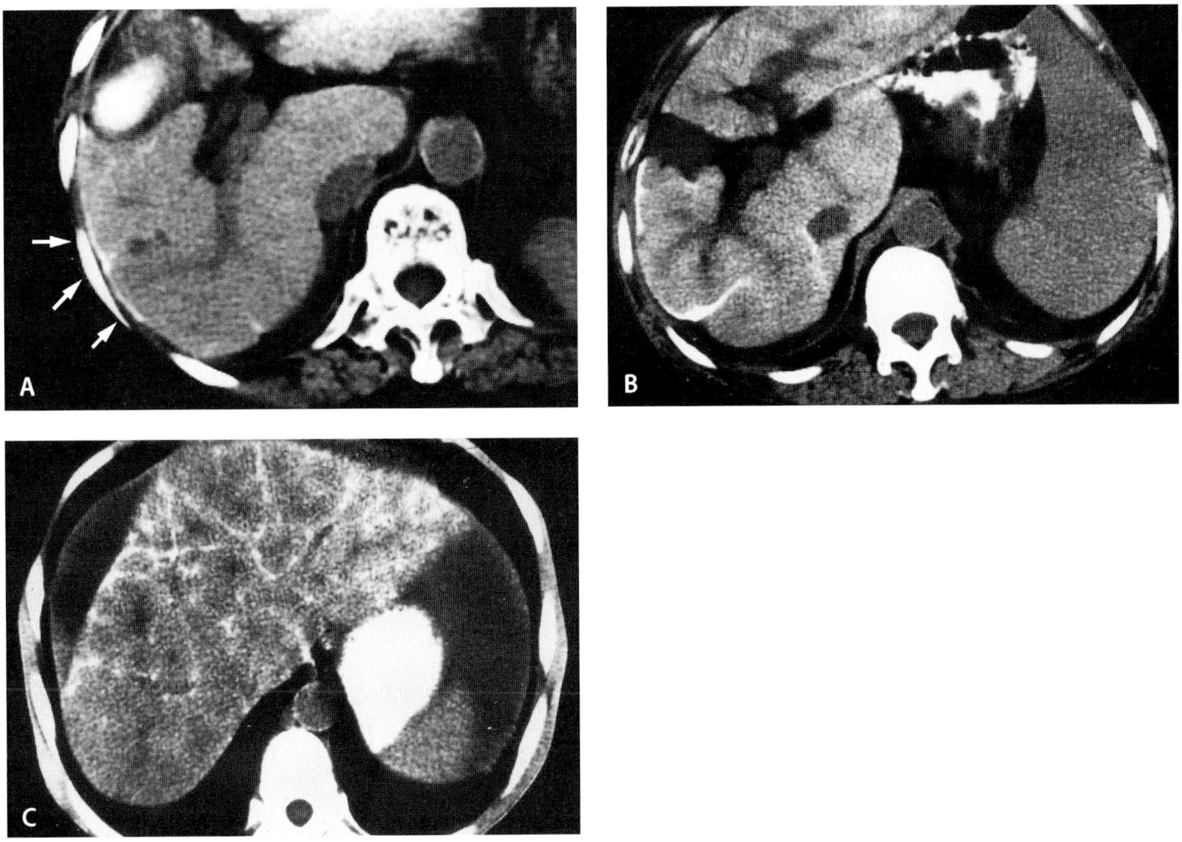

Fig. 2.51 A–C. Capsular calcification in *S. japonicum* can be quite dense, with or without septal calcification. **A** Calcification along the lateral aspect of the liver (*arrows*) seen on nonenhanced CT of a 65-year-old Japanese male with histologically proven schistosomiasis japonica. There is very little septal calcification. **B, C** Capsular and septal calcification in two patients from China, both with schistosomiasis japonica. (Courtesy of Prof. Xing-Rong Chen, Shanghai)

◀ **Fig. 2.50 A–F.** When the lobular calcification becomes extensive, the lobules become more clearly outlined and the characteristic pattern develops; this has been variously described as resembling a turtle or tortoise shell, a mosaic, or fish scales. The intervening liver parenchyma may still appear relatively normal. **A** Nonenhanced CT scan of a 79-year-old Japanese male with *S. japonicum* in the stool. **B** The cut section of a similar liver. AFIP 54-2663-5. **C, D** CT scans at different levels in a patient from China, showing an extensive calcified network. **E** Septal calcification with junctional thickening (notches), enhancing strongly with contrast. There is also capsular calcification. **F** An axial sonogram through the liver of a patient from Hong Kong with schistosomiasis japonica showing the same network-mosaic pattern. (E, F courtesy of Dr. H. Cheung, Hong Kong; F courtesy also of *Clin Radiol*, 1996)

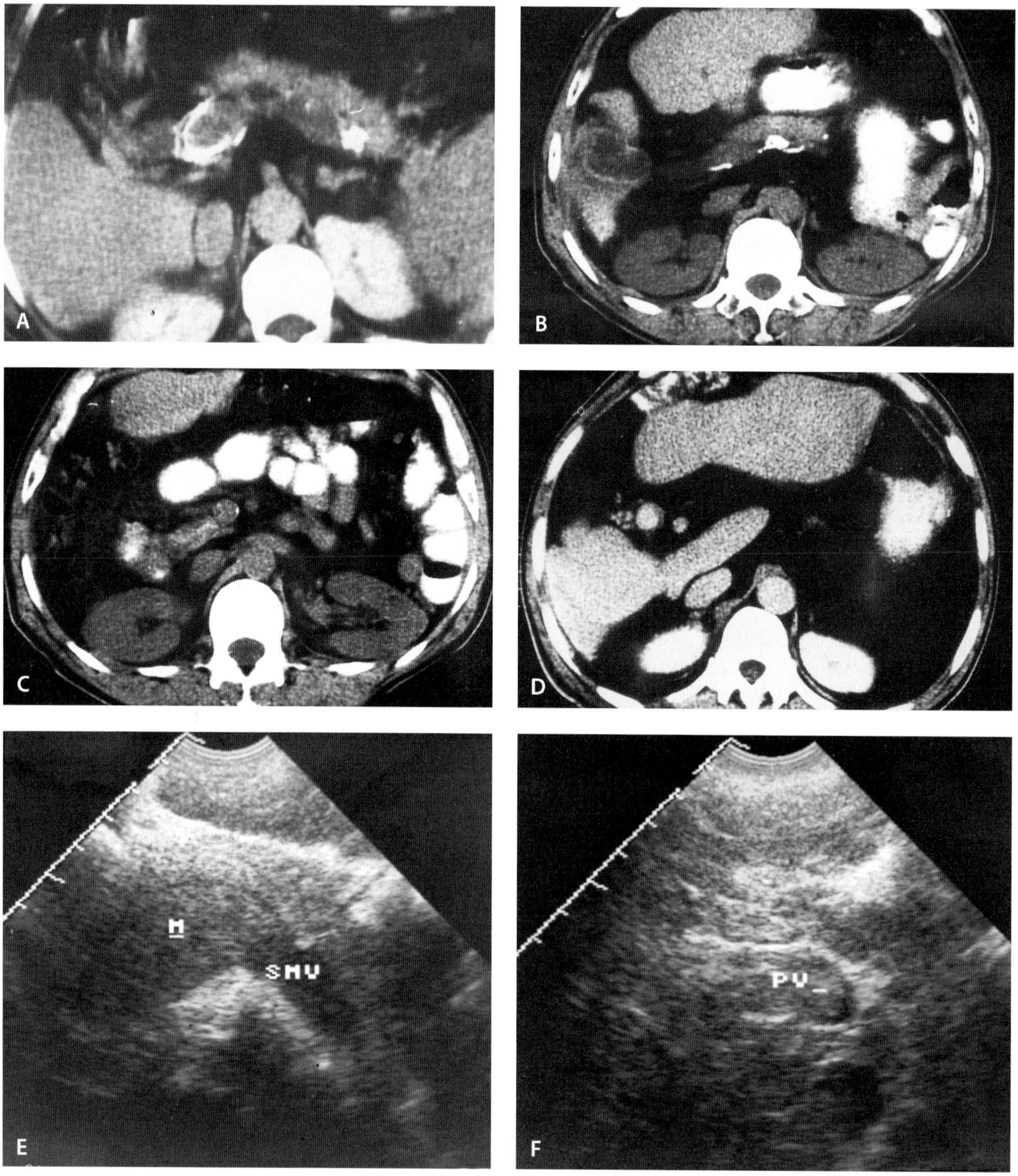

Fig. 2.52 A–F. Schistosomiasis japonica can also cause vascular calcification. **A** A CT scan showing calcification in the portal vein of a patient from China. **B** Another Chinese patient with calcification in both the portal and splenic veins. **C** Calcification in the wall of the superior mesenteric vein. Both **B** and **C**, and also **D**, show a decrease in size of the right lobe of the liver and some enlargement of the left lobe. This may be a little more common in *S. japonicum* infections in China than elsewhere. (**A–D** courtesy of Prof. Xing-Rong Chen, Shanghai) *S. haematobium* infections have not been reported as a cause of vascular calcification, but ultrasonography (or CT) may show thrombosis, as in these sonograms (**E**) of the superior mesenteric vein and (**F**) the portal vein of Africans from Zimbabwe. (Courtesy of Dr. Sam Mindel)

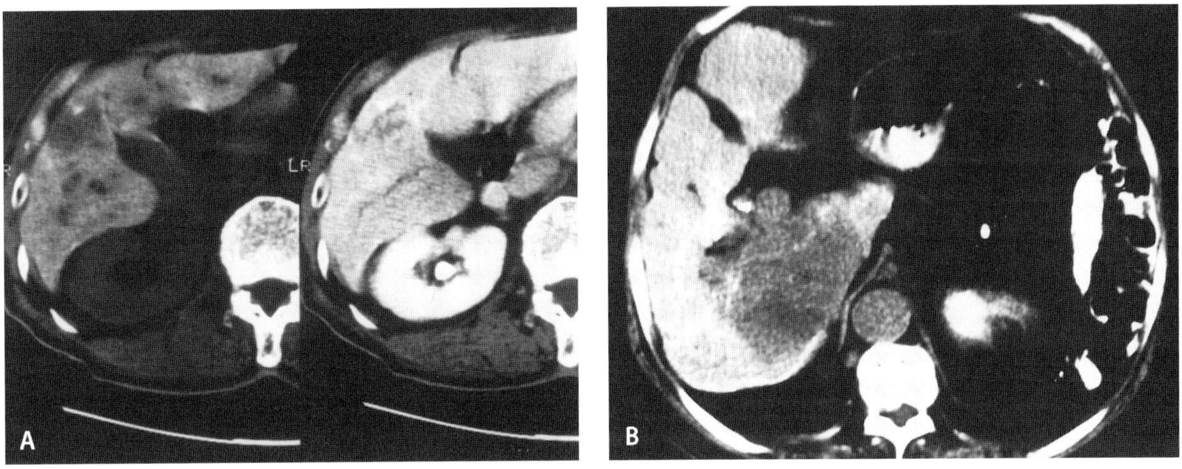

Fig. 2.53 A, B. In some patients with schistosomiasis japonica there may be focal liver lesions which resemble a tumor. **A** A localized hypoattenuating lesion with incomplete rim calcification which showed heterogeneous peripheral enhancement with contrast-enhanced CT, thought to represent a hepatoma. Biopsy showed *S. japonicum* eggs and increased liver iron. Such masses can also be mistaken for metastases. (Courtesy of Dr. H. Cheung, Hong Kong and *Clin Radiol*, 1996) There also seems to be a link between schistosomiasis japonica with hepatitis B infection and malignancy. **B** A hepatoma associated with the lobular pattern of schistosomiasis. (Courtesy of Prof. Xing-Rong Chen, Shanghai)

the iliac crest. There may be ascites. The liver enlarges as the infection progresses, but then shrinks as generalized hepatic fibrosis occurs. (This is more marked in *S. japonicum* infections; see pp. 246–252). Esophageal and gastric varices (Figs. 2.54, 2.55) may be identified with a barium upper gastrointestinal series. In some patients, mediastinal varices are so large that they cause displacement of the mediastinal stripe and widening of the mediastinum (best seen on the right side) on a chest radiograph. If the gastric varices are large enough, they cause undulating pressure on the gastric fundus and the upper third of the body of the stomach. The mucosa may appear serpiginous or there may even be a mass effect on the gastric fundus. In the majority of patients the diagnosis of schistosomiasis will have been made clinically and even confirmed by laboratory tests.

CT-Scanning

Plain radiographs may show calcification in the abdomen and even in the bowel, but it is more clearly seen on CT scanning. Although ultrasonography will provide most of the information which can be obtained from CT, there is a characteristic appearance on a CT scan. There will be low density, rapidly enhancing periportal areas, uniformly distributed throughout the liver. During a contrast examination, the low-density zones usually become hyperdense, but some will be isodense with the liver. In transverse section these low-density periportal areas are rounded, but in longitudinal section the pattern follows the portal vein and can be linear and occasionally branching. This is best seen in the central area of the liver because towards the periphery the veins are too small to be clearly demonstrated. It has been suggested that the rapid enhancement is due to the multiple small periductal vascular collaterals. It is also possible that there is increased hepatic artery circulation, particularly around small or medium obstructed portal veins, and this contributes to the enhancement. It has been described as angiomatous but this is perhaps somewhat misleading. As the fibrosis progresses, there is scarring and the periportal zones become less vascular. (The pattern in schistosomiasis japonica is different; see p. 195.) Measurement of the size of the hepatic and portal vessels may be used to grade the severity of the cirrhosis, but this is more commonly done with ultrasonography, aided by Doppler flow studies.

As already noted, CT can demonstrate the calcified eggs in the colon and rectum, and in the surrounding soft tissues. This does not have any clinical significance, apart from the diagnosis of schistosomiasis.

Isotope scanning

Isotope scintigraphy early in the disease shows a normal to moderately enlarged liver with either homogeneous or slightly mottled radioactive tracer uptake. The mottled pattern resembles that seen in Laënnec's cirrhosis and generally reflecting the extent of the liver damage. An enlarged spleen can also be visualized.

(Text continues on p. 184)

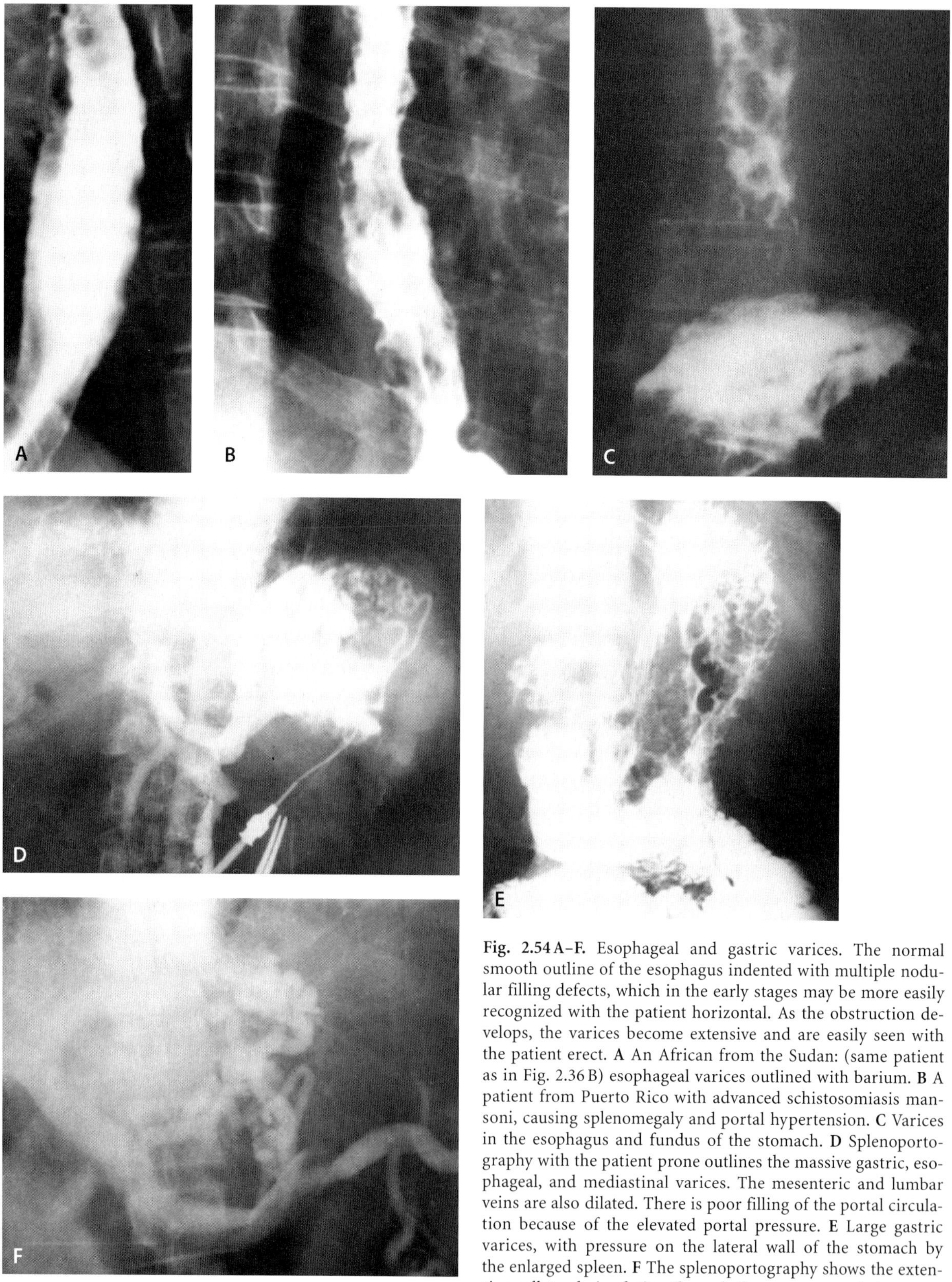

Fig. 2.54 A–F. Esophageal and gastric varices. The normal smooth outline of the esophagus indented with multiple nodular filling defects, which in the early stages may be more easily recognized with the patient horizontal. As the obstruction develops, the varices become extensive and are easily seen with the patient erect. **A** An African from the Sudan: (same patient as in Fig. 2.36 B) esophageal varices outlined with barium. **B** A patient from Puerto Rico with advanced schistosomiasis mansoni, causing splenomegaly and portal hypertension. **C** Varices in the esophagus and fundus of the stomach. **D** Splenoportography with the patient prone outlines the massive gastric, esophageal, and mediastinal varices. The mesenteric and lumbar veins are also dilated. There is poor filling of the portal circulation because of the elevated portal pressure. **E** Large gastric varices, with pressure on the lateral wall of the stomach by the enlarged spleen. **F** The splenoportography shows the extensive collateral circulation through the coronary and short gastric veins, leading up to the esophageal plexus. To outline the full extent of the collateral circulation it may be necessary to do contrast studies in both the supine and prone positions. (**B** courtesy of Dr. H. Pagan-Saez, San Juan; **C**, **D** courtesy of Dr. H. Moskowitz, Connecticut)

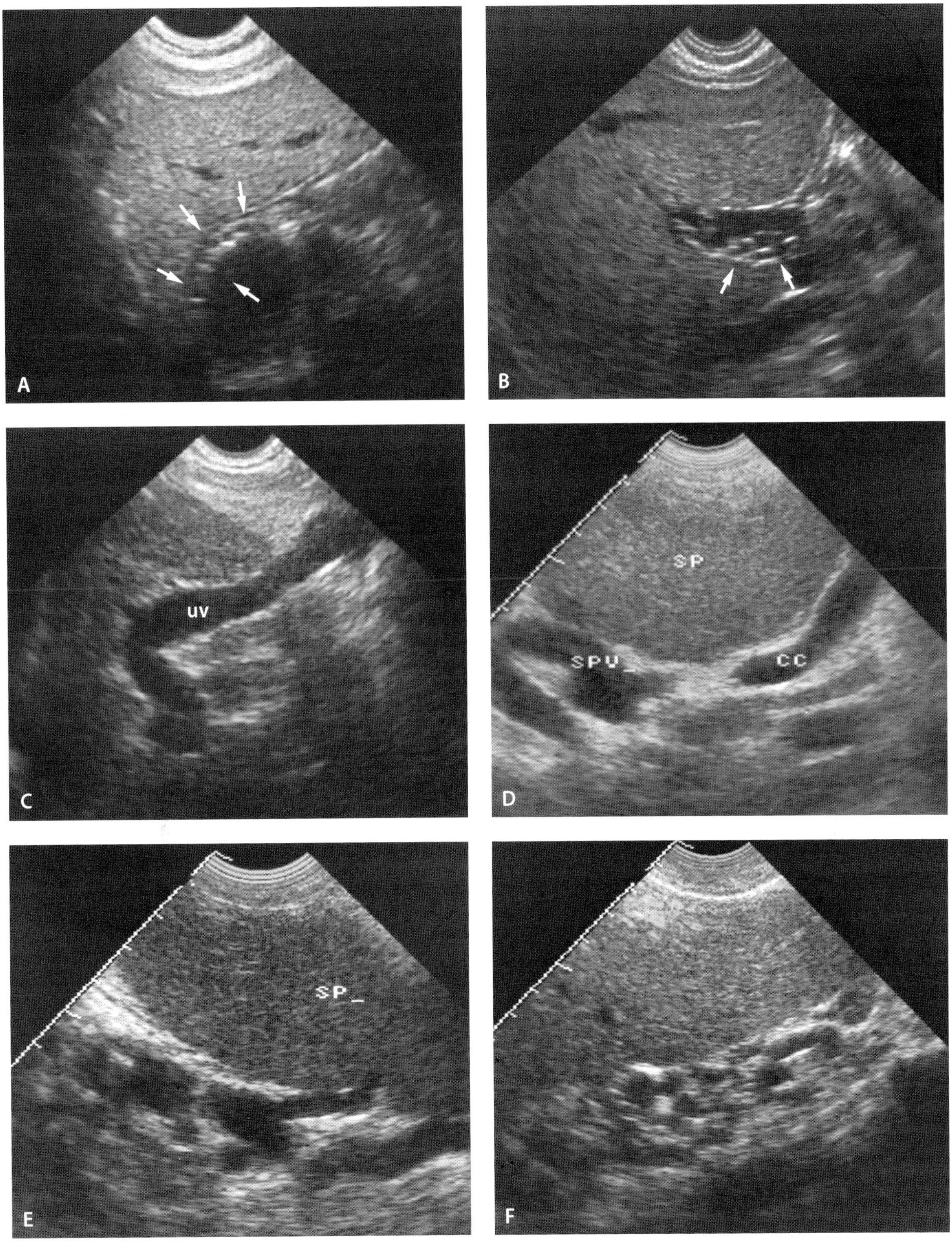

Fig. 2.55 A–F. Ultrasonography is an excellent way to demonstrate the varices which result from portal hypertension and an extensive collateral circulation in schistosomiasis. **A** Varices (*arrows*) in the gastric fundus (*F*). **B** Varices (*arrows*) in the porta hepatis. **C** A dilated patent umbilical vein (*uv*). **D** Splenomegaly with dilated splenic veins and collateral vessels. *SP* spleen; *SPV* splenic vein; *CC* collaterals. **E** Splenomegaly with multiple collateral vessels. *SP* spleen; **F** Multiple varices around the porta hepatis. All are African patients from Zimbabwe. (Courtesy of Dr. Sam Mindel)

Angiography

Where ultrasonography and Doppler are not available, splenoportography can reliably evaluate portal venous pressure due to the presinusoidal block. Even when ultrasonography is available, angiography may be valuable, particularly for demonstrating the anatomy of the collateral circulation before surgery. The full extent of the collateral circulation may be seen and the varicosities assessed. Arterial portography is safer but less informative than direct splenic contrast injection, and sometimes gives incomplete and inaccurate data. When the intrahepatic portal circulation is diminished, the splenoportogram will fail to show a normal hepatogram. The loss of peripheral branches within the liver produces the classical "pruned tree" appearance of cirrhosis. As a result, the sinusoidal phase may be diminished or absent.

Hepatic angiography cannot provide exact information early in the disease because the presinusoidal obstruction makes hepatic-wedge venous pressure unreliable. In end-stage disease, the hepatic-wedge pressure is more reliable and reflects portal venous pressure. Hepatic-wedge injection may demonstrate retrograde flow into the portal system. Celiac angiography will show a dilated splenic artery and stretched intrasplenic arterial branches within a markedly enlarged spleen. The hepatic arteries may also be large, but the liver is often smaller than normal. The arterial pattern within the liver shows slight dilatation but is otherwise unremarkable until late in the disease, when a corkscrew appearance may be noted due to the cirrhotic changes. Visualization of the splenic vein is difficult because the enlarged spleen soaks up the injected contrast medium.

Injection into the superior mesenteric artery demonstrates a normal arterial pattern and, on delayed films, may show reasonably good visualization of the superior mesenteric and portal veins as well as varicosities. If a splenorenal shunt is to be performed, an attempt should be made to ensure that the renal vein is suitable for anastomosis.

Postoperatively, ultrasonography is preferable to angiography and is a very reliable way to assess the result of a shunt. However, angiography may show that the varices have disappeared completely, and it can determine shunt patency and the portal hemodynamics (Fig. 2.57). This is best done by passing a preformed catheter through the right femoral vein into the inferior vena cava and the left renal vein (Fig. 2.57 C). It can then be passed through the anastomosis into the portal venous system so that pressure measurements can be obtained. It is also possible to inject contrast to visualize the anatomy, physiology, and flow pattern and to evaluate shunt patency. A patent splenorenal shunt is effective in decreasing portal hypertension when there are esophageal varices, but it is not without side-effects. Approximately 30% of patients develop incapacitating hepatic encephalopathy after a splenorenal shunt (Fig. 2.57 D).

Fig. 2.56. The development of collateral circulation in patients with schistosomiasis mansoni. **A–C** Natural decompression of the portal system occurs and opens the collateral circulation through the coronary and short gastric veins which connect to the esophageal plexus. Hepatofugal collaterals are established through the umbilical, retroperitoneal, lumbar, renal, and mesenteric veins. The intrahepatic portal system resembles a tree in winter, or after pruning, because many of the peripheral branches do not fill. Because of this, there is unlikely to be a normal hepatogram. When there is portal vein obstruction (**D–F**) decompression may be by retrograde flow into the large dilated umbilical vein (**D, E**), sometimes known as the Cruveilhier-Baumgarten syndrome. In **C** the proximal portal vein is blocked but in **D** it is patent, but both patients have developed extensive collaterals as well as the flow through the umbilical vein. In **F** there is an extensive network of collaterals which involves the retroperitoneal as well as the gastric and esophageal veins. All of these patients come from Puerto Rico and have advanced schistosomiasis mansoni. (**D, E** courtesy of Dr. H. Moskowitz, Connecticut) ▶

Magnetic Resonance Imaging

Magnetic resonance imaging can detect the broad periportal bands (Figs. 2.47, 2.49). On T1-weighted scans they may be isodense with the liver, but on T2-weighted scans they are markedly increased when the inflammation is active. As fibrosis becomes more significant, the difference will decrease and the bands are less obvious on T2-weighted scans. Eventually the central lucent line will be obliterated. The hepatic arteries usually remain normal and there are few parenchymal changes. MRI is a useful way to image early, active inflammatory stages.

Biliary Tract

When there is advanced portal fibrosis, ultrasonography or a T-tube, intravenous or percutaneous cholangiogram may show crowding and narrowing of the intrahepatic biliary radicals.

An extrahepatic granuloma can affect the biliary ducts and may cause constriction, of either the cystic or the common duct. This can happen at a relatively young age in endemic areas, and the patient may present with a tender, swollen gallbladder, with or without jaundice. The clinical diagnosis may well be that of an amebic abscess or, when jaundice is present, of *Ascaris* or *Clonorchis* in the common bile duct. Ultrasonography will exclude an abscess or the worms and demonstrate the distended gallbladder (see also p. 161).

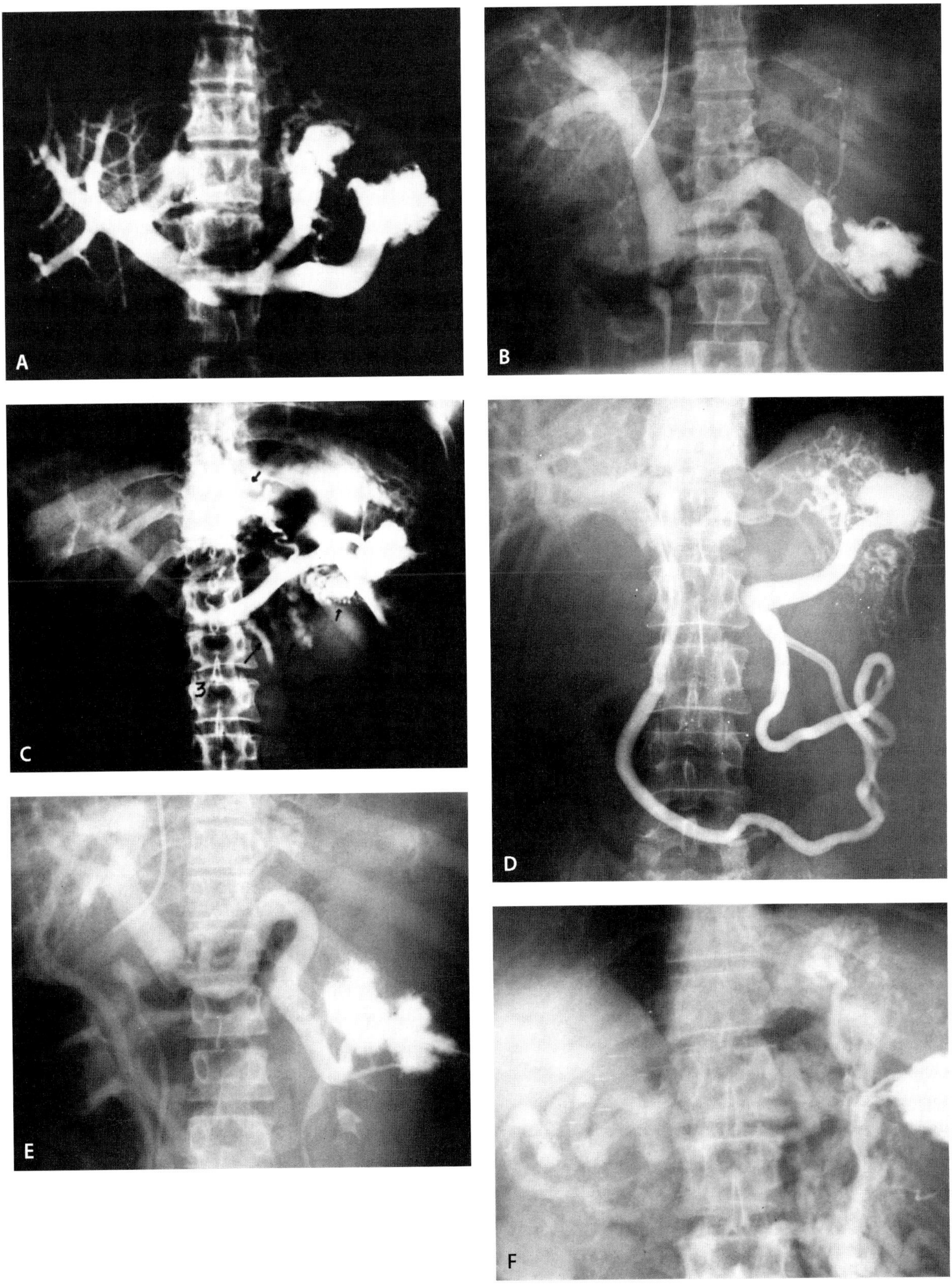
A
B
C
D
E
F

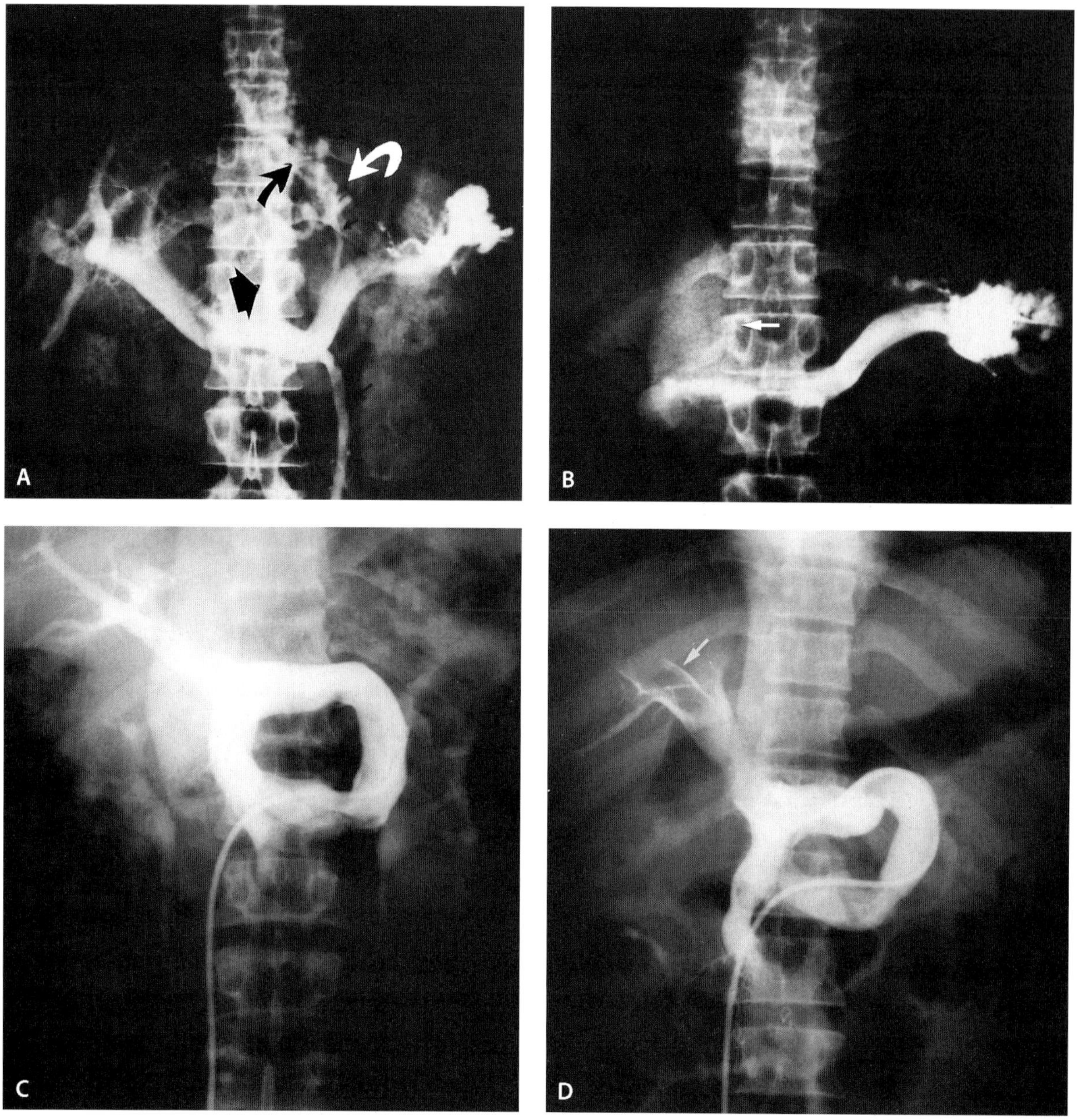

Fig. 2.57 A–D. Angiography is an excellent way to demonstrate the success (or failure) of portocaval shunting. This can be recognized with color Doppler ultrasonography, but angiography sometimes gives better anatomical visualization. **A** The preoperative splenoportogram shows extensive collateral circulation involving the coronary, short gastric, and esophageal plexi (*upper arrows*) and at the mesenteric vein (*arrowhead*): there is splenomegaly, but the liver is small. **B** Following a portocaval shunt there is no collateral circulation, but the contrast medium flows immediately into the inferior vena cava (*arrow*). **C** A normal splenorenal shunt. The catheter is in the inferior vena cava and into the left renal vein through the shunt. The anastomosis is widely patent. Contrast medium has run into the portal vein and the inferior vena cava. **D** This patient had developed severe hepatic encephalopathy; the shunt is widely patent but there is thrombosis of the portal vein (*arrow*)

Spleen

Either ultrasonography or CT can be used to demonstrate a fine, diffuse schistosomal fibrosis, which is quite common in Egypt and elsewhere in North Africa, but rare in Brazil. There are other variations; in some patients the spleens may be quite normal even when there is significant hepatic fibrosis. Splenic vein thrombosis may also occur, visualized by ultrasonography or contrast examination.

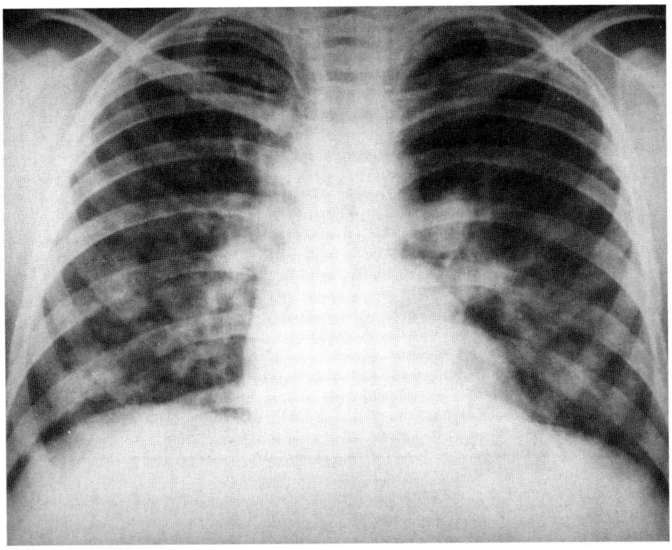

Fig. 2.58. The acute larval phase of pulmonary schistosomiasis; the patient's chest x-ray had been normal 2 months earlier. There is prominence of the hila with multiple soft patchy density throughout both lungs, particularly in the lower lobes. This corresponds to the passage of larvae through the lungs, the Katayama stage. (Courtesy of Dr. John Ebersole, Lancaster; see p. 122)

Differential Diagnosis of Hepatic Schistosomiasis

On scanning, the linear or circular pattern, depending on the section, of portal fibrosis is very characteristic. In transverse section, the multiple densities seen on scanning could be mistaken for metastases, but in longitudinal section the linear pattern removes that possibility, particularly when branching is observed. Nutritional or other cirrhosis must be considered, in which case the texture of the liver on scanning will be coarse with increased attenuation. There will be a nodular liver surface (compared with the smooth surface of schistosomiasis) and multiple regenerating nodules. This does not happen in schistosomiasis, which causes shrinkage of the liver. The perivascular and periportal thickening is less in cirrhosis and is usually seen in the main branches. Splenomegaly is less common, but there may be other reasons for an enlarged spleen (malaria, etc.). If the pattern of the portal veins and periportal fibrosis is carefully traced on scanning, the differential diagnosis will not be in doubt.

The thick-walled gallbladder may be mistaken for cholecystitis, but the pattern of inflammation is more ragged and there are likely to be gallstones. Jaundice is not a part of the syndrome of schistosomiasis. In acute hepatitis, the walls of the portal veins may be hyperechogenic, prominent, and echo bright. In schistosomiasis, the portal vein walls are much thicker, even up to 2 cm, and the brightness is less. The presence of calcified eggs in the abdomen helps the differential diagnosis.

Ascaris or *Clonorchis* affect the biliary system without the periportal fibrosis of schistosomiasis. Amebic or other abscesses are not likely to cause a differential diagnostic problem (Chap. 1).

Lungs

The lungs may be affected by *S. mansoni* both early and late in the infection.

In the initial phase of the disease, when the larvae pass through the lungs (the Katayama syndrome, Fig. 2.58 and p. 122) there is often a transient increase in lung markings, occasionally with some faint soft nodulation, more visible in the lower lobes, and enlargement of the mediastinal lymph nodes. If treatment is initiated, the reaction may be more obvious and spread throughout both lungs, probably due to an allergic alveolitis caused by reaction to the dead larvae. In either event the diagnosis of miliary tuberculosis, influenzal pneumonia, or other acute infection may be considered. Recovery is rapid and the chest radiograph will usually be normal thereafter. Although the pseudotubercles around the larvae may persist after the Katayama stage and calcify after treatment, this is not a common finding radiologically, nor does the resulting fibrosis show on the chest radiograph, though it may possibly be seen with high-resolution, thin-section CT.

The clinical and radiological manifestations of schistosomiasis mansoni involving the lungs probably depent not only on the number of eggs reaching the pulmonary circulation but also on the host reaction. Granulomas are an indication of delayed hypersensitivity, and previous infections result in markedly accelerated granuloma formation (Figs. 2.59, 2.60). Immunosuppression inhibits this process. Perhaps the variable immune status of the patients accounts for the geographic variation, because severe lung changes in schistosomiasis occur in Egypt and parts of South America and the Caribbean, and yet are uncommon in many regions of Africa, despite the prevalence of the infection.

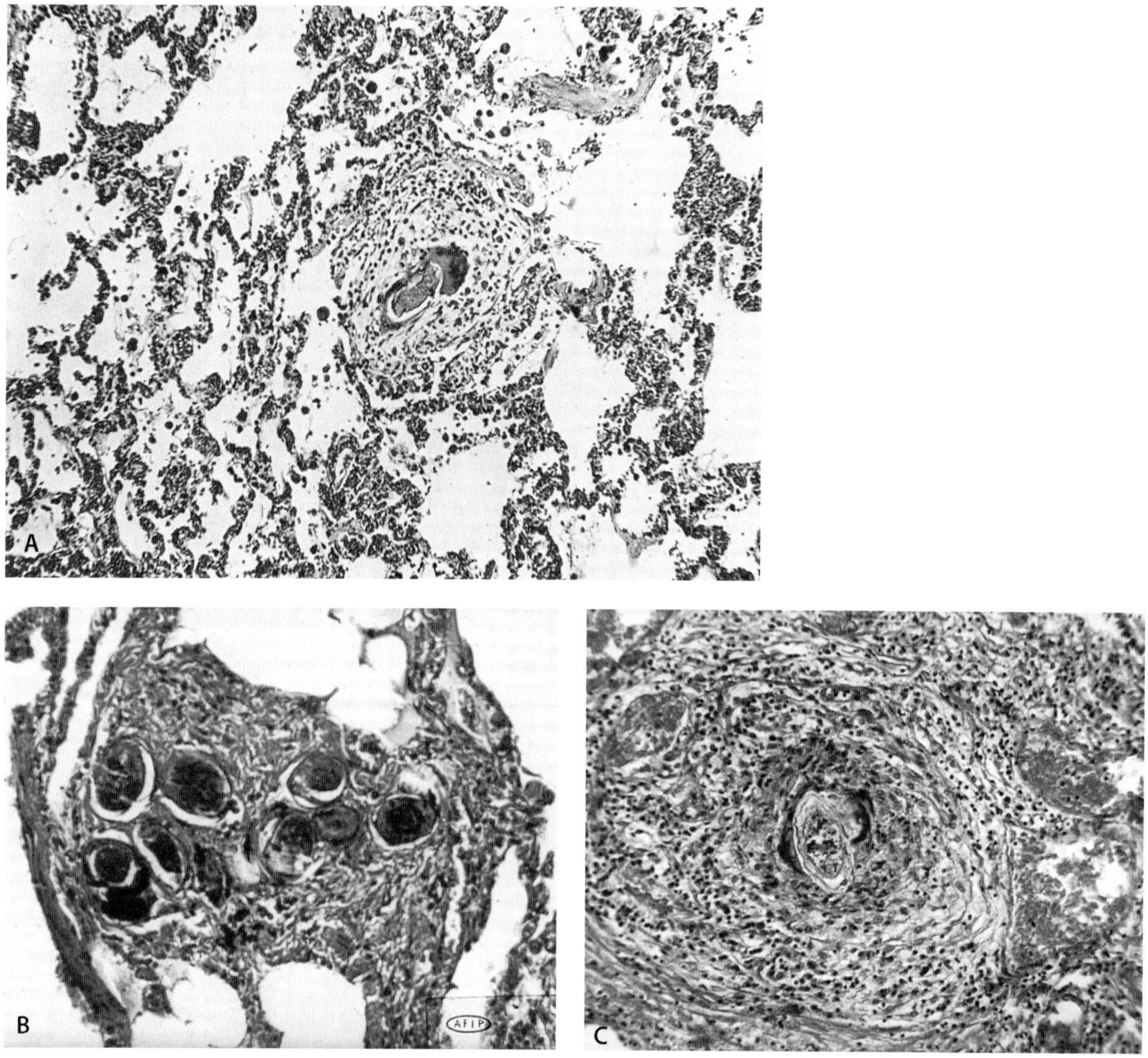

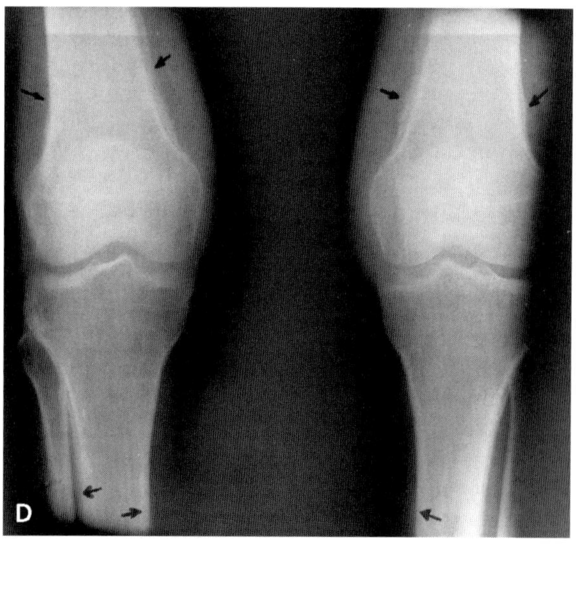

Fig. 2.59 A–D. All schistosomes cause pulmonary granulomas. **A** A pseudotubercle in the lung parenchyma; there is a multinucleated foreign body giant cell and small round cell inflammatory reaction surrounding an egg of *S. mansoni*. AFIP 729756. **B** Another lung granuloma containing multiple eggs of *S. mansoni* with a similar surrounding reaction and connective tissue proliferation. AFIP 68-4761-1. **C** This granuloma around an *S. mansoni* egg has replaced the lumen and extended through the wall of a pulmonary arteriole. There is a surrounding early angiomatoid, a new channel formation which diverts the flow of desaturated blood from the pulmonary arterioles into the pulmonary venules, creating a right-to-left shunt, with decompression of the pulmonary arteriole system and systemic desaturation. This results in the syndrome of cyanosis with normal pulmonary artery pressure and osteoarthropathy. **D** Hypertrophic pulmonary osteoarthropathy with periosteal new bone (*arrows*) along the lower end of the femora and tibia of a 42-year-old Egyptian, who also had schistosomal colonic polyposis. (**D** courtesy of Dr. Nabil Ayad El Mesery, Cairo)

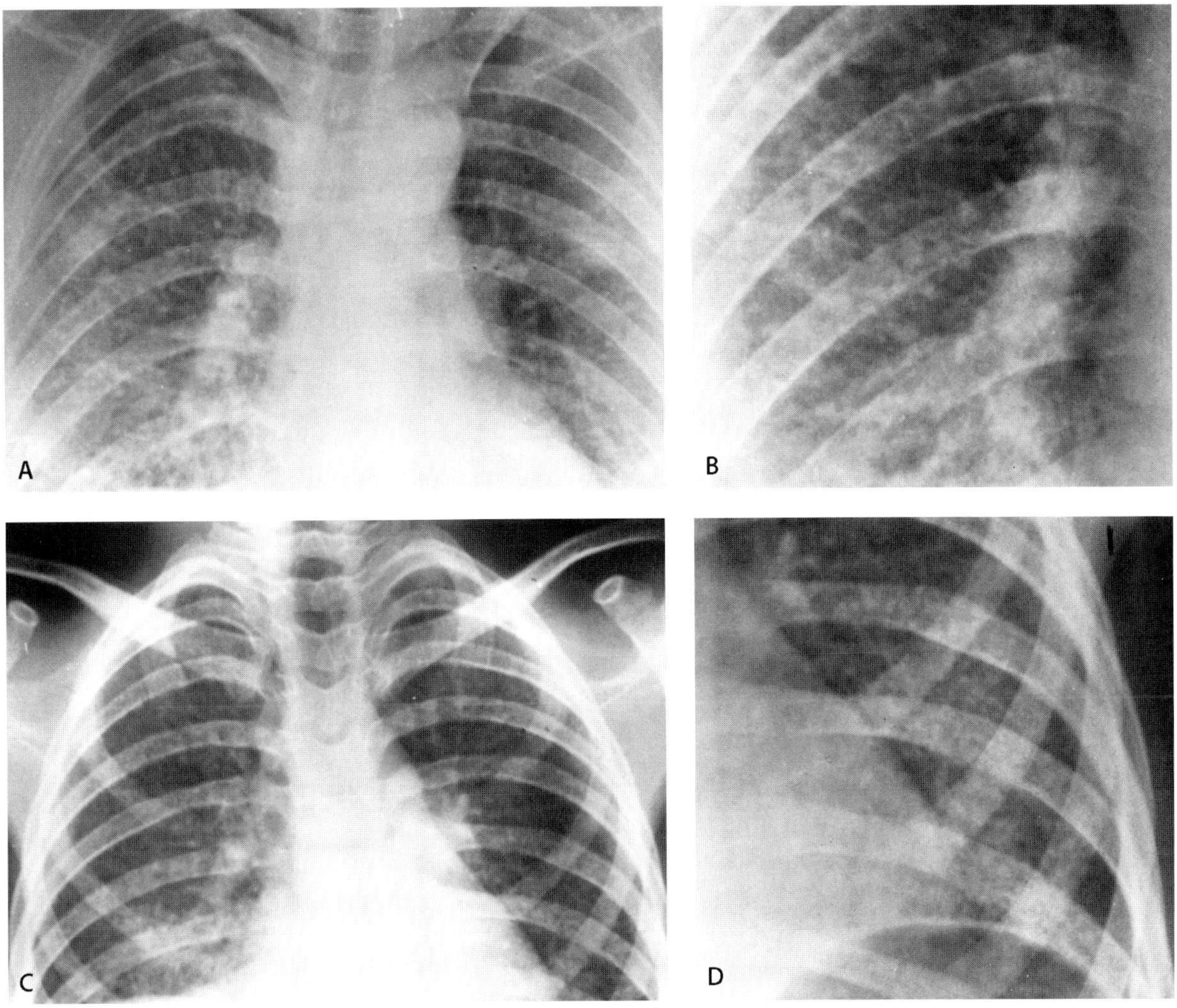

Fig. 2.60 A–D. Diffuse small nodular densities throughout both lung fields due to schistosomal granulomas. The right mid-lung field of **A** is enlarged in **B**. The left lower lung field of **C** is enlarged in **D**. (Courtesy of Dr. H. Pagan-Saez, San Juan)

It should be emphasized again that live adult schistosomes do not cause any host response and that many immature and dead eggs similary provoke little local response. The majority of patients with chronic schistosomiasis are asymptomatic; severe lesions are present in only a small percentage of the many millions of people who harbor this parasite. Nevertheless, in some unfortunate individuals there is eventual formation of a sufficient number of granulomas to produce anatomical and physiological alterations.

In the later phase, pseudotubercles develop in the lung parenchyma with small round cells surrounding the eggs of *S. mansoni* (Fig. 2.59 A–C). When numerous, these granulomas may cause a diffuse, fine reticulonodular pattern seen throughout the lungs on chest radiographs, but better demonstrated by high-resolution CT, which is also better at demonstrating the slight interstitial fibrosis that develops in some patients. This sometimes can be seen on a plain radiograph. Endovascular localization of the eggs, with intimal thickening and obliteration of the lumen of the small arterioles and extensive inflammation and granuloma formation, is a typical pathological finding as pulmonary schistosomiasis progresses (Fig. 2.61). This can often be seen on plain radiographs of the chest, as well as on CT scans. The differential diagnosis will include pneumonia, particularly eosinophilic pneumonia, and tuberculosis. In some patients a mass must be excluded. Such a mass will be due to a solitary pulmonary bilharzioma, and will resemble a tuberculoma or malignancy; there are no distinguishing features.

As the infection continues and more eggs are deposited in the pulmonary arterioles, with resulting arteriolitis and blockage of many small arteries, the changes become much more marked. The striking finding is dilatation of the central pulmonary arteries (Figs. 2.62, 2.63). The main pulmonary trunk, in particular, becomes enlarged and even aneurysmally dilated at times, and on fluoroscopy can be seen to pulsate vigorously. The sweep of both pulmonary arteries may be wider than usual. There will be accentuated second-degree arterial branches, and the basal arteries are usually wider and tortuous, also with visible pulsations fluoroscopically. There is no pulmonary plethora, however, and the peripheral vascular markings are normal, or more commonly, decreased. CT, with or without contrast, or selective pulmonary arteriography will show dilatation (which may be massive) of the main pulmonary artery and its central branches (Fig. 2.63) Peripherally there will be a "leafless tree with broken branches." In most patients there will be enlargement of the right ventricle and pulmonary conus, but the left heart will be normal.

There is usually a normal cardiac output and circulation time. Pulmonary hypertension is inevitable (Figs. 2.61–2.64), averaging from 18 to 65 mmHg, but at times reaching up to 110 mmHg. There is little correlation between the pulmonary pressure and the size of the pulmonary artery, because the latter is affected by direct granulomatous disease of the wall as well as by the pulmonary hypertension. The pulmonary hypertension is due to mechanical obstruction from the obliterative endarteritis, aggravated by an increased blood volume due to the liver disease and the portacaval shunts. There should be normal capillary pressure but some raised pulmonary vascular resistance, because in schistosomiasis the obstruction is at the arteriolar level (whereas in emphysema the obstruction is at the capillary level). Portal venography may rarely show shunting directly from the spleen through the diaphragm to the pulmonary veins and thence into the left atrium.

Bronchiectasis has been reported with schistosomiasis, but there is no causal relationship. The bronchiectasis is a coincidental finding and the report a little confusing! Chronic upper lobe pneumonia resembling fibrocaseous tuberculosis is a very rare manifestation, perhaps following inadequate anti-schistosomal therapy.

Myocardial damage due to schistosomiasis is rare. Although adult worms have been found in the coronay arteries and ova in the myocardium, cardiac failure is late and is almost always mechanical (Fig. 2.64). Although pulmonary artery aneurysms are not really uncommon, aortic schistosomiasis is rare and it can be difficult to know whether an aneurysm originated in the aorta or was the result of the spread of infection from neighboring lungs. In a single case report, schistosomal aneurysm involved the arch of the aorta in a 19-year-old African woman. CT scans showed the mass to be inseparable from the arch and descending thoracic aorta. A contrast examination showed that there was leakage, and aortography outlined the aneurysm completely. Histologically there were numerous eggs within the lung tissue, the visceral pleura, and the wall of the aneurysm. There were even eggs in the thrombus which had formed.

Central Nervous System

All *schistosome spp.* can affect the central nervous system, causing myelopathy or arachnoiditis. The granulomatous reaction can be demonstrated by MRI or CT scanning, and there may be a block on myelography (Figs. 2.65 and 2.66). Cerebral schistosomiasis has occurred, but is most common in schistosomiasis japonica. There is frequently a response to appropriate treatment but intramedullary granulomas, usually affecting the lower part of the cord and the conus, can be acute and necrotizing and may not respond to treatment. In the absence of CT or MRI, myelography is important, but may be normal. If there is acute paraplegia, surgical decompression may be required because the response to chemotherapy may not be immediate. (Refer also to the CNS in schistosomiasis japonica, pp. 196–200.)

Differential Diagnosis (S. mansoni)

When schistosomiasis affects the bowel, it may closely resemble ulcerative or especially granulomatous colitis. Fortunately, in most parts of the world where schistosomiasis is common, both of these conditions are rare and malignant disease of the large bowel is equally uncommon. A schistosomal granuloma might be mistaken for malignancy, but seldom occurs without other evidence of schistosomal colitis. The granulomas are frequently multiple and vary in size and shape; finding other lesions is additional evidence against malignancy, but follow-up after treatment will be necessary. It may be impossible to differentiate amebiasis radiologically: it is more common in the right colon, whereas schistosomiasis is more often in the left. Polyp formation is very rare in amebiasis and quite frequent in *S. mansoni* and *S. japonicum* infections. The real difficulty with colonic disease is that many patients will have both schistosomiasis and amebiasis. The radiological changes in the small bowel may be due to other parasites. The demonstration of calcified eggs by CT, or of the early changes of schistosomal liver disease, will influence the differential diagnosis.

(Text continues on p. 194)

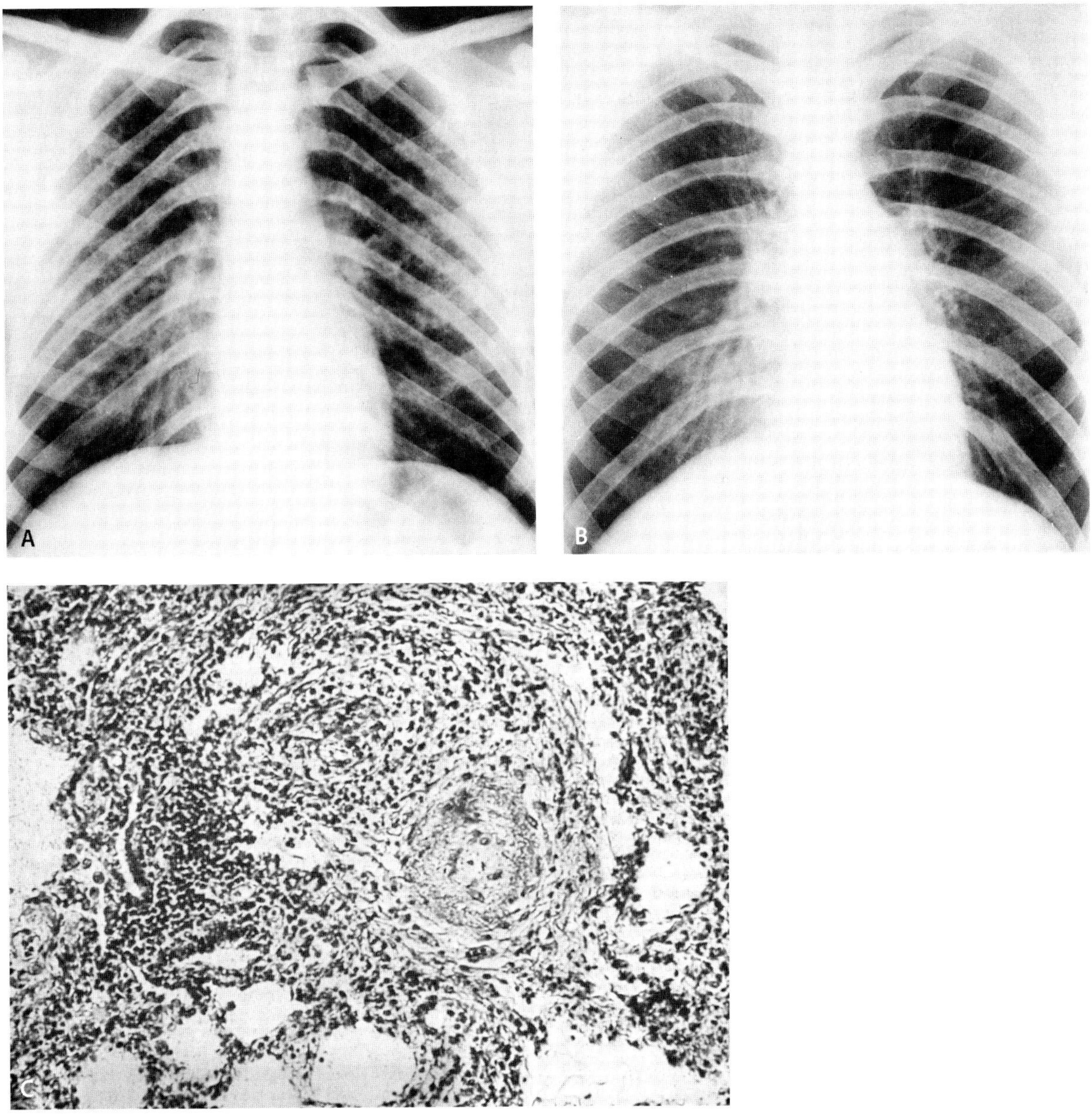

Fig. 2.61 A–C. Chronic schistosomiasis mansoni damages the cardiopulmonary system. In this Puerto Rican male there is (**A**) diffuse fine nodulation throughout both lungs because of numerous granulomas around the eggs in the parenchyma. At this stage the heart and pulmonary artery appear normal. A few years later (**B**), the miliary granulomatous pattern has cleared, leaving slight interstitial fibrosis. The main pulmonary artery segment has dilated and the central pulmonary artery has become prominent, while the peripheral arterial pattern has decreased. This indicates secondary pulmonary hypertension. **C** The lung of a different patient shows a pulmonary arteriole whose lumen has been virtually obliterated by marked intimal thickening, with an intense surrounding cellular reaction and early angiomatoid formation. H&E, ×196. (Courtesy of Dr. A. Chait and *AJR*, 1963) The diffuse endovascular, obliterative, granulomatous process blocks the pulmonary arteriole flow, which results in pulmonary arteriole hypertension, right heart strain, and cor pulmonale. Both the clinical and the radiographic findings depend on the number of eggs which reach the lungs and the formation of the extensive granulomas. In advanced pulmonary schistosomiasis there will be endovascular localization of the eggs, intimal thickening, and obliteration of the vascular lumen, with extensive inflammatory and granulomatous reaction

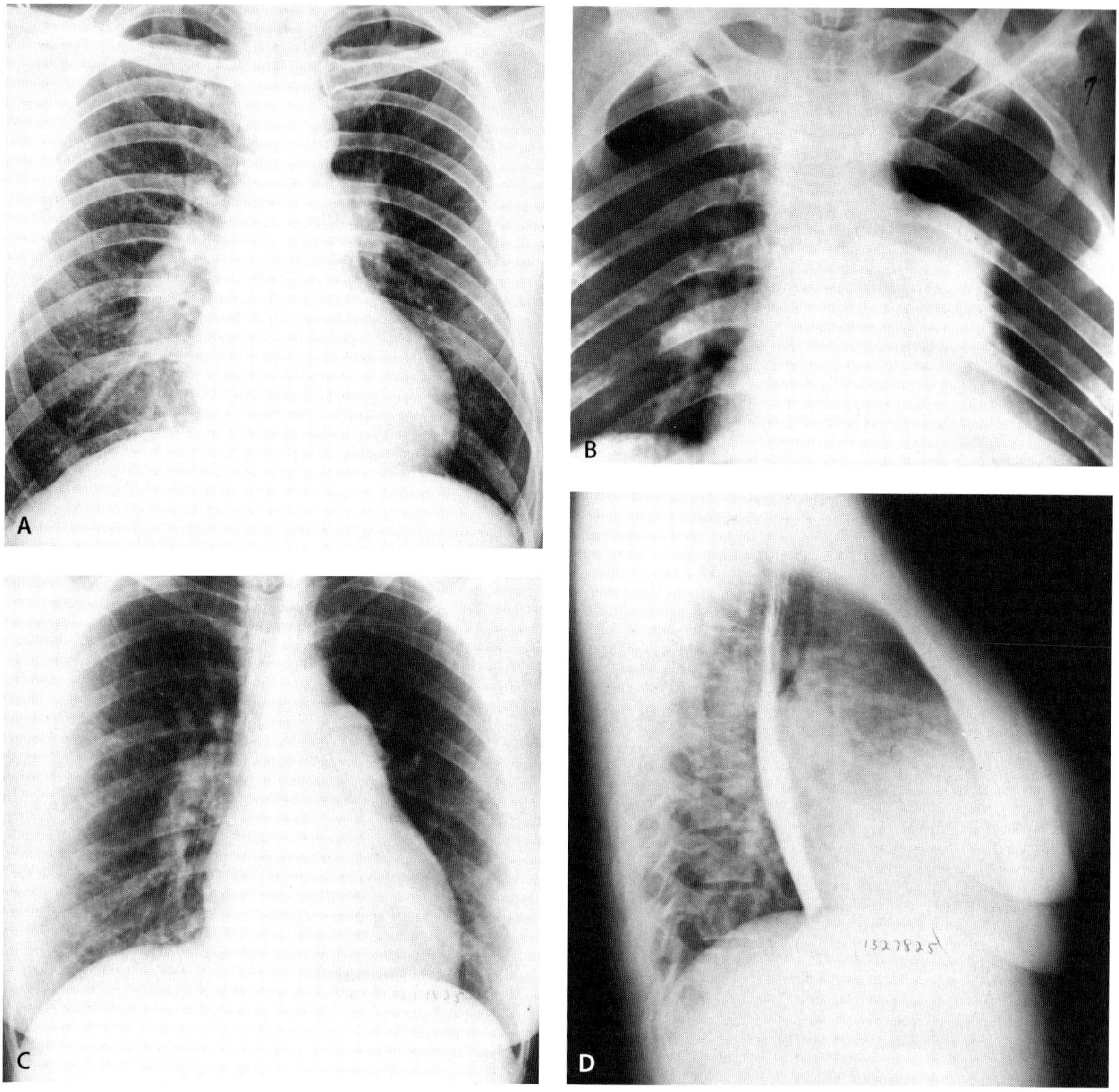

Fig. 2.62 A–D. The progress of pulmonary hypertension secondary to *S. mansoni.* **A** This PA chest radiograph of a Brazilian male shows prominence of the main pulmonary artery segment and the central pulmonary arteries, with tapering of the peripheral pulmonary arteries. There is right ventricular hypertrophy which has caused rounding of the cardiac apex. There are numerous small nodular densities in both lungs due to the schistosome granulomas. (Courtesy of Dr. J. Phillips et al. and *Radiology*, 1975) **B** In this young Puerto Rican male there is marked dilatation of the main pulmonary artery which, together with the left pulmonary artery, resembles a mass. The peripheral lung fields are clear, because the arterial circulation is diminished. (Courtesy of Dr. H. Pagan-Saez, San Juan) **C, D** PA and lateral chest radiographs of a 25-year-old Puerto Rican female showing marked right ventricular hypertrophy almost filling the retrosternal space in the lateral projection. The ECG provided confirmation. The main and central pulmonary arteries are prominent in both these projections. Cardiac catheterization did not demonstrate a left-to-right shunt: autopsy showed advanced hepatic and pulmonary schistosomiasis, right ventricular hypertrophy, and hypersplenism

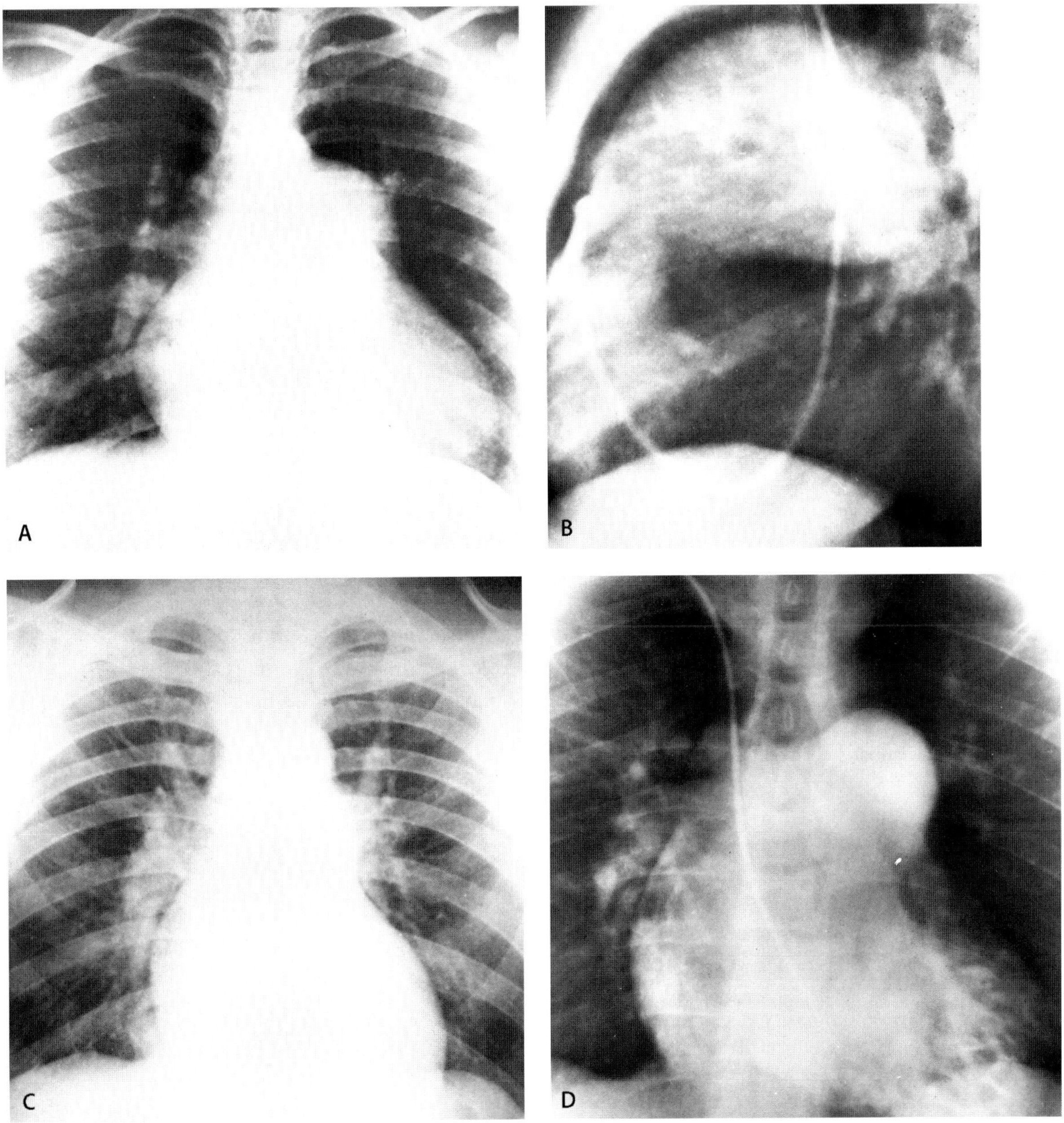

Fig. 2.63 A–D. As pulmonary hypertension worsens, the cardiovascular changes become more marked, even in quite young patients. **A** In this 21-year-old Puerto Rican female, there is marked dilatation of the main pulmonary artery and the central pulmonary arteries, with rapid tapering of the peripheral branches. There is moderate cardiomegaly mainly due to right ventricular enlargement. **B** Pulmonary angiography shows a massively dilated main pulmonary artery, with abrupt tapering of the peripheral arteries. (The tip of the catheter is near the origin of the pulmonary artery.) Her main clinical complaint had been epigastric pain and hematemesis for about 3 years. She had splenomegaly and esophageal varices and the ECG confirmed the radiographic findings. (Right ventricular pressure was 120 mmHg, end-diastolic pressure, 22 mmHg, and right atrial mean pressure, 12 mmHg.) **C** The chest radiograph of a 30-year-old Puerto Rican male shows right-sided cardiac enlargement, increased convexity of the right atrium, and rounding of the cardiac apex due to ventricular hypertrophy. The main pulmonary arteries are prominent due to pulmonary hypertension. In spite of this, pulmonary function tests were normal. Cardiac catheterization (**D**) showed right ventricular hypertrophy and dilatation, with markedly dilated main and central pulmonary arteries. There was tricuspid insufficiency with reflux back into the right atrium. Autopsy showed generalized schistosomiasis, aneurysmal dilatation of the main pulmonary artery, and diffuse atheromatosis. In the heart only the right ventricle was dilated. (Courtesy of Dr. A. Chait and *AJR*, 1963) Angiography is seldom necessary if echocardiography, CT, and MRI, are available

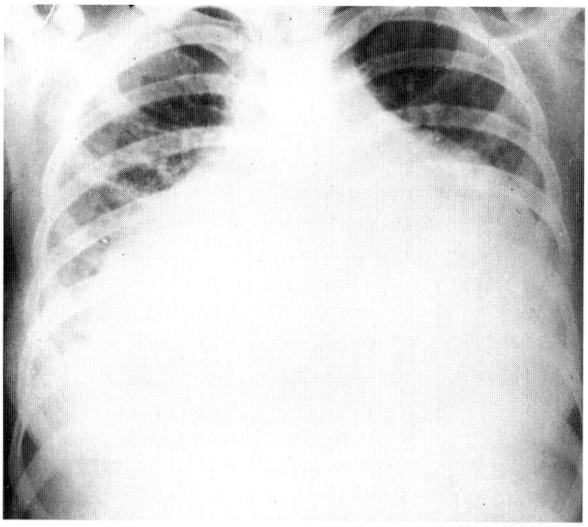

Fig. 2.64. The end stage of cardiopulmonary schistosomiasis. There is massive enlargement of the heart, and there are small bilateral pleural effusions, secondary to congestive cardiac failure. Pericardiocentesis removed 320 cc of straw colored fluid. Thoracotomy showed multiple tiny nodules in the lungs and thick fibrous plaques. The pericardium was greately thickened. Histology showed granulomas involving the lungs and pericardium and causing pulmonary arteriolities. There was no evidence of malignancy or tuberculosis. The patient, a female from Puerto Rico, was only 24 years old; she had hepatomegaly, right upper abdominal pain, and dyspnea, and had lost ten pounds in weight. She also had ancylostomiasis. (Courtesy of Dr. A. Chait and *AJR*, 1963)

Pulmonary schistosomiasis radiographed during the passage of the cercaria may resemble any pneumonia. During antischistosomal therapy there may be an allergic reaction of the Löffler type, resembling bronchopneumonia, which is constantly varying in distribution and which resolves within a few days. When there are granulomas and interstitial fibrosis they will require differentiation from all other possible causes of similar patterns.

The striking dilatation of the main pulmonary artery in advanced cases of cardiopulmonary schistosomiasis will often suggest the correct diagnosis in the proper clinical setting. The many other causes of pulmonary hypertension, as well as left-to-right shunts, pulmonary stenosis, and other entities which can cause pulmonary artery dilatation, will have to be differentiated.

The differential diagnosis of hepatosplenomegaly due to *S. mansoni* is discussed on p. 187.

Extreme Calcification in Schistosomiasis mansoni. There is one reported case of schistosomiasis mansoni in a 38-year-old man from Yemen in whom there was marked calcification (due to eggs) throughout the small bowel. This could be seen on a plain radiograph and might even have been mistaken for a barium contrast study. CT showed extensive submucosal calcification along the entire length of the small bowel. Biopsy confirmed that this was due to multiple calcified eggs of *S. mansoni*. There was no evidence of *S. haematobium* infection.

The liver showed similar advanced curvilinear calcification and this, too, could be seen on a plain abdominal radiograph. CT confirmed that there was extensive periportal egg deposition in the sleeve fibrosis, which is more usually found without many eggs. The only abnormal liver function test was a high (3× normal) serum alkaline phosphatase. The patient was anemic and there was a peripheral eosinophilia (Radhakrishnan et al. 1988).

Schistosomiasis japonica

The initial infection with *S. japonicum* can cause the Katayama reaction (see p. 122) and is more likely to give rise to CNS symptoms than the other varieties of schistosomiasis at this stage.

Schistosoma japonicum can produce 3000 eggs per worm per day, and the eggs are smaller than those of other schistosomes. It has been suggested that this may account for the somewhat different characteristics of schistosomiasis japonica. Others have disputed this but there is no doubt that the radiological findings are different.

The *S. japonicum* worms live in mesenteric veins and their eggs are deposited predominantly within small bowel venules and in the mesentery. CT has shown that in some patients the heaviest load is in the colon rather than in the small bowel. All the eggs are within the submucosal and subserosal layers of the intestine, and only a few are in the muscularis. They may also be found in the same layers in the appendix. In the later stages, fibrosis and constriction of the mesentery may occur, so that the loops of bowel, particularly the duodenum, may be deformed by adhesions as well as by the intrinsic granulomas.

Small Bowel

The mucosa of the duodenum and the upper jejunum becomes edematous, coarse and irregular; motility is decreased and there may be some dilatation. There is excess mucus secretion and flocculation of barium can occur. The terminal ileum may show similar changes (Fig. 2.36).

Colon and Rectum

Schistosoma japonicum infection produces changes very similar to those seen in schistosomiasis mansoni. The early changes include edema and spiculation of the mucosa; polyps are not uncommon: there may be a cobblestone appearance in the mucosa, in both the large and the small bowel, with less tendency to form large and multiple polyps. CT has shown that when the eggs calcify there can be either a curvilinear or a nodular pattern of calcification: in the sigmoid colon the calcification has been heavy enough to cause parallel lines. However, although the calcification may be more marked than in *S. mansoni*, there is usually less distortion of the colon (Fig. 2.33).

Retroperitoneum

Granulomas located in the retroperitoneal space may become large enough to resemble malignant disease. Although CT, and occasionally ultrasonography, can demonstrate multiple eggs, the exact differential diagnosis may only be possible by biopsy. Because such schistosomal granulomas are inflammatory, they have increased vascularity with many new vessels forming as collaterals bypass arterioles which have been obliterated. Ultrasonography, MRI, and even angiography can show that these are highly vascular masses. The response to appropriate antischistosomal therapy may be one way to make the correct diagnosis, but there are no specific features shown by any method of imaging.

Liver

The hepatic changes of schistosomiasis japonica are characteristic (see Figs. 2.45–2.53): rarely, similar changes may be found in other schistosomal infections. The background picture of periportal fibrosis is similar to *S. mansoni* infections, but the extent of hepatic calcification is quite different (Figs. 2.45–2.47).
Occasionally on plain radiographs, but especially on CT scanning, the pattern of the calcified eggs can be capsular or septal. Although described as "capsular," the eggs are actually subcapsular and may be arranged in a linear pattern all around the liver (Fig. 2.51). Within the septa, there is similar calcification, and the pattern has been described as a network or "turtleback" appearance (Fig. 2.50). The septal pattern, in particular, enhances on CT performed following contrast administration (Figs. 2.48, 2.49).
Another characteristic pattern is irregularity of the liver outline, caused by notching (Figs. 2.48–2.51). Where the focal fibrosis in the capsule joins the fibrosis in the septa, there is depression, macroscopically resembling a star or furrows if the retraction is sufficient. This notching has not been seen so clearly in any other schistosomal infection.
The third pattern is nodular, within the liver parenchyma. These macronodules, also due to fibrosis in the portal spaces, can be mistaken for macronodular cirrhosis or even metastases (Fig. 2.45).
Ultrasonography shows an echogenic network, and branching of the hyperreflective septa should be sought. Enclosed within these echogenic septa will be polygonal areas of apparently normal liver. When the fibrosis is incomplete, it causes a moderately fine sieve-like appearance. The fully developed septal changes in schistosomiasis japonica on ultrasonography are described as having a fish-scale or retiform pattern and may be found in 30% of patients, particularly those who have a high antibody titer (Fig. 2.50). The irregular notched surface of the liver can also be demonstrated by ultrasonography.
Although periportal fibrosis occurs in any type of schistosomiasis, in *S. japonicum* infections there is usually atrophy of the right lobe of the liver and some hypertrophy of the left and caudate lobes. This is another useful finding on either CT or ultrasonography (Figs. 2.50, 2.51).
There is an association of hepatic carcinoma with *S. japonicum* infections; it is possible that this is due to the increased incidence of hepatitis B infection, because carcinomas occur more commonly in mild schistosomiasis rather than in advanced cases. The tumors have been described as large, solitary, and nodular in pattern; some are even massive. Other partients may have multiple nodules. Differentiation may be possible by CT or MRI, but guided needle biopsy is usually required. In some series, there has been an increase in carcinoma of the stomach and even the duodenum, but whether this is a significant link is not yet established.
Although the imaging pattern of periportal fibrosis is easily recognizable, it is not entirely unique to schistosomiasis. Prominent periportal echogenicity occurs in patients with recurrent pyogenic cholangitis, rarely in acute cholecystitis, and occasionally in hepatocellular carcinoma.
Recurrent (oriental) cholangitis has a distinct history of fevers, and there will be dilatation of the intra- and extrahepatic ducts, often containing debris (see Chap. 21). In hepatocellular carcinoma the periportal echogenicity is predominantly vascular and can be imaged with MRI or angiography. In cholecystitis the cause is probably inflammatory and may be reversible.
Accompanying the hepatomegaly, there is often splenomegaly and, in many patients, ascites. The pat-

tern of vascular collaterals, including esophageal varices, is very similar to those that develop in *S. mansoni* infections. Thickening of the wall of the gallbladder can occur and may go on to fibrosis. There are seldom any biliary calculi or polyps. The assessment of portal hypertension is the same as for *S. mansoni* (see p. 169).

Lungs

The radiological findings in the lungs of patients with *S. japonicum* infections are very similar to those of *S. mansoni*. In many patients the chest radiograph appears normal and will remain so. In the acute stage, the pattern of the Katayama syndrome occurs; indeed, it was first described with *S. japonicum* infection. There is an increase in the pulmonary vascular and interstitial markings and enlargement of the hilar lymph nodes (see p. 187).
The lung changes may progress to fibrosis and occasionally scattered nodular calcification. As with other varieties of schistosomiasis, emphysema is not a major factor. In some patients *S. japonicum* infections progress to eventual pulmonary hypertension and dilatation of the pulmonary arteries, as occurs in *S. mansoni*, following the same pathological and radiological pattern (see p. 190).

Central Nervous System

Schistosomiasis in the CNS is asymptomatic in the majority of patients. Multiple ova and evidence of immune complex reaction, with, in some cases, small granulomas, may be found at autopsy but without clinically localizing signs.
The brain and spinal cord may be infected in all three varieties of schistosomiasis, but perhaps most frequently with *S. japonicum*.

Acute Infection

At the Katayama (acute) stage, cerebral infection presents with convulsions and seizures, with or without loss of consciousness. The clinical picture may resemble jacksonian epilepsy with an abnormal electroencephalogram, or intracerebral hemorrhage. Other patients will present with paraplegia, which may be severe or mild, complete or incomplete, and usually in the thoracic or lower lumbar area. The differential diagnosis may be confusing. The history of exposure to infected water a few weeks previously is very important. There is usually an accompanying fever, cough and sometimes urticaria, symptoms which are not usual with other cerebral or spinal illnesses. In this early (Katayama) stage, there may be no eggs in the stools and the serology may be negative. The patients may recover completely without specific antischistosomal therapy (although the cerebral swelling may need treatment). After a few months there may be eggs in the stool, the serology becomes positive and, if there is any doubt, liver biopsy will provide further evidence.
Computed tomography (and MRI) has shown large multifocal areas of low density or low signal intensity, with periventricular lucencies which enhance on CT performed following contrast administration. There may be a mass effect and raised intracranial pressure. There may be a similar mass effect in the spinal cord.

Chronic Infection

In chronic schistosomiasis, there may be cerebral or spinal involvement, often in young patients. It is possible that CNS involvement has been underdiagnosed and is now becoming more readily recognized with CT or MR scanning.
Infection of the brain presents clinically with a wide spectrum of signs and symptoms: headache, nausea, vertigo, visual and speech defects, rigidity, spasm, mental confusion, and hemiplegia have all been reported. The most common immediate diagnosis will be of a cerebral hemorrhage or brain tumor (and a subarachnoid hemorrhage has occurred in at least one patient). CT and MR have shown multifocal and

Fig. 2.65 A–G. Spinal cord schistosomiasis: *S. mansoni* granulomas can cause spinal cord symptoms. **A, B** PA and lateral radiographs from a myelogram showing partial extradural block and spinal cord compression at the T12-L1 level. (Courtesy of Dr. Ehrlich, San Juan) **C** A similar granuloma due to *S. haematobium*. This was a young African male with paraplegia of relatively sudden onset: he had early calcification in the bladder and his clinical condition responded to antischistosomal therapy. **D** A sagittal T2-weighted MR image shows enlargement of the conus medullaris with a central hyperintense signal. **E** A T1-weighted image following gadolinium injection reveals heterogeneous enhancement of the conus and confirms the enlargement. There was eosinophilia of the blood and CSF and intrathecal antibodies for *S. mansoni*. Four months after treatment the MRI was normal and there was no enhancement. (Courtesy of Dr. S. Grand et al. and *Clin Radiol*, 1996.) **F** The myelogram of a young Zulu male with spinal cord schistosomiasis. There is marked swelling of the conus medullaris. **G** The CT myelogram of the same patient. In many patients the cord swelling will resolve quite rapidly with treatment, usually with matching clinical improvement. However, in some patients the cord may shrink and there will be residual neurological changes. In others there may be the added complication of arachnoiditis. In a minority of patients atrophy of the cord occurs. (**F, G** courtesy of Prof. P. L. A. Bill, Natal) ▶

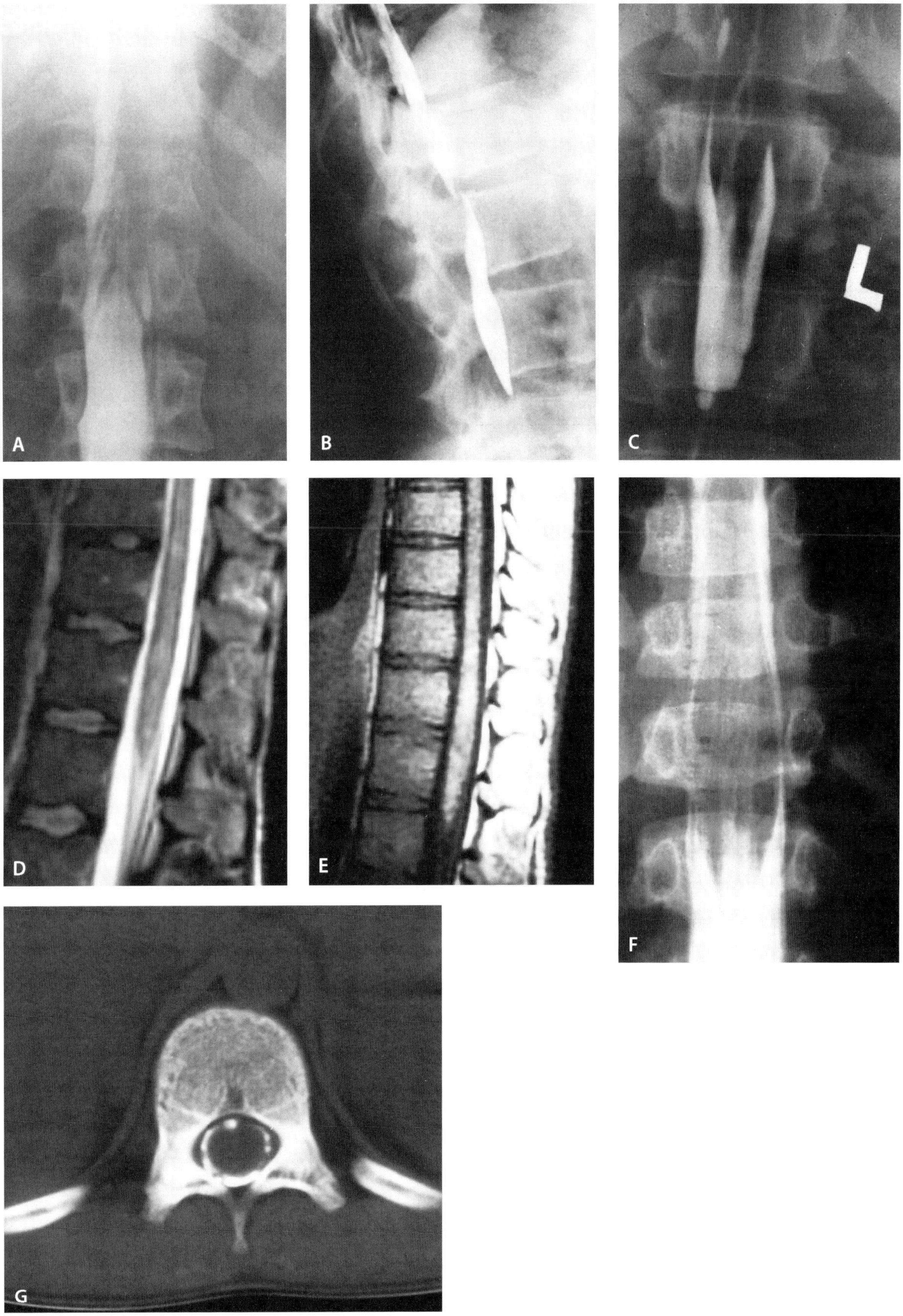
A
B
C
L
D
E
F
G

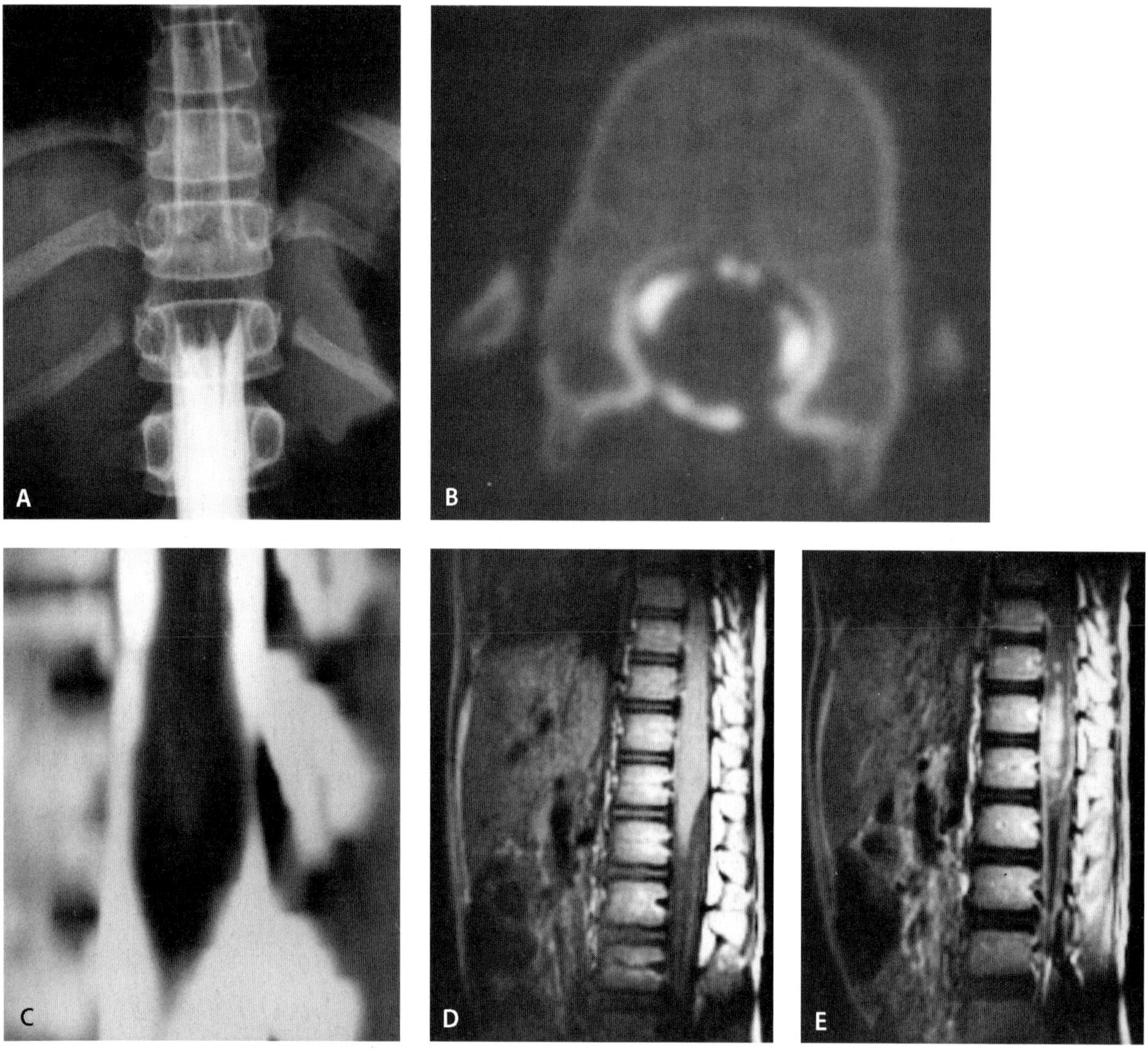

Fig. 2.66 A–E. Spinal cord schistosomiasis: a granulomatous intramedullary mass in a 7-year-old girl. **A** Myelography showing partial blockage at the level of T11–12. **B** Post-myelography axial CT scan showing the swollen cord, confirmed on the sagittal scan (**C**). **D** Pre- and **E** post-gadolinium sagittal T1-weighted MR scans show the markedly enlarged conus medullaris, with heterogeneous enhancement; the T2-weighted scans (not shown) had images with inhomogeneous signal intensity. None of these images provide a specific indication of schistosomiasis: the clinical history and examination need to be correlated in order to make the diagnosis. (Courtesy of Drs. R. Silbergleit and R. Silbergleit and *Am J Radiol*, 1992)

localized defects. T1-weighted MRI shows edema; T2-weighted and proton-density MR have shown nodular masses, sometimes iso-intense and surrounded by edema. Following specific treatment, scans return to normal and the clinical symptoms disappear.

In very chronic schistosomiasis mansoni, cerebral atropy has been reported (Fig. 2.67). Ultrasonography has shown a reduced brain mantle and dilated ventricles, confirmed by CT. In one series 36% of patients showed cortical atrophy and 12% showed central atrophy. Autopsy has confirmed multiple small granulomas in the cortex and gliosis after healing. Some patients have massive granulomas and blockage of several vessels by eggs.

When the spinal cord is infected, the patient complains of a low back pain and progressive CNS impairment, which may include paraplegia and urinary symptoms (Figs. 2.65, 2.66). Schistosomiasis causes localized granulomas or arachnoiditis or, in some cases, transverse myelitis. There is usually swelling of the cord, sometimes with an intramedullary mass. The transverse myelitis is probably due to vascular thrombosis, and when this occurs the response to treatment is poor. In other patients, the paraplegia

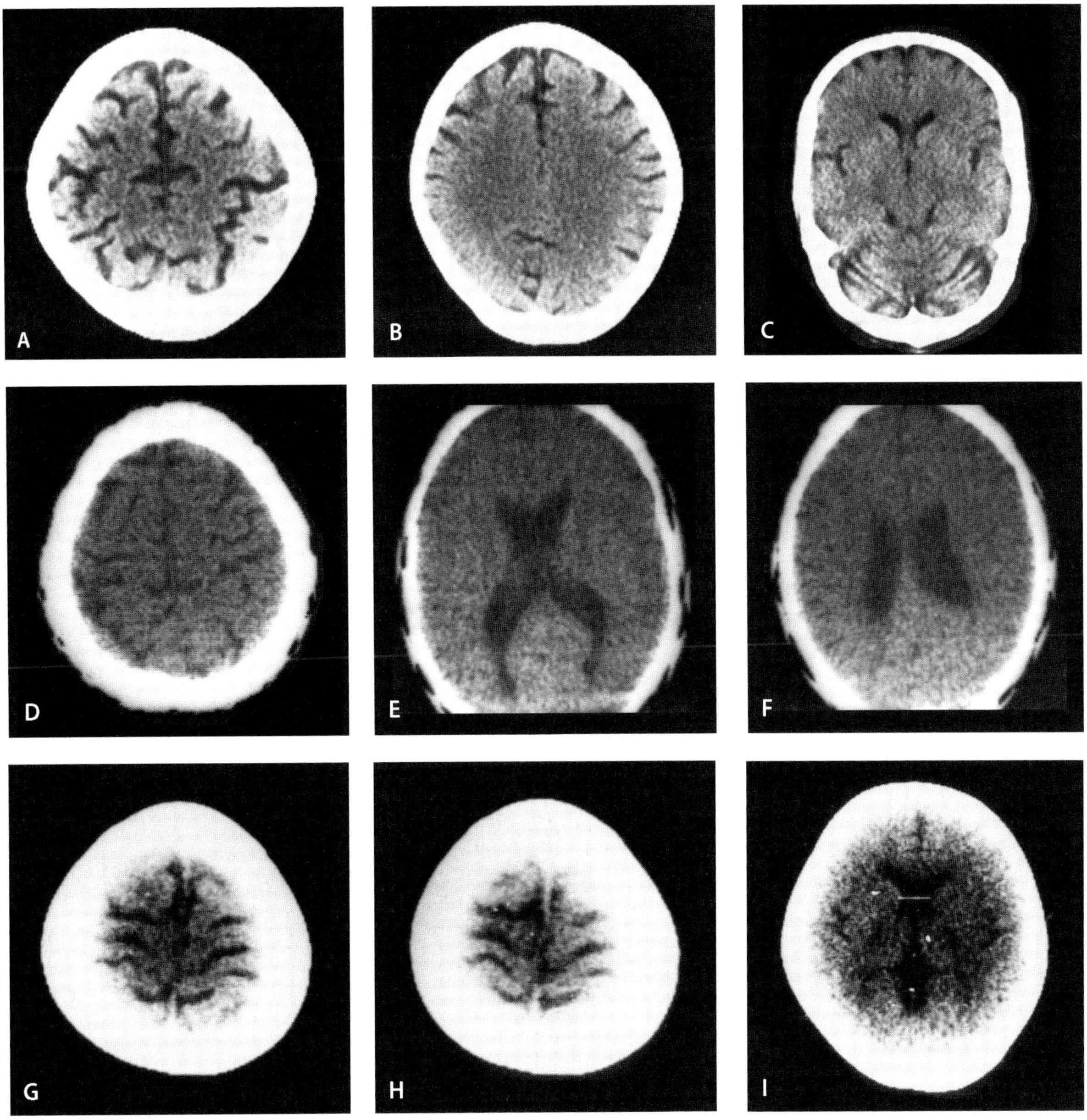

Fig. 2.67 A–I. Cerebral, schistosomiasis: cerebral atrophy following chronic schistosomiasis mansoni. CT scans of three Egyptian men who all had liver fibrosis, ascites, and splenomegaly. **A–C** Patient aged 35 years, with wide sulci and fissures including of the cerebellum. The ventricular system was normal. Assessed as mild cortical atrophy; sulci = 3 mm. **D–F** Patient aged 42 years with prominent cortical sulci and a normal ventricular system. This case was assessed as moderate cortical atrophy and mild cerebral atrophy. Sulci = 4 mm. **G–I** Patient aged 17 years who had undergone splenectomy and had cor pulmonale. Prominent sulci; normal ventricular system. This case was assessed as moderate cortical atrophy and mild cerebral atrophy. Sulci = 4 mm. All three patients clinically showed apathy, resignation, lack of activity, lack of curiosity, and a prolonged response time to simple questions. (Courtesy of Dr. H.H. Khalil and colleagues; scan in **B** and **C** courtesy of *Am J Trop Med Hyg*, 1986)

and other effects may resolve completely with specific treatment, though treatment is not always successful. Computed tomography and MRI have confirmed the swelling of the cord, which can be nodular or confluent and is usually enhanced with gadolinium. This is best seen on T1-weighted MR scanning, and on T2-weighted MR appears inhomogeneous, with a high signal intensity (Fig. 2.66). Intraoperative ultrasonography has shown a hyperechoic mass.

CT myelography can also demonstrate conus or cauda equina expansion and improvement after treatment (Figs. 2.65, 2.66). Irregularity and matting of the nerve roots may also be seen. In patients with myelitis (in some series, nearly half the patients) the myelogram may be normal.

If scanning is not available, contrast myelography will demonstrate obstruction or displacement of the cord but in some patients it will be normal in spite of the clinical symptoms.

The differential diagnosis can be extremely difficult, particularly in young patients with epilepsy or progressive paraplegia. Infection, e.g., tuberculosis or syphilis, must be excluded. Wherever schistosomiasis is endemic, the onset of these CNS symptoms, particularly if slow and otherwise unexplained, or the sudden onset of epilepsy in a teenager, should suggest the possibility of schistosomiasis: it is probably more common than usually thought.

Schistosomiasis in Other Parts of the Body

It is unlikely that the radiologist will be concerned with schistosomiasis elsewhere in the body. Cutaneous schistosomiasis may result from the asymptomatic deposition of eggs in the skin, commonly in the genital and perigenital areas. Similar lesions have been reported on the trunk and have resembled herpes zoster.

Occasionally, adult worms may be found in the skin. Schistosomal granulomas due to *S. japonicum* and *S. mansoni* have been found in the conjunctiva, particularly of children, and may undergo squamous metaplasia. The uvea, retinal vessels, and choroid have been affected. The lacrimal glands have also been damaged. A small painless lump has been found behind the right upper mandible, growing slowly over 10 years, due to *S. japonicum*. Such lesions are rare but, in theory, because of the numerous collateral circulations around the portal system in hepatosplenic schistosomiasis, granulomas can occur almost anywhere in the body. Unfortunate tourists have returned home from the tropics with hematospermia and have not been believed when they claim that it was simply a result of swimming in fresh water. We await with interest the first confirmed reports of schistosomiasis of bone!

Bibliography

Abdel-Halim RE, Al-Mashad S, Al-Dabbagh A: Fluoroscopic assessment of bilharzial ureteropathy. *Clin Radiol* 36:89–94, 1985

Abdel Latif EA, et al: Clinical and physiological studies in bronchopulmonary schistosomiasis. *J Egypt Med Assoc* 48:452–466, 1965

Abdel-Wahab MF: Ultrasound for detecting *S. haematobium* urinary tract complications. Comparison with radiographic procedures. *J Urol* 148:344–350, 1992

Abdel-Wahab MF, Strickland GT: Abdominal ultrasonography for assessing morbidity from schistosomiasis: 2 hospital studies. *Trans R Soc Trop Med Hyg* 87:135–137, 1993

Abdel-Wahab MF, et al: Characteristic sonographic pattern of schistosomal hepatic fibrosis. *Am J Trop Med Hyg* 40:72–76, 1989

Abdel-Wahab MF, et al: Sonographic studies of school children in a village endemic for *Schistosoma mansoni*. *Trans R Soc Trop Med Hyg* 84:69–73, 1990

Abdel-Wahab MF, et al: Grading of hepatic schistosomiasis by the use of ultrasonography. *Am J Trop Med Hyg* 46:403–408, 1992

Abdel-Wahab MF, et al: *Schistosoma haematobium* infection in Egyptian school children. Demonstration of both hepatic and urinary tract morbidity by ultrasonography. *Trans R Soc Trop Med Hyg* 86:406–409, 1992

Abdel-Wahab MF, et al: Ultrasonographic prediction of esophageal varices in *Schistosomiasis mansoni*. *Am J Gastroenterol* 88:560–563, 1993

Ahmed MM, Himaida MCS: Haemorrhoids in Khartoum. *East Afr Med J* 67:48–50, 1990

Aisen AM, Gross BH, Glazer GM: Computed tomography of ureterovesical schistosomiasis. *J Comput Assist Tomogr* 7:161–163, 1983

Al-Fawaz IM, et al: Schistosomiasis associated with a mediastinal mass. Case report and review of the literature. *Ann Trop Paediatr* 10:293–297, 1990

Al-Ghoarb MM, et al: Radiological findings of bilharzial (schistosoma) contracted bladder. *Urology* 11:303–305, 1978

Al-Hindowi, et al: Calcification of the large bowel in schistosomiasis demonstrated by computed tomography. *Br J Radiol* 63:357–360, 1990

Alvarez SA: Urogenital bilharziasis (apropos of 28 cases). *J Trop Med Hyg* 48:154–181, 1972

Anayi S, Al-Nasiri N: Acute mesenteric ischaemia caused by *S. mansoni* infection. *Br Med J* 294:1197, 1987

Andrade ZA, Rocha H: Schistosomal glomerulopathy. *Kidney Int* 16:23–29, 1979

Araki T, et al: Hepatic *Schistosomiasis japonica*. Identified by CT. *Radiology* 157:757–760, 1985

Araki T, et al: Computed tomographic detection of intestinal calcification of *Schistosomiasis japonica*. *Gastroenterol Radiol* 14:360–362, 1989

Bahar RH, et al: Chronic urinary schistosomiasis: patterns of abnormalities in radionuclide ^{99}Tc in DTPA diuretic renograms. *APMIS Suppl* 3:54–58, 1988

Bahia-Oliveira LMG, et al: Differential cellular reactivity to adult worm antigens of patients with different clinical forms of *Schistosomiasis mansoni*. *Trans R Soc Trop Med Hyg* 86:57–61, 1992

Barsooum RS: Parasitic glomerulopathies. *Proc RCP* Edin: 27:283–299, 1997

Bhagwandeen SB: The pathology of ureteric bilharziasis. *S Afr Med J* 41:950–955, 1967

Bittencourt AL, et al: Placental involvement in schistosomiasis mansoni. A report of 4 cases. *Am J Trop Med Hyg* 29:571–575, 1980

Bicalho SA: Pseudoneoplastic form of schistosomiasis mansoni. *Gastroenterology* 54:105–109, 1968

Blackie WK: *Service Memoirs, No 5.* London School of Hygiene and Tropical Medicine, 1932

Blair DM: The occurrence of terminal-spined eggs other than those of *S. hematobium* in human beings in Rhodesia. *Cent Afr J Med* 12:103–109, 1966

Blair DM, Weber WC: Multiple schistosome infections: an unusual case. *Cent Afr J Med* 15 (Suppl):9–10, 1969

Bland KG, Gelfand M: The influence of urinary bilharziasis on vesico-vaginal fistula in relation to causation and healing. *Trans R Soc Trop Med Hyg* 64:588–592, 1970

Bohrer SP, et al: Roentgenographic features of schistosomiasis in children. *Z Tropenmed Parasitol* 22:177–188, 1971

Brandt CT, et al: Surgical hepatosplenic schistosomiasis mansoni in children: a Doppler duplex study of the portal vein and hepatic artery. *Trans R Soc Trop Med Hyg* 89:70–71, 1995

Briers PJ: Schistosomiasis with particular reference to pulmonary and abdominal lesions (abridged). *Proc R Soc Med* 67:861–862, 1974

Bruguera CA, Corona RE, Colombato LO: Ultrasonografia Doppler Pulsado simultaneo (Duplex) an al evaluacion del paciente hipertenso portal pre y post operatorio. *Rev Argent Radiol* 3:151–161, 1987

Buchanan WM, Gelfand M: Calcification of the bladder in urinary schistosomiasis. *Trans R Soc Trop Med Hyg.* 64:593–596, 1970

Buck AA: Schistosomiasis in Adwa: an epidemiological pilot study. *Ethiop Med J* 3:84–92, 1965

Catto BA, et al: Cercaria-induced histamine release: a factor in pathogenesis of schistosome dermatitis. *Am J Trop Med Hyg* 29:886–889, 1980

Cerri GG, Alves VAF, Magalhaes A: Hepatosplenic schistosomiasis mansoni: ultrasound manifestations. *Radiology* 153:777–780, 1984

Cerri GG, Vezozzo DP: L'echographie des Schistosomiases hepatiques. *JEMU* 13:31–35, 1992

Cesmeli E, et al: Ultrasound and CT changes of liver parenchyma in acute schistosomiasis. *Br J Radiol* 70:758–760, 1997

Chait A: Schistosomiasis mansoni: roentgenologic observations in a nonendemic area. *Am J Roentgenol Radium Ther Nucl Med* 90:688–708, 1963

Chait A, Gannon WE: Schistosomiasis of the spinal cord. *Am J Roentgenol* 105:400–405, 1969

Chan EMT, Leong LLY, Chan FL: Prominent periportal echogenicity. Its sonographic evaluation and its significance. *Br J Radiol* 59:543–546, 1986

Chandra Chekkar K, Pathmanathan R: Schistosomiasis in Malaysia. *Rev Infect Dis* 9:1026–1037, 1987

Chaves E: Necrotizing and healing pulmonary arteritis in schistosomal cor pulmonale: a retrospective study of ten cases. *Am J Trop Med Hyg* 15:162–167, 1966

Cheever AW, Young SW, Shohata A: Calcification of *Schistosoma haematobium* eggs: relation of radiologically demonstrable calcification to eggs in tissues and passage of eggs in urine. *Trans R Soc Trop Med Hyg* 69:410–414, 1975

Chen MG: Relative distribution of *S. japonica* eggs in the intestine of man: a subject of inconsistency. *Acta Trop (Basel)* 48:163–171, 1991

Cheung H, et al: The imaging diagnosis of hepatic schistosomiasis sequelae. *Clin Radiol* 51:51–55, 1995

Ching HT, et al: MR imaging appearances of intracerebral schistosomiasis. *Am J Radio* 162:693–694, 1994

Chitiyo ME: Schistosomal involvement of the choroid plexus. *Cent Afr J Med* 18:45–47, 1972

Clarke VdeV et al: The Katayama syndrome: *Cent Afr J Med* 16:123–126, 1970

Corochan R, et al: Autochthonous case of *S. intercalatum* from Equatorial Guinea. *Am J Trop Med Hyg* 36:343–344, 1987

Dar J, Zimmerman LR: Schistosomiasis of the spinal cord. *Surg Neurol* 8:416–418, 1977

Davey WW: *Companion to surgery in Africa.* London, E & S Livingstone, London, 1968, pp 75–87

Davidson RN, Houston S, Kiire CF: Schistosomal periportal fibrosis in Zimbabwe: use of ultrasound in patients with oesophageal varices. *Trans R Soc Trop Med Hyg* 85:380–382, 1991

DeTavera MP, DeLeon EP: Pulmonary schistosomiasis in the Philippines. *Dis Chest* 53:154–161, 1968

Devidas A, et al: Ultrasonographic assessment of the regression of bladder and renal lesions due to *S. haematobium* after treatment with praziquantel. *Ann Soc Belge Med Trop* 69:57–65, 1989

Doehring E, et al: Morbidity in urinary schistosomiasis: relation between sonographical lesions and pathological urine findings. *Trop Med Parasitol* 36:145–149, 1985

Doehring-Schwerdtfeger E, et al: Sonomorphological abnormalities in Sudanese children, with *S. mansoni* infection: a proposed staging system for field diagnosis of periportal fibrosis. *Am J Trop Med Hyg* 41:63–69, 1989

Doherty JF, et al: Katayama fever: an acute manifestation of schistosomiasis. *Br Med J* 313:1071–1072, 1996

Dupuis MJ, et al: MR imaging of schistosomal myelitis. *Am J Neurol Radio* 11:782–783, 1990

Edington GM, et al: Pathological effects of schistosomiasis in Ibadan, Western Nigeria. *J Trop Med Hyg* 19:982–995, 1970

Edington GM, Nwabuebo I, Junaid TA: The pathology of schistosomiasis in Ibadan, Nigeria, with special reference to the appendix, brain, pancreas and genital organs. *Trans R Soc Trap Med Hyg* 69:153–162, 1975

Edington GM, et al: *Pathology in the tropics, 2nd edn.* Williams & Wilkins, Baltimore, 1976, pp 145–180

El-Afifi S: Intestinal bilharziasis. *Dis Colon Rectum* 7:1–13, 1964

El-Badawi AA: Bilharzial polypi of the urinary bladder. *Br J Urol* 38:24–35, 1966

El-BanLawy A, Elwan O, Taher O: Bilharzial granuloma of the conus medullaris and cauda equinae. *Paraplegia* 10:172–180, 1972

El-Basousy MM, et al: Radiological changes in the small intestine of children in bilharziasis. *Gaz Egypt Paediatr Assoc* 21:33–42, 1973

El-Bgai MEA: Bilharzial congestive gastropathy: ultrasound demonstration of gastric wall changes. SS-5-38. 19th International Congress of Radiology, Singapore, 1994

El-Masry NA, et al: Schistosomal colonic polyposis; clinical, radiological and parasitological study. *J Trop Med Hyg* 89:13–17, 1989

El-Sallab RA, et al: Angiographic appearances of bilharzial mass of the colon. *Br J Radiol* 40:151–153, 1967

Eltoum IA, et al: Predictors of upper gastrointestinal bleeding in patients with schistosomal periportal fibrosis. *Br J Surg* 81:996–999, 1994

Fataar S, Satyanath S: The radiographic evaluation of appendiceal calcification due to schistosomiasis. *Am J Trop Med Hyg* 35:1157–1162, 1986

Fataar S, et al: Radiographic spectrum of retrocolonic calcification from schistosomiasis. *Am J Roentgenol* 142:933–936, 1984

Fataar S, et al: Characteristic sonographic features of schistosomal periportal fibrosis. *Am J Radiol* 143:69–71, 1984

Fataar S, et al: CT of schistosomiasis calcification of the intestine. *Am J Roentgenol* 144:75–76, 1985

Fataar S, et al: CT of hepatic schistosomiasis. *Am J Roentgenol* 145:63–66, 1985

Fataar S, et al: CT of genitourinary calcification due to schistosomiasis. *Australas Radiol* 34:234–237, 1990

Fataar S, et al: Radiologically visible gallbladder calcification due to schistosomiasis. *Br J Radiol* 63:706–709, 1990

Fataar S, et al: Case report: calcified pancreas and bile ducts from schistosomiasis. *Br J Radiol* 69:1064–1066, 1996

Friis H, et al: Ultrasonographic organometry: liver and spleen dimensions among children in Zimbabwe. *Trop Med Int Health* 2:183–190, 1996

Garcia-Palmieri MR, Marcial-Rojas RA: The protean manifestations of schistosomiasis mansoni: a clinicopathological correlation. *Ann Intern Med* 57:763–775, 1962

Garcia-Palmieri MR, et al: Portal hypertension due to schistosomiasis mansoni. *Am J Med* 27:811–816, 1959

Gelfand M: Calcification of *Schistosoma haematobium* eggs. Editorial. *Cent Afr J Med* 22:123, 1976

Gendrel D, et al: *Schistosoma intercalatum* and relapses of *Salmonella*, infection in children. *Am J Trop Med Hyg* 33:1166–1169, 1984

Gilles HM, et al: *Schistosoma haematobium* infection in Nigeria. *Ann Trop Med Parasitol* 59:451–456, 1956

Girges MR: The syndrome of bladder-neck obstruction and ureteric fibrosis in *Schistosoma haematobium* infection. *J Trop Med Hyg* 69:187–188, 1966

Gjerde IO, Mark S, Hult G: Cerebral schistosomiasis presenting as a brain tumour. *Eur Neurol* 23:229–236, 1984

Goldsmid JM: Spurious parasites recovered from stools and urine in Rhodesia. *Cent Afr J Med* 16:173–178, 1970

Goldsmid JM, Rogers S: Observations on the diagnosis and treatment of schistosomiasis in an endemic area. *S Afr Med J* 51:29–33, 1977

Grand S, Movet E, LeBas JF: Case report: Spinal schistosomiasis. MRI findings. *Clin Radiol* 51:739–740, 1996

Guelrud M, et al: Wedged hepatic venography. A comparative study of cirrhosis and hepatic schistosomiasis. *Am J Gastroenterol* 62:504–508, 1974

Gundersen SG, Rann J, Haagensen I: Early detection of circulating anodic antigen (CAA) in a case of acute schistosomiasis with Katayama fever. *Scand J Infect Dis* 24:549–552, 1992

Hamada M, et al: Hepatic calcification in schistosomiasis japonica. *J Comput Assist Tomogr* 6:76–78, 1982

Hamash KA, et al: Predictive value of excretory urography, computerized tomography and liver and bone scans in the staging of bilharzial bladder cancer in Saudi Arabia. *Cancer* 54:172–176, 1984

Hammermann AM, Kotner LM, Doyle TB: Periportal enhancement of CT scans of the liver. *Am J Roentgenol* 156:313–315, 1991

Haribhai HC, et al: Spinal cord schistosomiasis. A clinical laboratory and radiological study. *Brain* 114:709–726, 1991

Hatz C, et al: Ultrasound scanning for detecting morbidity due to *S. haematobium* and its resolution following treatment with different doses of praziquantel. *Trans R Soc Trop Med Hyg* 84:84–88, 1990

Hatz C, et al: Ultrasound in schistosomiasis: a critical look at methodological issues and potential applications. *Acta Trop (Basel)* 51:89–97, 1992

Hatz C, et al: A review of the literature on the use of ultrasonography in schistosomiasis, with special reference to its use in field studies. *Acta Trop (Basel)* 51:15–28, 1992

Heurtier V, et al: Urinary tract lesions due to *S. haematobium* infection assessed by ultrasonography in a community based study in Niger. *Am J Trop Med Hyg* 35:1163–1172, 1986

Hillyer G, et al: The Circumoral precipitin test for the serodiagnosis of human schistosomiasis mansoni and haematobium. *Am J Trop Med Hyg* 30:121–126, 1981

Hira PR, Patel BG: Transmission of schistosomiasis in rural Zambia. *Cent Afr J Med* 27:244–249, 1981

Homeida M, et al: Diagnosis of pathologically confirmed Symmer's (periportal) fibrosis by ultrasonography: a prospective blinded study. *Am J Trop Med Hyg* 38:86–91, 1988

Homeida M, et al: Morbidity associated with *Schistosoma mansoni* infection as determined by ultrasound. A study in Gezira, Sudan. *Am J Trop Med Hyg* 39:196–201, 1988

Honey RM, et al: The urological aspects of bilharziasis in Rhodesia. *Cent Afr J Med* 6:199–212, 1960

Houpis J, et al: Acute schistosomiasis with transverse myelitis in American students returning from Kenya. *J Am Med Assoc* 252:1116–1123, 1984

Houston S, et al: Use of ultrasound in a study of periportal fibrosis in rural Zimbabwe. *Acta Trop (Basel)* 53:51–58, 1993

Hugosson C: Striation of the renal pelvis and ureter in bilharziasis. *Clin Radiol* 38:407–409, 1987

Hugosson C, Olsen P: Early ureteric changes in *S. haematobium* infection. *Clin Radiol* 37:501–503, 1986

Iarotski LS, Davis A: The schistosomiasis problem in the world: results of a WHO questionnaire survey. *Bull WHO* 59:115–127, 1981

Iarotski LS, Medvedev VF, Zal'Nova NS: Urogenital schistosomiasis in the People's Democratic Republic of Yemen and its clinicoroentgenological characteristics. *Med Parazitol (Mosk)* 46:485–487, 1977

Ihekwaba FN: Schistosomiasis of the testis. *Cent Afr J Med* 38:123–127, 1992

Joralf H, Lindstedt E: Urogenital schistosomiasis: CT evaluation. *Radiology* 157:745–749, 1985

Kane CA, Most H: Schistosomiasis of the central nervous system. *JAMA* 59:141–183, 1948

Kardoff R, et al: Ultrasonography of ureteric abnormalities induced by *S. haematobium* infection, before and after praziquantel treatment. *Br J Urol* 74:703–709, 1994

Kardorff R, et al: *S. mansoni*-related morbidity on Ukerewe Island, Tanzania. Clinical, ultrasonographical and biochemical parameters. *Trop Med Int Health* 2:230–239, 1997

Kark AW: Bile-duct strictures caused by schistosomiasis. *Br J Surg* 49:419–421, 1961

Khalil HH, et al: Cerebral atrophy: a schistosomiasis manifestation? *Am J Trop Med Hyg* 35:531–533, 1986

King CH, et al: Urinary tract morbidity in schistosomiasis haematobia: association with age and intensity of infection in an endemic area of Coast Province, Kenya. *Am J Trop Med Hyg* 39:361–368, 1988

Kirchoff LV, Nash TE: A case of schistosomiasis japonica: resolution of CAT-scan detected cerebral abnormalities without specific therapy. *Am J Trop Med Hyg* 33:1155–1158, 1984

Kongs A, et al: Clinical investigation of a population recently infected with schistosomiasis mansoni. *Trop Med Int Health* 2:191–198, 1996

Lambertucci JR, et al: Acute Manson's schistosomiasis: sonographic features. *Trans R Soc Trop Med Hyg* 88:76–77, 1994

Lechtenberg R, Vaida GA: Schistosomiasis of the spinal cord [abstract]. *Radiology* 125:856, 1977

Lee HF, et al: Human schistosomiasis in Thailand. *Am J Trop Med Hyg* 15:303–307, 1966

Lee RC, et al: Intestinal schistosomiasis japonica. CT-pathologic correlation. *Radiology* 193:539–542, 1994

Lichtenberg F: Lesions of the intrahepatic portal radicles in Mansoni schistosomiasis. *Am J Pathol* 31:757–771, 1955

Löffler TJP: Schistosomiasis in Lake Malawi [letter]. *Br Med J* 308:138, 1994

Macieira-Coehlo E, et al: The syndrome of portopulmonary schistosomiasis. *Am J Med* 43:944–950, 1967

MacSween RM, Williams HC: Seabather's eruption – a case of Caribbean itch. *Br Med J* 312:957–958, 1996

Marty AM, Andersen EM: Helminthology. In: Doerr W, Seifert G (eds) *Tropical pathology, 2nd edn.* Springer, Berlin Heidelberg New York, pp 801–982, 1995

Masson C, et al: Schistosomiase medullaire. Apport Del'imagerie per resonance magnetique. *Presse Med* 19:1223–1224, 1990

McCarten WG, et al: Schistosomiasis: evaluation of the indirect fluorescent antibody, complement fixation and slide flocculation tests in screening for schistosomiasis. *Exp Parasitol* 37:239–250, 1975

McKenna G, Schousboe M, Paltridge G: Subjective change in ejaculate as symptom of infection with *Schistosoma haematobium* in travelers. *Br Med J* 315:1000–1001, 1997

Medina J, et al: The roentgen appearance of schistosomiasis mansoni involving the colon. *Radiology* 85:682–688, 1965

Miller RL, et al: Paleoepidemiology of schistosoma infection in mummies. *Br Med J* 304:555–556, 1992

Monzawa S, et al: Schistosomiasis japonica of the liver. Contrast enhanced CT findings. *Am J Roentgenol* 161:323–327, 1993

Moriyasu F, et al: Measurement of portal vascular resistance in patients with portal hypertensin. *Gastroenterology* 90:710–715, 1986

Most H, et al: Schistosomiasis japonicum in American military personnel. Clinical studies of 600 cases during the first year after infection. *Am J Trop Med Hyg* 30:239–299, 1950

Mostofi FK (ed): *Bilharziasis.* International Academy of Pathology – Special Monograph. Springer, New York Berlin Heidelberg, 1967

Moyou SR, et al: Etude epidemiologique de la bilharziose urinaire dans le foyer des lacs Barombi, Cameroun. *Bull Soc Pathol Exotique Ses Filiades* 80:813–825, 1987

Nafeh MA, et al: Ultrasonographic changes in the liver in *S. haematobium* infection. *Am J Trop Med Hyg* 47:225–230, 1992

Nko'O-Amvene S, et al: Fibrose portale dans le schistosomiase à *S. mansoni.* Une étude ultrasonographique dans le foyer de Nkol bisson (Cameroun). *J Radiol* 74:269–274, 1993

Noix M, et al: Radiocinematographic study of the lower urinary tract in bilharziasis patients. Value of an endoradiocinematographic comparison. *Med Audiovision* 5:180–182, 1966

Nooman ZM, et al: Hepatosplenic disease caused by *Bilharzia haematobium* in upper Egypt. *J Trop Med Hyg* 77:42–48, 1974

Nouh MS, et al: Hepatitis-B virus vs. schistosomiasis and hepato-cellular carcinoma in Saudi Arabia. *East Afr Med J* 67:139–145, 1990

Owor R: Pathological aspects of schistosomiasis in Uganda, with particular reference to the West Nile district. *East Afr Med J* 48:399–405, 1971

Owor R, Madda JP: Schistosomiasis causing tumour-like lesions. *East Afr Med J* 54:137–141, 1977

Palmer PES: Pulmonary manifestations of schistosomiasis. In: Middlemiss H (ed) *Tropical radiology.* Heinemann, London, 1961, pp 103–107

Palmer PES: Tropical disease of the gastrointestinal tract. In: Simpkins KC (ed) *A textbook of radiological diagnosis, vol 4, 5th edn.* HK Lewis, London, 1988, pp 678–705

Paranagua-Vezozzo DC, Cerri GG: Duplex hemodynamic evaluation of hepatosplenic mansoni schistosomiasis. *Mem Inst Oswaldo Cruz* 87 (Suppl 4):149–151, 1992

Paul R: Pulmonary schistosomiasis. *Cent Afr J Med* 2:100–102, 1956

Pawar HN, Abdel-Dayen HM: Diuretic renography and urodynamic pressure studies in evaluating dilated bilharzial ureters. *Clin Nucl Med* 9:402–404, 1984

Pedroso ER, et al: Pulmonary schistosomiasis mansoni: post-treatment pulmonary clinico-radiological alterations in patients in the chronic phase: a double-blind study. *Trans R Soc Trop Med Hyg* 81:778–781, 1987

Pesigan TP: Brain schistosomiasis, a contribution to its pathogenesis. *Acta Med Philipp* 4:39–46, 1947

Phillips JF, et al: Radiographic evaluation of patients with schistosomiasis. *Radiology* 114:31–37, 1975

Pinto-Silva RA, et al: Sonographic features of portal hypertension in schistosomiasis mansoni. *Rev Inst Med Trop Sao Paulo* 36:355–361, 1994

Pi-Sunyer FX, et al: *Schistosoma haematobium* infection in Nigeria. *Ann Trop Med Parasitol* 59:304–310, 1965

Prata A, Schroeder S: A comparison of whites and Negroes infected with *Schistosoma mansoni* in a hyperendemic area. *Gazeta Medica Da Bahia* 67:92–98, 1967

Pulvertaft R, Hurst G: Bladder calcification in end stage renal failure. *Br J Radiol* 57:335–336, 1984

Rabello TAL, et al: Abdominal ultrasonography in acute clinical schistosomiasis mansoni. *Am J Trop Med Hyg* 50:748–752, 1994

Radhakrishnan S, et al: Hepatosplenic and small bowel calcification due to *S. mansoni* infection. *Dig Dis Sci* 33:1637–1640, 1988

Renand G, et al: Prevalence of vaginal schistosomiasis caused by *S. haematobium* in an endemic village in Niger. *Trans R Soc Trop Med Hyg* 83:7797–7798, 1989

Richter J, Feldmeier H: Hepatosplenic schistosomiasis. Part II: Diagnosis and staging using ultrasonography. *Hospimedica,* 26–29 January 1991

Rocha H, et al: Renal involvement in patients with hepatosplenic schistosomiasis mansoni. *Am J Trop Med Hyg* 15:108–115, 1976

Rosin IR, Todes GW: Bilharzial ulcer of the stomach. *Cent Afr J Med* 12:179–180, 1966

Rouguet P, et al: Hepatosplenic alteration determined by ultrasonography in a population recently infected with *Schistosoma mansoni* in Richard-Toll, Senegal. *Trans R Soc Trop Med Hyg* 87:190–193, 1993

Sabha M, Nilsson T: Urodynamic evaluation of calcified bilharzial bladder. *APMIS Suppl* 3:50–53, 1988

Sabour MS, et al: A clinical study of hepatic schistosomiasis. *J Trop Med Hyg* 6:85–93, 1966

Sadek AM, et al: Percutaneous transhepatic lymphography: evaluation in schistosomal hepatic fibrosis. *Lymphology* 9:47–52, 1976

Sadigursky M, Andrade ZA: Pulmonary changes in schistosomal cor pulmonale. *Am J Trop Med Hyg* 779–784, 1982

Sadun EH, et al: Susceptibility and comparative pathology of ten species of primates exposed to infection with *Schistosoma mansoni. Am J Trop Med Hyg* 17:705–718, 1966

Schaap HB, Den Dulk MO, Polderman AUR: Schistosomiasis in the Yemen Arab Republic. Prevalence of *S. mansoni* and *S. haematobium* infection among school children in the central highlands and their relation to altitude. *Trop Geog Med* 44:19–22, 1991

Schaberg T, et al: Intestinal protein loss in schistosomal polyposis of the colon. *Gastroenterology* 59:433–436, 1991

Schaberg T, et al: Pulmonary schistosomiasis resembling acute pulmonary tuberculosis. *Eur Respir J* 4:1023–1026, 1991

Schinski VD, Clutter WC, Murrell KD: Enzyme and ^{125}I-labeled anti-immunoglobulin assays in the immunodiagnosis of schistosomiasis. *Am J Trop Med Hyg* 25:824–831, 1976

Scrimgeour EM: Spinal cord disease due to *S. mansoni* successfully treated with oxamniquine [letter]. Br Med J 289:625, 1984

Scrimgeour EM, Gajdusek DC: Involvement of the central nervous system in schistosomiasis haematobia, and schistosomiasis mansoni infection: a review. *Brain* 108:1023–1158, 1984

Selwa IM, et al: Spinal cord schistosomiasis. A pediatric case mimicking intrinsic cord neoplasm. *Neurology* 41:755–757, 1991

Semin RM: Splenoportography and intrasplenic manometry in hepatic bilharziasis. *Gastroenterologia* 93:167–179, 1960

Sewez CH, Jeutzen H, Sanger R: Röntgenbefunde bei urogenital Bilharziose. *Radiol Diagn* 26:213–219, 1985

Shail E, et al: Neuroschistosomiasis myelopathy: case report. *Br J Neurosurg* 8:239–242, 1994

Shaw AFB, et al: Pathogenesis of pulmonary schistosomiasis in Egypt with special reference to Ayerza's diseaes. *J Pathol Bacteriol* 46:401–424, 1938

Shokier AA, et al: Urinary bilharziasis in upper Egypt (I & II). *East Afr Med J* 49:298–326, 1972

Silbergleit R, Silbergleit R: Schistosomal granuloma of the spinal cord: evaluation with MR imging and intraoperative sonography. *Am J Radiol* 158:1351–1353, 1992

Smith JH, Christie JD: The pathobiology of schistosomiasis haematobium infection in humans. *Hum Pathol* 17:333–345, 1986

Sniderman KW, Sos TA: Hepatic schistosomiasis: a case with intrahepatic shunting and extrahepatic portal vein occlusion. *AJR* 130:565–567, 1978

Sobh MA, et al: Schistosomal-specific nephropathy leading to end stage renal failure. *Kidney Int* 31:1006–1011, 1987

Sobh M, et al: Nephropathy in asymptomatic patiens with active *Schistosoma mansoni* infection. *Int Urol Nephrol* 22:37–43, 1990

Sparrow CH: Bilharziasis in the human eye – a report of a case. *Cent Afr J Med* 12:55, 1966

Stepanov EP: X-ray data in schistosomiasis of the urinary tracts. *Vestn Rentgenol Radio.* 4:72–76, 1976

Stephenson LS, et al: Regression of splenomegaly and hepatomegaly in children treated for *S. haematobium* infection. *Am J Trop Med Hyg* 34:119–123, 1985

Strickland GT, Abdel-Wahab MF: Abdominal ultrasonography for assessing morbidity from schistosomiasis. 1. Community studies. *Trans R Soc Med Hyg* 87, 1993

Suresh S, Indrani S, Vijayalakshmi S: Ultrasonography in tropical diseases. *Ultrasound Quarterly* 8:43–72, 1990

Thomas HM, Gage DP: Symptomatology of early schistosomiasis japonica. *Bull US Army Med Dep* 4:197–202, 1945

Truter PJ, van der Merwe JV: Transverse myelitis caused by schistosomiasis during pregnancy. *S Afr Med J* 71:184–185, 1987

Umerah BC: Evaluation of the physiological function of the ureter by fluoroscopy in bilharziasis. *Radiology* 124:645–647, 1977

Umerah BC: Less familar manifestations of schistosomiasis of the urinary tract [abstract]. *Radiology* 125:857, 1977

Vanker EA: Aortic aneurysm caused by schistosomiasis. *Thorax* 41:890–891, 1986

Vera C: Natural infection of *Bulinus senegalensis* by *Schistosoma haematobium:* characterizatioin by cercarial emergence patterns. *Trans R Soc Trop Med Hyg* 86:62, 1992

Vinhaes LS, et al: Pulmonary circulation in schistosomatic portal hypertension syndrome. Radiologic-hemodynamical interrelations. *Arq Bras Cardiol* 30:13–18, 1977

von Wechmar M, Vogel H: Blasenverkalkung durch Schistosomiasis. *Röntgenblätter* 42:435–436, 1985

Wang C, et al: Roentgenologic changes of small intestine in schistosomiasis japonica. *Chin J Radiol* 6:247–253, 1958

Weber MC, et al: The distribution of viable and non-viable eggs of *Schistosoma haematobium* in the urine. *Cent Afr J Med* 15:27–30, 1969

Wein-Min C, et al: Studies on ultrasonographic diagnosis of schistosomiasis japonica in China: a review of selected Chinese studies. *Acta Trop (Basel)* 51:37–43, 1992

Wittes R, et al: Three cases of schistosomiasis mekongi from Northern Laos. *Am J Trop Med Hyg* 33:1159–1165, 1984

World Health Organisation: Research and training in tropical disease. Proposal for a practical guide for the standardized use of ultrasound in the assessment of pathological changes in schistosomiasis. White report. WHO TDR/SCH/ultrason/19.3.1991

World Health Organization: Reports I & II of the WHO Expect Committee on the control of schistosomiasis. WHO Geneva, 1991, 1993

Yamigiwa K: Beiträge zur Aetiologie der Jacksonchen Epilepsie. *Virchows Arch* [A] 119:449–460, 1889

Zaky Y, et al: Duplex study of the portal vein in schistosomal hepatic fibrosis before and after shunt and non shunt therapy. S. 308 19th International Congress of Radiology, Singapore, 1994.

3 Hydatid Disease (Echinococcosis)

With Walther von Sinner and David Lewall

Hydatid disease was known to Hippocrates and Galen; it was well recognized by many physicians in the nineteenth century. It is not a truly tropical disease, since it is one of the few parasitic diseases that occur with far greater frequency in the temperate and subtropical zones of the world. Although it is most commonly seen in countries where sheep are raised, man and numerous other animals are frequently infected. Even the moose and the house mouse are intermediate hosts for this ubiquitous parasite. It is found throughout much of the world and must be considered in the differential diagnosis of a cyst or mass in virtually any patient who is residing in, or has traveled through, an endemic area. The prevalence is unknown because of underreporting and the probability that the majority of infections are undiagnosed. Many asymptomatic hydatid cysts have been first discovered by population surveys using ultrasound, as in Tunis and northern Kenya. In one series, 60% of hydatid cysts in the liver were clinically unsuspected; some are found by chance during a radiographic examination for an unrelated reason. The diagnosis can often be confirmed by direct cyst aspiration and treatment can be initiated. The disease is often managed more effectively in countries where it is known than in the United States and Europe, where it tends to be an exotic intruder. Among the many parasites infecting man, few are more serious in their consequences than the larval phase of hydatid disease.

There are two widely different principal varieties of the infection. The more widespread and better known cystic hydatid disease is caused by the larval form of the dog tapeworm *Echinococcus granulosus* and is characterized by the formation of one or more expanding unilocular cysts. The less common alveolar form is caused by *Echinococcus multilocularis* and produces destructive invasive lesions more closely resembling a malignancy than a parasitic infection. Because of the great disparity in the pathological, clinical, and radiological manifestations of these two varieties of hydatid disease, they will be discussed separately. The much less common *Echinococcus vogeli* and the very rare *Echinococcus oligarthus* have been responsible for occasional cases of polycystic hydatidosis: the first human infections with these hydatids were not recognized until 20 years ago.

Cystic hydatid disease is unusual in that rupture and its sequelae (biliary obstruction, infection, dissemination, and anaphylaxis) are more important than the mass effect of the cyst, despite the enormous size sometimes attained by the lesion. The natural progression from simple to complex cyst, and then to senescence and death, as well as rupture and its sequelae can be imaged noninvasively by ultrasonography (US), computed tomography (CT), and magnetic resonance imaging (MRI), and in some instances by plain radiographs. The gross appearance of hydatid cysts, even after rupture, is often appreciated better by the radiologist than by the pathologist, who usually receives only fragments of tissue (although even a fragment of the wall of a cyst has a characteristic gross and microscopic appearance and is diagnostic of hydatid disease).

Of the 20 or more classifications of cystic hydatidosis that have been proposed, most are based on imaging rather than on pathology of the lesion; many are not helpful in making outcome comparisons, nor are they ideal for planning surgical or medical treatment. A major problem is that, as imaging has improved over the past three decades, classifications have changed. The use of percutaneous drainage in addition to established surgical and medical therapy has increased the need for a consistent system of classification. In this chapter the pathophysiology of hydatid disease is reviewed and a pathology-based classification (Lewall 1998) with imaging correlation (von Sinner and Lewall) is presented.

Synonyms

Hydatid disease. Echinococcosis. Echinococciasis. Tapeworm disease. Hydatidosis. *Sp*: Hidatidosis. Equinocococia. *Fr*: L'echinococcose. Maladie hydatique. *Ger*: Beckenknochenechinokokkus. Echinokokkose. Blasenwurm-Krankheit. Echinokokken-Krankheit.

Table 3.1. The various forms of human echinococcosis and their causative agents. (Modified from Thompson and Lymbery 1995)

	Echinococcus granulosus	*Echinococcus multilocularis*	*Echinococcus vogeli*	*Echinococcus oligarthus*
Form of human echinococcosis	Cystic echinococcosis (hydatid disease)	Alveolar echinococcosis (alveolar hydatid disease)	Polycystic echinococcosis	*E. oligarthus* echinococcosis
Metacestode:				
Typical form	Unilocular (cystic)	Multivesicular (alveolar)	Polycystic	Polycystic
Organ site in humans	Visceral, primarily liver and lung	Visceral, primarily liver	Visceral, primarily liver and lung	Peripheral and visceral (heart, retro-ocular)
Main definitive hosts	Dogs and other canids	Foxes, other canids, cats	Bush dog, domestic dog	Wild felids
Main intermediate hosts	Primarily ungulates	Rodents	Paca, agouti, spiny rat	Paca, agouti, spiny rat
Geographic distribution	Cosmopolitan	Northern hemisphere	Central and South America	Central and South America down to the subantarctic

Definition

Hydatid disease is infection by larvae of the genus *Echinococcus* (Table 3.1). Four species can infect humans, but there are two main varieties, *E. granulosus* and *E. multilocularis*, with a widespread distribution. The uncommon *E. vogeli* and the rare *E. oligarthus* are found only in Central and South America.

Unilocular or Cystic Hydatid Disease (*E. granulosus*)

Geographic Distribution

As already noted, hydatid disease is an unusual parasitic disease in that it occurs much more commonly in the temperate than in the tropical zones of the world. The causative parasite of unilocular cystic hydatid disease, *E. granulosus*, is found in sheep-raising areas such as Australia, New Zealand, Tasmania, Iceland, England, Spain, Italy, Greece and other countries in Central, Eastern, and Southern Europe, Egypt, North, East, and southern Africa, Israel, the Arab countries of the Middle East, Russia, North China, the Philippines, and Japan (Fig. 3.1). In South America, it is especially prevalent in Uruguay, Argentina, and Chile. The disease occurs also in Canada and rarely in parts of the western United States and the lower Mississippi Valley. More than 1000 patients have been reported in the United States, but most of these were immigrants from countries where the disease is endemic.

Epidemiology and Pathology

To complete its life cycle, *E. granulosus* requires two hosts: a canine and a grazing animal (Figs. 3.2, 3.3). In the more common pastoral form, the primary host is the dog, while herbivores such as sheep, cattle, swine, or camels serve as intermediate hosts. In the less common sylvatic form, the wolf or fox is the primary host and reindeer or moose are the usual intermediate hosts. Humans are accidental intermediate hosts. There is a high degree of host specificity in the primary, but not in the intermediate host; the domestic cat, for instance, is not a primary host. The reasons for this unexplained specificity may include the microtopography of the host's intestine, biochemical and immunological factors, or the composition of the host's bile.
The adult parasite is a tiny tapeworm, 3–6 mm in length, hundreds or thousands of which may be found in the small intestine of a canine (Fig. 3.4 A). The worm is composed of four segments (Fig. 3.4 B, C): the head or scolex is pyriform with four suckers and a rostellum containing a double row of hooklets, enabling the worm to attach itself to the intestinal mucosa of the canine. Behind the short neck are three proglottids, the terminal and broadest of which is a gravid egg-containing segment. The shed gravid proglottids and/or eggs are

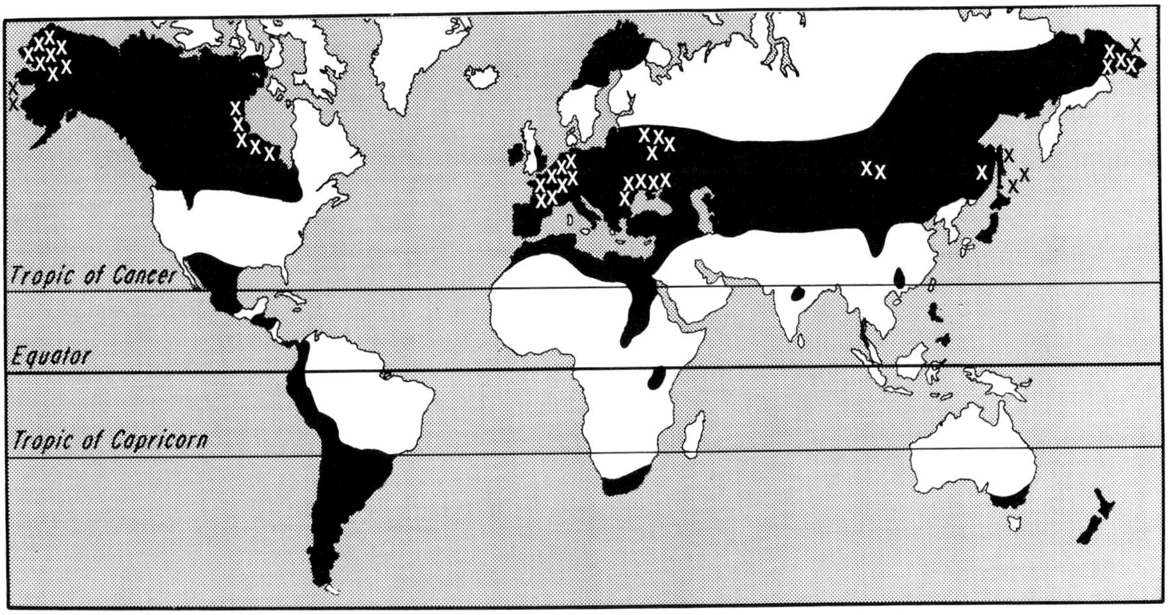

Fig. 3.1. Geographic distribution of hydatid disease [(*black areas*) *E. granulosus* and (*crosses*) *E. multilocularis*]. Note that both forms of hydatidosis are not truly tropical diseases, since they occur in more temperate zones. The highest frequency of cystic hydatid disease (*E. granulosus*) is in South America, North Africa, the Mediterranean littoral, Eastern Europe, and the Middle and Far East. The disease has been partially controlled in some areas which previously had a high incidence, such as Australasia, Greenland, and Cyprus

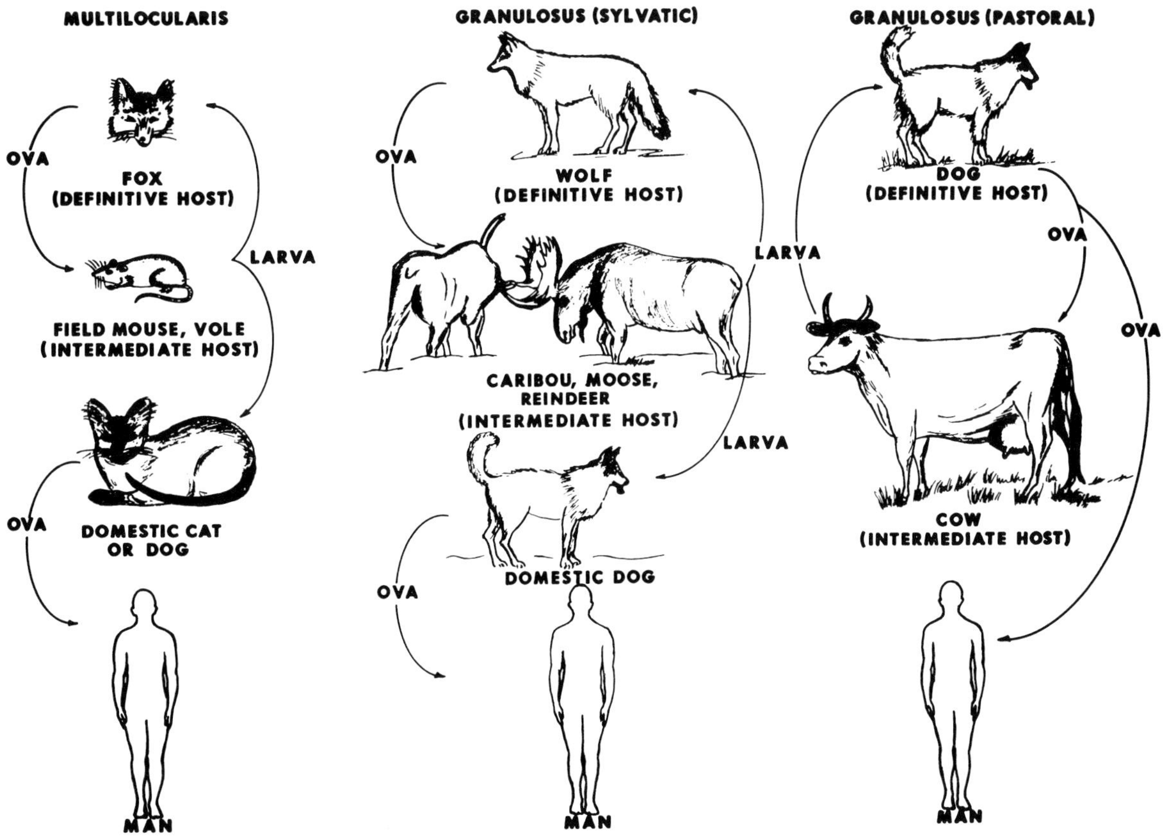

Fig. 3.2. Life cycles of the various forms of hydatid disease: *E. multilocularis* and *E. granulosus* (sylvatic and pastoral). The common hosts are represented

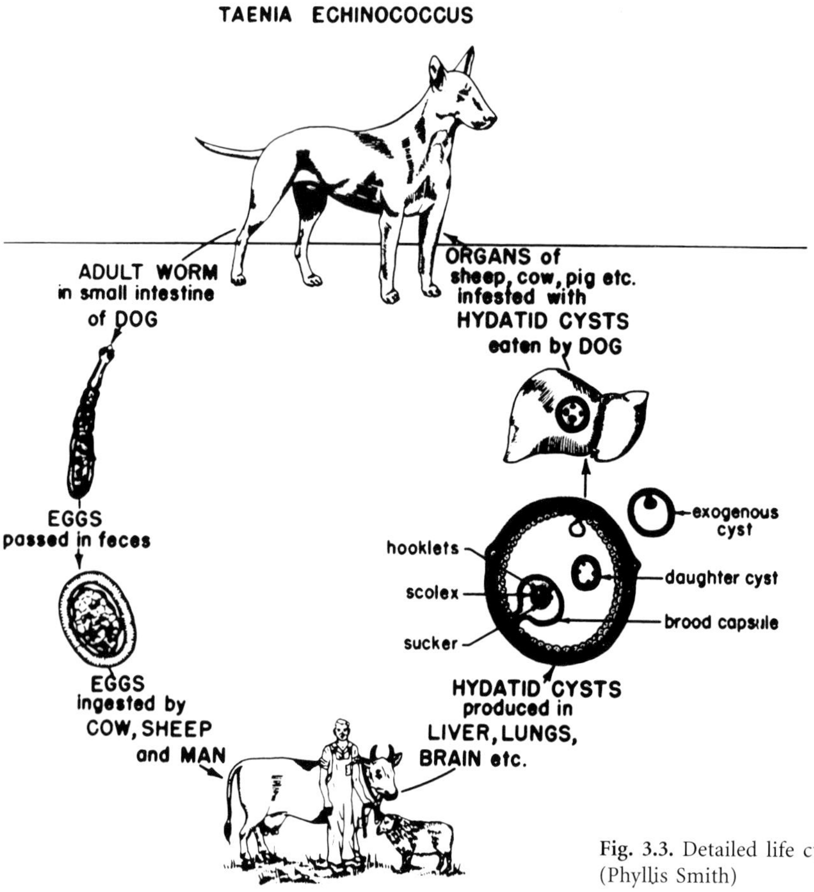

Fig. 3.3. Detailed life cycle of *E. granulosus*. AFIP 68-3573-15 (Phyllis Smith)

excreted in the feces of the primary host and contaminate the ground, including pastureland. They are subsequently ingested by intermediate hosts such as sheep, cattle, horses, pigs, goats, and camels. Monkeys, kangaroos, tapirs, moose, squirrels, and the house mouse are less common intermediate hosts.

Man may become accidentally infected with *E. granulosus* by contact with infected dogs or by ingesting food, water, or soil containing eggs deposited in the feces of the dog, wolf, or other canines. Children, shepherds, and agricultural workers whose play and leisure habits or duties promote intimate human-canine relationships are particularly vulnerable. Contaminated uncooked foods (e.g., watercress or other salad vegetables) may play an occasional part in transmission. There is indirect evidence that direct inhalation can occasionally cause lung hydatids in man, and it has been shown that eggs administered to sheep via a tracheostomy develop into lung cysts.

Once within man or other intermediate host, proteolytic enzymes in the digestive juices dissolve the external coats of the ingested eggs, which hatch in the duodenum to release oncospheres (true larvae) that attach to the jejeunal mucosa by hooklets and suckers. Oncospheres burrow into the submucosa by means of rhythmic muscular movements involving the body and hooklets, aided by secretions of the so-called penetration gland. Oncospheres then enter veins or lymphatics and those that travel in the portal system lodge in the capillary bed of the liver, which acts as an effective filter for most of the larvae; if, however, this barrier is overcome, the larvae pass through the inferior vena cava into the right side of the heart and then to the lungs. This accounts for the predominant involvement in those organs (liver approximately 50%–70%, lungs 15%–30%). If the worm is not trapped in either the liver or the lungs, or if it travels in lymphatics and bypasses the liver and lungs, it may lodge virtually anywhere in the body, most notably in the peritoneum, spleen, kidneys, heart, brain, spine, bony skeleton, and muscles. Not every larva develops; over 90% are overcome by the host reaction.

The encysted oncosphere grows 1–5 cm in diameter per year, depending on the density of the host tissue. The cyst produces protoscolices which are released when a carnivore ingests the viscera of the intermediate host. The swallowed protoscolices evaginate to become scolices which attach to the proxi-

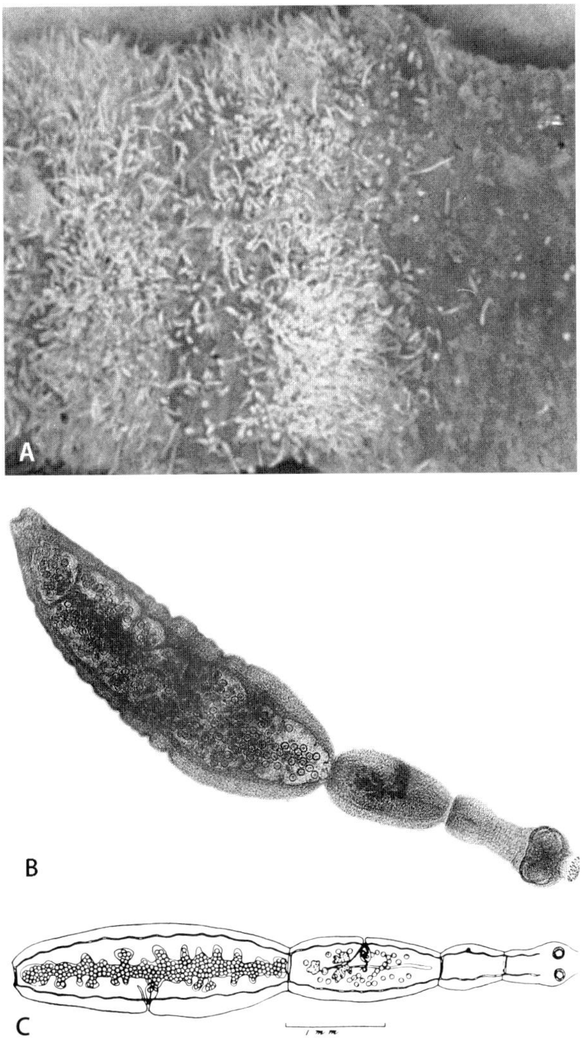

Fig. 3.4 A–C. The adult stage of *E. granulosus*. **A** Massive infection with thousands of tiny tapeworms in the small intestine of a dog. **B** The hooks on the scolex (*right*) appear as a dark ring. Numerous eggs are present in the terminal proglottid (*left*). **C** Line drawing of an adult *E. granulosus* showing the pyriform scolex or head (*right*), which contains four suckers and a rostellum with a double row of hooklets by which the worm attaches to the intestinal mucosa of the canine. Behind the short neck are three proglottids, the terminal and broadest of which is a gravid, egg-containing segment. AFIP 53-20053-1

mal small bowel of the primary host, completing the life cycle.

If the larva is not destroyed, it develops into a tiny cyst containing a small amount of clear fluid (Fig. 3.5). This mainly hollow cyst grows steadily over a period of years, at times reaching enormous proportions before it becomes clinically evident (Figs. 3.6–3.8). The average rate of growth varies from 1 to 5 cm a year, being partly determined by the pressure resistance of its anatomical location. Thus, its rate of growth is more rapid in the lungs than in the liver, spleen, or other solid organs, and slowest in bones. If the cyst has room to develop easily, as happens in the liver, lungs, or peritoneum, it almost always grows as the classic unilocular cyst. It can remain latent for a long period, a latency of up to 53 years having been reported.

The encysted oncosphere develops a delicate monocellular inner germinal layer which secretes a PAS-positive polysaccharide protein complex, the acellular laminated layer that forms around the germinal layer (Fig. 3.9). This endocyst grows up to 2 mm in thickness. Even though the laminated layer is delicate, it protects the inner more fragile germinal layer. The endocyst is the true wall of the cyst. The germinal layer produces clear fluid which attains a pressure of up to 300 mm of water, keeping the endocyst in intimate contact with the pericyst. The endocyst receives its sustenance from the pericyst.

Although hydatid fluid has been studied extensively, the mechanisms by which fluid and other substances are transferred into the avascular cyst are not well understood. It is certain, however, that transfer does take place since host proteins and some lipids that are not synthesized by *Echinococcus* are found in the cyst fluid. Diffusion, endocytosis, specific filter or transport mechanisms, and fissures in cyst membranes have been suggested to explain transport, although evidence for fissures is not convincing.

The inner germinal layer of the endocyst is the active part of the cyst, producing brood capsules which release protoscolices (after ingestion by the primary host the head of the protoscolex evaginates and the larva is then called a scolex) (Fig. 3.10). Most of the brood capsules and scolices pinch off from the germinal layer and precipitate to the bottom of the fluid to become hydatid sand, which is just visible to the naked eye. The hydatid sand floating within the cyst may contain as many as 400 000 protoscolices per millilitre and an average cyst contains up to 500 ml of such sand (Fig. 3.11).

Scolices, which are infectious miniature adult tapeworms, possess a dual potential. If they are ingested by a primary host the apical region of the scolex (suckers, rostellum, and hooklets) evaginates and the organism attaches within a crypt of Lieberkühn in the host's proximal small bowel, where it develops into the adult worm. However, if the scolex is deposited in a favorable milieu such as the peritoneal cavity or tracheobronchial tree after cyst rupture it may form a new hydatid cyst.

(Text continues on p. 212)

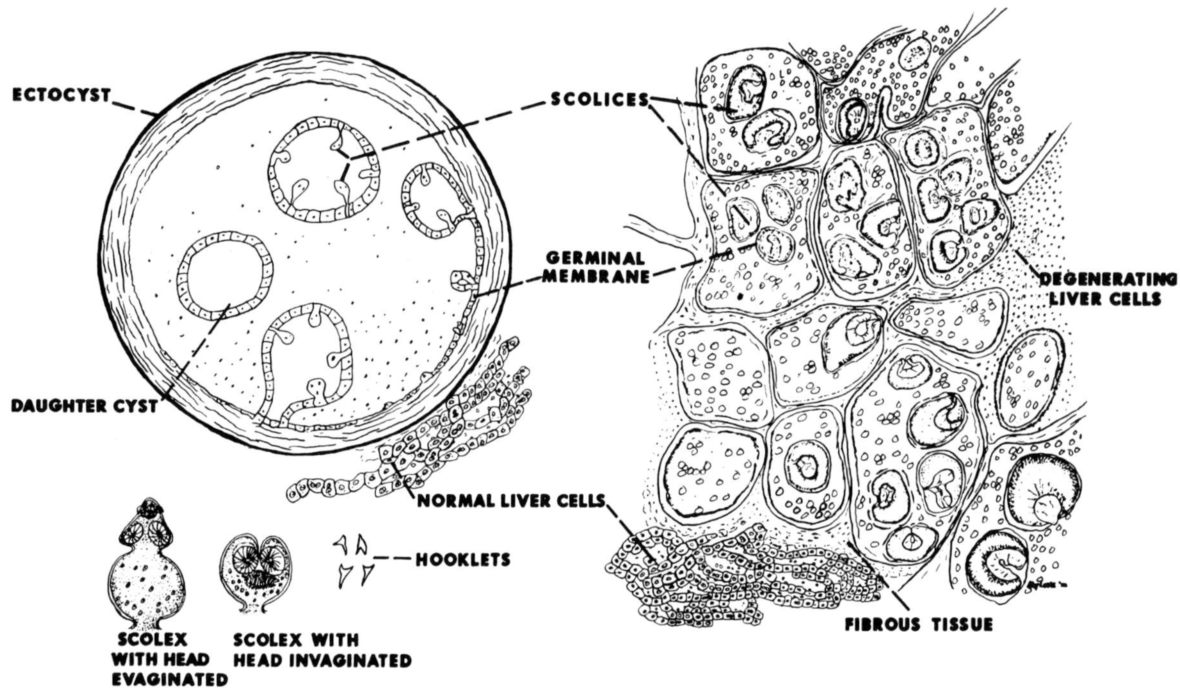

Fig. 3.5. Larvae of *E. granulosus* and *E. multilocularis*. In the *E. granulosus* larva (*left*), note the outer ectocyst, the acellular hyaline cuticle, the germinal membrane lining the endocyst, and, within the endocyst itself, the brood capsules with scolices and daughter cysts: note also the scolices with their heads evaginated or invaginated (*lower left*). By comparison, the *E. multilocularis* larva (*right*) buds outwards exogenously into the host tissue without the formation of an enveloping capsule. Note the numerous brood capsules containing invaginated scolices

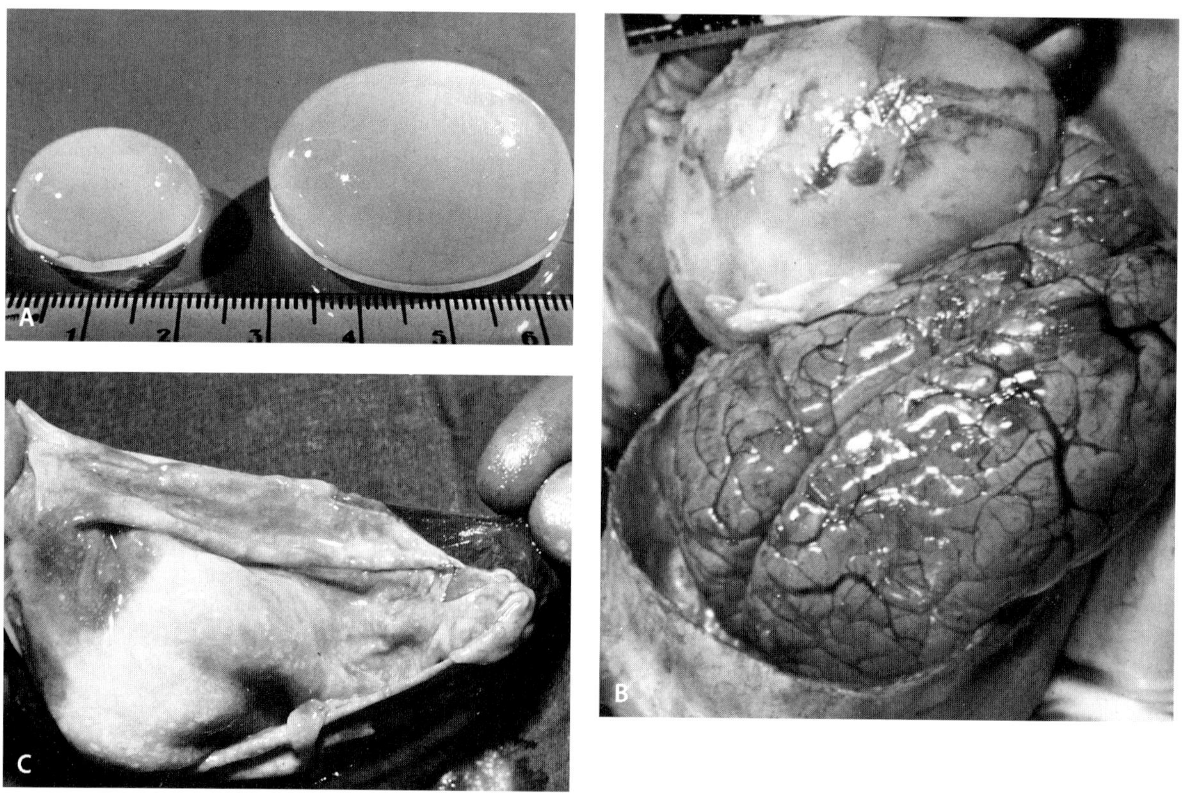

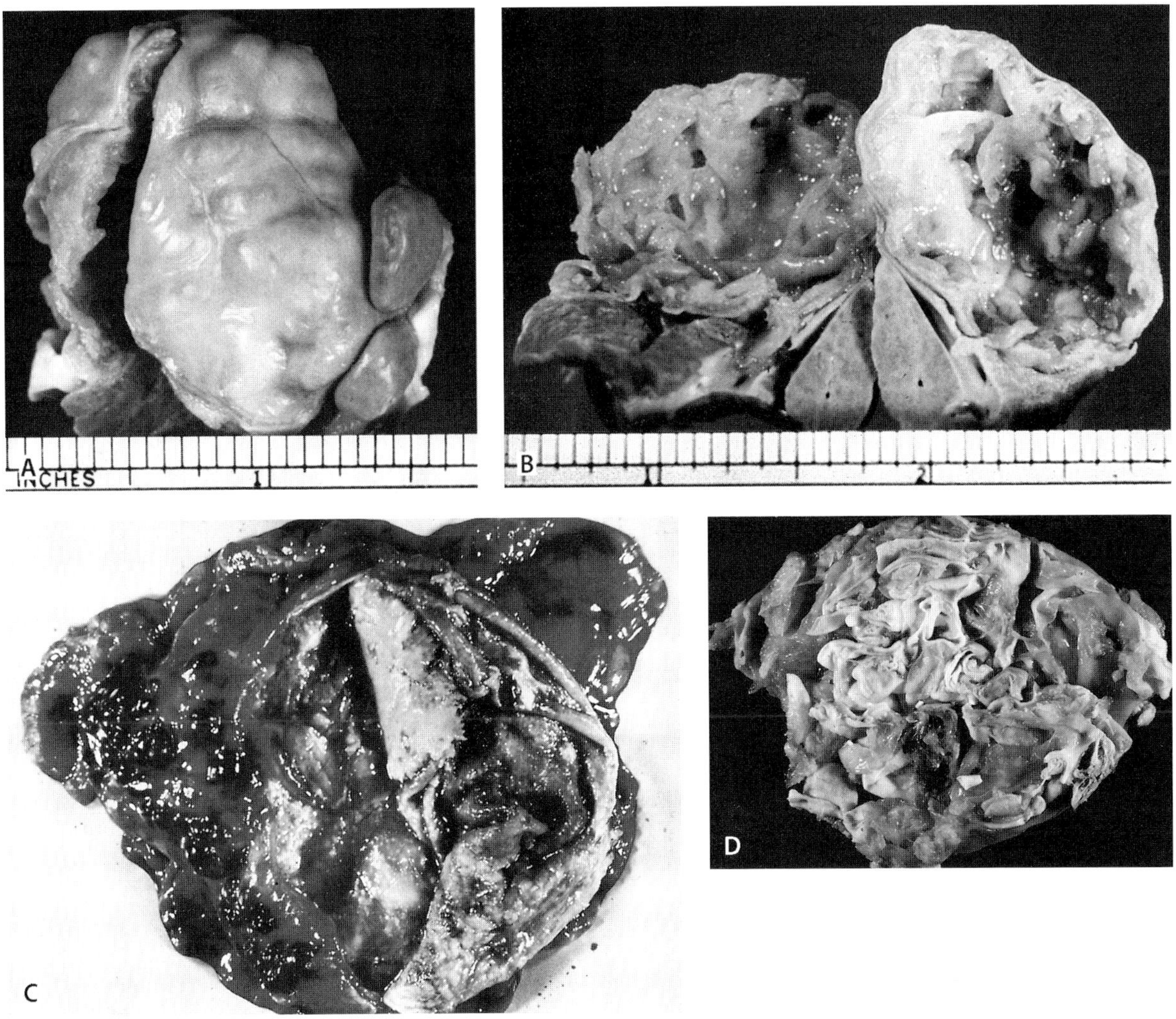

Fig. 3.7 A–D. *E. granulosus* cysts of the liver. **A** Gross specimen of a unilocular type I hydatid cyst of the liver showing a bosselated, nodular external surface. **B** The same cyst opened to show the glistening internal lining of the endocyst thrown into numerous folds. AFIP 66-11058-1 and 2. **C** Large unilocular cyst showing its glistening internal surface. **D** The gelatinous internal surface of another liver hydatid showing a markedly bosselated contour with brood capsules. AFIP 65-1843

◀ **Fig. 3.6 A–C.** Type 1 hydatid cysts. **A** Two intact unilocular hydatids. **B** A huge 250-g, 10×5 cm *E. granulosus* cyst bulging through the gray matter of the left cerebral hemisphere. An autopsy specimen from a 7-year-old Italian girl with vomiting, convulsions, headaches, intermittent drowsiness, fainting, and neck pain. She had neck stiffness, hyperactive knee jerks, positive Kernig and Babinski reflexes, and involuntary motions, and died after being in a deep coma for 2 days. (Courtesy of Dr. Howard Fink, Daytona Beach) **C** The inner lining of a large cerebral hydatid. The glistening membrane is studded with numerous tiny brood capsules containing scolices. **A** and **C** are from Africans in Zimbabwe

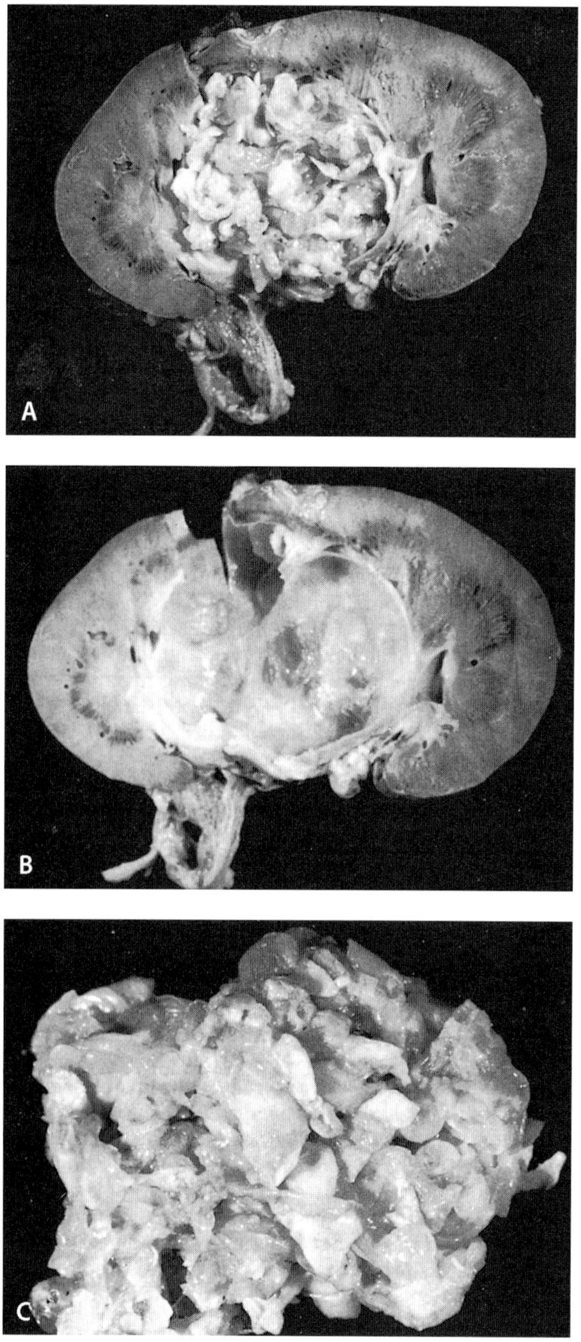

Fig. 3.8 A–C. A large unilocular type II hydatid cyst involving a kidney. **A** The kidney has been opened to show the renal pelvis with a large hydatid containing numerous daughter cysts. **B** The daughter cysts have been removed, revealing the glistening inner surface of the cyst. **C** The removed contents of the cyst showing numerous daughter cysts. AFIP 57-7659-1, 2 and 3

The hydatid's laminated membrane, which is white and slimy, is not elastic, yet its surface area increases and it becomes thicker as the hydatid sphere enlarges. It is not clear how such an acellular structure accomplishes this but presumably laminations are laid down to accommodate growth and repair. The host tissue adjacent to the cyst mounts a chronic inflammatory reaction. As this subsides, scar tissue forms arounds the cyst. This is the pericyst (ectocyst) and it protects the fragile hydatid much like a tire protects an inner tube. The pericyst, which is not demonstrable by ultrasonography or CT unless it is thickened or calcified (Figs. 3.12 A, 3.35 D), becomes thicker as the cyst enlarges. The pericyst around lung lesions is always quite thin, probably because the lung is less dense than liver. The thin pericyst allows the typical umbilication or notching of enlarging lung hydatids to occur where they contact bronchi and blood vessels. Blood vessels are obliterated within the developing pericyst, but bile ducts and bronchi are not. Eventually the increasingly substantial pericyst becomes a hindrance to further enlargement of the endocyst, forcing it to become redundant within the confines of the pericyst.

Those parts of the endocyst that become isolated from the nourishing hydatid fluid degenerate, forming a gelatinous amber-colored structure called matrix which may have a pseudotumoral appearance on ultrasonography or CT (Fig. 3.12). Because matrix is amorphous and yellow, it can be confused with pus by the surgeon. Matrix is most common in older patients who on average have harbored the parasite longer than the young. Lesions in the lung usually do not develop matrix, probably because enlargement of the cysts is relatively unrestricted until they become large enough that further growth is inhibited by the chest wall, mediastinum, or diaphragm.

Cysts and pericysts in the lung virtually never calcify for unknown reasons. Cysts in other sites, including the liver, spleen, kidney, mesentery, mediastinum, and pericardium, may calcify. Calcification of the pericyst, which can develop at all stages of the life cycle of hydatids, is found in nearly one-third of liver cysts (Fig. 3.12). Pericyst calcification does not always indicate that the cyst is dead, but calcification of the endocyst does (Fig. 3.13). Lesions in the spleen (Fig. 3.14) and kidney (Fig. 3.15) usually have a structure similar to those in the liver. Cysts in the peritoneal cavity elicit little pericyst reaction because they grow without compressing surrounding host parenchyma, which is the main source of pericyst tissue (Fig. 3.16). Brain cysts tend to be discovered before they develop daughters and matrix. Because they evoke little host reaction, brain lesions have an insubstantial pericyst (Fig. 3.17). Orbital hydatids cause unilateral exophthalmos and, if un-

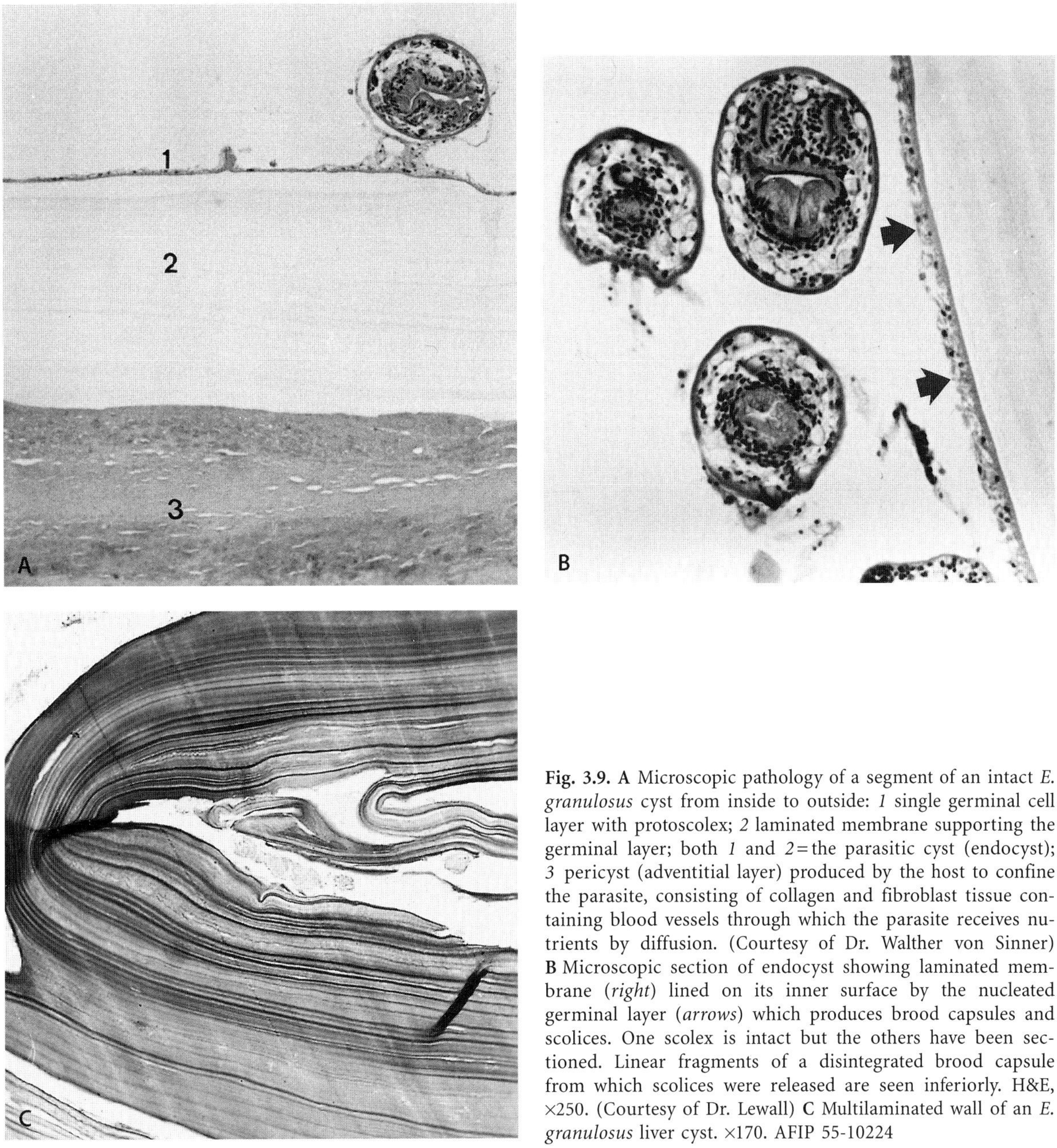

Fig. 3.9. **A** Microscopic pathology of a segment of an intact *E. granulosus* cyst from inside to outside: *1* single germinal cell layer with protoscolex; *2* laminated membrane supporting the germinal layer; both *1* and *2* = the parasitic cyst (endocyst); *3* pericyst (adventitial layer) produced by the host to confine the parasite, consisting of collagen and fibroblast tissue containing blood vessels through which the parasite receives nutrients by diffusion. (Courtesy of Dr. Walther von Sinner) **B** Microscopic section of endocyst showing laminated membrane (*right*) lined on its inner surface by the nucleated germinal layer (*arrows*) which produces brood capsules and scolices. One scolex is intact but the others have been sectioned. Linear fragments of a disintegrated brood capsule from which scolices were released are seen inferiorly. H&E, ×250. (Courtesy of Dr. Lewall) **C** Multilaminated wall of an *E. granulosus* liver cyst. ×170. AFIP 55-10224

treated, slowly compress the globe and enlarge the bony orbit, causing unilateral blindness (Fig. 3.18). Bone cysts occur most often in the pelvis, vertebral column, long bones, and skull and cause destruction without evoking bone reaction. A true pericyst develops only if cortical erosion allows involvement of soft tissue. This accounts for the often bizarre appearance of bony hydatids and possibly for their unusual propensity to cross joints and involve adjacent bones (Fig. 3.19).

Daughter cysts, which are thought to develop from scolices, are produced either synchronously with matrix or they may appear first (Fig. 3.20). They are generally considered an abnormal part of the parasite's life cycle. Many investigators theorize that daughter cysts are formed only when there is a threat to the continued existence of the hydatid in the form of mechanical, chemical, or bacterial insult. This may therefore be a defensive process of a damaged, degenerating, or dying cyst to guarantee survival. Even if the outer cyst is dead, daughter cysts may continue to survive and be infective, producing further daugher cysts, leading to the presence of multiple daughter and granddaughter cysts within a single unilocular hydatid cyst. The mother cyst and daughter cysts usually remain contained

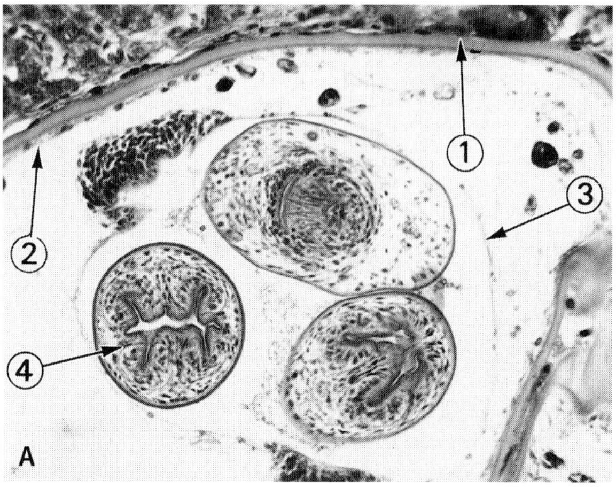

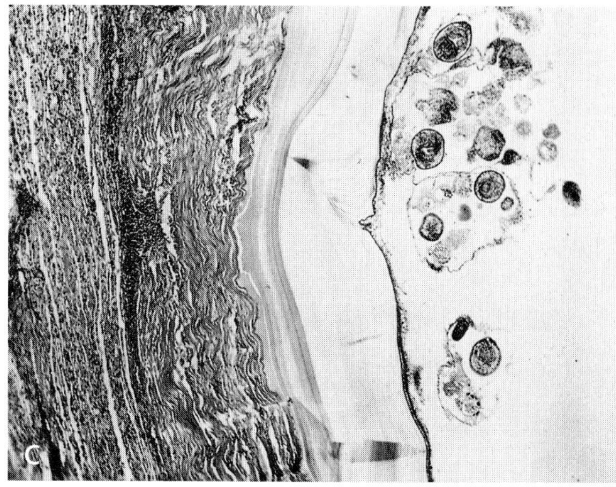

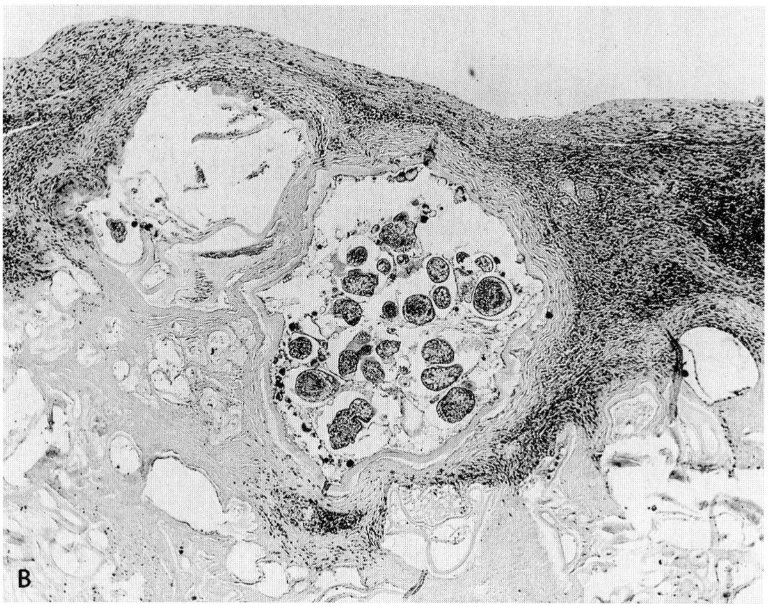

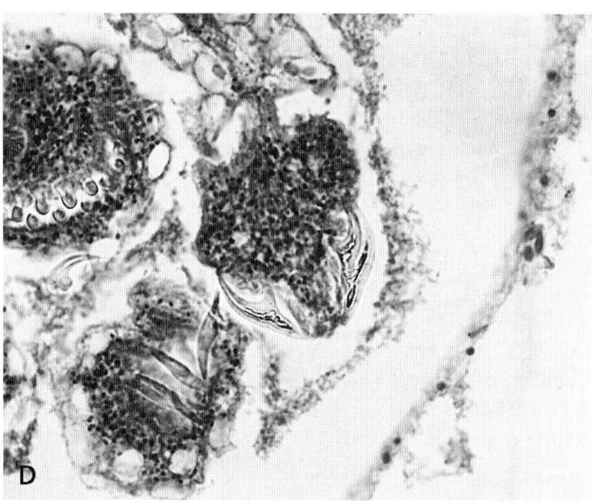

Fig. 3.10. A Microscopic section of a hydatid cyst showing brood capsules and scolices. This cross-section of a liver hydatid clearly reveals the acellular, hyaline, outer layer of the cyst (*arrow 1*) and the delicate inner layer or germinal membrane (*arrow 2*). A large brood capsule (*arrow 3*) arises from the germinal membrane as a vesicle one cell layer thick. Invaginated scolices (*arrow 4*) arise as buds from the inner surface of the brood capsule. AFIP 55-4985. **B** Hydatid cyst in the lung of a dog showing the thick pericyst, the thin germinal membrane of the endocyst, and several brood capsules containing multiple scolices. AFIP 56-11365. **C** A hydatid cyst of the liver showing the thick, acellular, adventitial layer, the thin germinal layer, and brood capsules with scolices. H&E, ×72; AFIP 65-2462. **D** Partially distintegrated brood capsules with scolices floating in the fluid of a hydatid cyst. Within the scolices can be seen the rostellum containing a double row of hooklets by which the worm attaches itself to the intestinal mucosa of a canine in its normal life cycle. The scolices arise as buds from the inner surface of the brood capsule, which in turn arises from the germinal epithelium of the endocyst (*right*). H&E, ×560; AFIP 65-2464

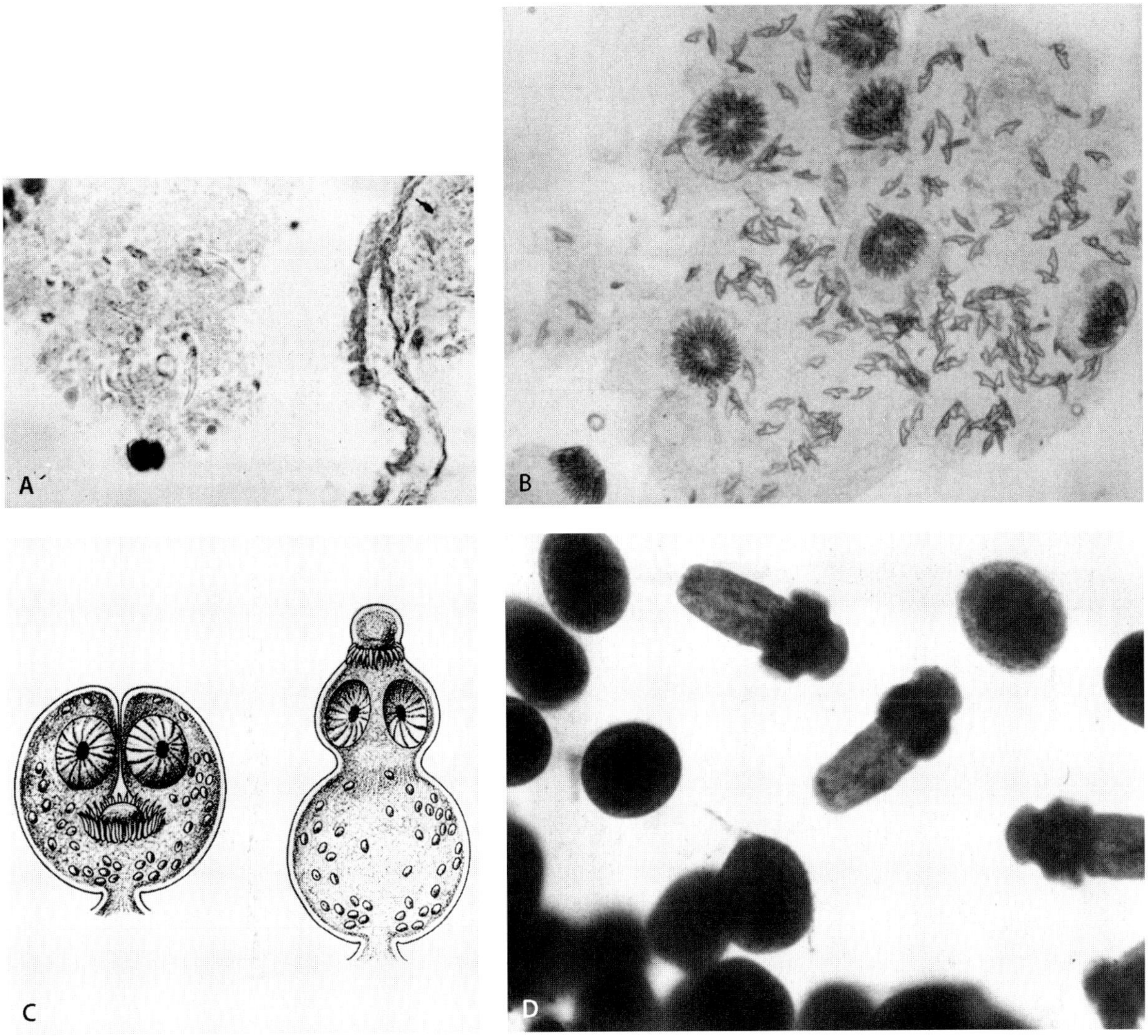

Fig. 3.11 A–D. Hydatid cysts contain "sand" or sediment with multiple scolices and hooklets. **A** The typical appearance of hydatid sand containing several scolices and hooklets floating free within the cyst fluid. The hooklets are birefringent and thus can be seen under polarized light. The germinal membrane lining the endocyst is on the right. AFIP 68-4760-2. **B** The sediment from a hydatid cyst containing numerous invaginated scolices with their hooklets, as well as free-floating, detached hooklets. **C** An invaginated scolex (*left*) and an evaginated scolex (*right*) showing the suckers and rostellum with its hooklets. AFIP 53-20053-6. **D** Numerous scolices, some free, some in cysts in the sediment at the bottom of a hydatid cyst. When the free scolices evert, the suckers may protrude to give a cross-like appearance

within the host-produced pericyst. Daughters replicate the structure of the mother cyst, but they do not stimulate production of their own pericyst as they are not in contact with host tissue. Cysts with a predominance of daughters are often erroneously thought to be septated (Fig. 3.21), but the "septa" are in fact the opposing walls of daughter cysts flattened by contact with one another. When the daughters are removed, the "septa" disappear.

All hydatid lesions start as purely cystic *type I* structures (Fig. 3.22), and if they develop daughter cysts or matrix (or both) they are termed *type II* cysts (Fig. 3.23). When the only remaining hydatid fluid is in daughter cysts, the lesion can be considered *hypermature* as it is probably nearing death by starvation (Fig. 3.23, 3.24). When formed elements completely replace the nourishing hydatid fluid, the type II lesion is starved, dies, and eventually becomes an end-stage calcified and biologically inert *type III* lesion (Fig. 3.25).

(Text continues on p. 221)

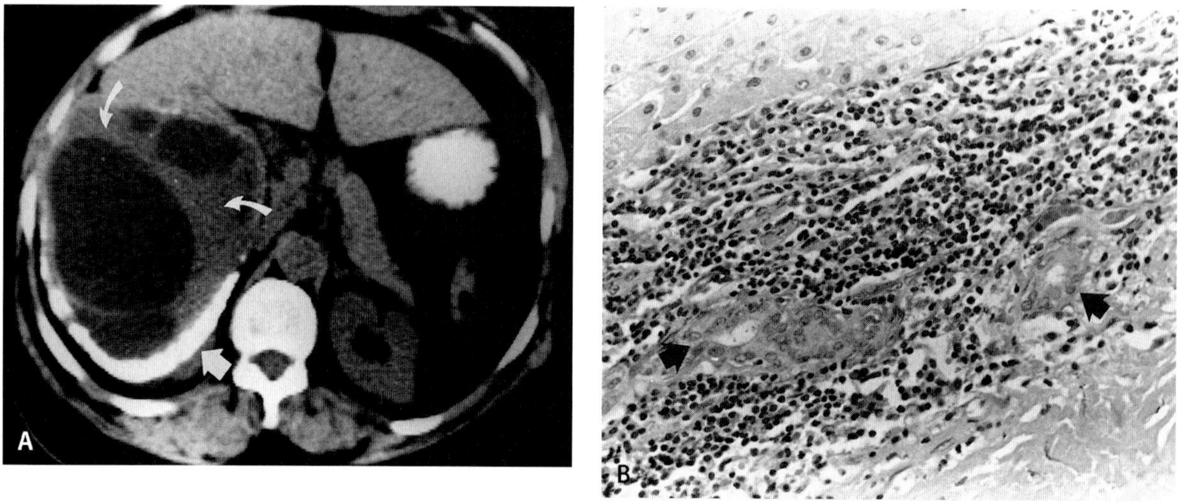

Fig. 3.12. **A** Transverse CT scan through liver showing type II hydatid with matrix (*curved arrows*) and daughter cysts. The pericyst is seen only where it is calcified (*broad arrow*). Pericyst calcification is usually neither as dense nor as asymmetrical as in this instance. On T2-weighted MR images the pericyst, whether calcified or not, appears as a zone of decreased signal intensity. **B** Photomicrograph of pericyst. Note hepatocytes in *upper left corner*. The highly cellular lymphoplasmacytic infiltrate contains bile ducts (*large arrows*) but not blood vessels. Collagen (*bottom right*), which is the toughest part of the pericyst, lies nearest to the parasite. The pericyst in the sampled region is not calcified. H&E, ×250. (Courtesy of Dr. Lewall and *Clinical Radiology*, 1998)

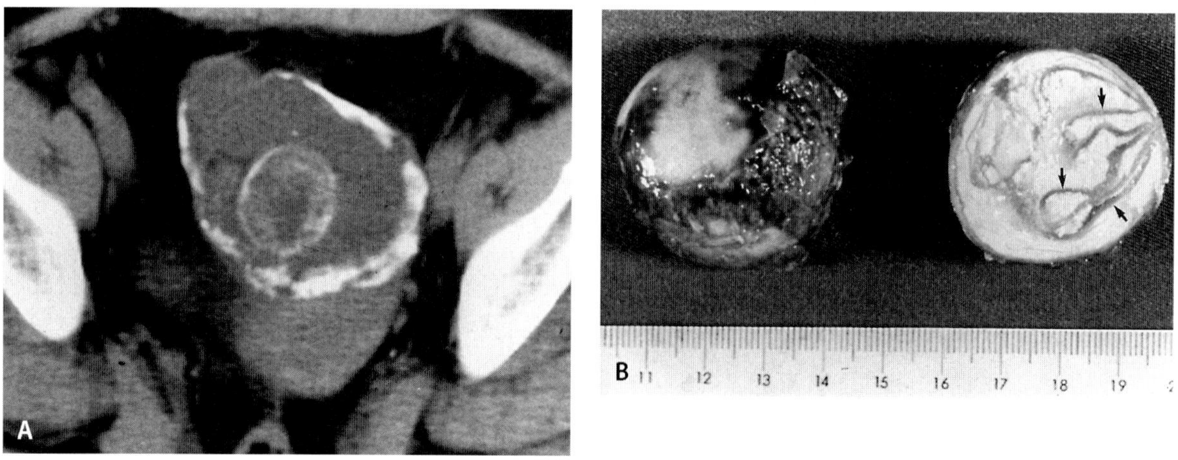

Fig. 3.13. **A** CT scan through true pelvis showing a type III hydatid. This was judged to be dead as the endocysts of both the daughter and the mother are calcified and the lesion has an irregular, nonspherical outline. Intraperitoneal hydatids evoke very little pericystic reaction because they do not compress host tissue as they do in the liver (Fig. 3.41). Thus, the peripheral calcification in this lesion is mainly endocystic, not pericystic. The indirect hemagglutination test for hydatid was negative and the lesion was not removed. In time it will probably become smaller and more densely calcified, to resemble the lesion in **B**. **B** Type III lesions are not normally resected, but as this one protruded beyond the liver edge it abraded the peritoneum as the patient breathed, causing pain. *Left*: external surface. *Right*: cut surface showing calcified matrix. Note the calcified laminated membranes (*arrows*). The remaining matrix, which is composed of older, more degenerated, and heavily calcified membranes, no longer has any discernible structure. The lesion was stony hard and had to be cut with a saw. (Courtesy of Dr. Lewall and *Clinical Radiology*, 1998)

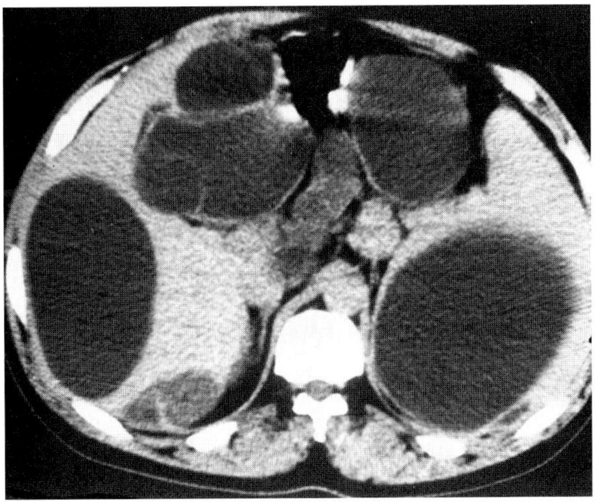

Fig. 3.14. Multiple hydatid cysts are identified on non-enhanced CT scan in the right and left lobes of the liver and in the spleen, most of which are type I except for a type II cyst in the anterior right lobe of the liver

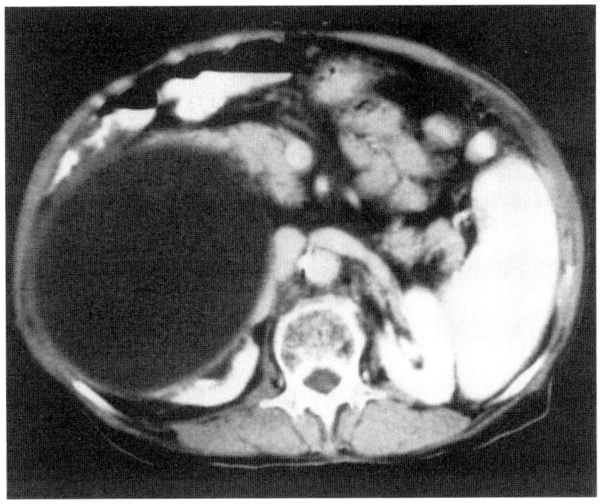

Fig. 3.15. CT scan through kidneys showing exophytic type I cyst of the right kidney. (Courtesy of Dr. Lewall and *Clinical Radiology*, 1998)

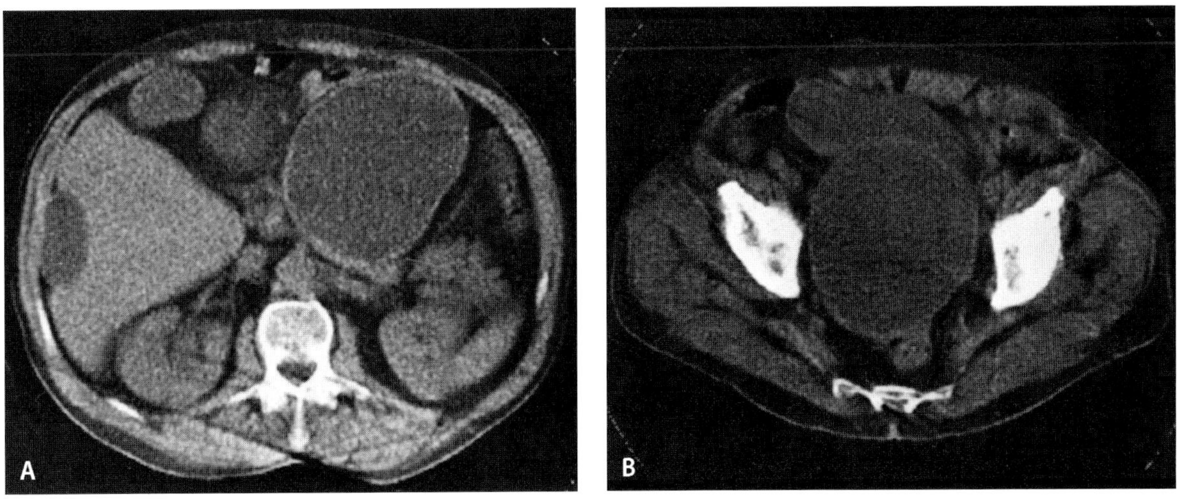

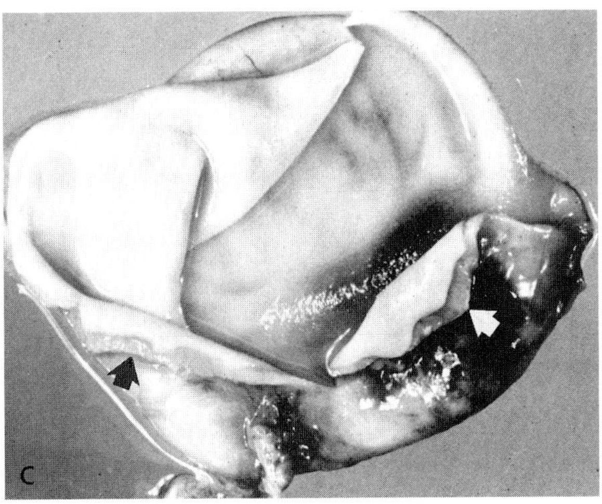

Fig. 3.16 A–C. Multiple type I hydatid cysts in the lateral aspect of the right lobe of the liver and the peritoneal cavity of the mid-abdomen (**A**) and pelvis (**B**). (Courtesy of Dr. John Haaga, Cleveland) **C** Opened type I intraperitoneal hydatid. Note the thin pericyst (*arrows*) formed mainly of fibrous tissue. The pericyst of intraperitoneal hydatids is so insubstantial that it is unwise to treat such lesions by percutaneous puncture for fear of provoking direct rupture. Purely medical treatment may be safer (see text). (Courtesy of Dr. Lewall and *Clinical Radiology*, 1998)

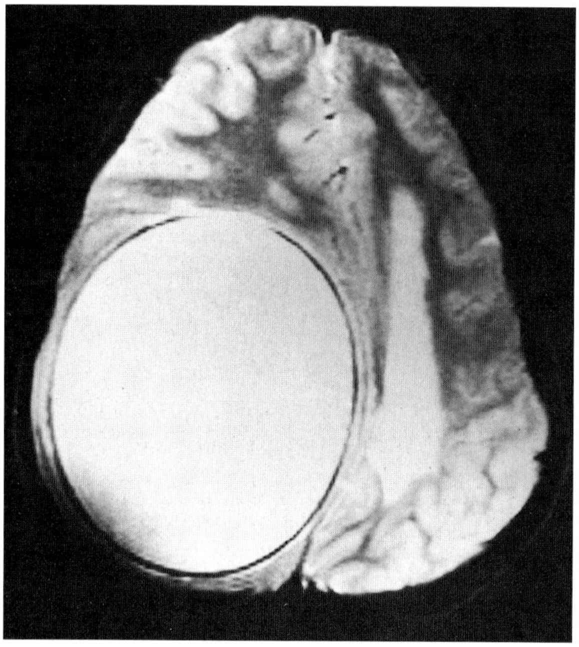

Fig. 3.17. Axial MR image (200/80) of right parietal hydatid cyst with peripheral rim of low signal intensity. (Courtesy of Dr. Walther von Sinner)

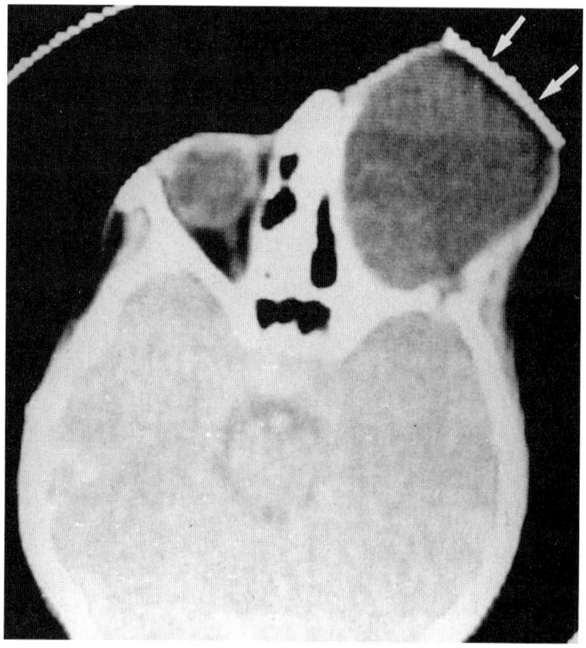

Fig. 3.18. CT scan of head showing a type I orbital hydatid cyst. The orbit is expanded but bone is not destroyed. The child arrived at hospital with her eyelids sutured together (*arrows*). (Courtesy of Dr. Lewall and *Clinical Radiology*, 1998)

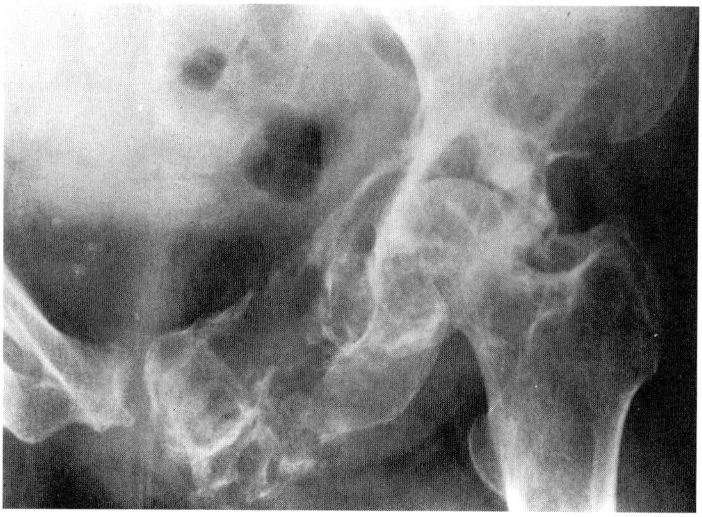

Fig. 3.19. Hydatid disease involving the left hemipelvis and hip. Although the bone is expanded and destroyed there is little evidence of attempted repair. The lesion crossed the hip joint and involved the femoral head and adjacent soft tissues (proven by CT and surgery). (Courtesy of Dr. Lewall and *Clinical Radiology*, 1998)

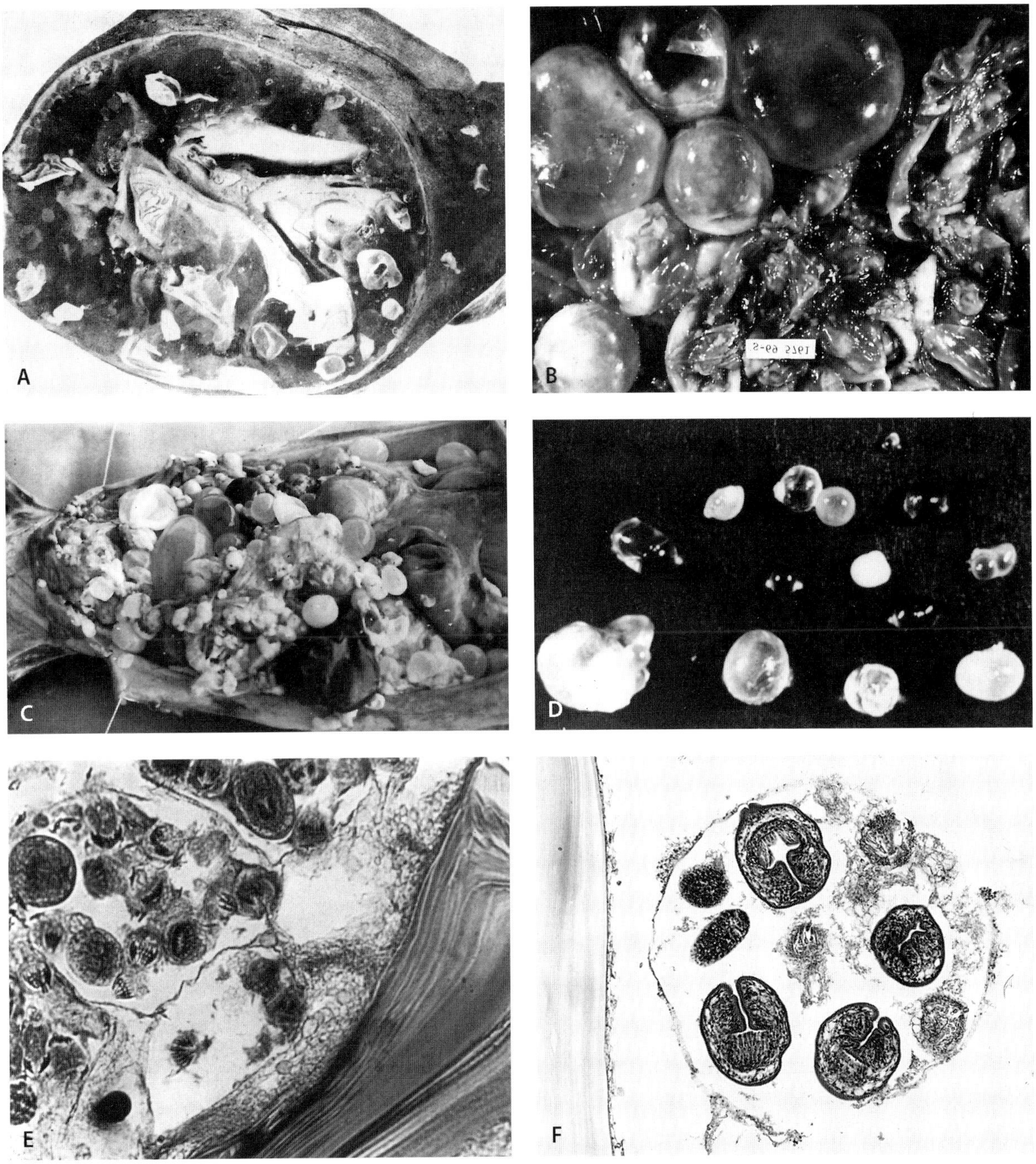

Fig. 3.20 A–F. The formation of daughter cysts in hydatid disease. Daughter cysts occur frequently in large, older unilocular cysts whose existence is threatened by some form of mechanical, chemical, or bacterial insult. These daughter cysts are thin-walled balloons formed from the detached germinal layer of the mother cyst or from brood capsule cells. **A** A large, unilocular hydatid cyst of the liver containing numerous daughter cysts which lie free in the cyst fluid. In this fluid there is also hydatid sand, containing free scolices and hooklets. AFIP N-31977. **B** Multiple daughter cysts lying free within a large unilocular hydatid. **C** Numerous daughter cysts in *E. granulosus* infection involving the abdominal cavity of a monkey. **D** Multiple small cysts taken from the vertebral column of a patient with signs and symptoms of lower cord compression. **E** Cyst of *E. granulosus* showing the characteristic laminated and proliferative layers. The daughter cysts contain scolices, many of which have degenerated as evidenced by the presence of free hooks. **F** A daughter cyst lying free within the mother cyst and containing multiple invaginated scolices. The germinal epithelium and laminated, acellular ectocyst of the mother hydatid are on the *left*. AFIP 65-2463

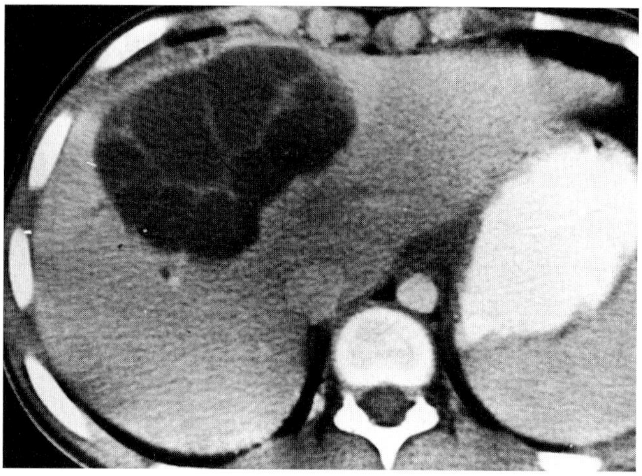

Fig. 3.21. CT scan of the liver showing a type II lesion with predominance of daughter cysts. The "septa" are the walls of daughter cysts flattened by contact with other daughters. (Courtesy of Dr. Lewall and *Clinical Radiology*, 1998)

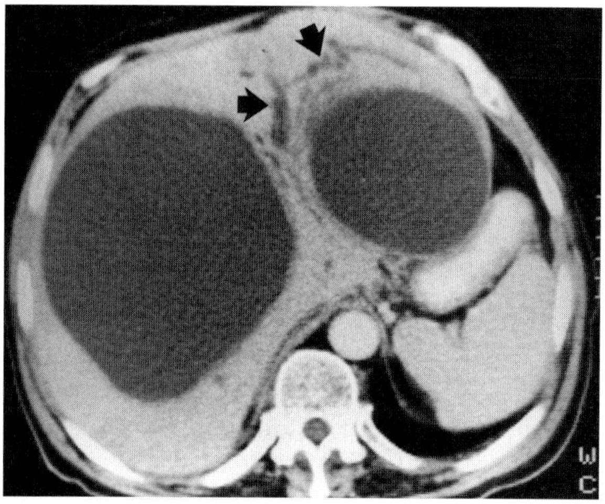

Fig. 3.22. Transverse CT scan through liver showing type I hydatid cysts. Hydatid sand, composed of brood capsules and scolices, settles to the dependent portion of the cyst but it cannot be resolved on CT images. However, sand can be shown by ultrasonography if the patient is rotated immediately before scanning so that the settling particles resemble a snow storm. An uncalcified pericyst and intact endocyst in intimate contact with the pericyst are not visible, but after rupture, a detached endocyst becomes visible by ultrasonography, CT and MRI (see Figs. 3.44 D, 3.45 D, 3.49). Note dilated pericystic ducts (*arrows*). (Courtesy of Dr. Lewall and *Clinical Radiology*, 1998)

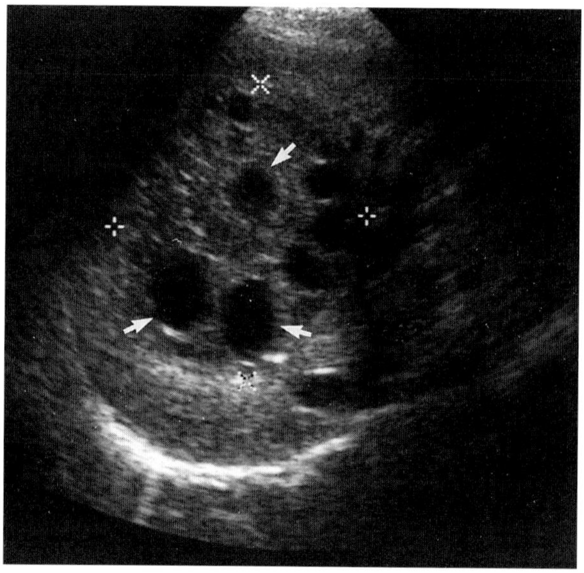

Fig. 3.23. Transverse ultrasound scan of a liver hydatid showing pseudotumoral appearance due to the abundance of echogenic matrix. The margins of the hydatid were defined by the sonographer with *crosses*. The fluid-containing daughter cysts (*arrows*) indicate the true nature of this hypermature type II cyst. (Courtesy of Dr. Lewall and *Clinical Radiology*, 1998)

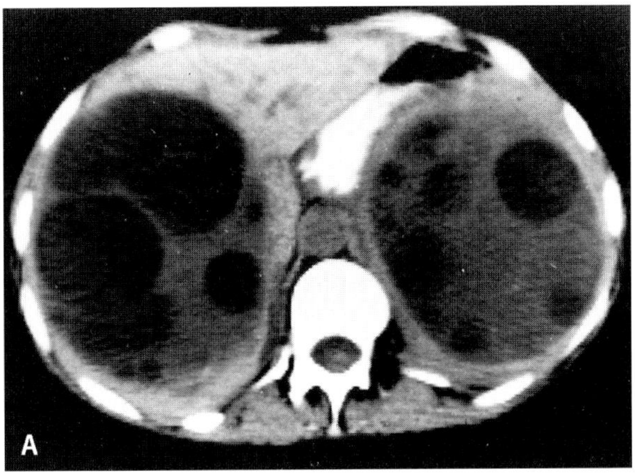

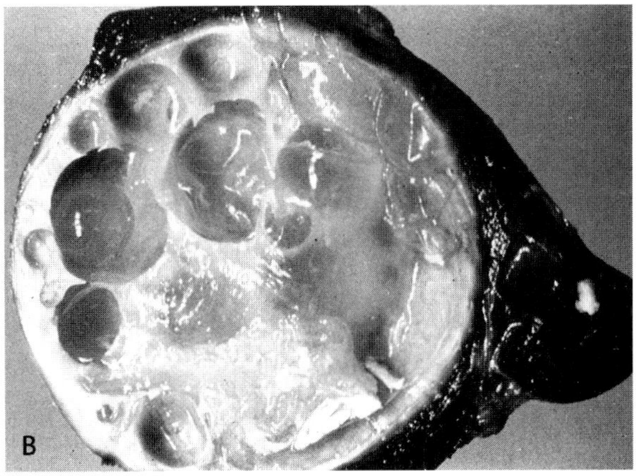

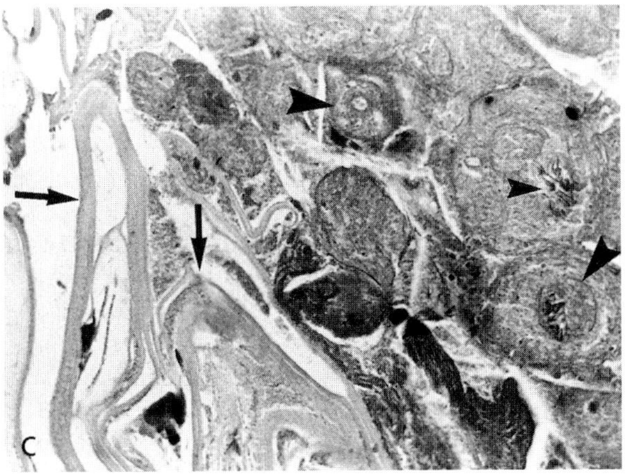

Fig. 3.24. **A** Transverse CT scan through liver and spleen showing hypermature type II hydatids in both organs with multiple daughter cysts and considerable matrix. Note dilated bile ducts anterior to the liver cyst. **B** Type II hydatid cyst in a cut spleen from another Saudi Arabian. Daughter cysts, which are embedded in matrix, originally completely filled the impressions in the matrix; the gaps between the two are artifactual due to dehydration of the daughters during formalin fixation. This is a hypermature lesion which probably would not have ruptured. **C** Photomicrograph of matrix (same patient). Note the folds of laminated membrane (*long arrows*), vestiges of scolices (*large arrowheads*), and hooklets (*small arrowhead*), all in advanced stages of degeneration. H&E; ×250. (Courtesy of Dr. Lewall and *Clinical Radiology*, 1998)

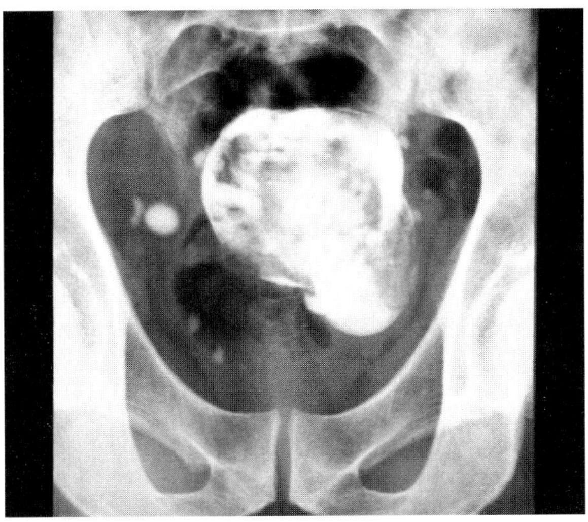

Fig. 3.25. Heavily calcified endocyst and pericyst of a biologically inert type III pelvic hydatid

The foregoing, which can be regarded as the natural history of hydatid cysts in the intermediate host, is often modified by rupture, which may cause biliary obstruction, infection, dissemination, and anaphylaxis, all of which are more important than the mass effect of the enlarging intact lesion. Type I lesions are more frequent than type II lesions. The incidence of type III lesions is unknown since these usually have no clinical importance and are rarely recorded, but personal experience (Lewall) suggests they are the most common type. The progression of hydatids from simple to complex is shown schematically in the column on the left side of Fig. 3.26.

It should be noted that Gharbi (1981), in his excellent report on 121 hydatid cysts of the liver seen in Tunisia, described five different types of ultrasound scans. This classification based on the sonographic analysis of the morphology and structure of liver hydatids, is still in use in many parts of the world but we prefer the classification described in this chapter, which is simpler and based on pathophysiology rather than a particular scanning modality. Gharbi's classification is as follows for comparison purposes: type I cyst: pure fluid collection; type II cyst: fluid collection

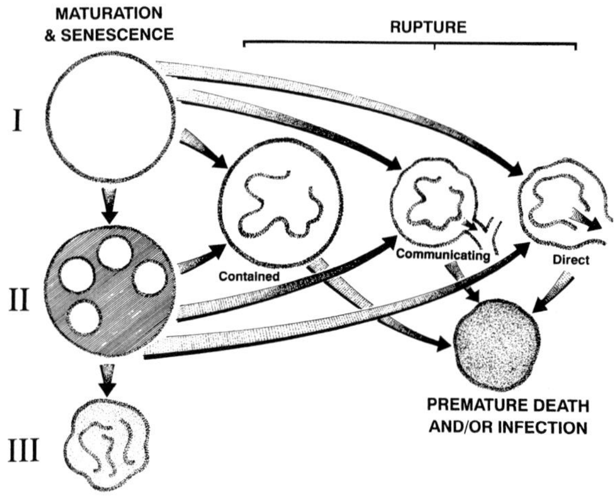

Fig. 3.26. Schematic representation of the natural history and complications of hydatid cysts. Cysts which have undergone contained rupture may die, but they do not become infected. The pericyst may calcify at any stage of maturation of the lesion and this does not imply that the lesion is dead. However, calcification of the endocyst and its contents is proof that the parasite has died. (Courtesy of Dr. Lewall and *Clinical Radiology*, 1998)

with a split wall; type III cyst: fluid collection with septa: type IV cyst: heterogeneous echo patterns; type V cyst: reflecting thick walls.

Degeneration by aging, trauma, toxins, chemotherapy, and lack of nutrients may lead to damage of the cyst wall with an increased risk of rupture. If this layer is damaged, infection nearly always occurs and the host may suffer hyperpyrexia and become severely ill; rarely, a fatal anaphylaxis may occur. If such a cyst is infected, it may transform into an abscess. After some time, the parasitic membranes are dissolved or destroyed. At this stage it is difficult to differentiate from other infected cysts or abscesses (e.g., amebic or bacterial). Sometimes the pathognomonic hydatid hooklets are still seen in infected cysts when all other evidence of parasitic material has been destroyed. When ruptured, the older mother cyst nearly always dies, but daughter cysts often survive. Perhaps 10%–30% of cysts die and disintegrate without treatment.

The increasing size of a cyst may lead to degeneration, causing the production of brood capsules or daughter cysts. In older and larger cysts, not only may indigenous daughter cysts develop from the germinal layer but some investigators contend that exogenous daughter cysts may develop also from herniation of a portion of the cyst wall into adjacent normal tissues. These are thought to separate entirely from the mother cyst to become secondary hydatid cysts, often in the mesentery and pelvis. Convincing histopathological proof for this contention is not available.

The severity of *Echinococcus* infection is governed by three basic factors: (1) the species; (2) the organ or body tissues in which the larva develops; and (3) whether or not secondary cysts develop. The *E. granulosus* unilocular cyst has only one cyst or several totally isolated cysts; each cyst is enclosed in its own solid laminated membrane, which acts as a barrier preventing the living germinal epithelium of the endocyst from invading adjacent normal tissue. The unilocular cyst induces formation of an enveloping fibrous capsule or pericyst. The *E. vogeli* polycystic or multilocular cysts, however, have many cysts embedded within a common adventitious membrane. The *E. multilocularis* alveolar cysts show an aggressive growth pattern within the liver with metastatic lesions elsewhere. A series of proliferating vesicles infiltrate into the surrounding host tissues, resembling malignancy. This type of hydatid disease will be discussed later (p. 333).

In many patients with *E. granulosus* infection, there are numerous cysts, depending on the number of ova ingested and the number that survive: two or more cysts may be present in the same or different organs. Estimates of multiple cysts vary widely: 5%–25% in some series, 30%–60% in others. On average, lesions are over twice as likely to be solitary as multiple and multiorgan involvement occurs in 10%–15% of patients. Multiple cysts are more common in the liver than in the lungs and elsewhere (except in metastatic hydatidosis), but, even when multiple, are distinct from the alveolar "malignant" cysts of *E. multilocularis.* Despite the frequency of multiple cysts, it should be remembered that a solitary cyst in any location within the body might well be a hydatid cyst (it may truly be the only cyst present or it may not be possible to recognize others clinically or by diagnostic imaging).

As already noted, the liver is the most common site of infection in echinococcosis, being involved in 50%–70% of all cases. The lungs are infected in approximately 15%–30% of all patients and are followed by the kidneys (4%), muscle (4%), spleen (3%), central nervous system (3%), soft tissues (3%), bone (2%), peritoneum and mesentery (2%), and heart, mediastinum, pleura, breast, thyroid, salivary glands, omentum, pancreas, orbit, and spinal canal (<1%–2%).

In one large series of 1350 hydatid patients, 250 had cysts in the lung, with 16 cases being bilateral. In children, however, there is some evidence from Australia that pulmonary hydatid disease may be as frequent as liver involvement there. Of 90 patients in a children's hospital in Sydney, 45 had pulmonary and 46 had hepatic cysts; of 72 pediatric patients from Melbourne, 36 had pulmonary cysts, 18 hepatic and 9 combined pulmonary and hepatic.

Complications

Rupture

The causes of rupture include trauma, medical treatment and degeneration of the endocyst. Three types of rupture are possible: *contained, communicating*, and *direct*.

Contained Rupture. A contained rupture occurs when the endocyst ruptures in a lesion in which patent biliary radicals (or bronchi in the case of pulmonary lesions) do not penetrate the pericyst (Fig. 3.27). The actual incidence of contained rupture is unknown since it is asymptomatic and is diagnosed fortuitously when sectional imaging shows floating membranes within the hydatid lesion. Lung hydatids are often not imaged by CT or MRI and virtually never by ultrasonography so contained rupture of lung lesions is probably underdiagnosed. Contained rupture does not invariably cause premature death of the cyst and does not predispose to secondary bacterial infection.

Communicating Rupture. Communicating rupture is possible when biliary radicals or bronchi perforate the pericyst in the liver or lung, allowing fluid and formed elements to escape into the biliary or bronchial tree (Fig. 3.28). Communicating rupture in the lung leads to expectoration of salty fluid and sometimes of fragments of endocyst, which the patient describes as "grape skins." If air enters the partially evacuated pericyst cavity, the "floating water lily sign" is seen on upright chest radiographs. Communicating rupture is apparently more common in lung than liver, presumably because of a higher incidence of bronchial than biliary patency through the pericyst. This is probably because bronchi are more robust than bile ducts and are less likely to be obliterated by the developing pericyst. Communicating rupture of lung cysts does not always kill the parasite. Because of the propensity of lung cysts to rupture, surgeons usually operate on lung lesions before they attend to those in the liver if the patient has both. Scolices probably do not survive in the hostile environment of the biliary tree, but scolices that were accidentally spilled into the tracheobronchial tree during resection of pulmonary hydatids were estimated to be the cause of secondary lung lesions in 0.61% of 650 patients. Thus, it is likely that spontaneous communicating rupture of lung cysts can lead to transbronchial spread of hydatid disease. The distinction between contained and communicating rupture is not always possible.

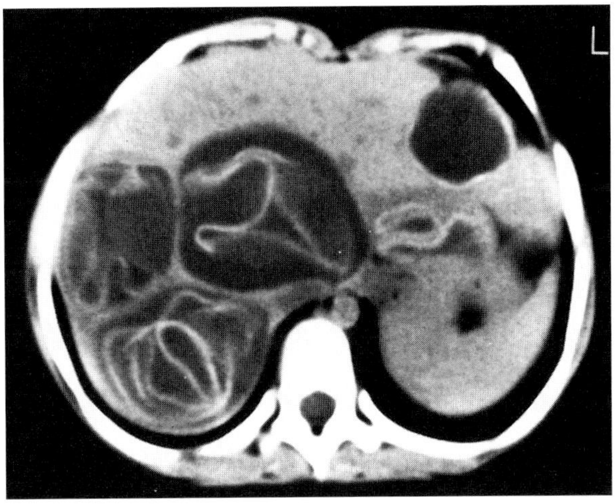

Fig. 3.27. Transverse CT scan through the liver showing ruptured type I hydatid cysts in a Saudi Arabian child who was treated medically with an oral antihelminthic which killed the cysts and caused spontaneous rupture. Because the cysts did not become smaller and there was no evidence of biliary obstruction, the rupture was assumed to be contained. Purely medical treatment is generally avoided in such cases because of the danger of provoking communicating or direct rupture. This patient was lost to follow-up. (Courtesy of Dr. Lewall and *Clinical Radiology*, 1998)

Direct Rupture. Direct rupture, which can have disastrous consequences, occurs when both endocyst and pericyst are torn. This usually happens to lesions near the edge of the liver, where the protective pericyst may be deficient and where there is little host tissue to offer support. In the lungs, the thin pericyst and compliant pulmonary parenchyma around cysts offer relatively poor protection to the endocyst. Fluid and infectious scolices spill into the peritoneal or pleural cavity causing seeding (Fig. 3.30) and often anaphylaxis, which is much more frequent after direct rupture than after communicating rupture, apparently as a result of antigenic hydatid fluid contacting a serosal surface.
Direct rupture into many sites has been reported, including the liver, bile ducts (Fig. 3.29), pleura, lung, gastrointestinal tract, and great vessels. Direct rupture into soft tissues almost certainly explains the development of small satellite lesions around a cyst. This type of rupture probably accounts for most reports of recurrence after surgery. Other causes of "recurrence" are small lesions that were not detected preoperatively, and growth of new lesions resulting from spillage of scolices during surgery. More complex explanations of recurrence such as exophytic growth do not seem tenable on biological grounds because there is no germinal layer on the outside of the endocyst. Bulging of part of the wall of the mother cyst, sometimes seen when cysts are near the edge of the liver or when they abut a fissure, must not be confused with exophytic budding.

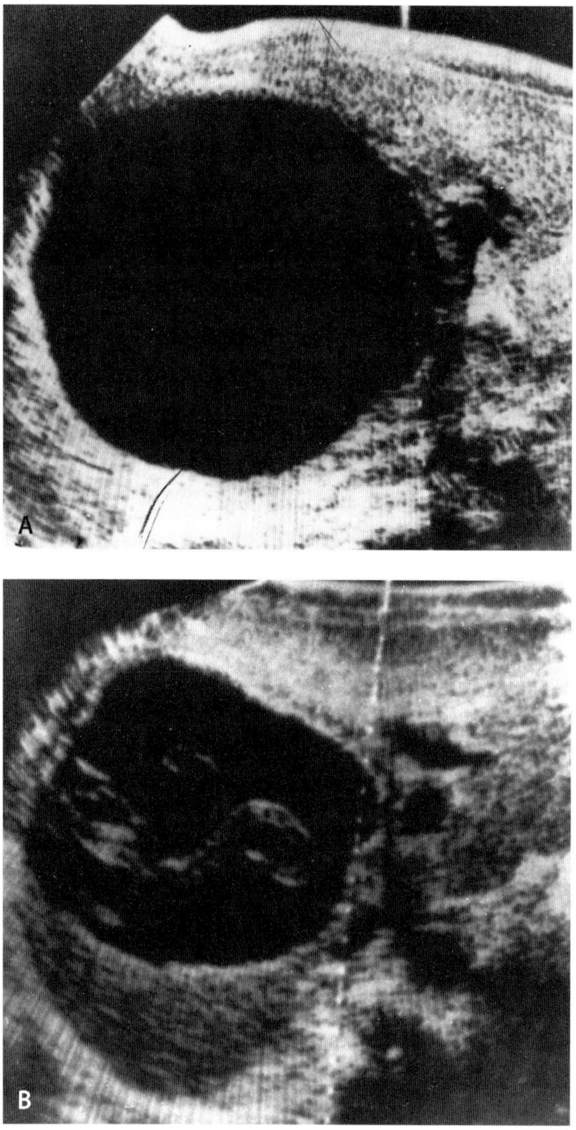

Fig. 3.28. **A** Longitudinal ultrasound scan of liver showing type I cyst prior to treatment. **B** Transverse ultrasound scan after treatment with an oral antihelminthic which caused the cyst to rupture. The fact that the cyst became smaller and less spherical proves that this is a communicating rupture even though dilated bile ducts are not demonstrable. Note the detached endocyst membranes on this transverse scan. A few days after this examination this Saudi Arabian patient developed biliary obstruction and required surgery. (Courtesy of Dr. Lewall and *Clinical Radiology*, 1998)

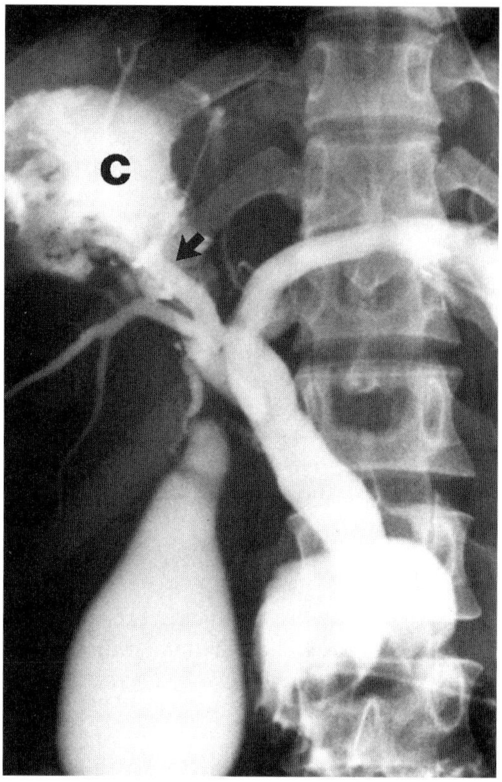

Fig. 3.29. Endoscopic retrograde cholangiopancreatography showing connection between the biliary tree and a type II cyst. During prolonged medical treatment before intended elective surgery the cyst ruptured and this Saudi Arabian patient developed biliary obstruction. Urgent surgery was performed to avoid the development of cholangitis. *C* collapsed pericyst. *Arrow* communicating bile duct. (Courtesy of Dr. Lewall and *Clinical Radiology*, 1998)

▶

Fig. 3.30. Transverse CT scan through false pelvis showing late sequel of spontaneous direct rupture into the peritoneal cavity. Secondary type I and II cysts developed from scolices that spilled into the peritoneal cavity. (Courtesy of Dr. Lewall and *Clinical Radiology*, 1998)

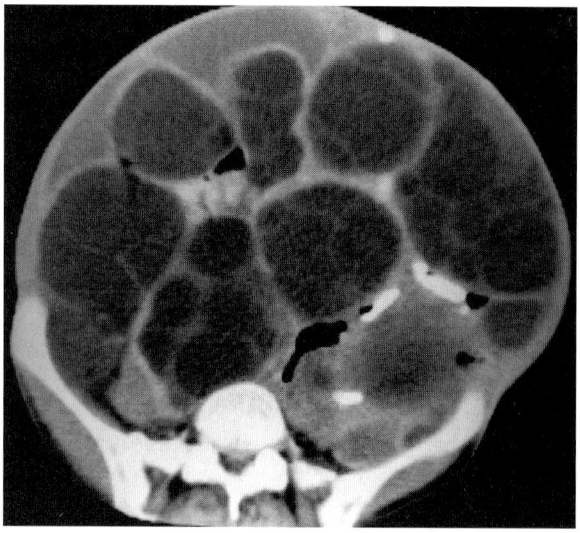

Biliary obstruction is usually not a feature of direct rupture because the cyst is quickly decompressed and solid elements are not forced into downstream ducts. Direct rupture usually leads to premature death of the cyst and theoretically can result in bacterial infection of the pericyst cavity.

Hydatid cysts in any site which result from rupture are termed *secondary cysts* (Figs. 3.30, 3.31). Most pleural cysts result from direct rupture of lung hydatids into the pleural space or from rupture of liver cysts through the diaphragm. Biliary-bronchial fistulae are a consequence of direct rupture of a liver cyst through the diaphragm and pleural membranes into the lung. The inflammatory reaction elicited by bile in the lung facilitates the biliary-bronchial connection. Cyst rupture is shown diagrammatically in Fig. 3.26.

Infection

Infection occurs only after communicating or direct rupture (usually the former) because bacteria-transporting blood vessels do not penetrate the intact pericyst. Infection associated with communicating rupture and biliary obstruction can result in an abscess within the pericyst cavity or in cholangitis, and probably always kills the parasite. Because of the danger of infection, biliary obstruction must be relieved promptly. Infection leads to loss of clarity of interior detail of the cyst, and fluid elements become echogenic by ultrasonography and denser by CT. The endocyst is usually seen to have detached from the pericyst, and occasionally gas is produced in the cyst.

Premature Death

Premature death is defined as death of the parasite that is not the result of starvation of a hypermature type II lesion; it may occur after rupture (Fig. 3.32), infection, or medical treatment. When a type I lesion dies prematurely after rupture it may develop directly into a type III lesion. However, a prematurely dead type I lesion followed for 30 months did not calcify (Lewall), so it is possible that such lesions are sometimes eventually resorbed. Unless infection produces gas, premature death and infection have identical appearances on CT and ultrasonography although they have very different clinical presentations. In both instances the fluid component becomes echogenic on ultrasonography and denser on CT (Fig. 3.32), and there is a loss of clarity of the internal detail of the lesion. With both methods of imaging the endocyst is usually seen to be detached from the pericyst. Premature death apparently does not produce a diagnostic change in the MR signal. Infection and premature death are indistinguishable with current imaging methods.

The proposed classification of the natural history and complications of hydatids (Fig. 3.26) is modified from two earlier classifications (Lewall).

Laboratory Diagnosis

The most satisfactory tests for hydatidosis currently in use are the indirect fluorescent antibody, immunoelectrophoresis, the enzyme-linked immunosorbent assay (ELISA), and the radioallergosorbent (RAST) tests. However, these tests are time-consuming and require a laboratory equipped with proper instruments and trained technicians. A new dot immunobinding assay for the detection of hydatid antigen-specific antibodies (HA-DIA) has been described (Mistrello et al., 1995). Correlation with ELISA-IgG and RAST-IgE was significant. HA-DIA (Echinostrip) has been demonstrated to be of good predictive value, allowing for speedy diagnosis of hydatid disease in the doctor's office and for large-scale screening of populations in developing countries, and helping to confirm the findings of epidemiological ultrasound surveys.

Overall sensitivity of tests for serum antibody detection in cystic echinococcosis remains in the range of 50%–80%. In individual patients the identification of IgG subclasses may allow the diagnosis of various clinical manifestations of the disease. Extensive studies from patients with cystic echinococcosis have shown that higher concentrations of IgG4 antibodies against *E. granulosus* antigen B correlate with illness, and a more or less active cyst, and to some extent provide an assessment of cyst viability.

The laboratory tests used in the diagnosis of hydatid disease formerly included the Casoni intradermal test and the Weinberg complement fixation test: these tests have been widely abandoned because of their unreliability. Intradermal tests are true-positive in approximately 65% of patients at best and more accurate when hydatids are in the liver rather than in lungs, brain, and other organs. The complement fixation test is reportedly positive in up to 70% of cases and remains positive for up to 2 years after surgical removal of a cyst. It is thus a somewhat unreliable indicator of residual cysts elsewhere in the body. False-positives are also possible as a result of cross-reaction by infection with other parasites (e.g., *Schistosoma*). A slight eosinophilia above 5% is present in about 20%–25% of patients with hydatid disease.

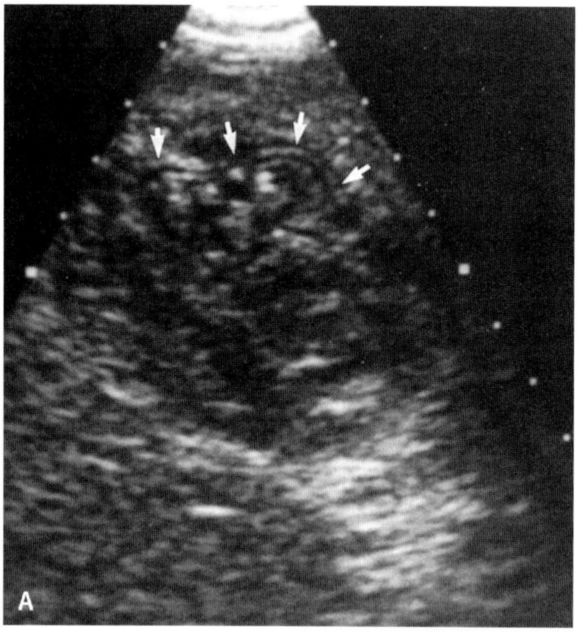

Fig. 3.31 A–E. Numerous secondary abdominal and pelvic hydatid cysts in a 19-year-old Saudi Arabian man. **A** Abdominal ultrasonography shows complex hepatic cystic changes with double-line structures representing collapsed parasitic membranes (*arrows*). **B** Nonenhanced CT reveals multiple hydatid cysts in the liver, spleen, and mesentery. **C** CT of the pelvis without contrast enhancement shows a large number of pelvic hydatids. **D** T1-weighted MR image, coronal view, right side (TR 850 ms, TE 20 ms), reveals a ruptured hydatid cyst with peritoneal spillage (*black curved arrows*). Observe also the prolapsed hydatid into the right lung base from the right liver lobe (*straight black arrows*). **E** T2-weighted MR image, axial view, right side (TR 2000 ms, TE 100 ms), reveals a ruptured hydatid cyst with discharge of cystic contents and peritoneal spillage (*large straight black arrows*). Note also the low-intensity rim (*small black arrows*) and pericystic reaction with edema (*curved open arrows*). (Courtesy of Dr. Walther von Sinner)

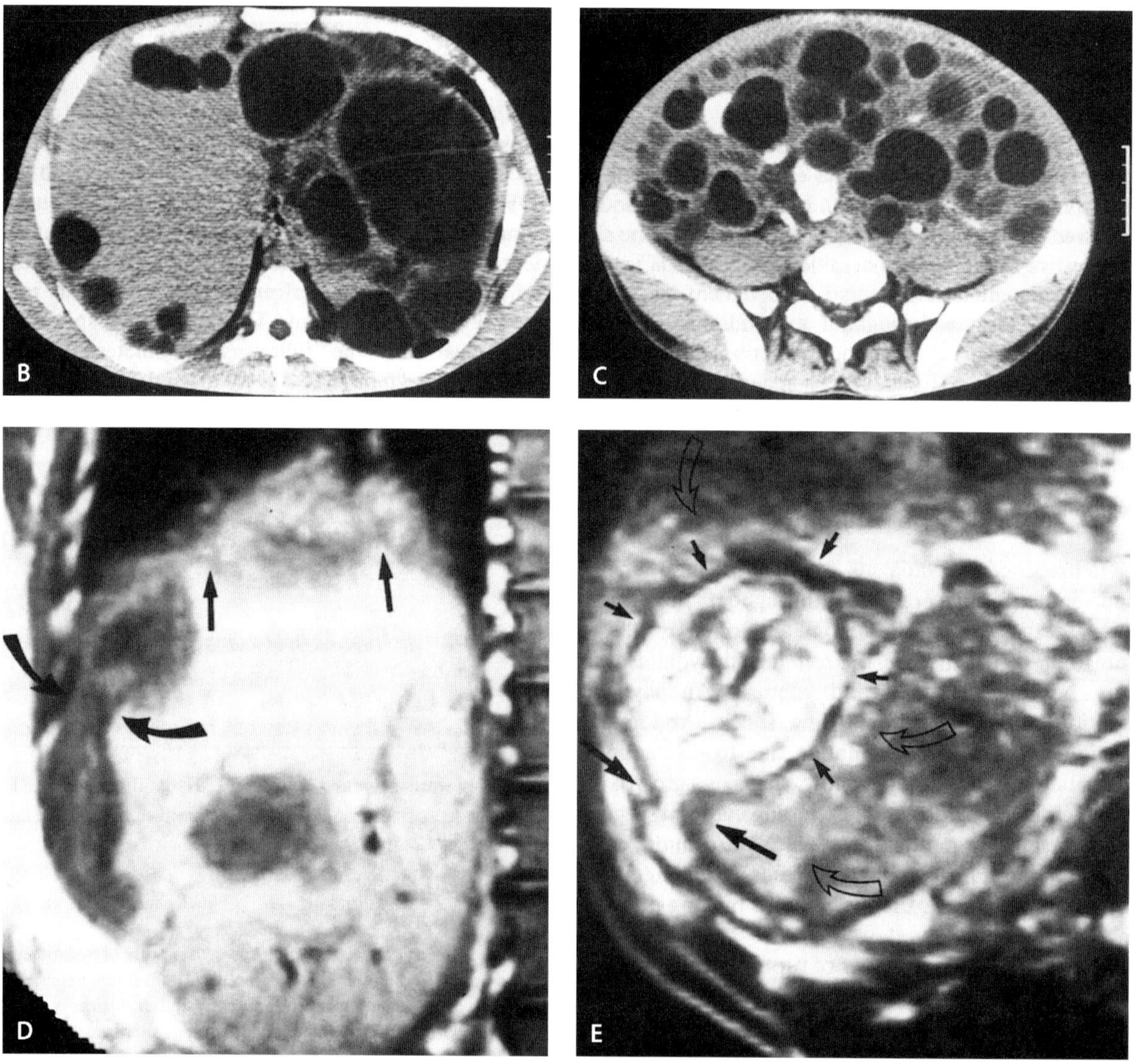

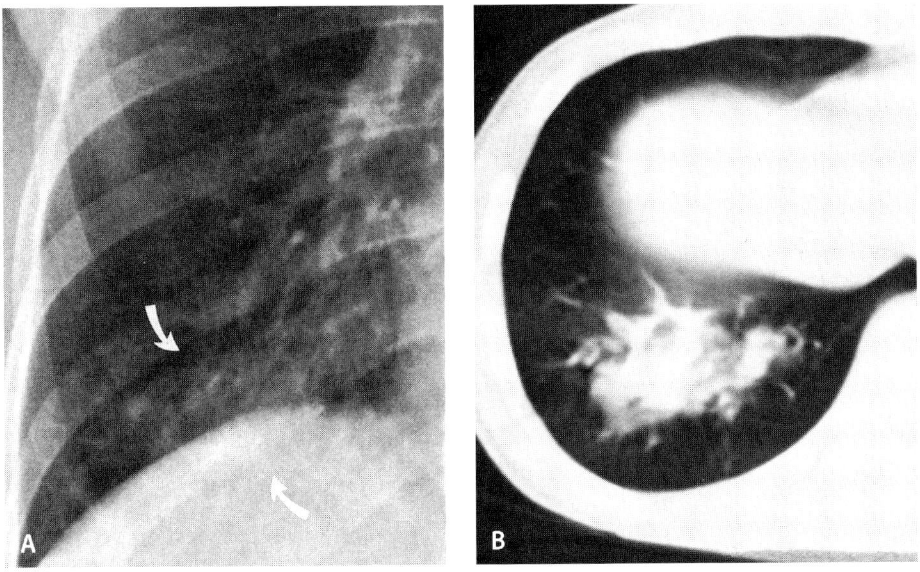

Fig. 3.32. **A** Hazy or fuzzy contour of an old dead and ruptured pulmonary hydatid cyst. **B** Nonenhanced CT scan reveals sunburst appearance of the same ruptured and collapsed pulmonary hydatid in the right lower lobe of a Saudi Arabian. Unless infection causes gas production, premature death and infection of a hydatid have identical appearances on ultrasonography and CT. The fluid component becomes echogenic on ultrasonography and denser on CT, and there is a loss of clarity of the internal detail of the lesion. (Courtesy of Dr. Walther von Sinner)

Clinical Characteristics

It is surprising how many cysts there may be in small children (and also in adults) or how large a single cyst can grow without any clinical complaints from the patient. The location of the cyst is clinically the important factor: in the chest or abdomen, cysts may remain silent for many years. In the brain, orbit, or spine they become clinically apparent much sooner. As a general rule, significant symptoms and physical evidence of the mass are unusual before the cyst has reached at least 10 cm in diameter: many deep cysts are not easily palpable until they are almost 20 cm in diameter. Hydatid cysts are long-lived and, in some human hosts, may remain viable for up to 53 years.

As already noted, the severity of the infection depends on the species, but clinically it is also the other two factors of location and spread which strongly influence the way hydatidosis will develop in any patient: clinical symptoms result from increasing pressure from the cyst(s) or from the sequelae of cyst rupture. In some patients, trauma will rupture a cyst and the symptoms then depend on the position of the cyst and which way it leaks. Thus, there may be acute abdominal pain if rupture occurs within the abdomen. Fever and an acute hypersensitivity reaction, including urticaria and, rarely, anaphylactic shock or death, may occur after direct cyst rupture at any site. Numerous scolices are discharged from the ruptured cyst to give rise to new daughter cysts (secondary hydatidosis) (Figs. 3.30, 3.31). If the primary cyst erodes into a vein, metastatic hydatidosis may develop in the lungs and other organs.

When a cyst ruptures in the lungs, there may be abrupt onset of coughing and expectoration. Cardiac hydatids may give rise to metastatic hydatids or cardiac tamponade; there may be dyspnea from mediastinal cysts compressing the trachea or a tension pneumothorax if rupture occurs into the pleura. Pressure symptoms such as bone pain, spontaneous fracture and deformity, hemorrhage due to erosion of a major vessel, and cerebral symptoms of epilepsy and blindness may all occur.

Many hydatids in the liver will remain clinically silent for a long time, but with gradual enlargement most patients will eventually have symptoms, which may vary from slight pain in the upper quadrant to severe biliary colic and jaundice following communicating rupture of the cyst and discharge of its contents into a major bile duct. Embolic obstruction of the biliary tract by daughters or fragments of the endocyst may result. Ruptured cysts may undergo suppuration and clinically mimic a hepatic abscess.

The clinical spectrum is wide and satisfactory imaging is only possible if the radiologist has a clear perception of the natural history of hydatid disease and what happens during treatment. It is equally important to know the capabilities of the different methods that are available to image hydatid disease, so that the best choice for the patient can be made.

Imaging Diagnosis

General Principles of Imaging

All imaging modalities can demonstrate some stages of hydatid cysts, but usually scanning (ultrasonography, CT, or MRI) provides the best images. All methods of scanning can provide images in multiple planes and no added contrast is necessary, except in CT imaging. Used alone, or in combination, and with knowledge of the laboratory test results, an almost 100% positive diagnosis of hydatid disease can be made in the majority of cases. Imaging may even provide a strong diagnostic probability when immunodiagnosis is equivocal or even (rarely) inaccurate.

In most suspected cases of hydatid disease, usually presenting with a cyst or a mass, ultrasonography should be the first method used to scan the patient, with a chest radiograph added. Ultrasonography is highly accurate (except in the chest, skeleton, and CNS), cost-effective, and does not need ionizing radiation. CT and MRI often provide additional valuable information, particularly when ultrasonography is anatomically unsatisfactory.

The approach to imaging hydatids thus depends on the availability of equipment and the site of the lesion. Except for lesions in the brain or spine, conventional radiography and ultrasonography are often sufficient for diagnosis and management. Pulmonary lesions are usually detected on the chest radiograph but, when it is available, CT is helpful for complete topographic evaluation. Evaluation of type I and type II lesions in solid organs requires ultrasonography and/or CT or MRI. If there are many cysts, CT is usually preferred by the surgeon. Brain hydatids can be imaged by either CT or MRI, but ease of imaging in all planes and detailed depiction of cerebral anatomy with MRI make this method particularly useful. Plain films are often adequate for imaging bone hydatids, but CT and MRI yield more information as to extent of the lesion and possible soft tissue involvement.

Angiography, Doppler sonography, and nuclear medicine are only occasionally useful in the diagnosis of cystic hydatid disease and are utilized only when the other modalities are unavailable.

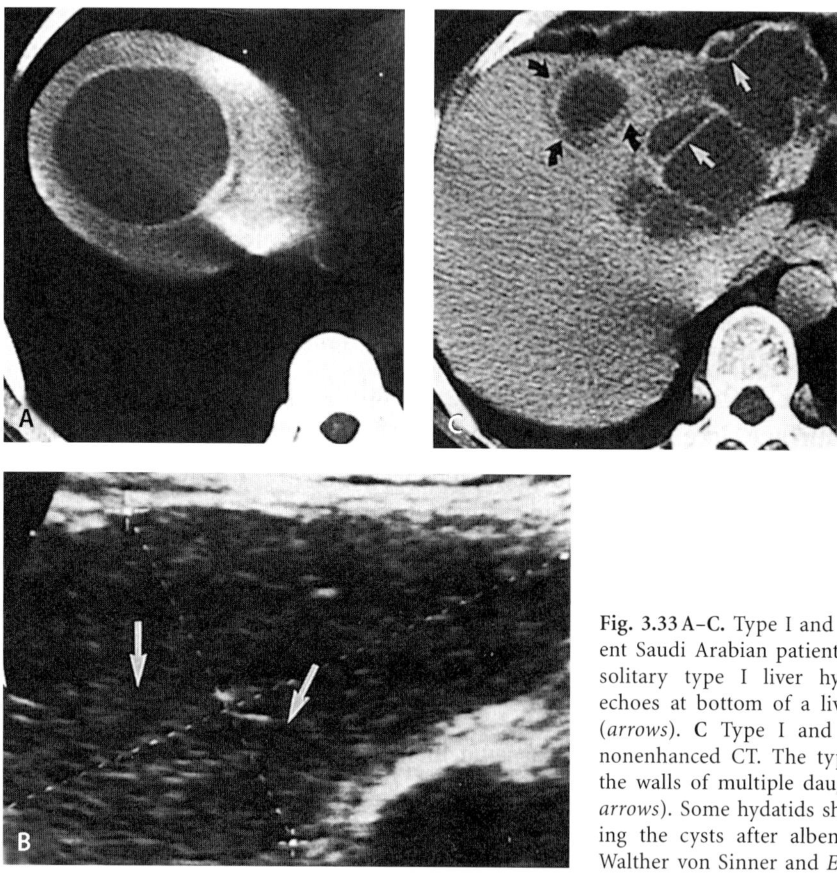

Fig. 3.33 A–C. Type I and II hydatid liver cysts in three different Saudi Arabian patients. **A** Nonenhanced CT scan shows a solitary type I liver hydatid. **B** Ultrasound scan reveals echoes at bottom of a liver hydatid caused by hydatid sand (*arrows*). **C** Type I and II hydatid cysts demonstrated on nonenhanced CT. The type II cysts appear septated because the walls of multiple daughter cysts abut one another (*white arrows*). Some hydatids show edema (*black arrows*) surrounding the cysts after albendazole treatment. (Courtesy of Dr. Walther von Sinner and *Eur J Radiol*, 1991)

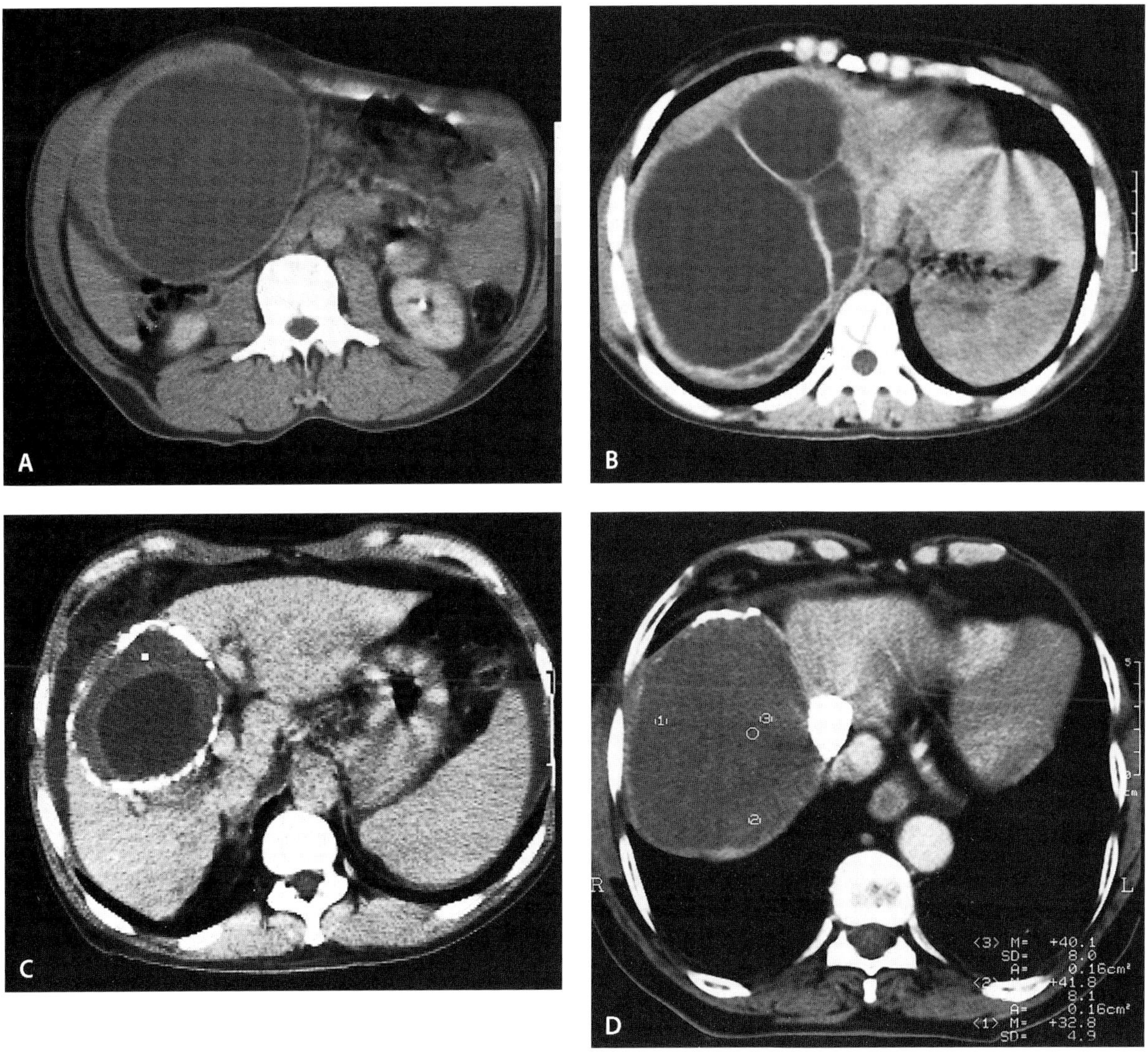

Fig. 3.34 A–D. Type I, II, and III unruptured hydatid cysts in four different patients from Tunisia. **A** Univesicular uncomplicated type I cyst in a 54-year-old man. **B** Multivesicular type II hydatid with multiple daughter cysts giving a septated appearance to the cyst in a 21-year-old woman. Dilated pericystic bile ducts are seen about the cyst periphery posteriorly. **C** Old hypermature liver hydatid in a 64-year-old man. Nonenhanced CT shows calcification in the cyst wall and matrix and fluid within the cyst, suggesting it is still evolving and not innocuous and should be treated. **D** Two hydatid liver cysts in a 75-year-old man. The larger pseudotumoral cyst has some calcification in its wall while the smaller type III cyst is totally calcified on nonenhanced CT. (Courtesy of Drs. Ben Cheikh and Gharbi, Tunis)

Imaging of Unruptured Cysts

Type I lesions have a nonspecific cystic appearance but if the patient is rotated immediately before ultrasound scanning, the settling hydatid sand produces signals which have been likened to falling snow (Fig. 3.33). The pericyst is rarely identified by ultrasonography (Fig. 3.35), and is seen by CT only if it is calcified (Fig. 3.34). However, it is demonstrable by MRI, particularly on T2-weighted images, which produce a low-intensity rim. Neither the cyst nor the pericyst enhance by CT or MRI as they are avascular. Lung hydatids are sometimes umbilicated on plain radiographs due to pressure on the cyst wall from adjacent blood vessels or major bronchi (see Fig. 3.83).

Type II lesions usually have a characteristic appearance due to daughter cysts, whether or not fluid or matrix is present (Figs. 3.12, 3.14, 3.21, 3.23, 3.24, 3.33–3.37). Hypermature type II lesions which lack daughters have a nonspecific appearance by ultrasonography and CT (Figs. 3.34, 3.35), but MRI is helpful as it shows the hypointense pericyst. Fluid in mother cysts has the same appearance as it does in daughters by all methods of cross-sectional imaging.

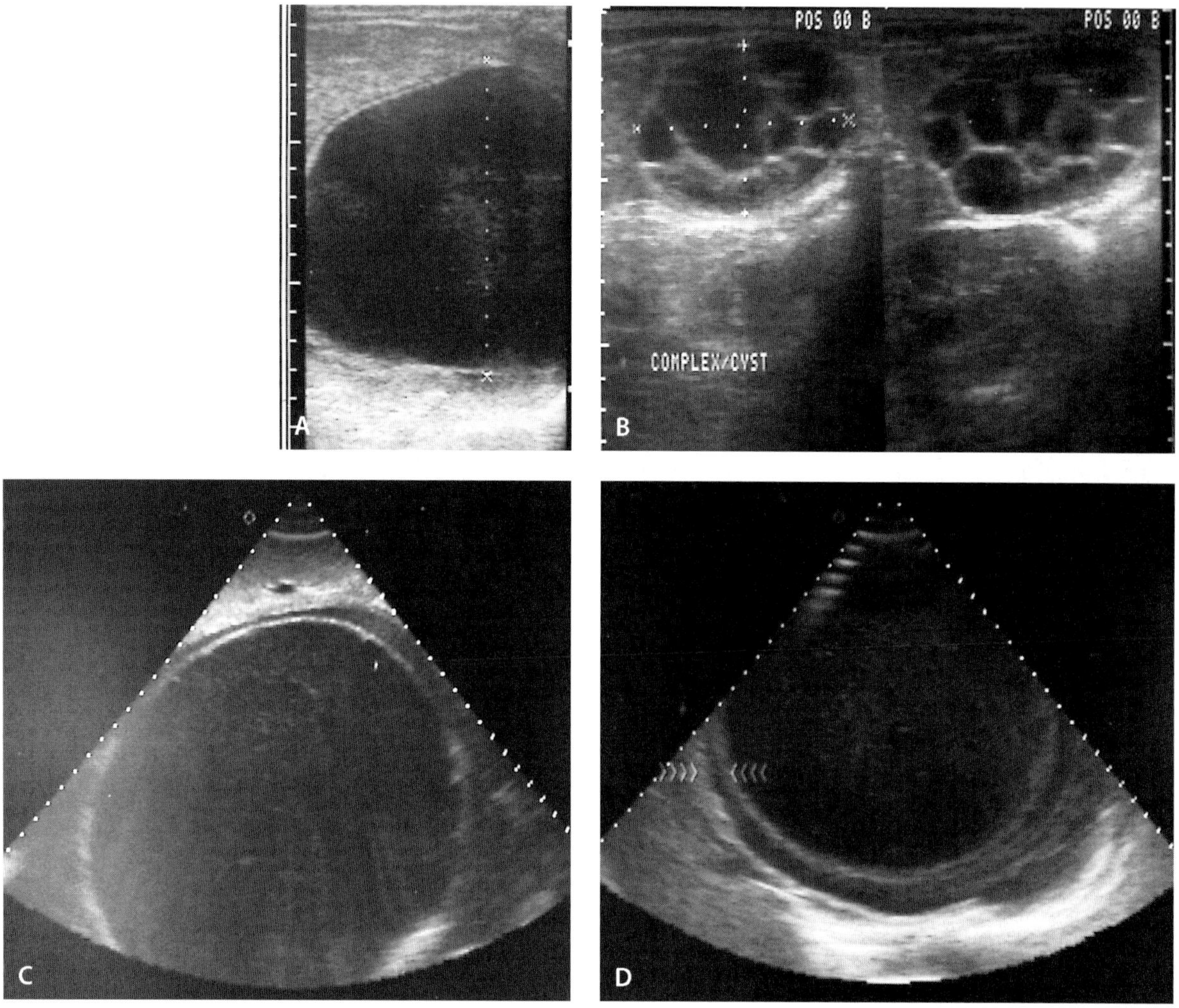

Fig. 3.35 A–D. Ultrasound identification of type I and II liver hydatid cysts in three different Kenyan patients. **A** Large simple type I liver hydatid with clear fluid. **B** Type II hydatid with multiple daughter cysts. **C, D** Large hypermature hydatid cyst filled with debris. Some detachment of the cyst wall from the host pericyst is noted. (Courtesy of Dr. M.W. Wachira)

Type III lesions are often discovered on plain films or CT scans (Figs. 3.13, 3.25, 3.34). They are densely and irregularly calcified and may reveal vestigial evidence of the antecedent type II lesion. Discovery of a type III lesion should provoke a search for uncalcified type I and II cysts in the liver and other organs.

Imaging of Ruptured Hydatids

Contained rupture makes the detached endocyst visible by all cross-sectional imaging methods. The lesion does not become smaller (Fig. 3.27).

Communicating rupture also produces a characteristic separation of endocyst from pericyst, and the cyst becomes smaller (Figs. 3.28 and 3.38). Biliary obstruction, if it occurs, may result in dilatation of *downstream* ducts. Occasionally daughter cysts or fragments of endocyst may be seen in the biliary tree by ultrasonography CT, or MRI. Endoscopic retrograde cholangiopancreatography (ERCP) shows filling defects within the biliary tree and may also reveal retrograde communication with the cyst cavity (Fig. 3.29). If air replaces some of the fluid in the pericyst cavity of lung lesions, the air meniscus and water lily signs are produced on upright chest radiographs (Figs. 3.39, 3.87–3.93).

Direct rupture of a liver lesion into the chest (identified by ultrasonography, CT, or MRI; Fig. 3.40) causes a pleural effusion and, if a bronchobiliary communication develops, it is demonstrable by bronchography or ERCP. Cyst rupture into the abdomen may produce a small amount of ascites and secondary cysts eventually develop in the peritoneal

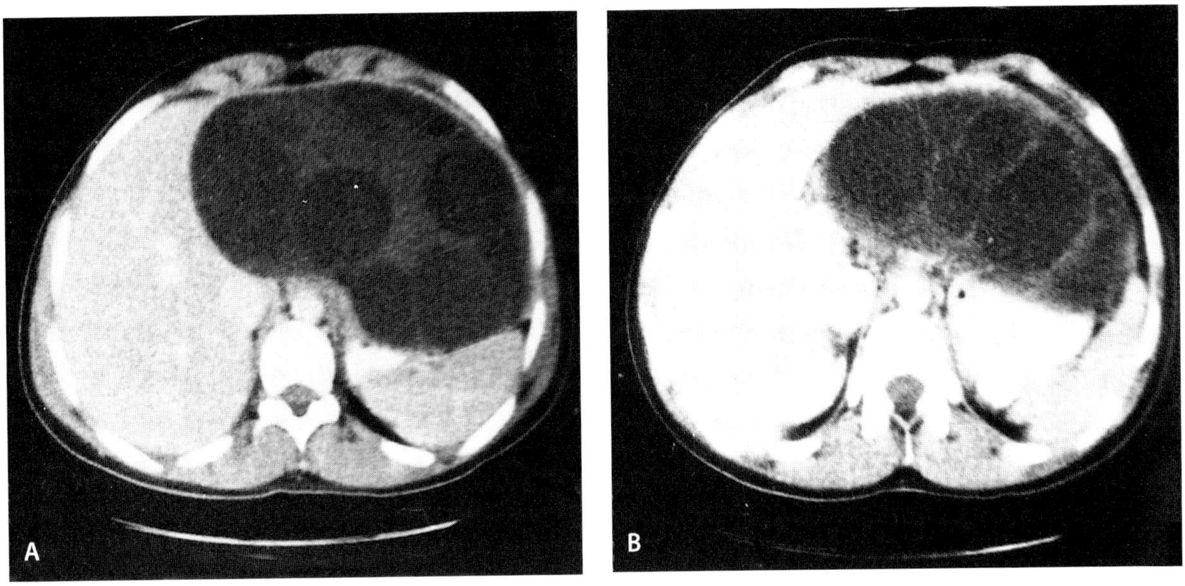

Fig. 3.36 A, B. Unruptured type II hydatid cyst in the left lobe of the liver of an Egyptian woman as seen on contrast-enhanced CT scan. Numerous daughter cysts are present

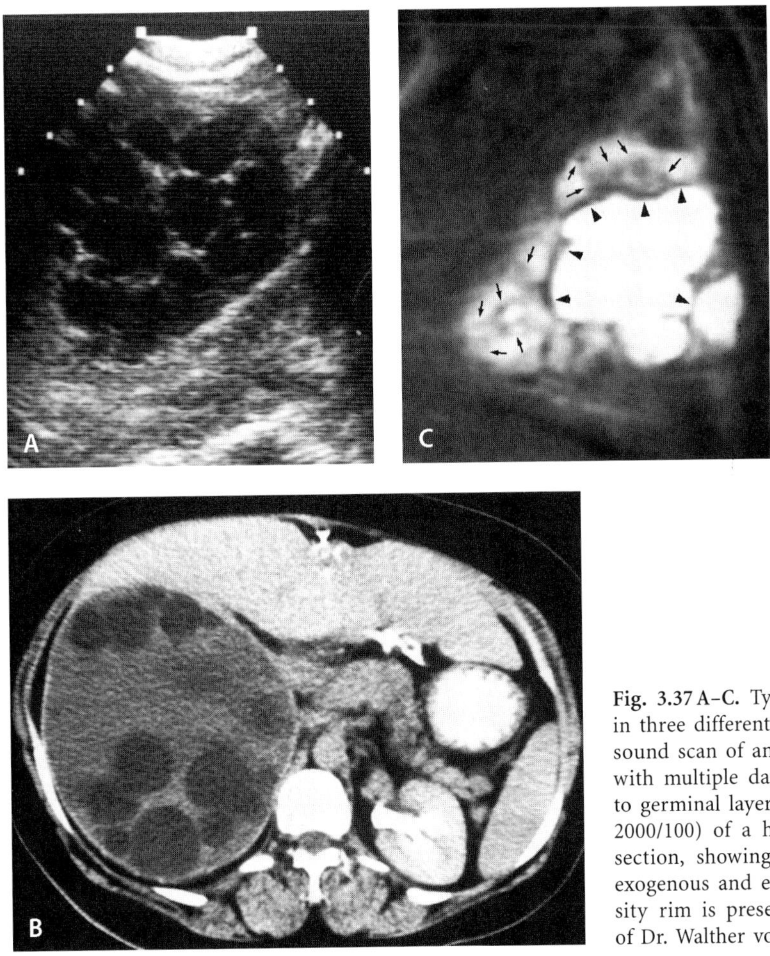

Fig. 3.37 A–C. Type II hydatids with multiple daughter cysts in three different Saudi Arabian patients as seen on: **A** ultrasound scan of an abdominal hydatid; **B** CT of a liver hydatid with multiple daughter cysts and brood capsules (connected to germinal layer) from endogenous proliferation; **C** MRI (SE 2000/100) of a hydatid cyst of the right chest wall, sagittal section, showing multiple daughter cysts (*arrows*); there is exogenous and endogenous proliferation. A low signal intensity rim is present around the cyst (*arrowheads*). (Courtesy of Dr. Walther von Sinner and *Eur J Radiol*, 1991)

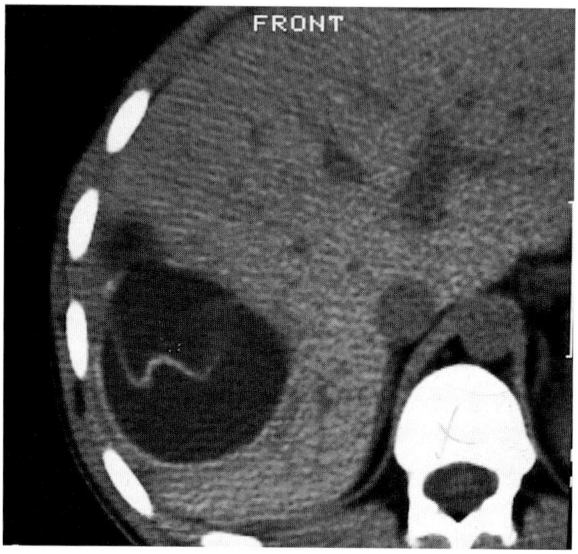

Fig. 3.38. Communicating rupture of a type I liver hydatid. Ultrasound scan in this 22-year-old Tunisian man shows partial rupture through the slightly calcified anterior wall of the cyst into the surrounding hepatic parenchyma. The "floating membrane sign" produced by detachment of the germinal membranes of the endocyst is well demonstrated. (Courtesy of Dr. Gharbi, Tunis)

cavity (Fig. 3.30). Direct rupture of a lung cyst into the lung parenchyma causes a local reaction which has been referred to as pericystic pneumonitis. Rupture into the pleural space induces a pleural effusion with or without pneumothorax. After direct rupture, cysts in all locations become smaller.

Premature death and infection are indistinguishable by ultrasonography and CT. Hydatid fluid becomes echogenic and daughter cysts become indistinct by ultrasonography. Hounsfield values of fluid increase and detail is lost on CT images (Fig. 3.32). Because it is difficult to distinguish between matrix and pus at surgery, some lesions that have been reported to be infected may actually have been sterile cysts containing matrix. The exact role of MRI in assessing infection and premature death is not yet clear. Some have concluded that distinction between cyst death and infection is not possible; others contend that it is not possible to distinguish between living and dead cysts, yet some have stated that cysts that are infected or communicate with the biliary tree produce a high-intensity proton density signal. The diversity of opinion probably reflects the fact that matrix (which is hyperintense on T2-weighted images) has sometimes been mistaken for hydatid fluid or sand.

As can be seen from the above discussion, each imaging technique has its inherent advantages and disadvantages which will now be discussed separately.

Conventional Radiography

Hydatid cysts present with a variety of radiological patterns, but frequently cannot be recognized, let alone positively identified, by plain radiography. The presence of other calcified or partially calcified cysts elsewhere in the body may suggest the diagnosis. Unfortunately, calcification in cysts in the liver is seen in only 16% of patients who are known to have hydatid cysts in other parts of the body. Nevertheless, the appearance is so characteristic that the discovery of a smooth, well-defined, round, oval, or lobulated "tumor" anywhere in the body, especially if there is rim calcification, should suggest hydatid disease in any patient who is living in, has visited, or has emigrated from an endemic area. Hydatid cysts may vary in diameter from 1 to 20 cm: there are often multiple cysts of different sizes in the same patient. Those in the liver (which is by far the most common site) often calcify (Figs. 3.41–3.43), as do those in other solid organs, e.g., the kidney and spleen. But calcification is extremely rare within lung hydatids and is not identifiable on plain radiographs within bone lesions or in most cerebral cysts.

Calcification of the cyst wall may have various patterns (Fig. 3.43). There may be a fine line of calcification that is well defined, usually sharp externally, but lacking clarity internally. Only part of the cyst wall may be calcified, giving a sickle-shaped or crescentic outline. Where the calcification is lacking altogether or is partial, inhomogeneous, or striped, there is the possibility of active growth: many believe this pattern is an indication for surgical removal of the cyst to prevent rupture, which could lead to biliary obstuction, disseminated hydatidosis, or even death from anaphylaxis. If the cyst calcification is total, with a dense thick wall and calcified endocyst, the cyst is dead (type III). Polycyclic calcification can be seen when both mother and daughter cysts have calcification within their walls; multiple daughter cysts are thought to indicate that the mother cyst's survival is threatened. A "crushed eggshell" or "sunburst" type of calcification may result from prior cyst rupture and collapse (see Fig. 3.77B). The polycyclic and crushed eggshell types of calcification are virtually diagnostic of hydatid disease, but can rarely indicate the end result of a hematoma or mycotic infection.

(Text continues on p. 237)

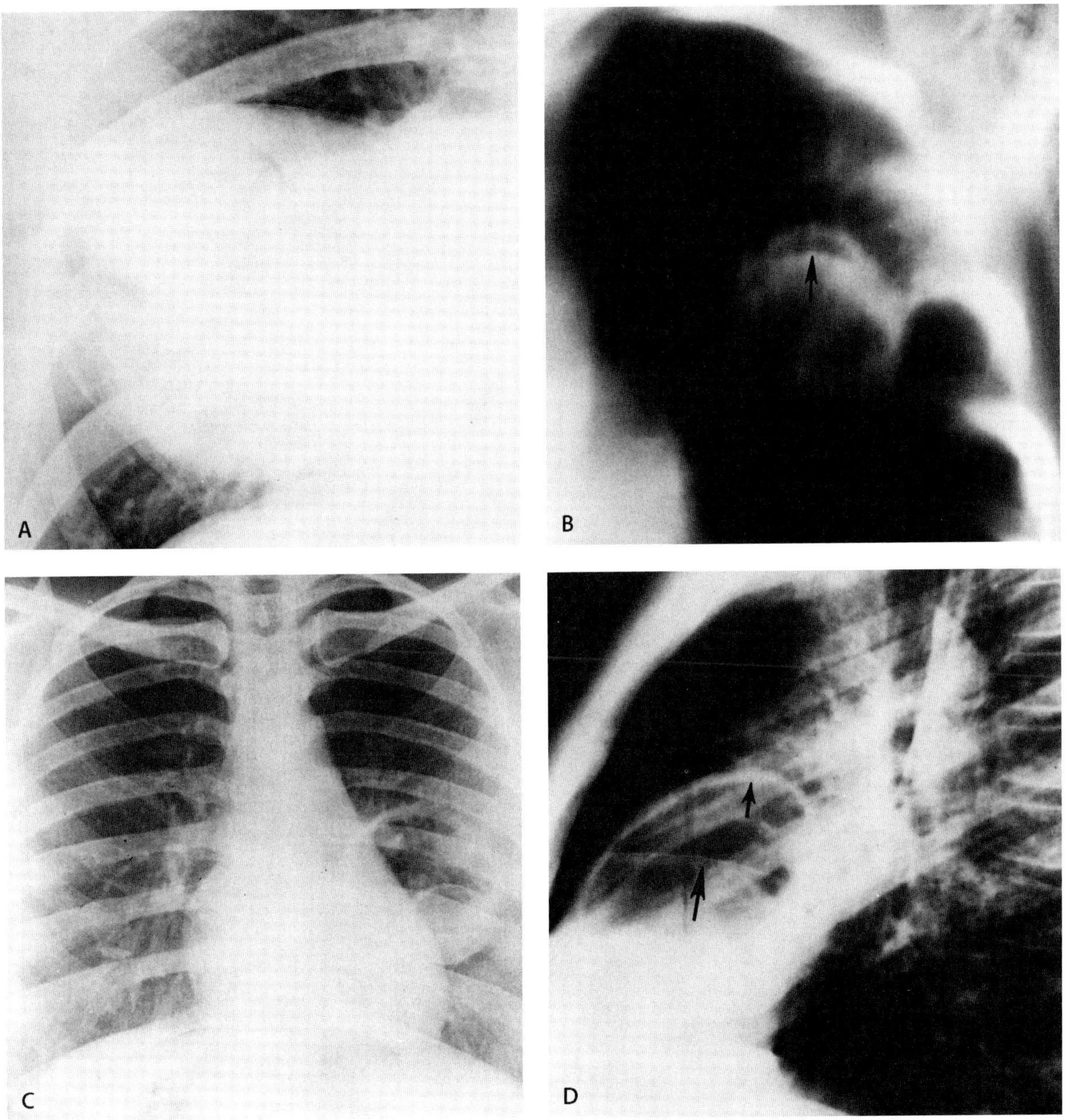

Fig. 3.39 A–D. Air meniscus and double arch signs in ruptured hydatid cysts of the lungs in four different patients. **A** A thin crescent of air is seen in a large hydatid cyst in the right lower lung of a Spaniard. The air has dissected the two walls of the cyst, one wall being the fibrous wall produced by the lung (pericyst) and the other being the wall produced by the parasite itself (endocyst). **B** Air meniscus in another pulmonary hydatid seen on AP tomographic cut. There is also air in the endocyst itself producing a double arch sign as well. **C, D** The double arch sign or "cyst-within-a-cyst" appearance (*arrows*) in a ruptured pulmonary hydatid. Once rupture of the cyst begins, a large opening may develop in the membranes and the shrinking cyst expels part or all of its fluid into the communicating bronchus. At this stage, air may enter the endocyst, producing an air-fluid level within the cyst that may itself be capped with a crescent of air between the pericyst and endocyst. The wall of the endocyst appears as an arch above the air-fluid level and the surrounding pericyst is visible as a larger arch

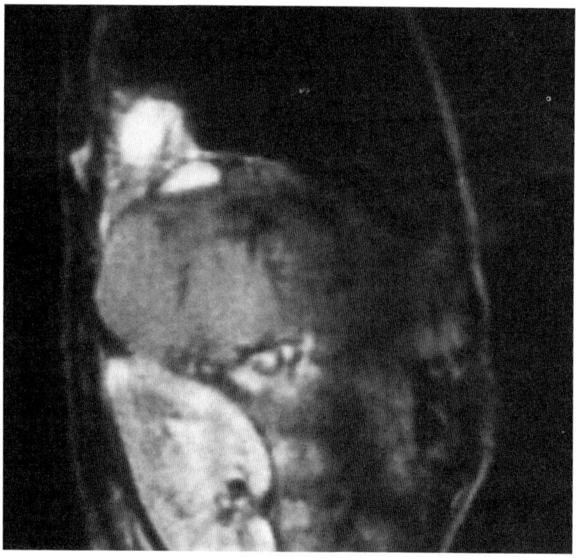

Fig. 3.40. Subphrenic and supradiaphragmatic spread of hydatid cysts, identified on T2-weighted sagittal MR image (SE 2000/100). Multiplanar imaging capability and excellent contrast resolution of MRI permit differentiation among the supradiaphragmatic lung cyst with surrounding reactive pulmonary and pleural changes, the left hemidiaphragm, and the subphrenic cyst. (Courtesy of Dr. Walther von Sinner et al and *AJR*, 1991)

◄

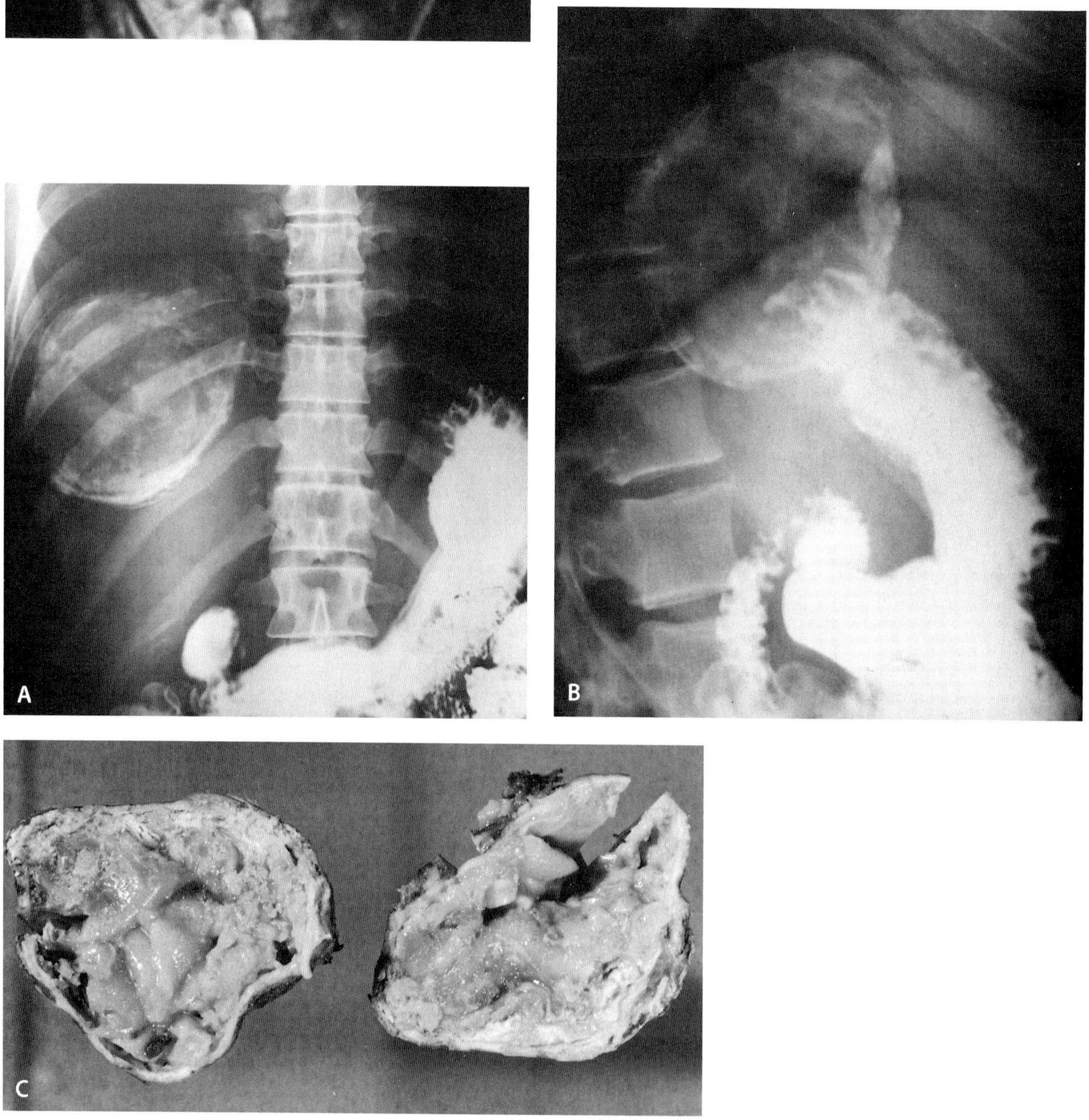

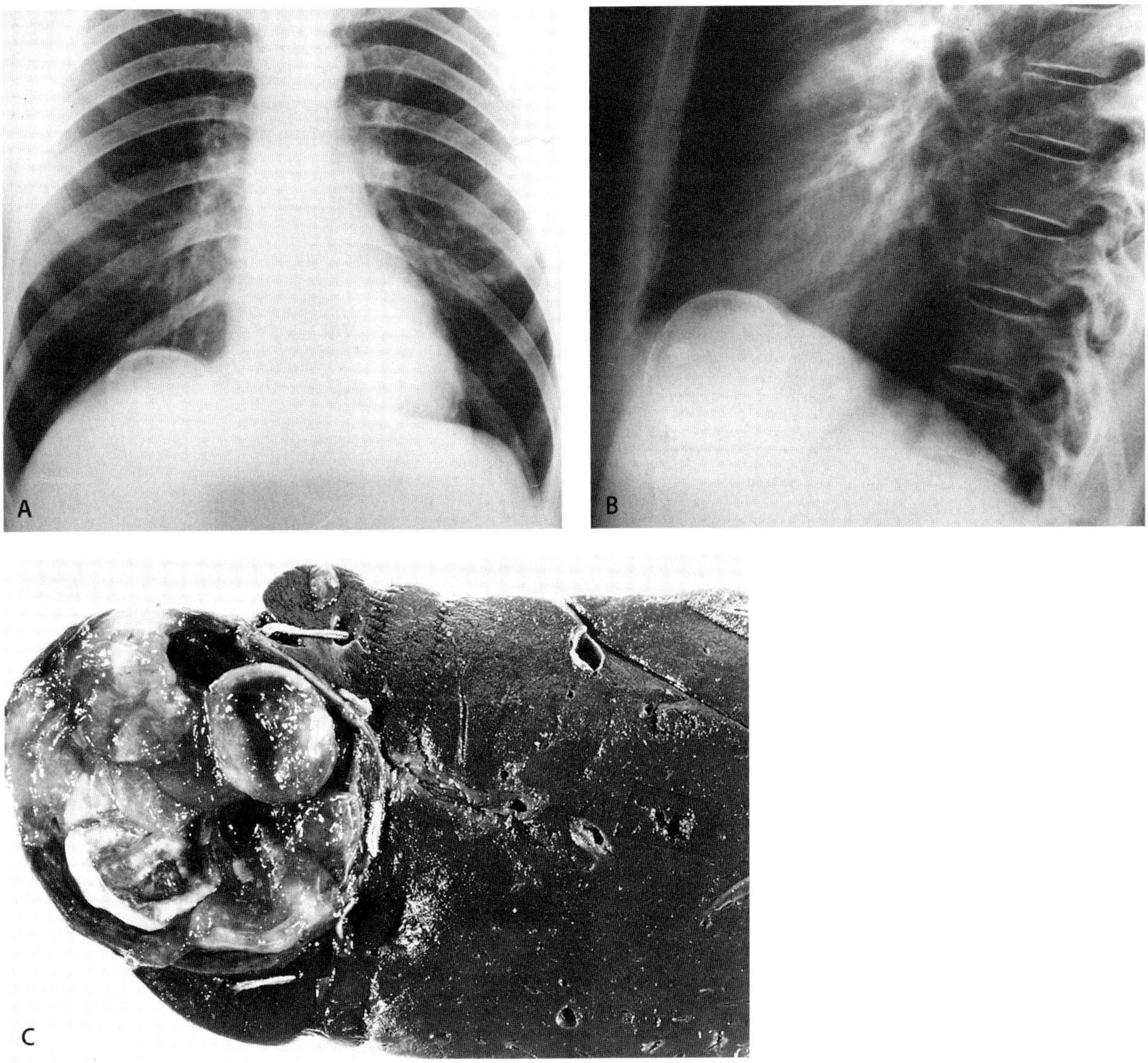

Fig. 3.42. A, B A solitary calcified liver hydatid causing a localized bulge in the anteromedial aspect of the right hemidiaphragm seen on posteroanterior (**A**) and lateral (**B**) views of the chest. Calcification in the hydatid wall completely encircles this smooth, round cyst. Whether calcified or not, hydatids which develop in the periphery of the liver beneath the dome often reveal their presence through a generalized or localized bulge in the diaphragmatic contour. This may be the only clue to the presence of a hydatid when there is no calcium in the cyst wall. (Courtesy of Dr. Douglas Sheft, San Francisco) **C** Gross specimen of a 5-cm unilocular hydatid cyst with multiple daughter cysts. The cyst is subcapsular and, if present beneath the dome of the diaphragm, would cause a bulge similar to that seen in **A** and **B**. AFIP 64-6538

Fig. 3.41 A–C. A large calcified unilocular hydatid cyst in the liver of a 37-year-old Basque woman. There are multiple small daughter cysts in the mother cyst. Calcification of the cyst wall is total and thick, as is much of the endocyst, indicating probable inactivity or death of the hydatid. There is elevation of the right hemidiaphragm on the anteroposterior (AP) view of the abdomen (**A**) and a localized bulge in the midportion of this diaphragm on the lateral view (**B**). **C** Gross specimen of a liver hydatid from another patient showing its glistening gelatinous inner surface and a portion of the cyst contents. In most hydatids, there is a rather dense fibrous outer wall (pericyst), as in this case. This correlates well with the thick calcified wall seen in **A** and **B**. AFIP 55-18468-1

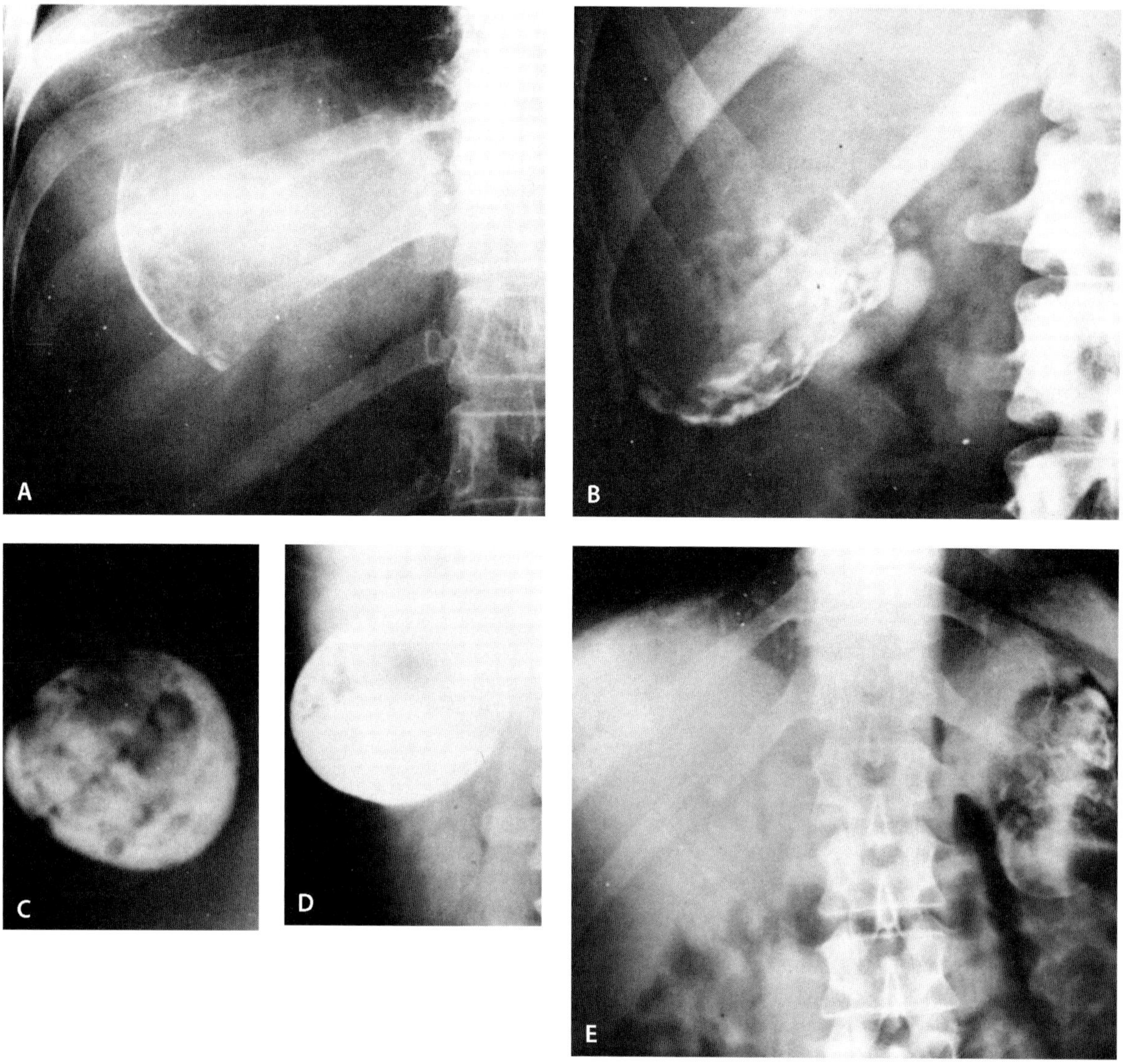

Fig. 3.43 A–E. Different types of calcification in a hydatid cyst may have diagnostic and prognostic significance. **A** Crescentic outline of a partially calcified *E. granulosus* cyst in a young Greek woman. Such a cyst is not harmless because it could still be viable and could rupture. **B** Moderately heavy calcification within a hydatid cyst in the right lobe of the liver containing many small calcified daughter cysts. The cyst shows a partial collapse with slightly compressed, irregular margins and calcification throughout the wall except for its superior aspect. (The gallbladder is incidentally opacified from an oral cholecystogram.) If a hydatid cyst should rupture and collapse, a crushed eggshell type of calcification may be seen. **C, D** Extremely heavy calcification of solitary hydatid liver cysts in two different patients. Such total calcification of a cyst indicates that the parasite has died and the cyst is inactive (type III). **E** Polycyclic calcification in an inactive type III hydatid cyst in the left lobe of the liver, a much less common location than the right lobe: there are numerous calcified small and large daughter cysts. There is a localized bulge in the medial aspect of the left leaf of the diaphragm due to the underlying large left lobe hydatid. (**E** courtesy of Dr. Douglas Sheft, San Francisco)

Ultrasonography

Ultrasonography is and should be the main imaging modality for hydatids, except in the lungs, brain, spine, or skeleton, because it does not need ionizing radiation and is inexpensive, yet can provide a very accurate multidimensional image of any cyst in solid organs or soft tissues. It is an accurate way to identify hydatid disease, particularly when "hydatid sand," daughter cysts ("septations") and/or calcifications are seen, and the parallel stripes due to reflections of sound waves from the endocyst and pericyst can be recognized (Fig. 3.44 A). Movement of the echogenic hydatid sand in the cyst, and of any membrane or debris, can be noted as the patient moves (Fig. 3.44 B). Similarly, the imaging of one or more cysts within a cyst provides a very strong diagnostic probability (Fig. 3.44 C). The linear appearance of a collapsed cyst or membrane is further evidence (Fig. 3.44 D).

Ultrasonography (provided a suitable unit is available) can also be used away from a clinic or hospital for valuable epidemiological surveys and the diagnosis and treatment of nomadic and migrant populations.

Computed Tomography

Computed tomography, particularly spiral (helical) CT with reconstruction, is a very accurate way to demonstrate hydatid cysts and show their regression after treatment. Nonenhanced CT may show minimal or partial calcification of the rim of hydatid cysts (Fig. 3.45 A). This is important, because a segmentally calcified cyst may still harbor a living parasite and therefore may be infective. Total rim calcification suggests degeneration and the parasite is usually, but not invariably, dead (Fig. 3.45 C); clinically, it can be observed rather than actively treated. CT can also demonstrate rupture of a cyst with detachment of the endocyst (Fig. 3.45 D), allowing the contents to leak into the surrounding tissues or cavities (direct rupture). Hydatid fluid has similar Hounsfield CT values to water and, because the cyst is avascular, these values do not change after intravenous contrast enhancement.

Contrast-enhanced CT (Fig. 3.46) may show ring enhancement around a cyst as a sign of superimposed infection, especially if there are air bubbles. Abscesses and fistulous tracts may develop. The contents of an infected cyst usually have higher attenuation values than a cyst that is not infected. Old hydatid abscesses may not be recognized as such if all the parasitic material has been resorbed: they may contain only amorphous calcification. However, hydatid hooklets are very resistant and often persist; they should be sought histopathologically if no other parasitic material can be found. Even a single hooklet found in pus from an abscess is convincing evidence of a disintegrated hydatid cyst.

Magnetic Resonance Imaging

Magnetic resonance imaging is an excellent technique to demonstrate the many different phases of hydatid infections, but cannot image small calcifications reliably.

There are five distinct phases seen on MR imaging (von Sinner et al.):

1. *Simple Viable Hydatid Cyst (Type I).* When the hydatid is intact, the two layers of the parasitic cyst (the endocyst and pericyst) cannot be separated on MR images. On T1-weighted spin-echo images, the cyst wall is isointense relative to the fluid in the cyst. On T2-weighted images, it appears as a low-intensity rim surrounding the high-intensity cyst contents (Fig. 3.47). A low-intensity ring is, however, not specific for the presence of a hydatid cyst, because it can also occur with other conditions, such as abscess and hepatocellular carcinoma.
2. *Hydatid Cyst with Daughter Cysts and/or Matrix (Type II).* Viable daughter cysts usually are isointense or slightly hypointense compared with the contents (hydatid sand) of the mother cyst on T1-weighted images (Fig. 3.48 A, C). On T2-weighted images, the mother and daughter cysts are both isointense (Fig. 3.48 B).
3. *Hydatid Cyst with Detached Parasitic Membranes (Type I or II Cyst with Contained Rupture).* Degeneration or damage of the cyst wall may lead to contained rupture of the parasitic membranes, causing detachment and allowing the membranes to float. These may occasionally be seen with conventional radiography, principally in lung hydatids, but MRI, as well as CT and sonography (Figs. 3.27, 3.38, 3.44 D, 3.45 D, 3.71 E), can demonstrate this event with great precision in cysts in all organs. On MRI these detached membranes are identified floating within the cyst and appear dark on both T1- and T2-weighted images and often present in a "snake-like" or "whirl-like" manner (Fig. 3.49). This "serpent" or "whirl sign" is virtually pathognomonic for a hydatid cyst and may allow the correct diagnosis of echinococcosis in an unknown cystic lesion. The pericyst is also dark on T2-weighted images, but tends to be isointense relative to normal liver tissue on T1-weighted images.
4. *Rupture of a Hydatid Cyst (Type I or II Cyst with Communicating or Direct Rupture).* When a cyst ruptures, the contents spill into the surrounding

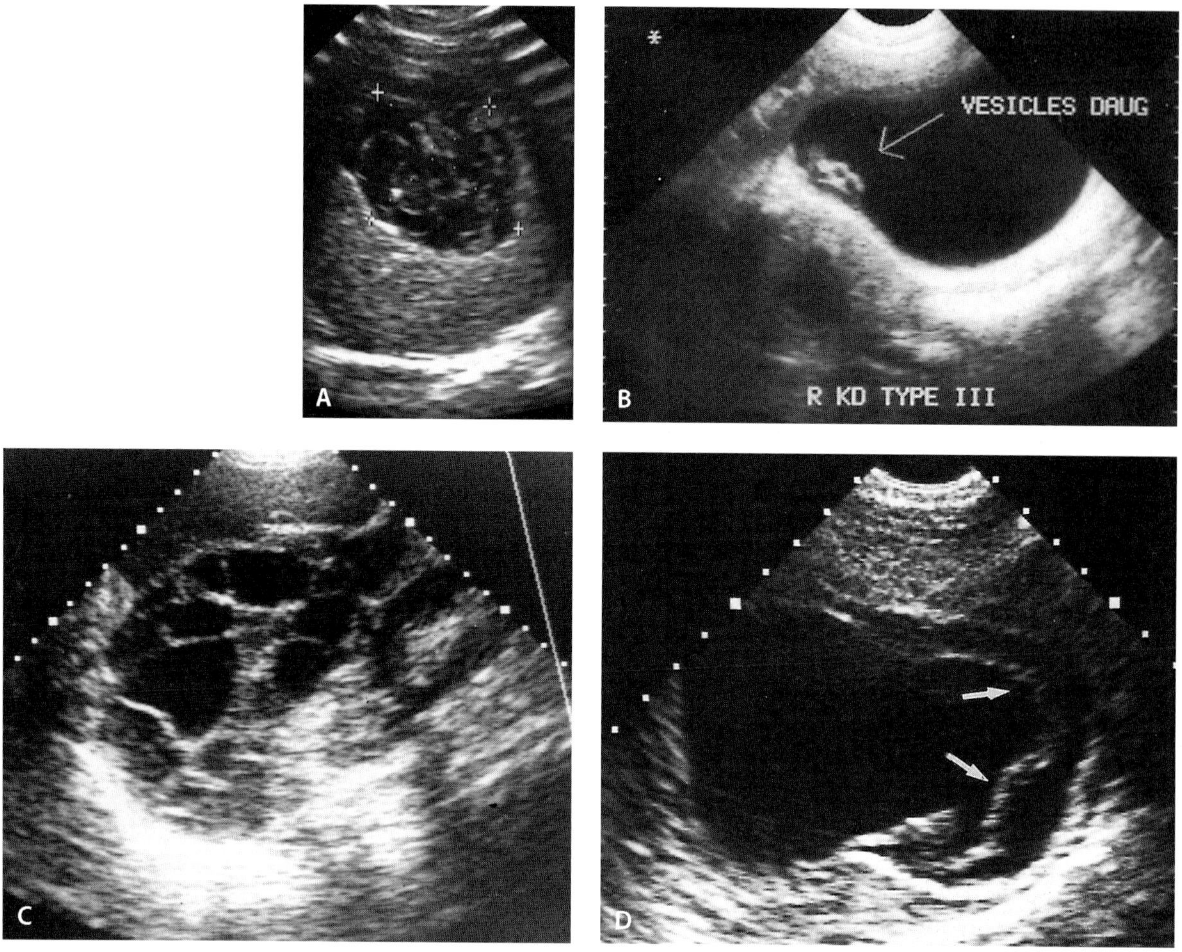

Fig. 3.44 A–D. The ultrasound appearance of various types of hydatid cysts. A Heterogeneous type III liver hydatid with calcifications in the cyst wall, and echogenic hydatid sand, membranes, and daughter cysts in the endocyst. B Type II hydatid cyst with daughter vesicles in a 39-year-old Tunisian man. (A, B courtesy of Dr. Gharbi, Tunis) (Note should be made that these cysts are typed using Dr. Lewall's pathology-based classification described in this text. Dr. Gharbi uses a different ultrasound-based classification described on pp. 221–222). C Type II liver hydatid containing a large number of different sized daughter cysts. D Large type I liver hydatid complicated by detached parasitic membrane, producing the snake or serpent sign (*arrows*). (C, D courtesy of Dr. Walther von Sinner and *Semin Roentgenol*, 1997)

tissues or cavities. In the liver, for instance, if rupture is communicating, biliary obstruction may ensue. A cyst may be ruptured by trauma and spill into the peritoneal cavity, pelvis, pleura, or pericardium. MR images will clearly show rupture of the cyst as an area of discontinuity of the low-intensity cyst wall, as well as the reaction in the pericystic tissues (Fig. 3.50). Following rupture, a serpent or snake sign may be demonstrated on MRI, CT, and ultrasonography. The actual event of cystic discharge resulting from spontaneous silent rupture of the wall of a bulging hydatid can also be visualized by MRI. If there has been seeding of scolices, there may be evidence of developing secondary cysts, especially in the abdomen and pelvis through peritoneal seeding (see Figs. 3.72, 3.75). In the lung, a cyst may rupture into the bronchial tree, with the patient coughing up cyst contents that may be aspirated, resulting in extensive reactive pneumonitis (Fig. 3.51). MRI may show a communication between the cyst and bronchial tree.

5. *End-Stage Calcified Cyst (Type III).* Late in the course of hydatid disease, spontaneous collapse and calcification of the cyst may occur. Partial calcification of the cyst wall represents degenerative changes that may be seen with living or dead parasites; total calcification of the endocyst indicates death of the hydatid. Calcifications are better visualized by CT, but they may be suggested on MRI by an area of signal dropout (Fig. 3.52).

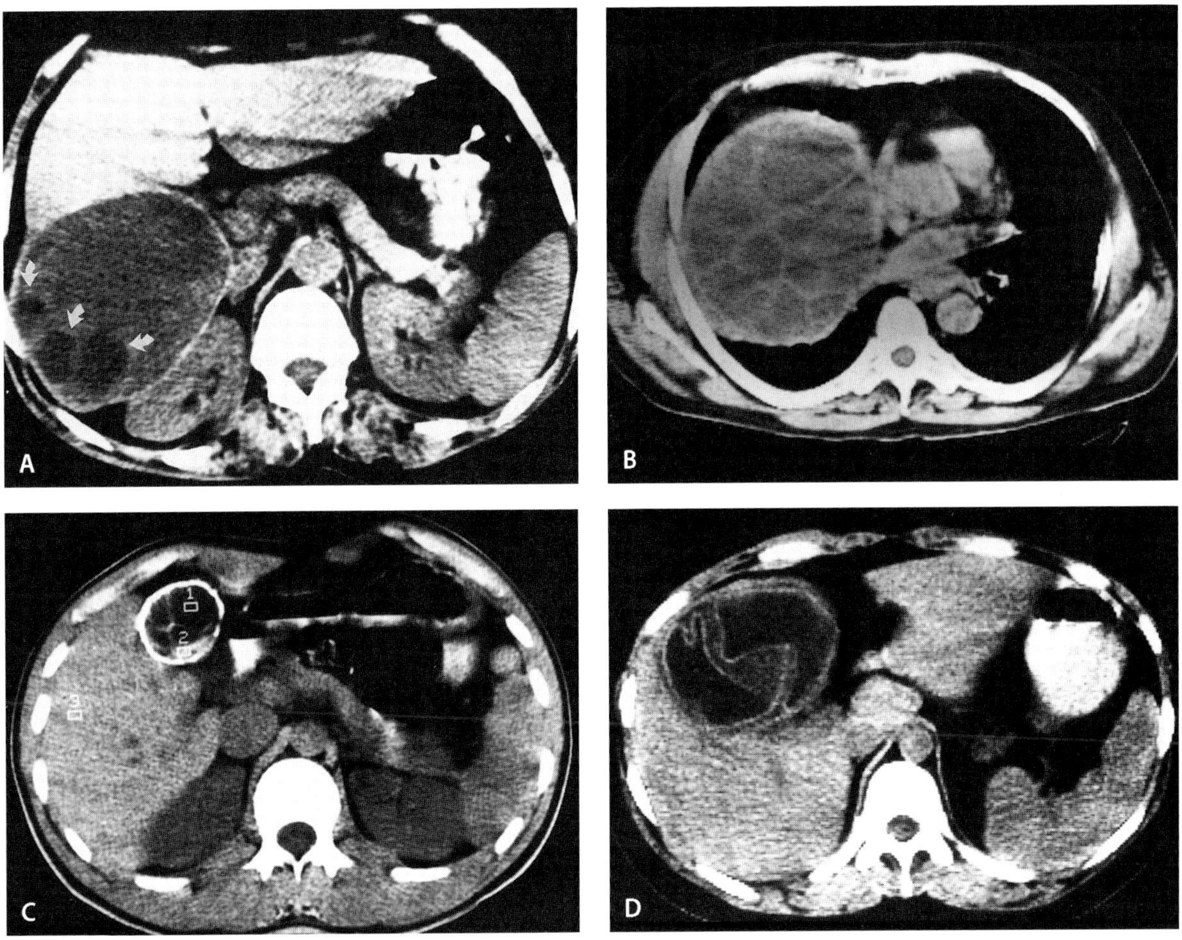

Fig. 3.45 A–D. Nonenhanced CT scans of the liver in four different patients with various types of hydatid cysts. **A** Large hypermature type II hydatid in the right lobe of the liver causing bulging of the liver capsule. The cyst wall is faintly calcified and there is abundant matrix and several daughter cysts (*arrows*) within the endocyst. (Courtesy of Dr. Walther von Sinner and *Semin Roentgenol*, 1997). **B** Large type II hydatid in the superior aspect of the right lobe of the liver protruding into the right lower hemithorax. There are numerous daughter cysts present within the mother cyst. (Courtesy of Dr. R. Dick, London) **C** Thick calcified wall of an old hypermature liver hydatid with daughter cysts. **D** Ruptured type I liver hydatid with detached internal membranes appearing as a "dancing hand" or a "serpent" within the cyst fluid. (**C**, **D** courtesy of Prof. Xing-Rong Chen, Shanghai)

Treatment or Recurrence. MRI can adequately assess the regression in size of hydatids and the changes in host tissue during chemotherapy (Fig. 3.53), and can show the residual debris after surgery or chemotherapy has destroyed a cyst. It is often possible, using serial scans, to recognize when any secondary infection is occurring or if treatment has been incomplete. (This is particularly important for alveolar hydatids caused by *E. multilocularis*, when incomplete removal is likely and will prove fatal without chemotherapy.)

(Text continues on p. 242)

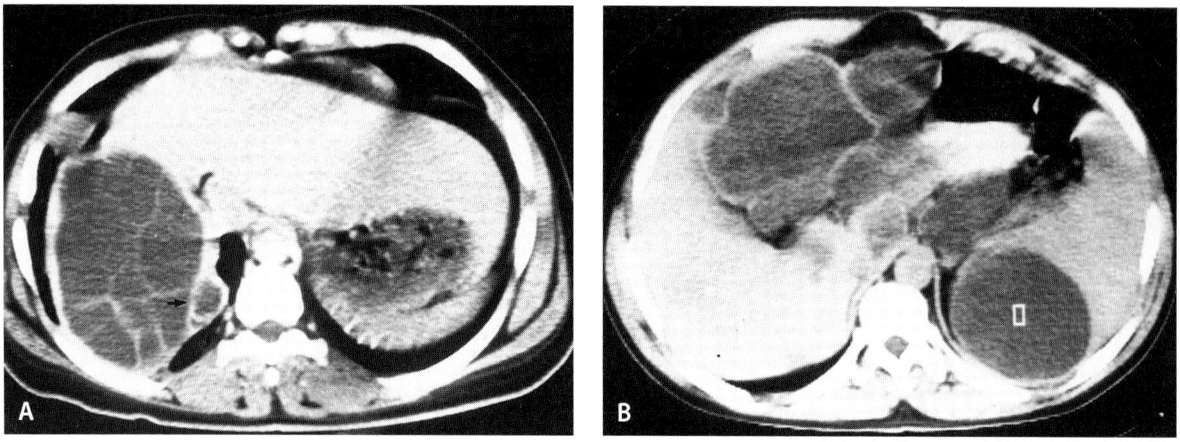

Fig. 3.46 A, B. Contrast-enhanced CT scans of liver hydatids in two different Saudi Arabian patients. **A** Type II hydatid cyst in right lobe of liver with multiple daughter cysts and thick contrast-enhanced cyst wall. There is one smaller medial cyst caused by outward proliferation. **B** Type II hydatid cysts in right and left lobes of liver and a type I hydatid in the spleen on contrast-enhanced CT scan. The large right lobe liver hydatid appears to be rupturing and collapsing. (Courtesy of Dr. Walther von Sinner)

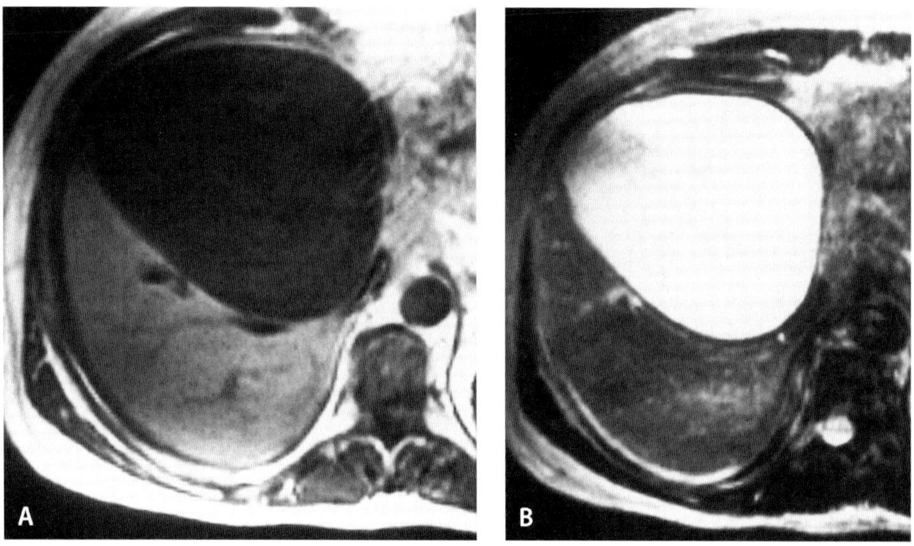

Fig. 3.47 A, B. MRI of a simple viable type I hydatid cyst of liver. **A** T1-weighted image (SE 733/20). The cyst wall is isointense relative to the cyst contents. **B** T2-weighted image (SE 2000/100). The cyst wall, consisting of both intact parasitic membranes and pericyst, is of low signal intensity compared with the high signal of cyst contents. (Courtesy of Dr. Walther von Sinner and *AJR*, 1991)

Fig. 3.49. **A** MRI of liver hydatid with detached parasitic membranes on T2-weighted image (SE 2000/100), producing the snake or serpent sign. Both detached parasitic membranes and pericyst are of low intensity. **B** MRI of another ruptured hepatic hydatid cyst showing the snake or serpent sign of detached membranes within the endocyst. The cyst wall (*black arrows*) is of low signal intensity relative to the cyst contents and the surrounding high-intensity host reaction and edema (*white arrows*). (Courtesy of Dr. Walther von Sinner and *AJR*, 1991)

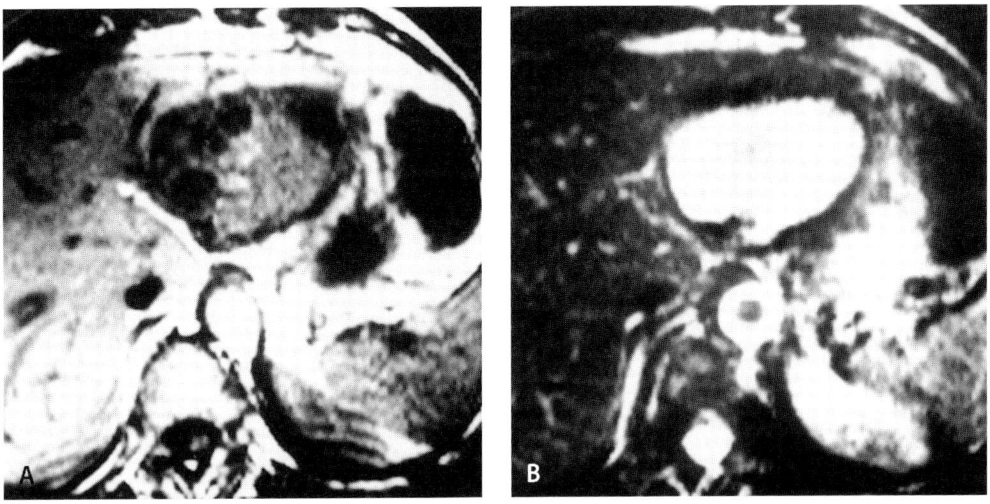

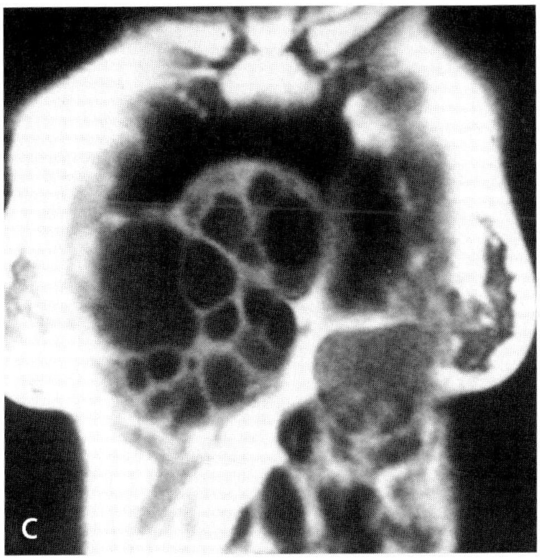

Fig. 3.48 A–C. MRI of type II hydatid cysts containing daughter cysts. **A** T1-weighted image (SE 640/20) shows multiple daughter cysts containing low-intensity fluid compared with intermediate signal of hydatid sand of mother cyst. **B** T2-weighted image (SE 2000/100). Contents of mother cyst and daughter cysts have same high signal intensity. **C** Coronal T1-weighted image (SE 640/20) in patient with large subdiaphragmatic hydatid containing numerous daughter cysts. (Courtesy of Dr. Walther von Sinner and *AJR*, 1991)

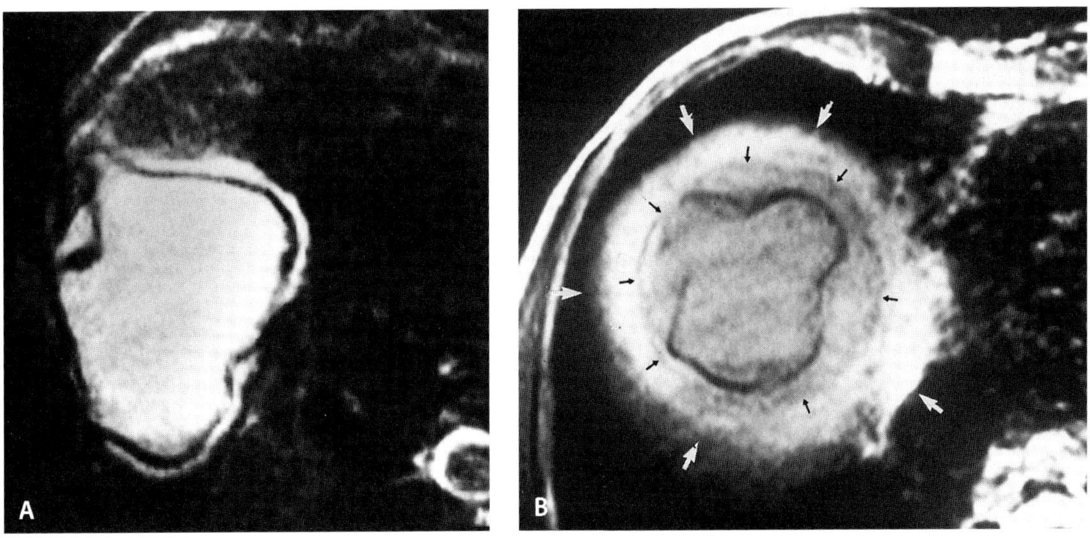

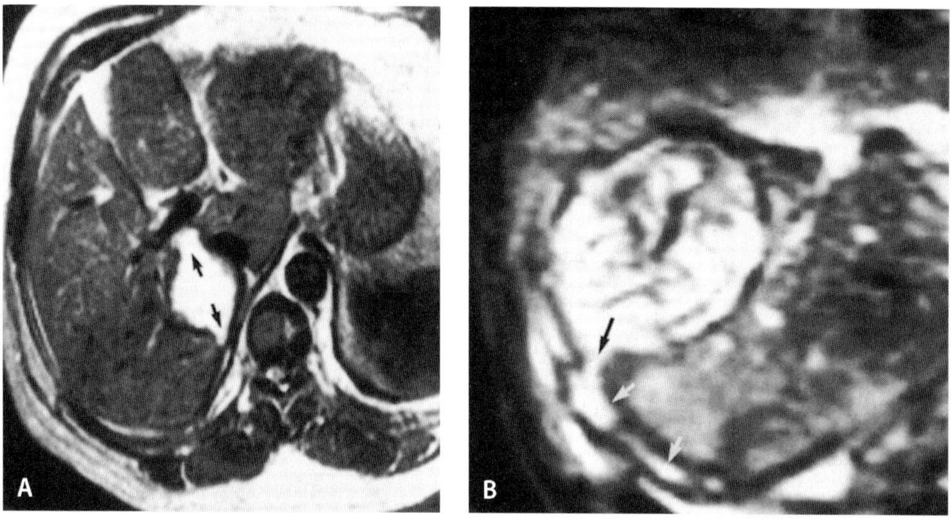

Fig. 3.50. **A** Intrahepatic rupture of liver hydatid on MR image (SE 2100/50). Low-intensity pericyst is disrupted, and fluid contents spill into liver parenchyma (*arrows*). **B** External rupture of liver hydatid. T2-weighted image (SE 2000/100) shows disruption of low-intensity rim of pericyst (*black arrow*) with spillage of fluid into perihepatic space (*white arrows*). (Courtesy of Dr. Walther von Sinner and *AJR*, 1991)

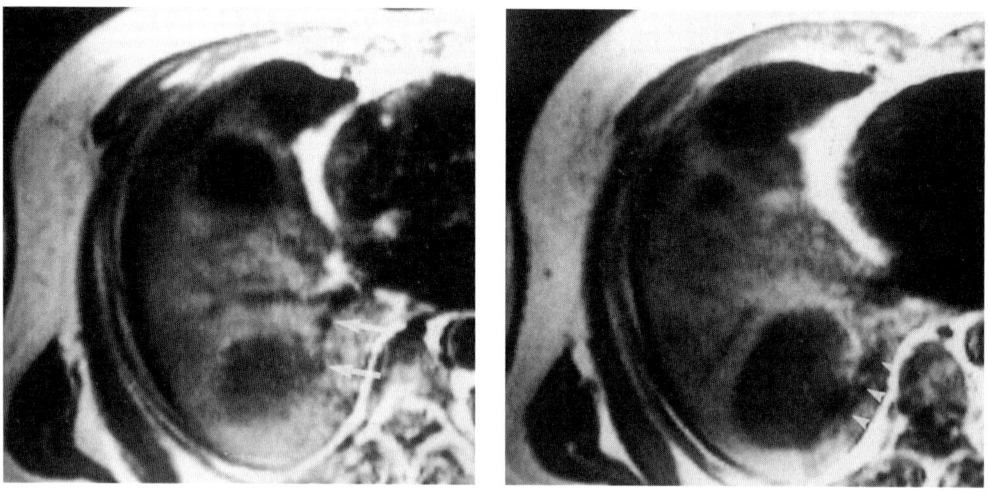

Fig. 3.51. Complicated hydatid cyst of lower lobe of right lung. MR image (SE 950/20) shows lower lobe bronchi in close contact with cyst wall (*arrows* and *arrowheads*). Spread of cyst contents into adjacent lung parenchyma caused infiltrates and reactive pneumonitis. (Courtesy of Dr. Walther von Sinner and *AJR*, 1991)

Radioisotope Scanning

Radioisotope scanning can be useful in identifying the location, number, and size of liver hydatids, if ultrasonography, CT or MRI are not available. In one series of 65 patients utilizing scans in three planes, the findings were as follows: (1) space-occupying "cold" lesions which were solitary in 44 patients, double in 16, and multiple in 5; 45 of the cysts were located in the right lobe; (2) morphological changes in hepatic size and shape with displacement or partial loss of the liver, and (3) occasional false-negative scans when the triplane technique was not used. As is the case with abscesses, the filling defects caused by liver hydatids are usually more sharply defined than those due to infiltrating primary or metastatic neoplasms, but the isotopic appearance is nonspecific.

Radioisotope scanning may also be used (if CT and MRI are not available) to show defects in the brain; these will be single or multiple, usually round and often causing ventricular displacement or even hydrocephalus. Apart from localizing a "space-occupying" mass, the scans are not specific.

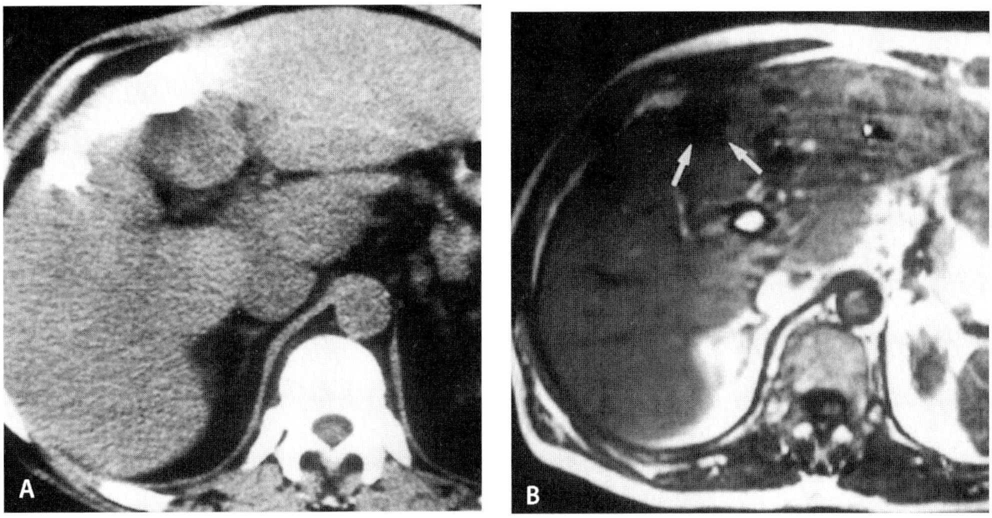

Fig. 3.52 A, B. End-stage collapsed calcified type III liver hydatid. **A** CT shows two calcifications in the liver. **B** T1-weighted MR image (SE 733/120) shows only larger calcified cyst as an area of signal dropout (*arrows*). (Courtesy of Dr. Walther von Sinner and *AJR*, 1991)

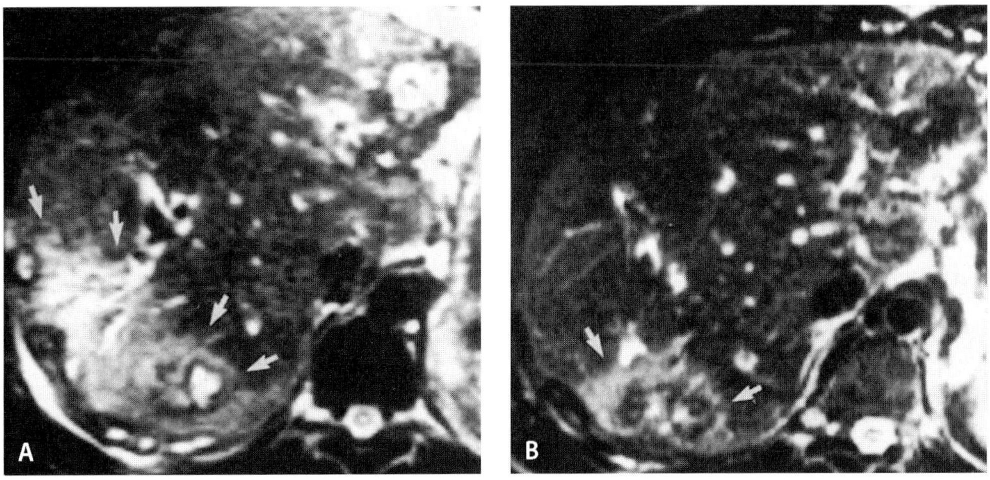

Fig. 3.53 A, B. MRI monitoring of response of liver hydatid to albendazole treatment. **A** MR image (SE 2100/100) obtained before therapy with albendazole. Excellent contrast resolution of MR allows delineation of extensive reactive edematous changes in liver surrounding hydatid cyst (*arrows*). **B** MR image (SE 2000/100) obtained after treatment shows decrease in size of hydatid and surrounding reactive changes (*arrows*). (Courtesy of Dr. Walther von Sinner and *AJR*, 1991)

Selective Celiac or Hepatic Angiography

Selective celiac or hepatic angiography (although rarely utilized today) can be useful in localizing hydatid cysts, in identifying unsuspected small cysts, and in planning the proper surgical approach. In the arterial phase, there will be displacement and stretching of the branches of the hepatic artery around one or more avascular cysts (Figs. 3.54, 3.55). In the capillary and venous phases, a circular, well-defined filling defect is seen on the hepatogram, and in most cases a rim of increased opacification measuring 0.5–4 mm surrounds the cyst. This represents compressed host vessels and is useful in differentiating hydatid cysts from nonparasitic cysts, primary neoplasms, and metastases. However, a liver abscess may show a wider, or similar, rim of increased vascularity due to inflammatory changes in its wall.

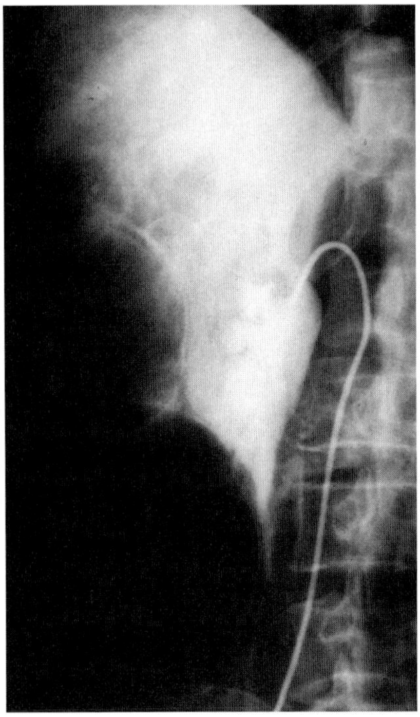

Fig. 3.54. Hepatic arteriography: noncalcified hydatid cysts are seen as large avascular filling defects in the inferior aspect of the right lobe of the liver, with hepatic artery branches stretched and displaced around them. In the capillary or hepatogram phase, there is often a thin rim of contrast medium in the surrounding pericyst. This aids in the differentiation of hydatid cysts from nonparasitic cysts, primary neoplasms, and metastases in the liver, but not from liver abscesses, which may show a similar rim or blush of increased vascularity

Endoscopic Retrograde Cholangiopancreatography

Endoscopic retrograde cholangiopancreatography is particularly useful when a hydatid cyst has ruptured into the biliary tract (Fig. 3.29). The cyst can often be localized and impacted hydatid material (daughter cysts, fragments of membranes) that may cause jaundice can be removed at the same time.

Follow-up After Treatment

Even if there are no clinical indications, it is a wise precaution to follow up all patients who have been treated for hydatid disease. This should be done after 1 year and again in another 2 years, to exclude both local recurrence (e.g., after surgery) and the growth of new cysts elsewhere in the patient. This is particularly important if the patient's laboratory tests have changed. Seroconversion from positive to negative usually occurs within 1 year after successful treatment, although it may take up to 4 years. The tests will become positive again when there is recurrence.

Ultrasonography and a chest radiograph will demonstrate any recurrent cysts except in the skeleton or CNS. If these are suspected, appropriate bone radiography or scintigraphy and CT or MRI scanning of the spine or brain will be needed.

Clinical and Imaging Correlation for Specific Organs and Regions

Abdomen

The majority of hydatid cysts occur within the abdomen (Figs. 3.56–3.58). The liver may harbor up to 70% of all hydatids, and various series from around the world indicate a frequency of 3%–9% for cysts within the spleen, 2%–4% within the kidney, and 2% to as high as 18% within the peritoneum. This wide variation in peritoneal involvement is probably a reflection of the fact that in some developing countries the primary liver cyst is not identified and treated and may eventually rupture into the peritoneum. The slow expansion of secondary cysts will in time lead the patient to medical attention.

Liver

Hydatids in the liver have a structure similar to lesions in other sites, but the host reaction (pericyst), which plays a role in the development of the cyst, is particularly intense in the liver. About 85% of liver hydatids occur within the right lobe, probably because this lobe is much larger than the left and has a greater portal venous circulation. Cysts in the liver may be superficial, near the capsule (Fig. 3.56 A), or lie deeply in the liver substance. Superficial cysts may enlarge in any direction, elevating the diaphragm or bulging into the peritoneal cavity. More deeply situated cysts may cause compression and atrophy of the surrounding hepatic tissues. They may cause biliary stasis and, if ruptured, reactive hepatitis. Secondarily infected ruptured cysts may cause cholangitis. Communicating or direct rupture may produce severe portal fibrosis and portal hypertension in some patients. If the cyst is located near the porta hepatis, there may be obstructive jaundice from compression of the main biliary ducts.

Central or deep hydatids may undergo direct intrahepatic rupture of the pericyst, resulting in the cyst contents no longer being contained and spilling into the liver parenchyma (Fig. 3.50). Sectional imaging of liver cysts which have undergone communicating rupture demonstrates detached endocyst floating in

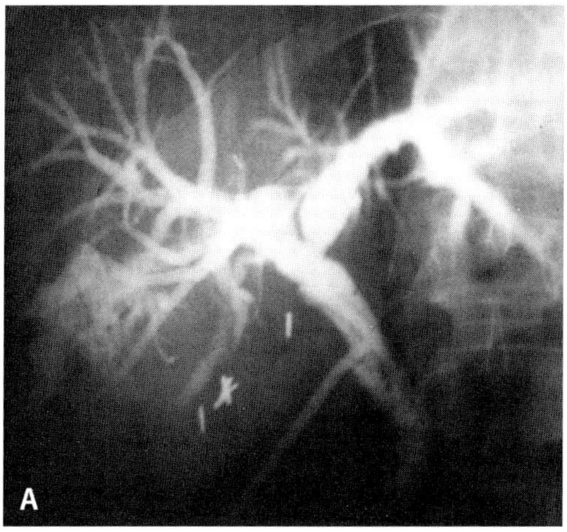

Fig. 3.55 A–C. Noncalcified liver hydatid identified on T-tube cholangiography and hepatic arteriography. **A** There is contrast filling of an irregular cyst cavity in the right lobe of the liver on a T-tube cholangiogram. This hydatid cyst had previously ruptured into one or more branches of the right hepatic duct, a situation which often leads to suppuration and gas formation within the cyst. **B** Late arterial and **C** capillary phases of a selective hepatic arteriogram showing at least two irregular, avascular filling defects in the right lobe of the liver, with stretching of hepatic artery branches around them. The irregular nature of these noncalcified hydatid cysts is best seen in the hepatogram phase (C). There is some increased uptake in the walls of these cysts, probably due in part to secondary inflammation as a result of cyst rupture and communication with the biliary tree

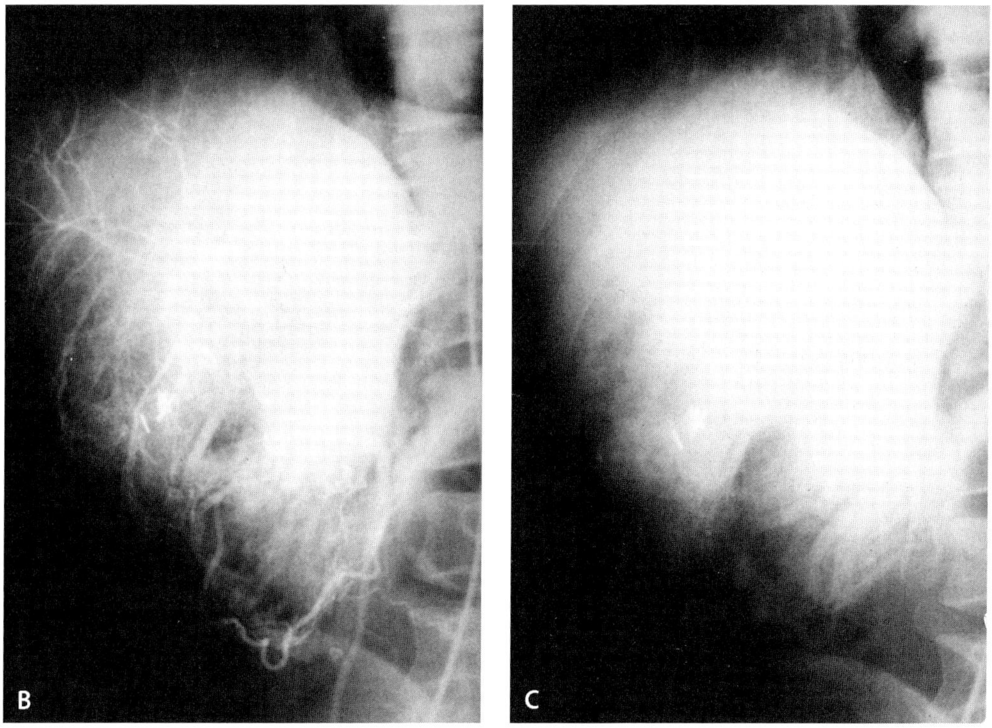

the remaining cyst fluid – the snake or serpent sign (Figs. 3.27, 3.44 D, 3.45 D, 3.49), which is the cross-sectional imaging counterpart of the floating water lily sign in the lung. The cyst may become appreciably smaller and less spherical (Fig. 3.28), and there may be evidence of downstream biliary obstruction. Communicating rupture may be diagnosed directly, by the demonstration of hydatid debris in the biliary tree, or when contrast enters the cyst cavity during ERCP (Fig. 3.29). Communicating rupture occasionally shows a fat-fluid level in the cyst cavity.

Dilated pericystic ducts, which are apparent in 25% of liver hydatids, are usually much more tortuous than blood vessels (Figs. 3.22, 3.34 B). A clear distinction between the two is possible only if CT scans are performed with intravenous contrast enhancement – a distinction that is not as easy on ultrasound examinations. Dilated bile ducts in the unruptured hydatid are always upstream (in terms of bile flow) of the cyst. The reasons for biliary dilatation and biliary perforation of the pericyst are probably related. Dilated bile ducts which perforate the pericyst and allow herniation of a small knuckle of delicate endocyst may predispose to rupture. Dilated ducts should be considered an indication that unseen communicating ducts exist downstream, threatening biliary obstruction after rupture. At the time of rupture, small daughter cysts and fragments of endocyst may be forced into the upstream ducts,

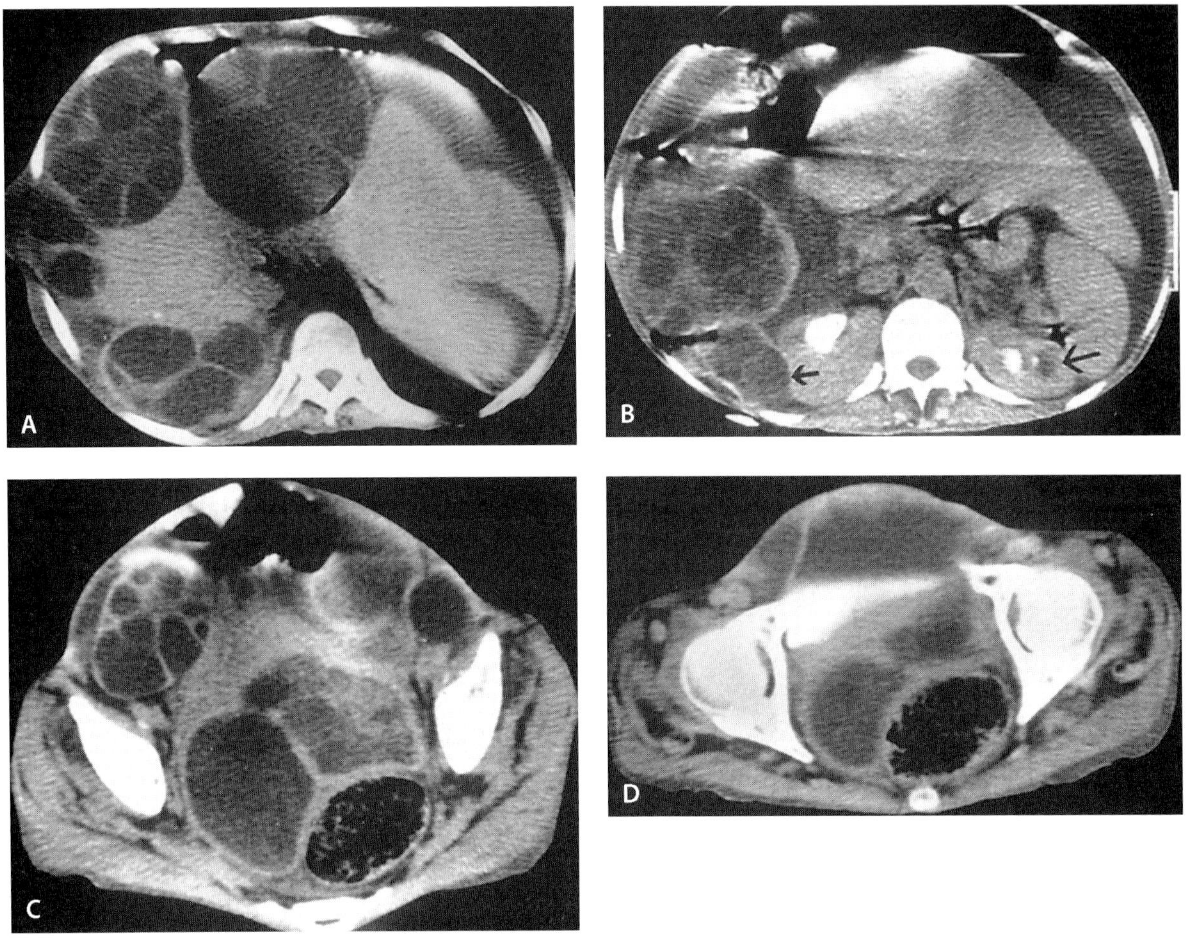

Fig. 3.56 A–D. Multiple hydatid cysts in the abdomen and pelvis demonstrated by CT after intravenous bolus of contrast medium in a Saudi Arabian patient. **A** Large type II hydatids with typical daughter cysts in both lobes of the liver. One cyst protruding through the right intercostal space later ruptured through the skin. **B** Hydatid cysts adjacent to the right kidney, causing an impression on the renal outline (*small arrow*). A small low-density lesion in the left kidney represents a simple or hydatid cyst (*long arrow*). Ascites and free abdominal gas are also noted. **C, D** Multiple type I and II hydatids in the pelvis with and without daughter cysts. (See Fig. 3.155, which shows the results of surgery and chemotherapy in this patient.) (Courtesy of Dr. Walther von Sinner)

but they do not cause obstruction as the pressure within the cyst cavity soon drops as hydatid fluid leaves via the downstream ducts. Bile flow then returns the debris to the pericyst cavity. The bile that floods the pericyst cavity probably always kills the parasite. Biliary obstruction, which occurs if formed elements enter downstream ducts, characteristically produces fluctuating jaundice which may disappear for short periods, presumably because of the compliance of the obstructing fragments.

Cysts located beneath Glisson's capsule protrude from the external surface of the liver, are dome-shaped, and may become pedunculated. Growing cysts at the dome of the liver or spleen exert pressure, leading to elevation or a local bulge of the hemidiaphragm and often restricted movement (Figs. 3.41, 3.42). This should not be confused with eventration or other abnormality of the diaphragm or prolapse of intra-abdominal organs into the chest. Other entities such as amebic abscess, subphrenic abscess, and primary or metastatic malignant disease must be distinguished. Unlike amebic or other subphrenic abscesses, unruptured liver hydatids confined to the hepatic parenchyma usually do not stimulate a pleural effusion or lung reaction. Rupture of an infected hydatid cyst located in the upper right lobe of the liver or in the spleen may, however, lead to a subdiaphragmatic abscess (Fig. 3.59). Rupture of a hydatid cyst, especially if direct, may be accompanied not only by abdominal pain but also by allergic phenomena, such as urticaria or asthma, and less often by collapse, and rarely by anaphylactic shock.

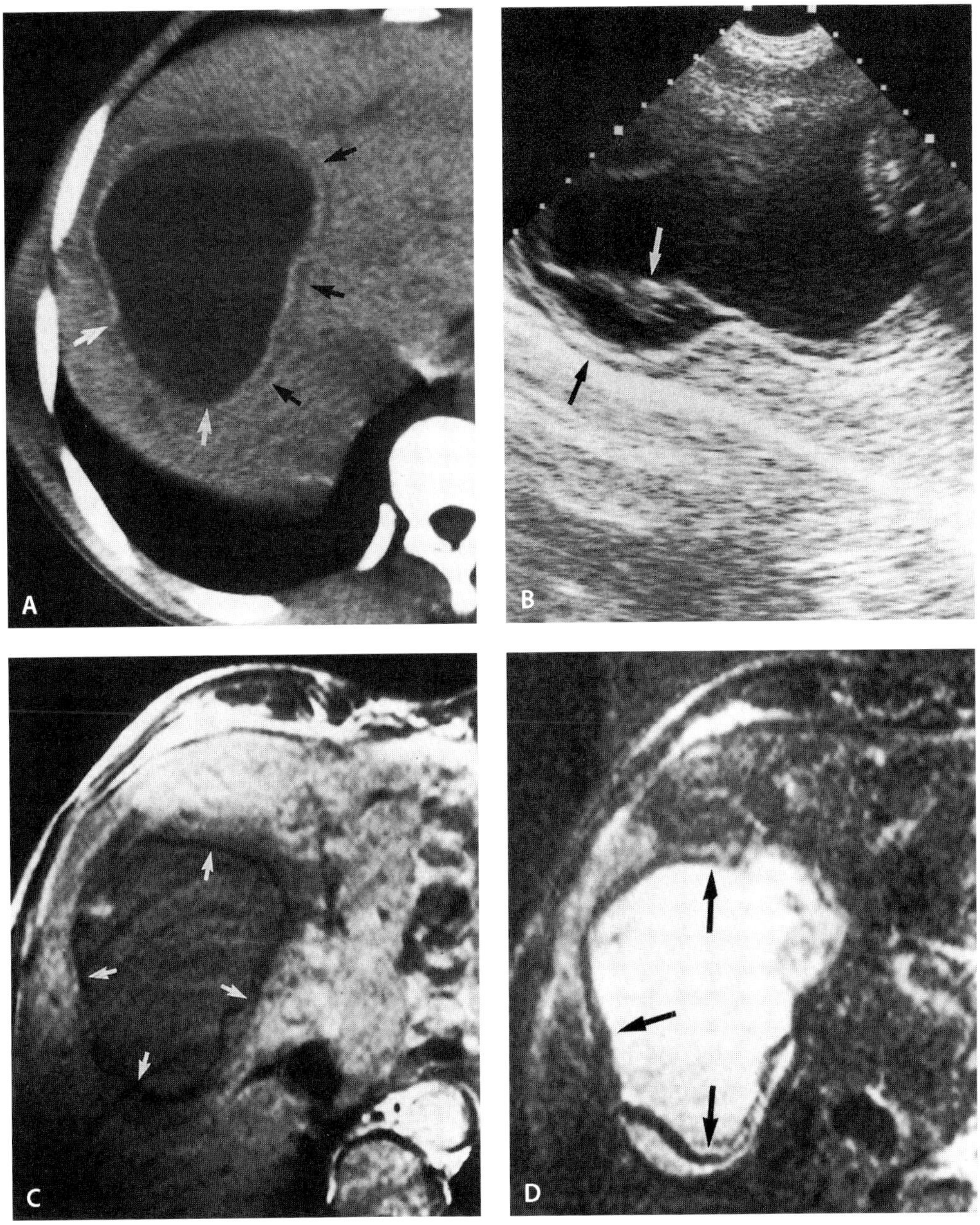

Fig. 3.57 A–D. A 40-year-old Saudi Arabian man with multiple hydatid cysts of the abdomen. Five years previously, he noted swellings in his upper abdomen, which disappeared 2 years later after a traffic accident. A year later he again noted abdominal distention, and at surgery hundreds of small hydatids were removed from his abdomen. He underwent mebendazole therapy for 3 years with unsatifactory results. Four months previously he had presented again with new abdominal swellings, and a large smooth nontender 8-cm mass was felt in his right hypochondrium, with a smaller mass in the left hypochondrium and a third mass in the right lumbar area. In his past history there was one episode of jaundice and abdominal pain. **A** Nonenhanced abdominal CT scan revealed a large hepatic hydatid cyst with a defective posterior cyst wall (*white arrows*) with a low-intensity rim (*black arrows*), suggesting possible imminent rupture. Three weeks later, an ultrasound study (**B**) of the right abdomen revealed the serpent or snake sign of detached parasitic membranes pathognomonic for hydatid disease, showing the cyst wall (*black arrow*) and collapsed membranes (*white arrow*). **C** At the same time, a T1-weighted axial MR image, right side (TR 850 ms, TE 20 ms) and **D** T2-weighted axial MR image (TR 2000 ms, TE 100 ms) demonstrated the serpent or snake sign of detached membranes (*arrows*). Following surgery, the patient made an uneventful recovery. (Courtesy of Dr. Walther von Sinner and *Eur J Radiol*, 1990)

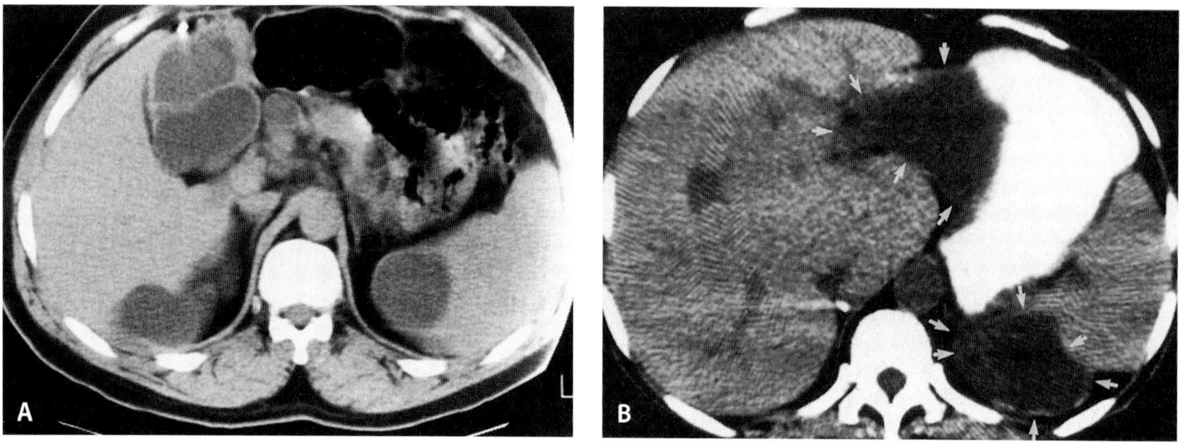

Fig. 3.58 A, B. Multiple type I and II hydatid cysts of the liver and spleen as seen on CT scans in two Saudi Arabian patients. In **B**, a 10-year-old boy, the hydatids of the left lobe of the liver and of the spleen (*arrows*) lie in close relationship to the barium-filled stomach. There is faint calcification in the wall of the splenic cyst. (Courtesy of Dr. Walther von Sinner and *Eur J Radiol*, 1990)

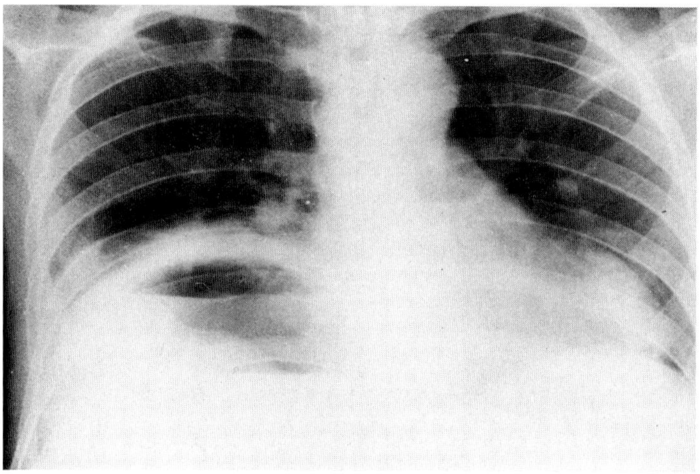

Fig. 3.59. A ruptured hydatid cyst of the dome of the right lobe of the liver which presented as a subdiaphragmatic abscess in a patient from India. An erect PA chest radiograph shows multiple fluid levels within the ruptured cyst beneath the right diaphragm, and large daughter cysts floating within the multiloculated fluid levels. The right hemidiaphragm appears thickened and moderately elevated and its movement was markedly restricted on fluoroscopy. (Courtesy of Dr. A. Chandrahasan Johnson)

Cysts growing towards the diaphragm may penetrate it and perforate into the pleura, pulmonary parenchyma, bronchi, or pericardium (this is one reason why cysts in the left lobe of the liver have a worse prognosis) (Fig. 3.60). Even if not infected, a slowly growing cyst may cause pressure atrophy of diaphragmatic muscle fibers and prolapse into the pleural cavity, accompanied by a pleural effusion. If there are extensive pleural adhesions, prolapse may even occur into the lung parenchyma. If the cyst ruptures, in addition to a marked pleural effusion, an allergic pneumonitis or even a tension pneumothorax may develop. The long-term damage, if no acute allergic reaction has occurred, may be secondary dissemination of echinococcosis in the pleura and lung parenchyma. Prophylactic treatment with effective chemotherapy is now available and should be considered in such cases.

Cysts growing in the direction of the peritoneal cavity may perforate into the peritoneum, duodenum, colon, or renal pelvis. A hydatid cyst, especially if large and bound by adhesions to a hollow viscus, may undergo direct rupture into that viscus. In some cases, daughter cysts and other parasitic material have been recovered from the stomach, urinary tract, and bowel (e.g., the rectum). If both the

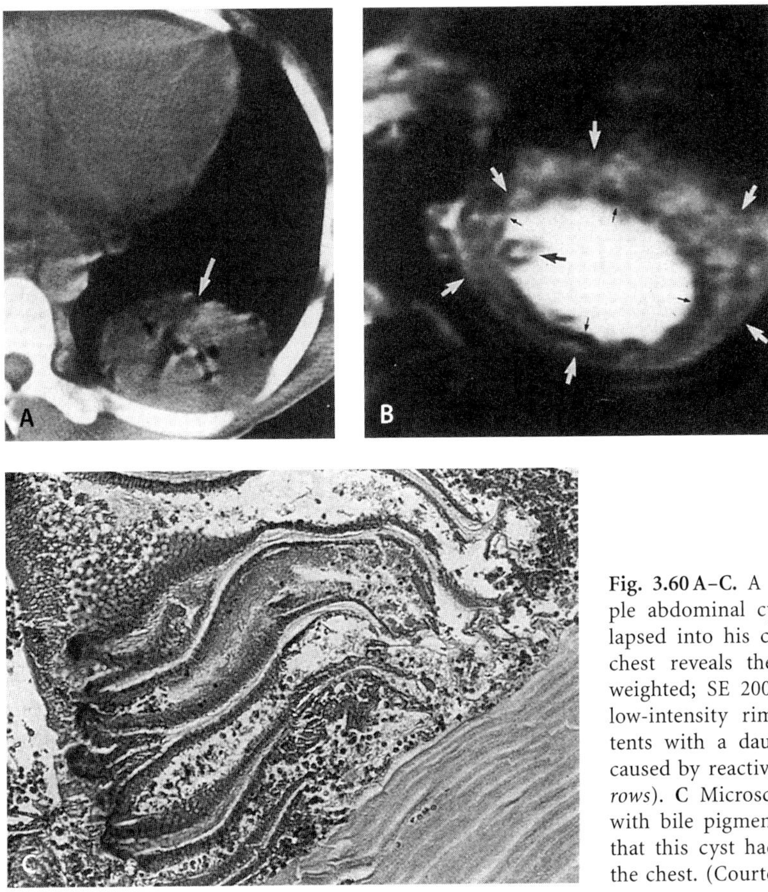

Fig. 3.60 A–C. A 24-year-old Saudi Arabian man with multiple abdominal cysts; one in the left lobe of the liver prolapsed into his chest. A Nonenhanced CT scan of the lower chest reveals the prolapsed hydatid (*arrow*). B MRI (T2-weighted; SE 2000/100) shows the prolapsed hydatid with a low-intensity rim (*small black arrows*), high-intensity contents with a daughter cyst (*large black arrow*), and a halo caused by reactive or compressed lung parenchyma (*white arrows*). C Microscopic pathology shows parasitic membranes with bile pigment from old biliary-cystic fistula, confirming that this cyst had originated in the liver and prolapsed into the chest. (Courtesy of Dr. Walther von Sinner)

cyst wall and the pericyst of the organ harboring the cyst rupture, spill of infective cyst contents into the peritoneal cavity usually occurs, leading to extensive intraperitoneal seeding (Fig. 3.30).

Plain film examination of the abdomen may show hepatomegaly with a slight generalized or localized bulge of the diaphragm, depending on the size and location of the cyst (Figs. 3.41, 3.42, 3.61). If there has been considerable destruction of one lobe of the liver, enlargement of the other lobe (usually the left) may develop solely from compensatory hypertrophy. The frequency of cyst calcification in the liver varies from 33% to 60% depending on the series and geographic area, and usually requires 5–10 years to develop. These calcified cysts, whether ruptured or unruptured, are not difficult to diagnose radiologically. The vast majority will be unruptured, have a spherical shape, and vary in diameter from 1 to 10 or more cm (Figs. 3.41–3.43, 3.62, 3.63).

The differential diagnosis will include calcification within a nonparasitic cyst, an old liver abscess (usually purulent, but occasionally amebic), hepatoma, vascular malformation, scar tissue, granuloma, or intrahepatic gallstones. Calcification within adjacent organs such as the gallbladder or adrenal

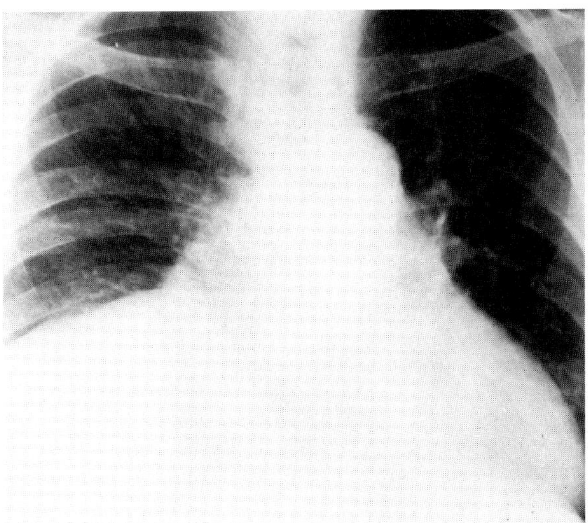

Fig. 3.61. Hepatomegaly causing generalized elevation of the right hemidiaphragm on plain film examination in a patient with large uncalcified hydatid cysts in the liver

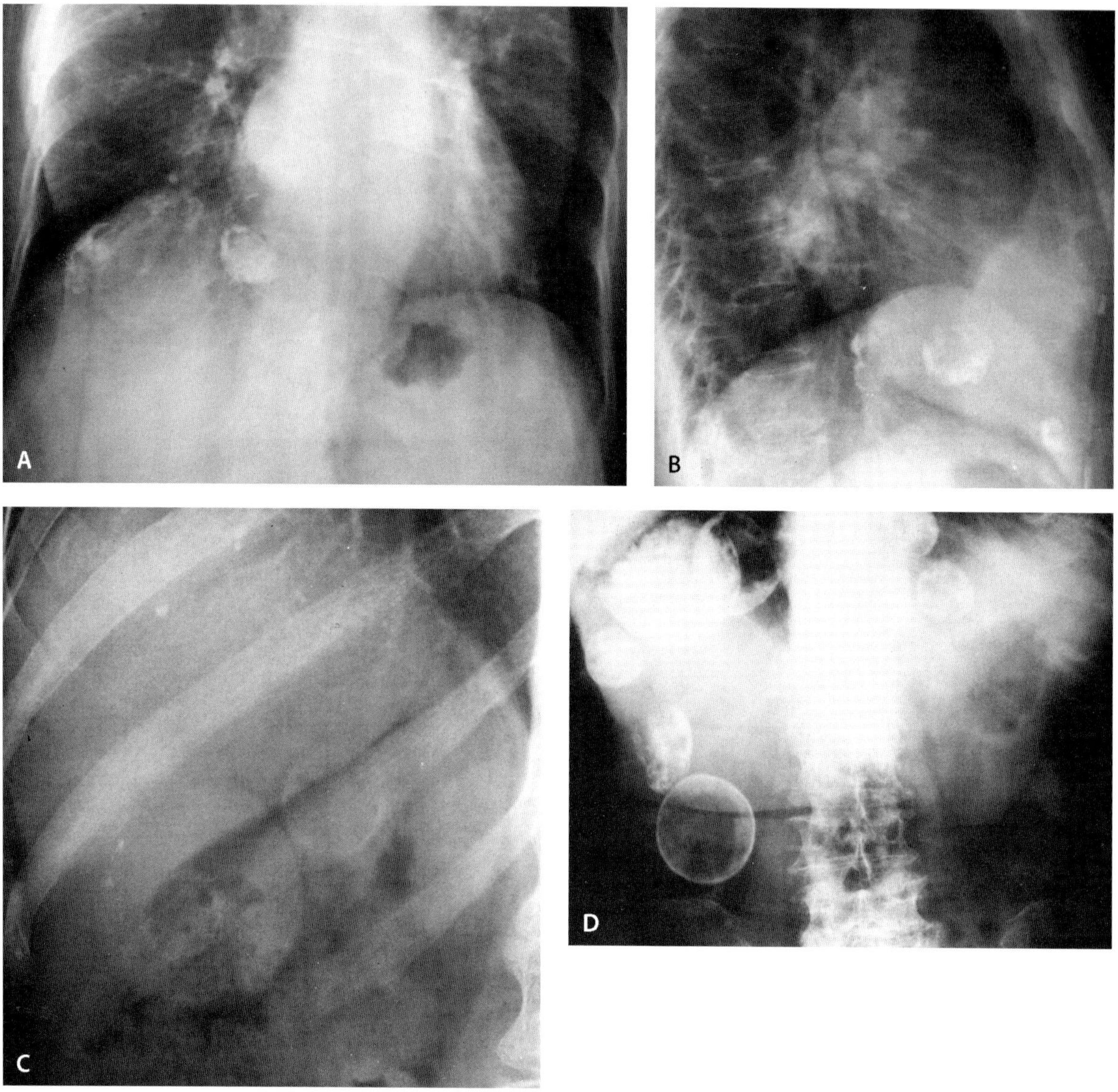

Fig. 3.62 A–D. Multiple calcified type III hydatid cysts of the liver. **A** PA and **B** lateral views of the chest and upper abdomen show three small, heavily calcified cysts within the liver as well as a rare hydatid cyst in the mediastinum, noncalcified and lying posterior to the right heart border in both projections. Two of the liver hydatids lie just below the slightly elevated right hemidiaphragm; the third and smallest calcified hydatid is in the midline and is probably in the left lobe of the liver. **C** Two hydatids in the right lobe of the liver which have faint calcification within the pericyst, permitting sharp delineation from surrounding normal liver parenchyma. There is a ring-like calcification overlying the larger of the two hydatids, which proved to be a partially calcified gallstone. The differential diagnosis between rim-like calcification in a hydatid versus other types of intra-abdominal calcifications such as gallstones can be difficult at times on plain radiographs: ultrasonography or CT will help to solve the problem. **D** Multiple thin- and thick-rimmed calcified hydatid cysts are seen throughout the right and left lobes of the liver. (**D** courtesy of Dr. William Thompson, Minneapolis)

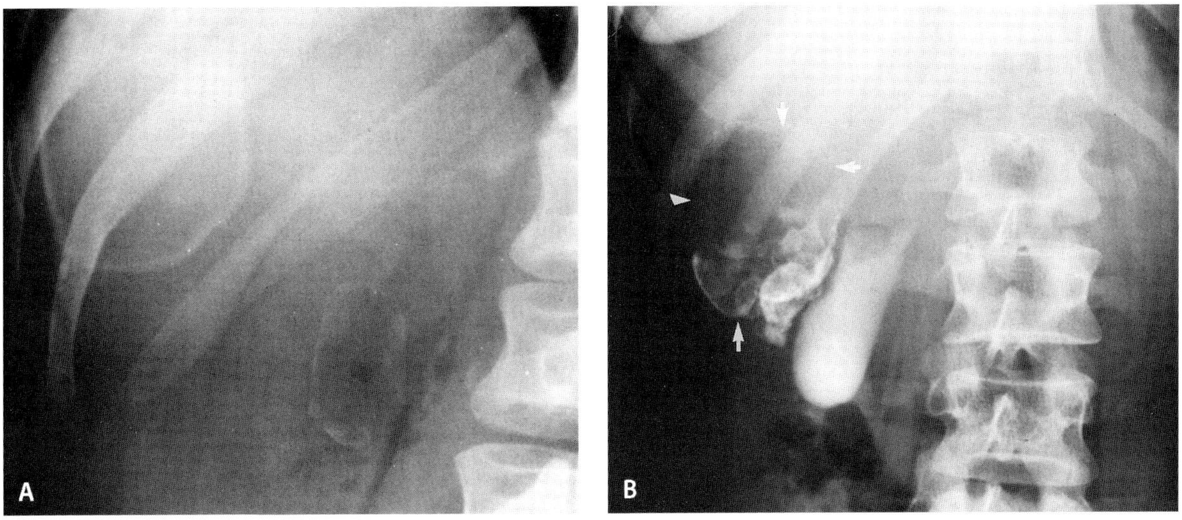

Fig. 3.63 A, B. Calcification in the walls of liver hydatids in two different patients. **A** There is rim calcification in a right liver lobe hydatid and in another hydatid overlying the right renal pelvis. **B** There is calcification in the wall of a collapsing hydatid cyst (*arrowheads*) in the right liver lobe with multiple calcified daughter cysts in the lower aspect of the mother cyst (*arrow*). The gallbladder is opacified with contrast medium

glands, and within renal or pancreatic cysts, calculi, or tumors, must be excluded.

The uncalcified hydatid in the liver or other solid organs can seldom be seen on a plain radiograph of the abdomen. Prior to the advent of modern cross-sectional imaging, such hydatids could only be identified by angiography or radioisotope scanning as avascular masses or filling defects (Figs. 3.54, 3.55). Occasionally, cholangiography will demonstrate communication with the bile ducts (Fig. 3.55 A): such communication with the biliary tract or neighboring organs may lead to suppuration or gas formation within the cyst. However, the vast majority of uncalcified cysts will remain undiagnosed unless demonstrated by modern scanning (ultrasonography, CT, or MRI), as discussed above under General Principles of Imaging. Numerous examples of cross-sectional imaging of liver hydatids are presented in Figs. 3.64–3.67. In the interest of completeness and because his classification based on the sonographic morphology of liver hydatids is still used in many countries, we have listed earlier the Gharbi classification of hydatid cysts, which differs from our own pathology-based classification used throughout this chapter.

Spleen

Hydatid cysts within the spleen behave in the same way as hydatids in the liver. They may be primary or secondary, solitary or multiple. Primary hydatids develop from larvae reaching the spleen via the arterial circulation. The first clinical indication of the presence of a splenic hydatid cyst is usually splenomegaly. If no typical calcification is present, an uncomplicated cyst may not be recognized. Single hydatid cysts may grow to a considerable size, almost totally replacing the splenic parenchyma. Multiple hydatid cysts of different sizes may also occur. Secondary hydatids of the spleen may result from extension of a peritoneal hydatid or metastases from other sites.

Clinically there may be pain or discomfort in the left upper quadrant and a palpable mass. Most cysts are painless, but when there is pain it usually results from communicating or direct rupture. Occasionally a cyst arising from the lower pole of the spleen may rupture into the peritoneum, leading to secondary peritoneal hydatids and sometimes causing an abdominal emergency. A splenic cyst can also rupture into the stomach, colon, or rarely the left kidney. Cysts arising from the upper pole of the spleen may rupture through the diaphragm into the pleura or lung (Fig. 3.68), causing secondary pleural or pulmonary hydatidosis. Such direct rupture may occur when there are adhesions between the pericyst and adjacent organ.

If there is calcification within the wall of a splenic cyst, it is usually recognizable on plain radiographs

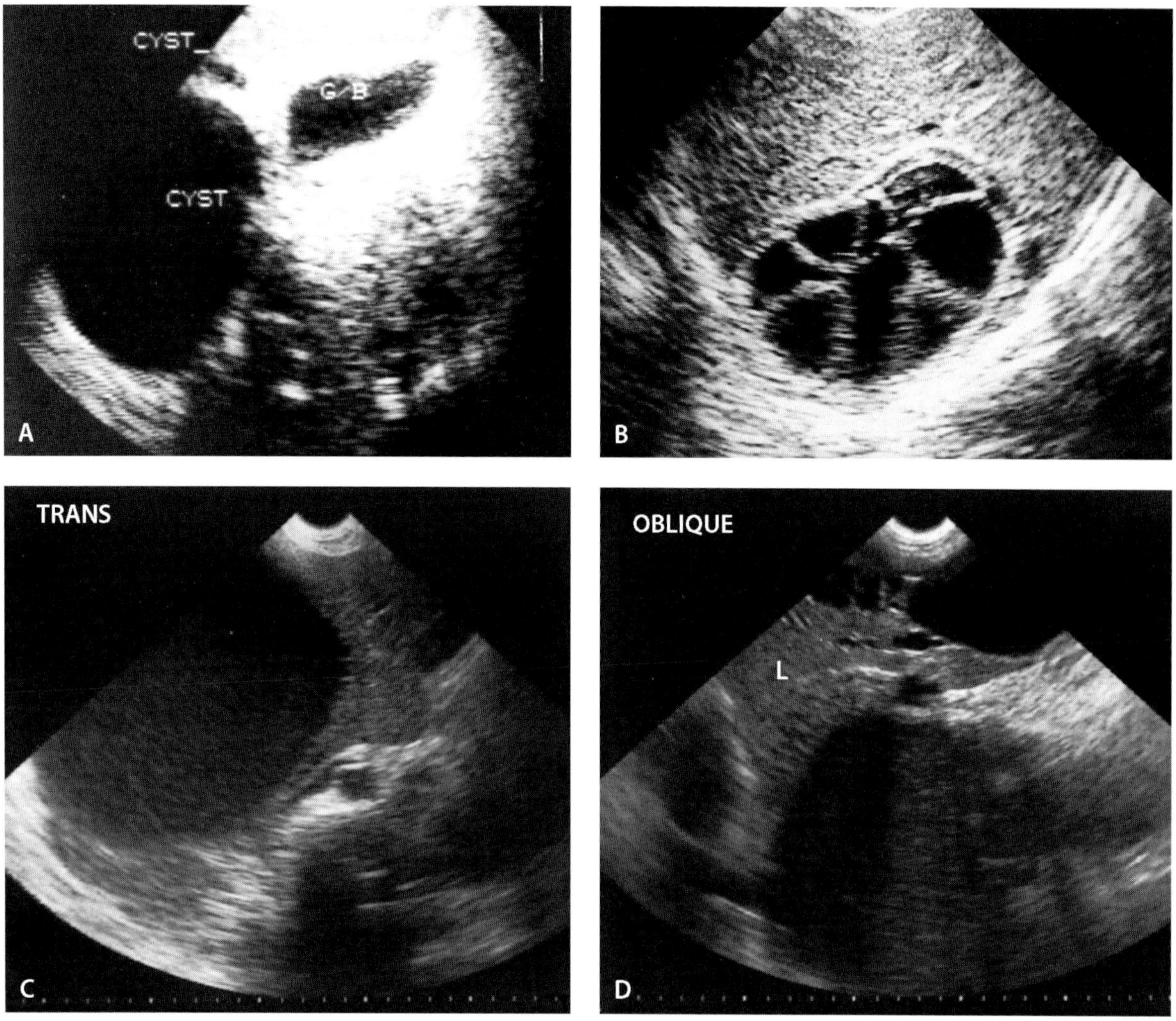

Fig. 3.64 A–D. Ultrasound examination of unruptured liver hydatids in three different patients. **A** Large type I cyst in right lobe of liver. Gallbladder (*G/B*) is also identified on this sagittal scan. **B** Type II cyst with multiple daughter cysts. **C** Transverse and **D** oblique scans (same patient) showing a large type I hydatid in the right lobe and multiple smaller cysts in the left lobe of the liver. (**C**, **D** courtesy of Dr. Sam Mindel)

of the abdomen and sometimes of the chest (Fig. 3.69). Where one or more large noncalcified hydatids are present, splenomegaly may be noted and may lead to accidental discovery of the cyst on ultrasonography (Fig. 3.70), angiography, or nuclear scanning. Hydatid cysts may also be accidentally discovered on CT and/or MRI done for other purposes (Fig. 3.71). All the imaging findings are similar to those described earlier for the liver and other organs.

Pancreas

Primary echinococcosis of the pancreas is rare, with a reported incidence of less than <0.2/100 cases. However, not all cases are reported and the incidence may be somewhat higher.

Clinical signs of pancreatic hydatids depend more on the size and stage of development than on location: they include abdominal pain, jaundice, weight loss, a palpable abdominal mass, and signs of portal hypertension. When a cyst ruptures into the peritoneal cavity, widespread dissemination may occur if not treated by chemotherapy. Surgery is still the method of choice for intact hydatid cysts and is curative in solitary cysts. The results of imaging (ultrasonography, CT and MRI) are not different from those in other organs. Ultrasound and CT scans may not always distinguish between ruptured and infected hydatid cysts and abscesses, complicated pancreatic pseudocysts, and cystic neoplasms of the pancreas.

(Text continues on p. 258)

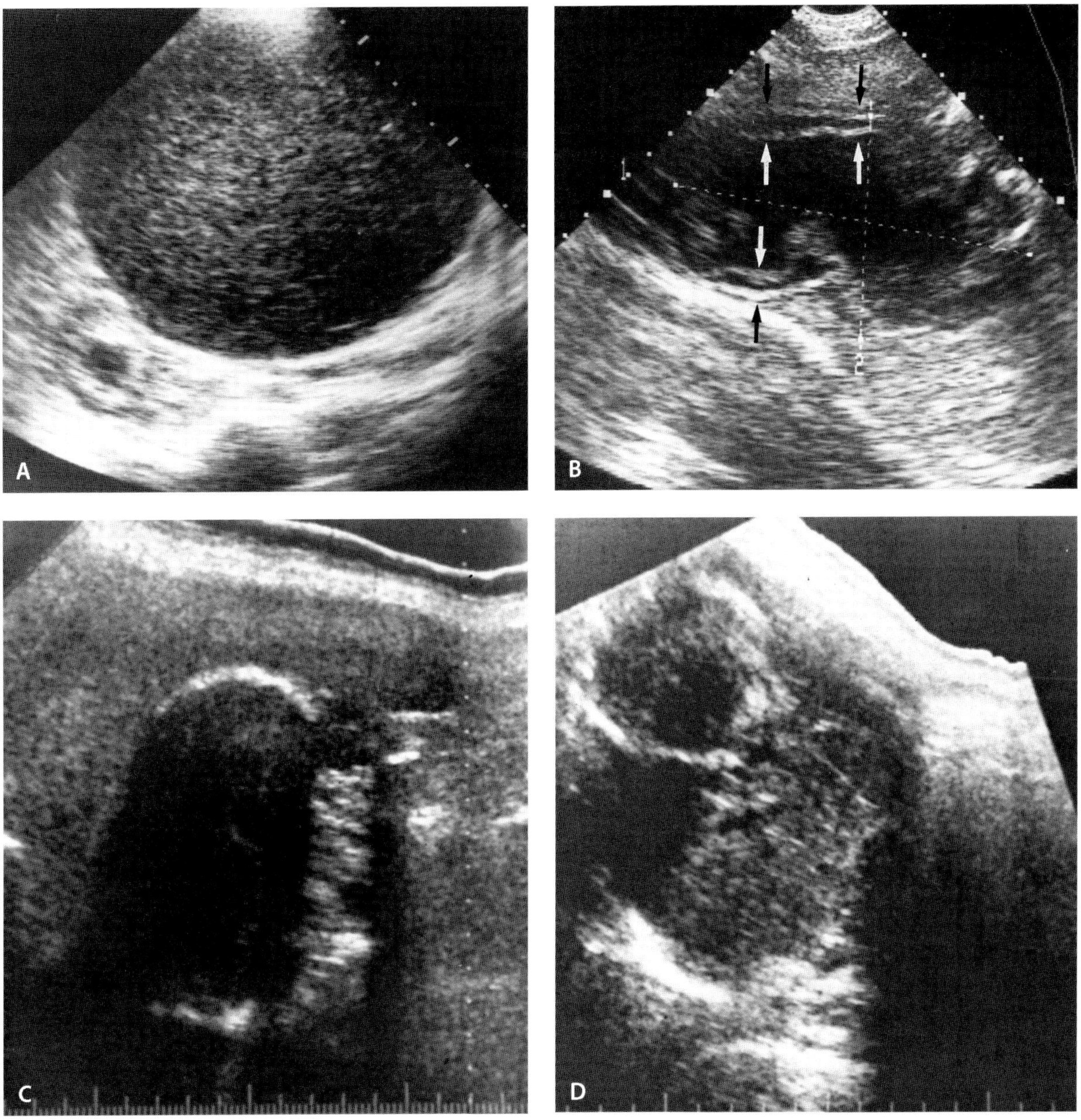

Fig. 3.65 A–D. Ultrasonography of complicated hydatid cysts of liver. **A** Transverse ultrasound scan of a prematurely dead type I hydatid. The appearance is identical to that of an infected hydatid cyst. (Courtesy of Dr. Lewall) **B** Ruptured and collapsing hydatid with parallel stripes indicating separation of parasitic membranes (*white arrows*) from the cyst wall (*black arrows*). (Courtesy of Dr. Walther von Sinner) **C, D** Calcification in the thickened walls of liver hydatids from two different patients. The internal echoes are caused by hydatid sand and degenerating membranes and matrix in the endocyst. These are old, probably inactive type III cysts, especially C. (Courtesy of WHO)

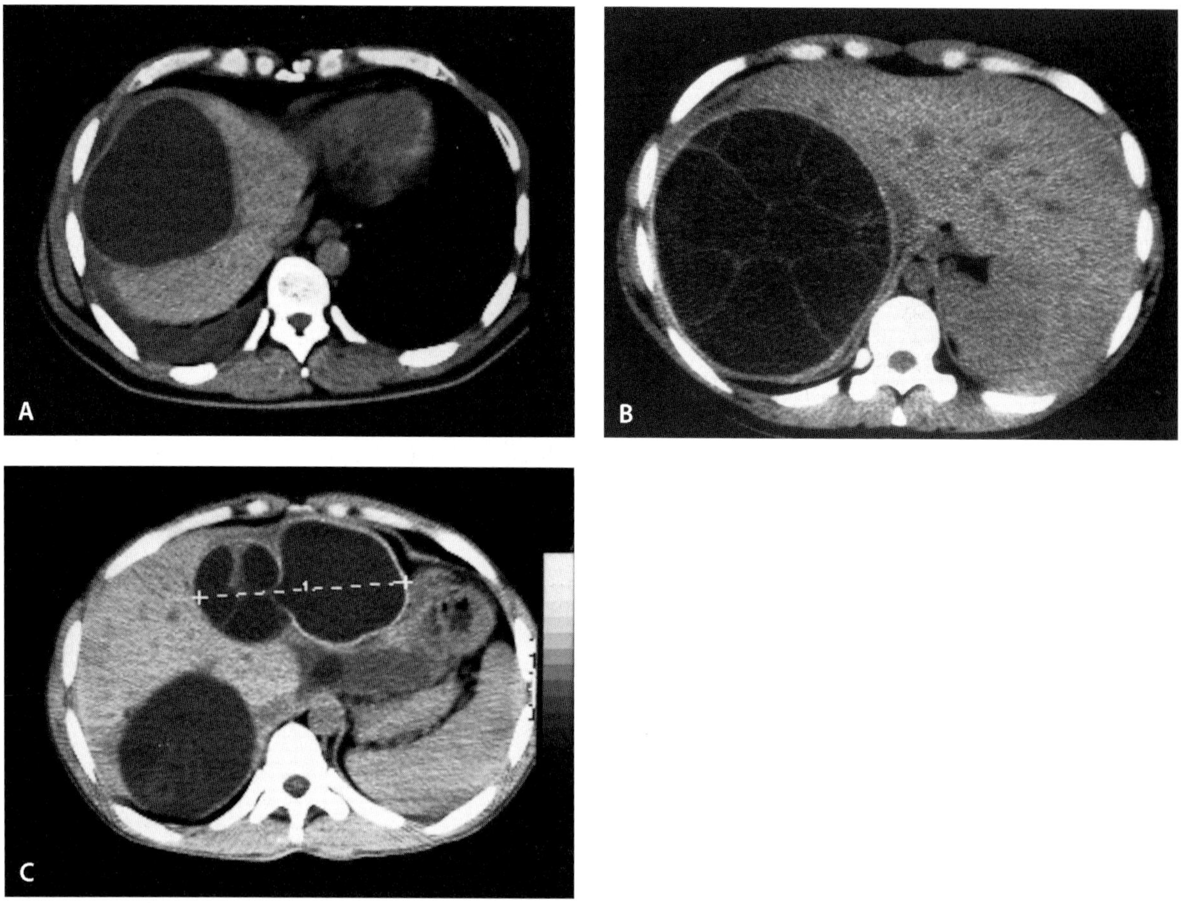

Fig. 3.66 A–C. Nonenhanced CT scans of liver hydatids in three different patients from Tunisia. **A** Type I hydatid in the dome of the right lobe of the liver of a 39-year-old man. A small right pleural effusion is present. **B** Type II hydatid in the right liver lobe with multiple daughter cysts giving a septated appearanced to the cyst. **C** Multiple hydatid cysts in both lobes of the liver of a 22-year-old man. Note the septated appearance and partially detached membrane in the right anterior cyst. (A–C courtesy of Drs. Ben Cheikh and Gharbi, Tunis)

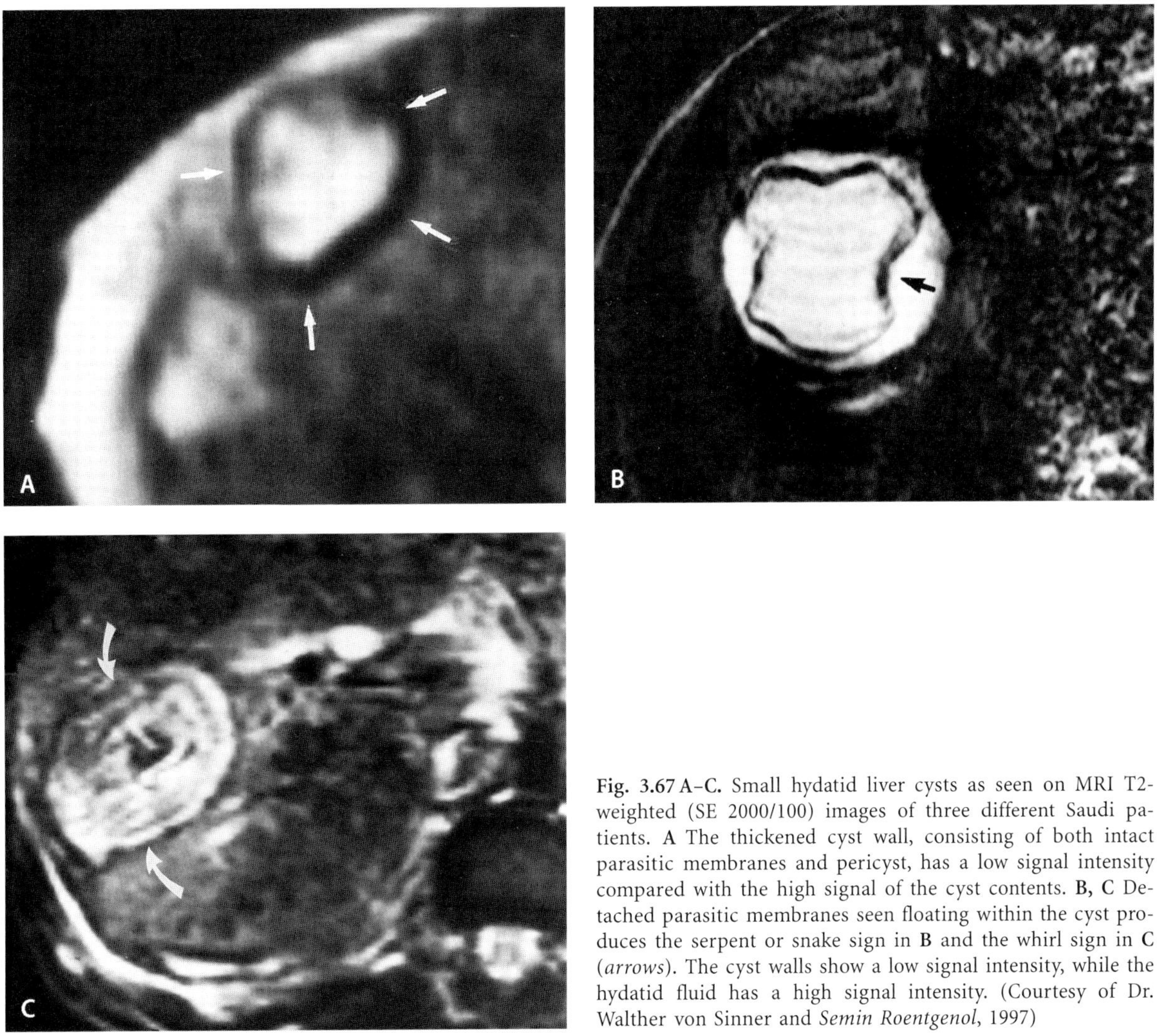

Fig. 3.67 A–C. Small hydatid liver cysts as seen on MRI T2-weighted (SE 2000/100) images of three different Saudi patients. **A** The thickened cyst wall, consisting of both intact parasitic membranes and pericyst, has a low signal intensity compared with the high signal of the cyst contents. **B, C** Detached parasitic membranes seen floating within the cyst produces the serpent or snake sign in **B** and the whirl sign in **C** (*arrows*). The cyst walls show a low signal intensity, while the hydatid fluid has a high signal intensity. (Courtesy of Dr. Walther von Sinner and *Semin Roentgenol*, 1997)

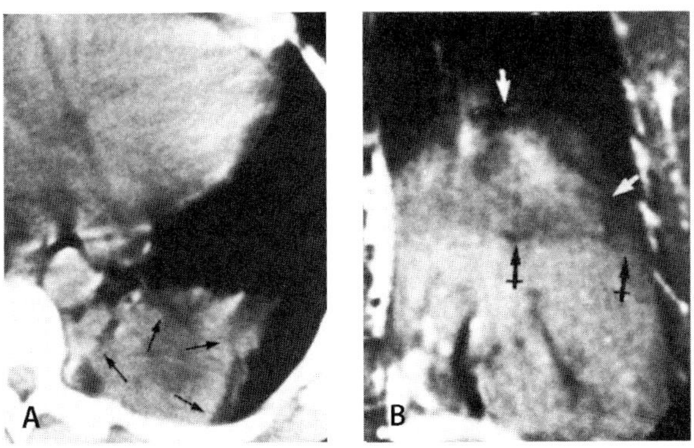

◀

Fig. 3.68 A, B. Hydatid cyst of the spleen. **A** Nonenhanced CT scan shows a ruptured hydatid cyst (*arrows*) prolapsed into the left lower hemithorax. **B** MRI, coronal plane, of same patient. A splenic hydatid has prolapsed into the left hemithorax. Level of left hemidiaphragm (*black arrows*). Hydatid pericyst of low signal intensity (*white arrows*) is noted with surrounding pulmonary parenchymal reaction. (Courtesy of Dr. Walther von Sinner and *Acta Radiol*, 1992)

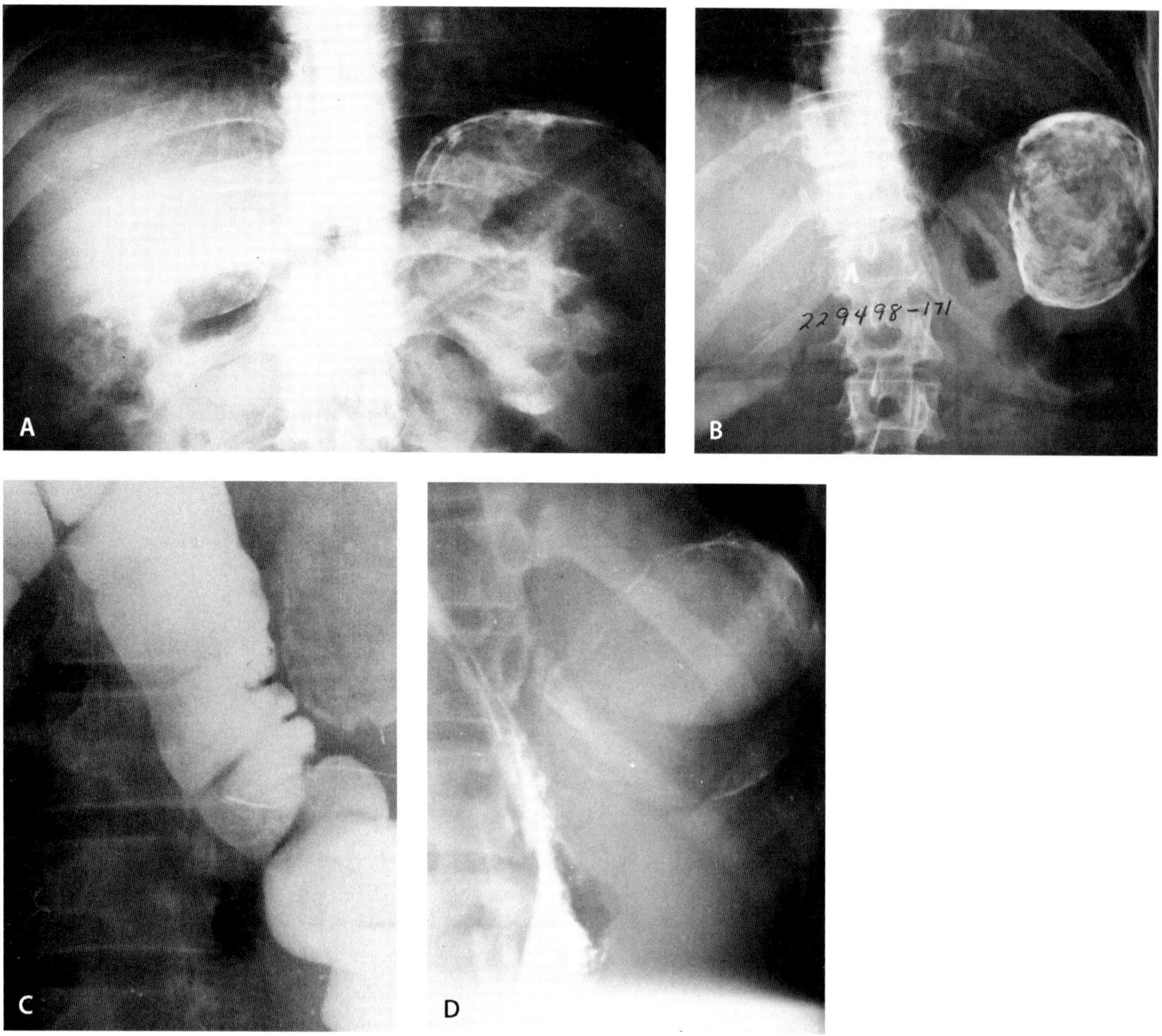

Fig. 3.69 A–D. Large calcified unilocular hydatid cysts of the spleen in four different patients. **A** In addition to the large calcified splenic cyst, there is a smaller calcified hydatid in the liver just to the right of the midline. **B** Dense calcification within a large splenic hydatid. **C** Calcified splenic hydatid with downward displacement of splenic flexure of colon on barium enema. **D** Large calcified splenic hydatid seen as a chance finding on barium swallow examination of a woman from Nairobi, Kenya

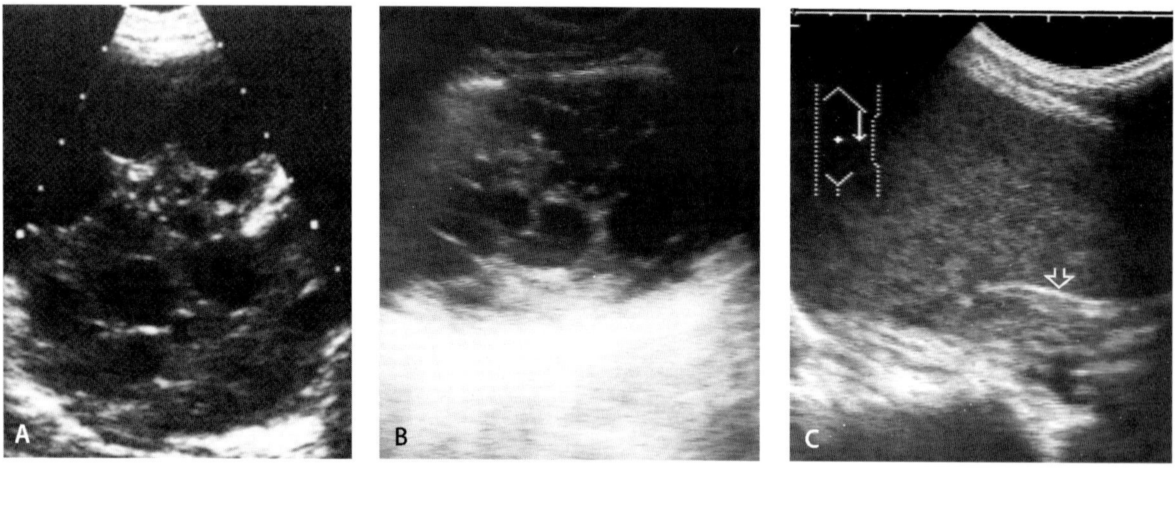

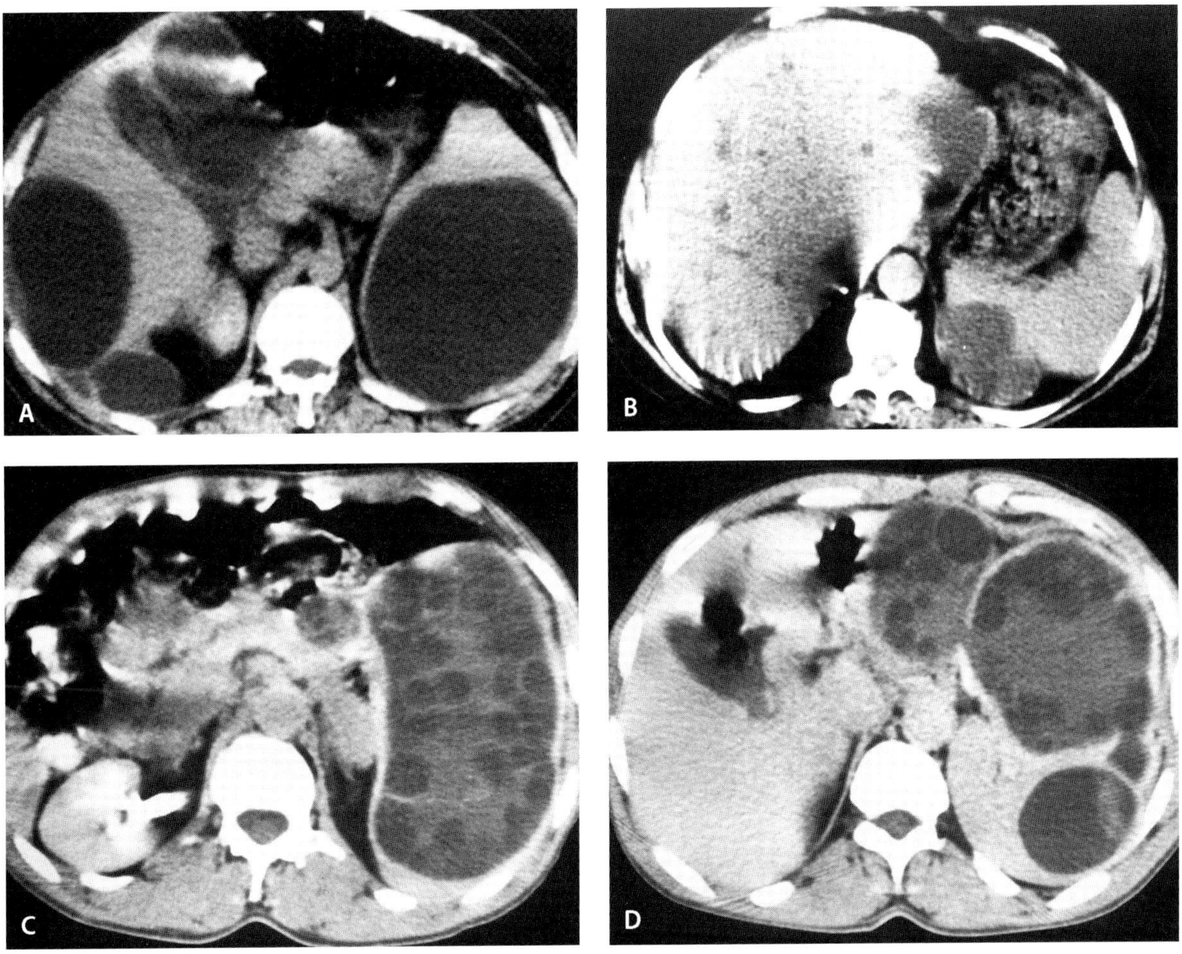

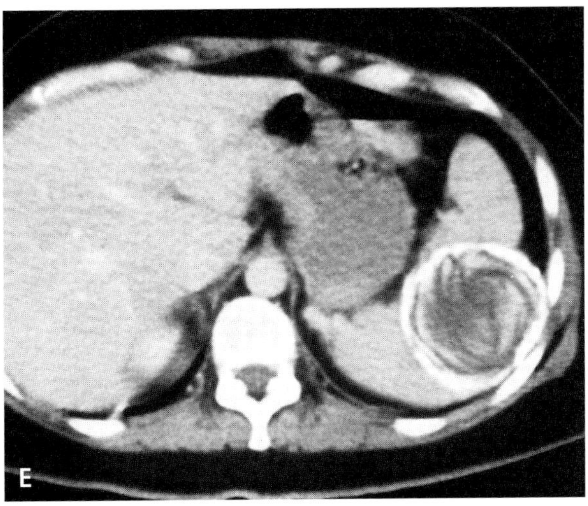

Fig. 3.71 A–E. CT scans of splenic hydatids in four different Saudi Arabian patients. **A** Multiple type I and II hydatids in both lobes of the liver and a solitary huge unilocular type I hydatid which has replaced most of the splenic parenchyma on nonenhanced CT scan. **B** Eccentrically located splenic hydatid causing a prominent bulge in the posterior splenic capsule on contrast-enhanced CT. Such a cyst can rupture into the retroperitoneum. **C** Contrast-enhanced CT scan showing a huge type II hydatid with numerous daughter cysts, which has replaced virtually the entire splenic parenchyma. **D** Multiple hypermature type II hydatids in the left lobe of the liver and in the spleen with multiple daughter cysts and considerable matrix on contrast-enhanced CT scan. The wall of the anterior splenic cyst is partially calcified. **E** Unilocular type III splenic hydatid. There is thick rim calcification of the pericyst and calcification of collapsed whirl-like parasitic membranes within the cyst. (Courtesy of Dr. Walther von Sinner and *Acta Radiol*, 1992)

◀ **Fig. 3.70 A–C.** Ultrasound scans of splenic hydatids. **A** Large hydatid cyst with a number of smaller cysts in a Saudi Arabian patient. Echoes from the bottom of daughter cysts indicate hydatid sand. (Courtesy of Dr. Walther von Sinner.) **B** Sixty-year-old woman from Tunisia with multiple hydatid cysts in the spleen. (Courtesy of Dr. Gharbi, Tunis) **C** Old calcified collapsed splenic hydatid (*arrow*) in a patient from Kenya. (Courtesy of WHO, Geneva)

Mesentery, Omentum, Peritoneum, Retroperitoneum, and Pelvis

Primary or secondary hydatids may be found anywhere along the omentum, mesentery, peritoneal cavity, retroperitoneum, or pelvis in at least 2% of patients. They may be palpable clinically or cause bowel or urinary complaints. When calcified, they may be detected radiologically on plain radiographs of the abdomen and pelvis (Figs. 3.72–3.74 A). Otherwise, they may be discovered, often as a chance finding, on ultrasonography, CT, or MRI (Figs. 3.74 B–E, 3.75).

Kidneys and Ureters

Renal hydatids are almost always primary, although direct invasion from the liver or spleen can occur. They stimulate pericyst formation and are similar to cysts in the liver. They are usually solitary and occur most commonly in the upper or lower poles and only occasionally in the central portion of the kidney (Fig. 3.76 A–D). The cyst may grow toward, and occasionally rupture into, the perirenal tissues and retroperitoneum or it may extend anteriorly into the peritoneum and adjacent organs. If the cyst ruptures into the renal pelvis, renal colic will occur

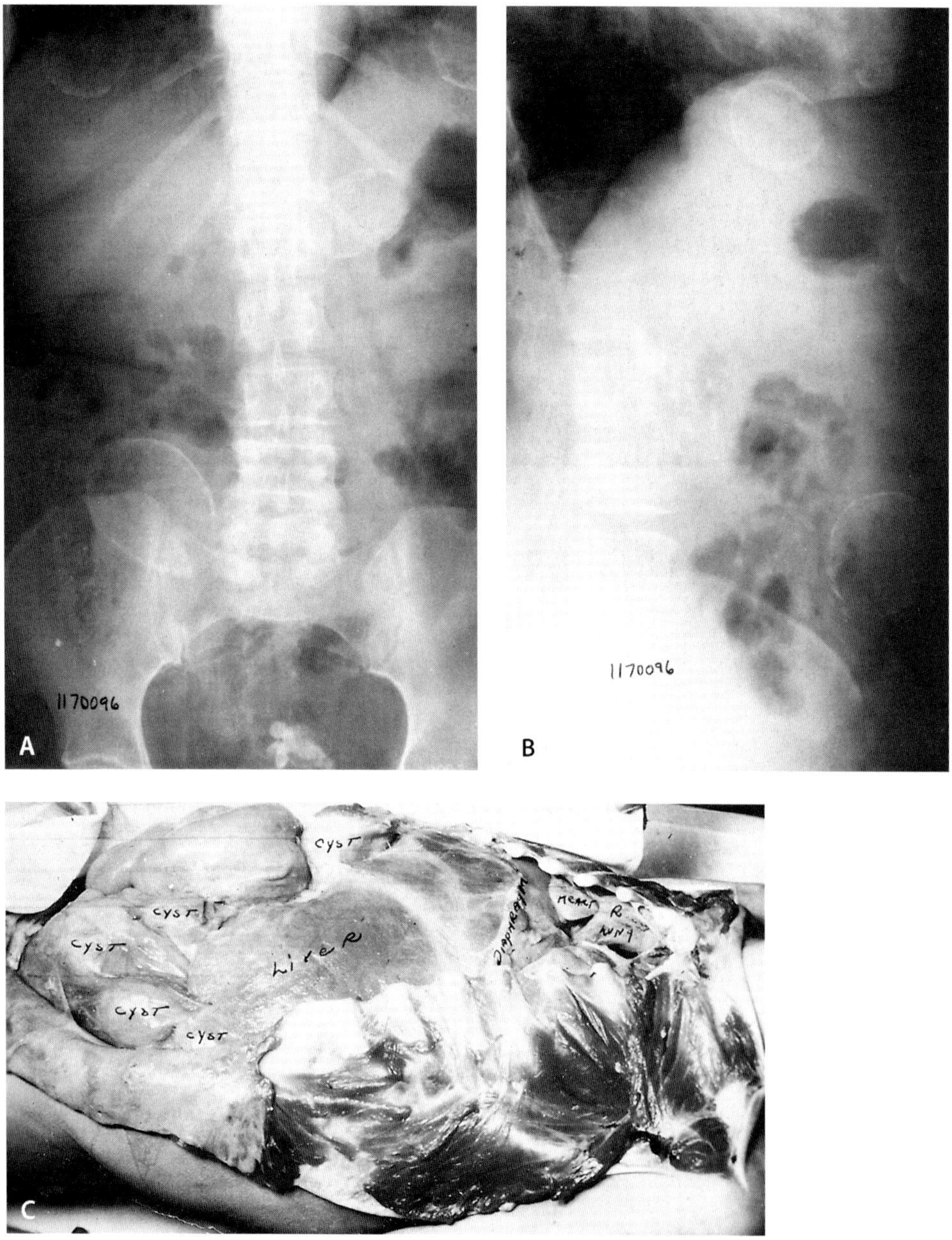

and portions of the cyst contents, as well as blood, will be seen in the urine. Secondary infections of the cyst and kidney usually ensue. Hydatid cysts of the urinary bladder and ureters (Fig. 3.76 E, F) occur rarely and can lead to obstructive hydronephrosis.

In a retrospective 15-year review of a population in an endemic area in central Spain, where 10 new cases of hydatid disease were identified per 100 000 people yearly, 52 patients were found with renal and retroperitoneal echinococcosis (Angulo et al., 1997, 1998). The kidneys were affected in 36 patients, with the lesion being solitary in 85% and bilateral in 6% of cases. Extrarenal disease was present in 16 patients; 13 had involvement of the psoas and quadratus lumbar muscles, and three involvement of the pararenal space. Other organs were involved in 44% of patients (29% liver, 15% lung, 3% spleen, 4% other). Preoperative diagnosis was made in 71% of cases, based on imaging in 62% (including urography, ultrasonography, and especially CT), serology in 45%, and hydatiduria in 2%.

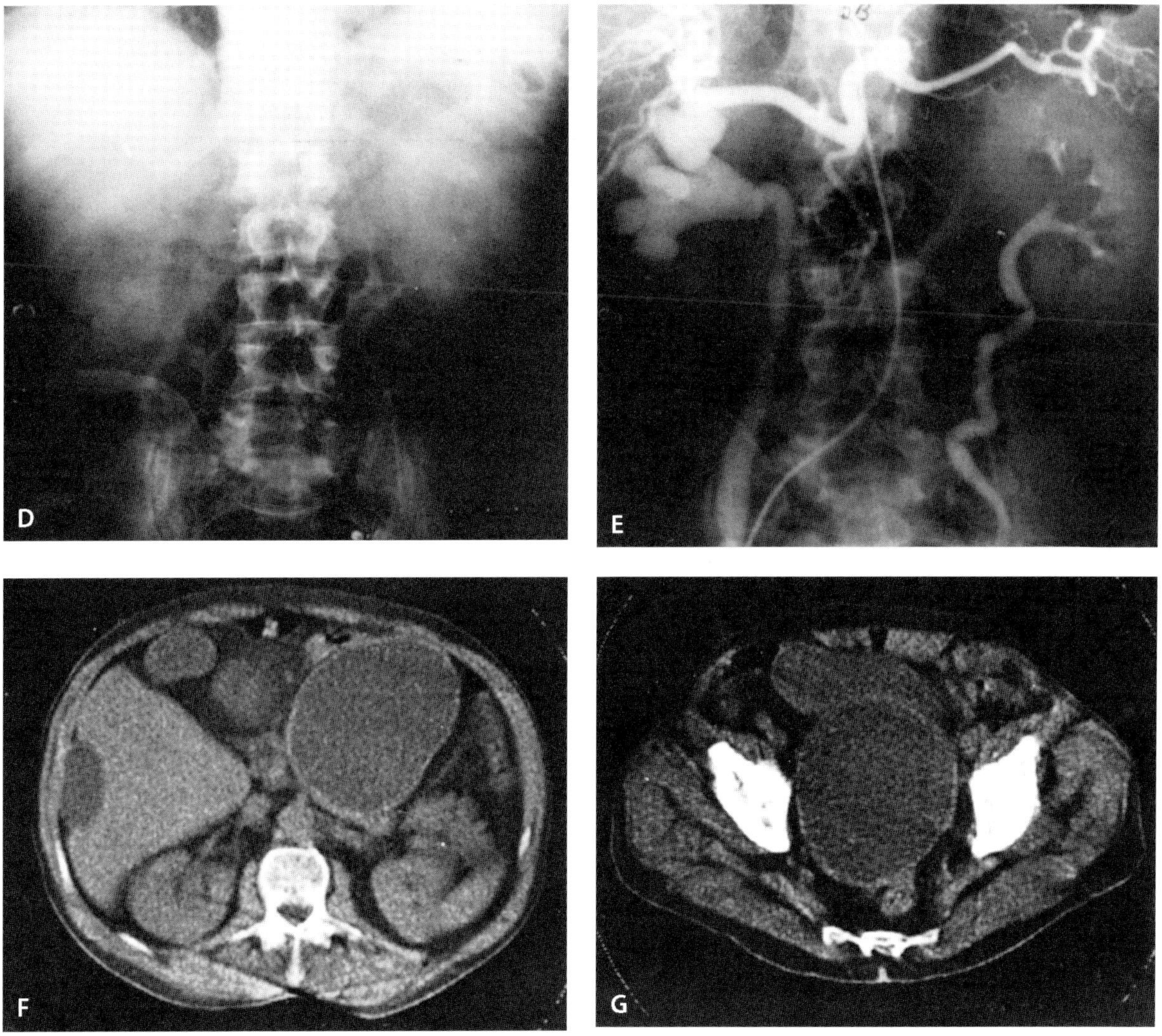

Fig. 3.72 A–F. Multiple calcified hydatid cysts in the liver, spleen, and mesentery. There are at least three calcified mesenteric cysts seen on AP (**A**) and lateral (**B**) views of the abdomen. **C** Multiple large mesenteric and peritoneal hydatid cysts seen in a cadaver. AFIP 53-20053-2. **D** A supine radiograph of the abdomen of another patient aged 66 years with multiple palpable "tumors." The patient had had abdominal swelling for several months. There is no calcification of the large left upper quadrant mass, but the stomach is displaced medially. Selective celiac arteriography (**E**) shows superior displacement of the gastric and splenic arteries, but there is no tumor blush and no abdominal neovascularity. The excretory urogram phase shows right hydronephrosis and bilateral hydroureter, due to pressure from the pelvic mass lying between the bladder and rectum shown clearly in (**G**). Other cysts are well shown, including one laterally in the right lobe of the liver (**F**). Hydatid disease should be suspected whenever there are multiple intra-abdominal cysts

(Text continues on p. 264)

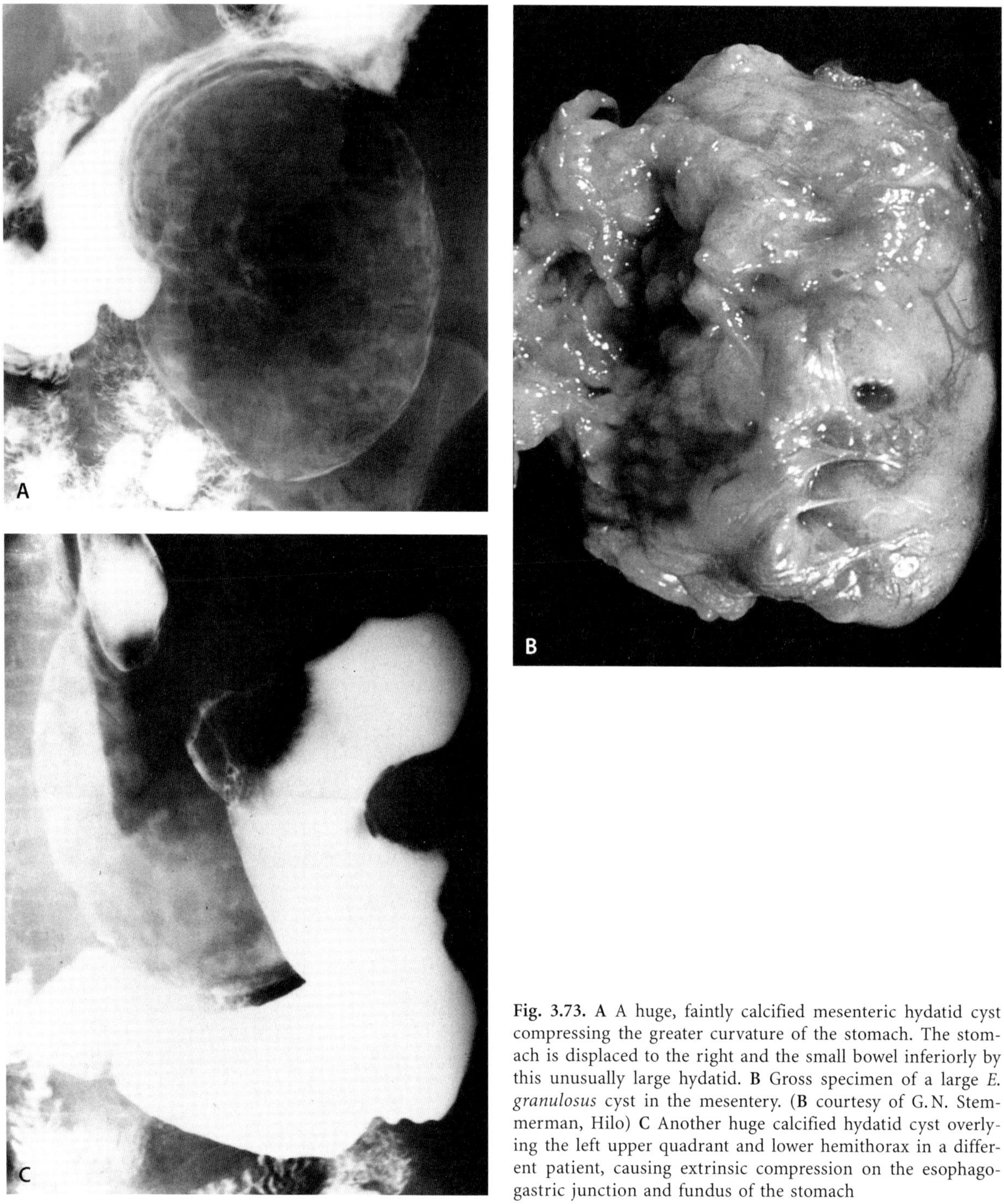

Fig. 3.73. **A** A huge, faintly calcified mesenteric hydatid cyst compressing the greater curvature of the stomach. The stomach is displaced to the right and the small bowel inferiorly by this unusually large hydatid. **B** Gross specimen of a large *E. granulosus* cyst in the mesentery. (**B** courtesy of G.N. Stemmerman, Hilo) **C** Another huge calcified hydatid cyst overlying the left upper quadrant and lower hemithorax in a different patient, causing extrinsic compression on the esophagogastric junction and fundus of the stomach

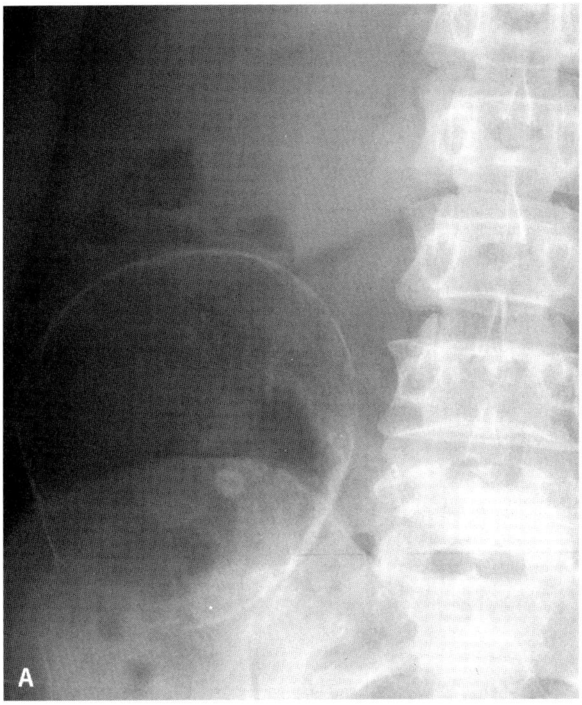

Fig. 3.74 A–E. Plain radiograph and sonograms of mesenteric, retroperitoneal, and pelvic hydatids in four patients from different parts of Africa. **A** Large calcified mesenteric hydatid with multiple calcified daughter cysts in the right mid-abdomen of a patient from Zimbabwe. **B** Ultrasound scan of the same patient showing a curvilinear echogenic rim with shadowing indicating calcium in the wall of the cyst. **C** Large mesenteric hydatid with probable daughter cyst in another patient from Zimbabwe. (**A–C** courtesy of Dr. Sam Mindel) **D** Retroperitoneal hydatid (*arrows*) in a Tunisian patient. (Courtesy of Dr. Gharbi, Tunis) **E** Large hydatid with daughter cyst seen on a longitudinal sonogram in the pelvis of another African

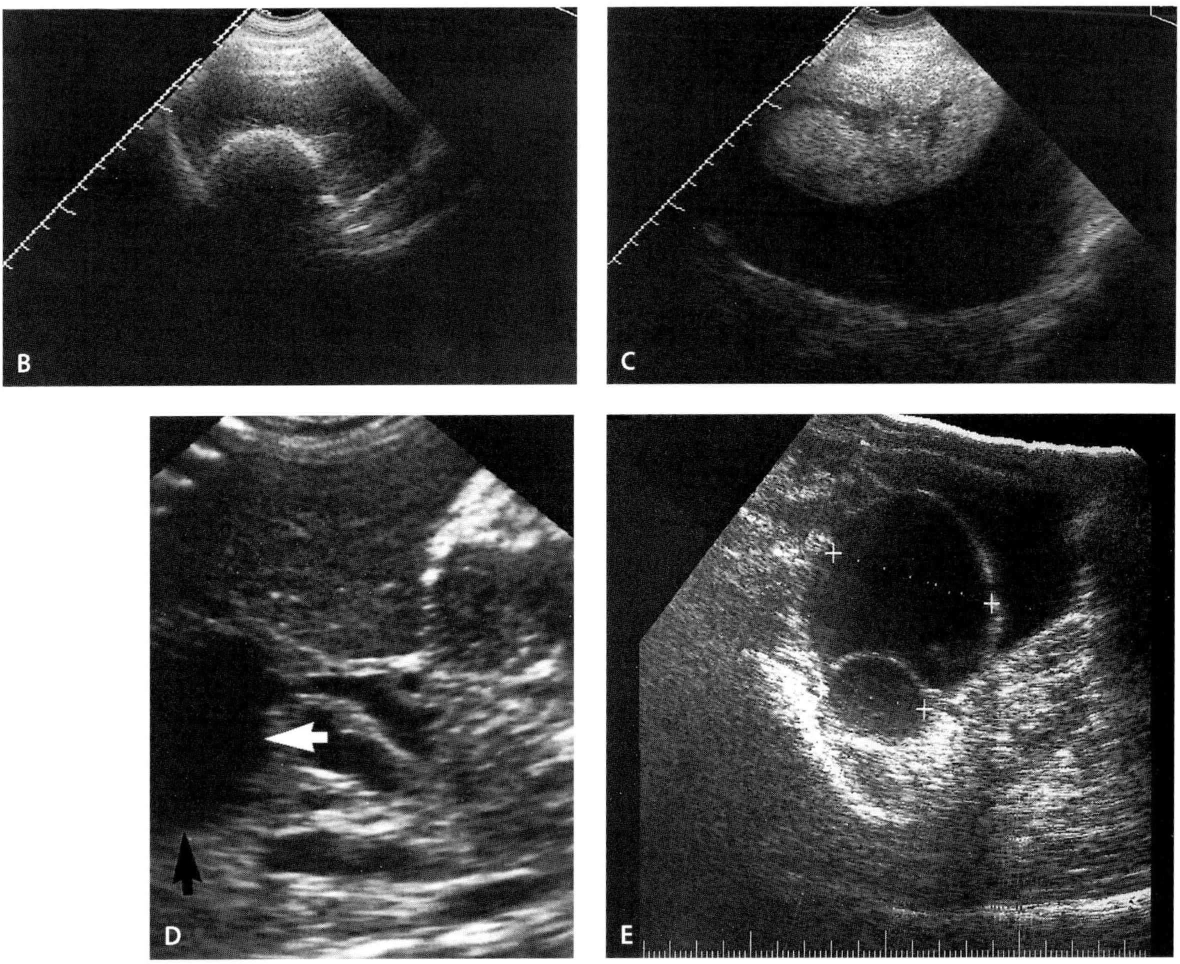

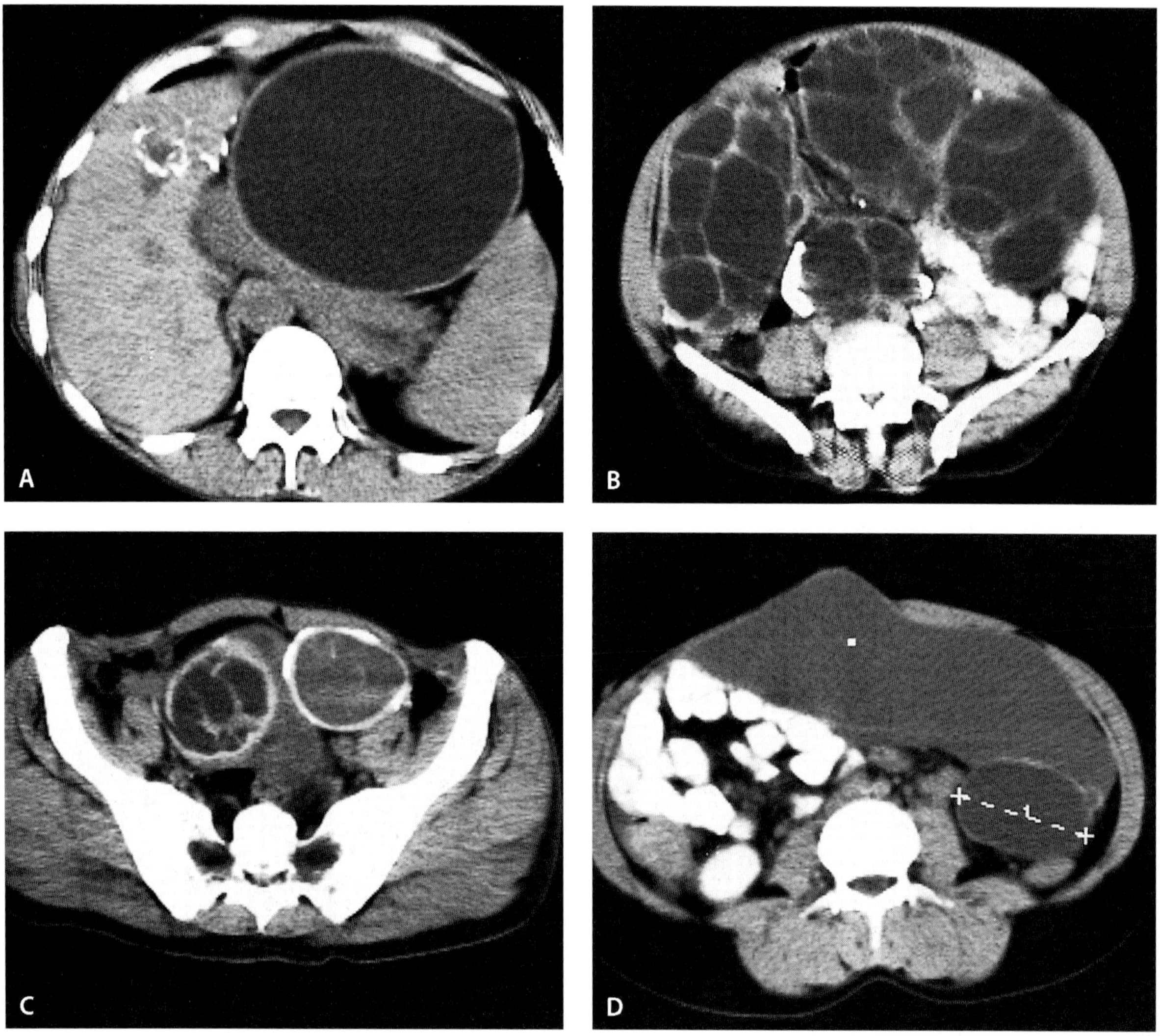

Fig. 3.75 A–D. CT scans of multiple peritoneal and pelvic hydatid cysts in four different patients from Tunisia. **A** Large type I peritoneal hydatid lying anteriorly in the upper mid-abdomen between the liver and spleen. There is also a small calcified and collapsed type III hydatid cyst in the liver of this 58-year-old man. **B** A 68-year-old man with multiple multivesicular type II hydatids with numerous daughter cysts in the pelvis. **C** A 50-year-old man with two old but evolutive pelvic hydatid cysts with calcification of the cyst walls and with daughter cysts, suggesting hypermature type II cysts. *Note:* In the Gharbi classification of hydatids based on cross-sectional (primarily ultrasound) imaging rather than the pathology-based classification of Lewall used in this chapter, these would be type V cysts; the cysts in patient B would be type III cysts, and the calcified, collapsing liver cyst in patient A would be a type IV cyst. **D** Hydatid cyst in the left lower quadrant of a 35-year-old woman. There is a large volume of peritoneal hydatid fluid septated as a complication of her hydatid disease, with bulging of the anterior abdominal wall in the midline of the lower abdomen. (Courtesy of Drs. Ben Cheikh and Gharbi, Tunis)

Fig. 3.76 A–F. Hydatid cysts of the kidneys and ureters. **A** Gross specimen showing bulging masses from the kidneys due to large hydatids. **B** A section through one of the renal hydatids showing the endocyst with numerous daughter cysts (type II cyst). **C** Another renal hydatid with numerous daughter cysts. (**A–C** courtesy of Dr. Herman Zaiman) **D** Microscopic section of a renal hydatid showing thick laminated cyst wall and the endocyst containing brood capsules and scolices. AFIP 60-2849. **E** Autopsy specimen of multiple hydatid cysts of both ureters causing bilateral obstructive hydronephrosis, more so on left side. AFIP 55-6075-2. **F** Multiple hydatid cysts involving a ureter. (**F** courtesy of J. Knaak, Montreal)

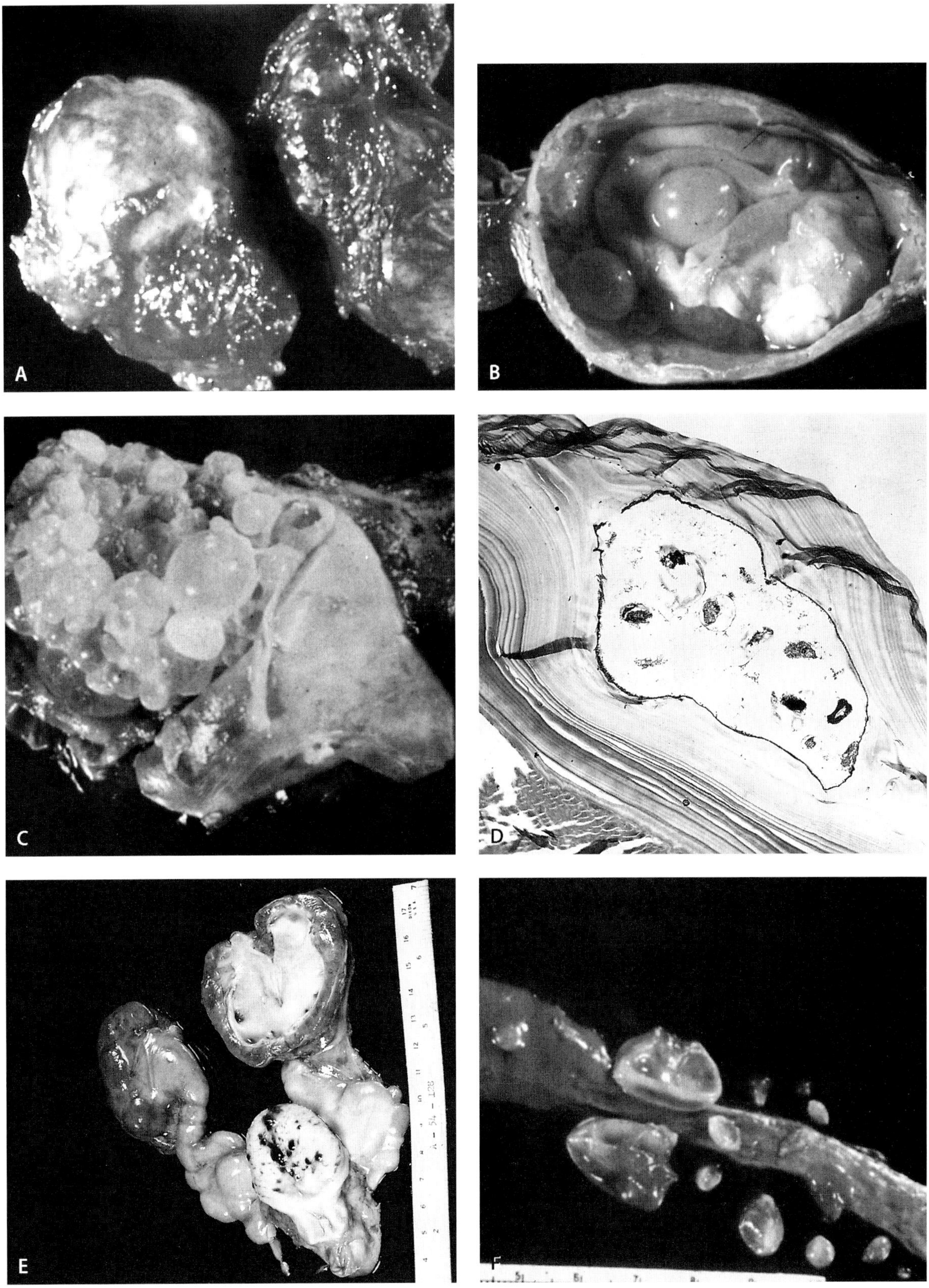
A
B
C
D
E
F

On *plain radiographs* of the abdomen, an intact hydatid cyst may appear as a localized bulge on the renal contour, without renal displacement; expansion occurs in the direction of least resistance, usually anteriorly. The cyst may be calcified (Fig. 3.77), but most often it is a chance finding on urography. The pattern of calcification in renal hydatids ranges from a delicate eggshell appearance to dense, reticular calcification (Fig. 3.77 C). Multiple ring-shaped calcifications within a larger calcified cystic lesion suggest the presence of daughter cysts. If a calcified hydatid cyst has ruptured and collapsed, it will have a typical crushed eggshell or sunburst appearance (Fig. 3.77 A, B), which at times may be confused with neoplastic or tuberculous calcification.

Distortion of the renal calyces, infundibula, or pelvis seen on intravenous or retrograde pyelography, or displacement of the renal vessels seen on *angiography*, is indistinguishable from any other cyst or avascular tumor (Figs. 3.78, 3.81 D). There is no neovascularity or intrinsic abnormality of the renal vessels, which show only displacement from an avascular mass; obliteration of one or more calyces or vessels can occasionally occur from pressure. If a vascular rim is found during the capillary or venous phase, a hydatid cyst should be seriously suspected.

There are basically three types of hydatid cysts which can be recognized on *intravenous or retrograde urography* (Fig. 3.79). *Closed hydatids (type I)* have an intact cyst lining and adventitia and do not communicate with the renal collecting system. The outline of the kidney may be enlarged, with a rounded mass (with or without calcification) causing elongation and splaying of the infundibula and calyces and, occasionally, obliteration of one or more calyces from pressure. These cysts, especially if not calcified, may be impossible to differentiate from other renal masses by pyelography, urography, or angiography, as already noted. Nephrotomography may show a thick cyst wall with an inhomogeneous lucent center.

With the *pseudoclosed or exposed type* of hydatid cyst, contrast media can interpose itself in crescent-like fashion in the space between the laminated ectocyst and the pericyst, producing the "goblet" or "wine-glass" sign (Surraco's sign) (Fig. 3.79).

When the cyst has ruptured and is communicating with the renal collecting system, contrast medium from either an intravenous or a retrograde urogram can spread around the cyst or fill it (Fig. 3.78 C): there is usually a residual "neck" where the communication exists. In other patients, there may be a renal cavity, indistinguishable from renal abscess, tuberculosis, or papillary necrosis. In this *open type* of hydatid cyst, an intermittent or permanent communication exists between the hydatid and the pyelocalyceal system so that contrast medium flows directly into the cyst. Usually there is a typical mottled appearance of contrast, insinuating itself among a mass of daughter cysts but, occasionally, if the cyst contents are tightly packed, the contrast will be compressed between the contents and cyst wall to produce an extensive false crescent sign.

In space-occupying lesions of the kidney or the urinary system in general, ultrasonography is used as the initial imaging method (Figs. 3.80, 3.81 C) since conventional radiography is often unsuccessful in determining the extent and cause of the disease. *Ultrasonography and CT* usually allow differentiation of cysts from tumors and their extension within the kidney (von Sinner et al., 1993). However, in some complex or atypical cystic masses, differentiation may be impossible. Precise assessment of relationships to neighboring organs and vascular structures generally is possible. In hydatid disease, characteristic structures such as daughter cysts or collapsed parasitic membranes may be seen. Ultrasonography and nonenhanced CT also may detect minor calcifications in the lesion (Figs. 3.81, 3.82).

The CT and sonographic appearances of renal hydatidosis have been amply described, with both studies yielding important and often quite similar information. The findings are not, however, pathognomonic in most cases. In its earliest stages of development, a round anechoic cyst is identifiable on ultrasonography, whose wall may be somewhat thicker than that seen with simple serous cysts (Fig. 3.80). Calcification is frequent, and "sand" may be encountered. Hydatid cysts tend to have a low CT attenuation value when unilocular but, as daugher cysts are formed, the CT appearance becomes heterogeneous (Fig. 3.82). The daughter cysts, however, which usually arrange themselves peripherally within the mother cyst, almost invariably exhibit a lower CT attenuation value than does the parent cyst, resulting in something of a rosette appearance. When daughter cysts are produced, CT or ultrasonography will reveal a multilocular structure with curvilinear "septa," which are actually the opposing walls of the daughter cysts (Fig. 3.82).

Parallel echogenic "stripes," caused by contact between the parasitic ectocyst and the pericyst of the host, are very suggestive of an echinococcal origin, and usually occur with undamaged or viable cysts. If the parallel stripes disappear and the parasitic membranes collapse (serpent sign), the hydatid cyst is damaged. In contrast-enhanced CT, secondary abscess formation may be recognized if there is ring enhancement of the pericyst or if air bubbles are present within the lesion or its surroundings.

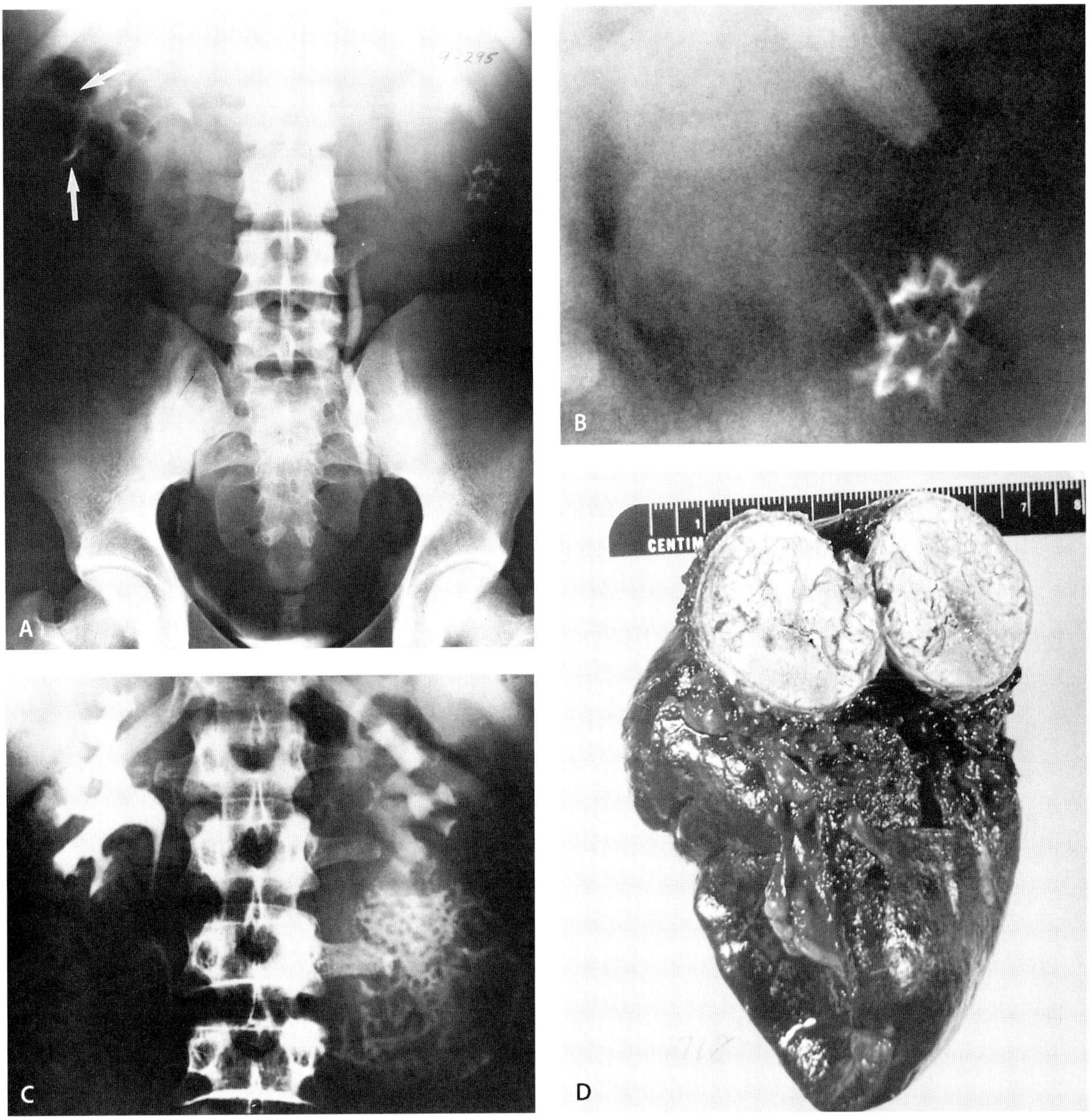

Fig. 3.77. A Calcified hydatid cysts in both kidneys. A supine radiograph taken during intravenous pyelography shows a mass with crescent-shaped calcification in its wall arising from the lateral margin of the right kidney (*arrows*). There is a ruptured, collapsed hydatid cyst in the lower pole of the left kidney with typical "crushed eggshell" or "sunburst" appearance. The right renal pelvocalyceal system appears relatively undisturbed by the hydatid cyst arising from the periphery of the renal cortex. The left renal pelvocalyceal system does not fill out well, although there is considerable contrast in the left ureter, indicating a functioning kidney. **B** Close-up of the crushed eggshell or sunburst calcification which strongly suggests a collapsed hydatid cyst. It may be mimicked at times by healed tuberculosis. **C** Calcified *Echinococcus* cyst of the kidney. An excretory urogram reveals a calcified mass extending inferiorly from the lower pole of the left kidney. This lacy or reticular pattern of calcification can be seen when daughter cysts and other contents of the cyst calcify. (**A–C** from P.E.S. Palmer and M.M. Reeder. In: H. Pollack: *Clinical urography, 2nd edn.* Philadelphia, Saunders, 1999.) **D** Gross specimen of a renal hydatid arising from the upper pole of the kidney of another patient

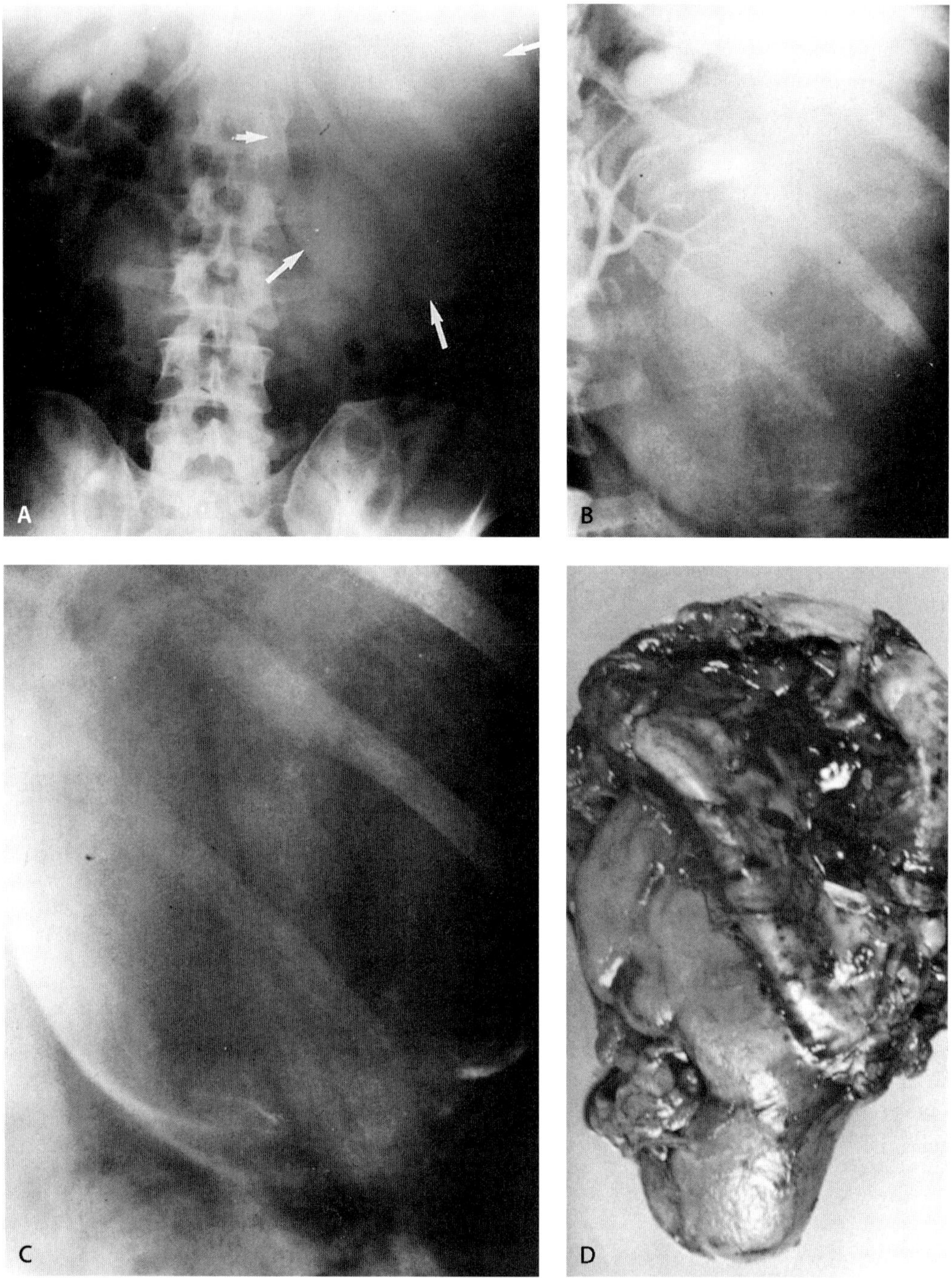

Fig. 3.78 A–D. Huge communicating hydatid cyst of the left kidney. **A** There is a large mass arising within the left kidney seen on intravenous pyelography (*arrows*). The right kidney and renal pelvocalyceal system appear normal. There is minimal contrast medium in distorted calyces in the upper pole of the left kidney. **B** Left renal arteriogram shows stretching of intrarenal branches around the large avascular mass. Some contrast medium is noted in blunted, distorted, and displaced calyces in the upper pole. **C** Contrast medium has spread around the large communicating hydatid cyst, outlining its contour. This may occur during either intravenous or retrograde urography or renal arteriography, when the cyst has ruptured and is communicating. At times, the contrast medium may fill the cyst rather than surround it. (**A–C** courtesy of Dr. John Evans, New York) **D** Gross specimen of a huge hydatid cyst occupying the central portion and upper pole of the kidney of another patient

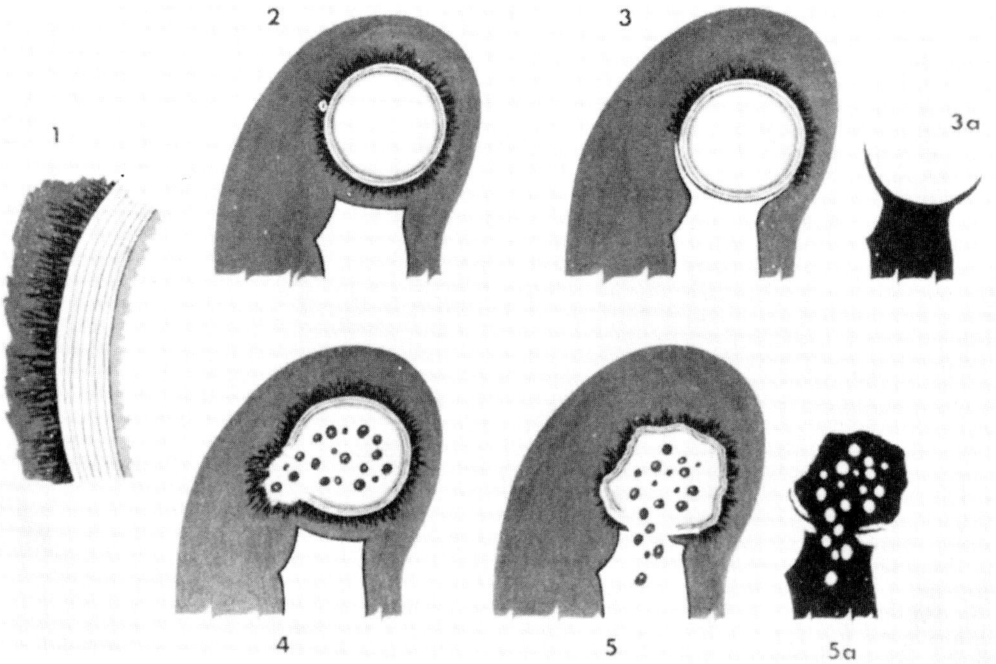

Fig. 3.79. The three layers of a renal hydatid cyst and its relationship to the collecting system are represented: *1* Endocyst, ectocyst, and pericyst constitute the wall of a hydatid cyst. *2* Closed cyst with all three layers intact, overlying a calyx. *3* Exposed cyst with absence of host adventitial layer or pericyst–cyst is in close contact with urine. *3a* Note goblet sign. *4, 5, 5a* Open cysts resulting from rupture and discharge of daughter cysts. (Courtesy of Dr. K. Kirkland and *Br J Urol*, 1966)

Ultrasonography and CT have been used to monitor the progress of hydatid cysts undergoing medical therapy. During treatment, the cyst may be seen to undergo a metamorphosis, changing from an anechoic to a complex, and finally a "pseudosolid" pattern on ultrasonography, owing to degradation of the cyst membranes (matrix formation) and the release of proteinaceous material. Under the effects of therapy, cysts may shrink notably and calcify, as demonstated by ultrasonography or CT.

Magnetic resonance imaging is not as accurate in discovering calcification as nonenhanced CT or ultrasonography, especially if the calcification is minimal. However, the previously noted typical signs of hydatid disease can be clearly demonstrated on T1- and T2-weighted MRI. A low-intensity rim on T2-weighted images is suggestive but not pathognomonic of hydatid disease. In selected cases, contrast-enhanced studies may be done.

Early discovery of hydatid disease of the kidneys or urinary system, and differentiation from tumors or tuberculosis, is important because endocystectomy or partial nephrectomy with preservation of kidney function may be possible. When surgery is contraindicated, chemotherapy may help to control the disease.

(Text continues on p. 270)

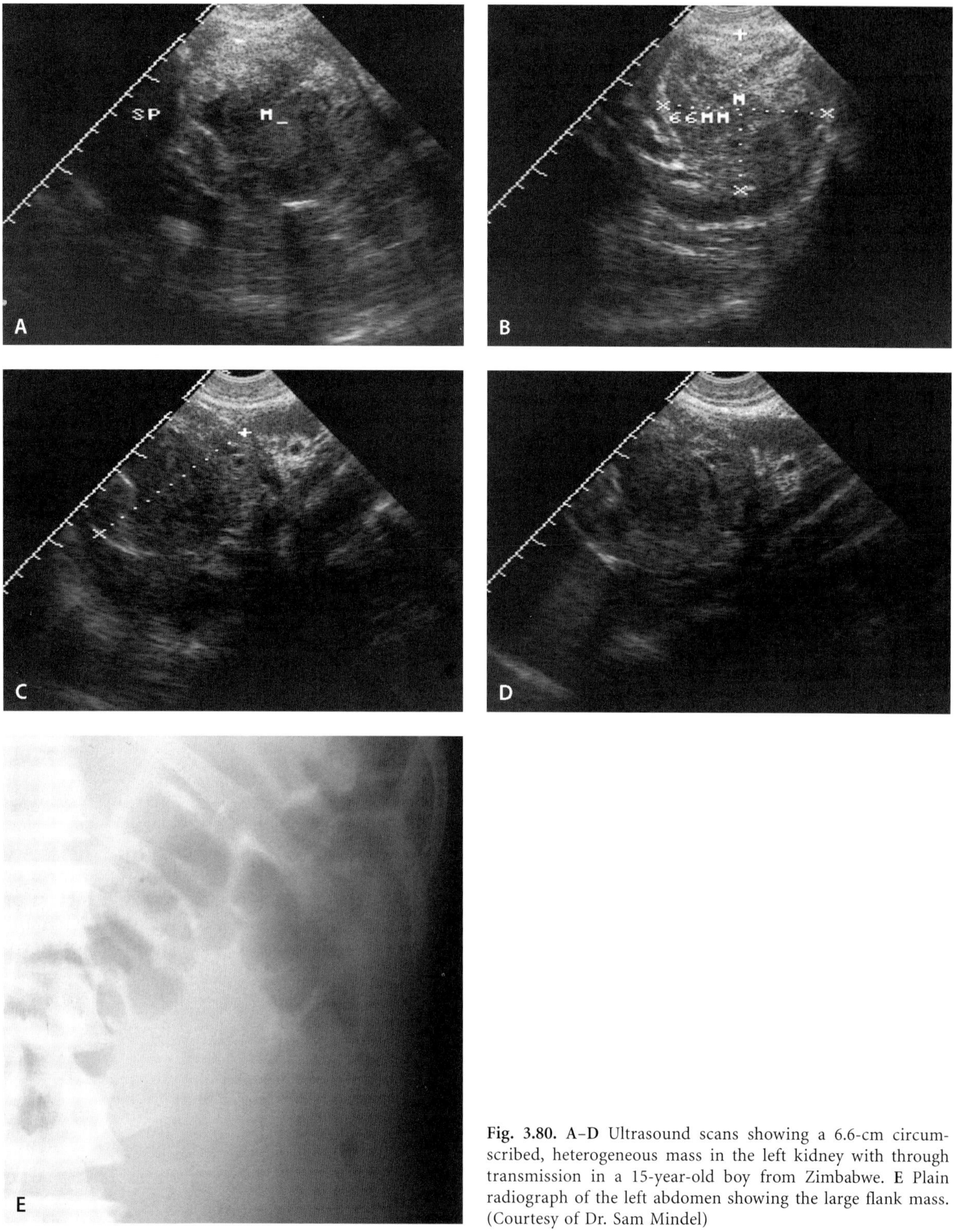

Fig. 3.80. A–D Ultrasound scans showing a 6.6-cm circumscribed, heterogeneous mass in the left kidney with through transmission in a 15-year-old boy from Zimbabwe. E Plain radiograph of the left abdomen showing the large flank mass. (Courtesy of Dr. Sam Mindel)

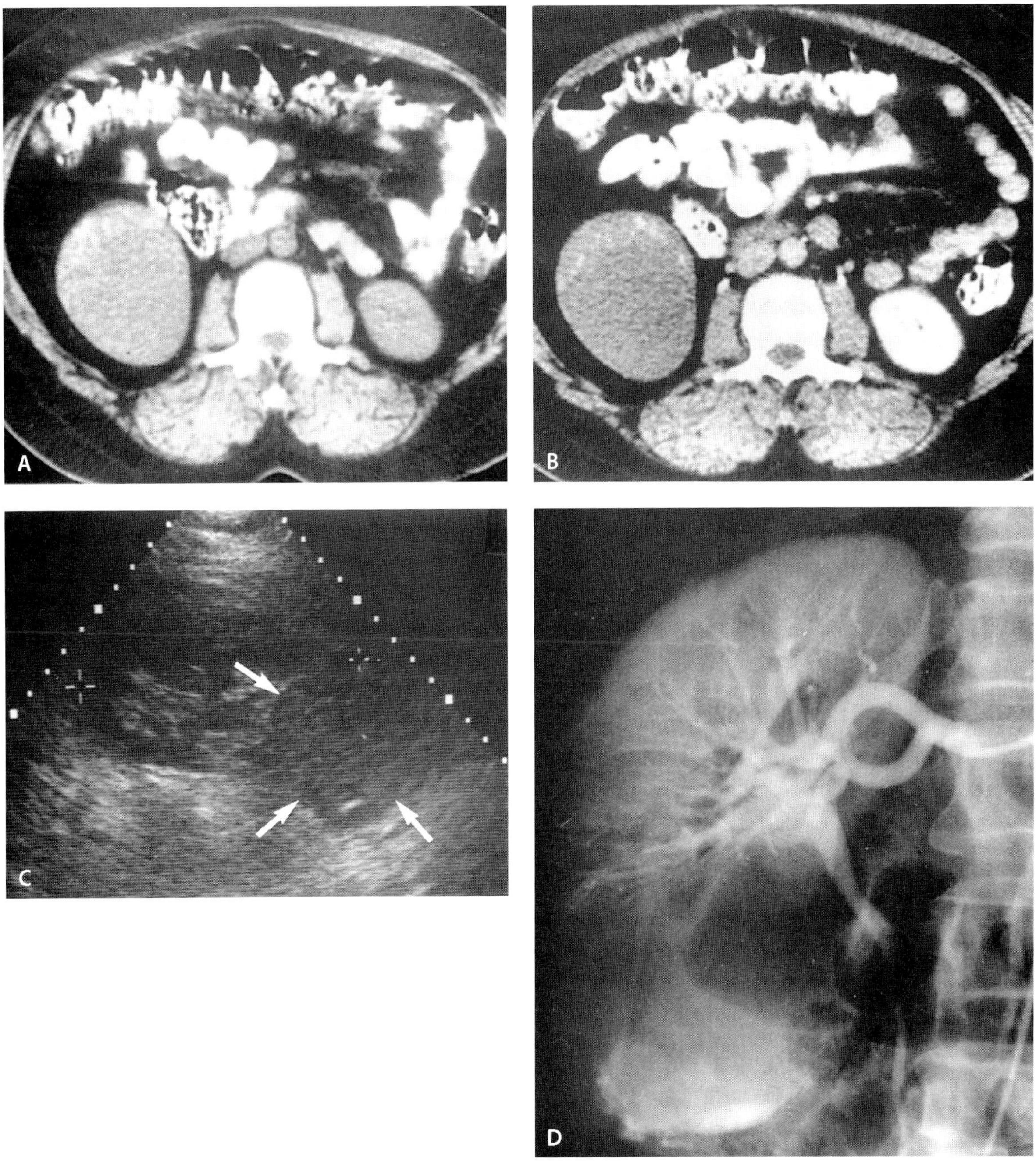

Fig. 3.81 A–D. Right renal hydatid in a 45-year-old Saudi Arabian woman who complained of right flank pain of 20 years duration. **A** Precontrast CT of the abdomen demonstrates a large 8×6.5 cm mass in the lower pole of the right kidney. The lesion is not typically cystic (density is 40 Hounsfield units.) Scattered calcifications are noted in the anterior part of the lesion. **B** After an intravenous bolus of contrast medium, the lesion's density remains unchanged, while the left kidney shows normal contrast enhancement. **C** Ultrasonography (sagittal view) of the right kidney reveals a low echogenic lesion (*arrows*) in the lower pole. **D** Selective right renal arteriography reveals a large avascular mass in the lower pole. Densities in the lower part of the lesion represent calcifications. *Echinococcus* titer and chest x-ray were normal, but a hydatid cyst was still suspected. Surgery was performed to rule out tumor. Preoperatively, the patient received 200 mg albendazole orally every 6 hours for 2 days and 3 g praziquantel the day before surgery. She was also premedicated with 100 mg hydrocortisone and 25 mg diphenhydramine hydrochloride to reduce the risk of an allergic reaction. The lower pole of the right kidney with the mass was then removed without leakage of cyst contents. Histopathology revealed a 9-cm cystic mass with a fibrous wall, which contained necrotic whitish-gray cheesy material with focal areas of hemorrhage, cholesterol, and calcification, as well as many hooklets, confirming hydatid disease. Postoperatively, she received 200 mg albendazole twice daily for 1 month and had an uneventful convalescence. (Courtesy of Dr. Walther von Sinner and *J Urol*, 1993)

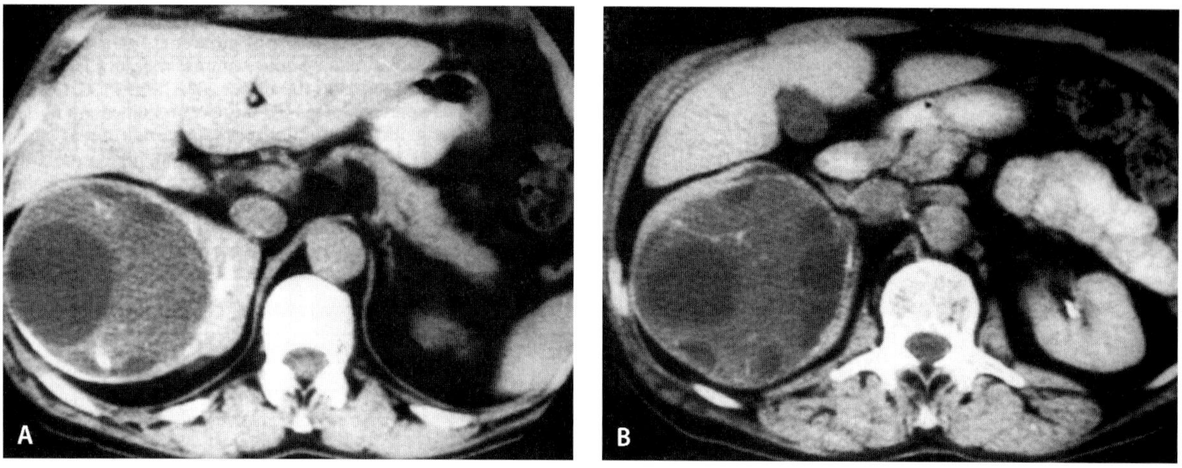

Fig. 3.82 A, B. CT appearance of hydatid cyst of the kidney in a 64-year-old man from Uruguay with palpable right flank mass. **A** Contrast-enhanced CT reveals a large right renal mass. The wall is densely calcified and discrete low-attenuation cysts are noted within a somewhat higher attenuation matrix. **B** A more caudal CT section reveals multiple daughter cysts arranged in rosette formation about the periphery of the mother cyst. Fine, delicate internal calcifications can be seen. Surgery revealed large hydatid cysts. No other intra-abdominal manifestations of hydatid disease were encountered. (Courtesy of Drs. Jose and Felix Lerborgne, Montevideo, and H. Pollack: *Clinical urography, 2nd edn.* Philadelphia, Saunders, 1999)

Thorax

Lungs

Intact hydatid cysts of the lungs are commonly solitary, well-circumscribed, homogeneous, uncalcified masses. They are usually round but may be oval, elliptical, or lobulated (Figs. 3.83–3.91). They can occur anywhere in the lungs, but are somewhat more common on the right side and in the basilar segments of both lower lobes. The majority of such cysts arise de novo within the lungs. Secondary cysts, which have spread through the diaphragm from the liver, can occur. Others result from rupture of a primary pulmonary hydatid into the bronchial tree with bronchogenic spread, or into a pulmonary blood vessel with metastatic spread. Multiple lung cysts are not uncommon (Figs. 3.85, 3.86). True daughter cysts are rare in the lung, because they usually develop only if a cyst becomes traumatized or infected, and a hydatid cyst in the lung is relatively protected from trauma.

As many as 16% of pulmonary hydatids are reported to be accompanied by concurrent liver cysts, but associated cysts within the mediastinum, pleura, rib cage, thoracic spine, and breast are uncommon. Involvement of the lung without hydatid disease in the liver may be due to inhalation of eggs excreted by the primary host, usually the dog. Eggs are quite resistant to drying and, because of their small size, could be carried in the wind. Direct entry of oncospheres into lymphatics rather than into the portal vein can also account for bypassing the liver.

The direction in which a cyst develops and its final shape depend largely upon its location within the lung relative to adjacent anatomical structures. Thus, a centrally located cyst tends to remain round, whereas others near the periphery may become polycyclic, lobulated, or umbilicated because of pressure from nearby vessels or bronchi (Fig. 3.83 A, B), or from adjacent cysts. Where there are multiple cysts, fusion is prevented by the host-derived pericyst around the hydatids.

Pulmonary hydatids vary from 1 cm in diameter to an enormous cyst of 20 cm or more, obliterating an entire lung and displacing the heart and mediastinum to the opposite side. Cysts may cause sufficient compression to cause death from asphyxia. Usually, however, the patient with an uncomplicated cyst will have few or no clinical symptoms and the cyst may be found accidentally on routine chest radiography. Only when the hydatid is of sufficient size will there be signs of compression, such as dyspnea, bronchitis, pleurisy, or distention of the thoracic wall. Other symptoms develop when the cyst becomes complicated by rupturing into either the bronchial tree or pleura. The coughing up of "grape skins" is pathognomonic of rupture of a hydatid cyst into a bronchus and may effect a natural cure or result in secondary hydatidosis via bronchial spread. If the cyst ruptures into the pleura, a hydropneumothorax, pyopneumothorax, empyema, or bronchopleural fistula may result. Residual pleural thickening and fibrosis may ensue, or multiple secondary pleural cysts may develop.

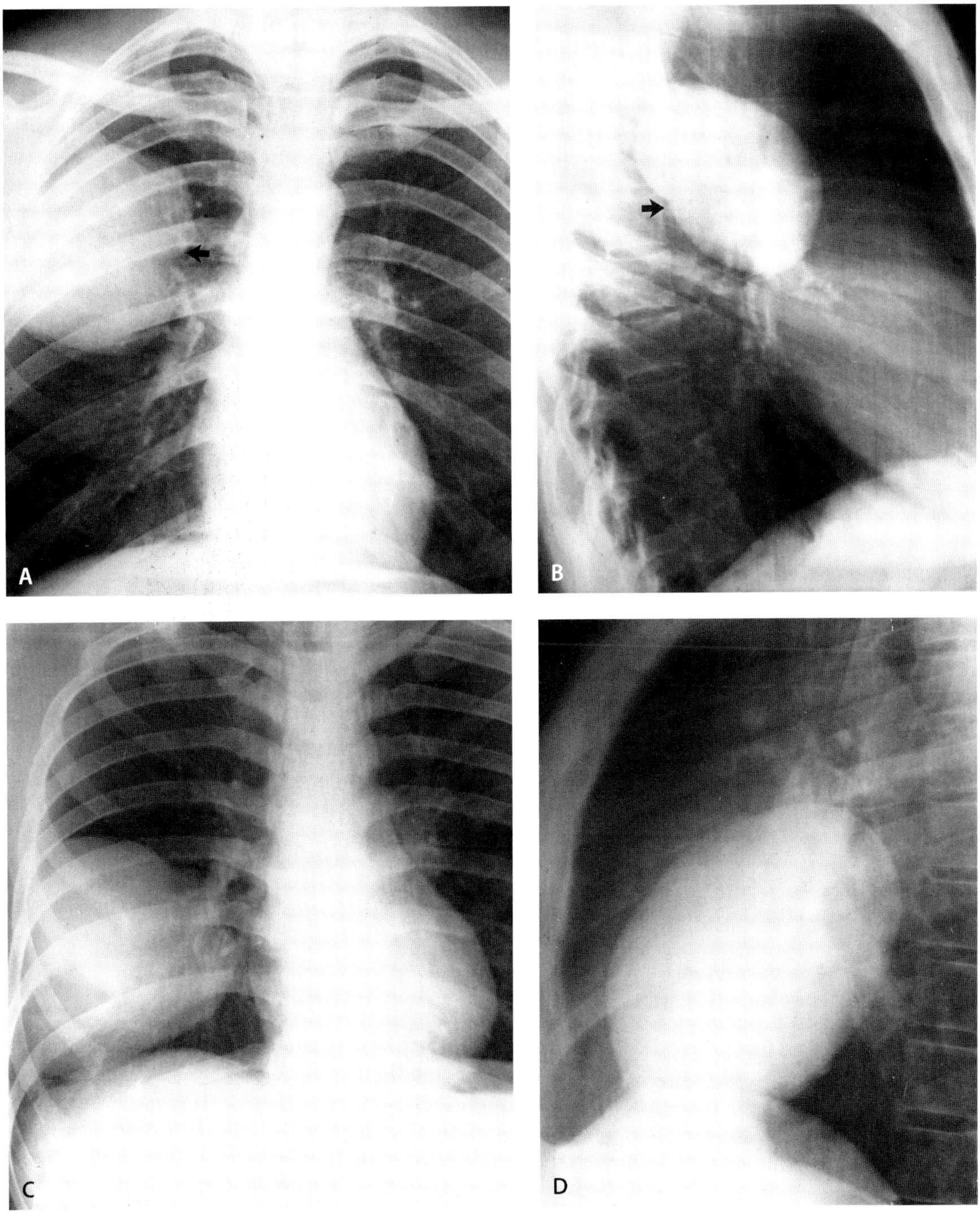

Fig. 3.83 A–D. Large solitary hydatid cyst of the lung in two different patients from Spain. When intact, pulmonary hydatids are usually solitary, well-circumscribed, homogeneous masses. They are usually round but may be oval, elliptical or lobulated in contour. **A** PA and **B** lateral views of the chest showing a lobulated, elliptical, homogeneous mass in the right upper lobe. There is umbilication or notching along the medial and posterior borders of this hydatid (*arrows*), caused by pressure on the cyst from adjacent vessels or bronchi. **C, D** A similar lobulated, elliptical mass in the right lower lobe of a second Spaniard. The elliptical or oval shape of some hydatids allows differentiation from benign or malignant neoplasms of the lung, which rarely show such a contour

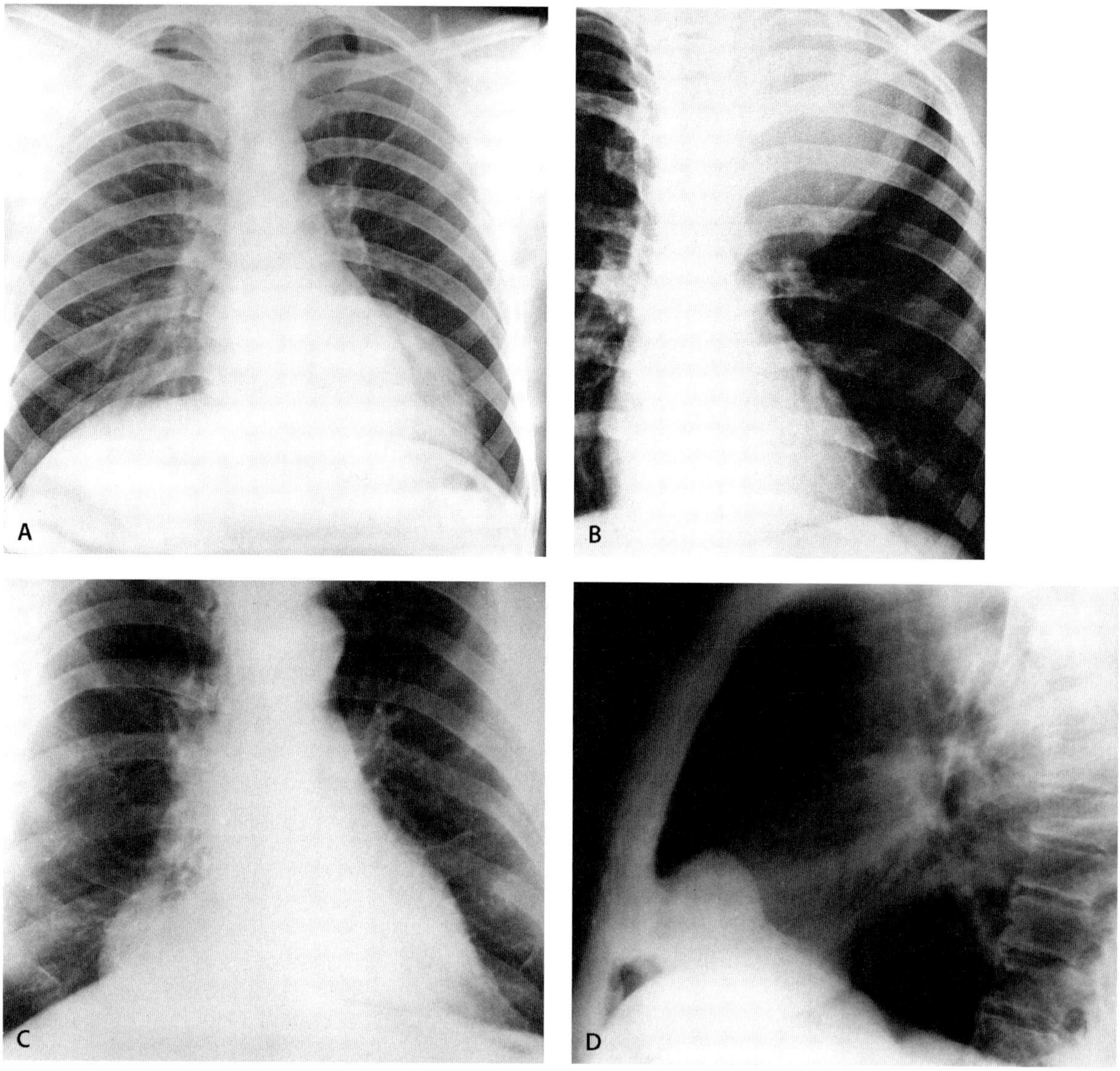

Fig. 3.84 A–F. Large, solitary, unruptured pulmonary hydatid cysts in four different patients. **A** There is a huge, well-circumscribed, round mass in the left lower lobe, partially concealed by the left heart border in a Peruvian Indian. **B** A large homogeneous mass in the left upper lobe of an 8-year-old child. **C, D** A smooth round mass in the right cardiophrenic angle with its medial border blending into the cardiac silhouette in a male patient from India. This was a hydatid cyst in the right middle lobe mimicking a pericardial cyst or foramen of Morgagni hernia. **E, F** see p. 273

As the pulmonary hydatid becomes older and larger, its sharp contour on chest radiographs may become hazy as the fibrous pericyst grows thicker and less regular. Localized compression atelectasis may further complicate its differentiation from other circumscribed pulmonary lesions. The correct diagnosis may be suggested radiographically only if there is evidence of umbilication (which can occur also with some primary or metastatic lung neoplasms) (Fig. 3.83 A, B) or if hydatid cysts are noted elsewhere within the liver or other organs. In prior decades, bronchography would demonstrate displacement of bronchi around the cyst with poor filling of the smaller bronchi because of compression (Fig. 3.92 C), but these findings were nonspecific and seen in other benign lung tumors or cysts.

There are, however, several radiographic patterns that are highly specific for a pulmonary hydatid once rupture is impending or has occurred. The pericyst of an enlarging cyst may communicate with an adjacent bronchiole and, when the patient coughs or strains, air may be forced between the pericyst and endocyst, producing a radiolucent air shadow in the form of a crescent or meniscus. This

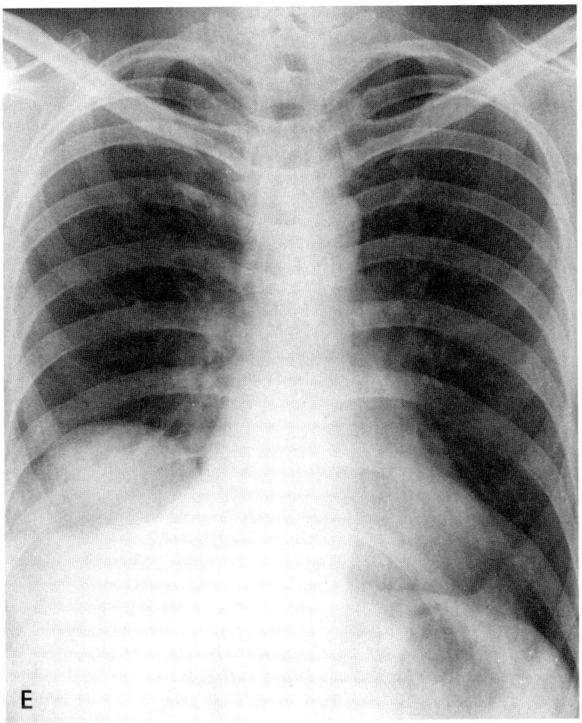

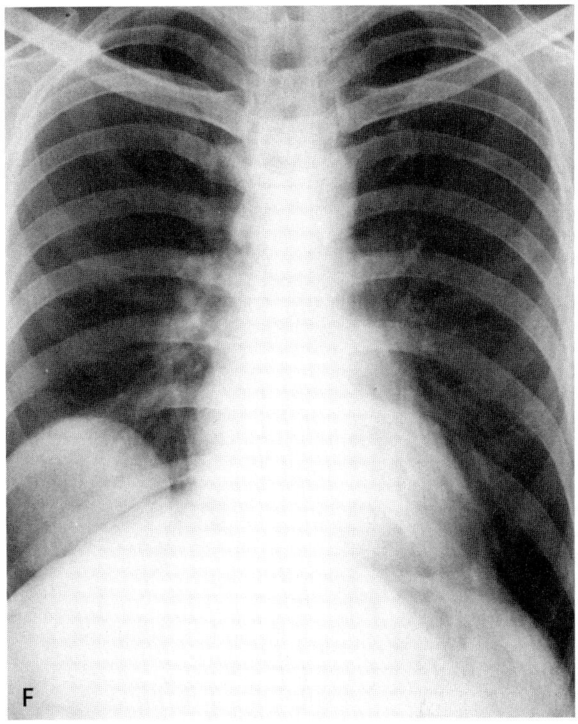

Fig. 3.84 (*continued*). **E** PA chest film in moderate inspiration shows a large round opacity in the right base of another Indian man. There is apparent flattening of the right hemidiaphragm with suggestion of possible pleural disease. There is tenting of the midportion of the left hemidiaphragm. **F** Chest film of the same patient taken in deeper inspiration demonstrates a smooth, round mass in the right base. The right hemidiaphragm now appears unaffected by this mass, which was an uncomplicated hydatid cyst in the right lower lobe. (**C–F** courtesy of Dr. A. Chandrahasan Johnson)

"sign of detachment" or "air meniscus sign" heralds the impending rupture of the cyst (Figs. 3.39, 3.87–3.90). This sign is highly reliable though not pathognomonic for a hydatid cyst. It may be mimicked occasionally by an intracavitary fungus ball or blood clot, usually in a bronchiectatic or tuberculous cavity.

Once a cyst ruptures, it leaks clear, salty fluid into the bronchus which is expectorated or disseminated further into the lungs. Air may enter the endocyst, producing an air-fluid level with the cyst (which may itself be capped with a crescent of air between the pericyst and endocyst). The endocyst is then seen as an arch above the air-fluid level and the pericyst is visible as a larger arch: this is the "sign of the double arch" or "Cumbo sign" (Figs. 3.39, 3.87 C).

As more hydatid fluid pours out of the cyst into the draining bronchus, paroxysms of coughing can occur, forcing more air into the hydatid. The radiographic appearance may now be that of a cavity with the collapsed wavy endocyst membranes floating on top of the remaining fluid to produce an irregular fluid level, described by South American authors as the water lily sign or "sign of the camalote" (or camelotte) because of its resemblance to a water plant found floating upon the Amazon and other South American rivers (Figs. 3.87 C, D, 3.91 C, 3.92 C, 3.93 C, 3.96 B). The double arch sign and the sign of the camalote are pathognomonic of a ruptured hydatid cyst. Conventional or computed tomography (CT) or MRI may be useful in some patients to identify the collapsed cyst membranes (Figs. 3.90, 3.93 D, 3.95, 3.96). When an uninfected cyst's contents are emptied by coughing, a large empty pericyst may remain (Fig. 3.95 H), closely resembling a congenital air cyst, bulla, or communicating infective cavity; secondary tuberculous infection of the empty pericyst cavity sometimes occurs.

Magnetic resonance imaging is also useful in showing pericystic parenchymal, pleural, and soft tissue reactions (Fig. 3.95 D); it is effective in demonstrating residual parasitic material after surgery and/or the response to chemotherapy. Recurrence of hydatid disease and extrapulmonary hydatid cysts can be more easily recognized.

(Text continues on p. 286)

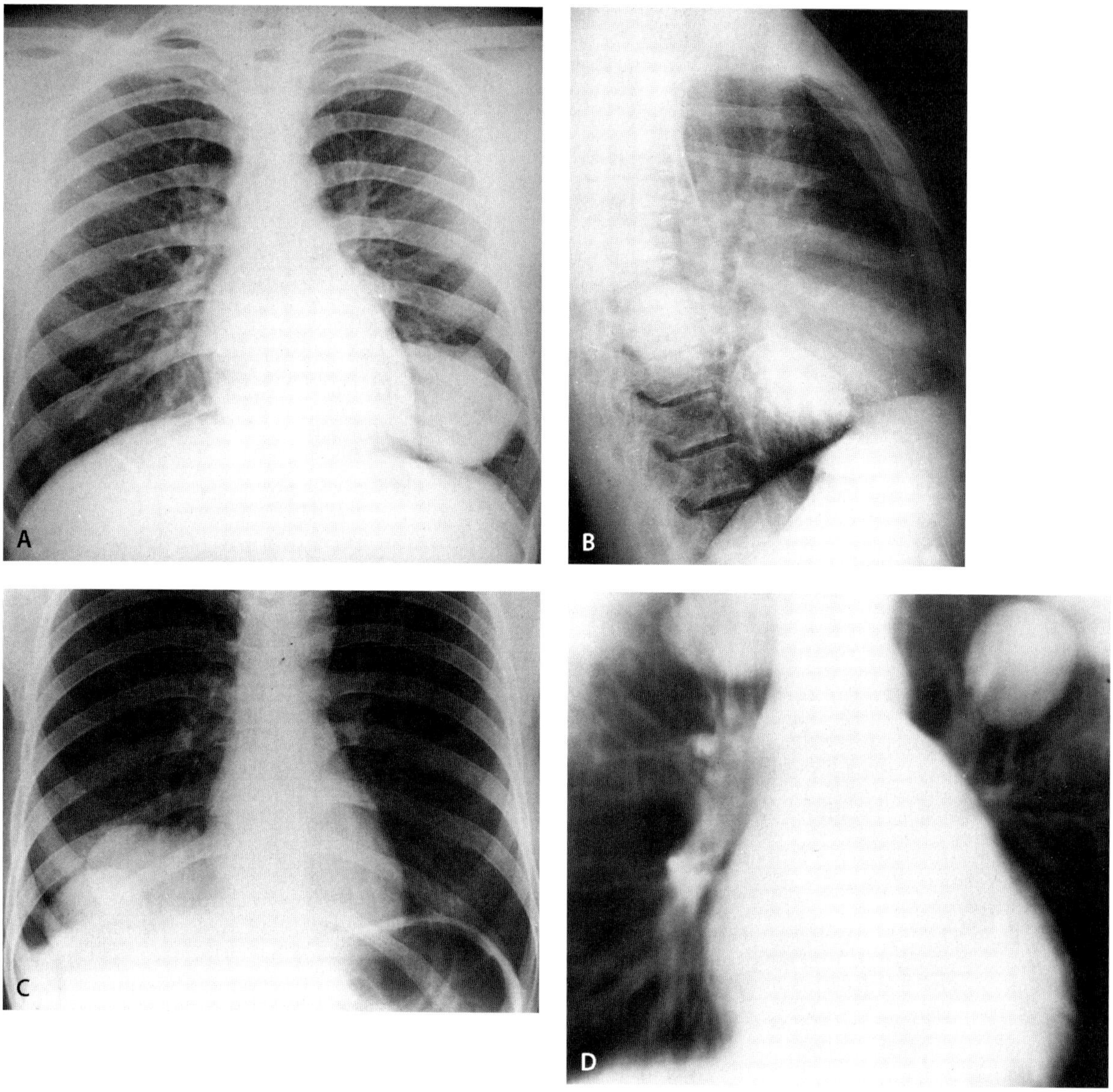

Fig. 3.85 A–D. Multiple hydatid cysts of the lungs. **A** PA and **B** lateral views of the chest show two large, slightly lobular, round masses in the left lower lobe. The mass in the superior segment of the left lower lobe is partially concealed by the left heart border in the frontal projection, but the lateral view clearly shows the two discrete masses. **C** There are two separate hydatid cysts in the right lung base partially superimposed on each other and obscuring the right hemidiaphragm of an African patient. There is a small right pleural effusion. **D** Two discrete round hydatids are present in the upper lobes of another patient

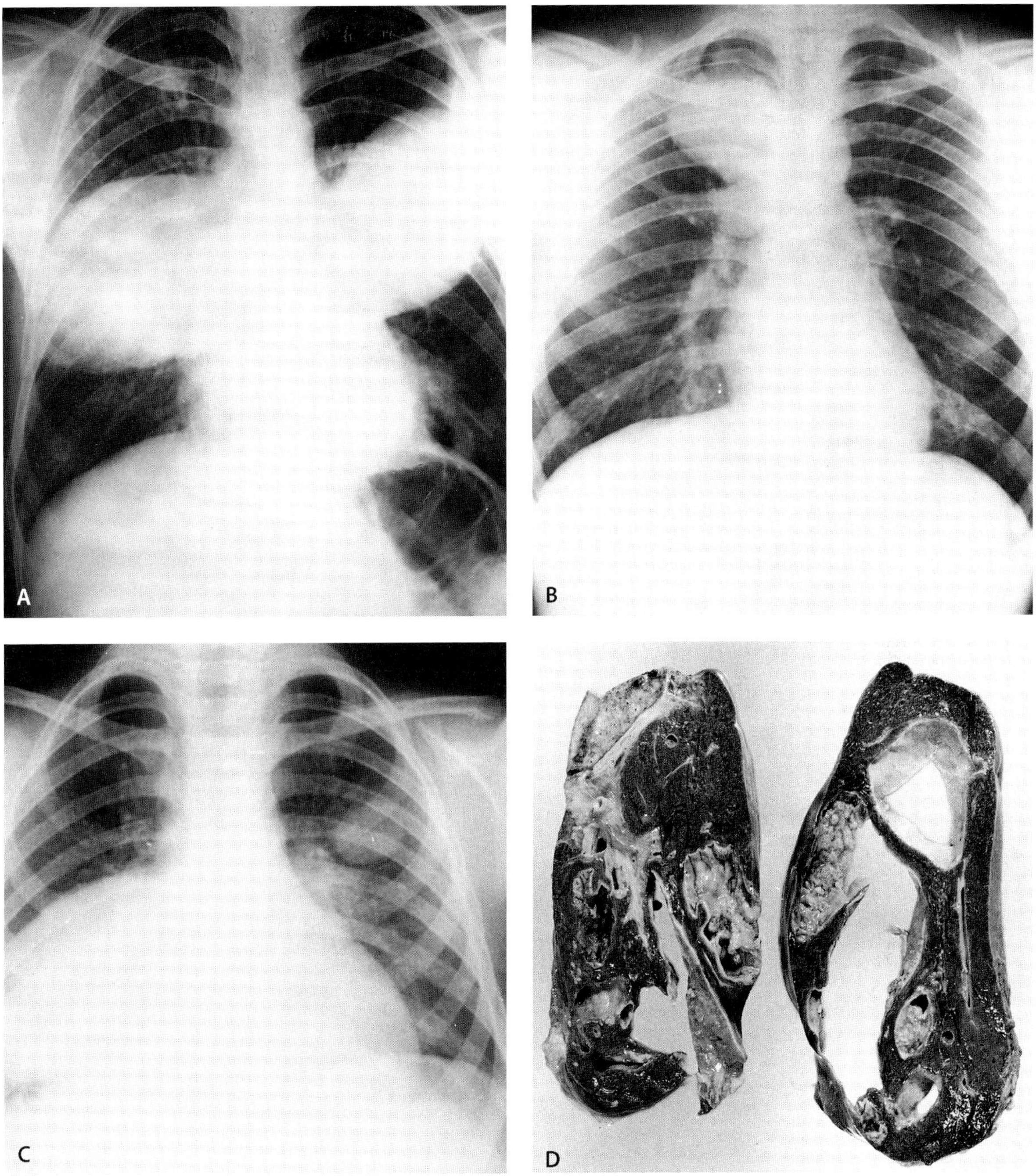

Fig. 3.86 A–D. Multiple hydatid lung cysts in three patients. **A** There are two large oval hydatids in the midportions of both lungs, giving a bizarre appearance to the chest on the frontal view. There is another hydatid at the left base which has ruptured and contains air and there are multiple small nodular and cavitary densities in the right upper lobe, which could be small metastatic hydatid implants or tuberculosis. The patient was an Inca Indian from the Andes Mountains of Peru. **B** Two hydatid cysts are present in the right upper lobe and suprahilar area of another man, and are partially superimposed on each other. **C** There is a large hydatid cyst occupying much of the right lower hemithorax with other smaller hydatids in the left perihilar area. **D** Autopsy specimens of multiple *E. granulosus* cysts of lung and liver. AFIP 57-15836-2

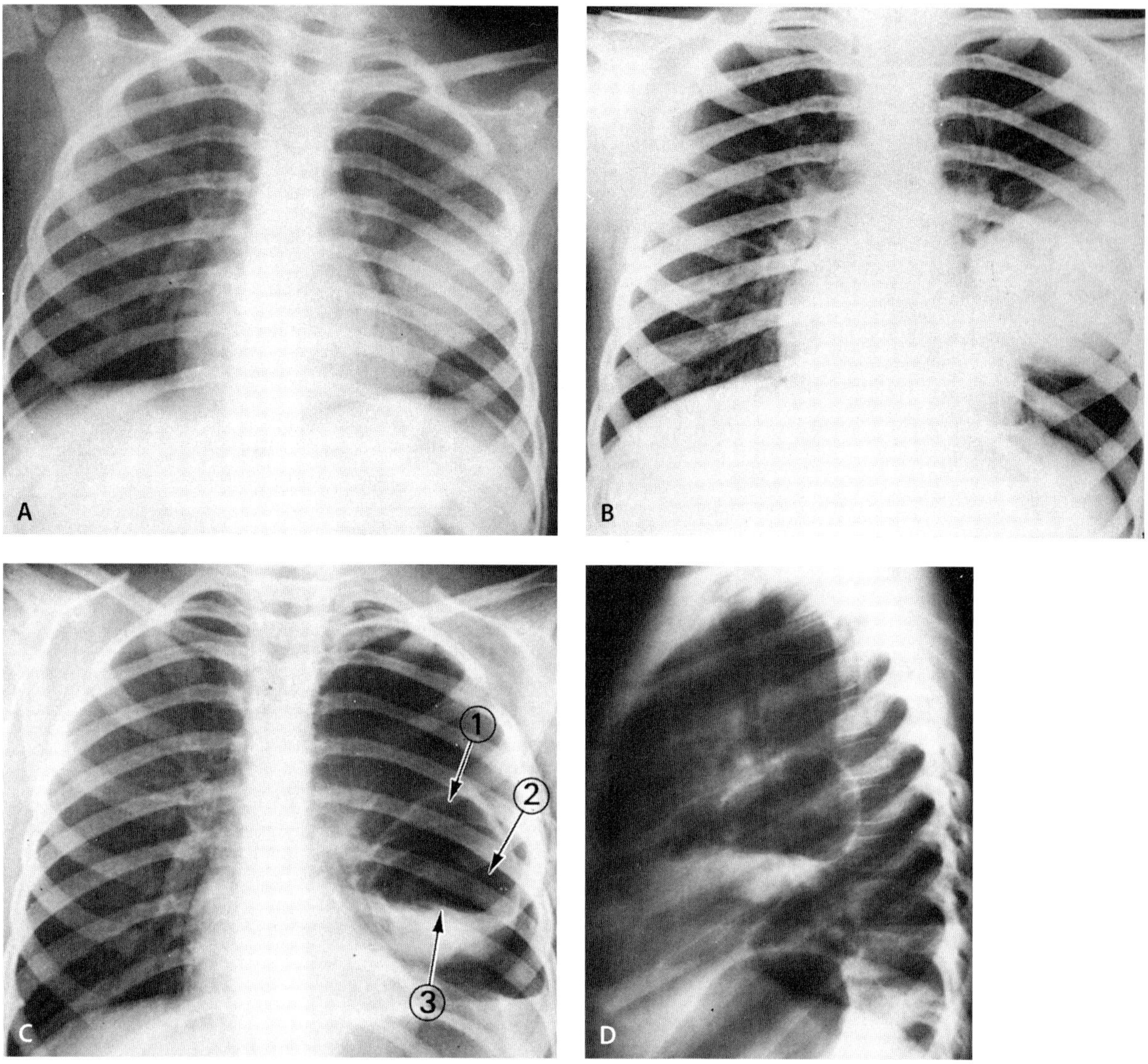

Fig. 3.87 A–D. Ruptured solitary hydatid cyst of the lung in a 4-year-old asymptomatic girl, showing the characteristic air meniscus, double arch, and floating water lily signs. **A** PA chest film shows a large solitary dense lesion in the left lingula, measuring approximately 4.5×5 cm in diameter. The mass is sharply circumscribed and roughly spherical. There is slight pleural-pericardial tenting along the left heart border. **B** A PA chest film a year later shows the lesion has grown considerably and is now 5×6 cm in diameter. The mass reaches the lateral chest wall and abuts against and obliterates part of the left heart border. **C** The correct diagnosis was not established until follow-up films showed the classical radiographic signs of a hydatid cyst that had undergone direct rupture. There is a 40% left pneumothorax and a left pleural effusion. The appearance of the cyst is diagnostic of a pulmonary hydatid that has ruptured into a bronchus or the pleura. The perivesicular air meniscus between the host adventitia and the parasitic endocyst (the so-called sign of detachment) (*1*) is clearly seen, as is a cyst within a cyst or sign of the double arch (*2*). The irregular wavy nature of the fluid level produced by the collapsed hydatid membranes floating on top of the residual hydatid fluid produces the pathognomonic floating water lily sign or sign of the camalote (*3*). **D** The lateral view of the chest shows the multilobulated outline of the ruptured cyst with its irregular fluid level. When a pulmonary hydatid ruptures into the pleura or into a blood vessel, metastatic hydatidosis frequently occurs due to the presence of numerous brood capsules and scolices in the hydatid fluid and sand. Formalin was injected into this cyst and the cyst wall was marsupialized (a common surgical procedure in treating hydatid disease of the lungs in the 1940s, but rarely used today). The present (1999) treatment of choice is surgical endocystectomy or occasionally removal of the affected segment or lobe, followed by chemotherapy when necessary. (Courtesy of Dr. Douglas Sheft, San Francisco; from Dr. M.M. Reeder and *Radiology*, 1970)

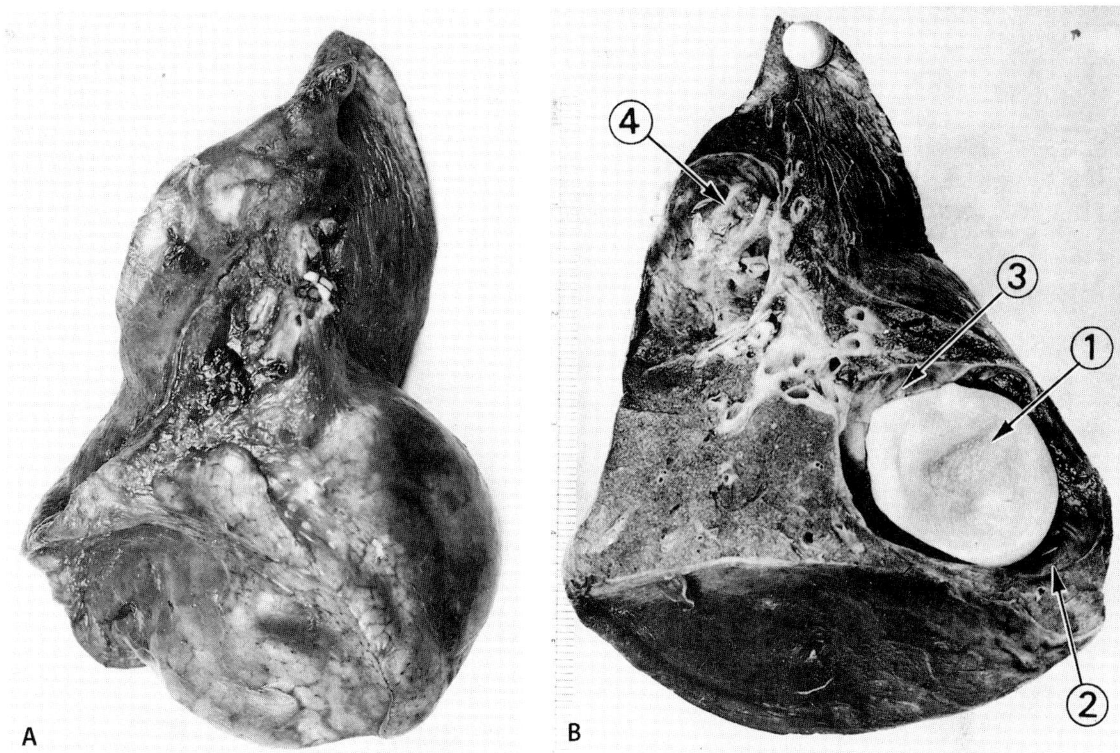

Fig. 3.88 A, B. A left lung containing three hydatid cysts, with the cut surface showing the different layers of the cysts and allowing correlation with the radiographic signs of a ruptured hydatid. **A** Two of the hydatids are causing marked bulging of the contours of the upper and lower lobes. AFIP 58-11739-E. **B** Cut surface of the same lung showing the hydatid endocyst (*1*) completely detached from the surrounding host adventitia or pericyst (*2*) in the large lesion in the left lower lobe. Air filling this space in vivo (*3*) would give the air meniscus sign or cyst-within-a-cyst appearance radiographically, depending upon the degree of separation of the endocyst from the pericyst. The endocyst and membranes have been totally removed from the second hydatid cyst (*4*), revealing the fibrous adventitial lining (pericyst) produced by the host tissues. A third, much smaller, intact cyst is present at the apex of the lung. AFIP 58-11739-D. (From Dr. M.M. Reeder and *Radiology*, 1970)

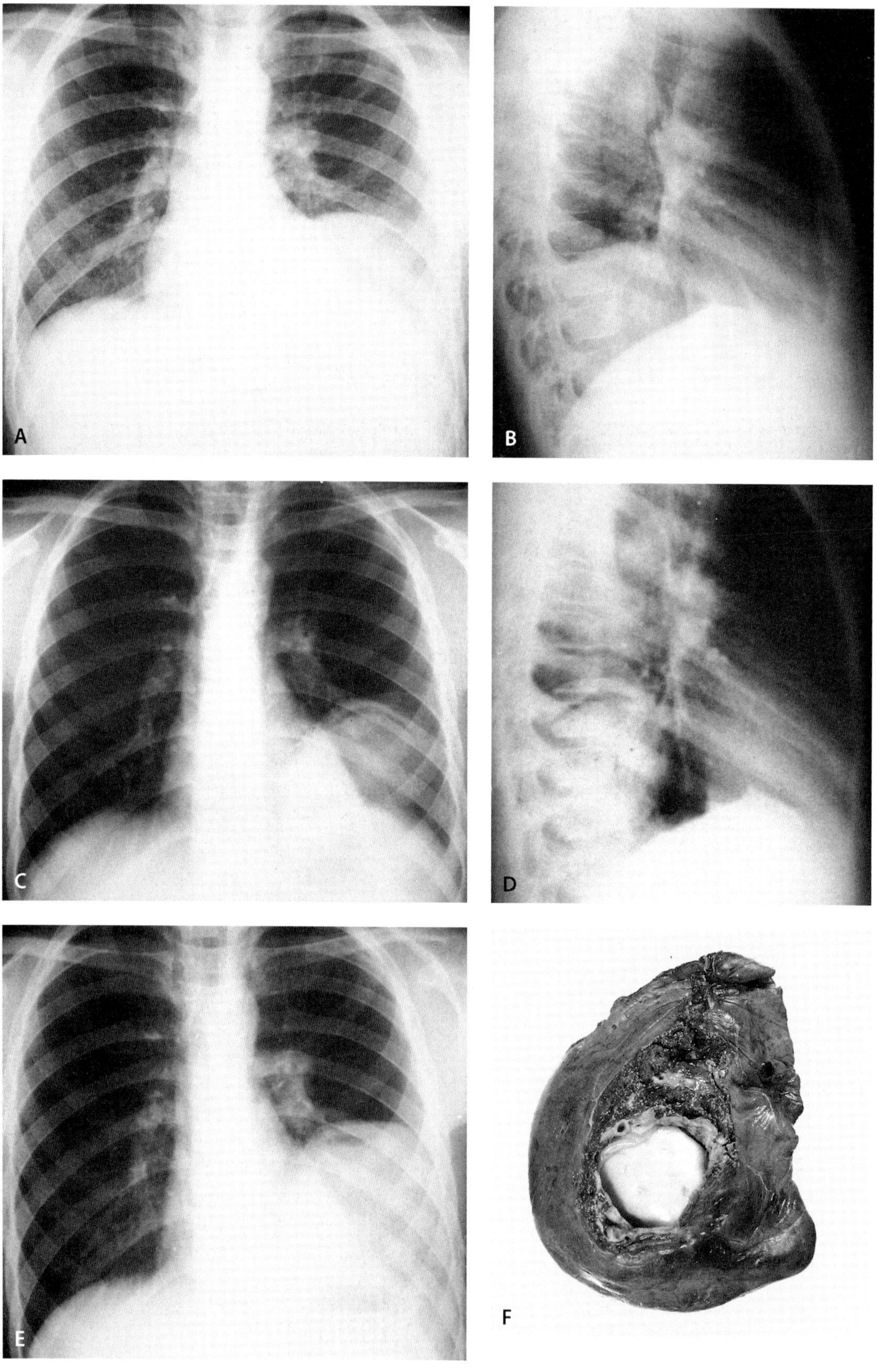
A
B
C
D
E
F

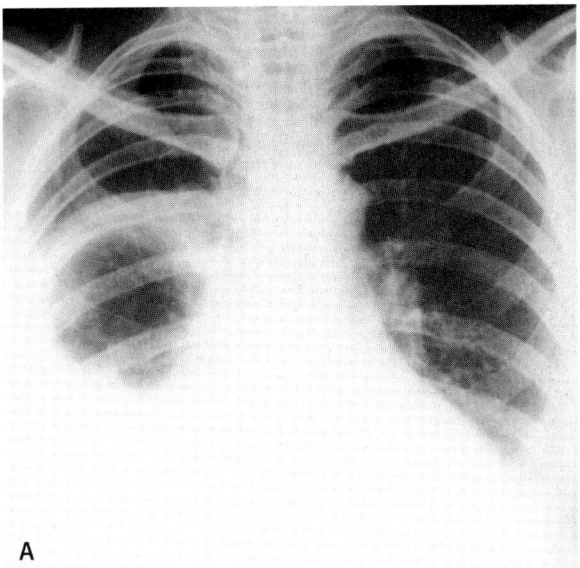

A

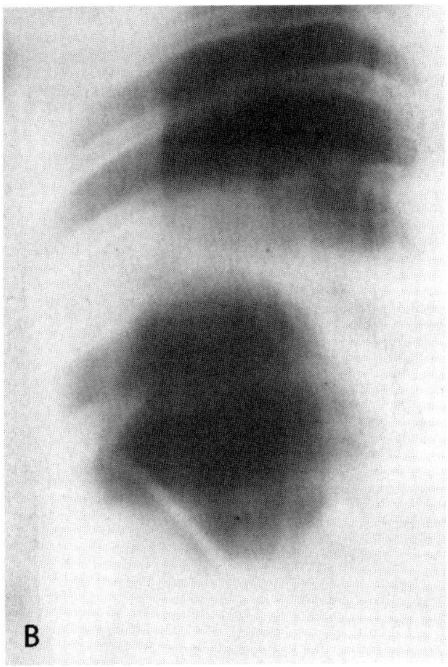

B

Fig. 3.90 A, B. The interior of a ruptured hydatid cyst and its collapsed membranes as seen on conventional tomography. A PA chest radiograph of a Spaniard showing a large ruptured hydatid cyst occupying most of the right lower lung. There is a thickened pericyst around this old hydatid. The diaphragm and lower lateral chest wall are obscured by pleural reaction and fluid. Secondary infection of such a ruptured hydatid may change its appearance to that of a pyogenic lung abscess. B However, an AP supine tomographic cut through the ruptured cyst clearly identifies collapsed hydatid membranes in its lower portion, thus establishing the true identity of this thick-walled cystic lesion. (Courtesy of Dr. Jose Bonmati, Madrid)

◀ Fig. 3.89 A–F. A hydatid cyst in the left lower lobe with subsequent rupture producing the air meniscus sign of detachment. The patient was a 10-year-old American boy who had lived in Iran for two years. A, B Initial PA and lateral views of the chest show a large round mass in the left lower lobe. C, D Follow-up PA and lateral chest films 7 weeks later show a classical air meniscus in the superior aspect of the lesion as a result of the enlarging cyst communicating with an adjacent bronchiole. This allowed a slight amount of air to enter between the pericyst and endocyst, producing the air meniscus (or air crescent) sign of detachment. E Subsequent PA chest film taken shortly thereafter shows a small air-fluid level within the cyst. F The gross specimen of a solitary large hydatid cyst in the lung of another patient shows the endocyst and surrounding pericyst adjacent to a bronchus. AFIP 138934-02281

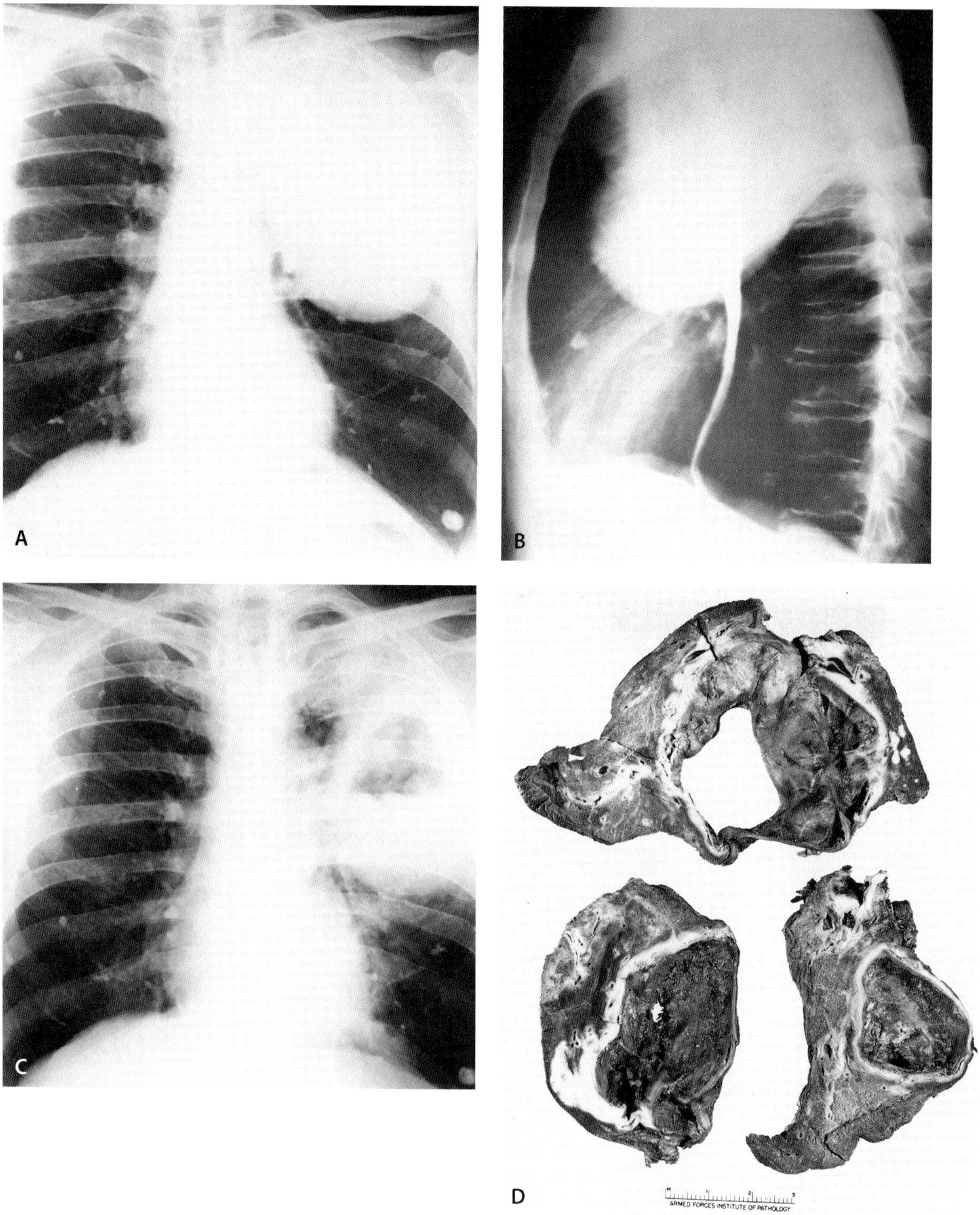

Fig. 3.91 A–D. Rupture of a huge, thick-walled hydatid cyst in the left upper lobe of an Inca Indian from Peru. **A** PA and **B** lateral views of the chest reveal a large oval mass occupying much of the left upper lobe. The oval contour of the mass suggests that it is more likely to be a hydatid cyst or lung abscess than a neoplasm. The scattered calcifications in the lungs are most likely the result of healed tuberculosis. **C** A follow-up chest radiograph 16 days later shows that the large hydatid has ruptured into a bronchus with expectoration of a portion of the cyst contents. Note the thick wall of the old cyst and the irregular fluid level within it due to the germinal membranes and cyst contents floating on top of the hydatid fluid (floating water lily sign or sign of the camalote). **D** A large hydatid cyst in the lung of another patient showing a thick outer layer or pericyst similar to that seen in **C**. AFIP 55-22877

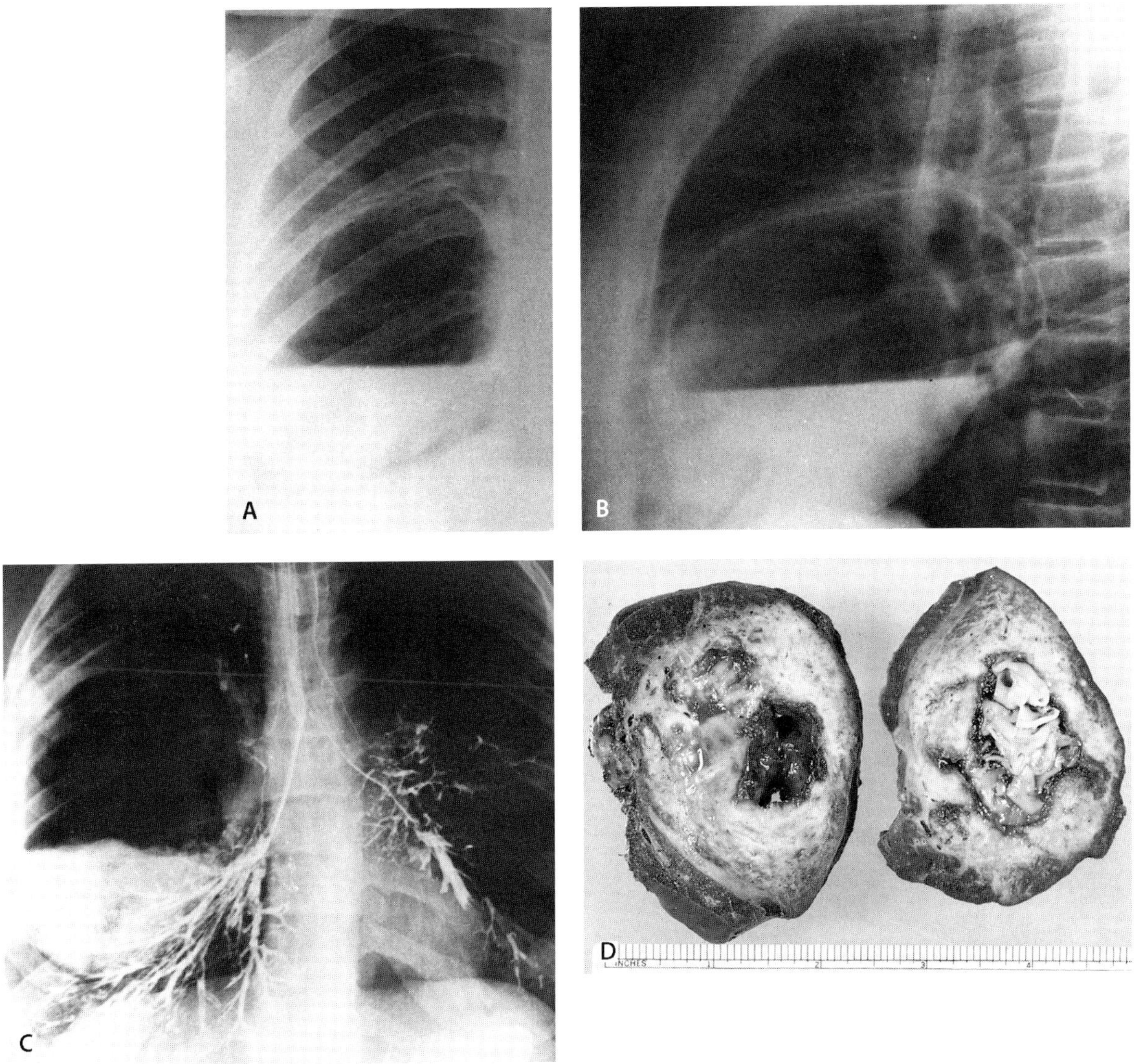

Fig. 3.92 A–D. Different types of air-fluid levels in ruptured hydatid cysts in two patients from India with cough and expectoration. **A** PA and **B** lateral views of the chest of the first patient show a huge ruptured hydatid cyst occupying the entire right middle lobe. The fluid level in this cyst is smooth, as might be seen in an infected nonparasitic cyst or abscess. **C** More commonly in a ruptured hydatid cyst, there is an irregular fluid level due to the collapsed membranes floating on top of the hydatid fluid (floating water lily sign). In this second patient, bronchography shows compression and displacement of the bronchi of the right lung by the huge pulmonary hydatid. Contrast medium may enter between the layers of the ruptured hydatid membrane, producing another pathognomonic sign of hydatid cyst. **D** The gross specimen of a large pulmonary hydatid from another patient showing clearly the wavy, gelatinous nature of the membranes and inner lining of the endocyst. When the cyst ruptures, these membranes may float on top of the residual hydatid fluid, producing the classic floating water lily sign or sign of the camalote. AFIP 556341-660-1

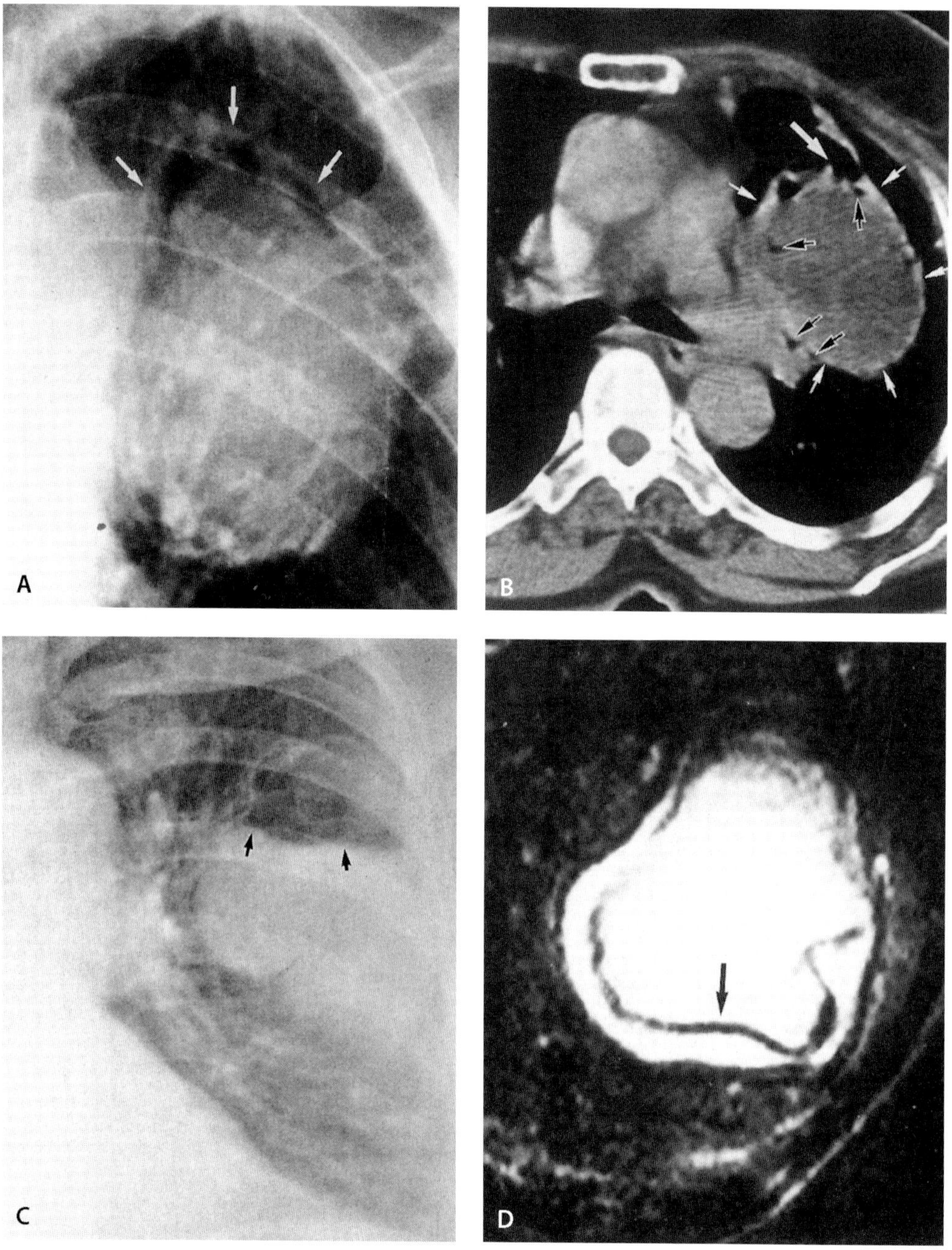

Fig. 3.93. A–C A 60-year-old Saudi woman with cough, hemoptysis, and hoarseness. **A** Chest radiograph reveals an air meniscus sign (*arrows*) in a large left upper lobe hydatid cyst. **B** Contrast-enhanced CT shows ring enhancement of the cyst wall (*small white arrows*); there is pericystic emphysema (*large arrow*) typical of an infected hydatid cyst containing air bubbles (*small black arrows*). **C** One week later, the water-lily sign (*arrows*) has appeared due to further cyst rupture and expectoration of more hydatid fluid. **D** MRI, 1.5 T (SE 2000/100), on another patient with hydatid lung cyst shows collapsed parasitic membrane causing the serpent sign (*arrow*)

Fig. 3.95 A–H. A 34-year-old Saudi man with ongoing hydatid cyst rupture. **A** Chest radiograph reveals a round mass in the right lower lobe corresponding to a closed type I hydatid cyst. **B** Two weeks later, there has been external rupture of the cyst with allergic parenchymal reaction mimicking pneumonitis. **C** CT scan taken at the same time as **B** and at the same level reveals a bronchocystic communication (*small white arrows*) with rupture and collapsed parasitic membranes (serpent sign, *small black arrows*); note also the direct rupture of cyst contents with parenchymal reaction (*curved white arrows*). **D** MRI, 1.5 T (SE 2000/100), taken the same day as **B** and **C** shows the collapsed parasitic membranes (serpent sign, *black arrows*) and pericystic reaction (*curved white arrows*) to better advantage. **E–H** see p. 284

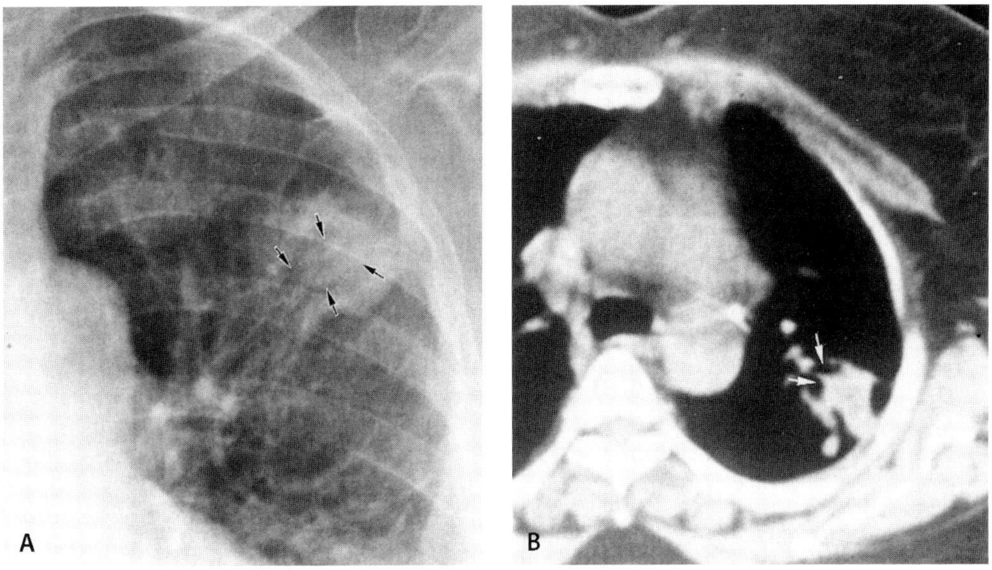

Fig. 3.94 A, B. A 39-year-old woman with hydatid cyst in the left upper lobe. **A** Chest radiograph shows "retained cyst sign" (*arrows*) caused by trapped, collapsed parasitic membranes after the pulmonary hydatid ruptured into the airways. **B** Contrast-enhanced CT reveals the retained cyst sign (*arrows*) showing trapped parasitic tissue in the airways after partial expectoration

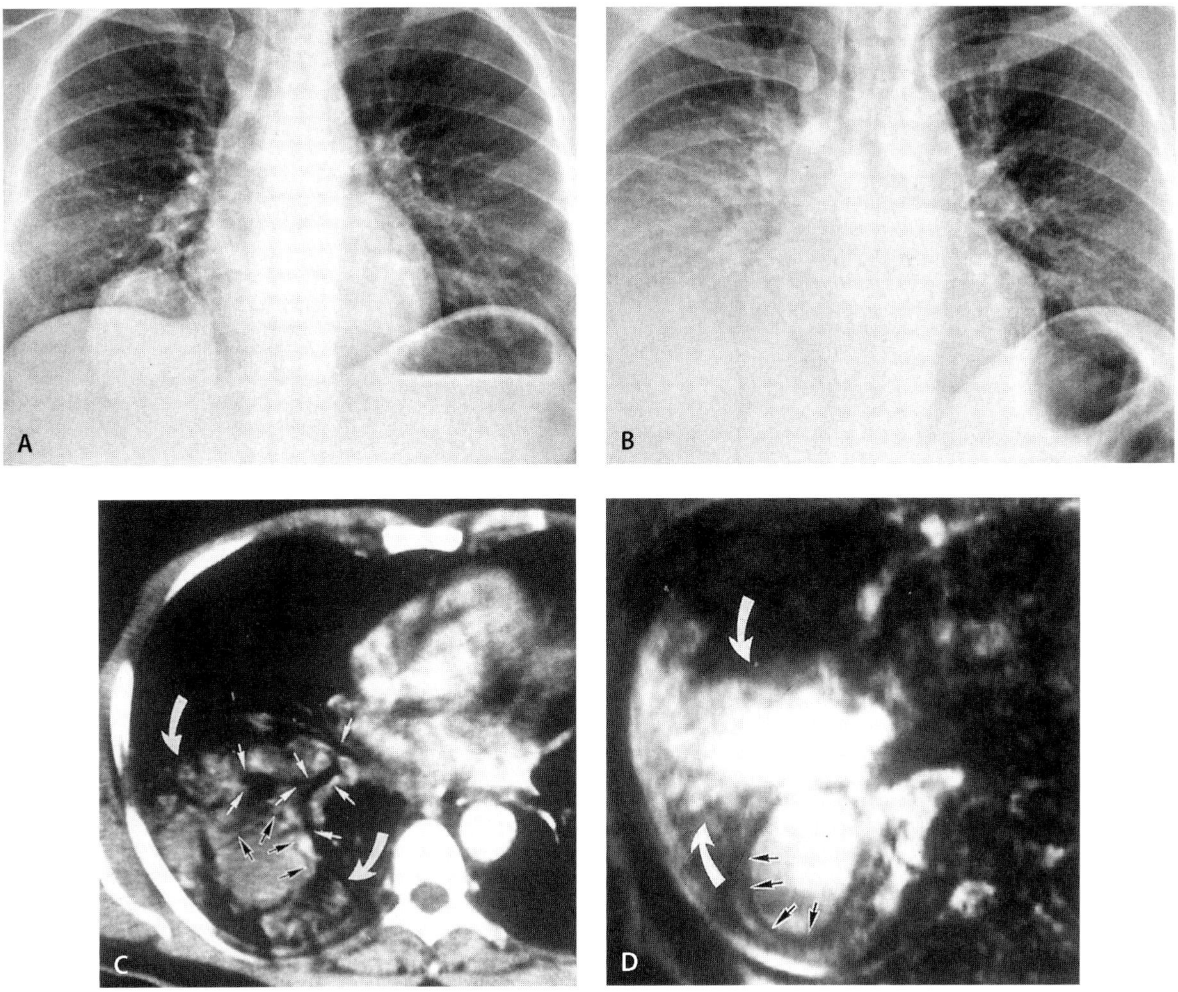

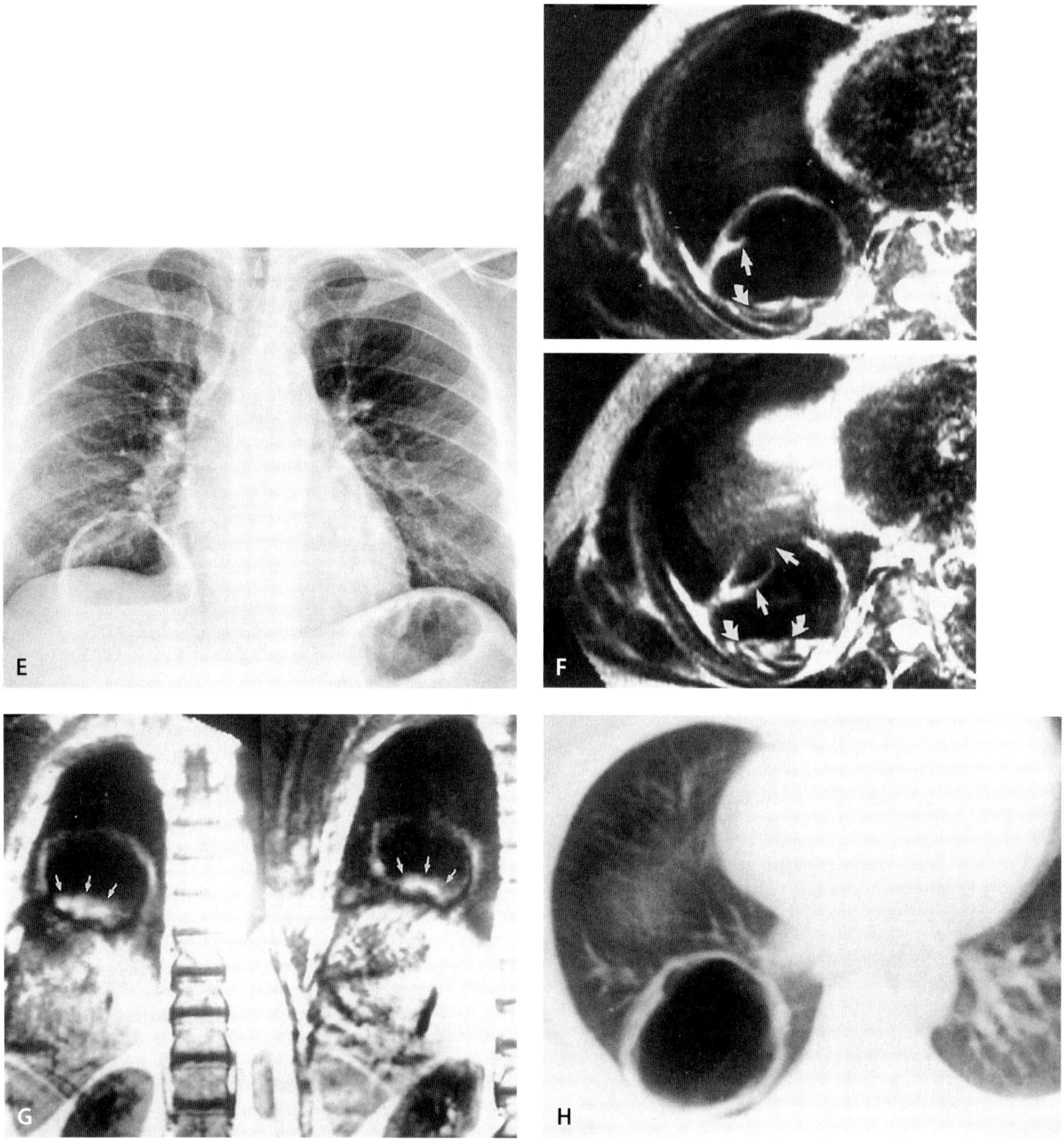

Fig. 3.95 (*continued*). **E** Chest radiograph a few days later shows the "cyst with a fluid level" mimicking an abscess. **F** MRI, 1.5 T (SE 850/20), taken at the same time as **E** demonstrates the serpent sign (*arrows*) and submerged parasitic membranes (*curved arrows*). **G** MRI, 0.5 T (SE 2000/100), coronal view, 1 week later reveals globular collapsed parasitic membranes at the bottom of the cyst producing the "sign of the rising sun" (*arrows*). **H** One month later, CT shows an "empty cyst" after complete evacuation of the parasitic membranes. (Courtesy of Dr. Walther von Sinner and *Eur Radiol*, 1993)

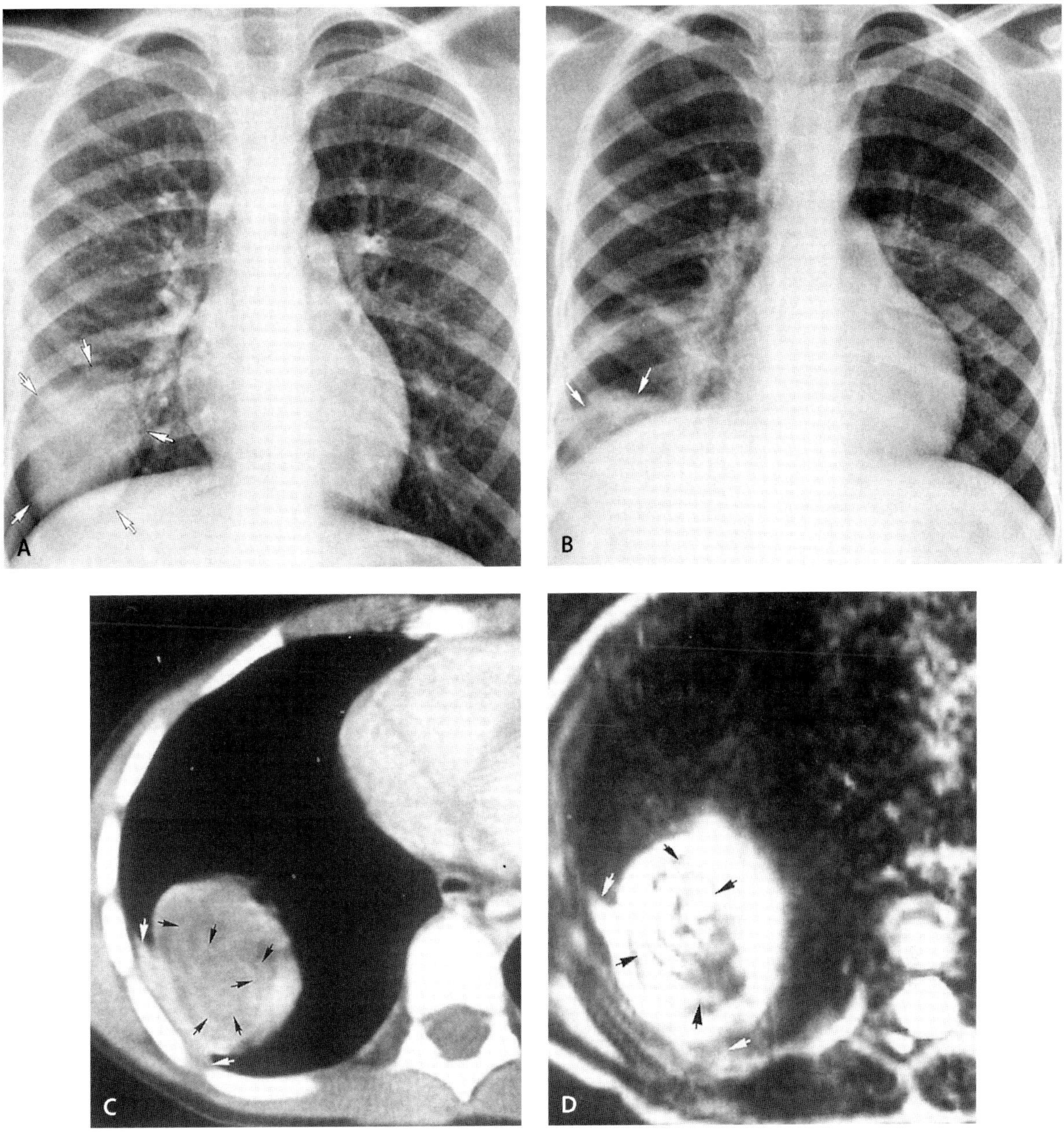

Fig. 3.96 A–D. A 9-year-old Saudi boy with ruptured pulmonary hydatid cyst. **A** Chest radiograph shows discrete pericystic hyperlucency around a mass in the right lower lobe (*arrows*), subsequently identified as a hydatid cyst. **B** Chest radiograph 2 weeks later demonstrates the "iceberg sign" indicating collapsed parasitic membranes which are partially submerged (*arrows*). **C** CT scan 1 week after **A** shows detached membranes (whirl sign, *black arrows*) with small pleural reaction (*white arrows*). **D** MRI, 1.5 T (SE 2000/100), obtained at same time as **C** shows the whirl sign to better advantage (*black arrows*) and pleural reaction (*white arrows*). (Courtesy of Dr. Walther von Sinner and *Eur Radiol*, 1993)

Thirty Saudi Arabian patients (18 female, 12 male) with thoracic hydatidosis caused by *Echinococcus granulosus* were studied by von Sinner (1993). The patients' ages ranged from 7 to 72 years with an average age of 35 years. CT without and/or with contrast enhancement (bolus and drip infusion) was performed in all patients. Findings from chest radiographs were compared with CT and in ten cases with MRI, using short TR/TE (700/20) and long TR/TE (2000/100) conventional spin-echo pulse sequences with 8 mm slice thickness. Pathological confirmation was obtained by surgery in 26 cases, and by noncomplicated fine-needle aspiration biopsy in four cases in which the appearance of the lesion initially mimicked neoplastic disease. The hydatid cysts were located in the lung (70%), mediastinum (6.7%), heart (10%), pleura (10%), and chest wall (3.3%). The radiographic, CT and MRI findings in unruptured and ruptured cysts at different stages of the disease are listed in Table 3.2 while the complications of pulmonary hydatids are listed in Table 3.3.

Unfortunately, the patterns cited in Table 3.2 do not always develop, especially if the cyst has become infected. Secondary infection of a hydatid cyst changes its appearance to that of a lung abscess, quite indistinguishable from an ordinary pyogenic abscess. A careful search of the sputum may demonstrate disintegrated scolices and hooklets.

Hydatid cysts which have undergone direct rupture may be surrounded by an allergic pneumonitis, which may develop into a bacterial pneumonia and bronchopneumonia (Fig. 3.98). Large cysts can cause compression, with resulting minor or segmental atelectasis or chronic pneumonia, eventually leading to dense scarring. Localized lung fibrosis and atelectasis (Fig. 3.99) can occur following cyst rupture.

The differential diagnosis of lung hydatids is essentially that of all round cystic or solid lung lesions. Scanning (CT, MRI, or rarely ultrasonography) can often shorten the list of possibilities, or even lead to a definitive diagnosis (Figs. 3.100–3.104). When there is a known or suspected neoplasm elsewhere in the body and multiple lesions are seen in the lungs on chest radiography, metastases will be erroneously suspected in many patients, only to discover that they in fact represent hydatid cysts as suggested by CT or MR scanning (Figs. 3.103–3.105).

Fig. 3.97 A–D. A 34-year-old Saudi man presented with a round homogeneous mass in his right lower lobe. **A** Chest radiograph 2 weeks later shows the hydatid cyst has ruptured with collapse of the parasitic membranes (*arrow*). **B** CT scan shows detached membranes producing the snake or serpent sign. **C** MRI T2-weighted (spin echo, 2000/100) image reveals detached membranes floating in the partially fluid-filled cyst with pleural reaction (*white arrows*), producing the serpent sign (*black arrow*). **D** MRI T1-weighted (spin echo, 950/20) image shows the lower lobe bronchus (*black arrows*) in close contact with the cyst wall (*white arrows*). Spread of cyst contents into the lower lobe caused infiltrates and reactive pneumonitis ▶

Table 3.2. Radiographic, CT, and MRI signs of hydatid cysts of the chest. (Courtesy of Dr. von Sinner and *Eur Radiol*, 1993)

Well-known radiographic signs include:

1. "Meniscus sign" (also called "crescent sign" or "sign of detachment") (Figs. 3.87–3.89, 3.93 A)
2. "Water-lily sign" (or "camalote sign") (Figs. 3.87, 3.91–3.93 C)

Less well-known imaging signs may reflect different stages of a ruptured hydatid cyst:

1. "Cyst with fluid level" (or "abscess") (Fig. 3.95 E, F)
2. "Iceberg sign" (Fig. 3.96 B)
3. "Double-arch or Cumbo sign" (Figs. 3.39, 3.87 C)
4. "Sign of the rising sun" (Figs. 3.95 G, 3.97 A)
5. "Serpent sign" (Figs. 3.93 D, 3.95 C, D, 3.97 B, C)
6. "Whirl sign" (Fig. 3.96 C, D)
7. "Retained cyst" (Fig. 3.94)
8. "Empty cyst" (Fig. 3.95 H)
9. "Calcification" (heart and mediastinum, rarely)

Table 3.3. Complications of thoracic hydatid cysts

1. Rupture and pericystic reaction (Figs. 3.95, 3.96)
2. Infection (Fig. 3.93 B)
   a) Air bubbles (Fig. 3.93 B)
   b) Abscess (similar to Fig. 3.95 E)
3. Rupture into airways (Figs. 3.94 B, 3.95 C)
   a) Expectoration of scolices or "grape skins" (daughter cysts), salty fluid, hemoptysis with or without suffocation, allergic reactions or shock
   b) Bronchocystic fistula (Fig. 3.95 B, C)
   c) Evidence of biliobronchial fistula
   d) Bronchogenic spread
4. Pleural perforation (Figs. 3.87, 3.99)
   a) Pleural effusion (Figs. 3.87, 3.96 C, D and 3.98) (may contain "hydatid sand" or "grape skins")
   b) Hydropneumothorax, pyopneumothorax, tension pneumothorax (Figs. 3.87, 3.99 A)
   c) "Rounded atelectasis" (Fig. 3.99 B)
5. Vascular spread (Fig. 3.102)
6. Overgrowth or spread to mediastinum

(Text continues on p. 292)

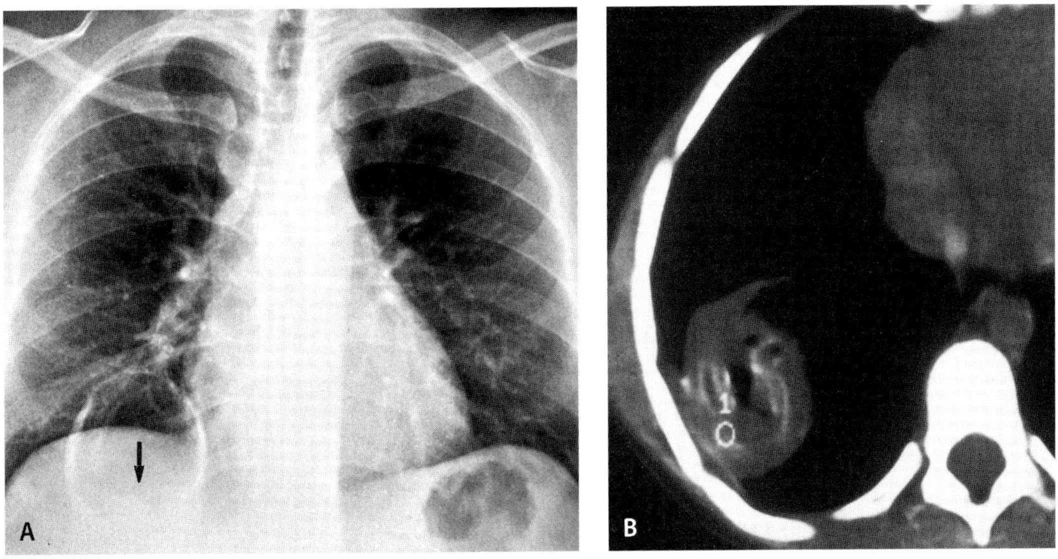

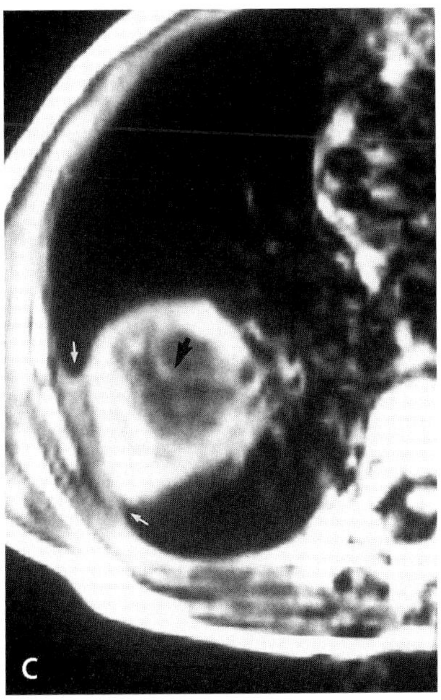

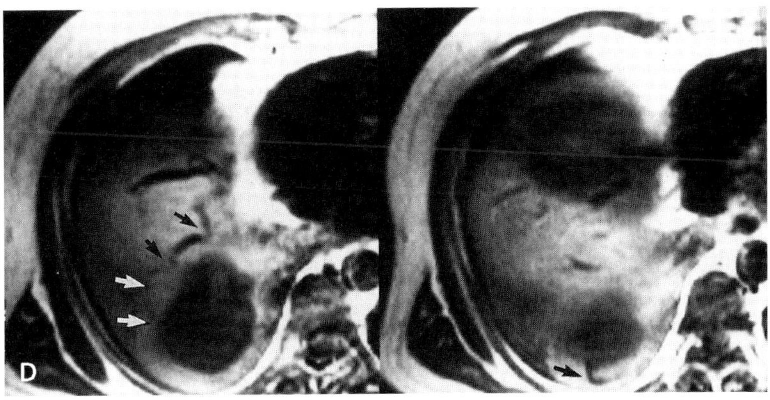

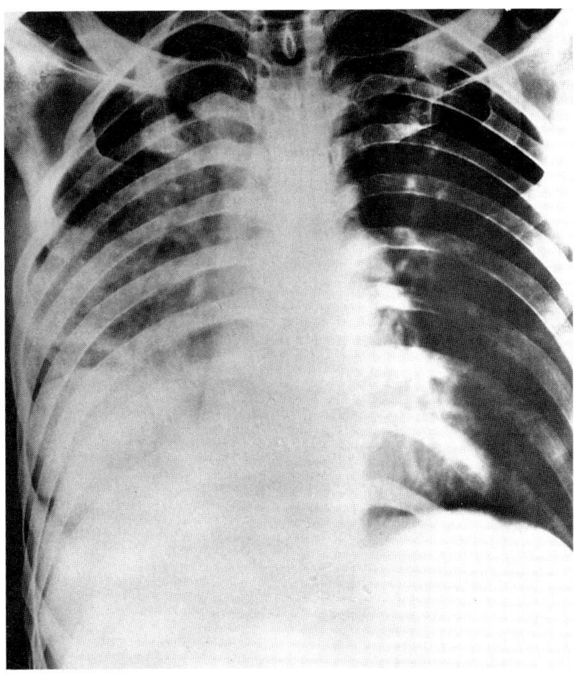

▶

Fig. 3.98. In the event of direct rupture of a lung hydatid, an allergic pneumonitis develops. This may proceed to a bacterial infection, as in this patient with a large hydatid in the right lower lung. Scattered areas of infiltrate are seen throughout the right lung. When a partially ruptured hydatid cyst becomes secondarily infected, it may be radiologically indistinguishable from a lung abscess

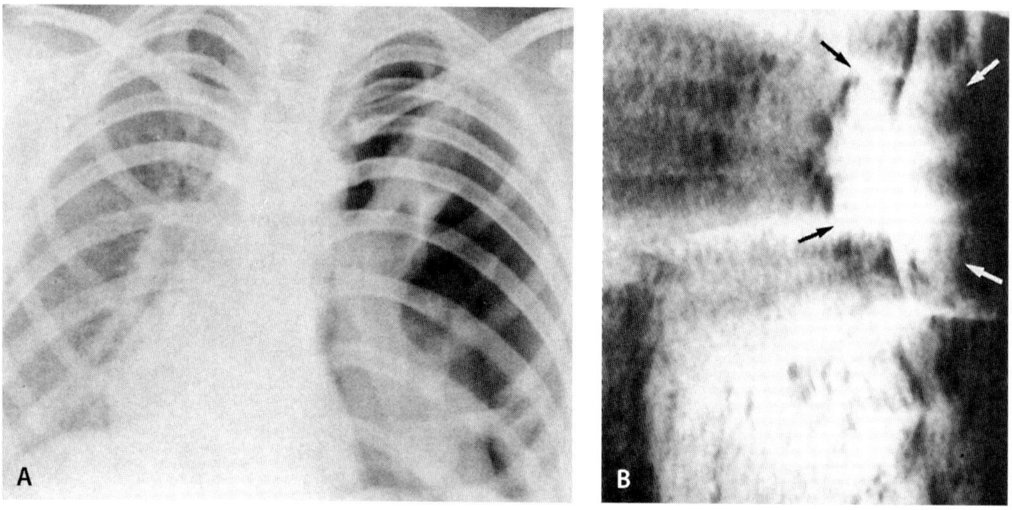

Fig. 3.99 A, B. A 28-year-old Saudi woman with a hydatid cyst that ruptured into the pleural space. **A** Chest radiograph reveals a tension pneumothorax after perforation of the lung hydatid into the pleural space. A chest tube was inserted through which parasitic material was recovered. **B** Ultrasound scan several months later shows that "rounded atelectasis" (*arrows*) has developed in the interval. (Courtesy of Dr. Walther von Sinner and *Eur Radiol*, 1993)

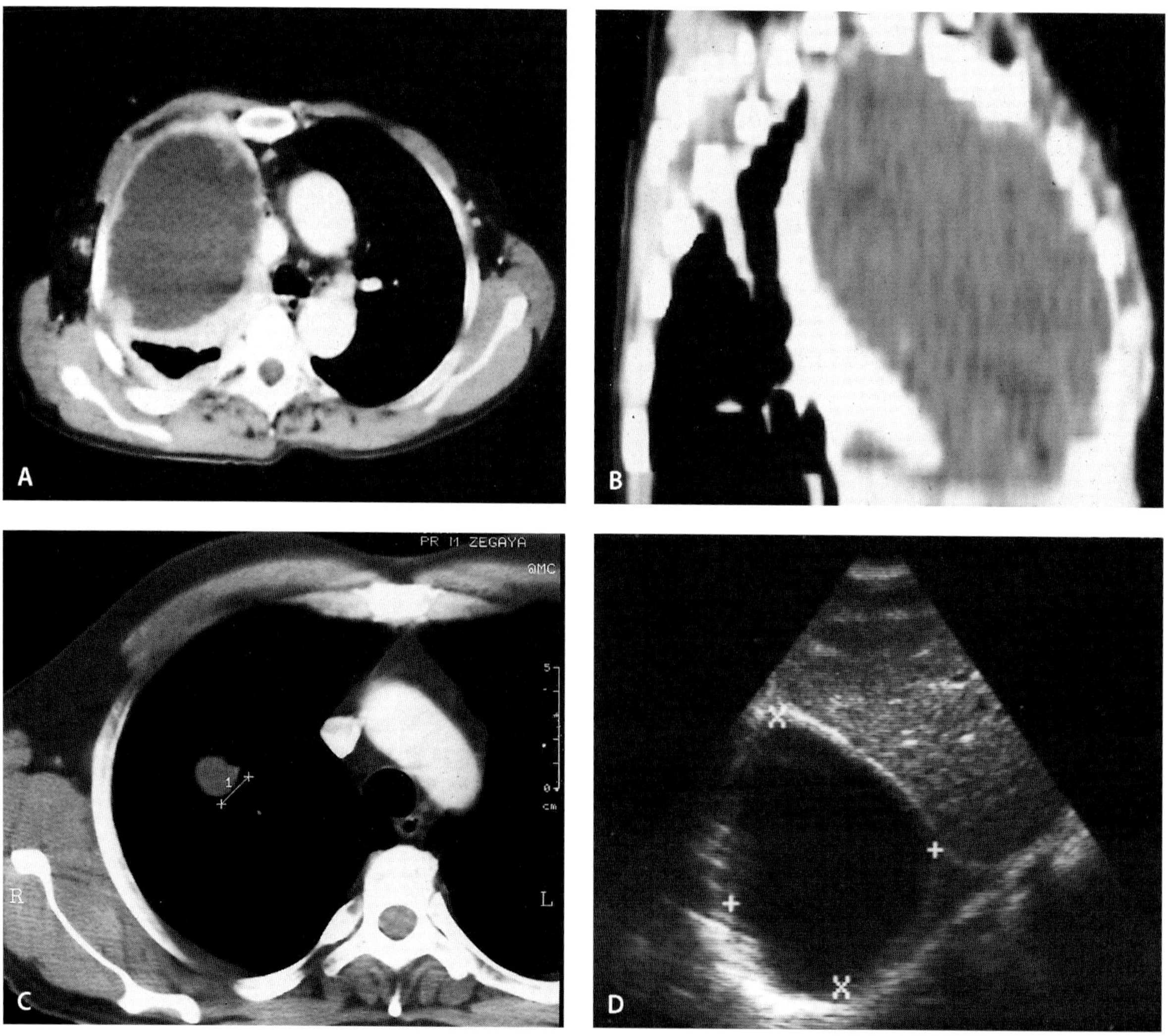

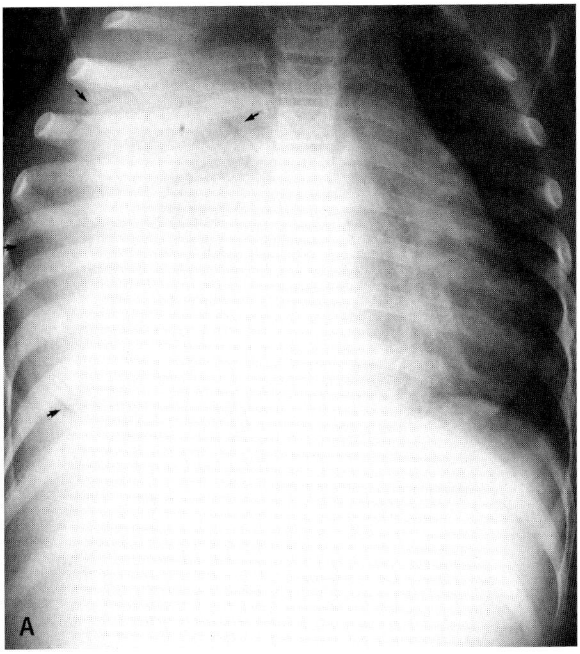

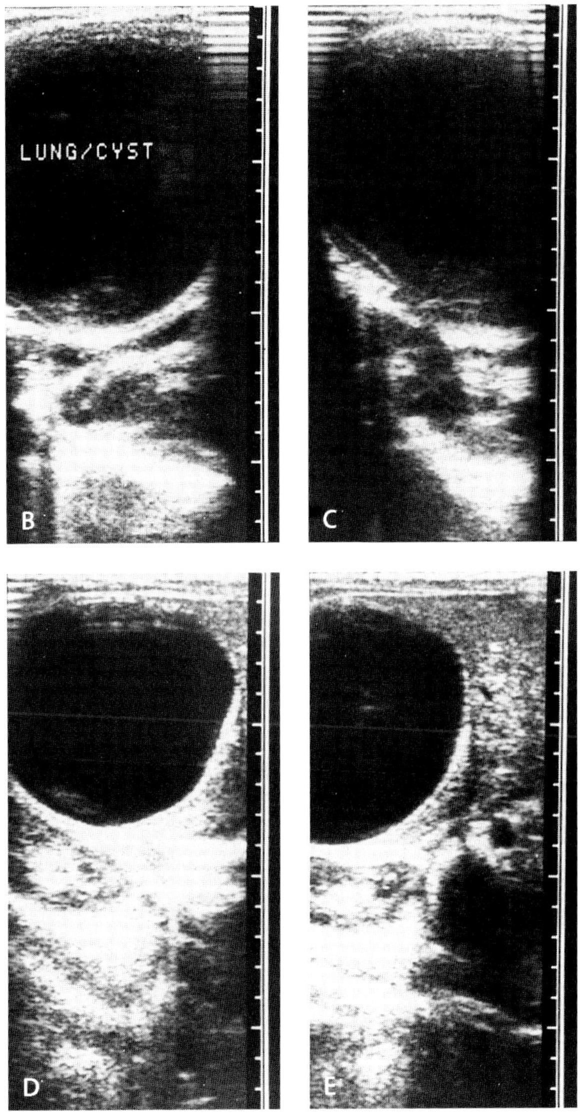

Fig. 3.101 A–E. Huge hydatid cysts in the lung and liver of a Kenyan child. **A** Chest radiograph reveals an enormous hydatid occupying most of the right lung. There is a thin rim of air outlining the cyst wall (*arrowheads*) with lung parenchymal reaction and compression atelectasis surrounding the cyst. **B–E** Ultrasound scans show the huge hydatids in the lung (**B**, **C**) and liver (**D**, **E**). Partial membrane detachment is seen in the lower aspect of the lung hydatid in **C**. (Courtesy of Dr. M.W. Wachira)

◀ **Fig. 3.100 A–D.** Three patients from Tunisia with thoracic hydatid cysts of varying sizes and locations evaluated with CT and ultrasound scanning. **A** Contrast-enhanced CT scan and **B** sagittal reconstruction of same scan in a 55-year-old woman showing a huge univesicular hydatid occupying most of the right hemithorax in the region of the right upper and middle lobes. Note the thick, enhancing pericyst. **C** Small uncomplicated 1.6-cm hydatid cyst on contrast-enhanced CT scan in a Tunisian man. **D** Ultrasound scan showing a huge type I hydatid cyst lying just above the liver and diaphragm in the right lower hemithorax of a 4-year-old boy. (Courtesy of Drs. Ben Cheikh and Gharbi, Tunis)

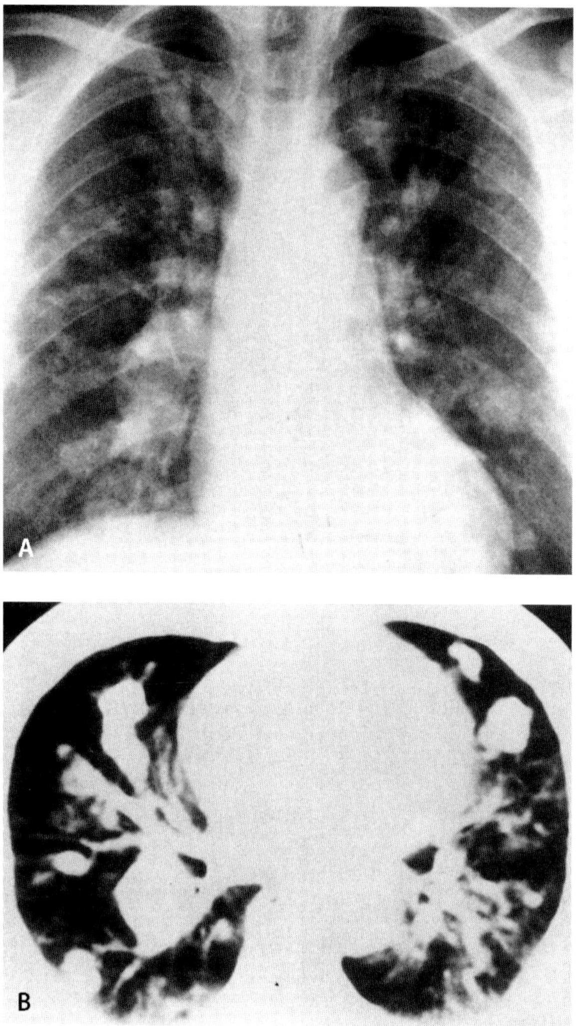

Fig. 3.102 A, B. A 60-year-old Saudi man with numerous pulmonary hydatids which could be mistaken for metastatic malignancy. **A** Chest radiograph shows multiple bilateral "nodules," some of which appear cavitated. Enlarged pulmonary arteries are visible, particularly the right interlobar pulmonary artery and some segmental arteries in the upper lobes. **B** CT scan was obtained at the same time. The nodules were later confirmed to be hydatid cysts. (Courtesy of Dr. Walther von Sinner and *Eur Radiol*, 1993)

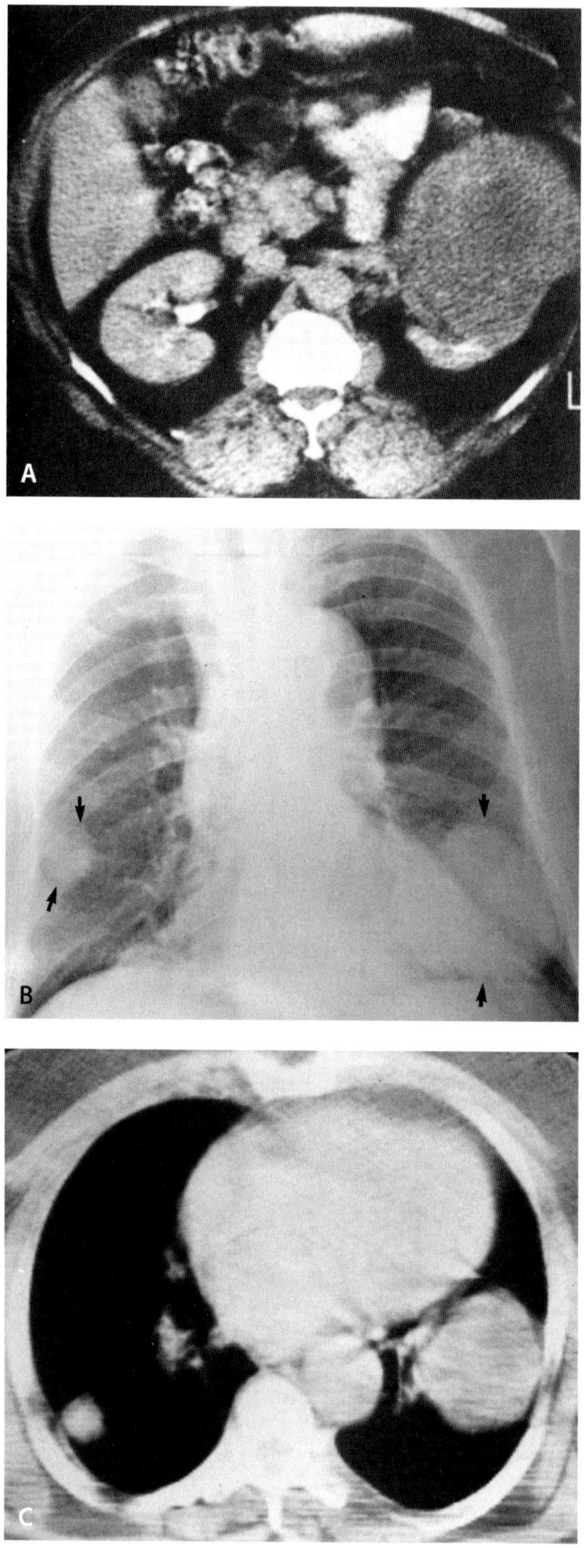

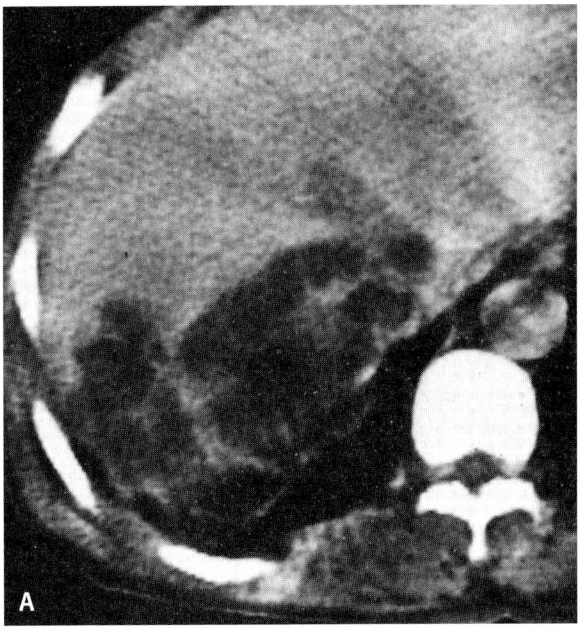

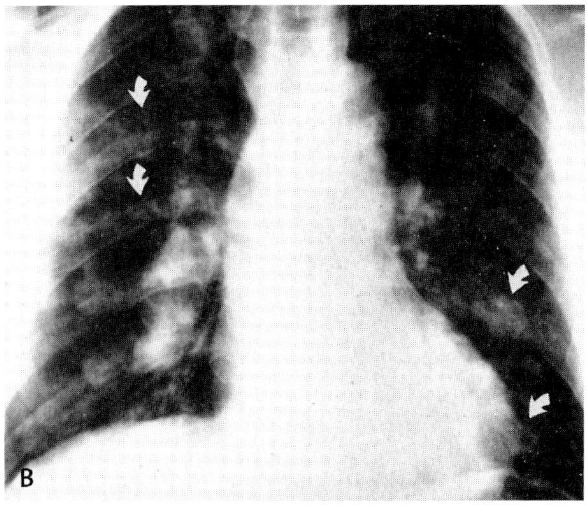

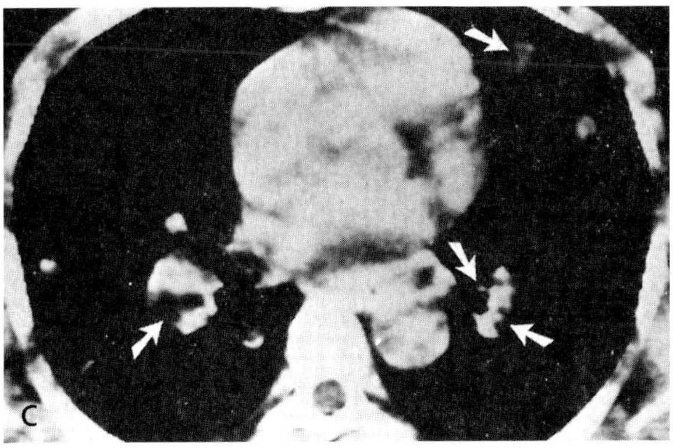

Fig. 3.104 A–C. A 46-year-old Saudi man with bilateral pulmonary "nodules" suggestive of metastatic disease, who had a large mass with cystic areas in the right lobe of the liver on ultrasonography and CT scan (**A**). Chest radiograph (**B**) showed bilateral nodules from 0.5 to several centimeters in diameter, thought to be metastases. The liver mass was wrongly though to be a cystic hepatocellular carcinoma. CT scan of the chest with soft tissue window settings (**C**) showed some of these lesions were air-filled and/or demonstrated "folding membranes" (*arrows*), suggesting the diagnosis of echinococcosis. Serological tests (indirect hemagglutinin – IHA) showed a highly elevated titer of 1:4096, confirming hydatid disease of liver and lungs. (Courtesy of Dr. Walther von Sinner and *Ann Saudi Med*, 1992)

◀ **Fig. 3.103 A–C.** Pulmonary hydatids masquerading as metastases in a 51-year-old Saudi man who had a 13-cm left renal mass with irregular density and a tiny calcification on contrast-enhanced CT scan (**A**). Fine-needle aspiration biopsy revealed a renal cell carcinoma. On preoperative chest radiography (**B**), two round bilateral densities were identified in the lower lobes and thought to be metastases, rendering the patient inoperable. CT scan of the chest (**C**), however, showed the lesions were cystic with a density of 10–20 HU. Serological examinations revealed very high echinococcal titers (IHA 1:2048; normal values up to 1:32), confirming hydatid disease in the lungs. (Courtesy of Dr. Walther von Sinner and *Ann Saudi Med*, 1992)

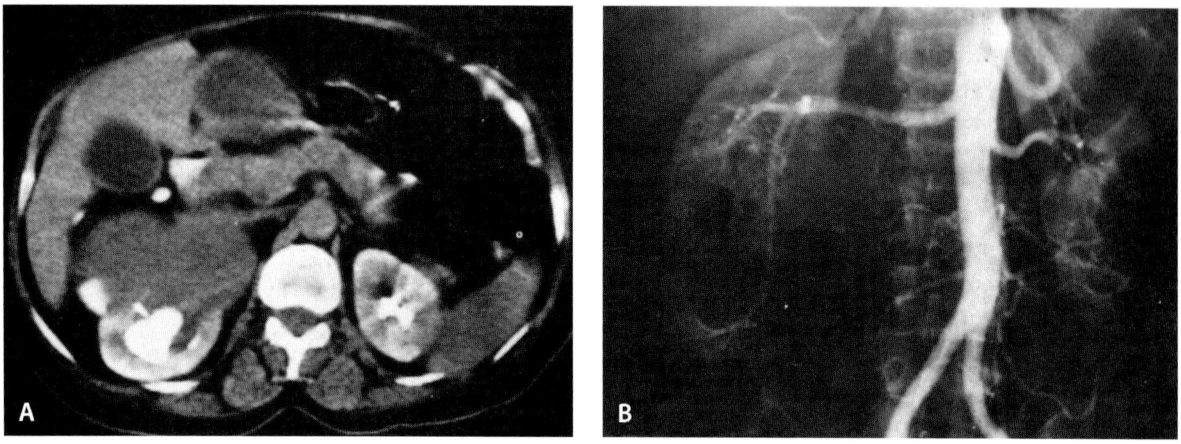

Fig. 3.105 A, B. A 51-year-old Saudi woman who presented with hypertension, angina, abdominal pain, and an enlarged liver. Abdominal radiographs showed hepatic calcifications. Hypoechoic lesions were seen in the left liver and right kidney on ultrasonography. Nonenhanced and contrast-enhanced CT scans (**A**) showed a 16-cm mass in the right kidney, presumably a cystic hypernephroma. Two other masses, thought to be cystic metastases, were seen in the left liver lobe and the cystic duct area with liver calcification. An abdominal angiogram (**B**) and selective renal arteriogram confirmed a hypovascular mass in the right kidney. At surgery, a right radical nephrectomy revealed a renal cell carcinoma, but hydatid cysts were found in the liver and cystic duct. A hydatid cystectomy with drainage of the hepatic cyst, which had ruptured into the left hepatic duct, was performed. A T-tube cholangiogram showed a communication between the cystic duct and the hydatid cyst, and microscopy confirmed the presence of scolices and daughter cysts. (Courtesy of Dr. Walther von Sinner and *Ann Saudi Med*, 1992)

Mediastinum

Primary hydatid disease of the mediastinum is rare, even in endemic areas. The incidence varies from less than 1% to about 4%. Conventional radiographic signs depend on the site, location, and stage of development of the disease, but uncomplicated hydatid cysts of the mediastinum usually cannot be differentiated from other cysts (e.g., bronchogenic or other duplication cysts or cystic tumors) on plain film radiography (Figs. 3.106, 3.107 A).

Computed tomography may be helpful in differentiating hydatid cysts from mediastinal tumors or other cysts because of differences in fluid densities due to degenerative changes, such as increased proteinaceous contents, inflammation, or bleeding. Apparent septation and rim or ring calcification are characteristic: daughter cysts and collapsed parasitic membranes are definitive findings (Figs. 3.107, 3.108 A). MRI can show all the characteristics of hydatid cysts to even better advantage (except for calcification, which is better seen on CT) and provides precise localization and relationships to neighboring structures or tissues (Fig. 3.108 B, C).

Heart

Primary cardiac hydatid disease is uncommon. It occurs in only 0.5%–2% of all human cases of echinococcosis. If undiagnosed, it is associated with an increased risk of severe or even lethal complications. Early diagnosis, using echocardiography, CT, or MRI, is crucial because surgical excision of hydatid cysts from the heart has low morbidity and mortality. If surgery is not possible for any reason, chemotherapy will usually improve the prognosis.

Primary involvement of the heart usually occurs via the coronary arteries. It has been estimated that it occurs (1) via the left coronary artery reaching the left ventricular wall in 70% of cases; (2) in the intraventricular septum in 7%; and (3) in the rest of the heart in 23%. Initially the cysts grow slowly between the cardiac fibers without causing symptoms or signs. However, after an asymptomatic period (which may last up to 5 or more years), major cardiac complications may develop, which are often fatal. These include rupture of a cyst into the pericardium or into the heart chambers, cardiac arrest, conduction disturbances including paroxysmal tachycardia and ventricular fibrillation or block, outflow tract obstruction, ischemic heart disease including angina and myocardial infarction, and aneurysm of the left ventricular wall with consequent thromboembolic disease.

Clinical complaints vary. After an asymptomatic period, patients may complain of precordial pain, dyspnea, palpitations, fever, severe abdominal pain, generalized itching, or a skin rash. Some patients present in cardiac failure, but in many this develops as the disease progresses.

There have been a number of reports of cardiac hydatid disease being recognized (often unexpectedly)

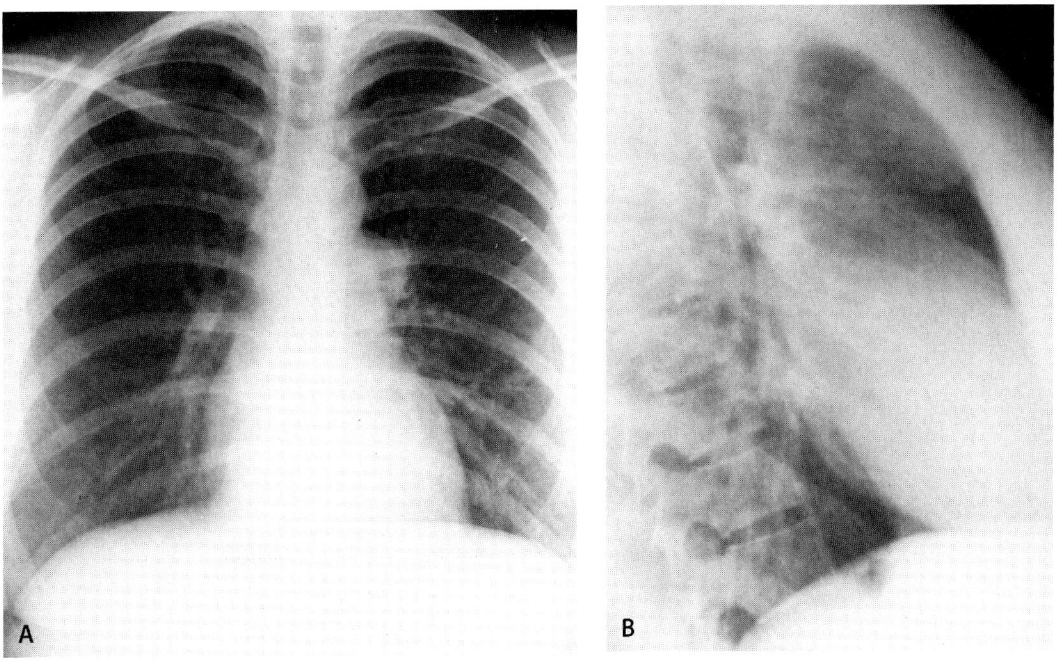

Fig. 3.106 A, B. A hydatid cyst within the mediastinum. This is an unusual site for a hydatid, especially when it occurs as a solitary lesion without other cysts in the lung parenchyma. In this Canadian Indian from northern Manitoba, there is a smooth, well-defined homogeneous mass overlying the left upper hilus on the PA chest film (A). On the lateral view (B) this mass is seen to lie in the anterior mediastinum. Its mediastinal location and etiology were proven at surgery. (Courtesy of Dr. Jack Tischler, Winnipeg)

on conventional chest radiographs (Fig. 3.109) because of calcification. Recognition will be enhanced with a very fast, high kV, grid technique because fine calcification will usually be blurred by the cardiac movement. The differential diagnosis will include pericardial calcification (e.g., tuberculosis or other infection) and cardiac aneurysms (see Chap. 25).

Echocardiography, especially transesophageal, is much more reliable in the diagnosis of cardiac hydatidosis, and both CT and MRI also provide further information. CT has the advantage of better resolution and better definition of anatomical details. Calcification, especially if small or discrete, is much better appreciated on CT than MRI (Figs. 3.110, 3.111). Extension of the disease can usually be well evaluated. MRI provides sophisticated differentiation between soft tissue structures such as the myocardium, endocardium, and pericardium (Figs. 3.110–3.115), but artifacts and signal dropout may limit MRI. Previous heart surgery such as valve replacement, pacemaker insertion or other metallic implants are contraindications for MRI. Nevertheless, in the absence of these limitations, it is the method of choice for multiple follow-up examinations to look for residual hydatidosis or early recurrence and to assess the effectiveness of long-term chemotherapy in inoperable patients.

Thoracic Wall

Hydatid cysts in the thoracic wall and soft tissues are uncommon (less than 1%). They are usually secondary, spreading from cysts in the lungs or bones of the thoracic cage. Superinfection, abscess formation, and fistulas may occur, but are not readily visualized in the early stages with conventional radiography alone. If there is strong clinical indication, CT or MRI will be helpful (Figs. 3.116, 3.117).

Breast

Hydatid disease of the breast is not common, but there are undoubtedly more than the approximately 55 cases so far reported. Many cysts are asymptomatic and have no specific local signs. They are found by the patient or physician accidentally as a smooth round mass in the breast. Neither clinically nor on mammography can an intact hydatid cyst in the breast be distinguished from any other benign cystic lesion. Several cases have been diagnosed cytologically after fine-needle aspiration of a cyst, a sometimes unexpected result.

(Text continues on p. 300)

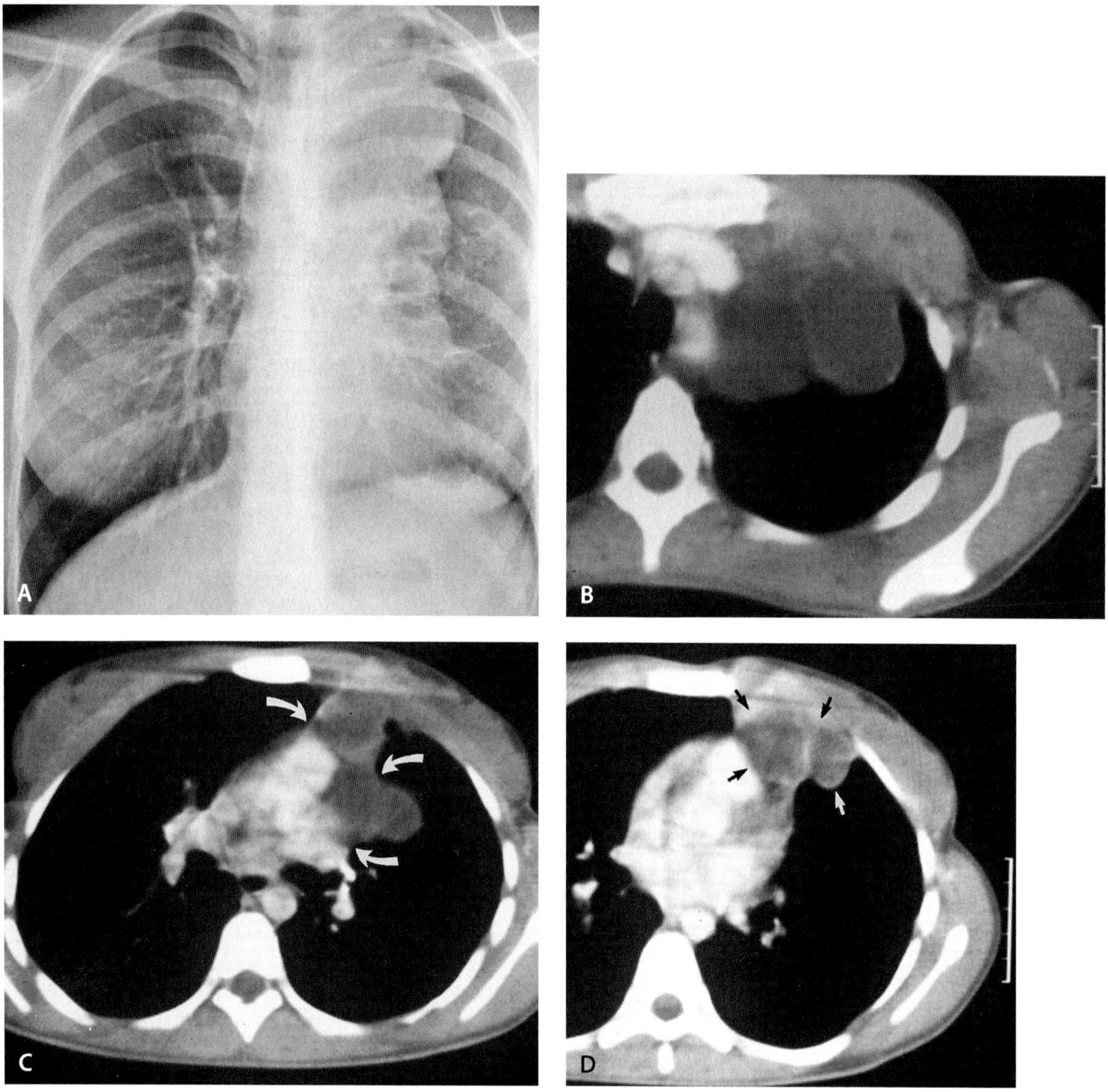

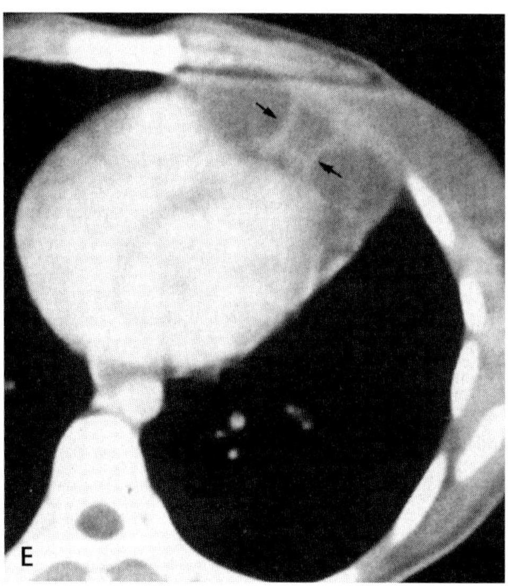

Fig. 3.107 A–E. A 17-year-old Saudi woman with an extensive hydatid cyst apparently originating in the lung and extending into the anterior mediastinum and pericardium. **A** Chest radiograph shows a huge lobulated left paramediastinal mass extending from the thoracic apex to the lower pericardial border. **B–E** Contrast-enhanced dynamic CT scans at various levels from superior to inferior in the chest show septated hydatid cysts (*arrows*) throughout the left anterior mediastinum from well above the aortic arch to the lower heart border. A cluster of hydatids (*arrows*) extend to the pericardium and compress the right and left ventricles (E). (Courtesy of Dr. Walther von Sinner)

Fig. 3.109 A, B. Large uncomplicated, univesicular type I hydatid cyst involving the pericardium and left ventricular wall of a 15-year-old Tunisian girl. **A** PA chest radiograph. **B** Chest CT scan. (Courtesy of Dr. Gharbi, Tunis)

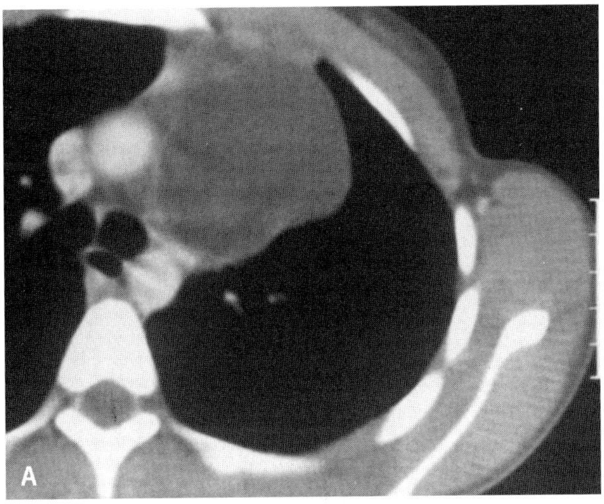

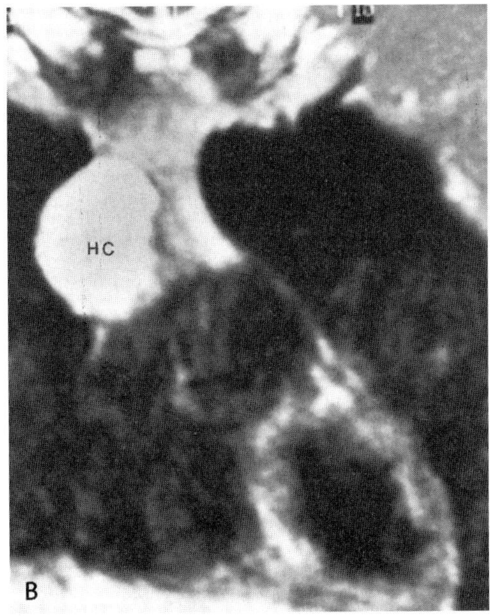

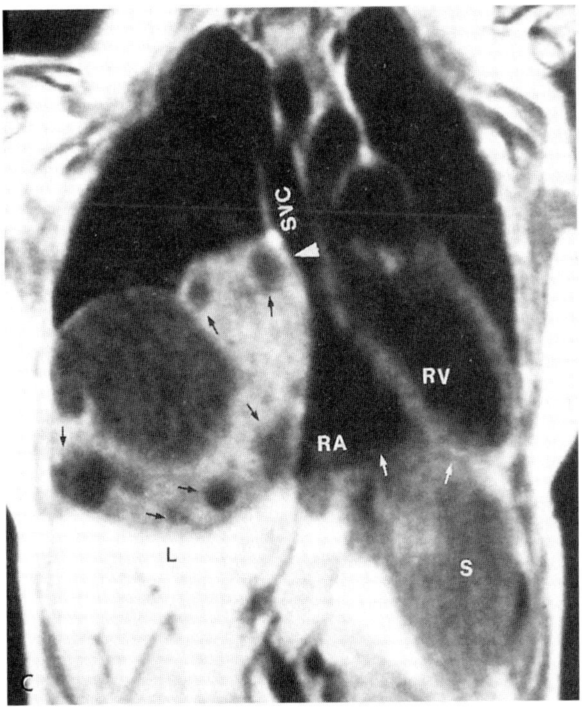

Fig. 3.108 A–C. Mediastinal hydatid cysts in three different Saudi Arabian patients. **A** Contrast-enhanced chest CT scan shows a large left anterior mediastinal hydatid at the level of the tracheal bifurcation along the left upper pericardial border. **B** A 15-year-old girl with a hydatid cyst arising primarily in the right upper anterior mediastinum and extending to the upper pericardium and superior vena cava. ECG-gated coronal MRI (1.5 T, SE 650/20 ms). *HC* hydatid cyst. **C** A 39-year-old woman with a large hydatid cyst arising from the dome of the liver (*L*) and containing multiple daughter cysts (*black arrows*). ECG-gated coronal MRI (0.5 T, SE 640/20 ms) shows extension of the cyst into the chest medially, compressing the right atrium (*RA*) and superior vena cava (*SVC*) (*arrowhead*) and displacing the heart to the left. There is also a second hydatid arising from the spleen (*S*) and involving the left hemidiaphragm at the inferior aspect of the right atrium (*RA*) and right ventricle (*RV*) (*white arrows*). (Courtesy of Dr. Walther von Sinner and *Eur Radiol*, 1995)

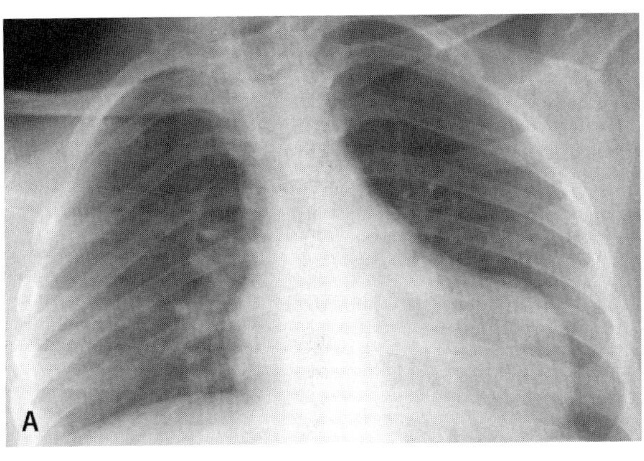

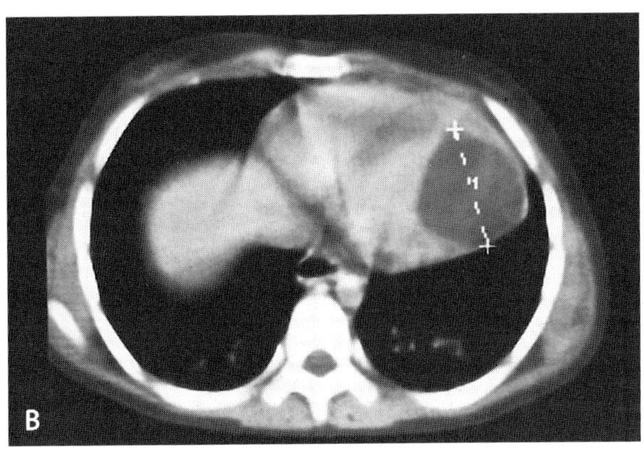

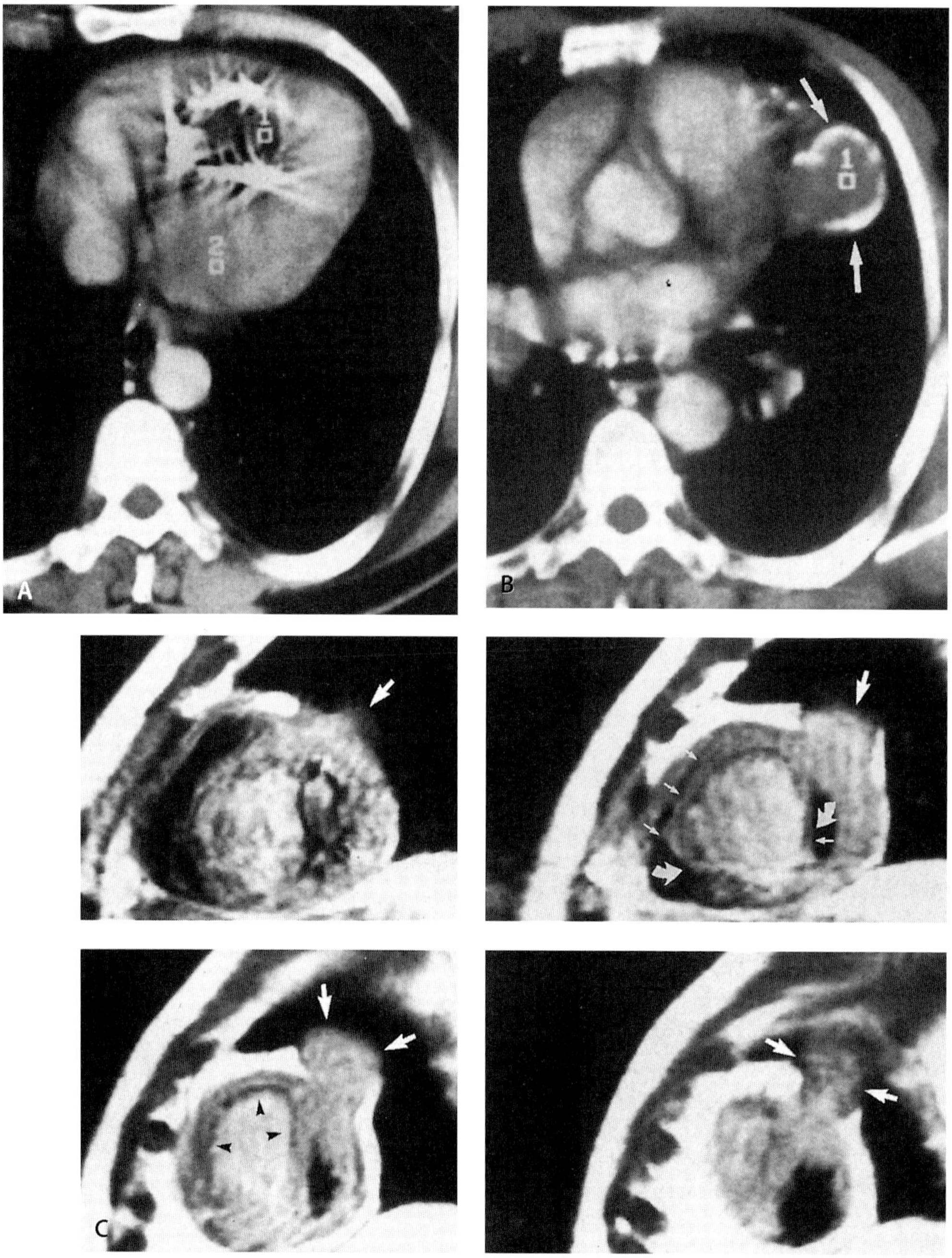

Fig. 3.110 A–C. A 52-year-old man with calcified hydatid cysts. **A** CT, showing "crushed eggshell" calcification projected over the left heart; its exact relationship to the heart chambers and septum is unclear. Calcifications (no. 1, 35 HU) are well seen. There is another suspected hydatid cyst (no. 2, 25 HU), with no evidence of calcification on this section and an indeterminate relationship with cardiac structures. The Hounsfield units (HU) identify these intracardiac masses as cysts with possible proteinaceous contents rather than solid masses (HU of water =0). **B** CT, on which a second hydatid cyst is now clearly visible (*arrows*), projecting from the left cardiac contour, with segmental ring calcification; the cyst is difficult to differentiate from the left ventricle or from a calcified aneurysm. **C** ECG-gated MRI, left anterior oblique section (SE 1800/50 ms), showing the expanded first hydatid cyst localised in the interventricular septum and surrounded by a low-density ring (calcified pericyst: *black arrowheads*) and the remaining thin layer of the interventricular septum (*small white arrows*), bulging into the right and left ventricles (*curved white arrows*). The second cyst is clearly seen in the upper part of the left ventricular wall and pericardium, interrupting the fat layer (*large white arrows*). Segmental calcification, however, is not visualized here (compare with **B**). (Courtesy of Dr. Walther von Sinner and *Eur Radiol*, 1995)

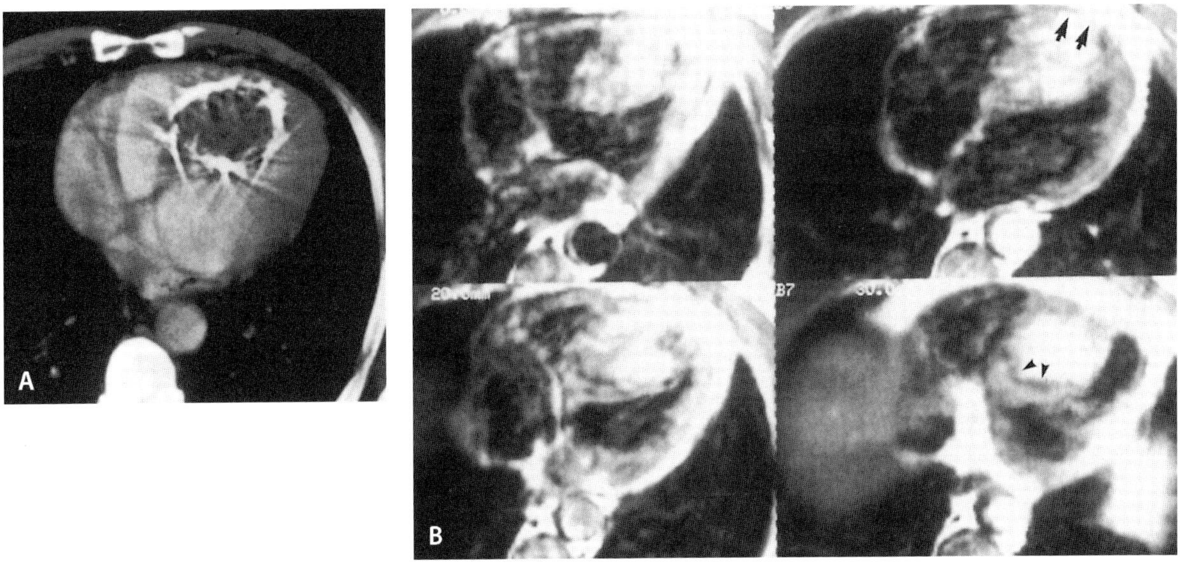

Fig. 3.111 A, B. Cardiac hydatid disease. **A** CT scan shows a calcified intracardiac cyst. **B** MR images (SE 1800/50) show low-intensity areas (*arrowheads*) probably corresponding to the calcifications seen on CT. The precise location of the cyst within the ventricular septum and its extension into the myocardium (*arrows*) are well demonstrated on MRI. (Courtesy of Dr. Walther von Sinner and *AJR*, 1991)

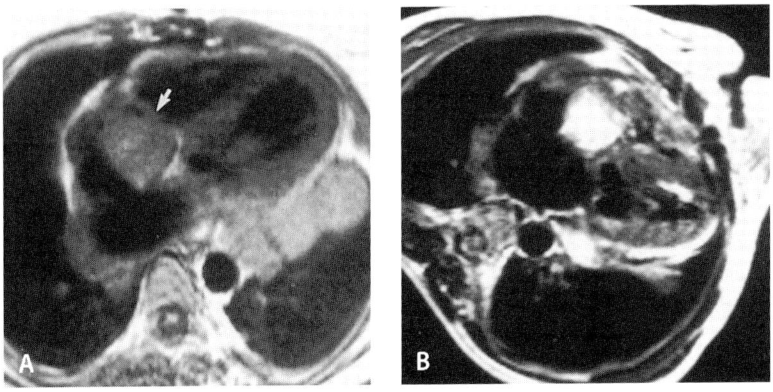

Fig. 3.112 A, B. Intracardiac hydatid cyst in a Saudi Arabian patient. **A** T1-weighted MR image (SE 750/30) shows a low-intensity mass in right atrium in close contact with tricuspid valve (*arrow*). **B** A second MR image (SE 1000/50) reveals a high-signal-intensity mass, suggesting the cystic nature of the lesion. (Courtesy of Dr. Walther von Sinner and *AJR*, 1991)

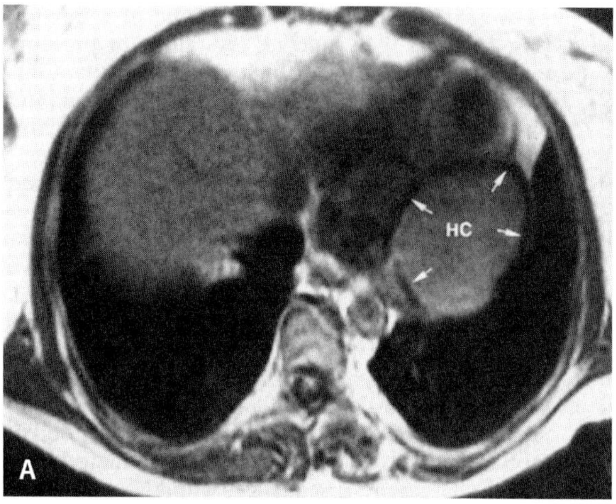

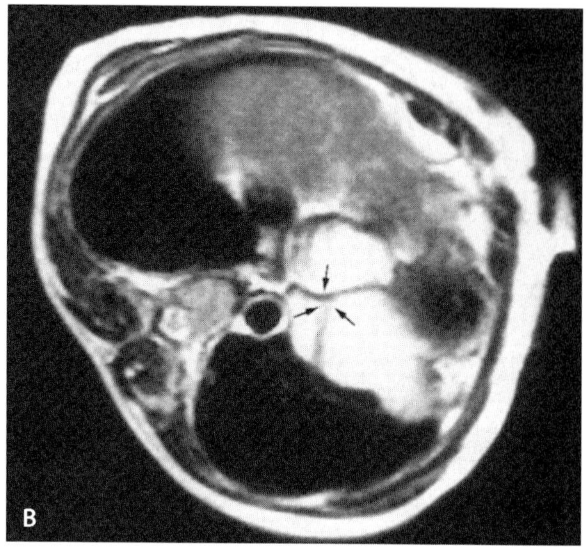

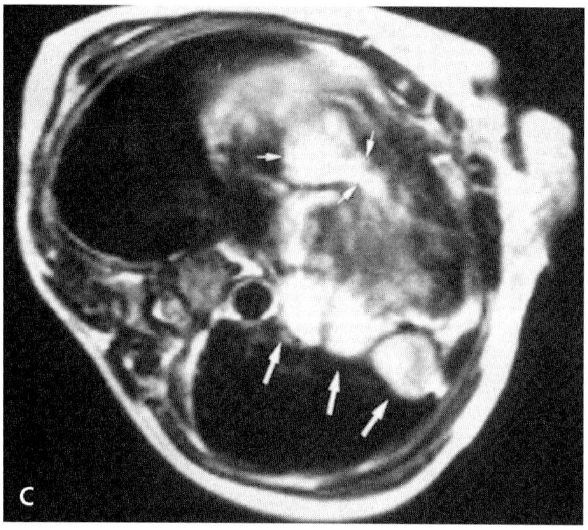

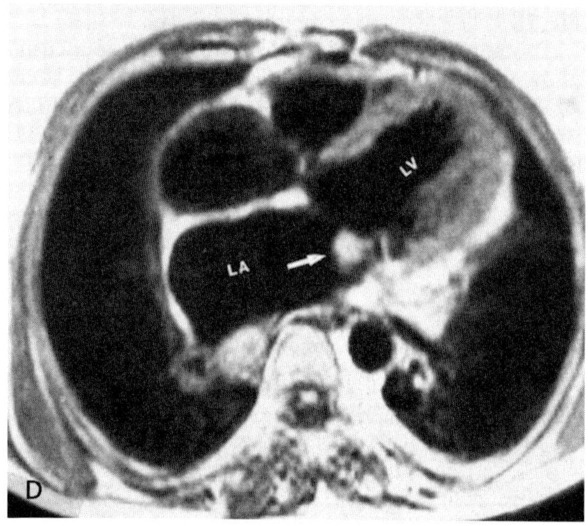

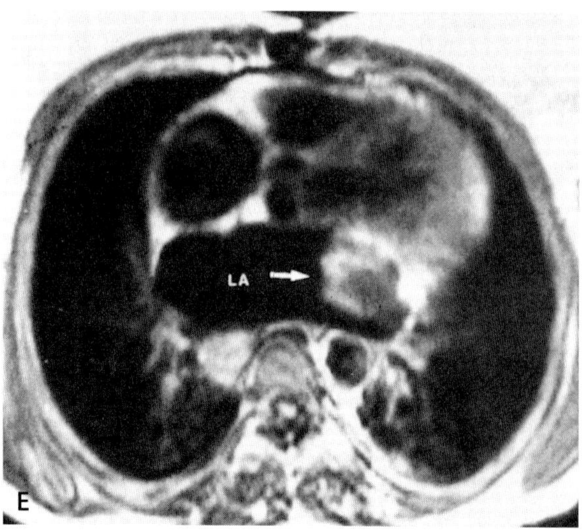

Fig. 3.113 A–E. A 30-year-old woman with hydatid cysts of the pericardium, left ventricle, and right atrium in close contact with the tricuspid valve, mitral valve, and left atrium. **A** ECG-gated MRI, transaxial view (0.5 T, SE 750/30 ms). Observe the large left pericardial "ringed" hydatid cyst (*HC*) consisting of homogeneous cyst contents surrounded by a low-intensity ring thought to be due to the ectocyst of the parasite and pericyst of the host (*arrows*). **B** ECG-gated MRI, transaxial view (0.5 T, SE 1000/150 ms), showing low-intensity partition of several cysts more clearly (*arrows*). **C** ECG-gated MRI, transaxial right anterior oblique view (0.5 T, SE 1000/50 ms), showing the heart in systole with the right atrial cyst demonstrating high signal intensity in close contact with the tricuspid valve protruding into the right ventricle (*small arrows*). Note also the pericardial and left ventricular wall extension of similar high-intensity cysts with low-intensity partition (*large arrows*). **D** ECG-gated MRI, transaxial view (0.5 T, SE 750/30 ms), showing a cystic mass close to the mitral valve (*arrow*). *LA* left atrium; *LV* left ventricle. **E** ECG-gated MRI, transaxial view (0.5 T, SE 750/30 ms), showing hydatid tissue protruding into the left atrium (*LA*) (*arrow*), mimicking a myxoma. (Courtesy of Dr. Walther von Sinner and *Eur Radiol*, 1995)

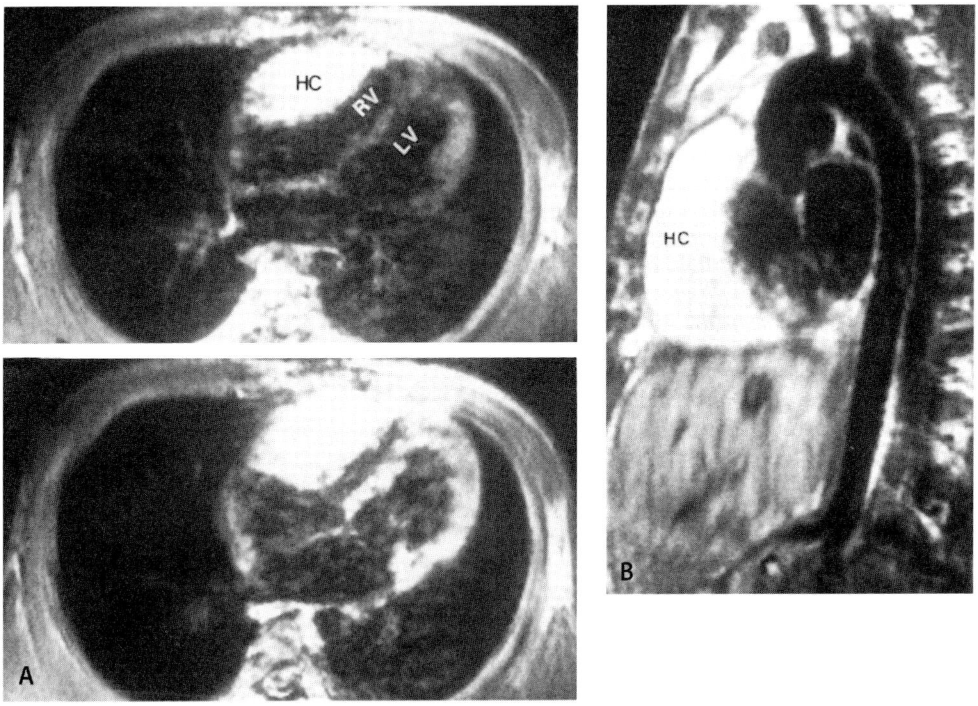

Fig. 3.114 A, B. A 20-year-old Saudi man with primary hydatid cyst (*HC*) of the pericardium and right ventricular wall. **A** ECG-gated MRI, transaxial view (1.5 T, SE 1523/20 ms), showing the hydatid cyst bulging into the right ventricular cavity (*RV*). *LV* left ventricle. **B** ECG-gated MRI, sagittal view (1.5 T, SE 1374/20 ms), showing the anterior, high signal intensity hydatid cyst to good advantage. (Courtesy of Dr. Walther von Sinner and *Eur Radiol*, 1995)

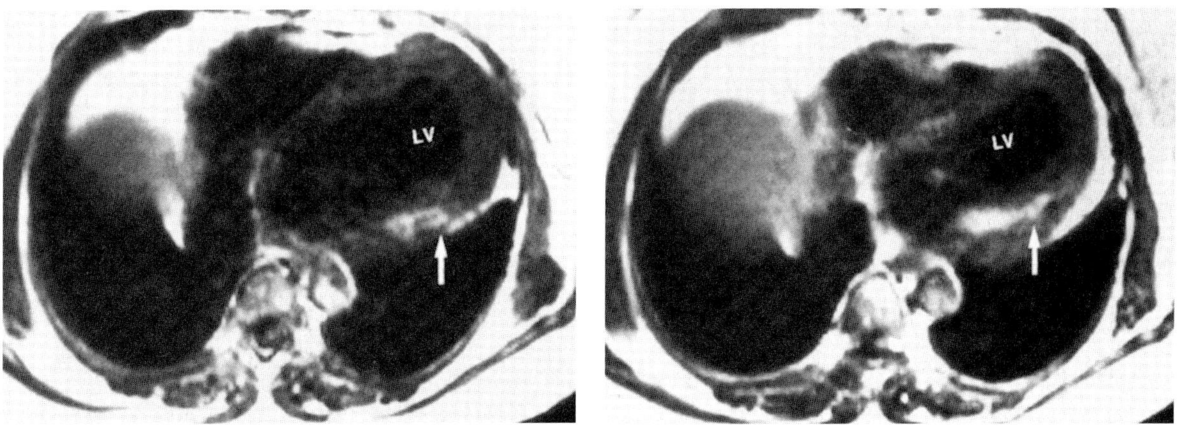

Fig. 3.115. A 49-year-old Saudi man with hydatid cyst after previous rupture of a pericardial hydatid into the pericardium, with bulging left ventricle (*LV*) after a myocardial infarction due to aneurysm with thrombotic masses. ECG-gated MRI, transaxial view (1.5 T, SE 600/20 ms), shows residual of ruptured hydatid cyst (*arrow*). (Courtesy of Dr. Walther von Sinner and *Eur Radiol*, 1995)

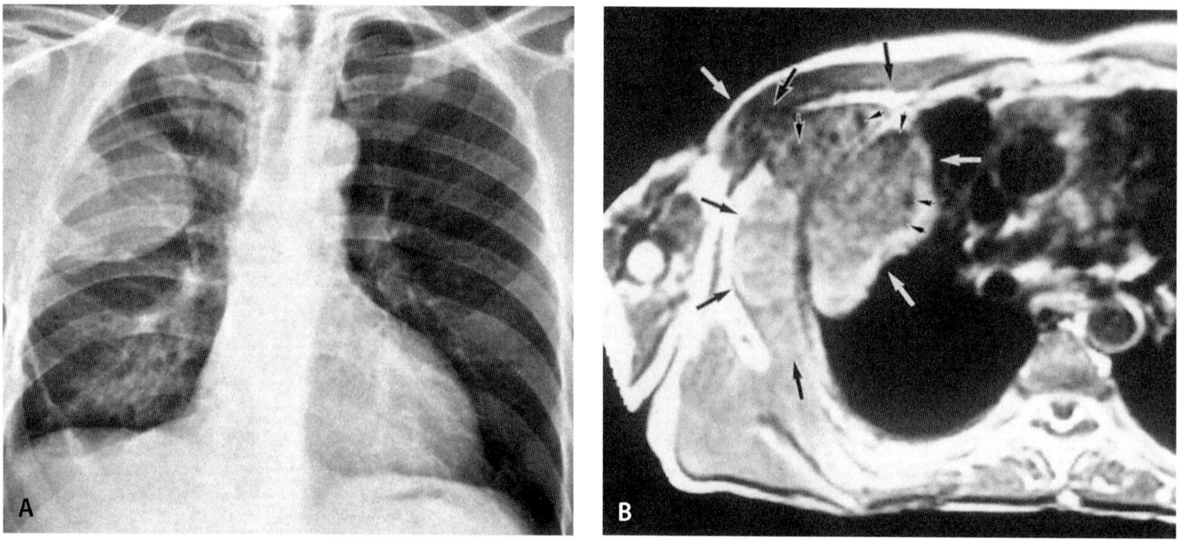

Fig. 3.116 A, B. A 66-year-old Saudi man with recurrent hydatid cyst after thoracentesis. **A** Chest radiograph shows recurrent lateral mass contiguous with pleura secondary to previous thoracentesis and removal of huge hydatid cyst several years earlier. **B** MRI (1.5 T, SE 850/20) axial view obtained at the same time as **A** reveals a cystic mass with subcutaneous extension (*large arrows*) containing multiple daughter cysts (*small arrows*). (Courtesy of Dr. Walther von Sinner and *Eur Radiol*, 1993)

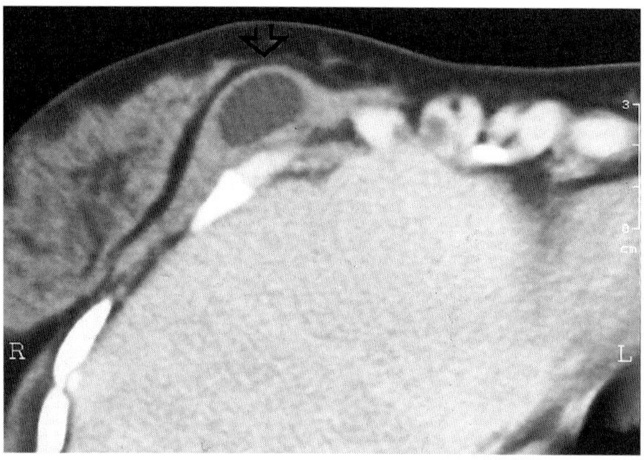

Fig. 3.117. CT scan showing a univesicular type I hydatid cyst (*arrow*) involving the thoracic wall musculature of a 28-year-old Tunisian woman. (Courtesy of Dr. Gharbi, Tunis)

The shell-like calcification of a hydatid cyst may mimic a fibroadenoma in the breast. If there are daughter cysts, hydatid sand, or collapsed membranes, the diagnosis can be made by mammography or ultrasonography (and also by CT and MRI). When the cyst is complex or multilocular with internal sonographic echoes due to debris, it is difficult to exclude added infection.

Brain

Intracerebral hydatids constitute 1%–4% of all cases of echinococcosis. The cyst is usually primary, developing from a larva carried to the brain via the arterial circulation, and is more often supratentorial than infratentorial in location. A cerebral cyst is generally smaller than a hydatid elsewhere in the body and becomes clinically manifest much earlier in life because symptoms of increased intracranial pressure from a space-occupying lesion occur relatively early in the disease. Thus, children with an average age of 10 years are the most commonly affected with a primary brain hydatid (Fig. 3.6 B). Secondary or metastatic cerebral hydatidosis, however, is seen in an older age group, usually middle-aged adults, similar to the manifestations of the disease in other organs; these metastatic hydatids may result from rupture of a primary cyst within the heart. Implantation of one or more embryos bypassing the liver and lungs is regarded as extremely rare, if not impossible with a normal circulation.
Most cerebral hydatids are in the white matter, usually in the parietal lobe (Fig. 3.118). They are most often solitary, and grow outward toward the cerebral cortex or inward toward the ventricles. Multiple intracranial hydatid cysts are rare and are usually caused by rupture of a single cerebral cyst (after trauma, surgery, or spontaneously) or they may be secondary implants from a ruptured primary extracranial cyst.

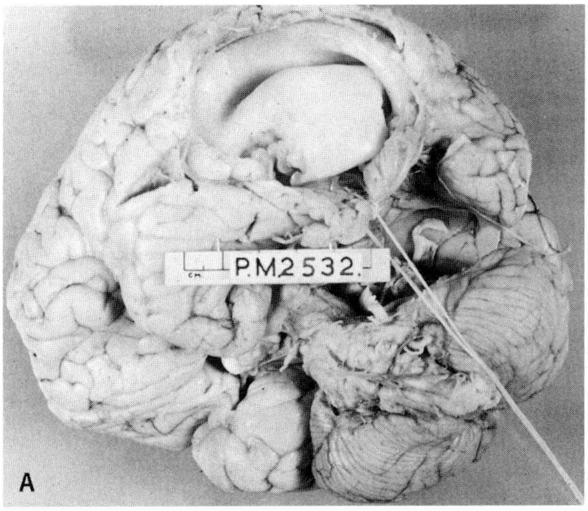

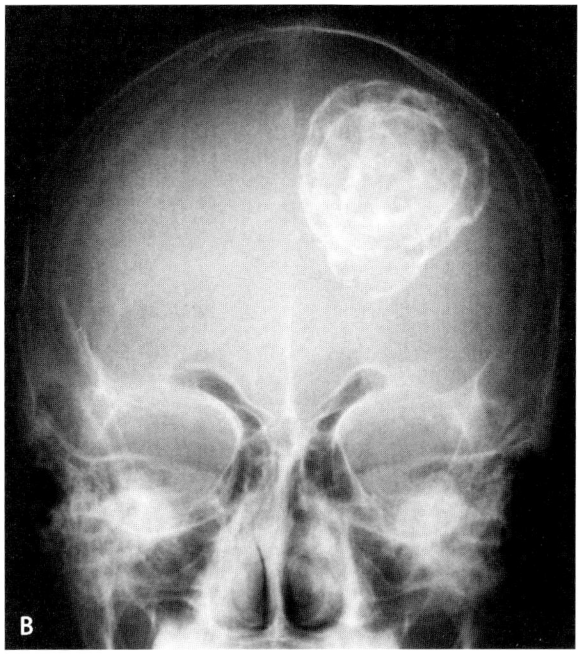

Fig. 3.118 A, B. Hydatid cyst of the brain. **A** Necropsy specimen from an Indian patient with large hydatid cyst in the parietal region of the brain. (Courtesy of Dr. A. Chandrahasan Johnson) **B** Large, calcified hydatid cyst of the left cerebral hemisphere in a 20-year-old man. (Courtesy of Dr. William Thomas, McLean)

Cerebral hydatid cysts can grow rapidly, but the prognosis is better than would be expected, except in very young children. Symptoms such as epilepsy or blindness may occur, depending on the location of the cyst. Calcification of the cyst may occasionally be seen on plain radiographs of the skull (Figs. 3.118 B and 3.119), but there is seldom any definitive clue on conventional radiography to identify the cyst if no calcification is visible.

Where CT and MRI are available, angiography is indicated only when surgery is considered and the details of the cerebral vascular supply are required. If scanning is not available, cerebral angiography will show a smooth, well-defined, avascular "tumor" (Figs. 3.119–3.121). There is seldom any surrounding vascular blush. If seen, this should suggest infection or leakage of the cyst contents.

On CT scanning there is often a large solitary spherical cyst, with a regular smooth border and a cyst content of fluid or water density similar to cerebrospinal fluid (CSF) (Figs. 3.122, 3.123 A). Calcification may be seen on nonenhanced CT, even if it is minimal. There is usually no rim enhancement or perifocal edema. With contrast, occasional lesions may show ring enhancement, suggesting inflammation. Infection (including tuberculosis) or abscess will have to be excluded, which can be difficult. Multiple cerebral hydatid cysts show the same characteristics, and are often quite different in size.

The differential diagnosis of an uncomplicated cerebral hydatid includes porencephalic cyst, arachnoid cyst, and cystic tumors. Arachnoid cysts are, however, not spherical and porencephalic cysts usually communicate with the lateral ventricles; a closed porencephalic cyst may present a differential problem on CT scanning. The CT density of cystic tumors differs from that of CSF, unlike hydatid cysts.

Magnetic resonance imaging studies of intracerebral cysts show a low signal intensity of the cyst wall, as found in liver and other hydatids. MRI is also more sensitive than CT in detecting perifocal edema. If present, a high-intensity halo or rim around the cyst on T1-weighted images (the rim is hypointense on T2-weighted images), with cystic contents on T1- and T2-weighted images similar to CSF (Fig. 3.123), constitutes a very significant combination for the diagnosis of cerebral hydatid disease.

Ventriculography is very rarely practiced today and seldom provides exact diagnostic information for hydatid disease. The cyst will show as a smooth space-occupying lesion, often causing quite marked ventricular displacement and, sometimes, hydrocephalus. Prior to 1975, pneumoencephalography would demonstrate similar findings.

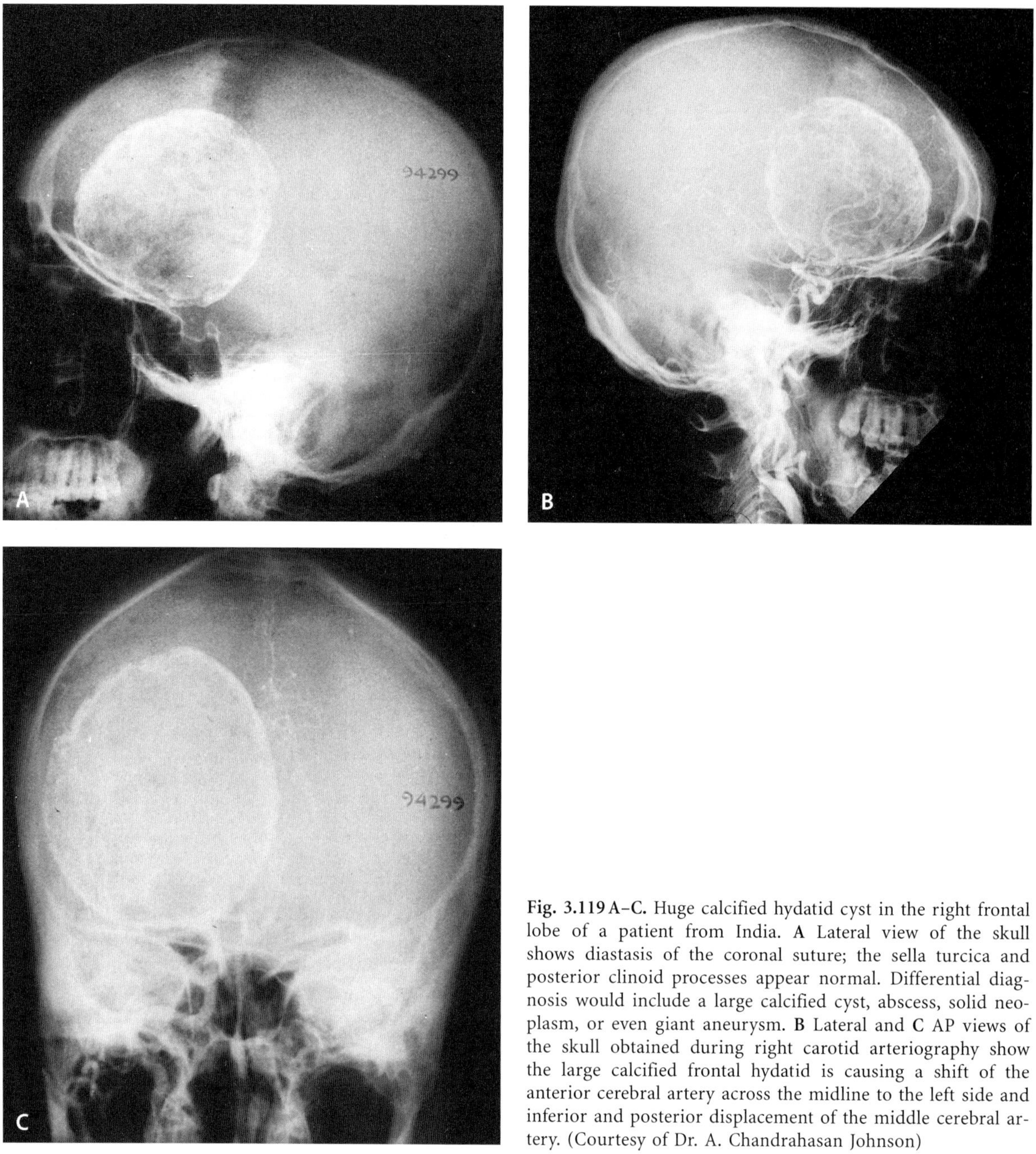

Fig. 3.119 A–C. Huge calcified hydatid cyst in the right frontal lobe of a patient from India. A Lateral view of the skull shows diastasis of the coronal suture; the sella turcica and posterior clinoid processes appear normal. Differential diagnosis would include a large calcified cyst, abscess, solid neoplasm, or even giant aneurysm. B Lateral and C AP views of the skull obtained during right carotid arteriography show the large calcified frontal hydatid is causing a shift of the anterior cerebral artery across the midline to the left side and inferior and posterior displacement of the middle cerebral artery. (Courtesy of Dr. A. Chandrahasan Johnson)

Skull and Facial Bones

Within the bones of the cranial vault, orbit, and mandible the pattern followed by osteohydatid disease is that described in the following section on the skeletal system. Any cystic or blowout expansile lesion of the cranial bones (Fig. 3.124), a unilateral tumor within the orbit, or a large expansile cyst within the mandible should cause consideration of hydatid disease in a patient from an endemic area. Cranial hydatids appear to be more common in the parietal and occipital regions of the skull.

Orbital Hydatid Disease. Orbital hydatid disease is not common, even in endemic areas. A preoperative diagnosis is important to avoid intraoperative cyst rupture resulting in dissemination. There is a preponderance of cases in children and young adults, typically causing painless unilateral proptosis in the superior quadrants. The extent of displacement of

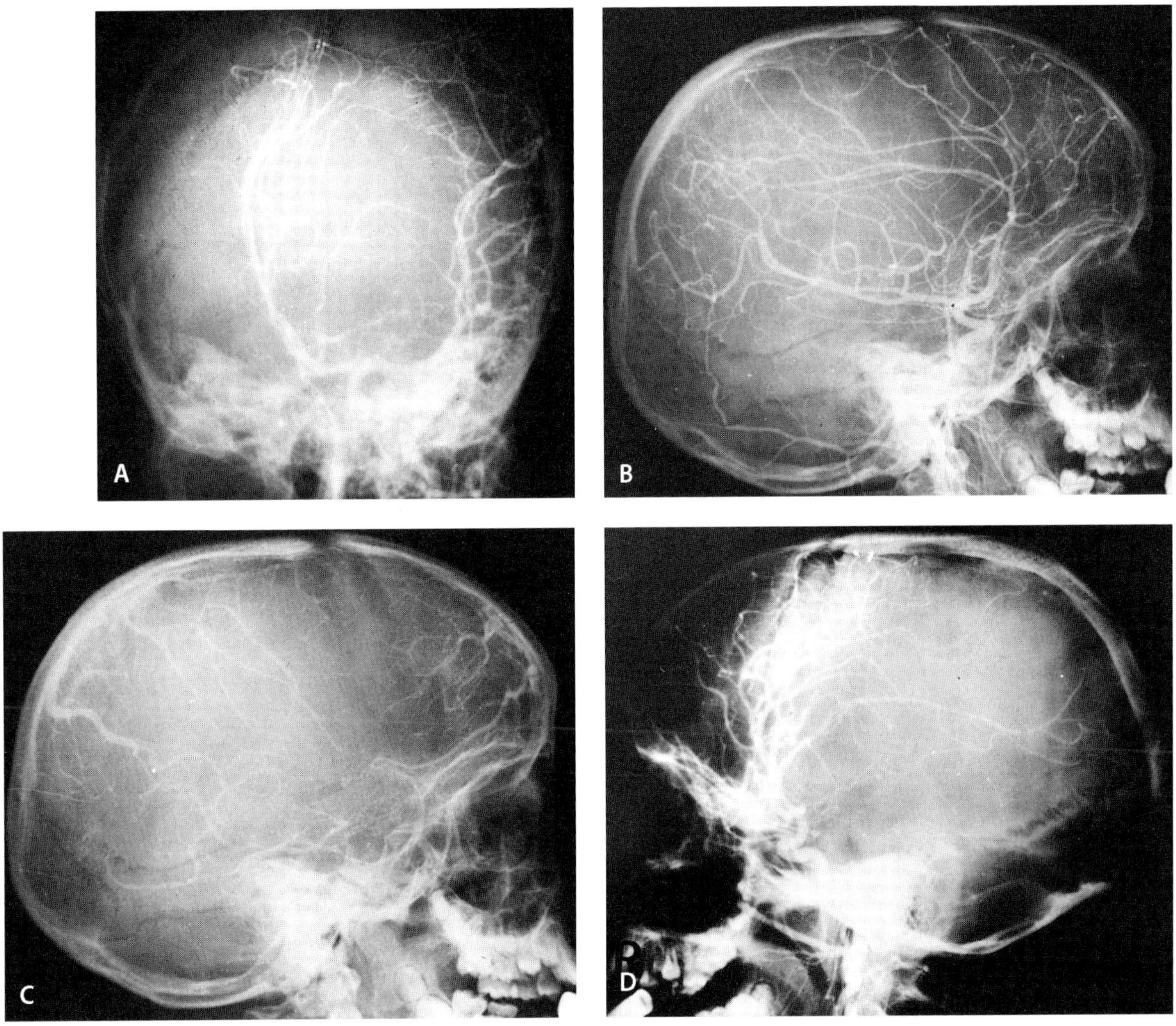

Fig. 3.120 A–D. Internal carotid arteriograms in two different patients with large hydatid cysts of the brain. In the first patient (A–C), there is a large non-calcified left frontoparietal hydatid which has caused diastasis of the cranial sutures, especially the coronal sutures. **A** AP and **B** left lateral views of the skull obtained during left carotid arteriography show marked shift of the anterior cerebral artery across the midline towards the right side as well as inferior displacement of the middle cerebral artery. No neovascularity is identified. **C** Lateral view of the skull of the same patient during the venous phase of the arteriogram shows the vein of Trolard is angulated and displaced posteriorly. **D** Lateral view of the skull obtained during carotid arteriography in another patient, a South African child with a huge temporal fossa hydatid cyst. The large mass extends into the parietal-occipital region with draping, stretching, and elevation of the middle cerebral artery. The anterior cerebral artery is also somewhat stretched, suggesting moderate hydrocephalus. There is slight diastasis of the coronal and lambdoidal sutures. (**D** courtesy of the University of Capetown Radiology Library)

the eye and degree of visual impairment varies. A solitary inferolateral lesion with palpable lower lid mass can occasionally occur.

Computed tomography in orbital hydatidosis shows unilateral, hypointense, nonenhancing cysts in 70% of patients. However, hyperintense cysts, probably caused by increased protein levels in the cystic contents, may also occur (30%); this makes them easily confused with "soft tissue tumors." In children in the tropics, Burkitt's lymphoma would have to be excluded. Occasionally, the cysts may be multifocal. Bony erosion of the orbital roof or floor and destruction of the lamina papyracea and bony displacement may occur as the cysts enlarge (Fig. 3.125).

As in hydatid cysts elsewhere, fine peripheral rim enhancement has been noted after contrast injection, especially if there are superimposed inflammatory changes.

(Text continues on p. 306)

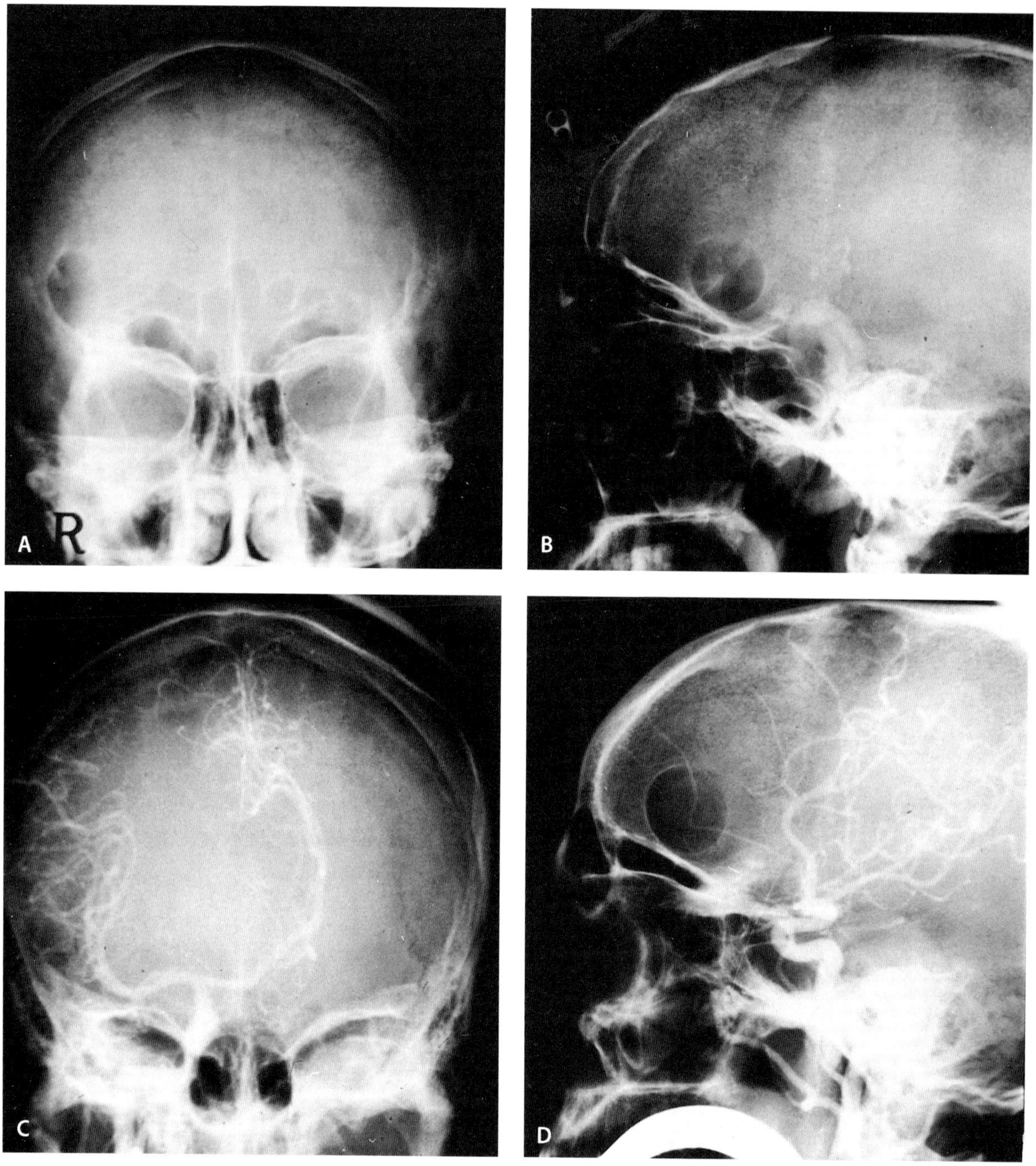

Fig. 3.121. A, B PA and lateral views of the skull of a South African patient show a well-defined rim of sclerosis about a small, round, lytic hydatid lesion involving the right frontal bone. C, D AP and lateral views from a right internal carotid arteriogram reveal marked displacement of the anterior cerebral artery across the midline on the AP view as well as posterior displacement on the lateral projection secondary to a right frontal cerebral hydatid cyst. (Courtesy of the University of Capetown Radiology Library)

Fig. 3.123 A–F. An 11-year-old Saudi Arabian boy admitted for suspected brain tumor. Medical imaging revealed a huge, simple unilocular type I hydatid cyst of the brain. A Axial CT scan of right parietal spherical hydatid, showing displacement of the ventricular system to the left. B MRI T1-weighted (spin echo, 950/20) axial image and C coronal image (600/20) show that the signal intensity of cyst contents is identical to that of CSF. D MRI T2-weighted (spin echo, 2000/80) coronal image and E (spin echo, 2000/40) axial image of the right parietal cyst reveal a peripheral rim of low signal intensity. F Intraoperative photograph of typical pearly white brain hydatid. (Courtesy of Drs. S. Coates, Walther von Sinner et al. and *AJNR*, 1990)

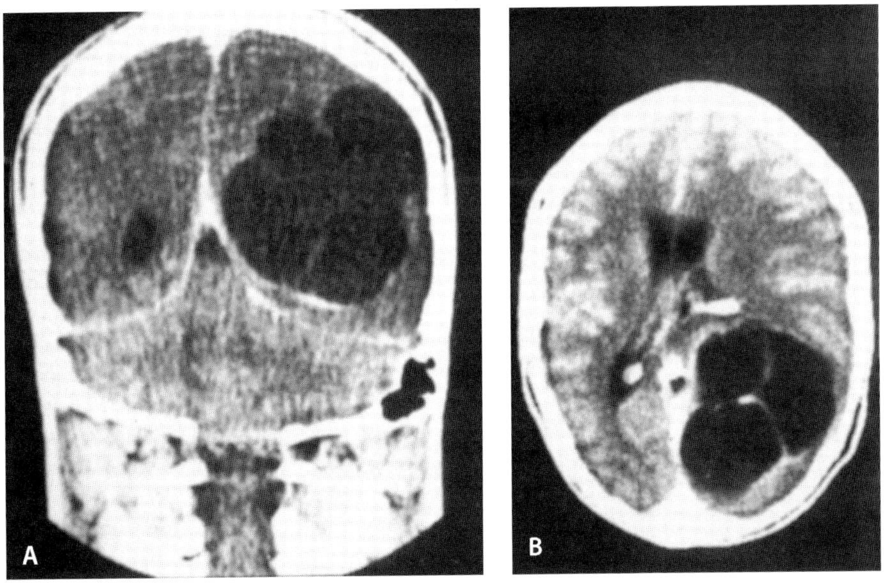

Fig. 3.122. Large left parietal hydatid cyst as seen on **A** coronal and **B** axial views of a CT scan. The cyst appears multilobulated and septated due to the presence of daughter cysts. The cyst contents have the same fluid density as the CSF. There is displacement of the falx and the ventricular system across the midline to the right with marked compression and displacement of the posterior horn of the left lateral ventricle

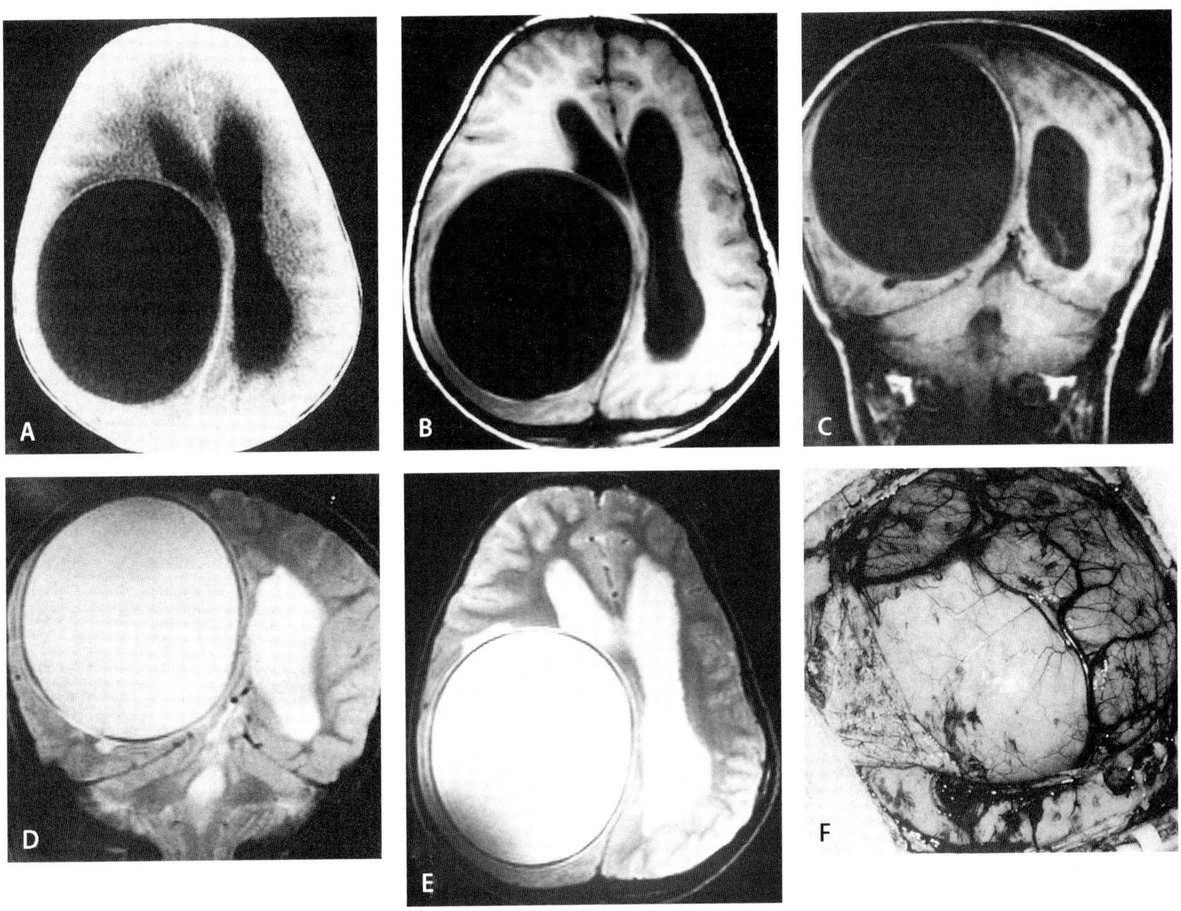

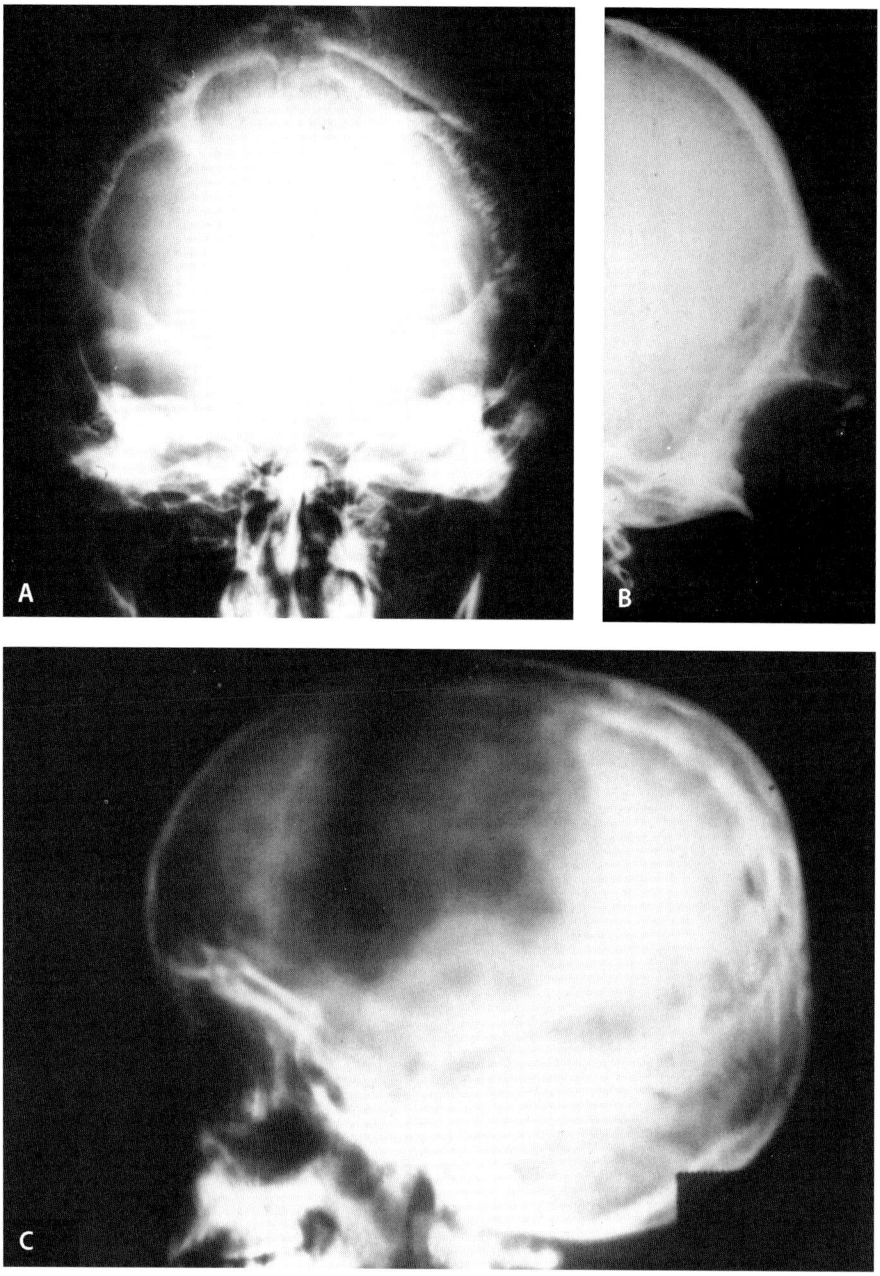

Fig. 3.124 A–C. Hydatid cyst of the skull in three different patients. A Grossly expansile blowout lesion of the cranial vault seen on AP view of the skull. B Blowout, expansile, destructive lesion of the occiput caused by a large hydatid cyst in another patient. C Large lytic lesion of the posterior frontal portion of the calvarium of a young child seen on lateral view

Musculoskeletal System

Bone

Hydatid disease in bone is uncommon. The world literature indicates an average incidence of 1.5% in bone. Sixty percent of all osteohydatid disease occurs in the spine, pelvis, and hip joint. Another 28% of cases are found in long bones (femur, tibia, and humerus) and 8% in the ribs and scapula. Isolated infections occur in the calvaria and phalanges. Hydatid cysts within bone are always primary, with the larva reaching the skeletal site via a systemic artery. Occasionally, there may be associated cysts in other organs, chiefly liver or lung.

The larval hydatid develops very slowly within the medullary portion of bone and almost always mani-

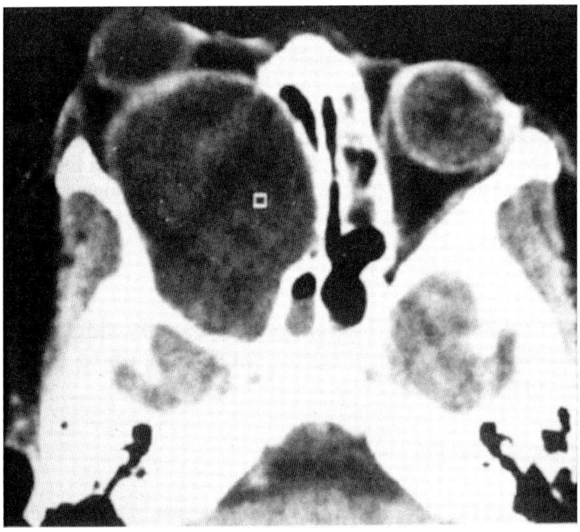

Fig. 3.125. Large hydatid cyst involving the right orbit with proptosis of the eye and compression erosion of adjacent bony structures and right ethmoid sinus

fests itself in adults rather than in children. In bone, because of the resistance of osseous tissue, the parasite is unable to follow its usual mode of development. There is a minimal response on the part of the bony tissues, and no adventitial wall forms as in other parts of the body. Instead of the single large cyst seen in other host tissues, microvesicles are produced by exogenous budding and spread throughout the spongiosa of the involved bone to create a lesion which initially molds itself to the rigid bony confines. The hydatid then develops multiple exogenous daughter cysts in the absence of any adventitial pericyst, and these insinuate themselves between the bony trabeculae, destroying them. The end result is extensive destruction of the medullary bone by a multivesicular cyst.

After destroying considerable cancellous bone and forming numerous daughter cysts, the hydatid may breach the cortex and periosteum and penetrate into adjacent soft tissues. An adventitial layer may form in the periosteum and soft tissues to surround the daughter cysts and produce a confluent multilocular cyst. The bony hydatid may penetrate through the articular cartilage of the epiphysis to invade the joint and cross the joint space to involve the opposite bone. Advanced destruction and pathological fractures almost invariably ensue.

Because the course of osseous hydatid disease is usually lengthy, symptoms may appear quite late. The clinical picture is vague, with pain occurring late in the disease; pain is usually secondary to a pathological fracture or follows rupture of the hydatid through the cortex and development of a soft tissue abscess and osteomyelitis. In the spine it is a serious condition, with a high incidence of neurological involvement and paraplegia and a relatively high mortality. Local recurrences are common at most skeletal sites because of the difficulty of eradicating the disease.

As in the case of clinical symptoms, there is a similar absence of radiological findings over a long period. According to the work of Bellini, there are three main stages in the development of radiographic findings. The first stage is *microvesicular infiltration*, in which the larvae are deposited in bone and cause destruction by mechanical pressure. As the vesicles or daughter cysts grow and enlarge, cyst-like spaces develop which are lined by thin trabeculae and produce a multilocular appearance resembling a "bunch of grapes." At this stage, there is no sharp demarcation of the lesion and no new bone formation or periosteal reaction. In the second stage, which occurs late in the disease, a *secondary infection* is engrafted on the hydatid process and produces an inflammatory osteitis. The prolonged irritation results in the development of sclerosis and hyperostosis in the involved bone, which gradually replaces the pre-existing mutilocular appearance. The third stage relates to the formation of the *ossifluent abscess* which occurs after the hydatid penetrates the cortex and breaks out with exuberant growth into adjacent soft tissues. The cysts that develop in the soft tissues are spherical, may reach several inches in size, and may subsequently calcify. Soft tissue hydatids may be identified by plain radiographs, especially if calcified (Fig. 3.126), but are better evaluated by ultrasonography, CT or MRI (Fig. 3.127). They may also cause complications by compression of neighboring structures such as ureters, resulting in obstruction; there may be overgrowth of the cyst to other organs and perforation into the spinal canal or veins, leading to dissemination. Additional stages and findings in musculoskeletal hydatid disease have been described in the past decade by von Sinner.

On conventional radiographs, early lesions in long bones appear as ill-defined, thin-walled areas of radiolucency which develop near the epiphyseal end of the bone and produce a multiloculated appearance. There is no sharp demarcation between these lesions and the surrounding normal bone. Later, well-defined cystic areas appear, which are circular or oval in the long axis of the bone: the margins now appear sharp and there is often surrounding bony sclerosis (Figs. 3.128, 3.129). Extension and coalescence of the cystic areas cause widening of the bone and thinning of the cortex and, in some patients, eventual spread of the hydatid process throughout the entire length of the bone (Figs. 3.129, 3.130). The overall loss in bone structure now resembles a large communicating cyst with a lattice-like trabecular pattern.

(Text continues on p. 310)

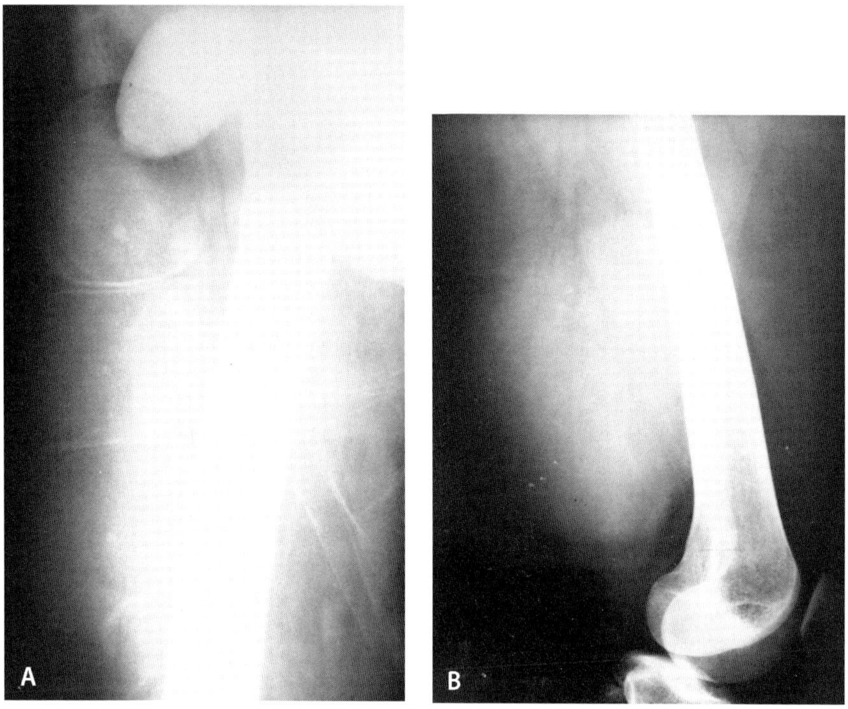

Fig. 3.126 A, B. Hydatid disease involving the soft tissues of the thigh in two different South African patients. A Multiple large, partially calcified, spherical cysts in the upper thigh of a 20-year-old man. B A huge noncalcified hydatid in the soft tissues of the midthigh, posterior to the femur in a young woman. Neither patient had any other demonstrable hydatid cysts. (Courtesy of the University of Capetown Radiology Library)

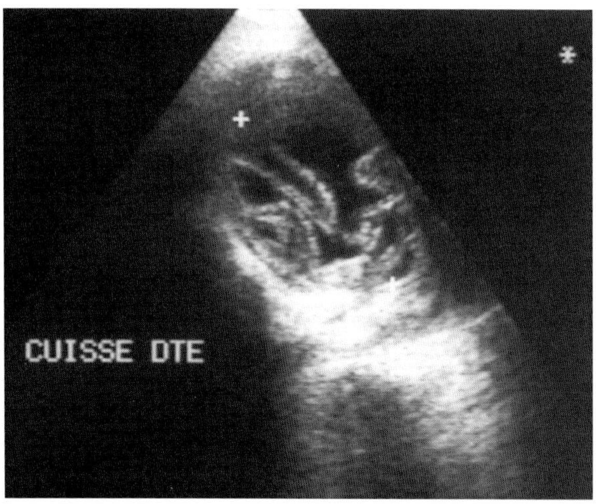

Fig. 3.127. Ultrasound scan of a 7-year-old Tunisian boy, showing a soft tissue hydatid cyst of the thigh muscles with detached parasitic membranes identified by the serpent sign. (Courtesy of Dr. Gharbi, Tunis)

Fig. 3.129 A–C. Hydatid disease of the tibia in two different patients. A There is extensive multilocular destruction of virtually the entire tibia. The extension and coalescence of multiple cystic areas has caused widening of the medullary cavity of the diaphysis and thinning of the cortex, especially along its medial aspect. The overall loss in bone structure resembles a large communicating cyst with a lattice-like network of residual bone; virtually all the fine trabeculae in the cancellous bone have been destroyed. There is some reactive sclerosis, but the bone is very soft and weak at this stage and pathological fractures are common. B AP and C lateral views of the lower leg of another patient show an extensive cystic lesion involving the midshaft of the tibia. There is some loculation, thinning, and erosion of the cortex medially and anteriorly. When there is such extensive destruction of cancellous bone and thinning of the cortex, pathological fractures commonly occur. This patient was a 49-year-old woman with complaints of intermittent pain and swelling of the right leg of 2 years' duration. (Courtesy of Dr. W. F. Hutchison et al. and *JAMA*, 1962) ▶

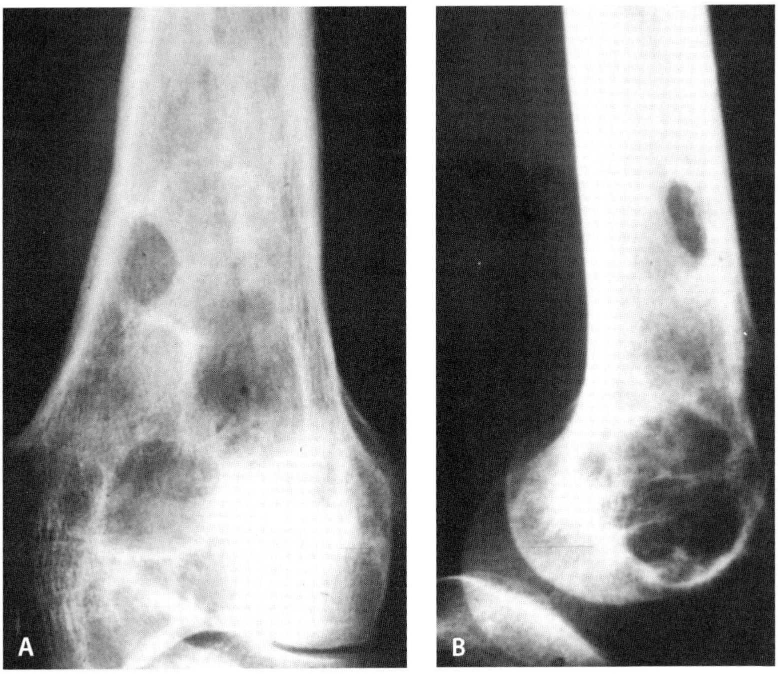

Fig. 3.128 A, B. Hydatid disease of the distal femur. **A** AP and **B** lateral views of the femur show well-defined cystic areas that are circular or oval in the long axis of the bone. The margins are sharp and there is moderate surrounding sclerosis, giving a multilocular cystic appearance to the femur. The cortex is slightly thinned in the diametaphyseal area and there is slight periosteal reaction along its lateral aspect, suggesting the presence of secondary infection, because hydatid disease alone does not cause periostitis. As in most cases of hydatid disease of long bones, this lesion began as thin-walled areas of radiolucency near the epiphysis and spread to involve the diametaphysis and shaft well into the midfemur

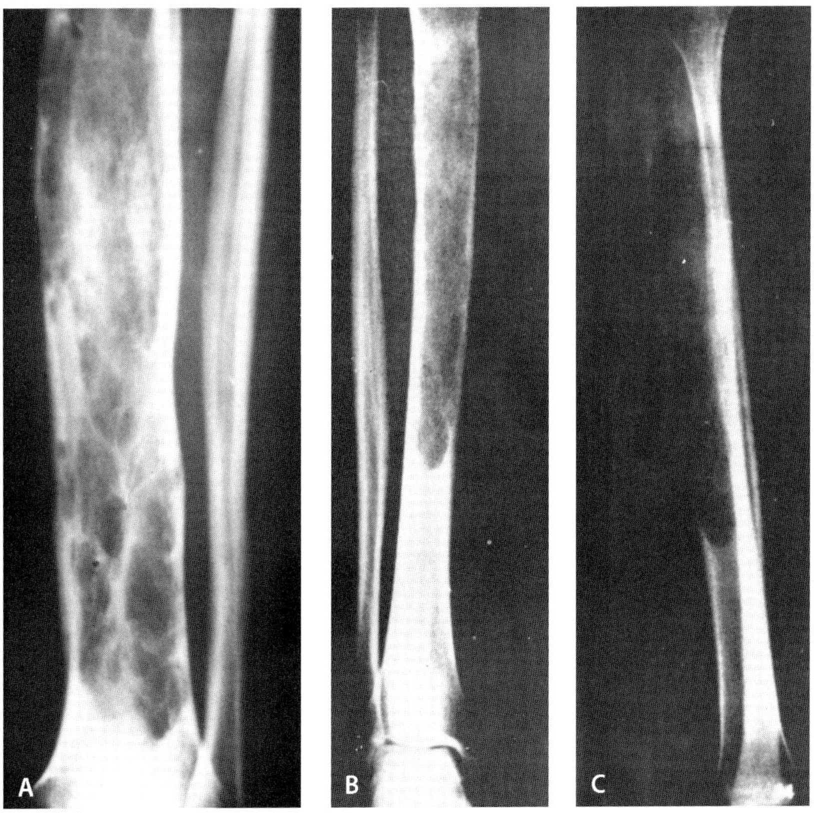

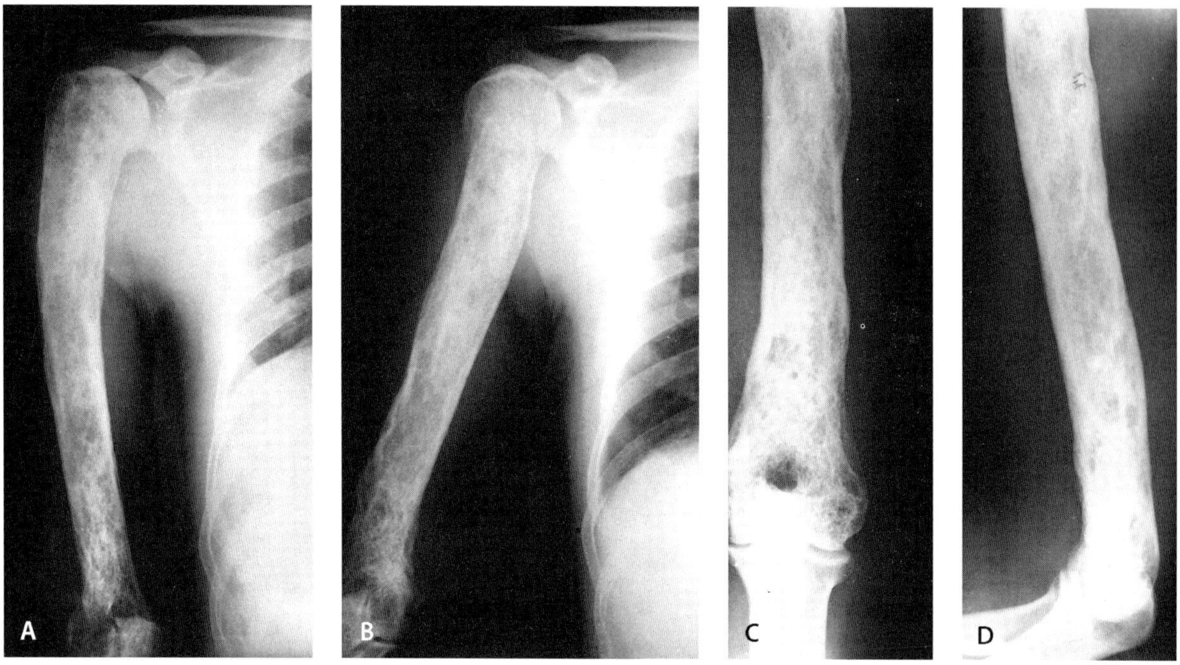

Fig. 3.130 A–D. Hydatid disease involving the entire humerus. AP views of the shoulder and humerus in internal and external rotation (**A** and **B**) together with AP (**C**) and lateral (**D**) views of the distal two-thirds of the humerus show that the hydatid process has spread throughout the entire length of the bone with overall loss of bone structure. The architecture is totally abnormal and has been replaced by multiple calcareous bubbles, giving a honeycomb appearance to the humerus. The medullary cavity is expanded and the cortices thinned; the bone has become markedly softened and weak with bowing of the proximal shaft. Because of the extensive destruction with thin cortices, the bone is fragile and may eventually fracture in one or more places

Pathological fractures often occur at this stage (Fig. 3.131). Secondary infection may further complicate the radiographic appearance in the older, more advanced lesion, resulting in the formation of areas of bony condensation, loss of cortical bone, and hyperostosis simulating the involucrum phase of osteomyelitis. Once these proliferative bony changes occur, the characteristic multilocular appearance is no longer identifiable.

When the hydatid lesion finally penetrates through the cortex and periosteum, an abscess is produced which appears radiologically as a smooth rounded mass in the adjacent soft tissues (Fig. 3.131 C). It should be remembered that periosteal reaction is never produced by hydatid disease alone and indicates either superimposed infection or some other process. In the final stages of advanced destruction, the hydatid process has spread so far that the bony architecture is totally abnormal and is replaced by multiple calcareous bubbles (Fig. 3.130). The bone may have expanded sufficiently to give a "blowout" appearance which, with associated pathological fractures, will result in considerable deformity.

The differential diagnosis of early hydatid lesions in long bones will include such varied entities as myeloma, primary or metastatic tumor, angioma, giant cell tumor, fibrous dysplasia, bone cyst, aneurysmal bone cyst, and other cystic lesions. When secondary infection has occurred later in the disease, the radiological findings may resemble an osteomyelitis. The various serological and other laboratory tests should confirm the diagnosis of hydatid disease of bone.

In bony hydatid disease, CT may be helpful in making the diagnosis and allowing the best choice of treatment. CT will clearly show the extent of the hydatid cyst and whether it has spread into neighboring tissues. When there is infection or abscess formation, contrast studies will probably show ring enhancement and there may be air bubbles in the lesion. CT is also useful in the follow-up of both surgery and chemotherapy for bone lesions. Recurrences can be recognized earlier and therefore more effectively treated, with increased prospects of cure and maximum preservation of function.

While the diagnosis of primary hydatidosis of bone in its early stages may be difficult or even impossible, the later stages are more easily recognized. There are many significant findings, such as the specific locations of cysts in bone, a bubbly or grape-like appearance, hypertrophy of trabeculae and molding of the cystic growth within the frame-

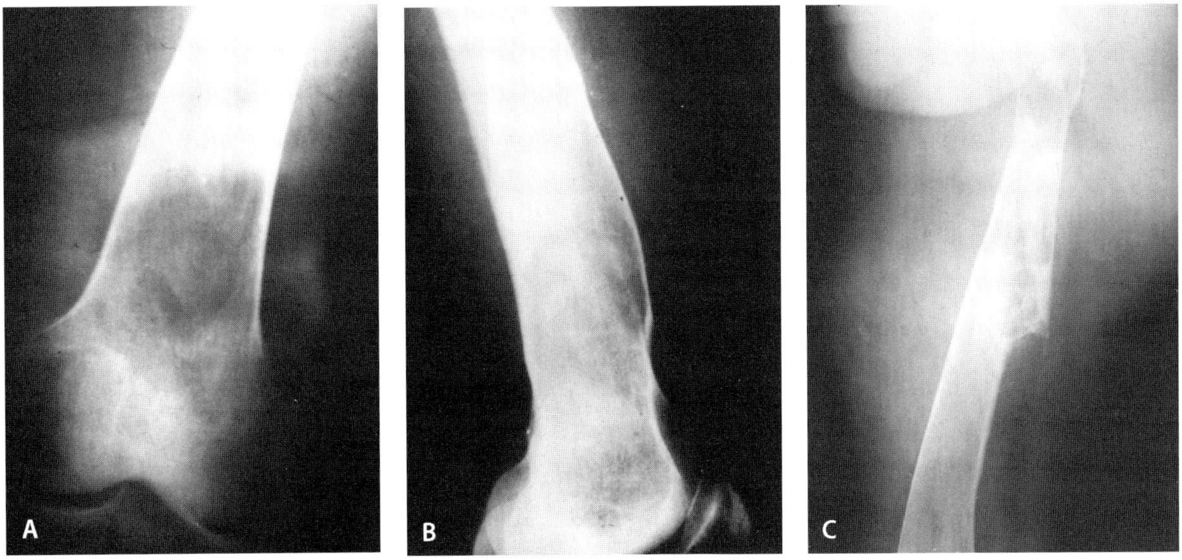

Fig. 3.131 A–C. Hydatid disease of the femur in two different patients with pathological fractures. **A** AP and **B** lateral views of the distal femur show an ill-defined destructive lesion with widening of the medullary canal and extreme thinning of the cortex. A pathological fracture through the anterior aspect of the distal shaft is seen on the lateral view (**B**). A well-defined 2-cm hole in the cortex is present at the fracture site on both views, where the hydatid process extended through the cortex into the soft tissues. **C** An oblique, complete, pathological fracture through the midshaft of the femur of another patient. There is widening of the medullary canal and thinning of the cortex of the femoral shaft with a multilocular cystic appearance of the lesion in the area of the pathological fracture. The hydatid lesion penetrated through the cortex and periosteum to produce not only a pathological fracture but also a large hydatid cyst and abscess in the adjacent soft tissues of the anterior and medial aspects of the midthigh

work of the bone, lack of calcification or capsules, "osteomyelitis without sequestration," pressure effect on the cortex leading to thinning, and finally breakthrough into neighboring soft tissue spaces, muscles, or subcutaneous tissue. A cystic expansile mass contiguous with a fractured bubbly or grape-like bony lesion is highly suspicious for primary hydatid disease of bone and has to be regarded as such until the contrary is proven, especially if it occurs in an endemic area of echinococcosis. Once the primary osseous cyst has broken through the cortex, causing fracture, the adjacent mass develops all the characteristics of any hydatid cyst. There may be a capsule, calcification, daughter cysts, rupture, infection, allergic inflammation of neighboring tissues, abscess formation, air bubbles, and fistulous tracts.

Magnetic resonance imaging shows primary osseous hydatidosis better than CT, except that minor osteolytic changes revealed on CT may not be seen on MRI. This is probably due to the better resolution and fewer motion artifacts on CT. On the other hand, compression and changes involving the spinal cord and canal over several levels are better demonstrated by MRI, and extraosseous changes, after the primary bone cysts have broken through the cortex, are well shown. However, calcifications are better seen on nonenhanced CT than on MRI.

Pelvis and Hip Joint

The pelvic girdle is a common site for the cyst wall and its laminated membrane to insinuate between the trabeculae and slowly spread within the cancellous bone, eventually eroding through the cortex into the surrounding soft tissues. Since the process may be asymptomatic for a long period, the initial radiographs usually show extensive destruction of bone (Figs. 3.132–3.135), although a solitary cyst-like or "bubbly cystic" lesion may be seen (Fig. 3.133 A). There may be one enormous solitary cyst, but more often there are numerous smaller cysts scattered diffusely through the pelvis, giving the characteristic appearance of "clusters of grapes" (Figs. 3.132 and 3.133 B). Since bony destruction proceeds at a slow rate, the skeleton can respond with the formation of dense reactive bone (Figs. 3.132 C–3.135). The resulting intermingling of large cystic spaces with coarse strands and islands of bone creates a bizarre appearance, which is often mistaken for a primary malignant bone tumor such as chondrosarcoma (Fig. 3.134). CT and especially MRI of primary pelvic hydatidosis, particularly if T2-weighted images are included, allow for easier recognition of cystic changes in bone, and their relationship to skeletal structures and soft tissues (Figs. 3.136, 3.137).

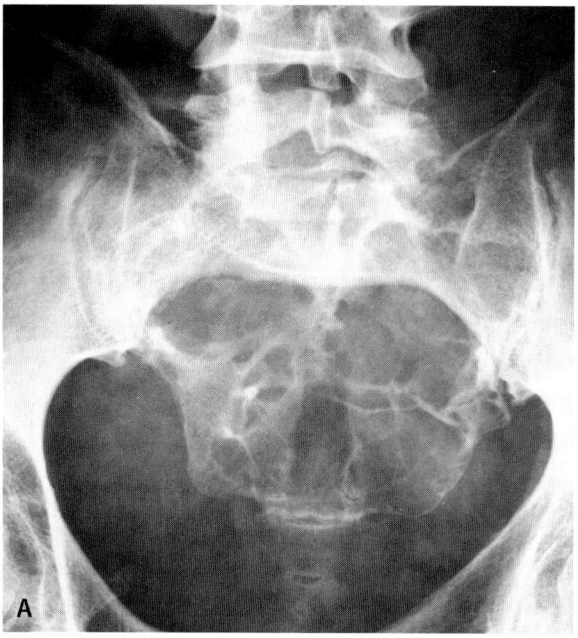

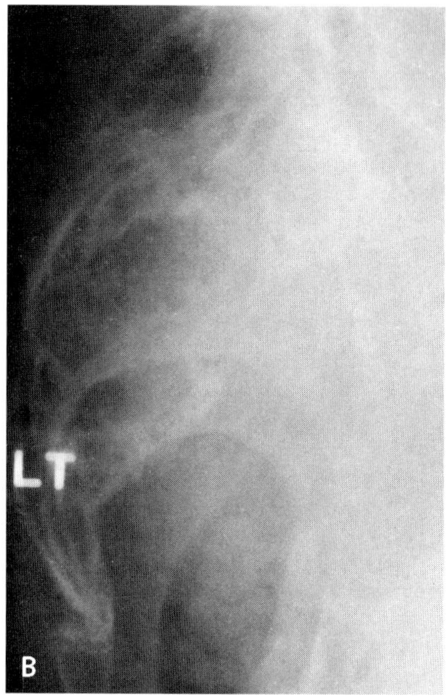

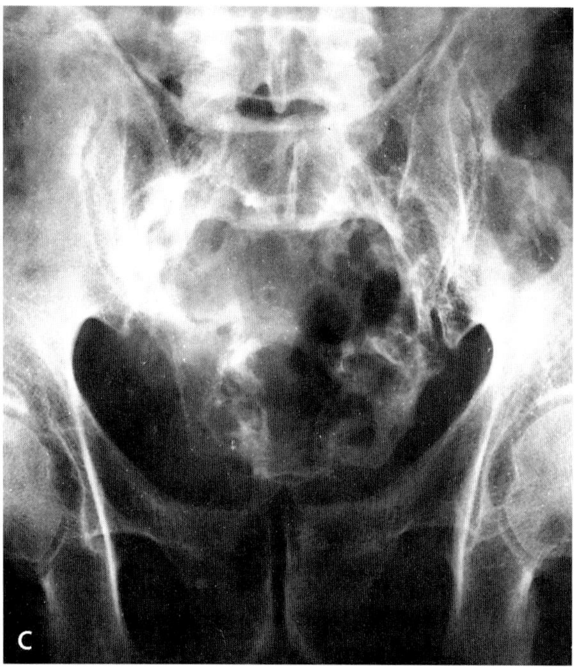

Fig. 3.132 A–C. Hydatid cyst of the sacrum in a 52-year-old man from the Mediterranean area. **A** The initial AP view of the pelvis in July reveals an extensive lytic destructive lesion involving most of the sacrum associated with a multilocular cystic appearance and expansion. In addition to being compatible with a hydatid cyst, the radiographic appearance is also suggestive of giant cell tumor, cyst, angioma, or myeloma. At this time, the patient had pain in the left hip referred down the leg, with numbness of the foot and toes of 18 months' duration. In May he had noticed swelling of the left gluteal region. By the time of the July radiograph, the swelling had developed into a large fluctuant, painful abscess which was drained 1 day previously of two quarts of thick, purulent material. At surgery, the cortex of the dorsal surface of the sacrum was penetrated and curettings were obtained; these consisted of small globular masses of homogeneous, dull, yellowish material, some of which contained individual pinhead-sized, clear cysts. Microscopic study initially showed granulomatous inflammation with some giant cells, and a giant cell tumor was suggested. However, examination of further material revealed an *Echinococcus* cyst. **B** Lateral and **C** AP views of the sacrum taken 3 years later in October show the expansile, bubbly cystic nature of the lesion, seen best on the lateral view (**B**). During the 3-year interval, there has been development of dense reactive bone surrounding and within the lesion, with coarse strands of dense bone particularly noticeable about the right upper and left lower wings of the sacrum. This represents attempted healing of the destructive process, which showed no further increase in extent in the 3-year interval. (Chemotherapy was not available when this patient was seen)

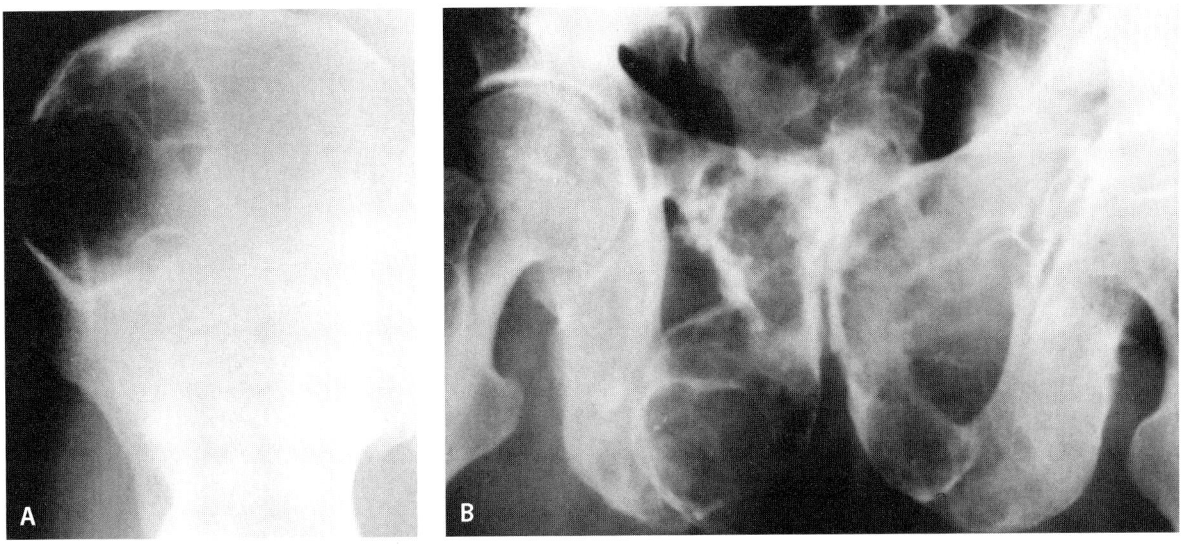

Fig. 3.133 A, B. Hydatid disease of the pelvis presenting as bubbly cystic, expansile lesions with surrounding reactive sclerosis. **A** A solitary large multilocular cyst in the right iliac bone. There is expansion of the iliac crest with cortical breakthrough and a thin reactive layer of bone sclerosis about the lesion. **B** Bubbly cystic, expansile lesion involving the pubis, ischium, and acetabulum on both sides of the pelvis. Hydatid disease may cross the pubic symphysis, as in this case, or the sacroiliac or hip joints

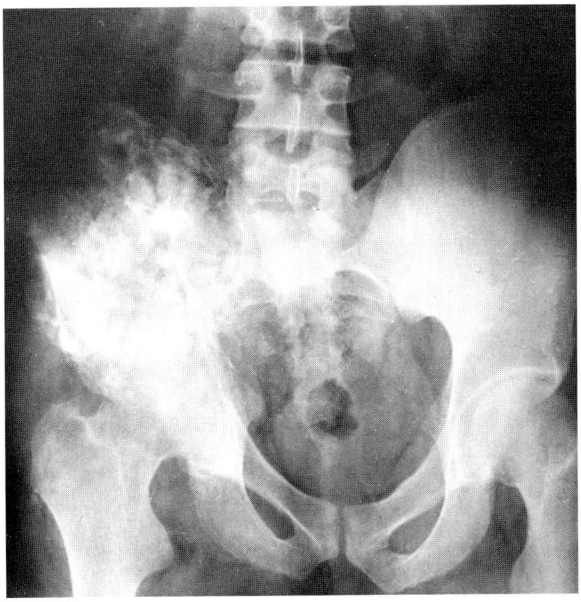

Fig. 3.134. Hydatid disease involving the right ilium and resembling chondrosarcoma. There is a diffuse multicystic type of bone destruction intermingled with irregular, coarse trabecular strands and islands of dense bone. The calcification, cortical destruction, and surrounding soft tissue mass produce an appearance that may be confused with chondrosarcoma. (From D. Wilner: *Radiological diagnosis of tumors in bone and allied disorders*. Philadelphia, Saunders, 1979)

The entire process may be quiescent for a year or longer, but as the hydatid is reactivated, interval radiographs show a progressive creeping type of bone destruction leading to complete osteolysis. The sacrum, ilium, ischium, and/or pubis may be completely destroyed, leaving only a shell of bone containing poorly defined trabecular strands and irregular calcifications (Figs. 3.135, 3.136). Pathological fractures often occur at this stage, allowing daughter cysts to escape into the soft tissues with hydatid abscess formation. Multiple dense, rounded masses become visible in the surrounding soft tissues, and occasionally calcification of the ectocyst is noted, implying demise of the parasite (Fig. 3.126). The widespread destruction of bone may extend across the sacroiliac joint, hip joint, and pubic synchondrosis (Figs. 3.136–3.138). The end result may be a complete deterioration of the pelvis on one or occasionally both sides, with crumbling and collapse of the innominate bone and dislocation of the femur, so that the femoral head migrates inwards to approximate itself against the sacrum (Figs. 3.137, 3.138). The head, neck, and trochanteric portions of the femur may be destroyed, and rarely the entire femur may show diffuse multicystic disease (Fig. 3.138 C). Despite the vast loss of bone structure in some patients, the complicating osteitis with dense bone formation tends to stabilize the process, although the end result is a crippling deformity (Fig. 3.135).

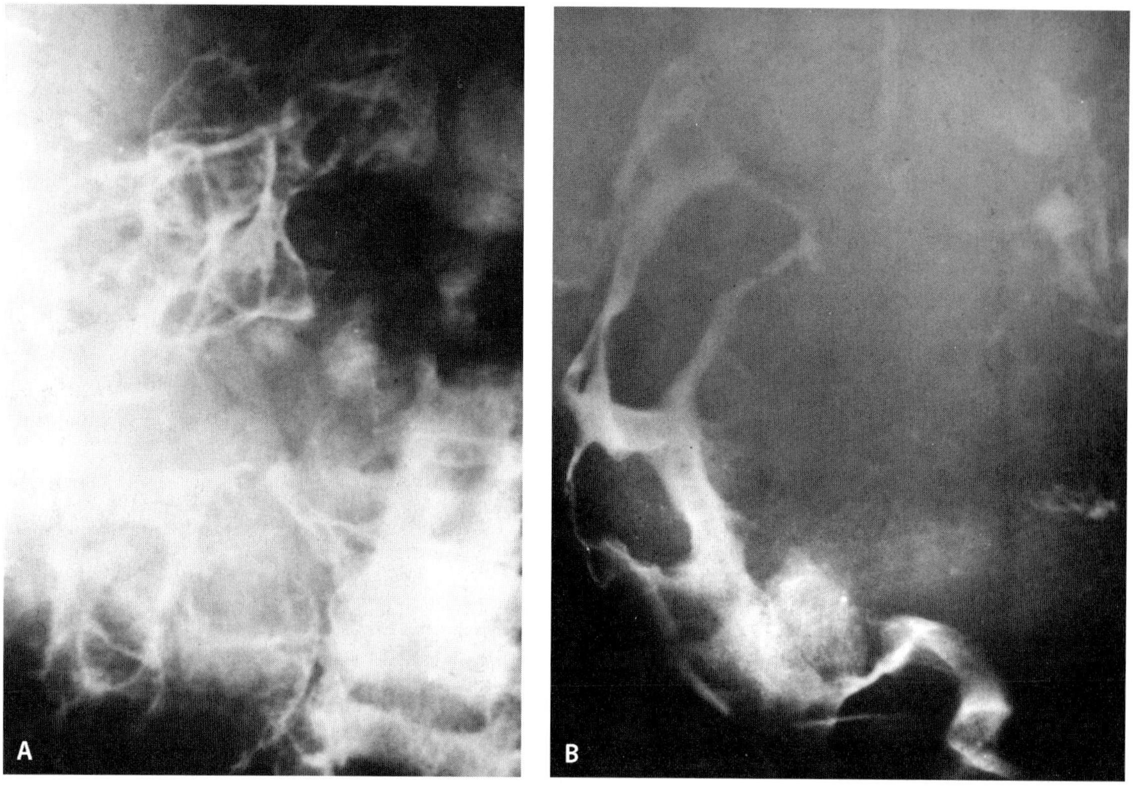

Fig. 3.135 A, B. Extreme destruction of pelvic bones by hydatid disease. There is gross osteolysis with expanded blowout lesions of bone involving the right hemipelvis in A and virtually the entire pelvis in B. The radiographic appearance at this end stage shows a massive destructive process so bizarre that no identifiable osseous features remain. The lumbar vertebral column can be seen to the right of the large expansile lesion arising from the right iliac bone in A. In B the upper sacrum with its spinous processes are barely discernible in the upper portion of the film. In both cases, there is little more than a shell of bone with reinforced trabecular strands and irregular calcifications in these grossly expansile, blowout lesions. Despite the vast loss of bone structure in such cases, the complicating osteitis with its dense reactive new bone formation tends to stabilize the process somewhat, although crippling deformities are obviously present

In the pelvis, the bubbly cystic, expansile pattern seen in many patients with osseous hydatid disease must be differentiated from myeloma, metastatic renal or thyroid carcinoma, angioma, giant cell tumor, fibrous dysplasia, bone cyst, aneurysmal bone cyst, and other cystic lesions. If the destructive process is extensive and is associated with a large soft tissue mass and calcification, it must be differentiated from a primary malignancy of bone such as chondrosarcoma. If there are coexisting round masses in the lungs due to pulmonary hydatid disease, the possibility of metastases from a bone sarcoma may be erroneously entertained. However, the chronicity of the process and the formation of sclerotic bone in the latter stages will exclude malignancy, and the pulmonary masses will grow very slowly.

Occasionally, there may be a soft tissue hydatid in the pelvis which does not originate in or destroy bone. It may be indistinguishable from other causes of pelvic soft tissue masses, even if it has calcium in its wall (Fig. 3.13).

(Text continues on p. 319)

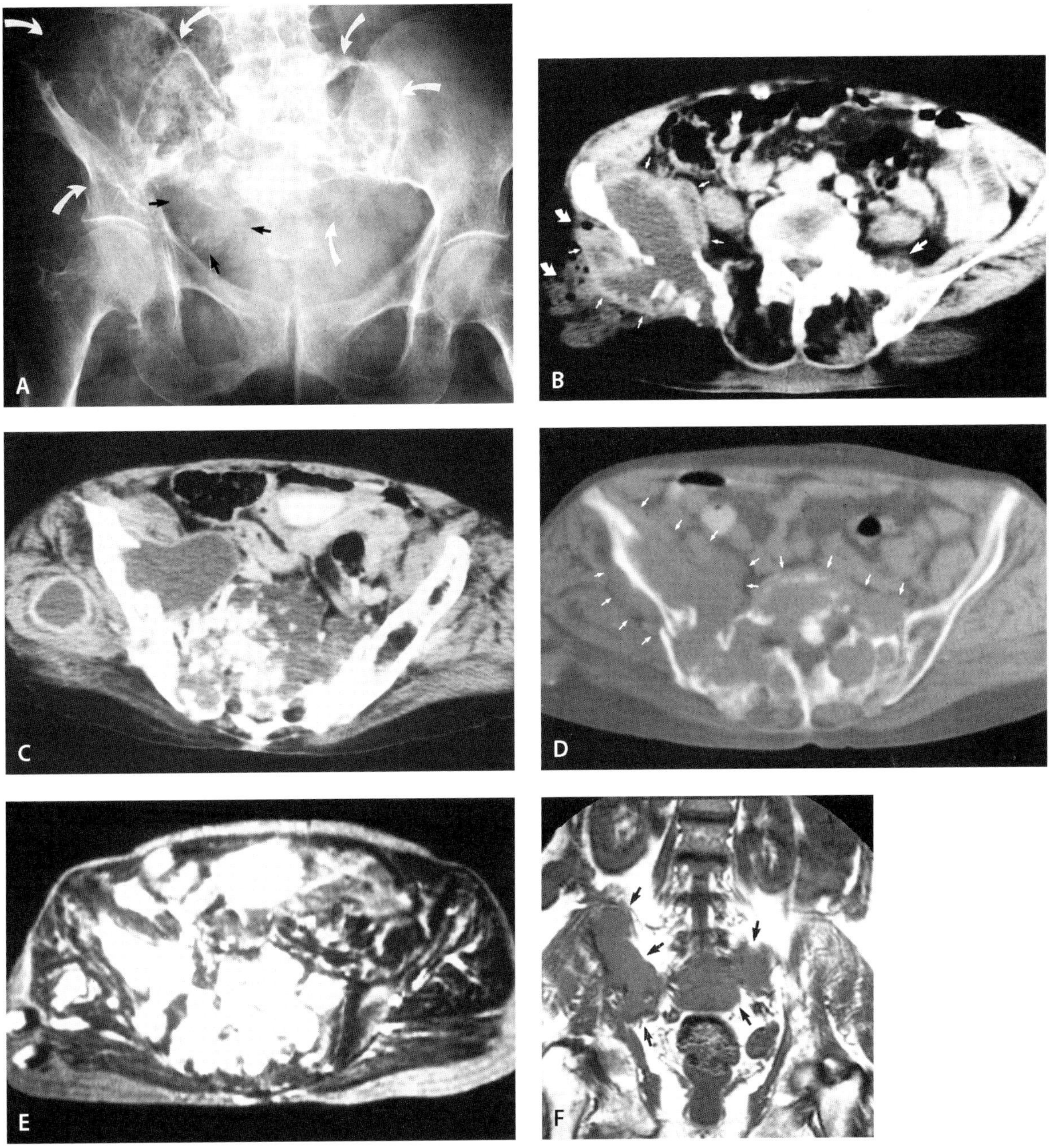

Fig. 3.136 A–F. A 72-year-old Saudi woman with primary osseous pelvic hydatid disease. **A** AP view of the pelvis reveals extensive destruction of the right ilium and sacrum (*curved white arrows*) with some extension into the adjacent soft tissues (*black arrows*). **B–D** Contrast-enhanced CT scans at different levels show destruction of the right ilium and sacrum by an expansile cystic process, and extensive soft tissue abscess formation (*small white arrows*) with multiple small gas pockets (*curved large white arrows*) in **B**. The sacrum, including its left wing and adjacent soft tissues, is also involved (*large white arrow*). The extent of soft tissue involvement is best seen in **D** (*arrows*). **E** MRI T2-weighted (spin echo, 2000/100) image shows cystic masses of high signal intensity replacing bone trabeculae and extending into the pelvis and subcutaneous tissues. **F** Coronal MRI reconstruction shows the destructive process in the right ilium, sacrum, and adjacent tissues (*arrows*). (Courtesy of Dr. Walther von Sinner and *Semin Roentgenol*, 1997)

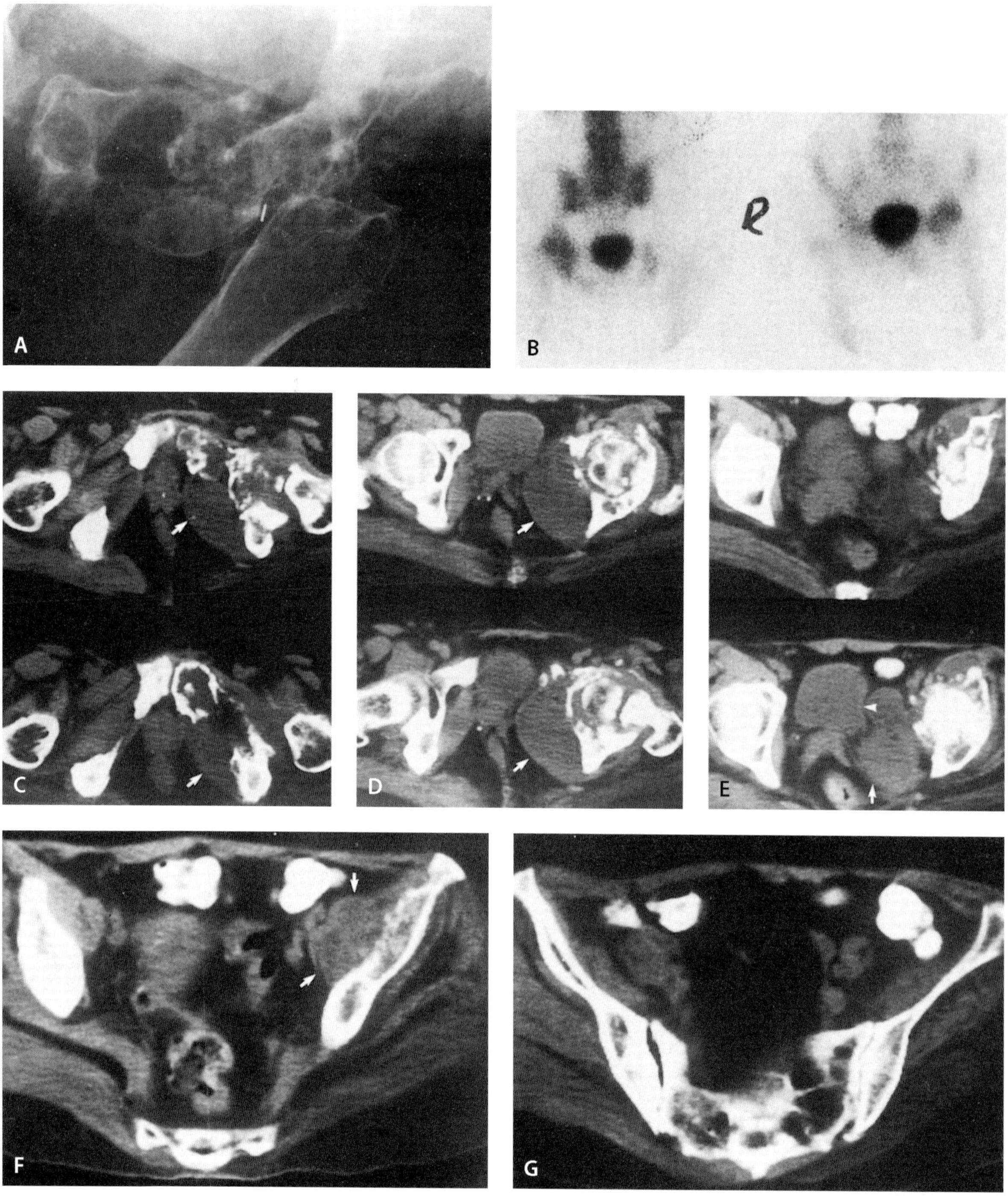
A
B
R
C
D
E
F
G

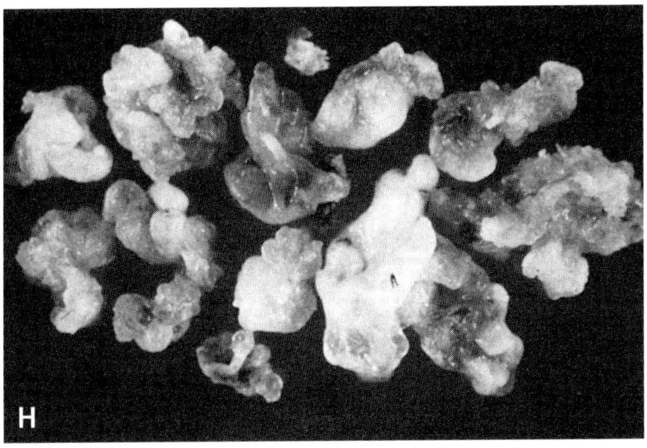

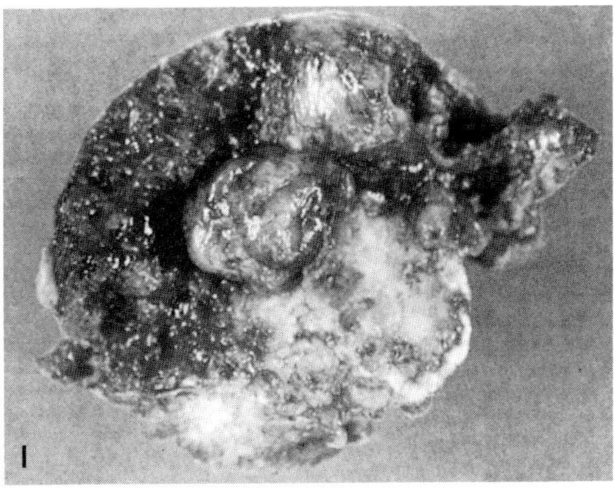

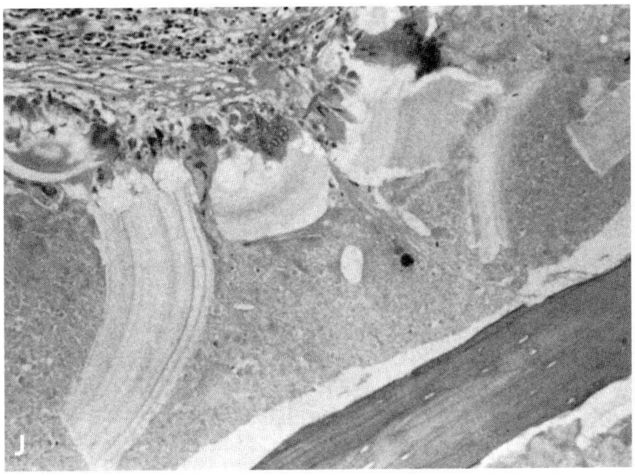

◀ **Fig. 3.137 A–J.** A 50-year-old Saudi woman with left pelvic pain of over 3 years' duration. A diagnosis of osteomyelitis was made elsewhere after purulent material was recovered from the left pubic bone, and she was treated with ampicillin. On admission, a painful left groin swelling was noted. Later, it was found the lesion was expanding despite antibiotics, and conventional radiography (**A**) showed extensive destructive lesions involving the left pubis, ischium, and ilium, as well as the left acetabulum and femoral head and neck. The hip joint cartilage is narrowed and the femoral head protrudes through the acetabulum medially. **B** A radionuclide bone scan (20 mCi technetium-99m methylene diphosphonate) shows increased uptake of isotope in the left innominate bone, especially in the ischium and acetabulum. **C–G** Six months later, nonenhanced CT scans at different levels show further extension of the destructive lesions in the area of the left pubis, trochanteric area and displaced proximal femur (**C**), left hip joint, femoral head and neck and acetabulum (**D**, **E**), ilium (**F**), and sacrum (**G**). In addition, a cystic soft tissue mass adjacent to bone protrudes into the pelvis (**C–F**, *arrows*) and impinges on the bladder (**E**, *arrowhead*). Ultrasonography of the abdomen showed no other lesions. Exploration of the left pelvis with curettage was performed. **H** Small irregular fragments of cystic, mucoid, glistening pieces of tissue from the iliac crest, some of which contained clear fluid as well as laminated membranes on microscopy suggestive of hydatid cysts. **I** The femoral head was loose and was extracted, with areas of necrotic material noted. The 3.5-cm specimen of the femoral head shows an irregular glistening 2-cm cyst on an uneven articular surface with fibrin deposits and loss of articular cartilage. **J** Microscopic examination shows several fragments of hyaline or laminated parasitic membranes but no germinal epithelium or scolices. (Courtesy of Dr. Walther von Sinner and *Skeletal Radiol*, 1990)

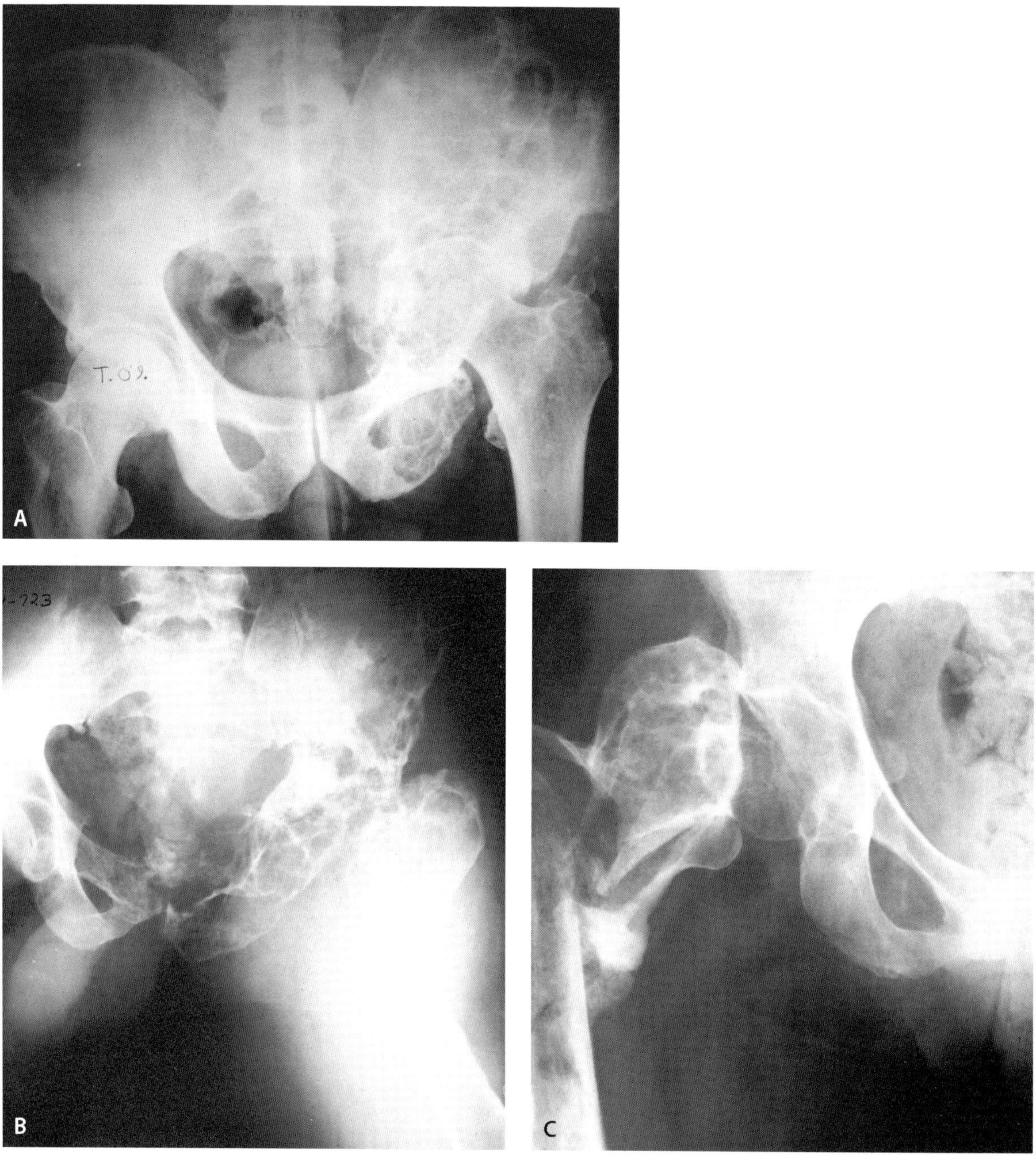

Fig. 3.138 A–C. Extensive hytadid disease involving the pelvis and hips in three different patients. **A** There is extensive bubbly cystic destruction of most of the left hemipelvis with a moderate degree of expansion. There has been collapse and crumbling of the innominate bone in the region of the acetabulum with inward dislocation of the femur so that the femoral head is driven deep into the pelvis in the direction of the sacrum. This extensive bubbly cystic pattern must be differentiated radiographically from other entities such as myeloma, metastatic thyroid or kidney carcinoma, angioma, giant cell tumor, fibrous dysplasia, unicameral bone cyst, or aneurysmal bone cyst. (Courtesy of Dr. Emanuel Levin, New York) **B** Extensive hydatid disease of the left hemipelvis and femur in a 50-year-old Iranian man with swelling and pain in his left thigh of 4 months' duration which began as a small, slightly painful mass and got progressively larger. The mass was nontender and mobile, and extended from the iliac crest to the gluteal fold. The AP radiograph of the pelvis and hips shows extensive bubbly cystic destruction of the left hemipelvis with moderate bone expansion. The process has extended across the pubic symphysis to involve the right pubis as well. The acetabulum is no longer recognizable and the hydatid infection has involved the entire proximal femur and shaft. The femoral head and neck are partially destroyed by the multilocular, expansile, destructive process and the femur is rotated and dislocated out of the acetabulum and lies superior and lateral to its normal position. There are huge soft tissue masses representing extension of the hydatid infection beyond the bones into the soft tissues of the left pelvis and thigh, with hydatid cysts and abscesses present there. Legend continues on p. 319

Spine

In the spine, the dorsal vertebrae are the most frequently affected with hydatid disease, especially the lower six thoracic vertebrae; over half of the cases with vertebral involvement occur in this area. About 30% of patients with vertebral hydatidosis will develop epidural extension of their disease with resultant compression of the spinal cord and paraplegia. There is usually pain and perhaps local swelling over the area. The pain and paraplegia occurs quite acutely. In the past, treatment has generally been unsatisfactory and, even in the unusual case where surgical resection appeared possible, recurrence was usually inevitable. Wounds failed to heal, sinuses developed, and continuing paraplegia and chronic invalidism were the end result (Fig. 3.139). Chemotherapy is helpful in many such cases today.

The spongy tissue of the vertebral body is a frequent site for hydatid bone disease. In the early stages, cystic areas may be seen in the vertebral body and often extend into the pedicle, lamina, and transverse process (Figs. 3.140, 3.141). Contiguous posterior rib involvement usually accompanies the vertebral disease in the thoracic area (Fig. 3.142 A, B). In many patients, however, instead of cystic areas, there is more generalized bone destruction, yet the vertebral height is usually maintained and the intervertebral disc space is spared. Later in the disease, especially when there is complicating secondary infection, partial collapse of the vertebra and narrowing of the disc space are not uncommon. Occasionally, a cystic lesion in a vertebra may cross the disc space to involve an adjacent vertebra, causing collapse of both vertebral bodies and disc space obliteration. When secondary

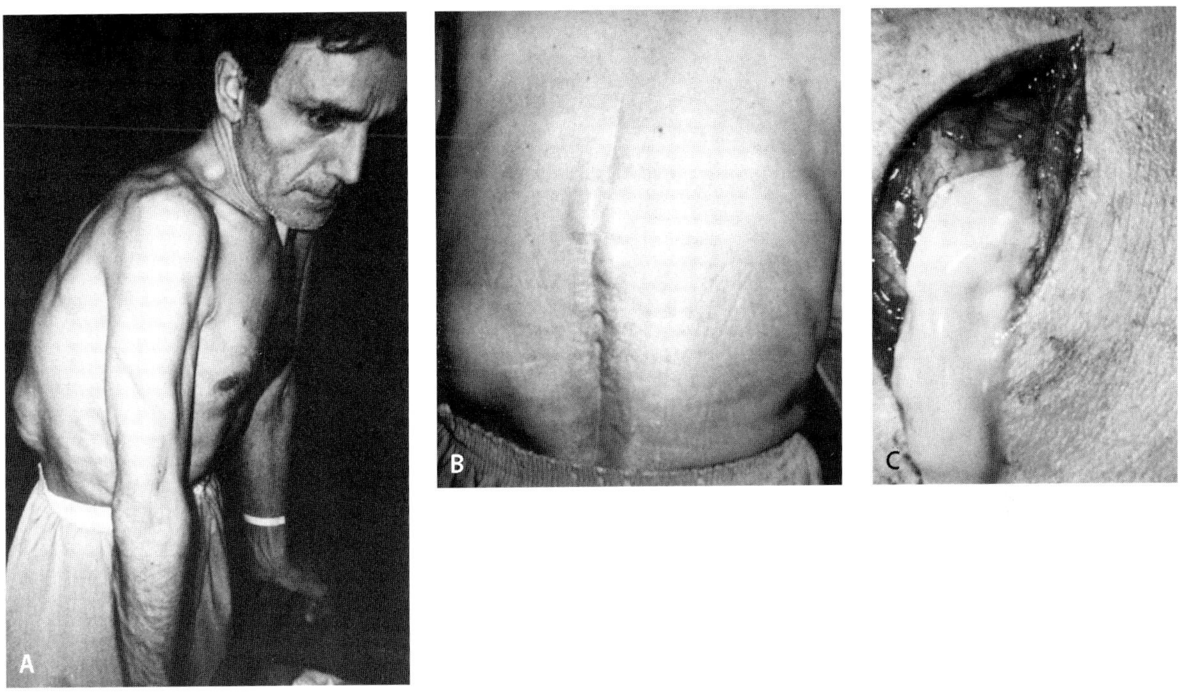

Fig. 3.139 A–C. Hydatid disease of the spine in a cachectic 53-year-old Italian man, who 10 years earlier was found to have hydatid cysts in the spine during a laminectomy to decompress his spinal cord. Dissemination to the pleura, lungs, and flank followed. The patient died several months after these photos were made. **A** There is a prominent kyphosis due to compression of vertebral bodies eroded by the cysts. Also note the bulge of the left flank caused by an underlying hydatid. **B** Posterior view showing scars from previous surgery, the large hydatid cyst bulging the left flank, and several smaller cysts near the upper end of the old midline surgical incision. **C** Incision into one of the hydatid cysts permitted escape of pseudopurulent material

◀ **Fig. 3.138** (*continued*). **C** Hydatid involvement of the proximal right femur and shaft in a 45-year-old Iranian woman. The patient had swelling of her right thigh, hip, and buttock as high up as the iliac crest of 20 months' duration. Hip movements were painful and limited. There is a pathological comminuted intertrochanteric fracture of the right hip with marked varus deformity and superolateral displacement of the femoral shaft with relation to the neck. There is a moderate degree of callus formation about the lower portion of the fracture site, but bony union is incomplete and a crippling deformity will persist. Note the honeycombed, lytic destruction of the femoral shaft and neck due to the underlying hydatid process. (**B**, **C** courtesy of Dr. Massoud Majd, Washington)

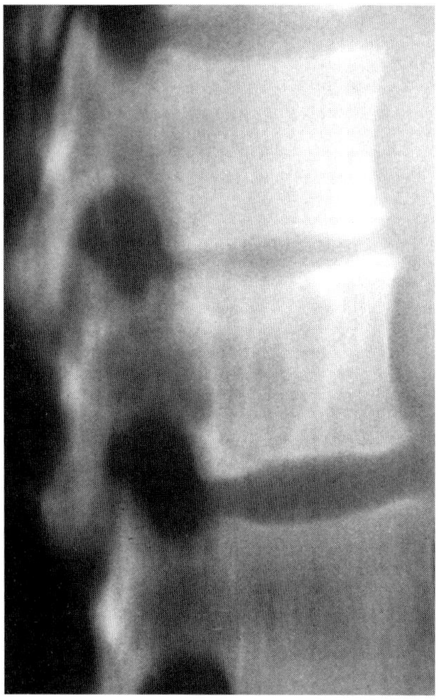

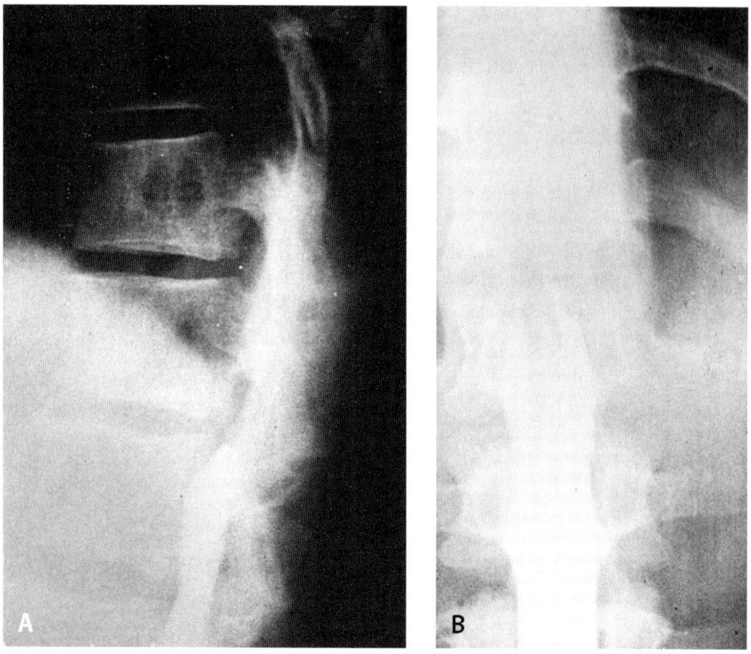

Fig. 3.140 (*left*). Hydatid disease affecting the body and neural arch of the second lumbar vertebra and the adjacent disc space. A lateral tomogram clearly shows the well-defined cystic area in the posterior portion of the vertebral body extending into the pedicle and lamina. There is narrowing of the L1–2 disc space as well. (Courtesy of the University of Capetown Radiology Library)

Fig. 3.141 A, B (*middle, right*). Hydatid disease involving T12 and L1 with extension posteriorly into the extradural space, causing complete block on myelography in a patient from India with signs of paraplegia. **A** Lateral and **B** AP views of the dorsolumbar spine obtained during myelography with the patient in a 70° Trendelenburg position show a complete block at L1 from an extradural hydatid mass. Cystic radiolucent defects are seen in the T12 and L1 vertebral bodies with a slight surrounding rim of sclerosis on the lateral view (**A**). There is minimal narrowing of the T12–L1 and L1–2 disc spaces compared with the normal discs above and below those levels. (Courtesy of Dr. A. Chandrahasan Johnson)

infection sets in, sclerotic changes develop in the affected vertebra, surrounded by hypertrophic bony overgrowth (Fig. 3.142 A).

Following perforation of the cortex and periosteum, the vesicles spill out into the adjacent soft tissues, causing a paraspinal abscess (Fig. 3.142) which must be differentiated from tuberculosis, malignancy, or mediastinal tumor (Fig. 3.143). This may in turn cause erosion of the lateral margins of the vertebral bodies, the pedicles, and posterior ribs. If the cysts break through into the neural canal, the hydatids may appear in the meninges and cause widening of the interpedicular space on the frontal view and scalloping of the posterior surface of the vertebral body on the lateral view (Fig. 3.144). In the past, myelography usually revealed a partial or complete block (compression myelopathy) at the site of the hydatid (Fig. 3.141). Today, CT and MRI, where available, have replaced, or are sometimes combined with, myelography and usually present a more complete evaluation of the true extent of the hydatid process within the spine and adjacent structures (Fig. 3.145).

The diagnosis of spinal hydatid disease is very difficult in the early stages and must be differentiated from a hemangioma or an inflammatory lesion, such as tuberculosis or brucellosis. Metastatic cancer must also be considered in the differential diagnosis, but preservation of the height of the vertebra and extension of the disease process to the adjacent posterior rib would favor hydatid disease (although tuberculosis can sometimes behave in the same way and mycotic infections will also spread to bone). When a hydatid abscess complicates hydatidosis of the dorsal spine and lies anterior or lateral to the spine, it will have to be differentiated from a pulmonary hydatid cyst or mediastinal tumor (Fig. 3.143). If CT and MRI are unavailable, a pneumothorax may be used to locate the mass more accurately. If located within the lung, it will collapse along with the lung; otherwise it will remain attached to the thoracic wall.

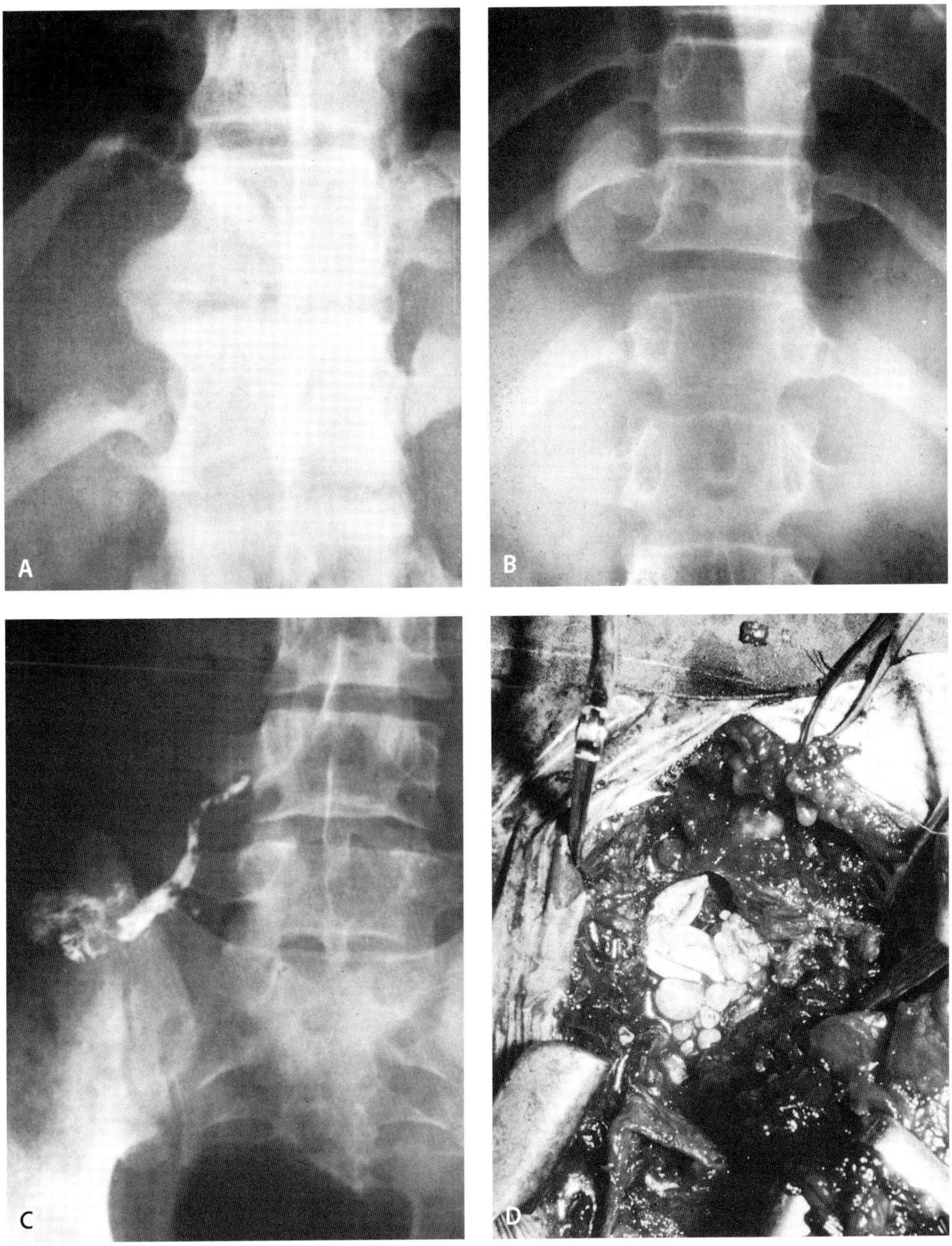

Fig. 3.142 A–D. Paraspinal abscesses due to extension of hydatid disease of the spine into the adjacent paravertebral soft tissues in three different patients. **A** A hydatid cyst arising from the lower thoracic spine with large paraspinal abscess extending from the top of T11 to the bottom of T12. The right pedicles and neural arches of T11 and T12 are involved and there is marked hypertrophic bony overgrowth on the right side of the T11–12 disc space, which is moderately narrowed. There is also erosion, splaying, and slight dislocation of the costovertebral aspects of the right 11th and 12th ribs. There is slight scalloping of the right lateral aspect of T12 due to erosion. **B** Hydatid disease involving the right lateral aspect of T11 with destruction of the pedicle and extension into the right paravertebral soft tissues, producing a well-defined paraspinal abscess at T10–11. There is dislocation of the costovertebral aspect of the right 11th rib and erosion with resulting scalloping of the lateral margin of T11. **C** Hydatid disease of the transverse process of L4 in a 30-year-old Syrian man with a sinus in the lumbar region. A sinogram shows the contrast medium leading to a lucent defect in the right transverse process of L4. **D** The appearance of hydatid disease of the lumbar spine at operation. Note the large number of daughter cysts and small vesicles around the dura mater, and invasion of the surrounding paravertebral muscles and soft tissues. (**C**, **D** courtesy of Dr. M.K. Booz and *J Bone Joint Surg* [*Br*], 1972)

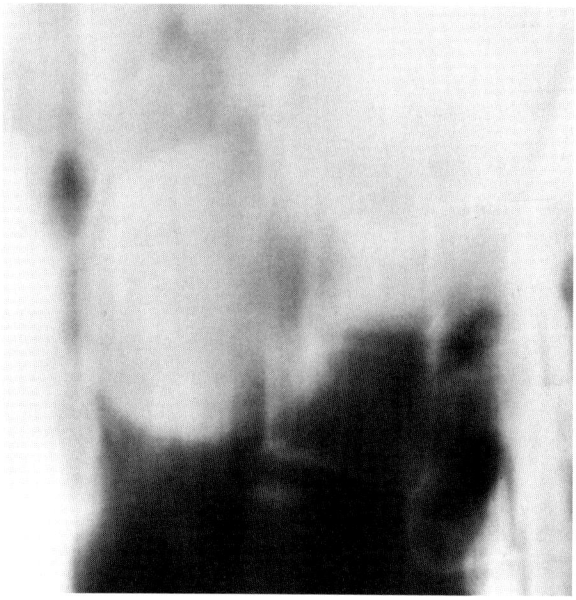

Fig. 3.143. Lateral tomogram of two large hydatid cysts involving the dorsal spine but presenting as mediastinal tumors. One cyst arises from the seventh thoracic vertebra, while the other overlies the anterior aspect of the mid-dorsal spine at a slightly lower level. Note the large erosive lytic defect in the anterior aspect of T7. (Courtesy of the University of Capetown Radiology Library)

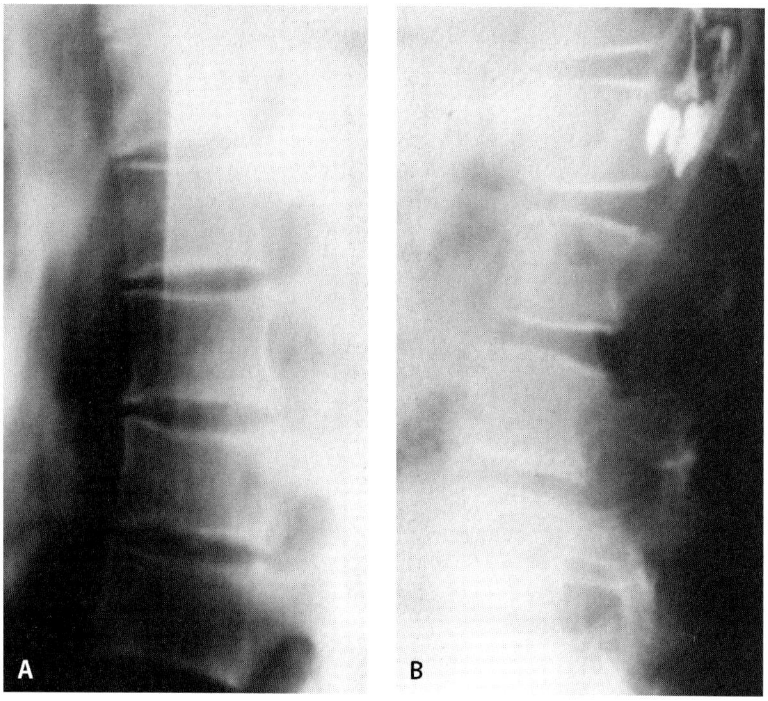

Fig. 3.144 A, B. Scalloping of the posterior surface of a vertebral body seen on lateral view of the spine in two different patients. As the hydatids break through into the neural canal they may appear in the meninges and cause widening of the interpedicular space on the frontal view and scalloping of the posterior aspect of the vertebral body on the lateral view. **A** Posterior scalloping of T7 vertebra. **B** Scalloping of the posterior aspects of L2 and L3 in another patient. (Courtesy of Dr. Harold Jacobson)

Ribs and Scapula

The ribs may become involved via the bloodstream or by direct extension from a lesion in the spine or lung. In its early stages, a primary rib lesion will appear as a multilocular cystic area with the cortex preserved. Later, the cortex is expanded and often perforated, permitting the hydatid tissue to break out from the bone and form a well-defined soft tissue mass (Figs. 3.146, 3.147). Rarely, a hydatid may break through the cortex and periosteum into the pleural cavity and reach a size of up to 9 cm, producing pressure erosion on the lateral aspect of the vertebral body and the pedicle (Fig. 3.146 D).

In the ribs, the radiological appearance of hydatid disease is far from pathognomonic and may be confused with many other lesions of bone, including fibrous dysplasia, simple bone cyst, aneurysmal bone cyst, angioma, myeloma, metastasis, eosinophilic granuloma, and even cystic tuberculosis.

Occasional patients with hydatid involvement of the scapula have been reported. These may present with a large multicystic area of bone destruction with a blowout appearance and with associated soft tissue mass (Fig. 3.148).

Fine-Needle Aspiration Biopsy of Hydatid Cysts

Until very fine aspiration needles became available, the percutaneous aspiration of fluid from hydatid cysts was generally regarded as extremely unwise because of the risk of anaphylactic reactions and possible dissemination of the disease. However, experience with unintended biopsies, where the diagnosis of hydatidosis was not suspected, has shown that complications, if they occur, are usually minor (urticaria, asthmatic symptoms, rash); anaphylactic shock can usually be medically controlled if the operator is prepared for this rare possibility. Today, careful fine-needle aspiration biopsy (FNAB) can be recommended, especially in patients in whom a precise pathological diagnosis is crucial, and can be combined with treatment (Figs. 3.149–3.152). Dissemination can be prevented by prophylactic medication with mebendazole or albendazole at least 12 hours, or preferably for 2–4 days, prior to biopsy.

Treatment

The role of surgery in the treatment of hydatid disease is diminishing, with increased indications for, and success with, chemotherapy and with the introduction of PAIR (puncture-aspiration-injection-reaspiration). The ability to treat hydatidosis with chemotherapy is an immense step forward in the management of this widespread disease. Guidelines for treatment in humans were published in 1996 by the World Health Organization (WHO). At that time surgery was recommended as the first choice for treatment wherever possible to totally remove the parasite (Fig. 3.153). However, chemotherapy with benzimidazole compounds (albendazole or mebendazole) or other suitable drugs, combined with diagnostic aspiration and the injection and reaspiration of sterilizing fluid when cysts cannot be removed, is a valid alternative therapy.

Patients are usually pretreated for a short time (10–14 days) with an antiscolicidal agent such as albendazole prior to definitive surgery or percutaneous drainage, and for several weeks after the procedure (see Fig. 3.81). An excessive period of pretreatment is dangerous as it may precipitate communicating or direct rupture (Fig. 3.29). Although various surgical methods have their advocates, centers with wide experience tend to favor the most conservative approach-endocystectomy. Many authors recommend that type II cysts should not be drained percutaneously because of the difficulty in removing daughter cysts and matrix; however, there are dissenting opinions, especially if only daughters are present as they can be punctured individually. Time and experience will tell whether uncomplicated hypermature type II cysts actually require resection. Hypermaturity is probably a terminal stage prior to death and conversion to a clinically insignificant type III lesion. Moreover, intuition suggests that hypermature lesions must be physically stable and resistant to rupture, especially if they are surrounded by substantial pericyst and organ parenchyma (the thickness of pericyst is difficult to estimate by CT or ultrasonography but MRI may be helpful).

Expansile lesions have sometimes been resected, even if the diagnosis of hydatid disease was not confirmed. However, in patients with multiple bilateral or multiorgan cysts, or when cysts have ruptured, disseminated, or recurred, surgery cannot cure the patient. In such cases, the diagnosis of hydatid disease must be confirmed (WHO Informal Working Group on Echinococcosis, 1996) because chemotherapy is not always without complications and has to be continued for several months or even years.

(Text continues on p. 329)

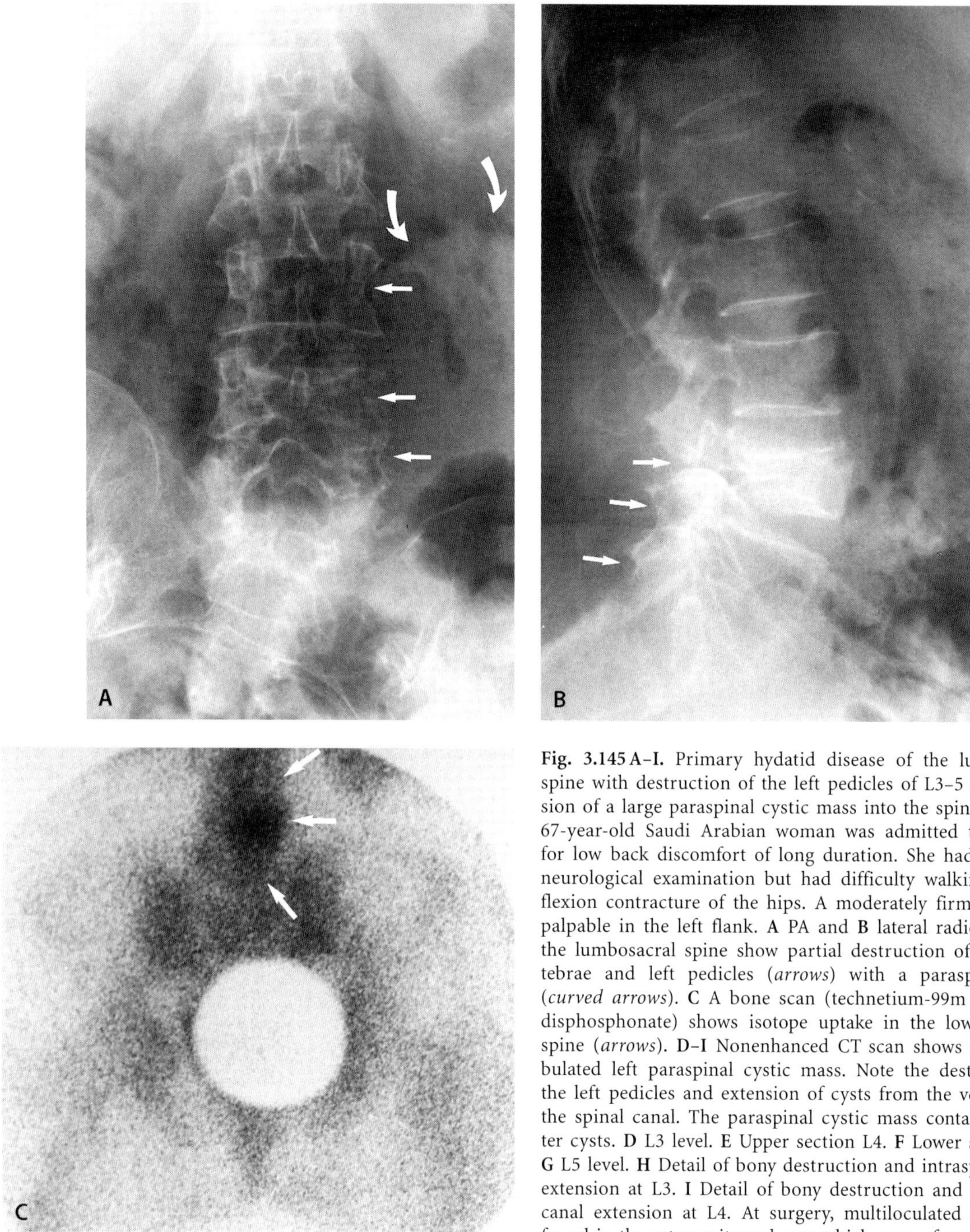

Fig. 3.145 A–I. Primary hydatid disease of the lumbosacral spine with destruction of the left pedicles of L3–5 and extension of a large paraspinal cystic mass into the spinal canal. A 67-year-old Saudi Arabian woman was admitted to hospital for low back discomfort of long duration. She had a normal neurological examination but had difficulty walking and no flexion contracture of the hips. A moderately firm mass was palpable in the left flank. **A** PA and **B** lateral radiographs of the lumbosacral spine show partial destruction of L3–5 vertebrae and left pedicles (*arrows*) with a paraspinal mass (*curved arrows*). **C** A bone scan (technetium-99m methylene disphosphonate) shows isotope uptake in the lower lumbar spine (*arrows*). **D–I** Nonenhanced CT scan shows a large lobulated left paraspinal cystic mass. Note the destruction of the left pedicles and extension of cysts from the vertebrae to the spinal canal. The paraspinal cystic mass contains daughter cysts. **D** L3 level. **E** Upper section L4. **F** Lower section L4. **G** L5 level. **H** Detail of bony destruction and intraspinal canal extension at L3. **I** Detail of bony destruction and intraspinal canal extension at L4. At surgery, multiloculated cysts were found in the retroperitoneal area which were of grape-like appearance and originated from the lumbar spine. Histological analysis confirmed hydatid disease. (Courtesy of Drs. Walther von Sinner and Akhtar and *Skeletal Radiol*, 1994) ▶

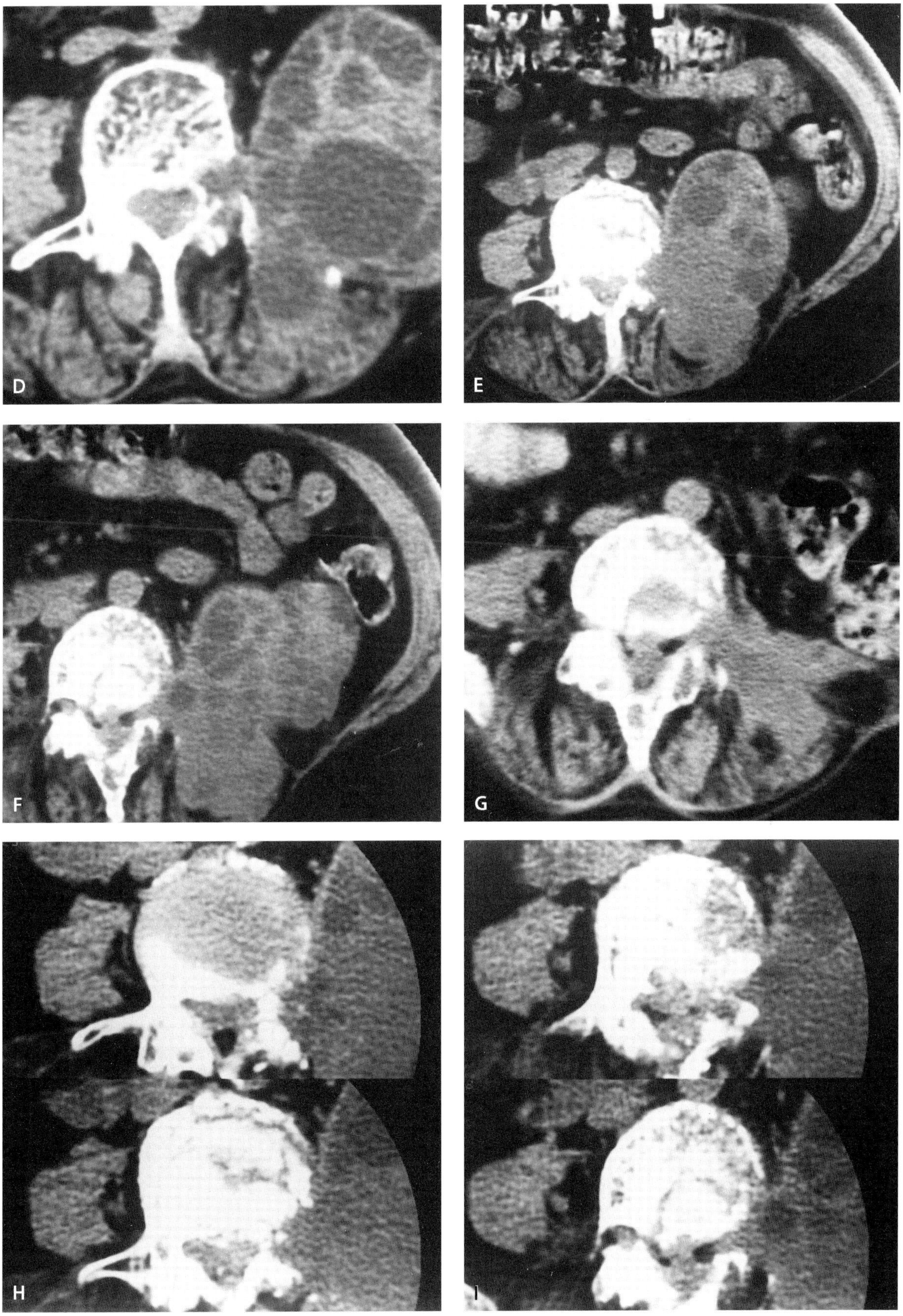
D
E
F
G
H
I

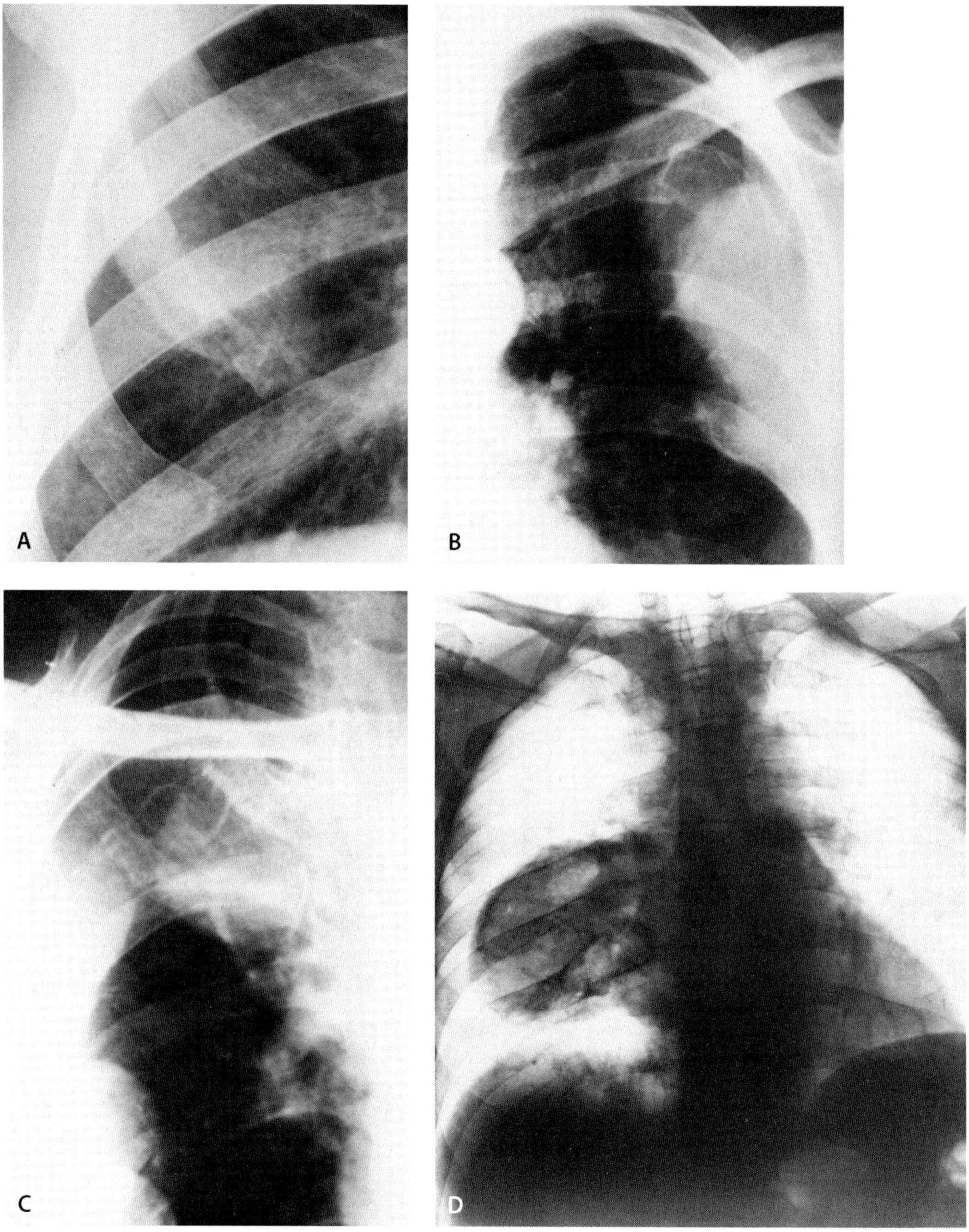

Fig. 3.146 A–D. Hydatid disease of the ribs. **A** A 46-year-old man with a cystic and sclerotic lesion in the anterior end of the right fifth rib. **B** A 50-year-old woman with a markedly expansile blowout lytic lesion of the posterolateral aspect of the left fifth rib. The hydatid lesion has broken through the confines of the rib to produce a well-defined extrapleural soft tissue mass. The lungs of the above two patients were clear and there were no other obvious hydatid cysts elsewhere in the body. **C** Hydatid cystic destruction and expansion of the right sixth rib with extension through the cortex and periosteum into the pleural cavity, producing large hydatid masses there. (Courtesy of Dr. Harold Jacobson) **D** A 57-year-old English sheep farmer who complained of cough, mucoid sputum, and pleuritic pain in the right chest of 9 months' duration. AP view of the chest (with reversed image) shows a multilocular, markedly expansile lesion involving the posterior right eighth rib. This large hydatid cyst produced pressure erosion of the right lateral border and right pedicle of T7. (Courtesy of Dr. K. Mendel and Dr. C. Evans and *Br J Radiol*, 1958, and Dr. Daniel Wilner, Boca Raton)

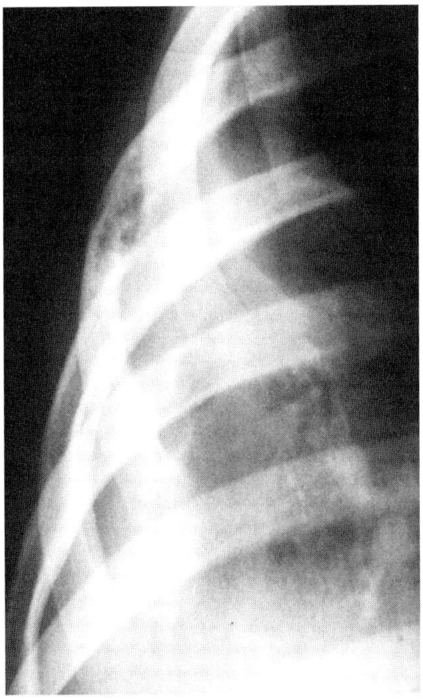

Fig. 3.147. Hydatid disease involving the lateral aspect of a rib with associated pleural extension

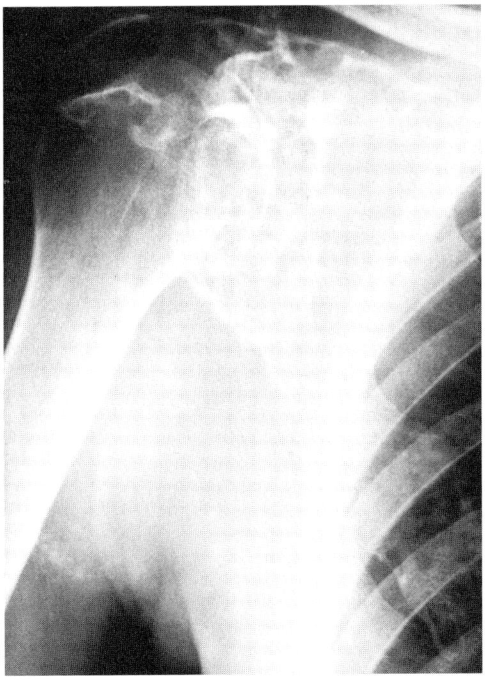

Fig. 3.148. Hydatid disease in the shoulder of a 69-year-old African. Virtually the entire scapula, including the glenoid fossa and acromion and coracoid processes, shows a bubbly cystic pattern of bone destruction with associated soft tissue mass and faint calcifications in the axilla. The head of the humerus is intact. (Courtesy of the University of Capetown Radiology Library)

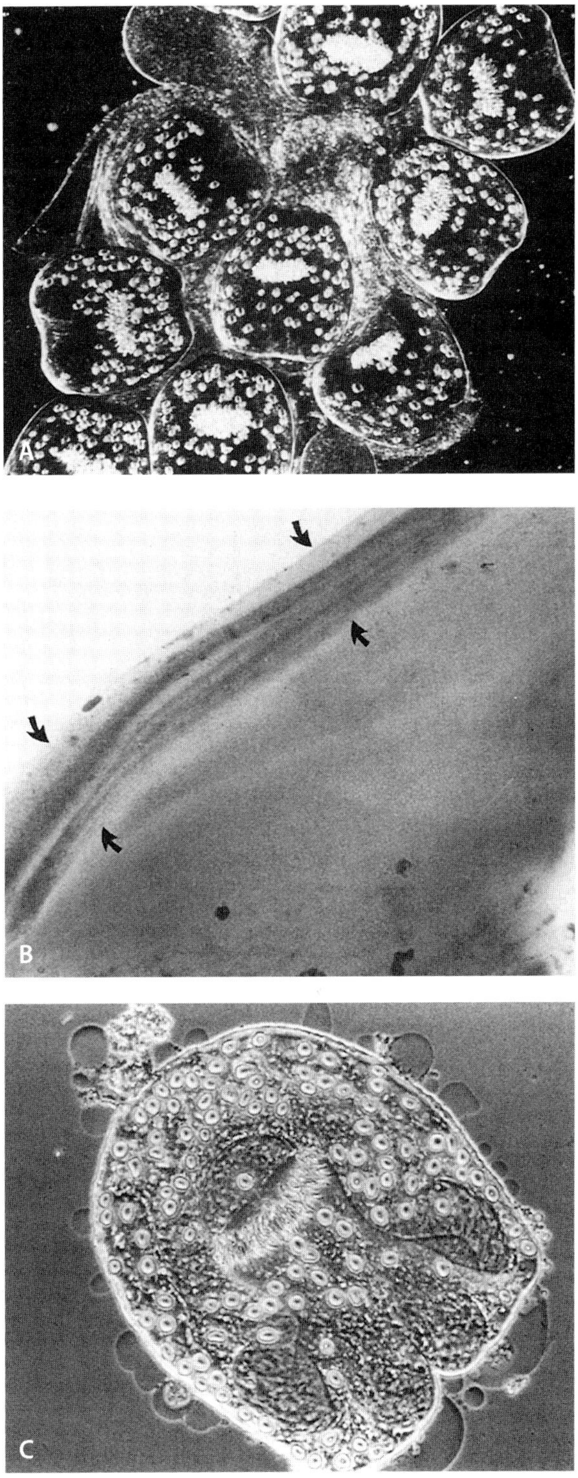

Fig. 3.149 A–C. Diagnostic parasitic material recovered by fine-needle aspiration biopsy (FNAB) from hydatid cysts. A A cluster of hydatid scolices. ×200. B Pieces of laminated parasitic membrane (*arrows*). H&E, ×200. C Fresh living embryo demonstrating invaginated head with crown of hooklets. ×300. (Courtesy of Dr. Walther von Sinner et al. and *Acta Radiol*, 1995)

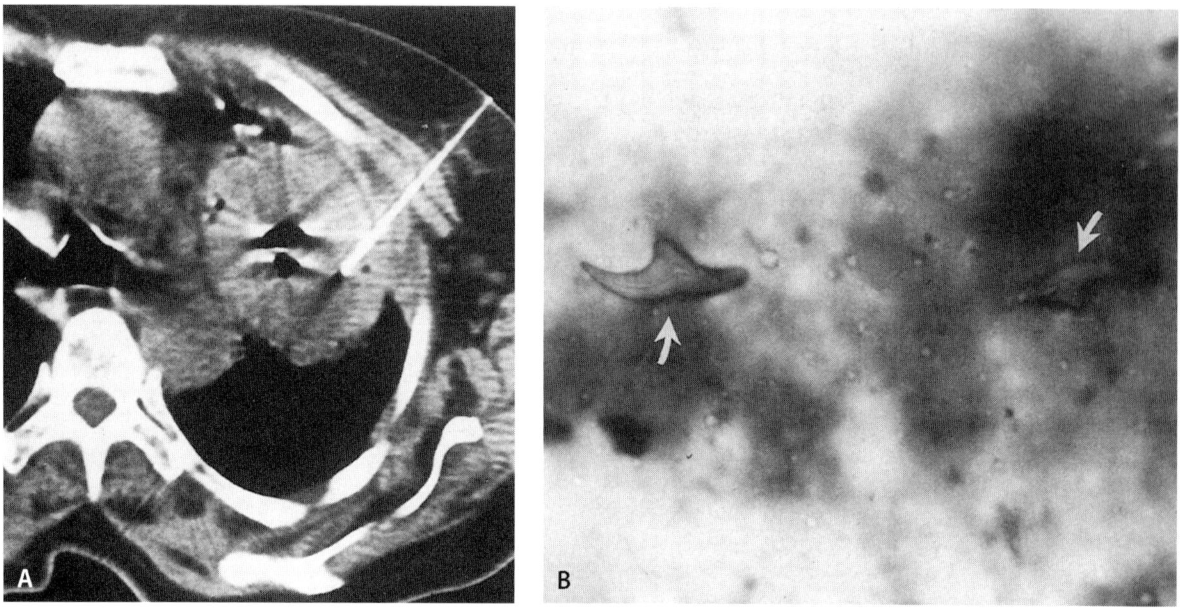

Fig. 3.150 A, B. A 55-year-old Saudi man admitted with mistaken diagnosis of bronchogenic carcinoma in the left upper lobe. **A** CT of chest during biopsy of the left upper lobe mass containing pockets of air. FNAB ×3 showed pus but no evidence of malignant cells, suggesting a lung abscess. **B** After a second look the FNAB sample revealed pathognomonic hooklets (*arrows*) for hydatid disease. H&E, ×300. (Courtesy of Dr. Walther von Sinner et al. and *Acta Radiol*, 1995)

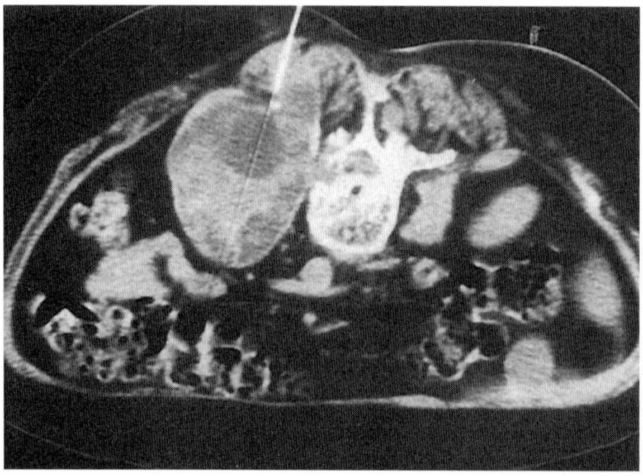

Fig. 3.151. A 50-year-old Saudi man with a mass destroying the lumbar spine with extension to the spinal canal and paravertebral area; the mass contains daughter cysts. FNAB showed hydatid material. (Courtesy of Dr. Walther von Sinner et al. and *Acta Radiol*, 1995)

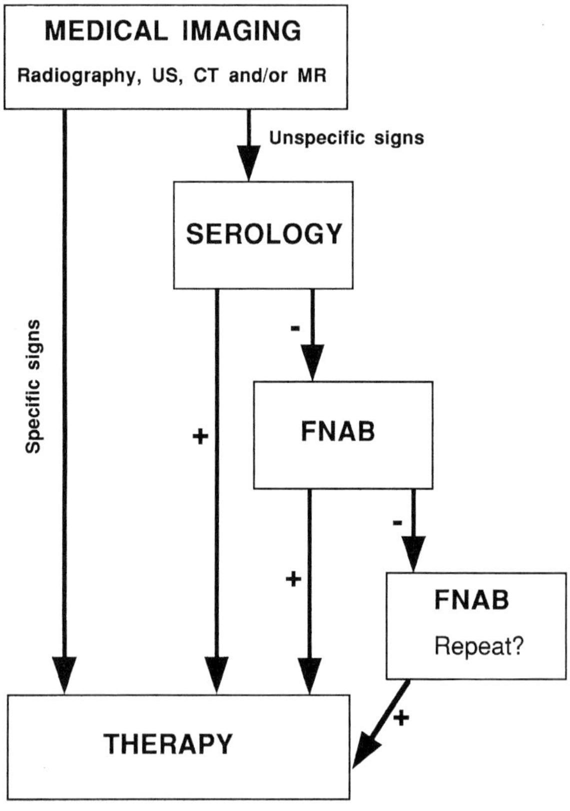

Fig. 3.152. Flow chart for the use of FNAB in suspected cystic hydatid disease. (Courtesy of Dr. Walther von Sinner et al. and *Acta Radiol*, 1995)

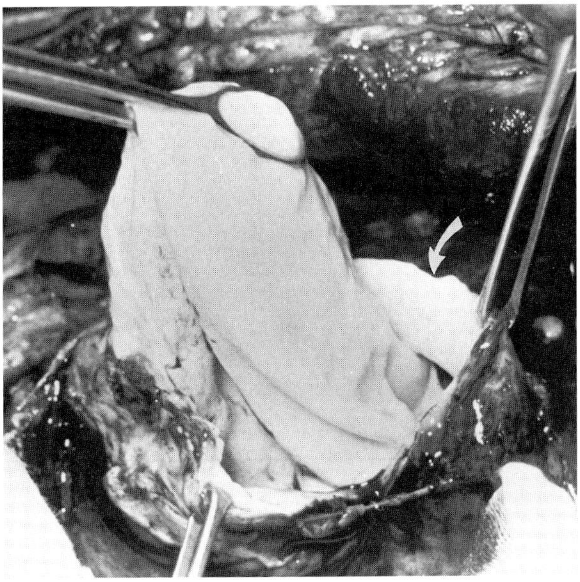

Fig. 3.153. Surgical removal of endocyst from the opened pericyst of a lung hydatid. The white endocyst is fragile and easily torn. When the surgeon opens the endocyst and hydatid fluid escapes, the endocyst falls away from the pericyst (*arrow*), as it does when a cyst ruptures. The surgeon must search for and oversew perforating bile ducts during endocystectomy of liver hydatids to prevent development of cystobiliary fistulas, but perforating bronchi in lung hydatids are usually not ligated. (Courtesy of Dr. Lewall)

When clinical findings, serology, and medical imaging are inconclusive, FNAB under the protection of antihelminthic prophylaxis should be considered to confirm the diagnosis. Ultrasonography- or CT-guided diagnostic cyst puncture (Figs. 3.150–3.151) should only be performed after other diagnostic methods have failed. The PAIR procedure consists in percutaneous puncture of cysts, aspiration of substantial amounts of cyst fluid, injection of protoscolicidal substances (such as 20% sodium chloride solution, cetrimide, or 95% ethanol) for a minimum of 15 minutes, and then reaspiration of the fluid cyst content. When properly performed by trained radiologists and physicians, PAIR has proven safe and effective; more than 500 favorable PAIR interventions have been reported with a 5-year follow-up period. The combination of risk, benefits, indications, and contraindications for surgery, chemotherapy, and the PAIR procedure are shown in Tables 3.4, 3.5, and 3.6, which are modified from WHO (1996) recommendations. Those of particular interest to radiologists can be summarized as follows:

The surgical complication rate postoperatively is 10%–25%. The operative mortality is probably less than 2%. The long-term recurrence rate after surgery is 2%–10%. Seroconversion (from positive to negative) after surgery usually occurs within 1 year but may take up to 4 years. When the infection recurs, the serology becomes positive again.

Table 3.4. Surgical aspects in the treatment of cystic echinococcosis (*E. granulosus*). (Courtesy of Dr. von Sinner and *Semin Roentgenol* 1997)

Indications	Contraindications	Choice of surgical technique	Choice of protoscolides	Concomitant drug treatment
Large, >10 cm diameter Single superficially situated liver cysts and potentially easy to rupture Infected cysts Cysts communicating with biliary tree Cysts exerting pressure on adjacent vital organs Some lung, brain, kidney cysts; spinal and bone cysts; and cysts in other organs and tissues	Inoperable cases Patients refusing surgery Patients at extremes of age Pregnant women Concomitant severe diseases Multiple cysts Difficult to access Dead cysts Very small cysts	Radical surgery Total pericystectomy Partial hepatectomy Conservative surgery Open cystectomy with or without omentoplasty Palliative surgery Simple tube drainage of infected cysts or communicating cysts	Effective with a relatively low risk of toxicity: 79% to 90% ethanol 15% to 20% hypertonic saline 0.5% cetrimide solution Potential communication with the biliary tree may cause chemical cholangitis leading to sclerosing cholangitis – do not use formalin Substances must be in contact with cysts ≥15 minutes	Preoperative chemotherapy with albendazole (ABZ) and mebendazole (MBZ) May be indicated to reduce risk of secondary echinococcosis Begin at least 4 days before surgery (ABZ) 1 month (MBZ) 3 months

Relates to the treatment of liver echinococcosis except where specifically indicated. Data from WHO (1996).

Table 3.5. Chemotherapeutic aspects in the treatment of cystic echinococcosis (*E. granulosus*). (Courtesy of Dr. von Sinner and *Semin Roentgenol* 1997)

Indications	Contraindications	Choice of antihelmintics	Benefits	Risks
Inoperable patients Primary liver or lung CE Patients with multiple CE Prevention of secondary echinococcosis Concomitant therapy recommended for PAIR	Large cysts with risk of rupture Inactive or calcified cysts Patients with chronic hepatic disease and bone marrow depression Early pregnancy	Albendazole (ABZ) Mebendazole (MBZ) Dosage: ABZ 10–15 mg/kg daily orally in several 1-month courses (up to 6 times) MBZ 40–50 mg/day orally for at least 3–6 months PZQ (praziquantel-isoquinaline derivative) – 40 mg/kg once a week, concomitantly with benzimidazoles	A noninvasive treatment Used in patients of any age Less limited by the patient's status (except pregnancy) than surgery	Adverse effects of benzimidazoles include: Hepatoxicity (transient increase of aminotransferase) Neutropenia Thrombocytopenia Alopecia

CE, cystic echinococcosis. Data from WHO (1996).

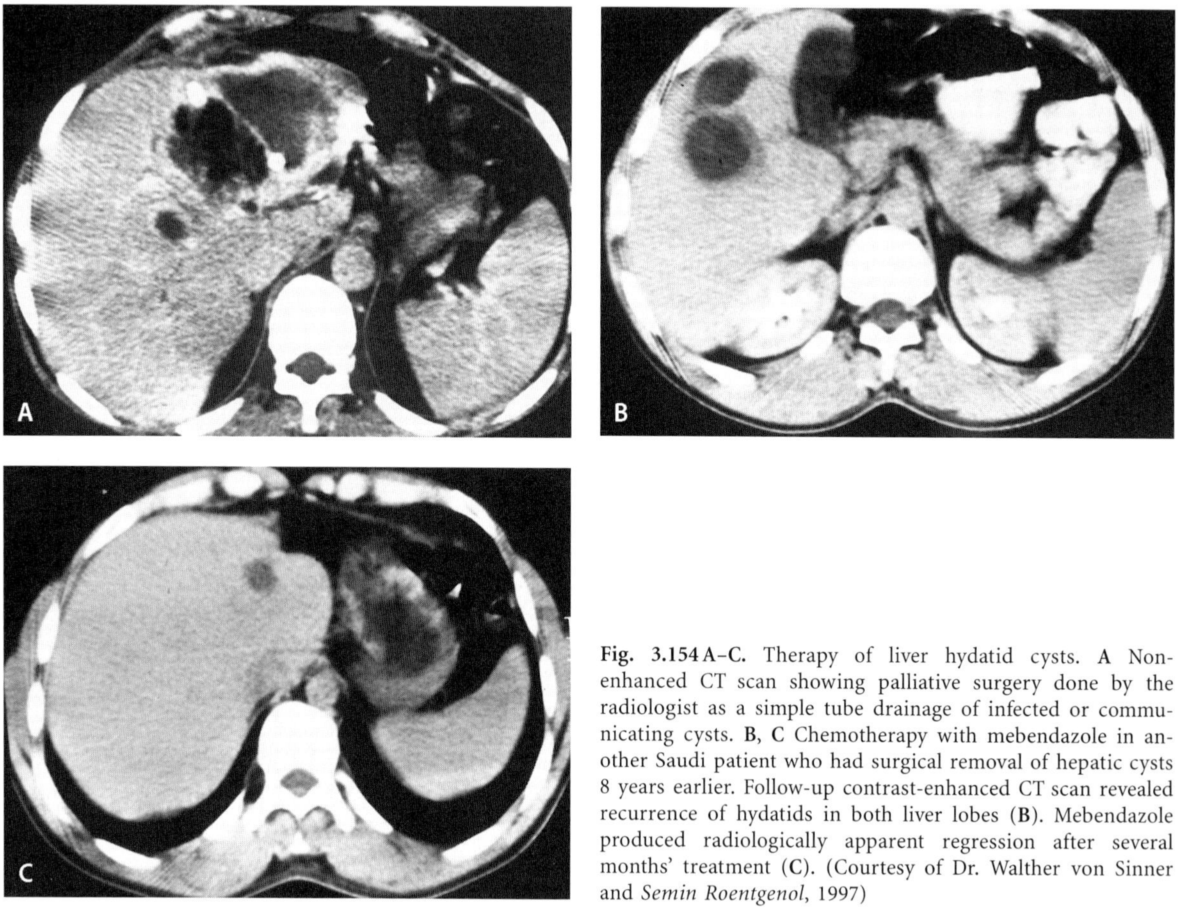

Fig. 3.154 A–C. Therapy of liver hydatid cysts. **A** Non-enhanced CT scan showing palliative surgery done by the radiologist as a simple tube drainage of infected or communicating cysts. **B, C** Chemotherapy with mebendazole in another Saudi patient who had surgical removal of hepatic cysts 8 years earlier. Follow-up contrast-enhanced CT scan revealed recurrence of hydatids in both liver lobes (**B**). Mebendazole produced radiologically apparent regression after several months' treatment (**C**). (Courtesy of Dr. Walther von Sinner and *Semin Roentgenol*, 1997)

Table 3.6. PAIR aspects in the treatment of cystic echinococcosis (*E. granulosus*). (Courtesy of Dr. von Sinner and *Semin Roentgenol* 1997)

Indications	Contraindications	Concomitant drug treatment	Benefits	Risks
Inoperable patients Patients who refuse surgery Cysts in the liver, abdominal cavity, spleen, kidney, and bones but not lung cysts Types of liver cysts: Anechoic lesions >5 cm diameter Cysts of types I and II (as classified by Gharbi et al.) Cysts with regular double laminated layer Cysts of >5 cm diameter with multiple septal division (Gharbi type III) except honeycomb-like cysts Multiple cysts 5 cm diameter in different liver segments (Gharbi types I, II, and III) Cases of relapse after surgery Failure to respond to chemotherapy Limited experience in pregnant women and children <3 years	Inaccessible or superficially located liver cysts (in the latter there is a risk of spillage of cyst content into abdominal cavity) Multiple septal divisions of cysts (honeycomb-like) Cysts with echogenic lesions Inactive cysts or calcified lesions Communicating cysts Lung cysts Aspirates should be analyzed for traces of bilirubin before injection of protoscolicides to avoid induction of chemical cholangitis Contamination with bile indicates direct communication with biliary ducts and a high risk of cholangitis after injection of protoscolicidal substances	Four days of treatment with benzimidazoles before PAIR is mandatory Albendazole at least 1 month or mebendazole 3 months after PAIR	Minimally invasive Less risky than surgery Confirms the diagnosis Removes a large number of protoscolices and antigens with aspirated cyst fluid Cost of PAIR and chemotherapy may be less than surgery, with fewer hospital days	Associated with any puncture: Hemorrhage Mechanical damage of other tissues Infections Anaphylactic shock or allergic reactions caused by leakage of cyst fluid Secondary echinococcosis due to spillage Other potential risks: Chemical sclerosing cholangitis Sudden intracystic decompression leading to biliary fistulas Persistence of satellite daughter cysts

Data from WHO (1996).

Drainage of type I cysts is gaining acceptance but it should be avoided if pericystic ducts are dilated (Figs. 3.22 and 3.154 A) because the inevitable communicating rupture may precipitate biliary obstruction. Even in the absence of visibly dilated ducts, aspirated fluid should be checked for bile and, as an additional precaution, a cystogram may be performed to ensure that the cyst does not communicate with the biliary tree. Communication is demonstrated more often at surgery than by noninvasive imaging, indicating that it is underdiagnosed preoperatively. Sclerosing solutions such as formalin or silver nitrate should never be injected into a liver cyst for fear of causing sclerosing cholangitis. Moreover, perforating bile ducts carry hypertonic saline to the gut, from where it is absorbed, causing hypernatremia and sometimes congestive heart failure. For this reason cetrimide has become the favored scolicidal agent in most, but not all, centers. Percutaneous drainage is not advisable if the cyst cannot be approached through normal parenchyma of the host organ or when the pericyst is insubstantial, because of the danger of direct rupture, dissemination, and anaphylaxis.

Purely medical treatment has been used occasionally when surgery is contraindicated or in widely disseminated disease, but the patient must be monitored closely because of the danger of communicat-

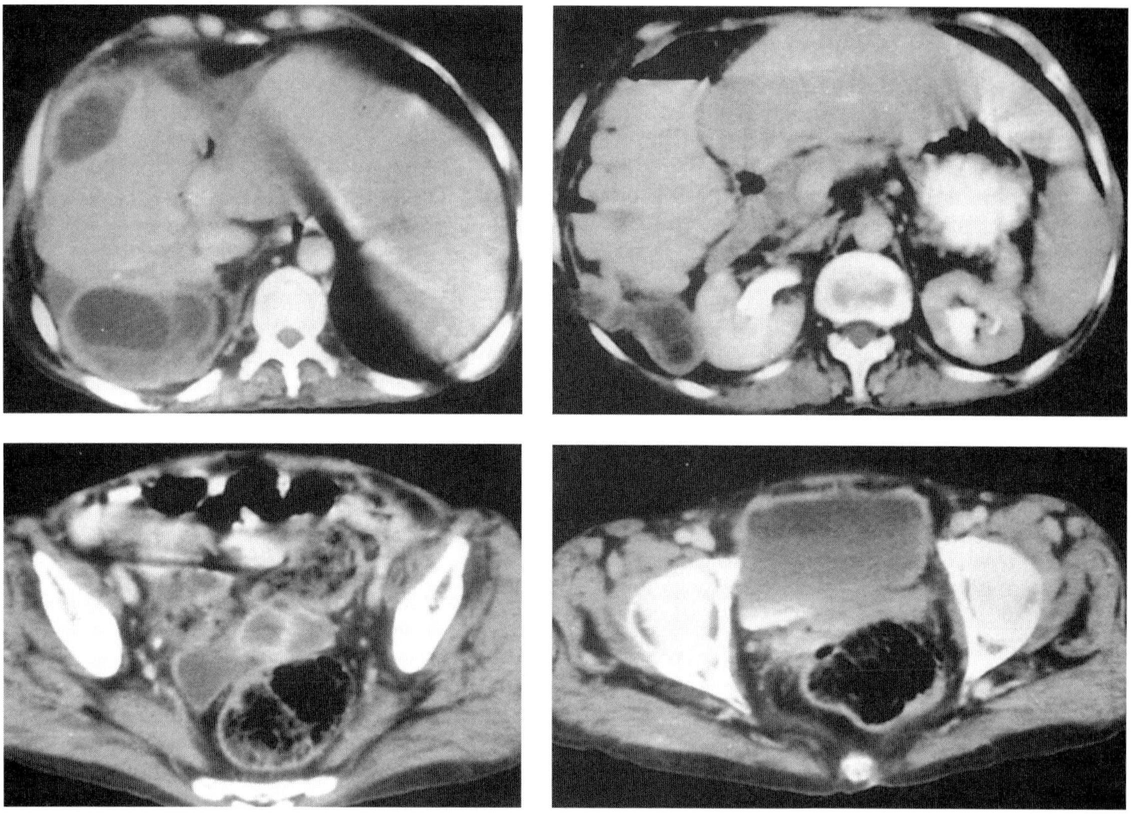

Fig. 3.155. Follow-up studies of the Saudi patient in Fig. 3.56 after surgery and chemotherapy. CT scans of the abdomen and pelvis 4 months after partial surgical resection and treatment with albendazole show marked improvement. Several remaining hydatid cysts are noted in the liver, abdomen, and pelvis. (Courtesy of Dr. Walther von Sinner)

ing or direct rupture. It is possible that direct rupture as a result of treatment of intraperitoneal and similar cysts may be a benign process since the ruptured cyst is probably sterile and the fluid probably has lost its antigenicity by the time of rupture. Furthermore, there is no danger of a biliary leak or bleeding after rupture of such lesions. This suggestion must, however, be tested in a controlled study before acceptance.

Evaluation of chemotherapy is gauged by the effectiveness of cyst response, as shown by ultrasonography, CT, MRI, and, in the chest in particular, conventional radiography. A successful response is disappearance or decrease in size of the cyst, or deformation and calcification of all cysts (Figs. 3.154 B, C, 3.155). A partially successful response is the above response in some but not all cysts, including increased density of cyst contents, hyperechoic structures, unsharpness of the cyst wall, collapsed parasitic membranes, or deformation of cysts and cyst wall with or without pericystic edema and calcification. An unsuccessful response is shown when there is no change in the appearance of cysts. Each cyst has to be evaluated separately.

Over 1000 well-documented cases of cystic hydatidosis have been treated with benzimidazoles (mebendazole and albendazole) as of 1997. After 12 months, 30% of patients show cyst disappearance (i.e., cure), 30%–50% show degeneration of cysts and/or significant size reduction (i.e., improvement), but 20%–40% exhibit no morphological changes in the cysts, indicating failure. Some of the treated patients suffer relapses, but these are sensitive to retreatment in a high proportion of cases (up to 90%). Local surgical drainage of cysts has also been successfully used (Fig. 3.154 A), but has largely been replaced by PAIR.

The PAIR method has been widely used by Italian groups and others in endemic areas in Africa, employing ultrasonography and serology (Echinostrip) for diagnosis. PAIR seems especially effective in developing countries where, in isolated areas, no equipment or facility for surgery exists, and ultrasonography combined with a simple technique of serology allows large-scale screening of populations without the need for a fully equipped laboratory. Nevertheless, PAIR should be performed only by experienced physicians and ideally with a surgical backup team prepared to deal with complications. PAIR treatment should be accompanied by chemotherapeutic coverage to minimize recurrence. However, further long-term, properly controlled studies are required to evaluate the efficacy and potential risks of this method.

Although hydatid disease is common, individual series are usually not large. For this reason an international medical hydatid registry employing uniform nomenclature and consistent reporting would be valuable for assessing the outcome of various forms of medical, surgical, and interventional management.

Polycystic Hydatid Disease (*E. vogeli* and *E. oligarthus*)

Polycystic hydatid disease is an infection caused by the larval stages of the tapeworm *Echinococcus vogeli* and, rarely, by *E. oligarthus*. *E. vogeli* infection is most common in rural areas of Panama, Ecuador, Colombia, Bolivia, Brazil, Argentina, Venezuela, and Costa Rica. It was first recorded in humans in Colombia in 1979. The first recorded human infection with *E. oligarthus* was an orbital cyst in a Venezuelan woman in 1989. *E. oligarthus* spreads further south than *E. vogeli*, as far as sub-Antarctica. Exact figures of incidence are perhaps unreliable because it is probable that some cases attributed to *E. oligarthus* were in fact first caused by *E. vogeli*.

The intermediate host is the paca (alpaca); this grazing mammal is one of the New World camels, many of which are domesticated. In one survey, 76% of pacas were infected with *E. vogeli*, and 3% with *E. oligarthus*. Domestic and bush dogs are hosts to *E. vogeli*, which together with *E. oligarthus* is also found in wildcats (ocelots, jaguar, puma). The life cycle of *E. vogeli* is similar to that of *E. granulosus*, but there are minor differences in size and particularly in the shape of the hooks. The larvae develop into relatively large fluid-filled cysts which are usually polycystic, unlike the unicysts of *E. granulosus*.

Polycystic hydatid disease is most common in the liver, followed by the lung, mesentery, spleen, and pancreas. Polycystic hydatid disease should be distinguished from a single cyst with multiple septa or daughter cysts, and from the many small grape-sized cysts of alveolar hydatid disease. Although they cannot be separated by serology, there is good reason to try to distinguish between *E. granulosus* and *E. vogeli* because the latter, the polycystic pattern, grows more rapidly and becomes clinically apparent sooner. *E. oligarthus* infection is very rare in humans, and has similar characteristics to *E. vogeli*.

Alveolar Hydatid Disease (*E. multilocularis*)

Alveolar hydatid disease is an infection caused by larval stages of the tapeworm, *Echinococcus multilocularis*. These larvae invade the infected organ, which in at least 90% of patients is the liver, and cause great destruction, resembling an infiltrating malignancy.

Geographic Distribution

This less common alveolar form of hydatid disease is seen chiefly in south central Europe in the area of the Alps, especially in France, Switzerland, Germany, and Austria, and throughout much of Russia and Siberia from the White Sea eastwards to the Bering Strait (Fig. 3.1). Other endemic areas in Asia extend from Turkey eastwards through Iran, Afghanistan, India, China, Mongolia, and northern Japan. In North America the parasite is present in subarctic Alaska and Canada, with recent expansion into several north central states of the United States. It has also been reported rarely from Australia, New Zealand, Argentina, Uruguay, and England.

Epidemiology and Pathology

Dogs, foxes, wolves, and cats are the usual definitive hosts for *E. multilocularis*, while field mice and other small rodents are the natural intermediate hosts (Figs. 3.2, 3.156). In the Arctic regions, especially among Eskimos, sled dogs are the usual source of human infection. In agricultural regions in central Europe and elsewhere, man may become infected by eating fruits or vegetables contaminated by the feces of foxes or other canines (Fig. 3.156), by handling contaminated soil, or by intimate association with infected dogs or cats.

For many years there was a controversy as to whether alveolar hydatid disease represented a separate entity. It was first described in 1855 as an "ulcerating multilocular hydatid of the liver." The larva of *E. multilocularis* is multiloculated rather than unilocular. Its growth is invasive and destructive, in part because the human host cannot develop an intact enveloping pericyst. This larva therefore behaves like a malignant neoplasm and is very difficult to eradicate surgically. The liver is the primary organ of involvement in over 90% of human infections. Larval growth is exogenous with spread by budding, and the affected tissue is honeycombed by the alveolar hydatid (Figs. 3.5, 3.157). Once the cystic mass has developed to a certain size, it undergoes central necrosis, forming an abscess-like cavity

(Text continues on p. 336)

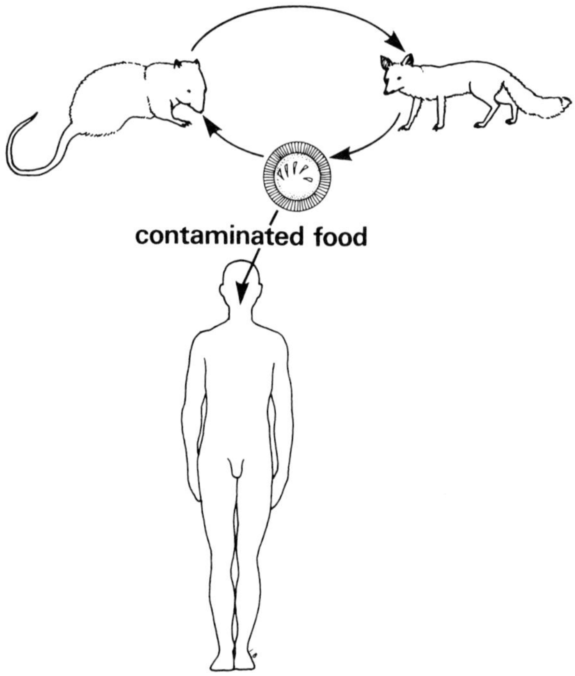

Fig. 3.156. Mode of transmission of *E. multilocularis* in agricultural regions in Central Europe and elsewhere. See also Fig. 3.2 for alternate modes of transmission of the parasite

Fig. 3.157 A–D. Alveolar or *E. multilocularis* hydatid disease of the liver. **A** Experimental infection in the liver of a muskrat. The multicystic nature of the parasite is well demonstrated in this formalin-fixed specimen. **B** *E. multilocularis* cyst in a gerbil liver. **C** *E. multilocularis* infection in a vole liver. Note the many cysts of the parasite. Numerous brood capsules and invaginated scolices are present. The small dark granules are calcareous bodies. **D** H&E-stained section from the liver of an Eskimo who died of *E. multilocularis* infection. The parasites appear as irregularly lined cystic spaces (*left and center*) with hepatic and inflammatory cells on the *right*. (**A**, **C**, **D** courtesy of R.L. Rausche) ▶

Fig. 3.158 A, B. Terminal alveolar hydatid disease in a cachectic woman from India. The abdomen is markedly protuberant from massive hepatomegaly and ascites. Generalized wasting of the patient is obvious. *E. multilocularis* is rarely seen in India, whereas *E. granulosus* infection is not uncommon. (Courtesy of Dr. A. Chandrahasan Johnson)

▼

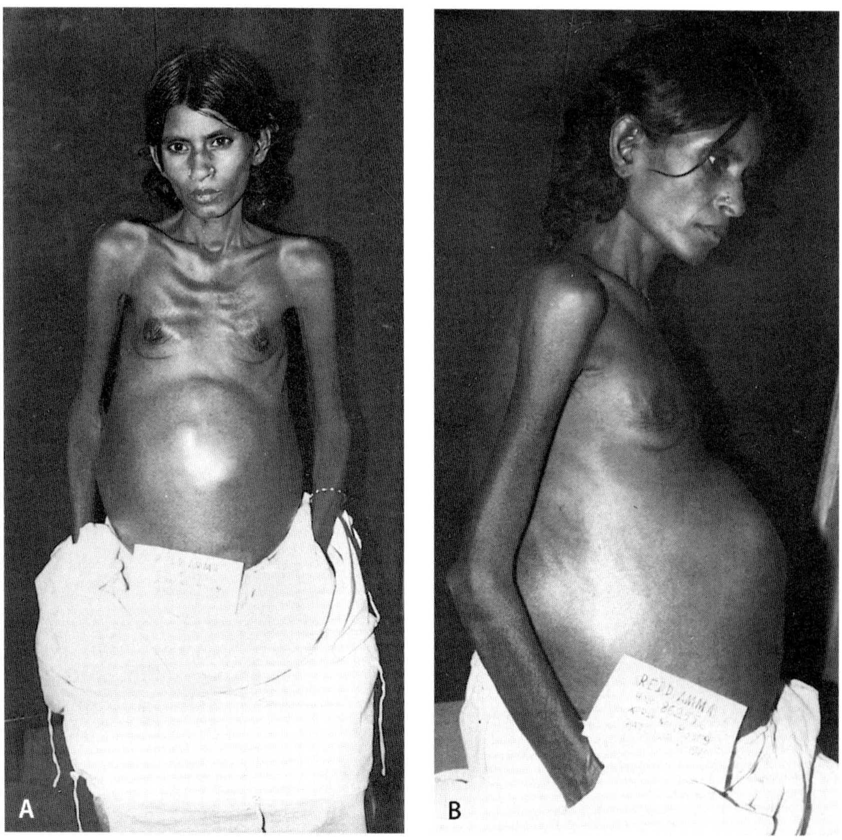

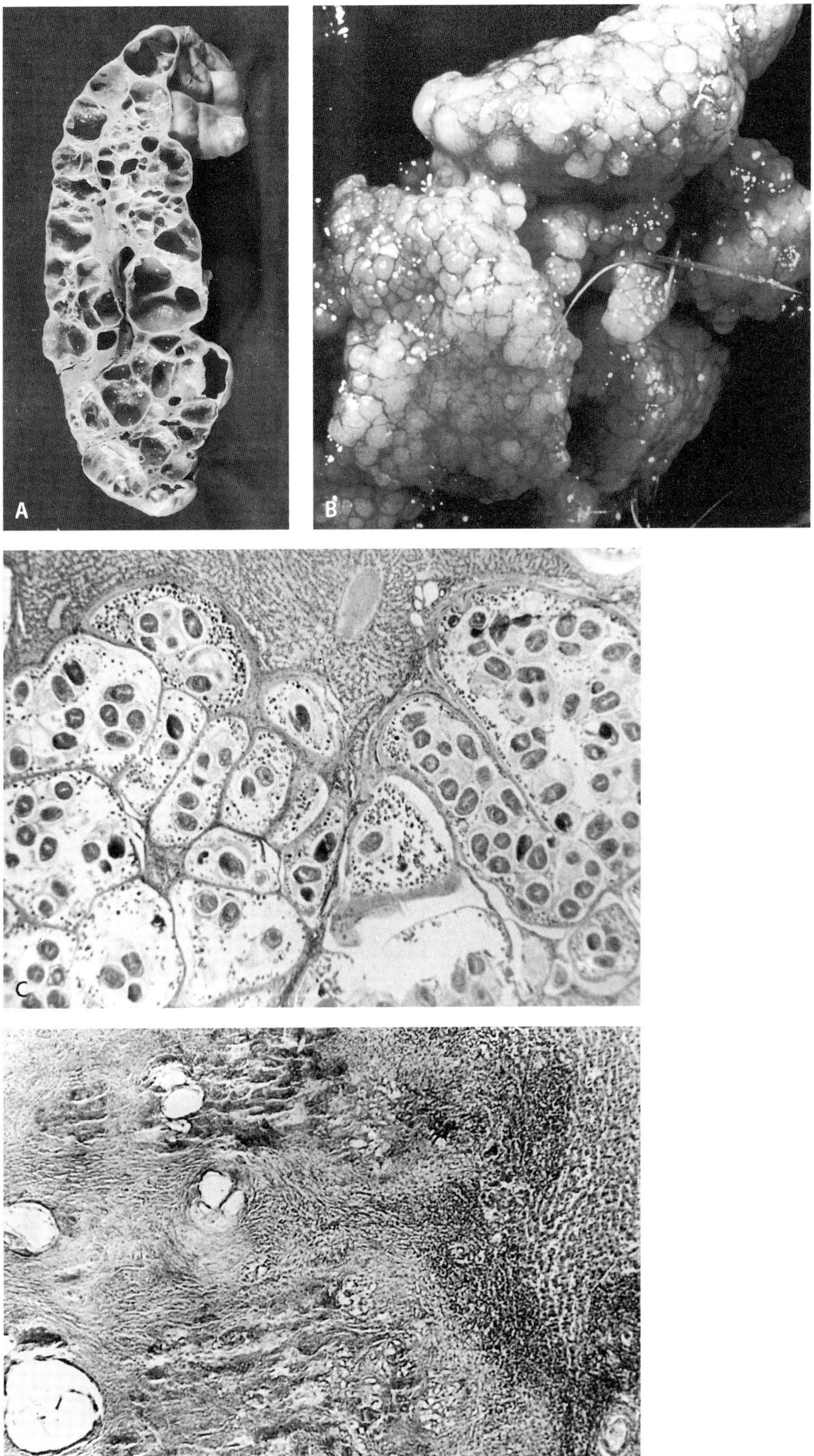
A
B
C
D

while the more peripheral cysts continue to multiply. The infection may spread by direct extension to adjacent organs and lymph nodes or hematogenously to produce metastatic foci in the lungs or distant organs.

Although the disease runs a chronic, afebrile course in most patients, the outcome is usually fatal. The patient will have hepatomegaly, with clinical signs of an enlarging mass within the liver, and portal hypertension, splenomegaly, jaundice, and ascites (Fig. 3.158). It is usually very difficult to distinguish clinically between alveolar hydatid disease and carcinoma of the liver. The diagnosis is established by histological examination of biopsy specimens, although radiographic examination may be quite helpful when the peculiar calcifications seen in the majority of cases of alveolar hydatidosis are present.

Imaging Diagnosis

The chronic granulomatous reaction which occurs in alveolar hydatid disease of the liver, with central necrosis and cavitation, may eventually result in characteristic calcifications. In 19 patients with alveolar hydatidosis from Alaska (Thompson et al.), there was hepatomegaly in 42% and hepatic calcifications in 68%. Typically, the latter are small spheres with central radiolucencies and range from 2 to 4 mm in diameter (Figs. 3.159–3.163).

As with the more common unilocular cystic hydatid disease, there are many different ways to image alveolar cystic lesions in the liver. Ultrasonography, CT, MRI, and radionuclide scanning can be supplemented by selective hepatic or celiac arteriography, inferior vena cavography, and cholangiography. Each modality has a selected diagnostic role.

Scanning (ultrasonography, CT, or MRI) is the most effective way to identify the one or more masses which may develop within any part of the liver. As the lesions grow older, the wall thickens and a necrotic center develops, filled with debris. All methods of scanning may show displacement of the common bile duct and/or the right and left hepatic ducts and their branches within the liver caused by one or more alveolar hydatid masses (Figs. 3.162, 3.163). Since these lesions are often of considerable size, the displacement of the biliary duct system may be pronounced. Contrast medium may leak during cholangiography from the bile ducts into a large necrotic lesion, partially outlining its ragged interior (Figs. 3.162, 3.163).

Fig. 3.159 A–F. *E. multilocularis* calcifications in the liver of an asymptomatic 42-year-old Alaskan Eskimo woman who had skinned many foxes; there were also many dogs in her village. Except for occasional postprandial epigastric discomfort, she was otherwise asymptomatic. She had a diffusely nodular and slightly tender liver palpable 5 cm below the right costal margin. There was an 8% blood eosinophilia. *Echinococcus* hemagglutination and flocculation titers were strongly positive. **A** AP radiograph of the right upper quadrant shows the characteristic small radiolucencies surrounded by calcification, forming spheres measuring 2–4 mm in diameter (*arrow*). These calcifications were visible on a lumbosacral spine radiograph taken 4 years earlier and had increased in size in the interval. A radioisotope liver scan showed a large area of decreased uptake anteriorly in the region of the porta hepatis. Cholelithiasis was noted on oral cholecystogram and the calcified mass was anterior to the gallbladder. Hepatic arteriography showed an anterior avascular mass in the liver, possibly involving both lobes. At cholecystectomy, a pedunculated hydatid lesion was attached to the anterior inferior edge of the liver involving the right and left lobes without extensive parenchymal invasion in the bulk of the liver. **B** A radiograph of the surgically resected specimen showed both scattered, amorphous, nondiagnostic calcium and the small radiolucencies surrounded by calcium thought to be diagnostic of alveolar hydatid disease (*arrow*). The resected hepatic tissue measured 10×8×8 cm and was virtually replaced by a large cyst with a thick irregular wall. At the periphery of this large cyst, there were multiple small cysts 5–6 mm in diameter, many of which budded from the wall of the large cyst while some were discrete within the adjacent liver parenchyma. The large cyst was filled with thick, white, pasty material and contained translucent membranes, forming small 2-to 4-mm translucent spheres. The small peripheral cysts were lined by such membranes and many contained clear fluid. **C** Section of the resected hydatid lesion showing necrotic, diffusely stippled (with finely divided calcium), amorphous material (center of lesion) containing pale eosinophilic, laminated membranes which were acellular, PAS positive, and diastase resistant. The small peripheral cysts (bottom of lesion) were also lined by laminated membranes and surrounded by fibrous walls, which were separated from the liver parenchyma by a thin rim of granulation tissue and inflammatory cells. The calcification associated with these small cysts was primarily between the parasitic membranes and the adjacent fibrous wall, both as finely divided calcium and as somewhat larger granules. Focally, there were small calcific deposits between laminae of the parasitic membrane. There were also granulomas with necrotic centers surrounded by epithelioid cells, giant cells, and other inflammatory cells. No germinal epithelium or scolices were identified. **D** Enlargement of the cysts at the periphery of the multilocular lesion. **E** Photomicrograph showing a portion of one cyst with the cyst wall (*right*) and surrounding reactive tissue (*center*). Several liver cells are seen (*lower left*). H&E, ×45. (**A–E** courtesy of Dr. W. Thompson et al and *AJR*, 1972.) **F** Gross photograph of liver of another patient with alveolar hydatidosis, showing multiple cysts on the cut surface. (Courtesy of Drs. R.L. Rausch and Daniel H. Connor)

(Text continues on p. 341)

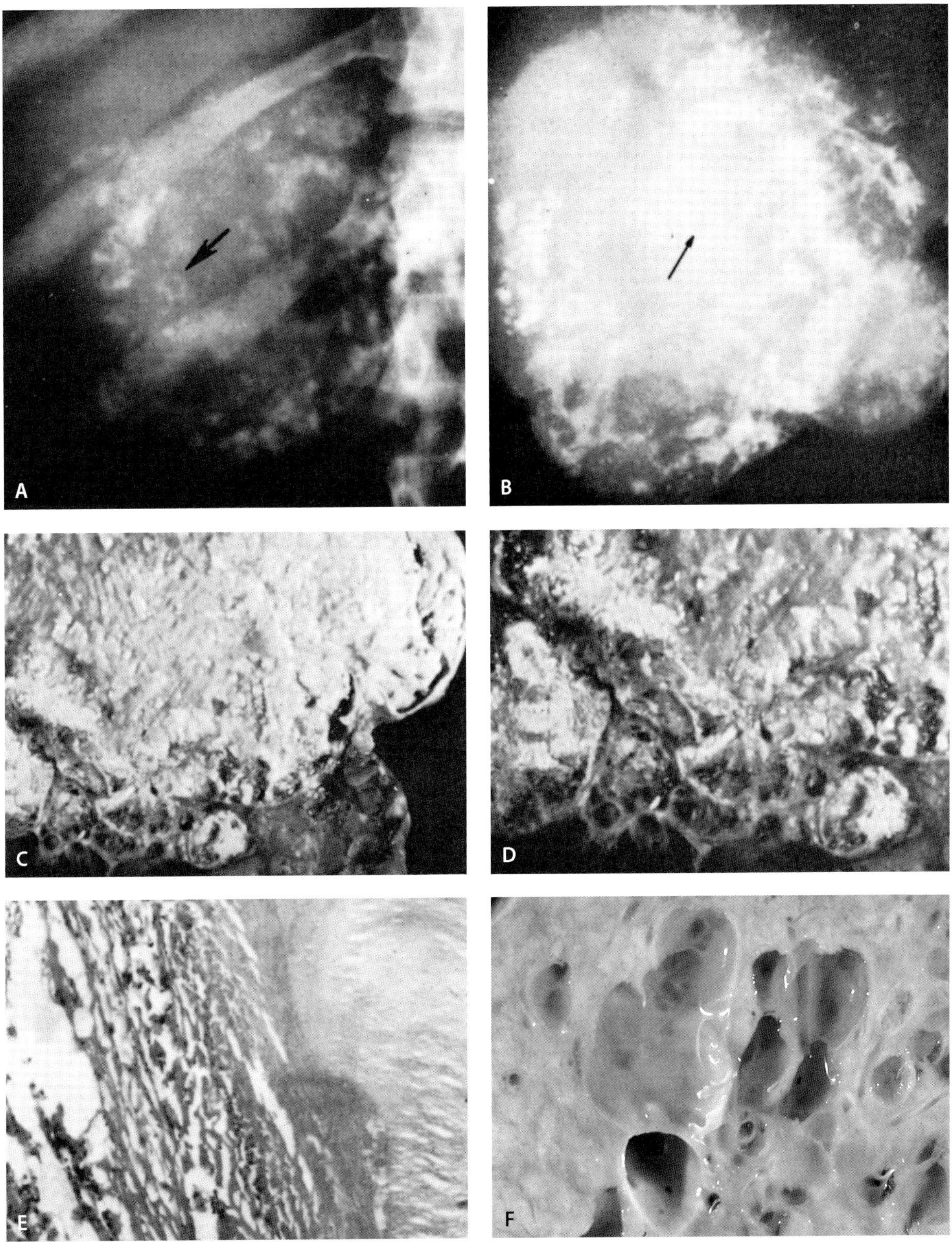
A
B
C
D
E
F

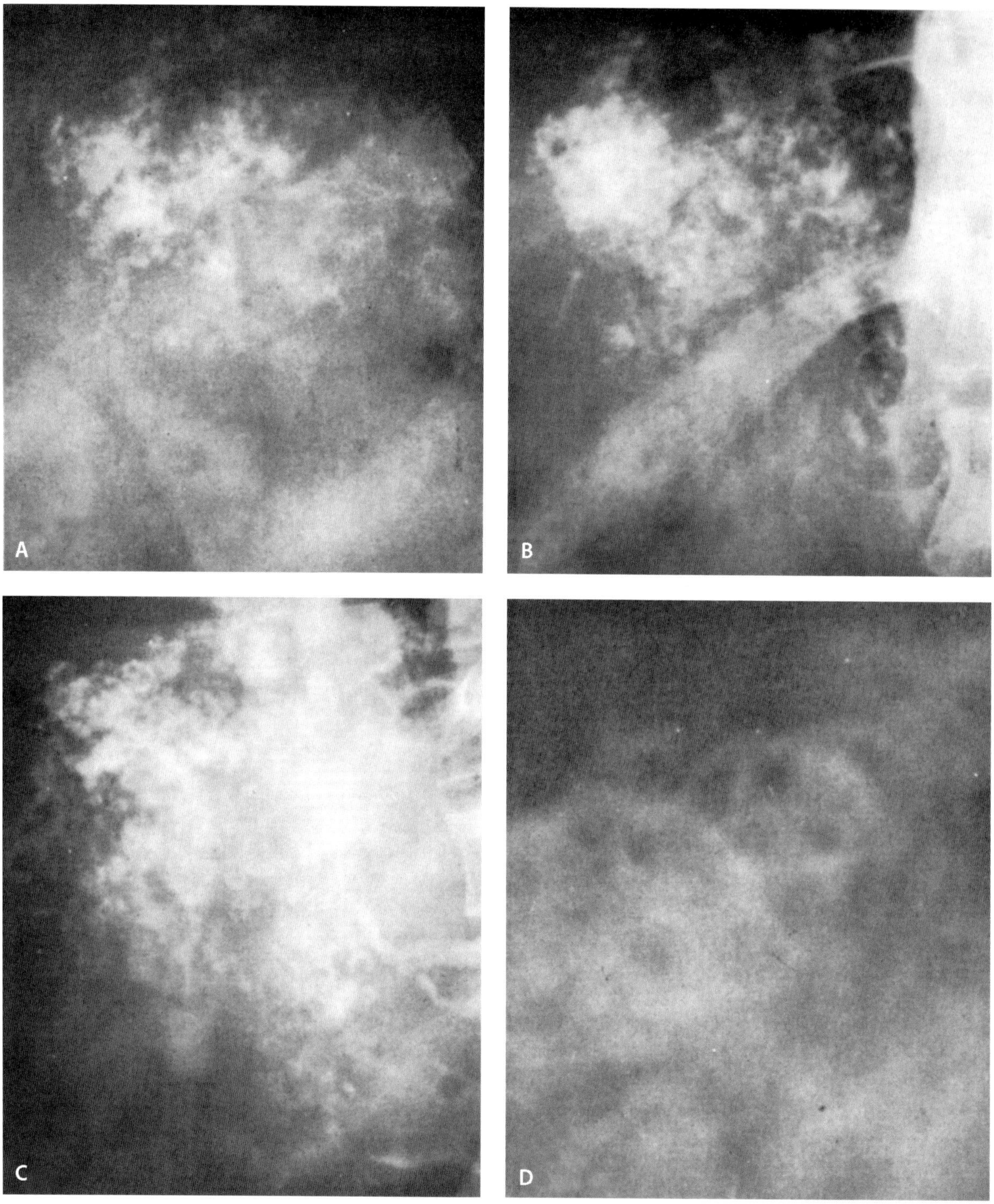

Fig. 3.160 A–D. Typical *E. multilocularis* calcifications in the liver of a patient with surgically proven alveolar hydatid disease. **A** Oblique radiograph of the right upper quadrant. **B** The calcifications have shown some increase in extent 6 years later. **C** After another 6 years there is further increase in the amount of calcification. **D** Enlargement of an area in **C** shows numerous small radiolucencies surrounded by calcification, a finding felt to be diagnostic of alveolar hydatid disease. (Courtesy of Dr. William Thompson et al. and *AJR*, 1972)

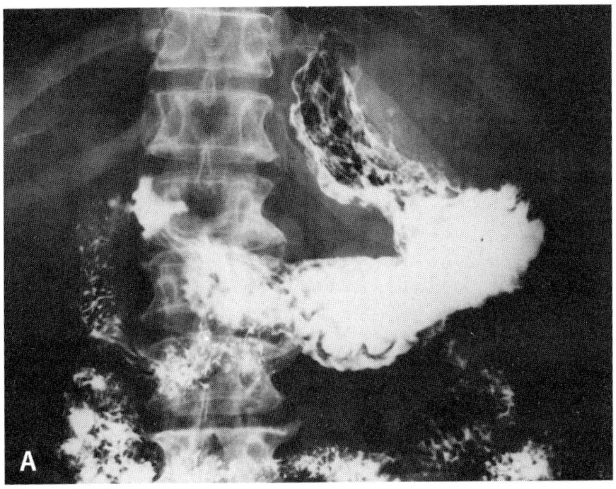

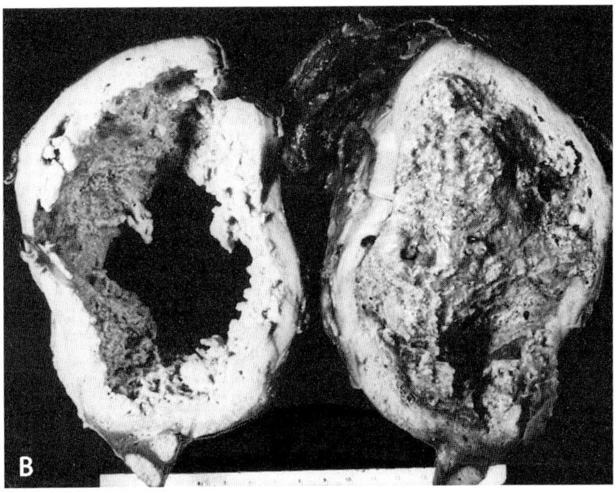

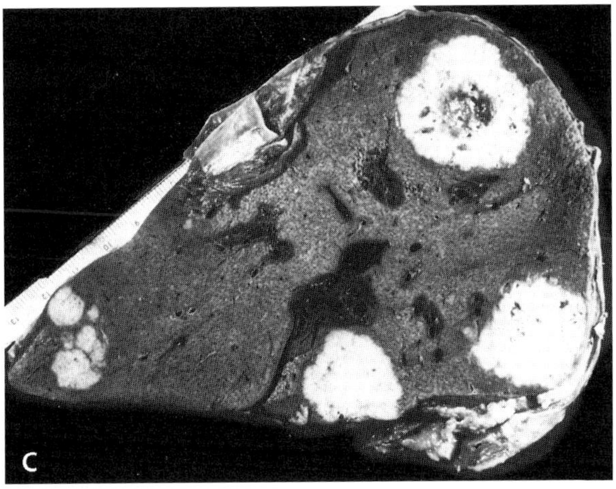

Fig. 3.161 A–C. Alveolar hydatid disease involving both lobes of the liver in a 61-year-old Eskimo woman from northwestern Alaska. She was admitted to the hospital in 1970 for the fifth time for neurological evaluation. Six weeks previously, she had an episode of clouded sensorium and bizarre behavior but returned to normal in a few days. Later she experienced a grand mal seizure. In 1960, she had a presumptive diagnosis of alveolar hydatid disease made at laparotomy: prior echinococcal titers had been positive. Upper gastrointestinal series in 1965 and 1968 showed enlargement of the left lobe of the liver and calcifications in both lobes (**A**). Radioisotope liver scans showed hepatomegaly with gross enlargement of the left lobe, in which there was a large mass with a central area of diminished uptake. When admitted, she was cachectic but oriented. She had a mild fever of 100° F and slight lateral nystagmus and ataxia. The liver was enlarged, chiefly in the epigastrium, but was not tender. The albumin-globulin ratio was reversed at 3.2:4.5 mg/ml. Echinococcal hemagglutination and flocculation titers were 1:4096 and 1:320, respectively. Several lumbar punctures revealed normal pressures, 550–2500 white blood cells per mm^3, of which 80% were lymphocytes, and protein which increased from 430 to 730 mg/100 ml. A pneumoencephalogram showed atrophy of cortical tissue and enlargement of the lateral ventricles and basilar cisterns. The fourth ventricle was not demonstrated. She had been on triple tuberculosis chemotherapy and steroids, but she gradually deteriorated and terminally developed left third, fourth, and seventh cranial nerve palsies. At autopsy, the liver was markedly enlarged and the entire left lobe was replaced by a large cyst with a white fibrous wall 2–3 cm thick, lined by shaggy, yellow material, and with a large necrotic center (**B**). Hemisection of the right lobe of the liver revealed numerous white, somewhat lobulated, gritty nodules measuring 1–5 cm in diameter, one of which showed a necrotic center (**C**). A tumor-like mass was found in the left cerebellar-pontine angle and a similar lesion extended around the brain stem, deforming the midbrain and pons. These lesions resembled those in the liver and histologically showed the characteristic features of alveolar hydatid disease. (Courtesy of Dr. William Thompson et al. and *AJR*, 1972)

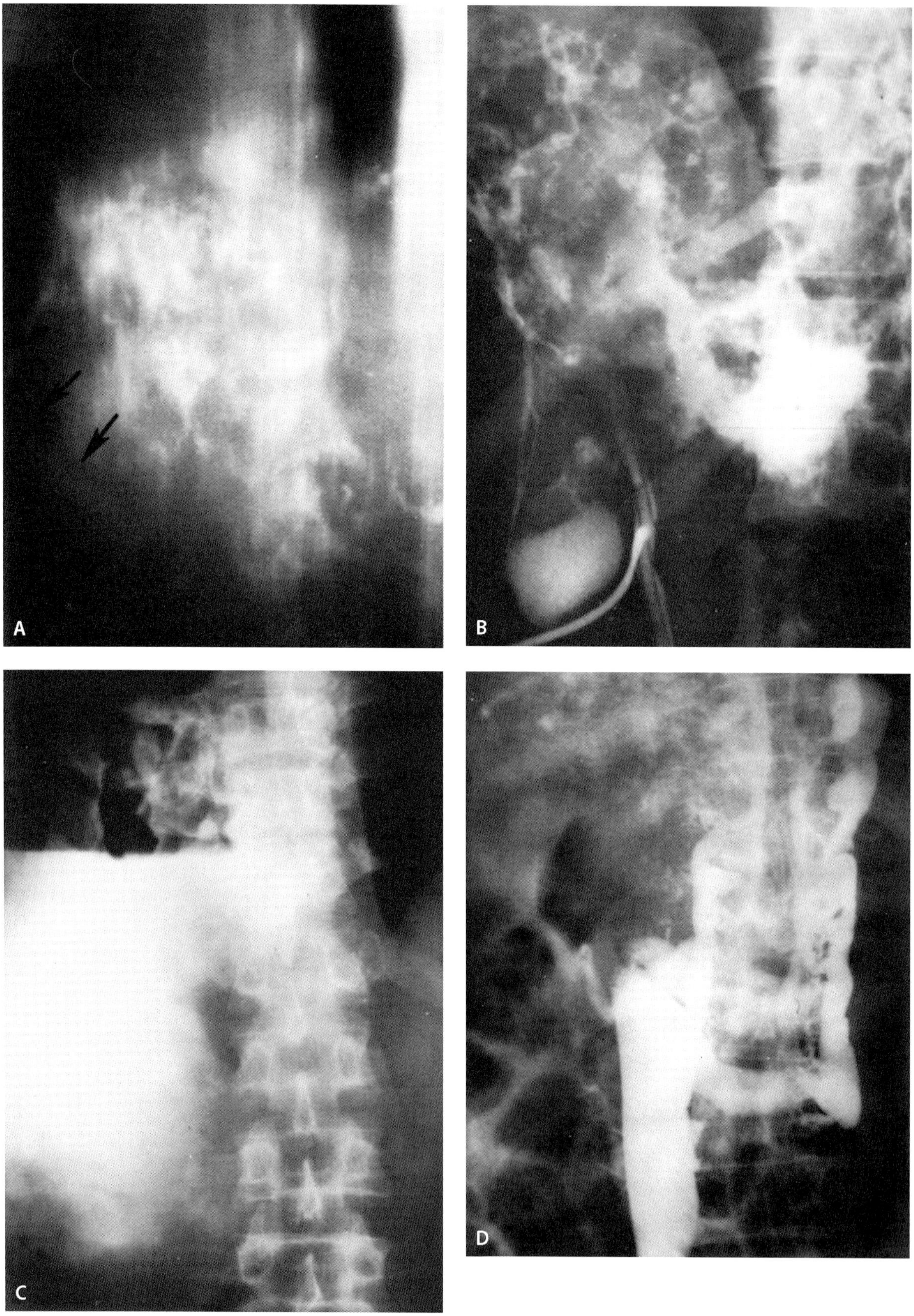
A
B
C
D

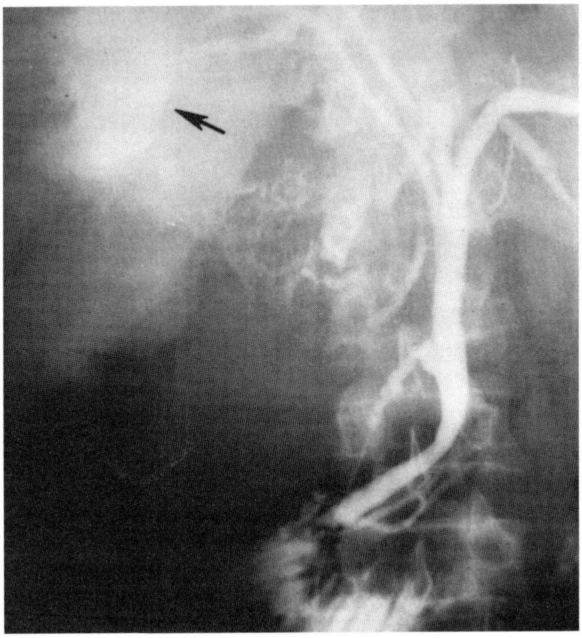

Fig. 3.163. Cholangiogram showing marked displacement of the common bile duct and right hepatic ducts towards the midline by a huge alveolar cystic lesion of the liver in an Eskimo. Some of the contrast medium has entered the necrotic lesion (*arrow*) via a branch from the right hepatic duct. The cystic duct and pancreatic ducts are well outlined. A few bizarre ring-like and irregular calcifications are seen within a portion of the liver lesion just to the right of the patient's midline (*center of photo*). (Courtesy of Dr. William Thompson et al. and *AJR*, 1972)

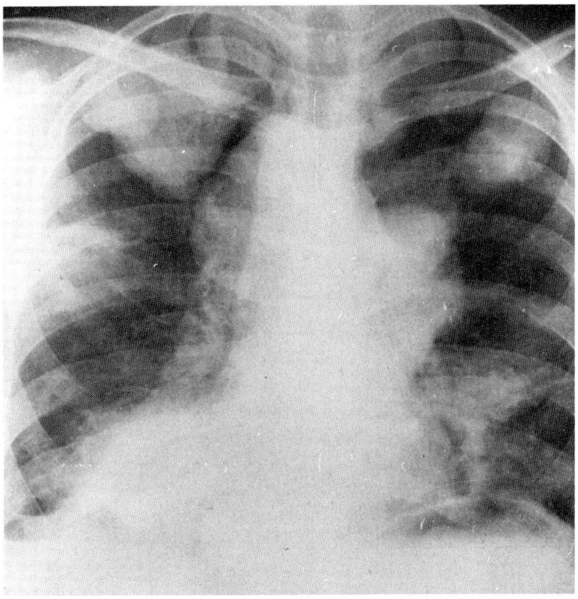

Fig. 3.164. Multiple large hydatid cysts of varying sizes and shapes throughout both lungs and the mediastinum in a patient from India. The appearance resembles metastatic neoplasm, but these were in fact metastatic hydatids. Air is present within several cysts that have ruptured, especially at the lung bases, and there are several air-fluid levels in the right lower hemithorax. Several of these masses have indistinct, irregular margins, suggesting infiltration into the surrounding lung, or pneumonitis adjacent to the lesions. Although *E. granulosus* infection is by far the most common form of hydatid disease in India, this reportedly was a fatal case due to *E. multilocularis*

◀ **Fig. 3.162 A–D.** Huge necrotic alveolar hydatid lesion in the liver of an Alaskan Eskimo who died from hepatic failure 6 months after these studies. **A** Tomogram of the right upper quadrant during an intravenous cholangiogram shows diffuse irregular calcifications within a huge mass in the midline of the liver which is displacing the common bile duct laterally (*arrows*). **B** A T-tube cholangiogram shows contrast medium has leaked from one of the hepatic ducts into this extensively necrotic, irregular, cystic lesion of the liver. Several branches of the right hepatic duct are filled, as well as the cystic duct and gallbladder (*lower left*). **C** An erect radiograph of the upper abdomen shows a prominent air-contrast level within this large lesion which has replaced most of the right lobe of the liver. The air above the contrast level shows the irregular necrotic nature of the lesion to good advantage. The right hemidiaphragm is markedly elevated. **D** An inferior vena cavogram shows complete obstruction of the inferior vena cava at the L2 level with collateral flow through dilated azygos, hemiazygos, and lumbar veins. The irregular calcifications typical of *E. multilocularis* infection are again identified within the large liver lesion, which had extended posteriorly to block the vena cava. (Courtesy of Dr. William Thompson et al. and *AJR*, 1972)

Selective arteriography will likely show displacement of the hepatic artery branches around one or more avascular, often irregular filling defects in the liver; abrupt narrowing and cut-offs of arteries can be seen due to the diffuse infiltrating process. An inferior vena cavogram may reveal partial or complete obstruction of the inferior vena cava with collateral circulation via the azygos, hemiazygos, and lumbar venous plexus, if the liver mass has extended posteriorly or metastasized to regional lymph nodes, blocking the vena cava (Fig. 3.162 D). While the liver is the primary and most often involved organ (99%), hematogenous dissemination may occur to other organs such as lungs (Fig. 3.164), brain, and bone in up to 5% of patients. Liver lesions vary from minor foci to large areas of infiltration of 15–20 cm diameter or more. Any part of the liver may be infiltrated.

In most countries, ultrasonography will be the primary imaging tool for diagnosing hepatic alveolar echinococcosis (Figs. 3.165–3.168). Weill has described in detail the sonographic findings, noting

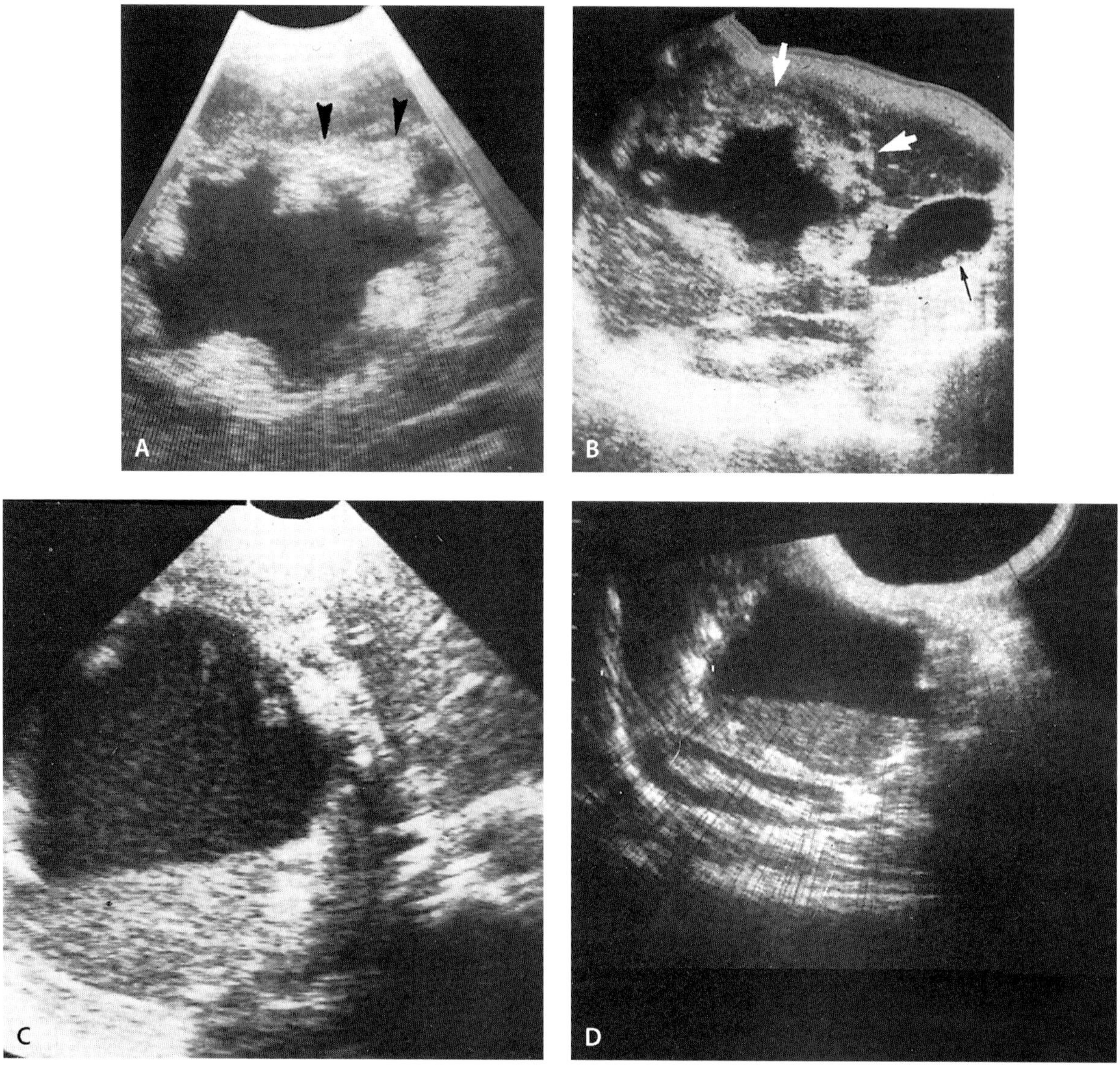

Fig. 3.165 A–D. Sonograms of hepatic alveolar echinococcosis. **A** A right coronal section and **B** a sagittal section show the typical massive necrosis of the large irregularly marginated lesion with shaggy borders and abnormal adjacent parenchyma (*arrowheads and arrows*). **C, D** A second patient with marked necrosis of a huge lesion with dependent debris within the cavity and heterogeneous hyperechoic areas bordering the cavity. (From Weill 1990)

that necrosis and resulting cyst formation occur in 30% of patients. The necrotic debris, when present, causes a heterogeneous appearance; the lesions are usually much more irregular than those of cystic hydatid disease caused by *E. granulosus* and do not have a well-defined wall (Figs. 3.165, 3.166). The multiple cystic complexes are surrounded by abnormal hepatic parenchyma and their outlines are often craggy, so that they may simulate the snowstorm or complex pattern of metastatic disease. Scattered hyperechoic foci are often the result of calcifications, better seen with plain films or CT scanning. The infiltrating character of the disease causes postobstructive dilatation of multiple biliary ducts (Figs. 3.166, 3.167) as well as narrowing of portal and hepatic veins and, at times, the inferior vena cava (Fig. 3.168), all of which can lead to jaundice and portal hypertension which may require liver transplantation, if available.

The principal sonographic signs of alveolar hydatid disease elaborated by Weill are as follows:

- Hepatomegaly
- Hyperechoic foci
- Calcifications
- Cystic, often craggy, necrosis
- Dilatation of the biliary tree
- Deformity and narrowing of portal and hepatic veins

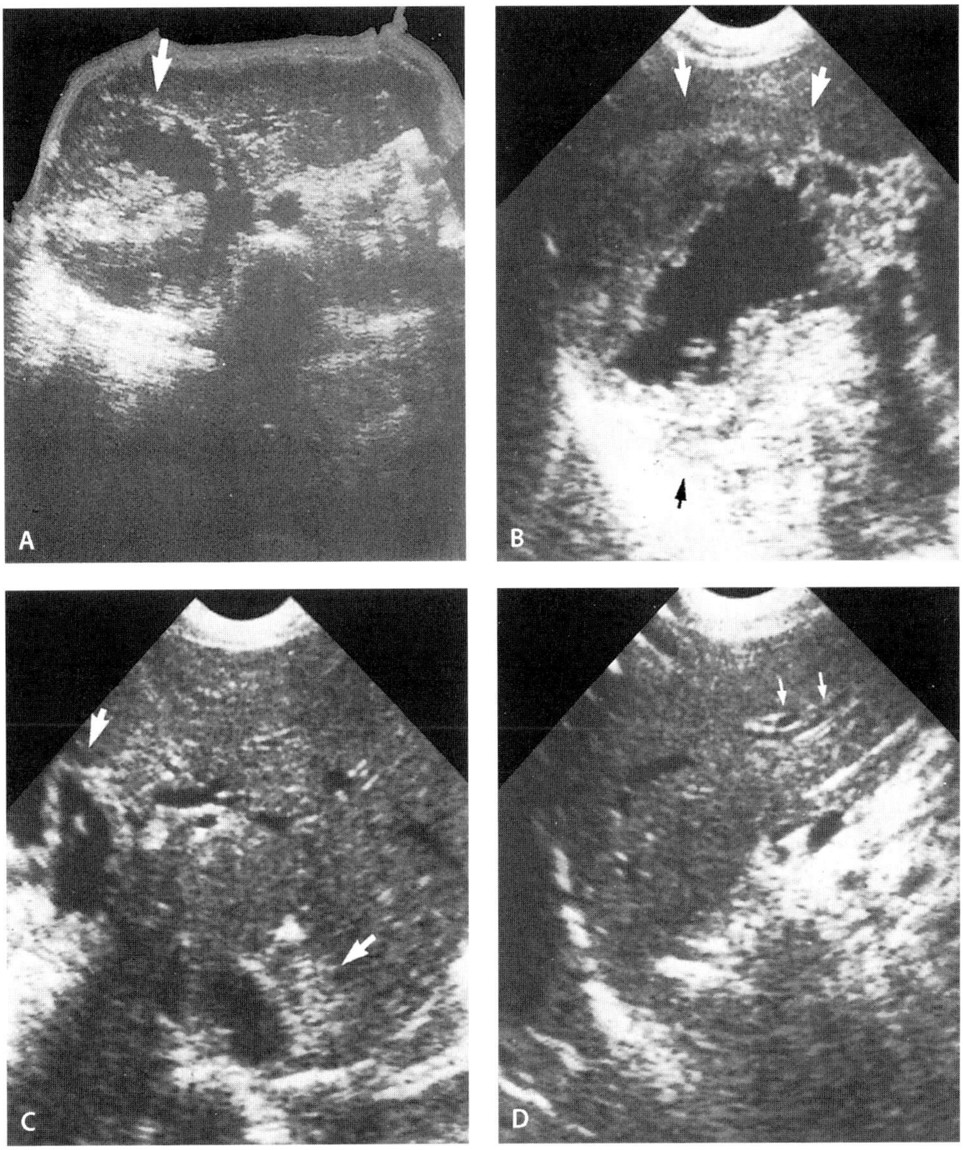

Fig. 3.166 A–D. Hepatic alveolar echinococcosis. **A** Transverse sonogram shows a huge, partially necrosed lesion of the right liver lobe (*arrow*). **B, C** Oblique and sagittal sections reveal the complex heterogeneous, often hyperechoic nature of the lesions near the dome of the liver (*arrow*). **D** Sagittal section of the left lobe shows localized dilatation of bile ducts (*arrows*). (From Weill 1990)

The following CT findings and staging of hepatic alveolar echinococcosis, adapted from Rozanes et al. (1995) (Fig. 3.169), correlate well with the surgical findings and seem to be useful for therapeutic planning.

Stage 1: Lesion measuring less than 3 cm in diameter
Stage 2: Lesion greater than 3 cm, confined to less than three hepatic segments
Stage 3 a: Lesion with invasion of more than three hepatic segments
Stage 3 b: Invasion of the liver hilum or suprahepatic vena cava
Stage 4: Invasion of surrounding organs and/or distant metastases

As noted above, the ultrasound and CT findings of hepatic alveolar hydatidosis include hepatomegaly and heterogeneous geographic invading lesions with irregular margins. On contrast-enhanced CT, these present as low-density masses which may be combined with amorphous or nodular calcifications (Fig. 3.169). This pattern may suggest alveolar hydatidosis rather than hepatocellular carcinoma, but biopsy of the lesions is often required to exclude hepatic malignancy: no complications have been re-

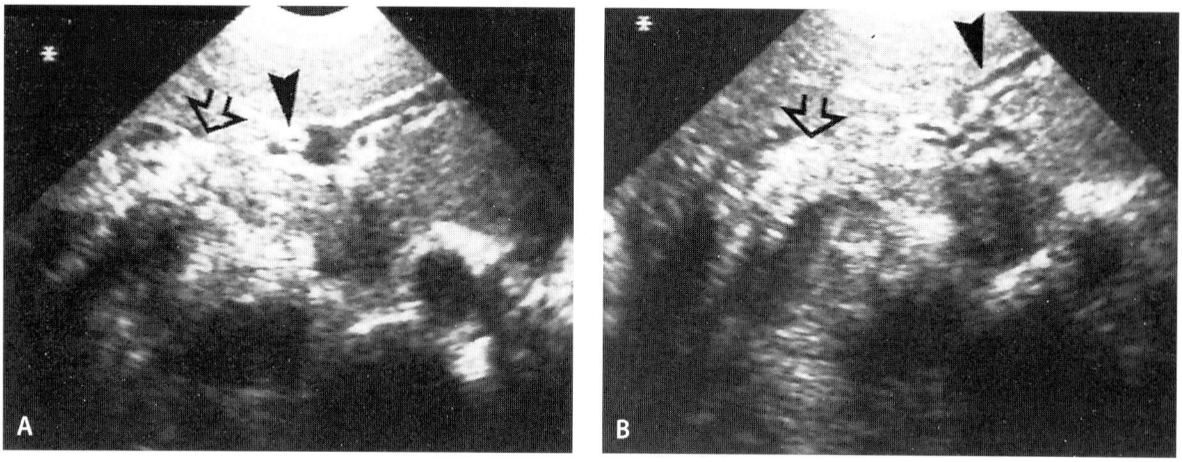

Fig. 3.167 A, B. Hepatic alveolar echinococcosis. **A** Hyperechoic lesion contains calcifications (*open arrow*) and obstructs the portal branch (*arrowhead*). **B** Parallel section also shows hyperechoic calcifications (*open arrow*) with posterior acoustic shadowing and dilated intrahepatic ducts (*arrowhead*). (From Weill 1990)

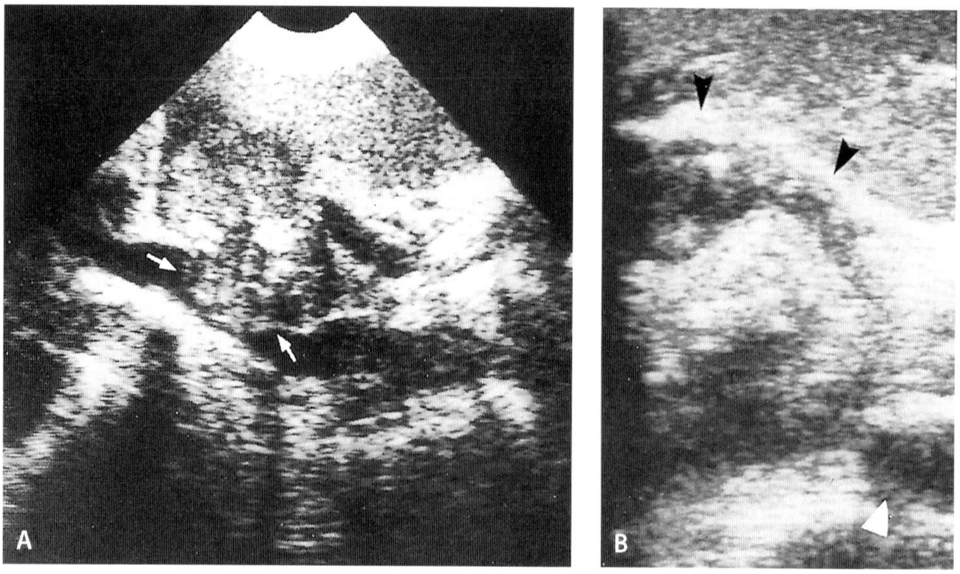

Fig. 3.168. **A** Sagittal sonogram shows heterogeneous hyperechoic hepatic lesion of *E. multilocularis* invading the inferior vena cava (*arrows*). **B** Transverse intraoperative sonogram shows the lesion (*black arrowheads*) obstructing the lumen of the vena cava whereas the lumen of the aorta (*white arrowhead*) is clear. (From Weill 1990)

ported in those cases where fine-needle aspiration biopsy was performed.

By the time alveolar hydatids are detected in the liver, the parasitic growth has usually caused stenosis, local dilatation, or displacement of the bile ducts, and given rise to portal vein and inferior vena cava thrombosis and/or thrombosis of hepatic veins and arteries. It is therefore not surprising that mortality rates in untreated or inadequately treated patients are high: in one series of 66 patients, 70% died within 5 years, and 94% within 10 years after diagnosis. In a recent study of 21 patients, the average survival time was 5.3 years after diagnosis, and 100% died within 14 years (Ammann and Eckert, 1995).

When the lungs are involved with alveolar hydatids, conventional chest radiography shows multiple irregular, spherical and lobulated masses, 1.5–3 cm in diameter, mainly in the lower lobes and in a peripheral subpleural position (Fig. 3.164). Chest CT shows central hypodensity and, in some cases, amorphous peripheral calcification within these masses.

Metastatic alveolar hydatids in the brain may appear as late as 10 years after onset of the disease. In 11

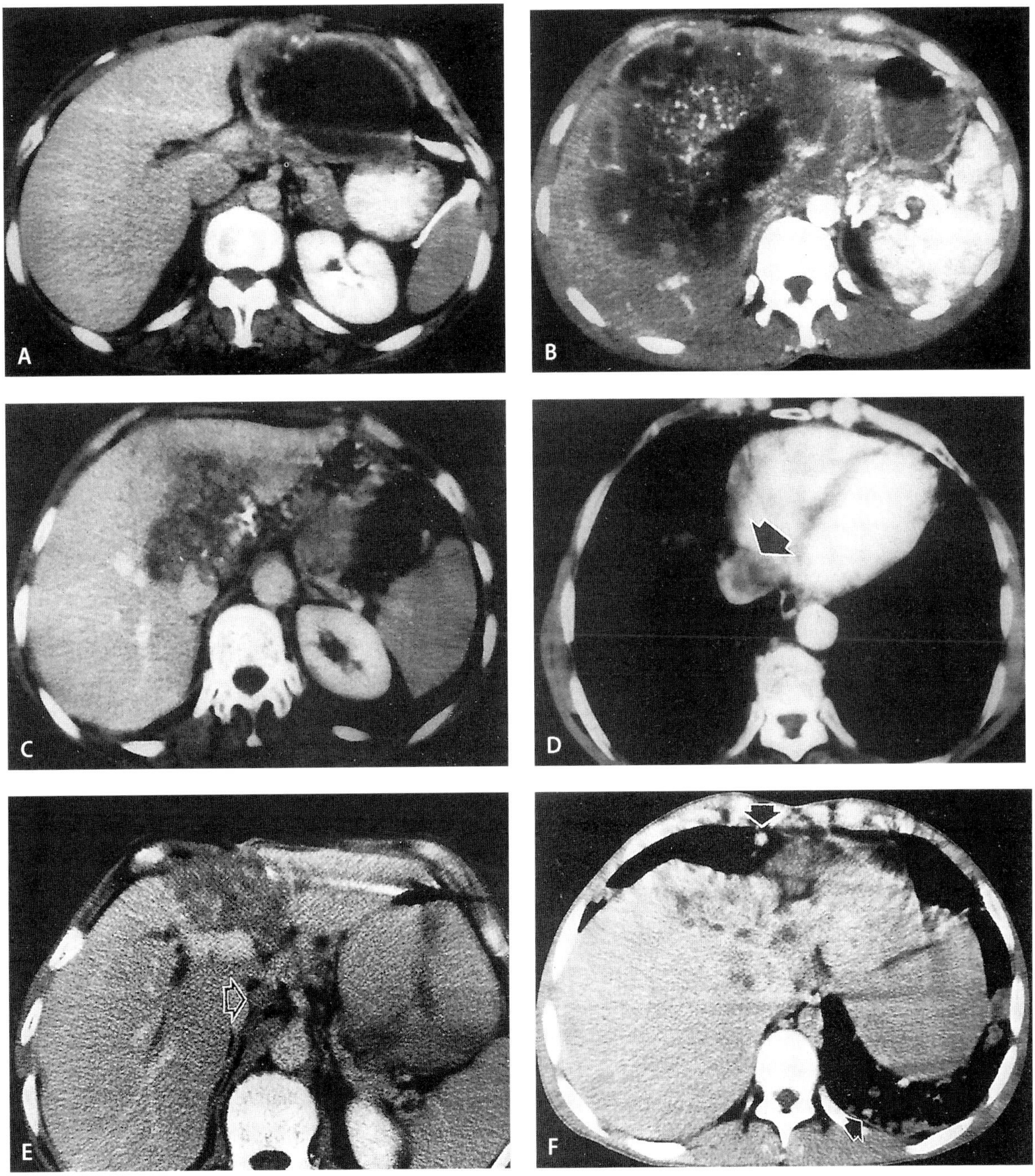

Fig. 3.169 A–I. CT staging of alveolar hydatid disease of the liver in multiple patients. **A** Stage 2 lesion with several calcific foci and large pseudocystic zone confined to the lateral segment of the left liver lobe. **B** Stage 3a lesion with multiple calcifications, pseudocystic necrotic areas, and invasion of more than three hepatic segments. **C** Stage 3b lesion with invasion of the inferior vena cava. **D** Same patient with tumor thrombus in the suprahepatic vena cava extending into the right atrium (*arrow*). **E** Stage 3b lesion with invasion of the liver hilum. Dilatation of intrahepatic bile ducts in both lobes of the liver is present, as well as lymphadenopathy in the liver hilum (*arrow*). **F** Stage 4 lesion with invasion of the liver dome associated with multiple pulmonary and pleural metastases (*arrows*). **G–I** see p. 346

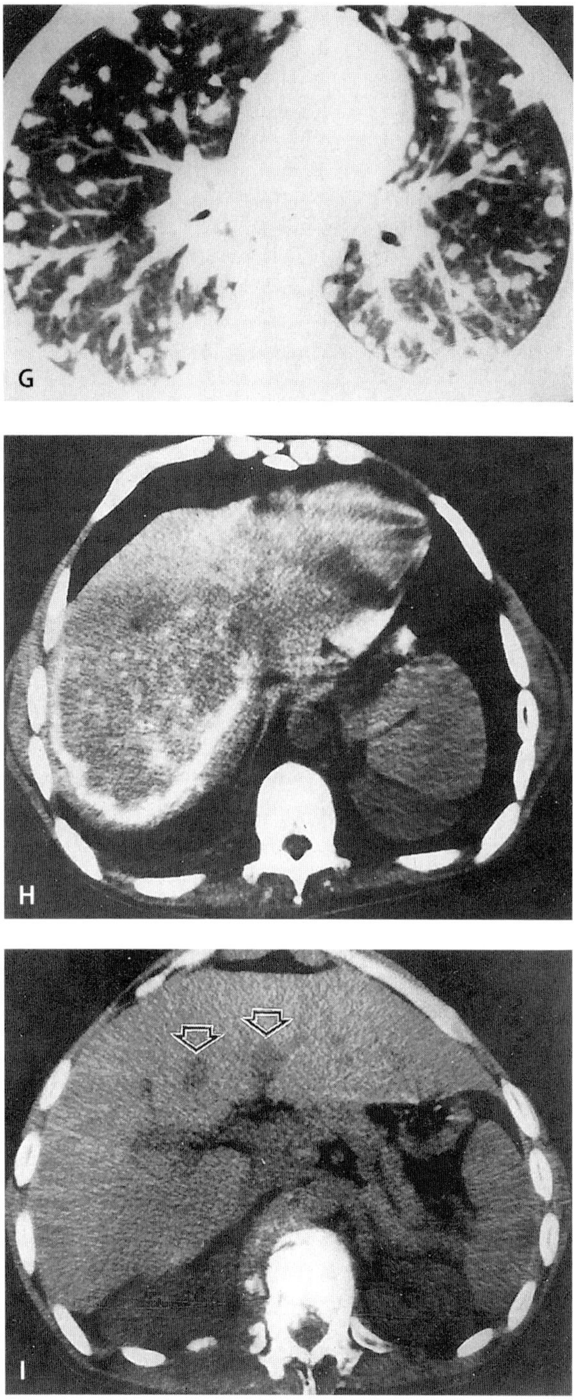

Fig. 3.169 (*continued*). **G** Numerous pulmonary metastatic nodules are seen in the lung window. **H** Another patient with a stage 4 lesion with numerous mottled calcific foci and prominent rim calcification in the right lobe of the liver. **I** Metastasis to the T12 vertebra with bony destruction, invasion of the epidural space, and paravertebral soft tissue thickening and calcification. Two metastatic nodules are present in the left liver lobe (*arrows*). (Courtesy of Dr. I. Rozanes and *Eur Radiol*, 1995)

patients, Bensaid et al. (1994) found alveolar hydatids in these locations: four parietal, three temporal, and four in the frontal or posterofrontal areas. Two features were different from alveolar hydatids in the liver: (1) extirpation of masses in the brain is easier due to better defined margins and (2) protoscolices are found more often in brain than in liver lesions. These alveolar cysts of the brain appear on CT and MRI as grape-like, multilocular cystic masses with definite margins; calcification and surrounding edema is common (Figs. 3.170, 3.171). Contrast enhancement occurs with inflammatory reaction around the cysts. If there is ring enhancement, bacterial abscess, tuberculoma, or cysticercosis have to be excluded; otherwise, glioma, especially oligodendroglioma, must be included in the differential diagnosis.

Early diagnosis and treatment significantly improves the prognosis of alveolar echinococcosis. It is therefore important to discover this very serious disease in an early stage. In highly endemic areas or in a highly exposed population, serological or ultrasound screening of the abdomen may be justified. In selected cases, this may be combined with CT and/or MRI. For serological screening, a highly sensitive and specific Em2 plus ELISA kit is now commercially available.

Treatment

1. Surgical resection of the parasite in all organs
2. Long-term chemotherapy of inoperable patients
3. Long-term complementary chemotherapy in patients with incomplete surgical resection, and at least 2 years of chemotherapy in patients after radical surgery or liver transplantation for alveolar echinococcosis (Bresson et al., 1991)

Contraindications for chemotherapy (with mebendazole and albendazole, as of 1999) are few due to relatively low toxicity, but some patients show severe drug intolerance in the final clinical stages, and certain precautions and modifications of drug administration are necessary. About 60% of the patients under treatment showed clinical improvement (increased body weight, regression of cholestasis, decrease in liver lesion size), 20% showed stabilization, and 20% progression. The 10-year survival rate in a group of 70 treated patients was 89% as compared to 6% in untreated patients (Eckert et al., 1995). Recurrences are frequent after discontinuation of long-term treatment of inoperable patients; however, they seem to respond favorably again following renewal of therapy.

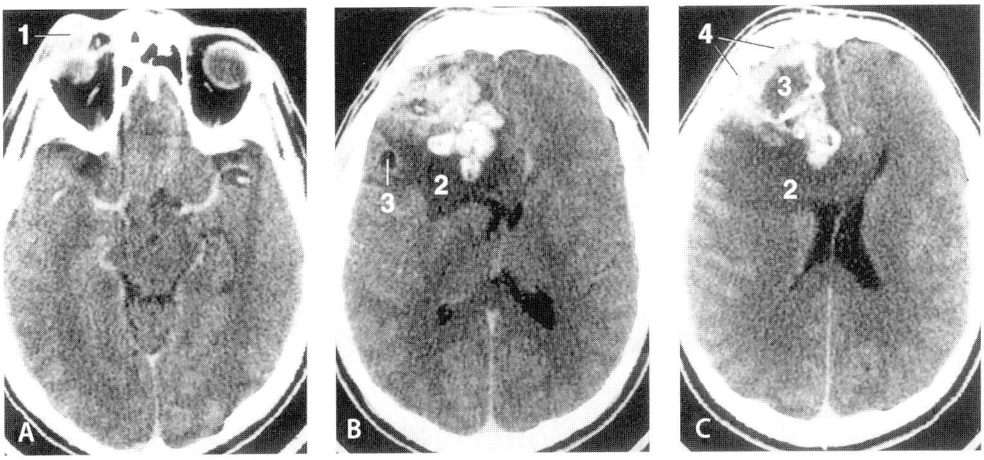

Fig. 3.170 A–C. *E. multilocularis* involvement of the orbit and brain of a patient from Alsace, France. **A** Contrast-enhanced CT reveals a round right palpebral mass (*1*). **B** A large right frontal lobe mass is present with posterior displacement of the corpus callosum, posterior and contralateral displacement of the right frontal horn, and contralateral displacement of the falx cerebri. Nodular and ring-like calcifications are seen within the mass, which shows partial contrast enhancement and is surrounded by edema (*2*). Nonenhancing and noncalcified areas represent alveolar hydatid cysts (*3*). **C** The inner table of the skull (*4*) is irregular anterior to the mass. (Courtesy of Dr. J. L. Dietemann, Strasbourg and *Neuroradiology*, 1994)

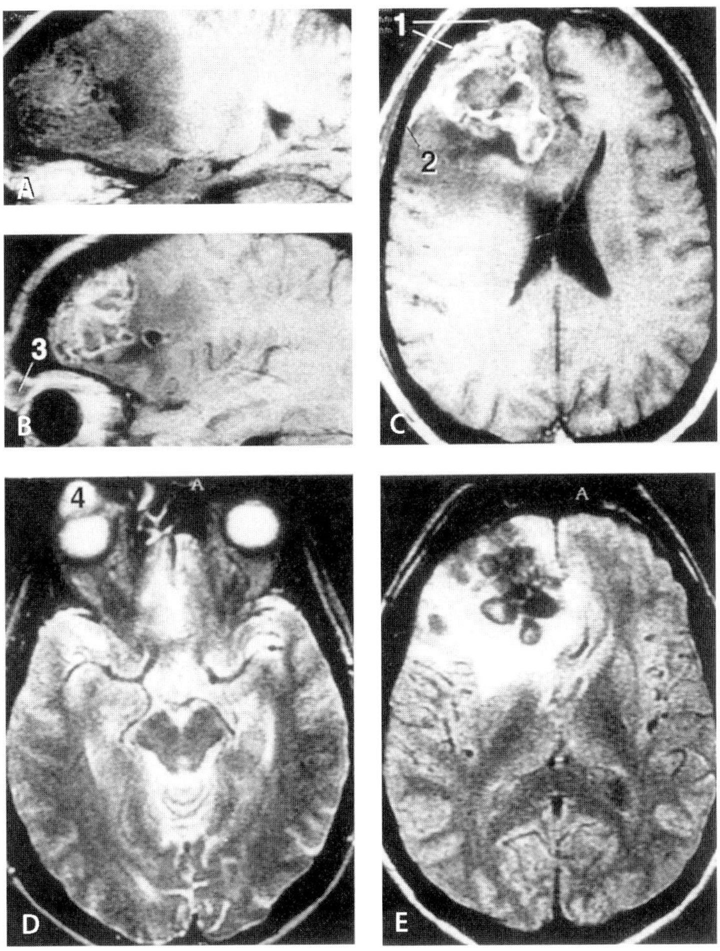

Fig. 3.171. **A** T1-weighted MR image on the same patient reveals a heterogeneous low signal within the right frontal lobe mass. **B, C** Heterogeneous contrast enhancement is present within the mass. The inner table of the cranial vault appears irregular (*1*) and there is dural enhancement (*2*). The calcified areas show low signal intensity. There is ring enhancement of the low-intensity palpebral mass (*3*), which shows high signal (*4*) on a T2-weighted image (**D**). On proton density (**E**) and T2-weighted images a grape-like low-signal right frontal mass was identified, surrounded by high signal edema. (Courtesy of Dr. J. L. Dietemann, Strasbourg and *Neuroradiology*, 1994)

Bibliography

Acunas B, Rozanes I, Acunas G, et al: Hydatid cyst of the liver: identification of detached cyst lining on CT scans obtained after cyst puncture. *AJR* 156:751, 1991

Acunas B, Rozanes I, Celik L, et al: Purely cystic hydatid disease of the liver: treatment with percutaneous aspiration and injection of hypertonic saline. *Radiology* 182:541–543, 1992

Aggarwal ML: Hydatid disease of the lung. *Indian J Radiol* 10:10–17, 1956

Akhan O, et al: Percutaneous treatment of abdominal hydatid cysts with hypertonic saline and alcohol; an experimental study in sheep. *Invest Radiol* 28:121–127, 1993

Akhan O, Ozmen MN, Dincer Sayek I, Gocmen A: Liver hydatid disease: long-term results of percutaneous treatment. *Radiology* 198:259–264, 1996

Akoglu M, Davidson BR: A rational approach to the terminology of hydatid disease of the liver. *J Infect* 24:1–6, 1992

Al Karawi MA, et al: Advances in diagnosis and management of hydatid disease. *Hepatogastroenterology* 37:327–331, 1990

Alldred J, Nisbet NW: Hydatid disease of bone in Australasia. *J Bone Joint Surg [Br]* 46:260–267, 1964

Alparslan L, Kanberoglu K, Peksayer G, et al: Orbital hydatid cyst: assessment of two cases. *Neuroradiology* 2:163, 1990

Alper A, et al: Intramural hydatid cysts of pulmonary arteries: CT and MR findings. *Eur Radiol* 5:666–668, 1995

Ameli M, et al: Surgical treatment of hydatid cysts of the heart: report of six cases. *J Thorac Cardiovasc Surg* 98:892–901, 1989

Ammann R, Eckert J: Clinical diagnosis and treatment of echinococcosis in humans. In: Thompson RCA, Lymbery AJ (eds) *Echinococcus and hydatid disease*. CAB International, Oxon, 1995, pp 411–463

Angulo JC, Sanchez-Chapado M, Diego A, et al: Renal echinococcosis: clinical study of 34 cases. *J Urol* 157:787–794, 1997

Angulo JC, Escribano J, Diego A, Sanchez-Chapado M: Isolated retrovesical and extrarenal retroperitoneal hydatidosis: clinical study of 10 cases and literature review. *J Urol* 159:76–82, 1998

Ayuso LA, de Peralta GT, Lazaro RB, et al: Surgical treatment of pulmonary hydatidosis. *J Thorac Cardiovasc Surg* 82:569–575, 1981

Babcock DS, Kaufman L, Cosnow I: Ultrasound diagnosis of hydatid disease (echinococcosis) in two cases. *AJR* 131:895–897, 1978

Bakir F: Serious complications of hydatid cyst of the lung. *Am Rev Respir Dis* 96:483–493, 1967

Bakir F, Al-Omeri M: Echinococcal tension pneumothorax. *Thorax* 24:547–556, 1969

Bakri YN, von Sinner WN, Khougeer F: Choriocarcinoma presenting as pulmonary hydatid disease. Letter to the Editor. *Int J Gynecol Obstet* 38:315–316, 1992

Balikian JP, Mudarris FF: Hydatid disease of the lungs. A roentgenologic study of 50 cases. *AJR* 122:692–707, 1974

Baltaxe HA, Fleming RJ: The angiographic appearance of hydatid disease. *Radiology* 97:599–604, 1970

Barriga P, Cruz F, Lepe V, et al: An ultrasonographically solid, tumor-like appearance of echinococcal cysts of the liver. *J Ultrasound Med* 2:123–125, 1983

Bartoloni C, et al: The efficacy of chemotherapy with mebendazole in human cystic echinococcosis; long term follow-up of 52 patients. *Ann Trop Med Parasitol* 86:249–256, 1992

Beggs I: The radiologic appearances of hydatid disease of the liver. *Clin Radiol* 34:555–563, 1983

Beggs I: The radiology of hydatid disease. *AJR* 145:639–648, 1985

Belghiti J, Benhamou J-P, Houry S, et al: Caustic sclerosing cholangitis. A complication of the surgical treatment of hydatid disease of the liver. *Arch Surg* 121:1162–1165, 1986

Bensaid AH, et al: Intracranial alveolar echinococcosis: CT and MRI. *Neuroradiology* 36:289–291, 1994

Berenson MM, et al: Traumatic intrahepatic rupture of an echinococcal cyst. *J Trauma* 14:798–804, 1974

Bezzi M, Teggi A, De Rosa F, et al: Abdominal hydatid disease: ultrasound findings during medical treatment. *Radiology* 162:91–95, 1987

Binford CH, Connor DH: *Pathology of tropical and extraordinary diseases*. Armed Forces Institute of Pathology, Washington DC, 1976, pp 530–533

Bloomfield JA: Protean radiological manifestations of hydatid infestation. *Australas Radiol* 10:330–343, 1966

Bobrowitz ID: Round densities within cavities; lung lesions simulating the pathognomonic roentgen sign of *Echinococcus* cyst. *Am Rev Tuberc Pulm Dis* 50:305–312, 1944

Bonakdarpour A: Echinococcus disease. Report of 112 cases from Iran and a review of 611 cases from the United States. *AJR* 99:660–667, 1967

Booz MK: The management of hydatid disease of bone and joint. *J Bone Joint Surg [Br]* 54:698–709, 1972

Borrie J: Fifty thoracic hydatid cysts. *Br J Surg* 50:265–287, 1962

Borrie J, Shaw JHF: Hepatobronchial fistula caused by hydatid disease. *Thorax* 36:25–28, 1981

Borrie J, Gemmell MA, Manktelow BW: An experimental approach to evaluate the potential risk of hydatid disease from inhalation of *Echinococcus* ova. *Br J Surg* 52:876–878, 1965

Bouras A, et al: The value of computed tomography in osseous hydatid disease (echinococcosis). *Skeletal Radiol* 12:192, 1984

Boyd DP: Bronchobiliary and bronchopleural fistulas. *Ann Thorac Surg* 24:481–487, 1977

Braithwaite PA, et al: Vertebral hydatid disease. Skeletal Radiol 6:408, 1981

Bresson Hadni S, et al: Orthotopic liver transplantation for incurable alveolar echinococcosis of the liver: report of 17 cases. *Hepatology* 13:1061–1070, 1991

Brett PM, Fond A, Bretagnolle M: Percutaneous aspiration and drainage of hydatid cysts in the liver. *Radiology* 168:617–620, 1988

Can Basalkar A: Hydatid cysts in children: report of 88 cases. *J R Coll Surg Edinb* 36:166–169, 1991

Capurro FG: Osseous hydatid disease. *Acta Radiol Interam* 6:137–142, 1956

Chambers WL: Echinococcus cyst of the lung in native born Americans. *Am J Surg* 108:655–659, 1964

Charles RW, et al: Echinococcal infection of the spine with neural involvement. *Spine* 13:47, 1987

Christie HK: Hydatid cysts in both lungs. *Aust NZ J Surg* 8:373–378, 1939

Chrysospathis P: Echinococcus cysts of the lung. *Chest* 49:278–283, 1966

Cifarelli FP: Radiological diagnosis of hydatidosis. *Acta Radiol Interam* 5:17–27, 1955

Claudon M, Bessieres M, Regent D, et al: Alveolar echinococcosis of the liver: MR findings. *J Comput Assist Tomogr* 14:608–614, 1990

Coates R, von Sinner WN, Rahm B: MR imaging of an intracerebral hydatid cyst. *AJNR* 11:1249–1250, 1990

Cockshott P, Middlemiss H: *Clinical radiology in the tropics.* Churchill Livingstone, Edinburgh, 1979

Cosme A, et al: CT findings of pancreatic hydatid disease. *J Comput Assist Tomogr* 20:815–816, 1996

Czerniak P, et al: Radioisotopic scanning in liver echinococcosis. *Radiology* 83:690–696, 1964

Davis A, Dixon K, Pawlowski ZS: Multicentre clinical trials of benzimidazole-carbamates in human cystic echinococcosis (phase 1). *Bull WHO* 64:383–388, 1986

Davis A, et al: Multicentre clinical trials of benzimidazole-carbamates in human cystic echinococcosis (phase 2). *Bull WHO* 67:503–508, 1989

Dawson JL, Stamatakis JD, Stringer MD, et al: Surgical treatment of hepatic hydatid disease. *Br J Surg* 75:946–950, 1988

De Arzua Zulaica E: Radiology of calcified hydatid cysts of the liver. *Rev Clin Esp* 73:53–58, 1959

DeBernardi E: Pulmonary hydatid disease in man. *Acta Radiol* 36:234–240, 1951

De Rosa F, Teggi A: Treatment of *Echinococcus granulosus* hydatid disease with albendazole. *Ann Trop Med Parasitol* 84:467–472, 1990

Desnos M, Brochet E, Christofini P, et al: Polyvisceral echinococcosis with cardiac involvement imaged by two-dimensional echocardiography, computed tomography and nuclear magnetic resonance imaging. *Am J Cardiol* 59:383–384, 1987

Deve F: *L'Echinococcose primitive.* Masson, Paris, 1949

Dew HR: *Hydatid disease: its pathology, diagnosis and treatment.* Australasian Medical Publishing Co, Sydney, 1928

Diamond HM, et al: Echinococcal disease of the kidney. *J Urol* 115:742–744, 1976

Dogan R, et al: Surgical treatment of hydatid cysts of the lung: report on 1055 patients. *Thorax* 44:192–199, 1989

Eckert J, Pawlowski ZS, Dor FK, et al: Medical aspects of echinococcosis. *Parasitology Today* 11:273–276, 1995

Elkouby A, et al: Cardiac hydatidosis. Review of recent literature and report of 15 cases. *Ann Chir* 44:603–610, 1990

Ellis ME, von Sinner WN, Ali A, et al: Echinococcal disease and mycobacterial infection. *Ann Trop Med Parasitol* 85:243–251, 1991

Ellis ME, von Sinner WN, Al-Hokail A, Sieck JO: A clinical-radiological evaluation of benzimidazole compounds in the management of *Echinococcus granulosus* cysts. *Scand J Infect Dis* 24:1–13, 1992

Esfahani F, Rooholamini SA, Vessal K: Ultrasonography of hepatic hydatid cysts: new diagnostic signs. *J Ultrasound Med* 7:443–450, 1988

Fahl M, et al: MRI in intradural and extradural spinal echinococcosis. *Clin Imaging* 18:179–183, 1994

Fawzy ME: Hydatid disease of the heart. *Br Heart J* 38:307–308, 1076

Filice C, et al: Parasitologic findings in percutaneous drainage of human hydatid cysts. *J Infect Dis* 161:1290–1295, 1990

Filice C, Pirola F, Brunetti E, et al: A new therapeutic approach for hydatid liver cysts. *Gastroenterology* 98:1366–1368, 1990

Filice C, Maurizio S, Brunetti E, et al: Percutaneous drainage of hydatid liver cysts. Letter to the Editor. *Radiology* 184:579–580, 1992

Fitzpatrick SC: Hydatid disease of the lumbar vertebrae. *J Bone Joint Surg [Br]* 47:286, 1965

Fraiji EK Jr, Connor DH: Echinococcosis. In: Connor DH, Chandler FW, et al (eds) *Pathology of infectious diseases,* vol 2. Appleton & Lange, Stamford, Conn., 1997, pp 1405–1413

Franquet T, Lecumberi T, Joly M: Hydatid heart disease: case report. *Br J Radiol* 57:171–173, 1984

Frayha GJ, Haddad R: Comparative chemical composition of protoscolices and hydatid cyst fluid of *Echinococcus granulosus (Cestoda). Int J Parasitol* 10:359–364, 1980

Frider B, Losada CA, Larrieu E, DeZavaleta O: Asymptomatic abdominal hydatidosis detected by ultrasonography. *Acta Radiol* 29-4:431–434, 1988

Fyfe B, Amazon K, Poppitti RJ, et al: Intraosseous echinococcosis: a rare manifestation of echinococcal disease. *South Med J* 83:66–68, 1990

Garcia FJ, Marti-Bonmati L, Menor F, et al: Echogenic forms of hydatid cysts: sonographic diagnosis. *J Clin Ultrasound* 16:305, 1988

Gargouri M, Ben Amor N, Chehida FB, et al: Percutaneous treatment of hydatid cysts (*Echinococcus granulosus*). *Cardiovasc Intervent Radiol* 13:169–173, 1990

Garrett WJ, et al: Gray scale ultrasonic investigation of focal defects on ^{99m}Tc sulfur colloid liver scanning. *Radiology* 119:425–428, 1976

Gharbi HA, et al: Rare sites of hydatid disease in children. *Ann Radiol* 20:151–157, 1977

Gharbi HA, Hassine W, Brauner WM, et al: Ultrasound examination of the hydatid liver. *Radiology* 139:459–463, 1981

Gharbi HA, et al: Parasitoses pulmonaires. *Encyclopedie Medico-Chirurgicale (Paris)* 32-470-A-10, 1993

Gilsanz V, Campo C, Cue R, et al: Recurrent pulmonary embolism due to hydatid disease of the heart: study of three cases with intermittent tricuspid valve obstruction (atrial pseudomyxoma). *Br Heart J* 39:553–558, 1977

Giorgio A, Tarantino L, Francica G, et al: Unilocular hydatid liver cysts; treatment with US-guided, double percutaneous aspiration and alcohol injection. *Radiology* 184:705–710, 1992

Gottstein B, Reichen J: Echinococcosis/hydatidosis. In: Cook GC (ed) *Manson's tropical diseases, 20th edn.* Saunders, London, 1996, pp 1486–1508

Grunebaum M: Radiological manifestations of lung echinococcus in children. *Pediatr Radiol* 3:65–69, 1975

Gupta SK, et al: Case report: multiple intracranial hydatid cysts with postoperative dissemination. *Clin Radiol* 44:203–204, 1991

Guthrie JA, et al: Case report: the MR appearances of primary intramuscular hydatid disease. *Clin Radiol* 51:377–379, 1996

Gutierrez Y: *Diagnostic pathology of parasitic infections with clinical correlations.* Lea & Febiger, Philadelphia, 1990

Hadidi A: Ultrasound findings in liver hydatid cysts. *J Clin Ultrasound* 7:365–368, 1979

Hadidi A: Sonography of hepatic echinococcal cysts. *Gastrointest Radiol* 7:349–354, 1982

Haertel CF, Fretz CH, Fuchs WA: Computed tomography in the diagnosis of echinococcosis. *Fortschr Roentgenstr (Rofo)* 133:164–170, 1980

Hankins J, Werner D, Kobout E: Surgical treatment of ruptured and unruptured hydatid cysts of the lung. *Ann Surg* 167:336–341, 1968

Harris A, Heath DD, Lawrence SB, et al: *Echinococcus granulosus:* ultrastructure of epithelial changes during the first

8 days of metacestode development in vitro. *Int J Parasitol* 19:621–629, 1989

Harris JD: Rupture of hydatid cysts of the liver into the biliary tracts. *Br J Surg* 52:210–214, 1965

Hendaoui L, et al: Hydatid cyst of the aorta. *Clin Radiol* 43:423–425, 1991

Hoff FL, Aisen AM, Walden MR, Glazer GM: MR imaging in hydatid disease of the liver. *Gastrointest Radiol* 12:29–42, 1987

Hutchison WF, et al: Osseous hydatid (*Echinococcus*) disease. Report of an indigenous case. *JAMA* 182:81–83, 1962

Ismail MA, Al Dabagh MA, Al-Tanabi TA, et al: The use of computerized axial tomography (CAT) in the diagnosis of hydatid cysts. *Clin Radiol* 31:287–290, 1980

Ivanissevich O, Ferrari RC: Diagnostico Radiologico de los quistes hidaticos del pulmon. *Sem Med* 2:825–831, 1937

Jain AK, Gupta NC, Gupta PD, et al: Sonographic appearance of hepatic hydatid disease. *Australas Radiol* 33:373–375, 1989

Jain AK: Primary spinal echinococcosis causing paraplegia; case report with MR and pathologic correlation. *AJNR* 12:560, 1991

Jesiotr M, Romanoff H: Pneumothorax following rupture of a primary pleural hydatid cyst. *J Thorac Cardiovasc Surg* 63:594–598, 1972

Kalovidouris A, Gouliamos A, Demou L, et al: Post-surgical evaluation of hydatid disease with CT: diagnostic pitfalls. *J Comput Assist Tomogr* 10:1114–1119, 1984

Kalovidouris A, Pissiotis C, Pontifex G, et al: CT characterization of multivesicular hydatid cysts. *J Comput Assist Tomogr* 10:428–431, 1986

Kalovidouris A, Voros D, Gouliamos A, et al: Extracapsular (satellite) hydatid cysts. *Gastrointest Radiol* 17:353–356, 1992

Kalovidouris A, Gouliamos A, Demou L, et al: MRI of abdominal hydatid disease. *Abdom Imaging* 19:489–494, 1994

Kapila K, Verma K: Aspiration cytology diagnosis of echinococcosis. *Diagn Cytopathol* 6:301–303, 1990

Karak PK, Mittal M, Bhatia S, et al: Isolated cerebral hydatid cyst with pathognomonic CT sign. *Neuroradiology* 34:9, 1992

Karavias D, Panagopoulos C, Vagianos C, et al: Infected echinococcal cyst. A common cause of pyogenic hepatic abscess. *Ups J Med Sci* 93:289–296, 1988

Kattan YB: Intrabiliary rupture of hydatid cyst of the liver. *Br J Surg* 62:885–890, 1975

Katz AM, Pan CT: Echinococcus disease in United States. *Am J Med* 25:759–770, 1958

Katz M, et al: *Parasitic diseases*. Springer, New York Berlin Heidelberg, 1982

Kegel RFC, Fatemi A: The ruptured pulmonary hydatid cyst. *Radiology* 76:60–64, 1961

Khuroo MS, Showkat AZ, Mahajan R: *Echinococcus granulosus* cysts in the liver: management with percutaneous drainage. *Radiology* 180:141–145, 1991

Khuroo MS, et al: Percutaneous drainage versus albendazole therapy in hepatic hydatidosis: a prospective, randomized study. *Gastroenterology* 104:1452–1459, 1993

Khuroo MS, Wani NA, Javid G, et al: Percutaneous drainage compared with surgery for hepatic hydatid cysts. *N Engl J Med* 13:881–887, 1997

Kilani T, Horchani H, Daoues A: L'hydatidose pulmonaire secondaire bronchogenetique. *Ann Chir Thorac Cardio-Vasc* 46:160–164, 1992

King DL: Ultrasonography of echinococcal cysts. *J Clin Ultrasound* 1:64–67, 1973

Kirkland K: Urological aspects of hydatid disease. *Br J Urol* 38:241–254, 1966

Kourias B: Apropos of 2000 cases of operated hydatid cysts. Brief considerations of a statistical and surgical nature. *Presse Med* 69:165–168, 1961

Kurul S, Tenekeci N, Topuzlu C: Case report: an unusual mass in the breast: the hydatid cyst. *Clin Radiol* 50:869–870, 1995

Langer JC, Rose DB, Keystone JS, et al: Diagnosis and management of hydatid disease of the liver. A 15-year North American experience. *Ann Surg* 199:412–417, 1984

Latham WJ: Hydatid disease. *J Fac Radiol Lond* 5:65–81, 1953

Lewall DB: Hydatid disease: biology, pathology, imaging and classification. *Clin Radiol* 53:863–874, 1998

Lewall DB, McCorkell SJ: Hepatic echinococcal cysts: sonographic appearance and classification. *Radiology* 155:773–775, 1985

Lewall DB, McCorkell SJ: Rupture of echinococcal cysts: diagnosis, classification and clinical implications. *AJR* 146:391–394, 1986

Lewall DB, Nyak P: Hydatid cysts of the liver: two cautionary signs. *Br J Radiol* 71:37–41, 1998

Lewall DB, Bailey TM, McCorkell SJ: Echinococcal matrix: computed tomographic, sonographic and pathological correlation. *J Ultrasound Med* 5:33–35, 1986

Lo Casto A, Salerno S, Grisanti M, et al: Hydatid cyst of the liver communicating with the left colon. *Br J Radiol* 70:650–651, 1997

Luntz MH: Hydatid cysts of the orbit demonstrated by pneumotomography. *S Afr Med J* 31:286–287, 1957

Lupetin AR, Dash N: Intrahepatic rupture of hydatid cyst: MR findings. *AJR* 151:491–492, 1988

Magistrelli P, Masetti R, Coppola R, et al: Value of ERCP in the diagnosis and management of pre- and postoperative biliary complications in hydatid disease of the liver. *Gastrointest Radiol* 14:315–320, 1989

Magistrelli P, Masetti R, Coppola R, et al: Surgical treatment of hydatid disease of the liver. *Arch Surg* 126:518–523, 1991

Malaika S, Attayeb A, Sulaiman S, Reddy JJ: Human echinococcosis in Saudi Arabia. *Saudi Med J* 2:77–84, 1981

Marani SAD, Canossi GC, Nicoli FA, et al: Hydatid disease: MR imaging study. *Radiology* 175:701–706, 1990

Marti-Bonmati L, Serrano FM: Complications of hepatic hydatid cysts: ultrasound, computed tomography, and magnetic resonance diagnosis. *Gastrointest Radiol* 15:119–125, 1990

Martin J, et al: Hydatid disease of the soft tissues of the lower limb: findings in three cases. *Skeletal Radiol* 22:511–514, 1993

Martinez Peralta CA: A warning to surgeons who occasionally see hydatid cysts. Letter to the Editors. *Surgery* 105:570, 1989

Marty AM, Andersen EM: *Echinococcus granulosus, E. multilocularis,* and *E. vogeli.* In: Doerr W, Seifert G (eds) *Tropical pathology, 2nd edn.* Springer, Berlin Heidelberg New York, 1995, pp 857–862

Massenti S, Racugno V: Hydatid cyst causing a Pancoast syndrome. *Radiol Med (Torino)* 43:63–67, 1957

Matossian RM, et al: Immune status during albendazole therapy for hydatidosis. *Ann Trop Med Parasitol* 86:67–75, 1992

McCorkell SJ: Unintended percutaneous aspiration of pulmonary echinococcal cysts. *AJR* 143:123–126, 1984

McCorkell SJ, Lewall DB: Computed tomography of intracerebral echinococcal cysts in children. *J Comput Assist Tomogr* 9:514–518, 1985

McGreevy PB, Nelson GS: Larval cestode infections. In: Strickland GT (ed) *Hunter's tropical medicine, 6th edn.* Saunders, Philadelphia, 1984, pp 771–782

McLoughlin MJ, Hobbs BB: Selective angiography in the diagnosis of hydatid disease of the liver. *Can Med Assoc J* 103:1147–1151, 1970

McManus DP: A biochemical study of adult and cystic stages of *Echinococcus granulosus* of human and animal origin from Kenya. *J Helminth* 55:21–27, 1981

McNulty JG: Angiographic manifestations of hydatid disease of the liver. A report of two cases. *AJR* 102:380–383, 1968

Meltzer H, et al: Echinococcosis in North American Indians and Eskimos. *Can Med Assoc J* 75:121–128, 1956

Mikhael MA, et al: MR imaging in spinal echinococcosis. *J Comput Assist Tomogr* 9:398, 1985

Mistrello G, et al: Dot immunobinding assay as a new diagnostic test for human hydatid disease. *Immunol Lett* 47:79–85, 1995

Montero JVM, Carcia JA, Lafuente JL, et al: Fat-fluid level in hepatic hydatid cyst: a new sign of rupture into the biliary tree? *AJR* 167:91–94, 1996

Morales AG, Croxatto JO, Crovetto L, et al: Hydatid cysts of the orbit: a review of 35 cases. *Ophthalmology* 95:1027–1032, 1988

Morris D, Skene-Smith H, Haynes A, Burrows FGO: Abdominal hydatid disease: computed tomographic and ultrasound changes during albendazole therapy. *Clin Radiol* 35:297–300, 1984

Morris DL, Dykes PW, Marriner S: Albendazole – objective evidence of response in human hydatid disease. *JAMA* 253:2053–2057, 1985

Morris DL, Buckley J, Gregson R, et al: Magnetic resonance imaging in hydatid disease. *Clin Radiol* 38:141–144, 1987

Morshed AA: Hydatid disease of the spine. *Neurochirurgia* (Stuttg) 20:211–215, 1977

Mottaghian H, Saidi F: Postoperative recurrence of hydatid disease. *Br J Surg* 65:237–242, 1978

Mueller PR, et al: Hepatic echinococcal cyst: successful percutaneous drainage. *Radiology* 155:627–628, 1985

Musacchio F, et al: Primary renal echinococcosis: a case report. *Am J Trop Mod Hyg* 15:168–171, 1966

Myers NA: Hydatid disease in a children's hospital. *Med J Aust* 47:806–808, 1960

Nahmias J, et al: Three to seven year follow-up after albendazole treatment of 68 patients with cystic echinococcosis (hydatid disease). *Ann Trop Med Parasitol* 88:295–304, 1994

Niron EA, Ozer H: Ultrasound appearances of liver hydatid disease. *Br J Radiol* 54:335–338, 1981

Noah MS, El-Din Hawass N, Joharjy I, Abdel-Hafex M: Primary cardiac echinococcosis: report of two cases with review of the literature. *Ann Trop Med Parasitol* 82:67–72, 1988

Novick RJ, Tchervenkov CI, Wilson JA, et al: Surgery for thoracic hydatid disease: a North American experience. *Ann Thorac Surg* 43:681–686, 1987

O'Leary P: A five-year study of human hydatid disease in Turkana district-Kenya. *East Afr Med J* 53:540–544, 1976

Oosthuizen SF, Fainsinger MH: Hydatid disease. *Radiology* 53:248–254, 1949

Ozgen T, et al: The use of computerized tomography in the diagnosis of cerebral hydatid cysts. *J Neurosurg* 50:339–342, 1979

Ozturk C, Agildere M, Cila A, et al: Pulmonary arterial embolism secondary to hydatid cyst of the liver. *Can Assoc Radiol J* 43:374–376, 1992

Palmer PES, Reeder MM: Parasitic diseases of the urinary tract. In: Pollack H (ed) *Clinical urography, 2nd edn.* Saunders, Philadelphia, 1999

Pardal HC, et al: Hydatid mesaortitis in the abdominal aorta: case report. *Angiology* 1:889–894, 1985

Pawlowski ZS: Critical points in the clinical management of cystic echinococcosis. In: Andersen FL, et al (eds) *Compensium on cystic echinococcosis with special reference to the Xingjiang Uygar autonomous region of the People's Republic of China.* Brigham Young University, Provo, Utah, 1993, pp 119–131

Piaggio Blanco RA, Garcia Capurro F: *Equinococcosis pulmonar: estudio anatomoclinicoradiobroncografico y terapeutico.* El Ateneo, Buenos Aires, 1939

Poole JB, Marcial-Rojas RA: Echinococcosis. In: Marcial-Rojas RA (ed) *Pathology of protozoal and helminthic diseases.* Robert E. Krieger, Huntington NY, 1975, pp 635–657

Porat, et al: Hydatid disease of the spine causing paraplegia. *Spine* 9:648, 1984

Ptasnik R, Hennessy OF: Pelvic hydatid disease presenting as urinary retention. *Br J Radiol* 61:164, 1988

Pumar J, et al: Multiple intracranial hydatid cysts: MR findings. *Eur Radiol* 2:385–387, 1992

Qian Z: Thoracic hydatid cysts: a report of 842 cases treated over a thirty-year period [abstract]. *Radiology* 171:882, 1989

Rakower J, Milwidsky H: Hydatid pleural disease. *Am Rev Respir Dis* 90:623–630, 1964

Ramos L, Hirnandez-Mora M, Klanas M, et al: Radiological characteristics of perforated pulmonary hydatid cysts. *Radiology* 116:539–542, 1975

Reeder MM, Hamilton LC: Radiologic diagnosis of tropical diseases of the gastrointestinal tract. *Radiol Clin North Am* 7:57–81, 1969

Reeder MM: RPC of the month from the AFIP (hydatid cyst of the lung). *Radiology* 95:429–437, 1970

Reeder MM: Tropical diseases of the liver and bile ducts. *Semin Roentgenol* 10:229–243, 1975

Reeder MM, Palmer PES: *The radiology of tropical diseases with epidemiological, pathological and clinical correlation.* Williams & Wilkins, Baltimore, 1981

Reittner P, et al: Systemic manifestations of *echinococcus alveolaris* infection. *J Comput Assist Tomogr* 20:1080–1082, 1996

Rizk GK, et al: The angiographic changes in hydatid cysts of the liver and spleen. *Radiology* 99:303–309, 1971

Ross RM, Coghlan CJ: Hydatid disease of the lung. *East Afr Med J* 48:646–649, 1971

Rozanes I, Acunas B, Celik L, et al: CT in lobar atrophy of the liver caused by alveolar echinococcosis. *J Comput Assist Tomogr* 16:216, 1992

Rozanes I, Acunas B, Celik L, et al: Grading of liver lesions caused by *Echinococcus granulosus*. *Eur Radiol* 3:429–433, 1993

Rozanes I, Acunas B, Emre A, et al: CT staging of alveolar echinococcosis of the liver. *Eur Radiol* 5-3:259, 1995

Sagin HB, et al: Hydatid cyst of the breast diagnosed by FNAB. *Acta Cytol* 38:965–967, 1994

Saint Martin GA, Larrieu E, Chiesa JC, et al: Ultrasound scanning as a screening technique for hydatidosis in developing countries. *JCU* 16:233, 1988

Saksouk FA: Extrapleural extraosseous costal echinococcosis. *Br J Radiol* 52:918–919, 1979

Saksouk FA, Fahl MH, Risk GK: Computer tomography of pulmonary hydatid disease. *J Comput Assist Tomogr* 10:226–232, 1986

Sanchez FA, Sanchez AC: Estudios de algunas propriedades fisicas y componentes quimicos del liquido y pared germinativa de quistes hidaticos de diversas especies y de diferente localizacion. *Revista Iberia de Parasitologia* 31:347–366, 1971

Saremi F, McNamara TO: Hydatid cysts of the liver: Long-term results of percutaneous treatment using a cutting instrument. *AJR* 165:1163–1167, 1995

Schaefer JW, Khan MY: Echinococcus (hydatid disease): lessons from experience with 59 patients. *Rev Infect Dis* 13:243–247, 1991

Schlanger PM, Schlanger H: Hydatid disease and its roentgen picture. *AJR* 60:331–347, 1948

Schrumpf J, Hoffer PB: Cerebral echinococcal cyst demonstrated on radionuclide angiogram. Case report. *Radiology* 125:170, 1977

Sciarrino E, Virdone R, LoIacono O, et al: Ultrasound changes in abdominal echinococcus treated with Albendazole. *J Clin Ultrasound* 19:143–148, 1991

Sener RN: Hydatid cyst in the infratemporal fossa: MRI demonstration. *Clin Imaging* 18:213–215, 1994

Sener RN, et al: Multiple hydatid cysts. *AJR* 154:1126–1127, 1990

Shapiro SZ, Bahr GM, Hira PR: Analysis of host components in hydatid fluid and immunoblot diagnosis of human *Echinococcus granulosus* infection. *Ann Trop Med Parasitol* 86:503–509, 1992

Shawket IN, et al: Hydatid cysts of the kidney simulating similar kidney lesions. *Br J Urol* 46:371–376, 1974

Simonetti S, et al: Percutaneous treatment of hepatic cysts by aspiration and sclerotherapy. *Cardiovasc Intervent Radiol* 16:81–84, 1993

Sperryn CW, Corr PD: CT evaluation of orbital hydatid disease: a review of 10 cases. *Clin Radiol* 49:703–704, 1994

Spruance SL: Latent period of 53 years in a case of hydatid cyst disease. *Arch Intern Med* 134:741–742, 1974

Srouji M, et al: Hydatid cyst of the lung with bronchographic evaluation of treatment by internal suture of the pericyst. *J Thorac Surg* 35:779–794, 1958

Stampfel G: Anaphylactoid reaction: a rare complication after fine-needle biopsy of the lungs [in German]. *Radiologe* 19:329–330, 1982

Suwan Z: Sonographic findings in hydatid disease of the liver: comparison with other imaging methods. *Ann Trop Med Parasitol* 89:261–269, 1995

Taneja K, Gothi R, Kumar K, et al: Peritoneal *Echinococcus multilocularis* infection: CT appearance. *J Comput Assist Tomogr* 14:493, 1990

Taourel P, Marty-Ane B, Charasset S, et al: Hydatid cyst of the liver: comparison of CT and MRI. *J Comput Assist Tomogr* 17:80–85, 1993

Taylor KJW, et al: Gray scale ultrasound imaging; the anatomy and pathology of the liver. *Radiology* 119:415–424, 1976

Tellez G, Nojek C, Juffe A, et al: Cardiac echinococcosis: report of 3 cases and review of the literature. *Ann Thorac Surg* 21:425–430, 1976

Teymoorian GA, Bagheri F: Hydatid cyst of the skull: report of four cases. *Radiology* 118:97, 1976

Thompson RCA, Lymbery AJ (eds) *Echinococcus and hydatid disease, 2nd edn.* CAB International, Oxon, UK, 1995, pp 6–8, 233–331

Thompson WM, et al: Plain film roentgenographic findings in alveolar hydatid disease – *Echinococcus multilocularis. AJR* 116:345–358, 1972

Thumler J, Munroz A: Pulmonary and hepatic echinococcosis in children. *Pediatr Radiol* 7:164–175, 1975

Todorov T, Vutova K, Mechkov G, et al: Chemotherapy of human cystic echinococcosis: comparative efficacy of mebendazole and albendazole. *Ann Trop Med Parasitol* 86:59–66, 1992

Tompkins RK: Management of echinococcal cysts of the liver [editorial]. *Mayo Clin Proc* 66:1281–1282, 1991

Topal U, Parlak M, Kilic E, et al: CT and MRI findings in cerebral hydatid disease. *Eur Radiol* 5:244–247, 1995

Torricelli P, Martinelli C, Biagini R, et al: Radiographic and computed tomographic findings in hydatid disease of bone. *Skeletal Radiol* 19:435, 1990

Treugut H, Schulze K, Hubener KH, Andrasch R: Pulmonary involvement by *Echinococcus alveolaris. Radiology* 137:37–41, 1980

Vachier E, Hillman DC: Solitary pulmonary hydatid cyst: report of a case and discussion of its differential diagnosis. *Pediatrics* 35:699–703, 1965

van Sonnenberg E, et al: Percutaneous abscess drainage: current concepts. *Radiology* 181:617–626, 1991

Varela-Diaz VM, et al: Evaluation of four variants of the indirect hemagglutination test for human hydatidosis. *Am J Trop Med Hyg* 24:304–311, 1975

Vega A, et al: Hydatid cyst of the breast: mammographic findings. *AJR* 162:825–826, 1994

Venkateswara Rao R: X-ray diagnosis of hydatid cyst of the lung: its rupture into the bronchus and spontaneous healing. *J Indian Med Assoc* 34:353–354, 1960

von Sinner WN: Hydatid disease involving multiple bones and soft tissue. Case report 616. *Skeletal Radiol* 19:312–316, 1990

von Sinner WN: Successful treatment of disseminated hydatid disease using albendazole monitored by CT. *Eur J Radiol* 1:232–233, 1990

von Sinner WN: Pleural complications of hydatid disease (*Echinococcus granulosus*). *Fortschr Roentgenstr (Rofo)* 152:718–722, 1990

von Sinner WN: Ultrasound, CT and MRI of ruptured and disseminated hydatid cysts. *Eur J Radiol* 11:31–37, 1990

von Sinner WN: A case of primary osseous pelvic hydatid disease (*Echinococcus granulosus*). *Fortschr Roentgenstr (Rofo)* 155:88–90, 1991

von Sinner WN: New diagnostic signs in hydatid disease: radiography, ultrasound, CT and MRI correlated to pathology. *Eur J Radiol* 12:150–159, 1991

von Sinner WN: Hydatidosis mimicking metastases. *Ann Saudi Med* 12:316–320, 1992

von Sinner WN: Radiographic, CT and MRI spectrum of hydatid disease of the chest: a pictorial essay. *Eur Radiol* 3:62–70, 1993

von Sinner WN: CT and MRI findings of cardiac echinococcosis. *Eur Radiol* 5:66–73, 1995

von Sinner WN: Advanced medical imaging and treatment of human cystic echinococcosis. *Semin Roentgenol* 32:276–290, 1997 von Sinner WN, Stridbeck H: Hydatid disease of the spleen: ultrasonography, CT and MR imging. *Acta Radiol* 33:459–461, 1992

von Sinner WN, Akhtar M: Primary spinal echinococcosis (E.g.) of lumbosacral spine with destruction of the left pedicles of L3-5 and extension of a large paraspinal cystic mass into the spinal canal. Case report 833. *Skeletal Radiol* 24:220–223, 1994

von Sinner WN, Rifai A, te Strake L, et al: MRI of thoracic hydatid disease: correlation with radiography, ultrasonography, CT and pathology. *Acta Radiol* 31:59–62, 1990

von Sinner WN, Linjawi T, Al-Watban J: Mediastinal hydatid disease; correlations with clinical findings, radiography, CT and pathology: report of three cases. *J Can Assoc Radiol* 41:79–82, 1990

von Sinner WN, te Strake L, Clark D, Sharif H: MR imaging in hydatid disease. *AJR* 157:741–745, 1991

von Sinner WN, Hellstrom M, Kagevi I, et al: Hydatid disease of the urinary tract. *J Urol* 149:577–580, 1993

von Sinner WN, Nyman R, Linjawi T, et al: Fine needle aspiration biopsy of hydatid cysts. *Acta Radiol* 36:168–172, 1995

Vuitton DA, et al: The natural history of alveolar echinococcosis in patients before and after the era of benzimidazoles. In: Uchino J (ed) *Proceedings of the International Symposium on Alveolar Echinococcosis of the Liver.* Hokkaido University Press, Sapporo, Japan, 1997

Waddel N: Pulmonary hydatid disease. A review of 479 cases reported in the Louis Barnett Hydatid Registry of the Royal Australasian College of Surgeons. *Aust NZ J Surg* 19:273–290, 1950

Warambo MW: Hydatid disease of the spleen. *East Afr Med J* 47:286–287, 1970

Wea K, et al: Initial observation on albendazole in combination with cimetadine for the treatment of human cystic echinococcosis. *Ann Trop Med Parasitol* 88:49–52, 1994

Weill FS: *Ultrasound diagnosis of digestive diseases, 3rd edn (revised).* Springer, Berlin Heidelberg New York, 1990

Weri H, et al: Diagnosis and treatment of human hydatidosis. *Br J Clin Pharmacol* 35:565–574, 1993

WHO Informal Working Group on Echinococcosis: guidelines for treatment of cystic and alveolar echinococcosis in humans. *Bull World Health Organ* 74:231–242, 1996

Wilner D: *Radiological diagnosis of tumors in bone and allied disorders.* Saunders, Philadelphia, 1979

Wolcott MW, Harris SH, Briggs JN, et al: Hydatid disease of the lung. *J Thorac Cardiovasc Surg* 62:465–469, 1971

Wolfgang RW, Poole JB: Echinococcus disease in Northwestern Canada. *Am J Trop Med Hyg* 5:869, 1956

Woodli W, Bircer J, Witassek F, et al: Effect of plasma mebendazole concentrations in the treatment of human echinococcosis. *Am J Trop Med Hyg* 34:754–760, 1985

Xu Ming-gian: Hydatid disease of the lung. *Am J Surg* 150:568–573, 1985

Zargar SA, Khuroo MS, Khan BA, et al: Intrabiliary rupture of hepatic hydatid cyst: sonographic and cholangiographic appearances. *Gastrointest Radiol* 17:41–45, 1992

4 Chagas' Disease (American Trypanosomiasis)

With LUIZ FELIPPE MATTOSO

There are few diseases confined to one continent. Fortunately for the rest of the world, Chagas' disease occurs only in the central and southern half of the Western hemisphere, from Texas to Patagonia. Restricted though it is, there are 90 million people at risk of infection and 18 million infected individuals according to the 1998 World Health Report issued by the WHO. It is thus one of the most important public health problems in many South American nations. In Brazil 20% of the population in the endemic areas are infected. Once a disease of the rural poor, the increased migration of rural workers to the cities has made it an urban disease as well. Sao Paulo, with over 350 000 infected persons, accounts for most of the new cases seen in Brazil each year. A recent national study revealed that there are between 5 and 6 million people with Chagas' disease in that country and that 30% of all adults with clinical evidence of chronic Chagas' disease die as a result of their infection.

Chagas' disease presents with many different manifestations in both its acute and chronic stages. In the acute phase it may cause acute diffuse myocarditis and encephalitis; in the chronic form, in addition to serious myocardiopathy, there is a decrease in the number of ganglion cells in the central and peripheral autonomic nervous system. This may lead to marked enlargement of the heart, esophagus, colon, and other hollow viscera. The heart is the organ most commonly involved and, in both the acute and chronic phases, myocarditis accounts for greater morbidity and mortality than does involvement of all other organs. Despite research since 1909, when it was first described by Carlos Chagas, it remains a puzzling and incurable disease with many unresolved problems. Campaigns against the disease have often been half-hearted since it affects mostly the poor, although the spraying of insecticides to kill the reduviid bug vectors and the increased testing of blood to eliminate transmission by infected blood transfusions offer some hope for partial control.

Synonyms

Chagas' disease/syndrome. American trypanosomiasis. Chagas-Cruz disease. Barbeiro fever. Careotrypanosis. Opilation. *Sp*: Enfermedad de Chagas. Opilacao. Schizotripanosomiasis. Tripanosomiasis. *Fr*: Trypanosomose de Cruz. Maladie de Chagas. Schizotrypanose. *Ger*: Chagas-Krankheit. Chagassche Krankheit. Amerikanische Schlafkrankheit.

Definition

Chagas' disease is an acute, subacute, or chronic infection by *Trypanosoma cruzi*, a flagellated protozoan that circulates in the blood of man and other hosts.

Geographic Distribution

Chagas' disease is confined to North and South America from Texas to Patagonia (Argentina) (Fig. 4.1). It is hyperendemic in eastern Brazil, Argentina, Uruguay, Chile, and Venezuela. It is found chiefly in rural areas, and human infections have been reported from every country in the Western Hemisphere except Canada. Several children with Chagas' disease have been reported from Texas and infected triatomes (the insect vectors) and wild rodents have been discovered elsewhere in the southern and western United States.

Today several million immigrants from countries where the disease is endemic live in the United States and Europe, creating a renewed interest in the study of Chagas' disease around the world.

Epidemiology and Pathology

Chagas' disease is primarily an infection of children and young adults living in mud huts in rural areas. *T. cruzi* is transmitted by several species of reduviid bugs (especially triatomes) and has been found in

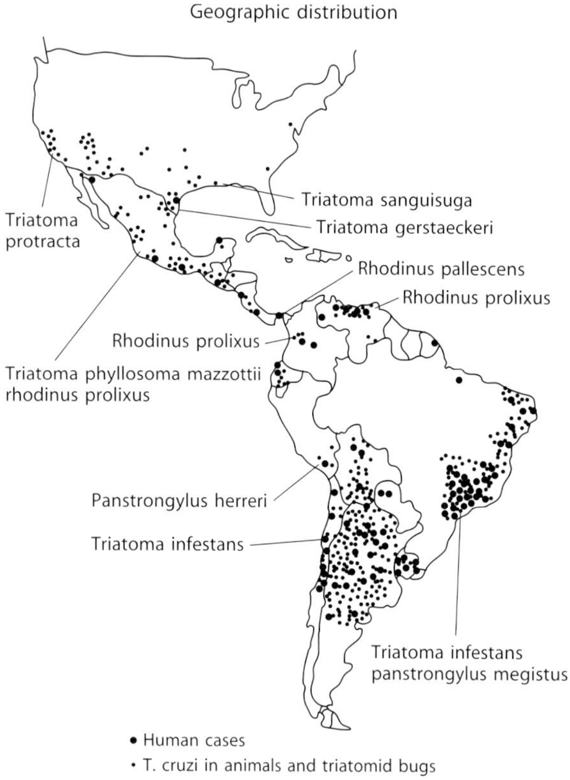

Fig. 4.1. Geographic distribution of Chagas' disease, showing human cases as well as *T. cruzi*-infected animals and *Triatoma* vectors

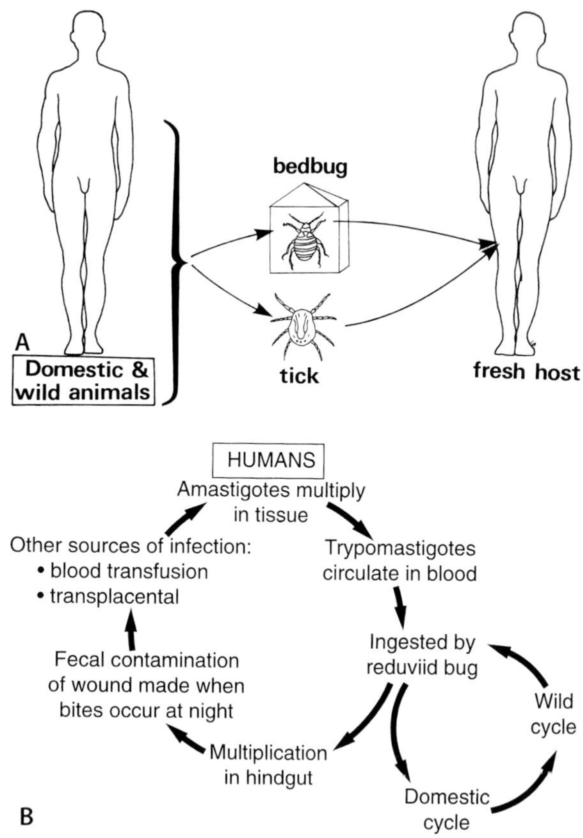

Fig. 4.2 A, B. Transmission of Chagas' disease

some bedbugs and ticks. The most important South American species are *Triatoma infestans, Rhodnius prolixus,* and *Panstrongylus megistus* (Fig. 4.1). They become infected after feeding on man, an armadillo, or other animal host (Fig. 4.2). There are many local names for the insect, such as kissing bug, assassin bug, Mexican bedbug, cone-nose bug, and wild bedbug. Most of these bugs, by preference, bite sleeping children around the face at night. Some species have a painless bite, but others have a powerful salivary toxin which produces intense local pain. The bugs live in cracks in the walls and thatched roofs of rural homes made of mud, adobe, or cane, and also in the burrows of armadillos and the nests of opossums (Fig. 4.3). Reduviids have also been found in stables, in pigsties, and in wood piles within, or adjacent to, houses.

The natural reservoirs of *T. cruzi* are man and domestic and wild animals. Approximately 150 animals harbor *T. cruzi* but the most important of these in hyperendemic areas appear to be domestic dogs and cats, and sylvatic opossums and armadillos; skunks, pigs, monkeys, guinea pigs, rats, raccoons, and bats also carry the organism. The reduviids become infective within 8–10 days after ingesting trypomastigotes of *T. cruzi* during a blood meal from one of the animal reservoirs and may remain infective for 2 years. The parasites multiply by binary fission within the digestive tract of the bugs and are transformed first into crithidia or epimastigotes. By the 10th day, these differentiate into infective metacyclic trypomastigotes in the insect's rectum and are passed in its feces. Man becomes infected when the feeding site becomes contaminated by the bug's feces which are loaded with trypomastigotes. Because the bug's bite causes irritation and itching, usually at night when a child or other victim is asleep, the person may rub the contaminated feces into the site of the bite or into the eye. *T. cruzi* may also penetrate directly through the mucous membranes of the lips or conjunctiva.

Transmission of Chagas' disease can occur by blood transfusion, and this is becoming increasingly important since many blood donors in hyperendemic areas are already infected. One of the most useful tests for detecting Chagas' disease is the enzyme-linked immunoabsorbent assay (ELISA) method, but a 1990 report showed that only 60% of Brazil's 5.5 million blood transfusions each year use blood that has been so tested. The poor, who need blood trans-

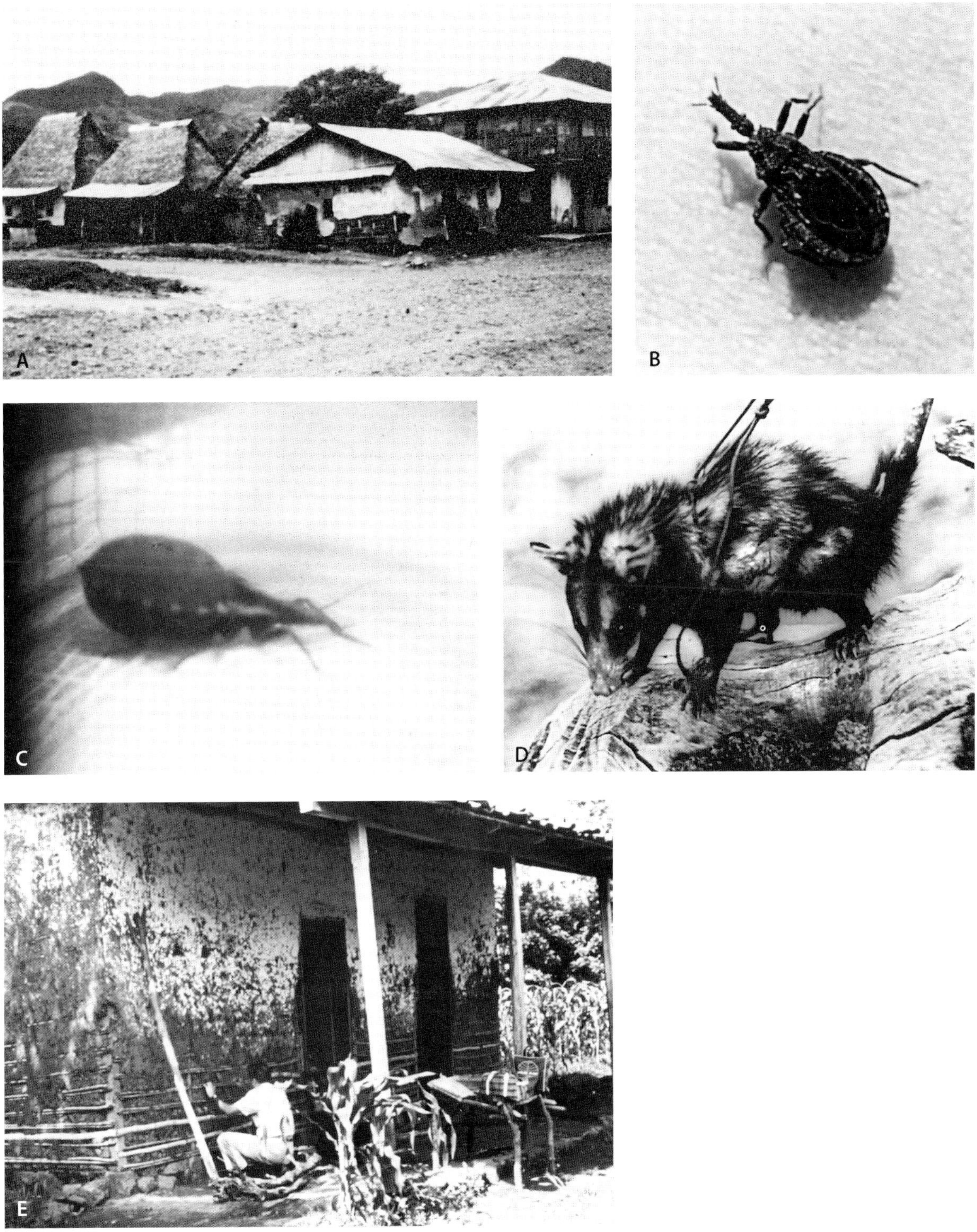

Fig. 4.3 A–E. Epidemiology of Chagas' disease. **A** Primitive housing in an area outside Panama City showing thatch-roofed adobe and mud huts which are the typical breeding grounds for Chagas' disease. Reduviid bugs, especially triatomes (**B**, **C**), or bedbugs are found in the burrows of armadillos and the nests of opossums (**D**) and in the cracks of walls of rural homes made of mud, adobe, or cane, where the bugs concentrate near sleeping areas (**E**). In **C** the triatome vector is taking a blood meal from a guinea pig. The proboscis is penetrating through the gauze mesh and the abdomen of the bug is greatly swollen by blood that it has ingested during feeding. The opossum in **D** is a *Didelphis* caught near one of the adobe houses in the upper Maranon River valley of Peru. This animal was naturally infected with *T. cruzi, T. rangeli*, and numerous helminths

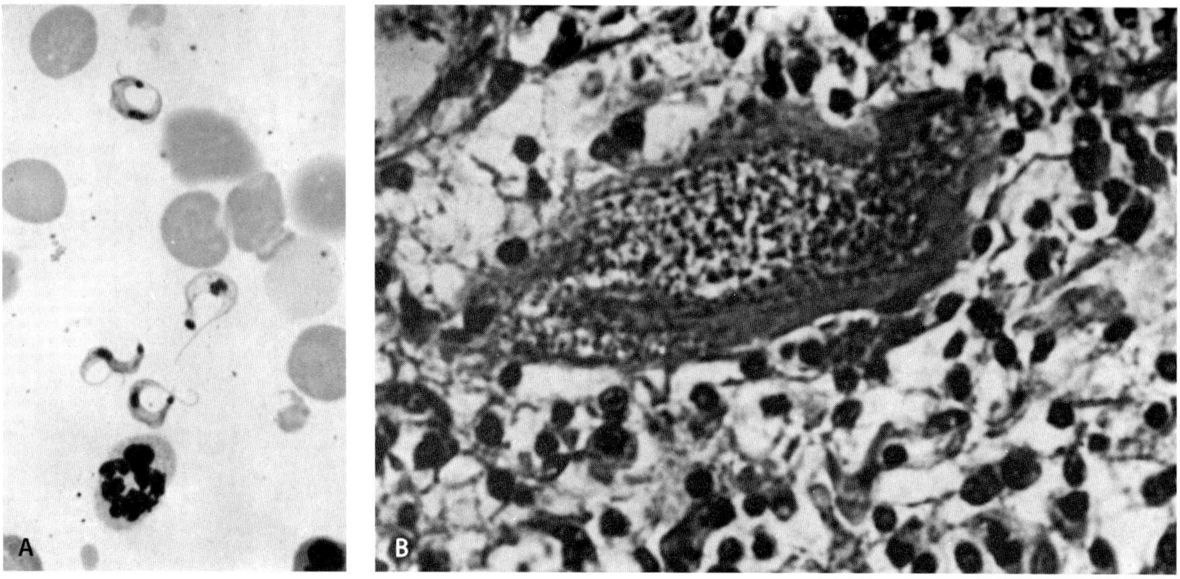

Fig. 4.4. **A** Photomicrograph of a blood smear containing several trypomastigotes. The parasite can be recognized by its large anteriorly placed kinetoplast and its C or U shape, which distinguish it from the parasite of African trypanosomiasis which has an S shape and a small kinetoplast. ×1020; AFIP 56-3455. **B** High magnification of myocardium in acute Chagas' myocarditis. A mononuclear cell infiltrate surrounds a degenerating myofiber in which large numbers of amastigotes are enclosed within a pseudocyst. The heart was extensively involved with a pancarditis

fusions after surgery or trauma, cannot afford to pay for this tested blood; in the worst areas 10% of blood was found to be infected. Poorer countries, such as Bolivia with more than 500000 infected people in a population of over 7 million, have few resources available to test blood for Chagas' disease carriers. Rarely, transmission may occur through food contaminated by feces or urine from an infected animal. Fetuses may be infected by transplacental transmission during either the acute or chronic phase of Chagas' disease. Sequelae from such an infection may include spontaneous abortion, intrauterine growth retardation, myocarditis, neurological changes, and perinatal death. Transmission may also occur by organ transplantation and, in these cases, infection is more severe due to immunosuppressive therapy.

Trypanosoma cruzi was first described by Carlos Chagas in the state of Minas Gerais, Brazil, in 1909. It is a tiny pleomorphic protozoan (16–22 µm long) which divides its life cycle between man (and animals) and the bug vectors. Trypomastigotes, the flagellated forms of trypanosomes, circulate in the blood of infected individuals. In stained blood smears they appear as C- or U-shaped flagellated organisms (unlike African trypanosomes responsible for sleeping sickness, which are S-shaped) (Fig. 4.4A). Amastigotes, also called leishmanial forms, are intracellular. When a trypomastigote invades the host tissues it enters the host cells, especially reticuloendothelial cells, muscle, and glia. In so doing, it loses its flagellum and undulating membrane and rounds up into an amastigote, a tiny round body 3–5 µm in diameter (Fig. 4.4B). Division occurs by successive binary fission to form intracellular masses of amastigotes (pseudocysts). When the cell ruptures or disintegrates, amastigotes are transformed to trypomastigotes which invade more host cells and enter the blood.

This multiplication occurs rapidly at the site of inoculation, causing a severe localized inflammatory reaction consisting of neutrophils, eosinophils, interstitial edema, and focal lymphangitis (a chagoma). This is followed by lymphatic spread to regional lymph nodes to produce a primary complex in the first or second week of infection. Amastigotes multiply within the cells over a 5-day period, and evolve into highly motile trypanosomes, rupture the cell membranes, and disperse to either enter a new cell or return to the blood. The fact that *T. cruzi* multiplies within the host cell cytoplasm and not in the bloodstream makes Chagas' disease especially difficult to treat.

This parasitemia results in dissemination of the disease and invasion of multiple host tissues. Amastigotes can be found in virtually any organ or tissue but there is a distinct predilection for smooth and striated muscle (especially cardiac muscle) and glial and nerve cells. In heavy infections, where many amastigotes are released, there may be destruction of other cells, such as myofibers, liver cells, and adipose cells. This occurs primarily in the acute phase

of the disease, when the parasitemia and invasion of tissues is most pronounced and before specific immunity has developed.
With progression of the disease and development of partial immunity, the acute inflammatory process abates and is followed by a chronic inflammatory reaction consisting of histiocytes, lymphocytes, plasma cells, and, later, epithelioid and multinucleated giant cells. The lesions become more localized with occasional development of distinct granulomas. Adjacent nonparasitized cells may exhibit hyaline degeneration with partial or complete disappearance of cross-striations and necrobiosis. Marked degeneration and lysis of ganglion cells occurs in the tissues surrounding ruptured pseudocysts, especially in the heart and brain. As the amastigotes degenerate, the ganglion cells in their immediate vicinity rapidly disappear without cellular reaction. Köberle believed that destruction of the ganglion cells is due neither to parasitism of the nerve cells themselves nor to the marked inflammatory reaction, but rather to cytotoxic and necrolytic substances (i.e., a toxin or enzyme liberated or elaborated after disintegration of the amastigote forms outside the ruptured pseudocyst). However, no such substance has yet been found, and the etiology of the extensive nerve cell destruction seen in Chagas' disease remains a mystery.
This is the basic pathological process during the *acute and subacute phases*, but the pathogenesis of Chagas' disease involves at least three distinct phases, each with its own pathological processes. Once defense mechanisms have developed, the disease passes into a *latent phase* for many years, usually several decades, during which the parasites are difficult to demonstrate, both in the bloodstream and in body tissues. The *third or chronic* (late) stage of the disease provides the Chagas' syndromes which are the end result of the destruction of ganglion cells in the central or peripheral nervous system. The lesions may be widespread, but are most severe in the heart, muscles, nervous system, and gastrointestinal tract, particularly the esophagus and colon.
The three stages of the disease, although of one etiology, are clinically and radiologically distinct. The middle latent period is clinically silent; the acute and late stages can be severe and dramatic.

Laboratory Diagnosis

There is a complement fixation test (Machado-Guerreiro reaction) which becomes positive in the acute stage at 1 month postinfection and remains positive thereafter. The Machado-Guerreiro reaction may present a high incidence of false-positives and -negatives, resulting in a low sensitivity and specificity test.
There is a precipitin test (hemoagglutination reaction) which is 95% positive in the early stages. The immunofluorescence and ELISA tests are highly sensitive and specific, although false-positive reactions with malaria, leprosy, and leishmaniasis can occur. The xeno test is diagnostic: uninfected laboratory-raised bugs are fed on a patient, then examined 30 days later for metacyclic trypanosomes in their hindgut or feces. Xenodiagnosis can be used to check serology, isolate strains, and evaluate medical (chemo) therapy.
Direct microscopic search for *T. cruzi* in peripheral blood smears may be attempted only in the first few weeks of the acute stage (Fig. 4.4 A). It is rare to find the parasites in the blood after the 6th week. They are seldom identified during the chronic stage. In the acute stage, there is a leukocytosis with marked lymphocytosis or monocytosis, a moderate eosinophilia, and an elevated sedimentation rate.

Acute Chagas' Disease

The characteristic pathological process is the chagoma. This can be a primary lesion at the site of inoculation or a secondary lesion with the same pathogenesis. The principal and most important findings are in the heart and central nervous system.
In the heart, a multifocal myocarditis is invariably present and is more intense than other types of myocarditis. The heart is flabby and enlarged, with dilatation being a more predominant feature than hypertrophy, often accompanied by thinning of the ventricular walls (Fig. 4.5 A, B). Focal areas of inflammation and hemorrhage may occur in the endocardium (rarely leading to mural thrombosis) and in the epicardium, giving rise to pericardial effusion. Microscopically, there is a severe diffuse interstitial and interfibrillary edema, congestion, and numerous swollen myofibers containing leishmania (Fig. 4.5 C). There is degeneration of the myofibers and infiltration by lymphocytes, plasma cells, and other mononuclear cells (Fig. 4.5 D). In addition, there is hyaline necrosis of isolated cardiac fibers and some fibers have dark bars of clumped fibrils arranged tranversely on their longitudinal axis. This change, seen in sections stained with iron hematoxylin or in silver-impregnated sections (the "Magarinos-Torres' lesion"), is characteristic and perhaps specific for acute Chagas' myocarditis. The cardiac valves are not involved.
In patients with encephalitis or meningoencephalitis, examination of the brain, spinal cord, and meninges may show similar inflammatory infiltrates

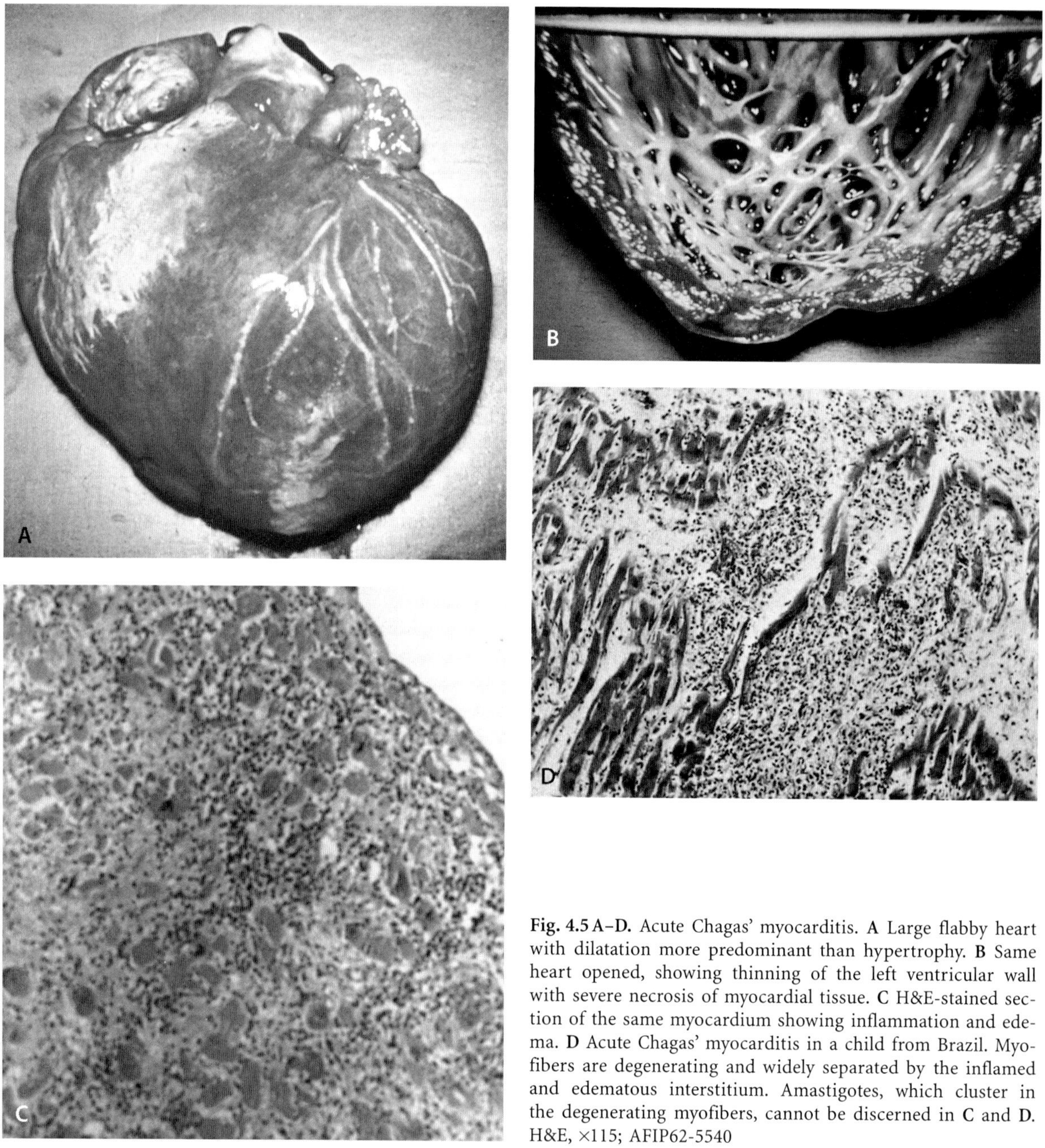

Fig. 4.5 A–D. Acute Chagas' myocarditis. **A** Large flabby heart with dilatation more predominant than hypertrophy. **B** Same heart opened, showing thinning of the left ventricular wall with severe necrosis of myocardial tissue. **C** H&E-stained section of the same myocardium showing inflammation and edema. **D** Acute Chagas' myocarditis in a child from Brazil. Myofibers are degenerating and widely separated by the inflamed and edematous interstitium. Amastigotes, which cluster in the degenerating myofibers, cannot be discerned in **C** and **D**. H&E, ×115; AFIP62-5540

with mononuclear cells, congestion, perivascular inflammation, small hemorrhages, and neuronophagia. Chagas described these parasitic nodules in the cerebrum, cerebellum, basal nuclei, pons, and spinal cord. The parasites may be present within the reticulum cells of the meninges as well as in the glial cells and neurons. Lesions may be found elsewhere in the body, such as the liver, spleen, prostate, and testes, but parasites are rare and must be diligently searched for, sometimes at great length.

Clinical Characteristics

Acute Chagas' disease may occur at any age, but is most frequent in the first years of life, especially during the summer. It has been estimated that, in the initial stage of infection (first 2 months), only 1% of those infected will develop recognizable clinical signs; therefore the vast majority of infections go undiagnosed. In previous years, the mortality during this stage was thought to approximate 50% in some areas, but currently is less than 5% in most areas and, when subclinical cases are considered, the overall mortality falls below 1%. Less than 5% of patients will present in the acute phase with meningoencephalitis or heart failure, both of which indicate a bad prognosis. The mortality from acute myocarditis or meningoencephalitis varies from 2% to 10%. In Laranja's series of 235 acute patients, the mortality was 9.4%, with death from congestive heart failure, convulsive seizures, or secondary infection. Acute Chagas' disease occurs in AIDS patients, causing severe encephalitis or myocarditis.

The incubation period of acute Chagas' disease varies from 1 to 2 weeks depending on the portal of entry, the size of inoculum, and the patient's age. Clinical signs include a high continuous fever up to 104° F, which may persist for 1 or more months, malaise, muscle pains, sweating, anorexia, vomiting, and diarrhea. In about 50% of patients the trypanosomes enter through the conjunctiva, causing elastic edema of the upper and lower eyelids, chemosis of the conjunctiva, and enlargement of the preauricular lymph nodes (Romaña's sign) (Fig. 4.6). In 25% of patients a portal of entry can be identified by a nodular or ulcerative skin lesion (chagoma) at the site of inoculation with accompanying regional lymph node enlargement. The presence of Romaña's sign and/or a chagoma is quite helpful in the clinical diagnosis of acute Chagas' disease; these signs may disappear within 30 days. The lymphadenitis, which at first is localized to the area of the primary lesion, later becomes generalized. A firm nonpitting edema may develop in the legs and feet and become generalized; this is probably related to hypoproteinemia and usually disappears in about 3 weeks. The liver and spleen frequently enlarge after several weeks. Parasitic-induced lesions in the lungs may result in pneumonia from secondary infection. Symptoms of meningoencephalitis may be the primary manifestation of Chagas' disease, but are more frequently noted after onset of other clinical signs.

Some cardiac involvement probably occurs in virtually all patients with acute Chagas' disease, but is usually unrecognized. The clinical manifestations resemble myocarditis from other causes. Most patients have transient cardiac insufficiency with slight to moderate reversible cardiac enlargement. More severe right- and left-sided failure may occur with pulmonary and systemic congestion, tachycardia, gallop rhythm, Stokes-Adams syndrome, premature ventricular contractions, hypophonetic heart sounds, and a systolic murmur in the mitral area. The systolic blood pressure and pulse pressure are decreased.

Echocardiography, serial chest radiographs, and electrocardiograms provide the most accurate methods of detecting acute myocarditis and of assessing the degree of involvement. ECG abnormalities were noted in 78 of 180 patients with acute Chagas' disease studied by Laranja; 21 of these patients died. The most common findings include a prolongation of the P-R interval, primary T-wave changes, low-voltage QRS, prolonged Q-T interval and associated ST-T changes.

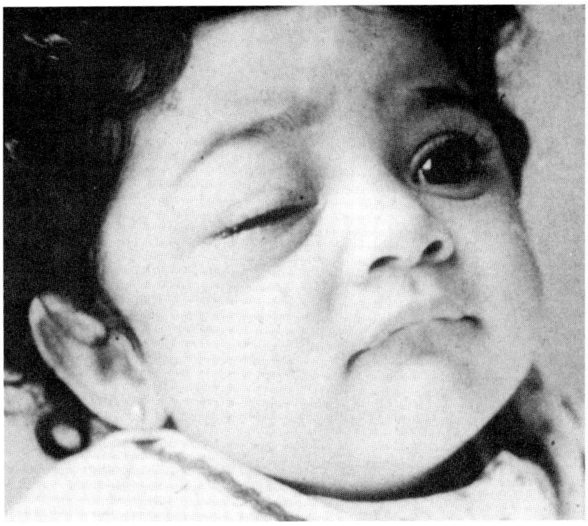

Fig. 4.6. Child with Romaña's sign: unilateral conjunctivitis, palpebral and periorbital edema, and preauricular lymphadenopathy. AFIP 62-3934-6

These changes are usually reversible and, in most patients, symptoms disappear within 2–3 months, although some patients (probably 15%) continue to have residual ECG abnormalities. The fever usually subsides within 4–5 weeks; the parasites disappear from the peripheral blood and as mentioned above, Romaña's sign and the chagoma disappear within 1 month, but hepatosplenomegaly may persist for 1–5 months after onset of the disease. Serology is not useful in this early stage.

Imaging Diagnosis

In the acute phase ultrasonography may help in detecting enlarged regional or disseminated lymph node involvement and occasionally may show in patients with hepatosplenomegaly a hyperechoic liver due to fatty infiltration. No focal lesions are detected in the liver or spleen.

The heart changes are very well seen in echocardiograms that display to advantage anatomical and functional alterations, such as decreased cardiac performance usually found in myocarditis. Pericardial effusions are easily identified. MRI is also accurate but more expensive.

In patients with clinical evidence of acute myocarditis, echocardiography and radiographs of the chest show moderate or marked diffuse cardiac enlarge-

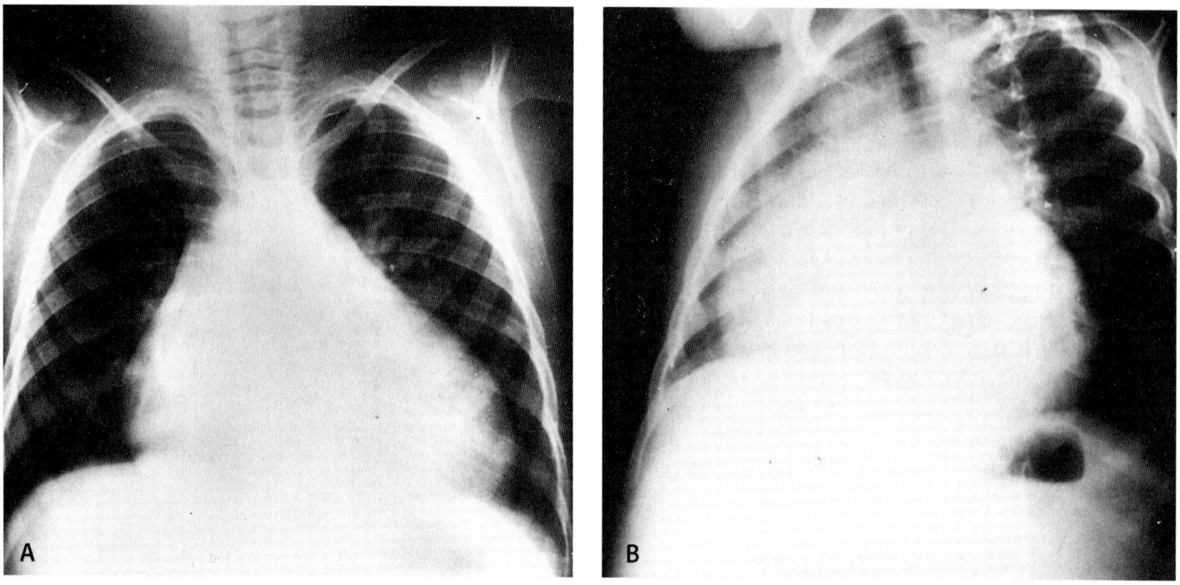

Fig. 4.7 A, B. Acute Chagas' myocarditis in a 6-year-old Brazilian boy. Posteroanterior (PA) (**A**) and left anterior oblique (LAO) (**B**) views of the chest show marked generalized cardiac enlargement with dilatation of all chambers. The hilar areas are not prominent and the lungs show no evidence of vascular congestion. Fluoroscopically the cardiac pulsations were decreased. The child had had dyspnea and abdominal pain for 4 months and pitting edema in the lower legs for 2 months. The jugular veins were distended and the heart sounds were weak, with a systolic murmur in the mitral area. The liver was palpable 10 cm below the right costal margin. Chagas' serology was positive. (Courtesy of Dr. Clovis Simao, Sao Paulo)[1]

ment (Fig. 4.7). Ultrasonography or fluoroscopy will show decreased cardiac pulsations, especially at the left apex. A radiographic "cardiac series" will demonstrate enlargement of all chambers; the normal outline of the cardiac silhouette and the interventricular groove are lost. The right ventricle abuts against the sternum on the lateral view and the left ventricle overlaps the spine. The left atrium displaces the esophagus posteriorly and the left main bronchus superiorly. Oblique views confirm the atrial and ventricular enlargement. The lung fields are usually clear without evidence of congestion or edema.

Subacute Chagas' Disease

Several investigators (Laranja, Oliveira, and Andrade) have described a subacute cardiac form of Chagas' disease. This is seen rarely in young patients and is characterized by severe rapid heart failure. These patients fail to respond to the usual therapeutic modalities and do not have fever or other signs of acute Chagas' disease. Large numbers of parasites are present in the cardiac fibers and perhaps in the peripheral blood as well. Microscopically, there is an intense diffuse myocarditis with exudative changes, marked interstitial inflammation, and often degenerative changes in the cardiac fibers, at times with the Magarinos-Torres' lesion.

Latent (Indeterminate) Chagas' Disease

The acute stage of Chagas' disease usually resolves completely in a few weeks or months, but may pass into a latent subacute or chronic stage. Patients who recover from the acute disease, as well as millions of people in endemic areas who have never had clinical evidence of Chagas' disease, have a positive complement fixation test (Machado-Guerreiro reaction). Others have a positive xeno text. Since spontaneous cures have not been seen in patients with *T. cruzi* infection, the assumption has been made that in the latent phase a patient may harbor the infection without symptoms and with a normal physical examination and ECG, chest radiograph, barium swallow, and barium enema but a positive serum or blood test. It is unknown whether these patients have a host-parasite equilibrium without developing additional lesions or whether, in fact, they have slowly progressive lesions.

This latent stage has also been called the "indeterminate or undetermined phase" and 2%–5% of these patients become symptomatic each year so that, between 10 and 20 years, about 4% of this

[1] The authors wish to express their apprecution to Dr. Clovis Simao, Sao Paulo who participated in writing this chapter for the first edition of this book. Many of his fine illustrations have been used in developing the current chapter.

group will become symptomatic, with the figure rising to 70% in 40 years. Reactivation may occur when HIV-positive patients develop AIDS.

In one follow-up study of 72 patients with acute disease over a 4- to 10-year period, 15% had ECG changes indicating an active myocarditis. Diminution in the number of ganglion cells in the Auerbach plexi of the digestive tract is occasionally found in patients with a positive complement fixation test, who are ill or dying of causes other than trypanosomiasis. In patients with the "latent" phase of Chagas' disease, changes in esophageal motility have been diagnosed by barium swallow studies or by placing a balloon within the esophagus and recording peristaltic activity. Thus, a person with a positive complement fixation test or positive xenodiagnosis probably should not be placed in the latent category unless the ECGs are normal and function of the alimentary tract is also found to be normal.

More recently, echocardiograms of this group have shown a high incidence of ventricular wall dyskinesis and hypokinesis, mainly in the apical region, which helps to differentiate this myocardiopathy from others. Minor cardiac involvement may be seen, with dilatation of the heart but normal motility; the systolic volume is increased but ventricular function is preserved. Alteration of myocardial contraction may be noted with the use of isoproterenol and isotonic effort maneuvers. The future will probably show whether these patients will become symptomatic in a shorter period and whether they will have a poorer prognosis.

Chronic Chagas' Disease

After a period of many years or decades, and probably after repeated infections with the trypanosomes, the systemic changes of the chronic stage may develop. These occur commonly in the esophagus, rectosigmoid colon, and heart, and less often in the central nervous system (CNS). CNS involvement may be the late result of the acute phase or due to reactivation, e.g., in the immunosuppressed.

Gastrointestinal Tract

Brasil suggested that the name "aperistalsis" be applied to chronic Chagas' disease to denote the pathophysiological disturbances of motor incoordination and defective esophageal and colonic motility, together with disturbed or absent peristalsis without propulsive efficiency. Köberle and others demonstrated that the quantitative and qualitative reduction in the number of ganglia throughout the entire gastrointestinal tract, especially in the colon and esophagus, causes aperistalsis and atony, which in turn result in dilatation of these hollow viscera. The complement fixation and hemagglutination tests are positive in 95% and the immunofluorescence test is 100% positive in this group. The age range is from 2 to 75 years with an average of 33 years. Although there is deficiency of ganglion cells throughout the gastrointestinal tract in chronic Chagas' disease, radiographically and clinically the esophagus and rectosigmoid colon show by far the greatest distention, probably because they are subjected to greater mechanical pressure. The gallbladder, bronchi, ureters, and bladder may rarely be dilated.

Esophagus

In the esophagus, early changes of motor dysfunction are hypercontractility and increased tone and hypertrophy of the circular muscle layer, often resulting in dysphagia. Later, as denervation progresses, there is decompensation, dilatation, and stasis. Food may become lodged in the esophagus and cause local irritation, leading to inflammation, ulceration, bleeding, perforation, and fistulae.

The earliest radiographic manifestations of Chagas' disease in the esophagus are those of motor dysfunction. Initially, tone is maintained and there is little or no dilatation. Gradually increasing disturbances in tone, rhythm, and motility over a number of years give the appearance of bizarre, dysrhythmic contractions on barium swallow (Fig. 4.8). In severe infections, however, there may be an extremely dilated and flaccid esophagus with a transverse diameter of 7 cm or more, exhibiting marked loss of tone with weak, uncoordinated contractions. The appearance of advanced megaesophagus both on plain radiographs of the chest and on barium swallow is remarkably similar to that of achalasia. In both entities the dilated esophagus appears as a vertical density along the entire right paramediastinal border on frontal films, usually distended with air and sometimes with an air-fluid level if the patient has recently ingested liquids (Figs. 4.9–4.12). A tapered distal esophageal segment down to the cardiac sphincter is seen in Chagas' megaesophagus, similar to that seen in achalasia. There may be some delay in passage of food through this area because of failure of relaxation and motor incoordination at the level of the sphincter, as well as lack of propulsive peristalsis throughout the esophagus.

Carcinoma of the esophagus, sometimes with rupture into the mediastinum and abscess formation, develops in about 7% of patients with Chagas' megaesophagus (Fig. 4.13). Intraesophageal ultraso-

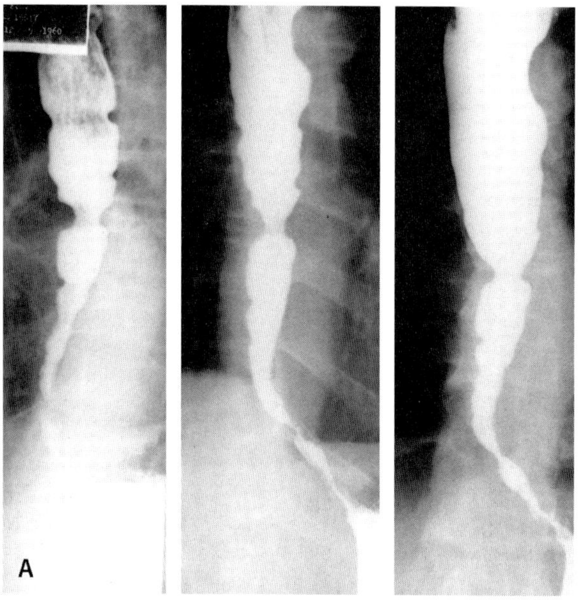

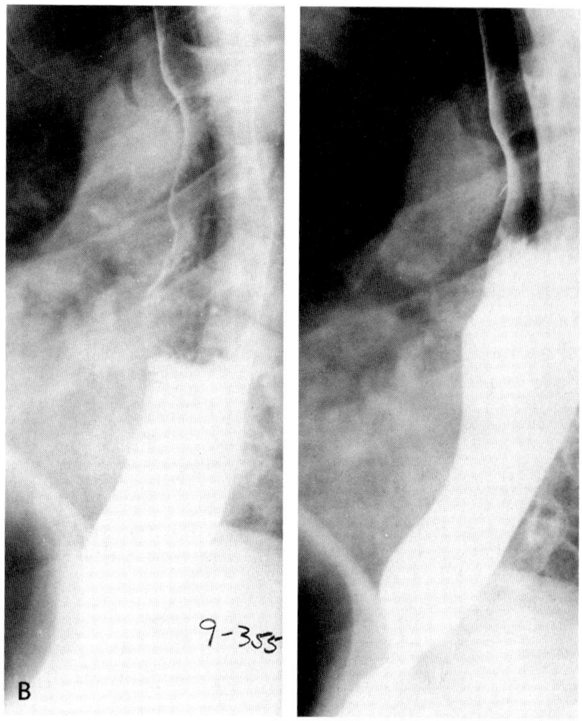

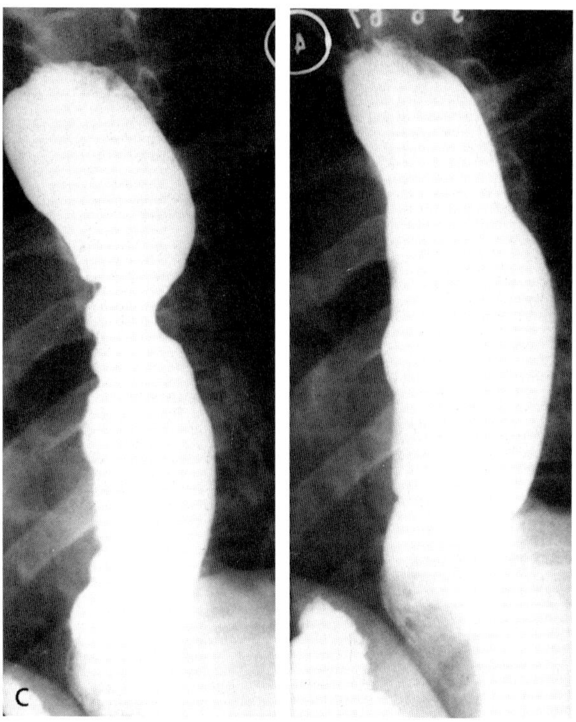

Fig. 4.8 A–C. Chagas' megaesophagus in three different Brazilian patients showing dysrhythmic contractions, disturbance of tone, and moderate dilatation of the esophagus. Note the marked alteration of persistalsis with local incoordinate, bizarre, nonpropulsive contractions in patient **A**. Patient **B** was a 48-year-old man with bowel constipation for 18 years and bowel movements every 18–20 days. He also complained of heart palpitations and dysphagia for dry foods. A systolic murmur was heard in the mitral area. Serological test for Chagas' disease was positive. Radiographic evaluation revealed myocardiopathy as well as typical megacolon and megaesophagus of Chagas' disease due to aganglionosis. (**A**, **B** courtesy of Dr. Clovis Simao, Sao Paulo.) Patient **C**, a 34-year-old man from the state of Bahia, lived in a clay house infested by numerous barbeiro (*Triatoma infestans*). He had no difficulty in swallowing but had severe constipation, with 15 days between bowel movements. The Machado-Guerreiro complement fixation test was postive. There is considerable esophageal dilatation with dysrhythmic contractions and a spastic distal segment at the esophagogastric junction

nography may help detect and stage carcinoma in association with megaesophagus by allowing grading of the mural involvement and by showing transmural extension of the tumor to the mediastinum. Computed tomography (CT) and magnetic resonance imaging (MRI) studies are also excellent imaging modalities for demonstrating the extent of the tumor and detecting mediastinal and nodal involvement when carcinoma develops in Chagas' megaesophagus, or for detecting evidence of mediastinitis after esophageal perforation. They will also show an uncomplicated megaesophagus (Fig. 4.14), but barium studies are much easier and cheaper for this purpose.

(Text continues on p. 369)

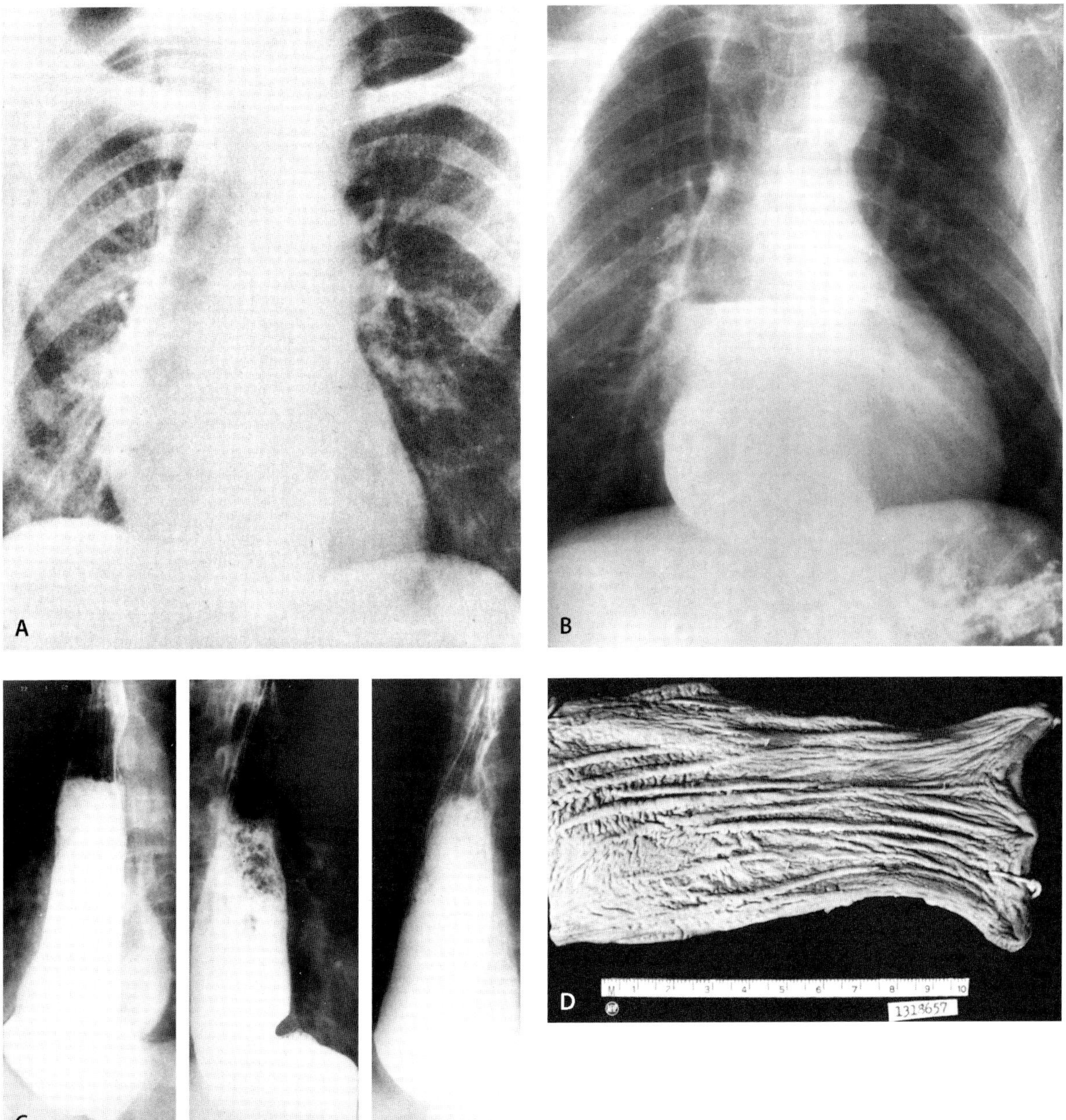

Fig. 4.9 A–D. Megaesophagus in three different Brazilian patients. **A** Fifty-year-old black man with difficulty in swallowing dry foods for 15 years. He felt that food stopped behind his sternum. The dysphagia became progressively worse until he could no longer swallow fluids. The entire esophagus is dilated from the diaphragm to the thoracic inlet, with a resultant air-filled vertical soft tissue density widening the entire right paramediastinal border. The appearance is identical to advanced achalasia of the esophagus on plain film examination of the chest. **B** Fifty-year-old white man with dysphagia of 20 years' duration with frequent regurgitation and increased salivation. For the past year he had postprandial epigastric pain. Barium swallow shows both barium and air within a grossly dilated esophagus widening the right paramediastinal border. There is a tapered distal esophageal segment at the esophagogastric junction. Radiographically, this appearance is indistinguishable from achalasia. This chest film was obtained 5 min after ingestion of barium and shows a prominent air-barium fluid level in the dilated mid-esophagus. **C** Thirty-six year old white man with dysphagia for dry foods of 16 years' duration. He had almost complete incapacity to swallow food. In addition he had a systolic murmur in the mitral area: his ECG showed right bundle branch block and left axis deviation. Barium swallow showed moderate dilatation of the esophagus down to a somewhat contracted esophagogastric junction. The three films in this patient were obtained 30 seconds, 5 minutes and 30 minutes, respectively, after ingestion of barium and indicate markedly delayed emptying of the esophagus due to loss of effective peristalsis and a failure of the cardiac sphincter to relax. All three patients had a positive serological reaction for Chagas' disease. (**A–C** courtesy of Dr. Clovis Simao, Sao Paulo) **D** Gross specimen of Chagas' megaesophagus. AFIP 69-6536

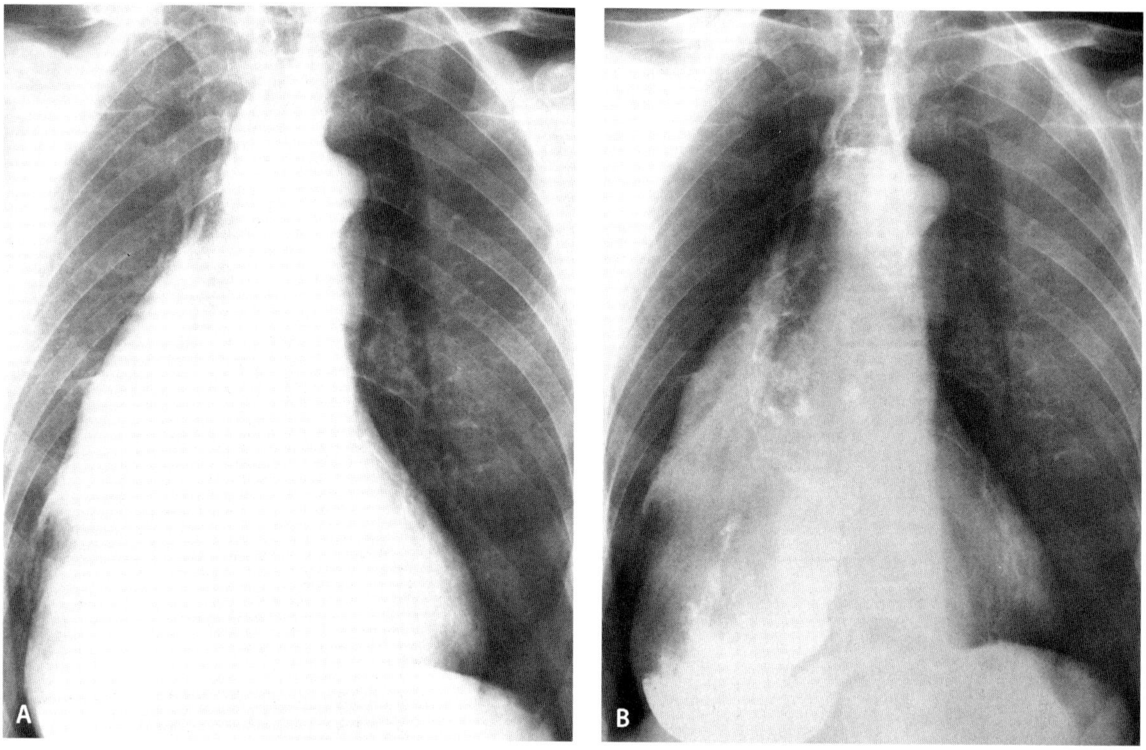

Fig. 4.10 A, B. Massive megaesophagus in an adult Brazilian man with chronic dysphagia. **A** A soft tissue mass widens the right paramediastinum and projects almost to the lateral chest wall. The esophagus is distended with fluid and a minimal amount of air. **B** Barium swallow shows the full extent of the markedly dilated mid and lower esophagus with barium having settled to the bottom of the fluid column. The contracted distal esophageal segment follows a tortuous course to the esophagogastric junction. This PA film of the chest was taken 30 minutes after ingestion of barium, indicating marked delay in esophageal emptying due to virtually complete loss of peristalsis within the dilated, atonic esophagus

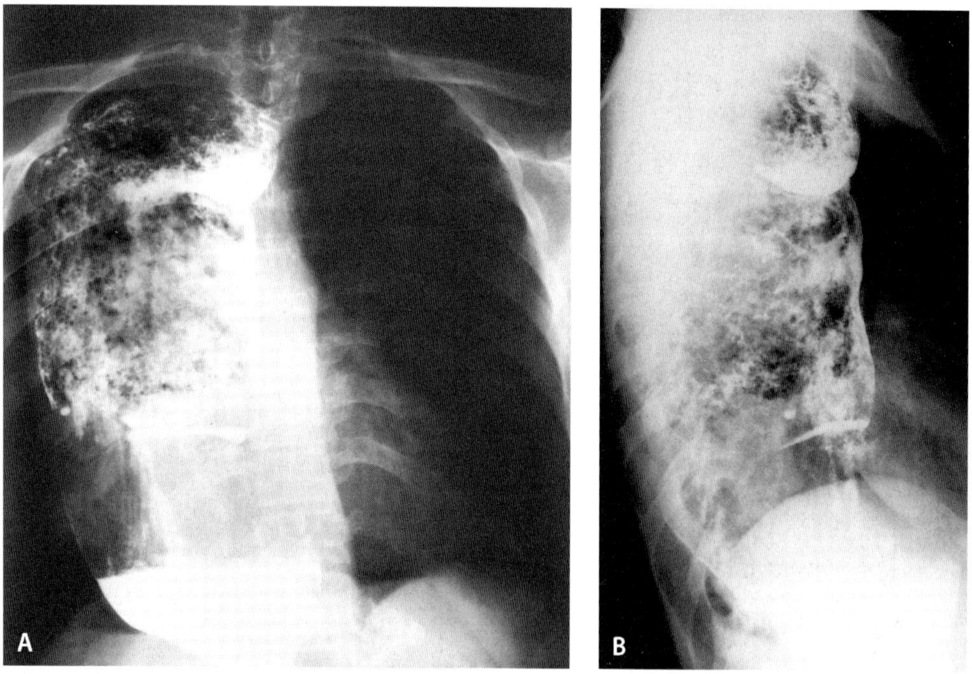

Fig. 4.11 A, B. Megaesophagus in a Brazilian man. Massive dilatation of the esophagus is seen on frontal (**A**) and oblique (**B**) views of the chest following barium swallow. Food residue, barium, and fluid fill the entire distended esophagus down to the tapered esophagogastric junction. (Courtesy of Dr. Clovis Simao, Sao Paulo)

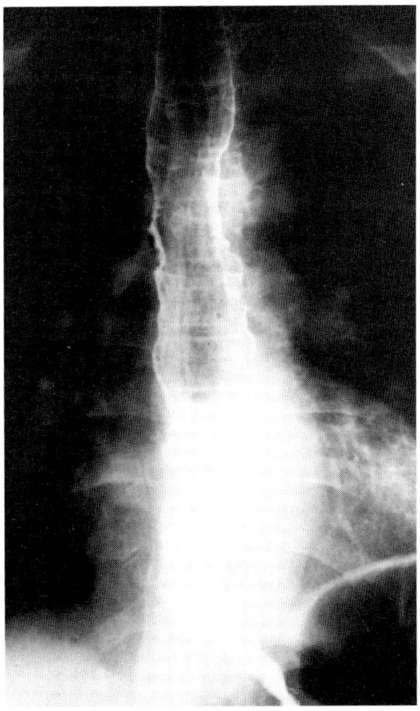

Fig. 4.12. Chagas' megaesophagus in an adult Brazilian man showing only slight dilatation of the esophagus but multiple shallow ulcerations with a ragged contour of the mid-esophagus. Note the tapered distal esophageal segment. (Courtesy of Dr. Clovis Simao, Sao Paulo) ▶

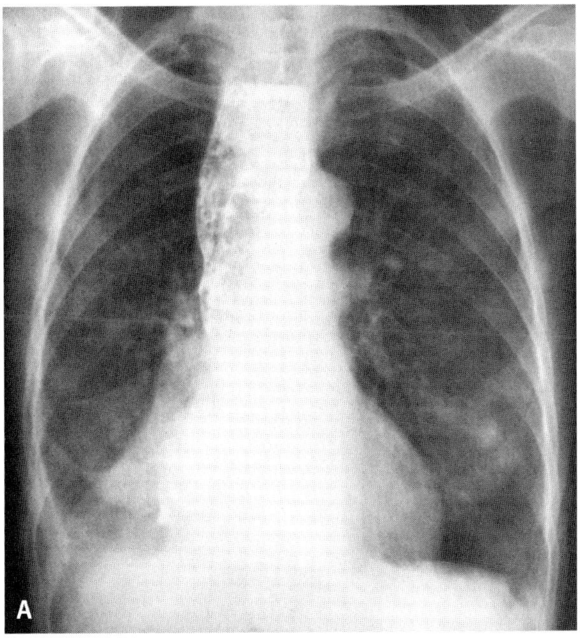

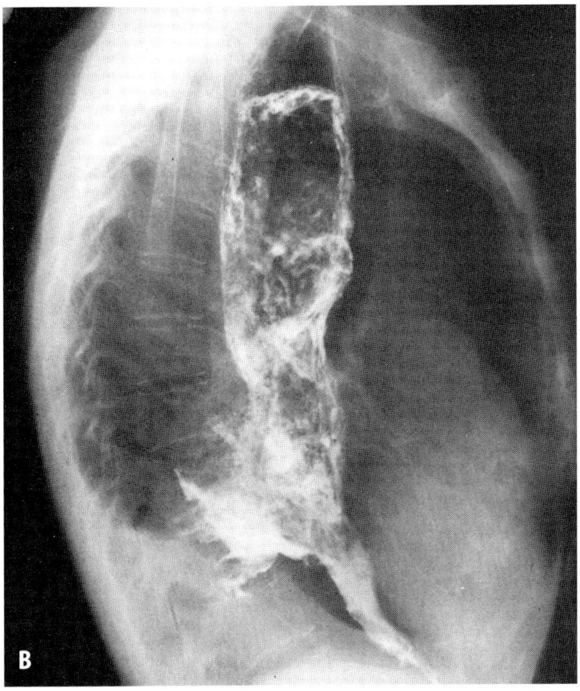

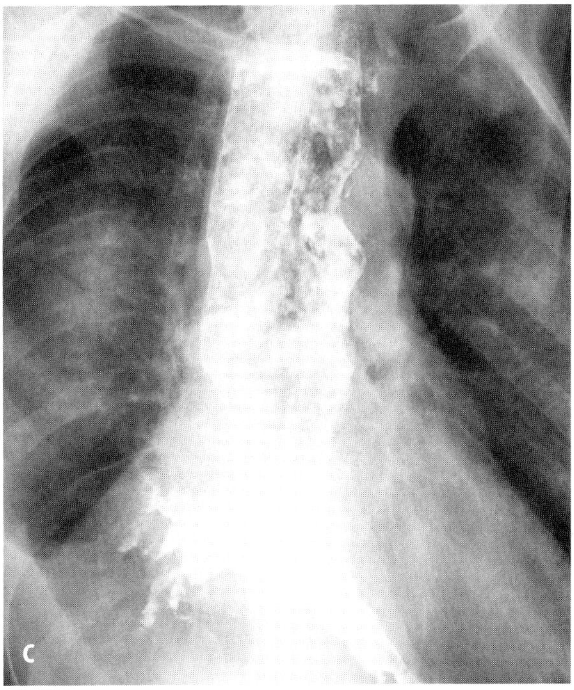

Fig. 4.13 A–C. Chagas' megaesophagus in an adult Brazilian man. There is development of carcinoma in the distal third of the esophagus, with perforation to form a large abscess extending into the right lower lobe and pleural space (**A**). Note the irregularity and thickening of the esophageal wall at the junction of the middle and distal thirds of the esophagus. Barium enters the mediastinal and right lower lobe abscess, seen best on lateral (**B**) and RAO (**C**) views. There is considerable pleural fluid (empyema) at the right base posteriorly and laterally. Carcinoma is a complication in 7% of patients with Chagas' megaesophagus. (Courtesy of Dr. Clovis Simao, Sao Paulo)
▼

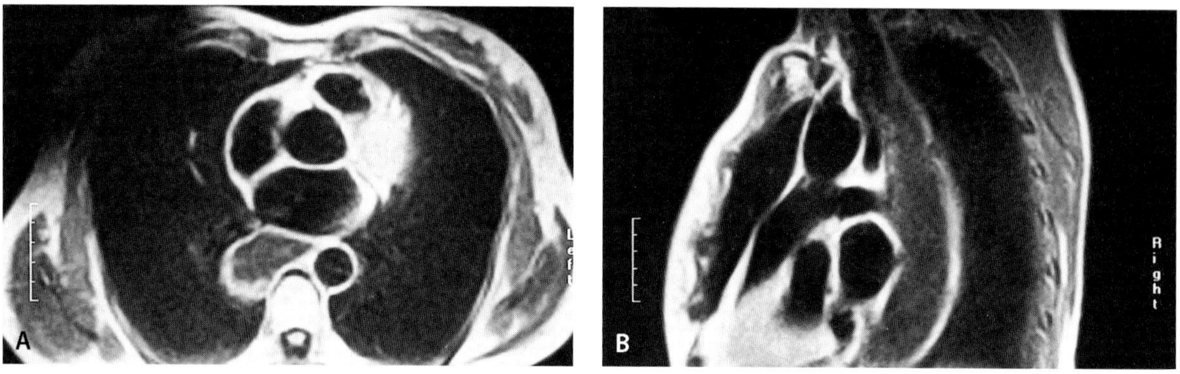

▲

Fig. 4.14. T1-weighted MR images showing a megaesophagus from Chagas' disease in axial (**A**) and sagittal-oblique (**B**) planes

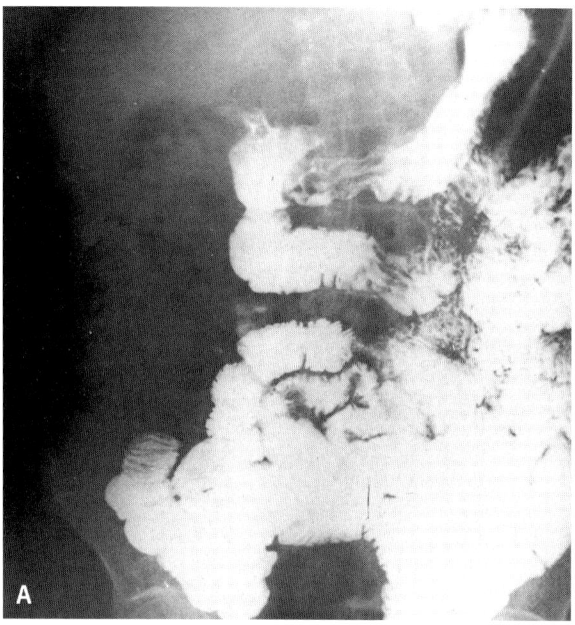

Fig. 4.15 A–C. Chagas' disease with megaduodenum in a 57-year-old Brazilian black man. The patient had epigastric burning and pain for 1 year which was unrelated to meals but improved with alkali agents. He also complained of occasional nausea and vomiting but no hematemesis or melena. Ten months later he had the same problems and an ECG showed sinus bradycardia. Serological test for Chagas' disease was positive. A gastrojejunal anastomosis was performed, and at surgery the duodenum was found to be dilated throughout its length, but there were no ulcers and no tension from adjacent aorticomesenteric vessels. (Courtesy of Dr. Clovis Simao, Sao Paulo)

▼

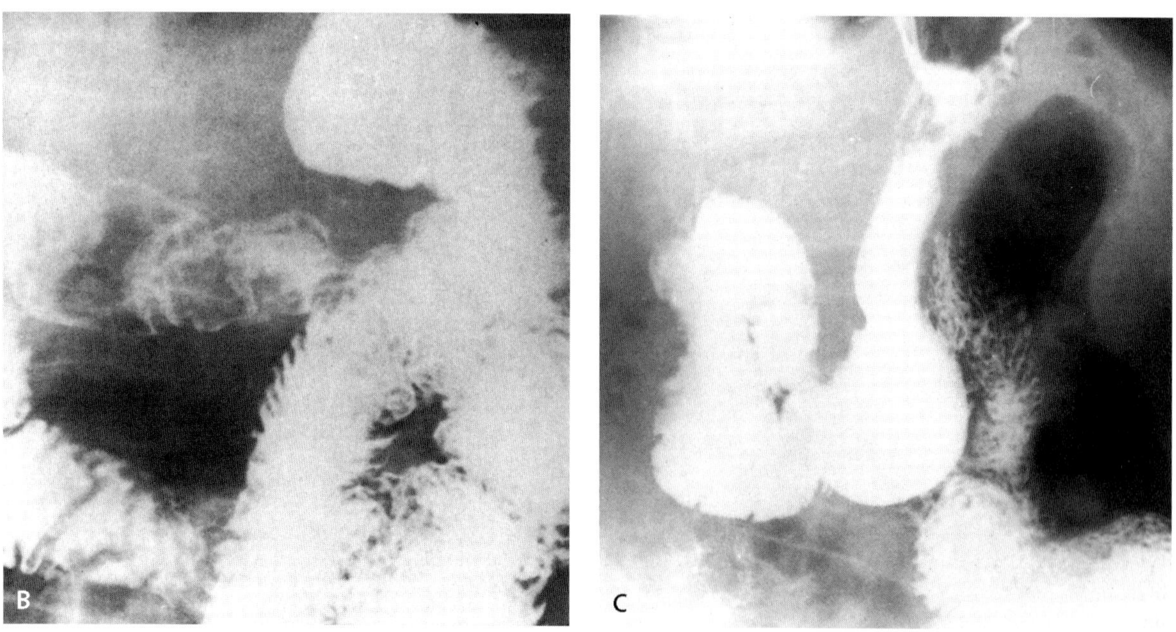

Stomach and Small Bowel

There are seldom abnormal radiographic changes in the stomach or small intestine other than occasional instances of megastomach, megaduodenum or megajejunum (Fig. 4.15). Gastric emptying due to dysfunction of the pylorus can be evaluated by ultrasonography instead of fluoroscopy and radiography. Pyloric dysfunction is seen in up to 22% of patients with intermediate or advanced stage megaesophagus and is diagnosed if gastric emptying does not occur within 2 hours. Duodenal dysfunction is also present in a minority of patients with megaesophagus, sometimes involving only a dilated bulb (1st part), but usually causing dilatation of the entire duodenum to the ligament of Treitz. The jejunum and ileum are rarely dilated but either acceleration or delay in transit time through the small bowel may sometimes be seen.

Colon

In patients with megacolon, the outstanding symptom is chronic obstipation, with bowel movements occurring at intervals from 8 days to 5 months. Large boluses of desiccated feces may become impacted in the dilated, atonic rectosigmoid colon, leading to inflammation and stasis ulceration. Another serious complication of megacolon is sigmoid volvulus, which occurs in approximately 10% of patients and is often the presenting manifestation of the disease.

In the colon, the chief radiographic manifestations are striking elongation and dilatation, especially of the rectosigmoid and descending colon (Fig. 4.16). Changes are often readily identified on plain radiographs, where large fecaliths may be seen within a markedly dilated, often redundant colon (Fig. 4.17). A grossly distended splenic flexure or even a redundant sigmoid loop may at times slightly elevate the left hemidiaphragm on plain films of the chest and abdomen (Fig. 4.18). The appearance simulates the splenic flexure syndrome.

Barium enema studies, using diluted barium and without colon cleansing, reveal a decrease in the number and depth of the haustra or their complete disappearance. Poor contractility and emptying ability of the colon are also noted (Figs. 4.19, 4.20). A hive-like mucosal pattern (urticarial wheal or intestinal hives) is occasionally seen within a portion of the dilated colon, probably due to chronic obstipation and stasis ulceration of the mucosa from chronic fecal impactions or due to a hypersensitivity or autoimmune phenomenon (Fig. 4.21); rarely a diffusely ulcerated bowel may complicate Chagas' megacolon (Fig. 4.22).

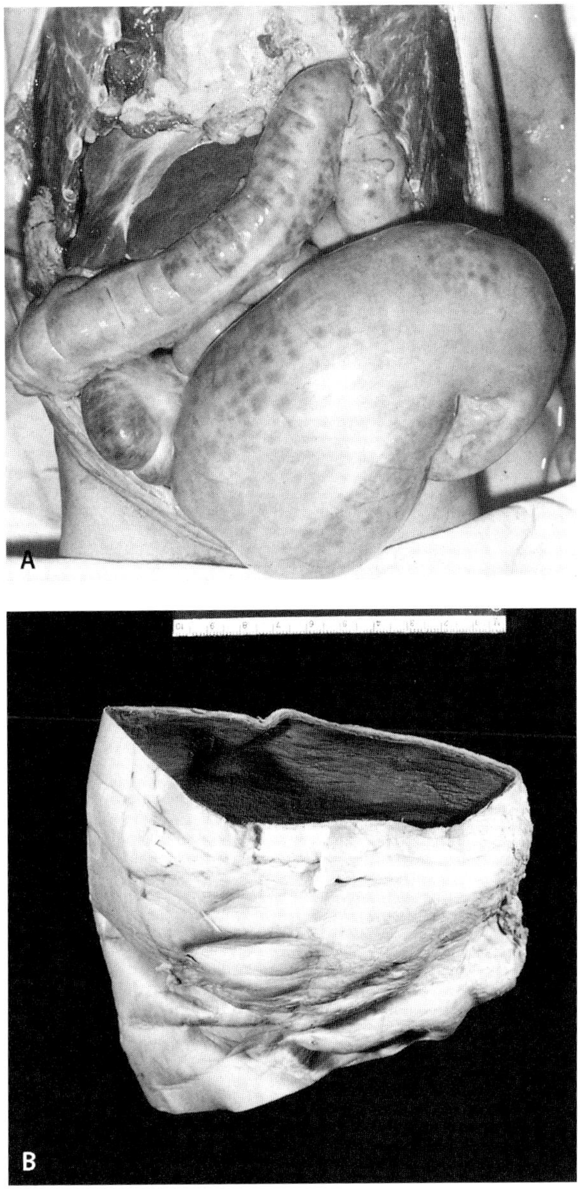

Fig. 4.16. **A** Chagas' megacolon in an adult Brazilian man at necropsy, showing massive dilatation and elongation of the rectosigmoid and distal descending colon. The proximal colon is nearly normal in caliber. AFIP 68-3269-1. (Courtesy of Dr. Clovis Simao, Sao Paulo) **B** Section through a Chagas' megacolon showing the great diameter of the intestinal lumen and the relatively thin intestinal wall. AFIP 69-6534

(Text continues on p. 373)

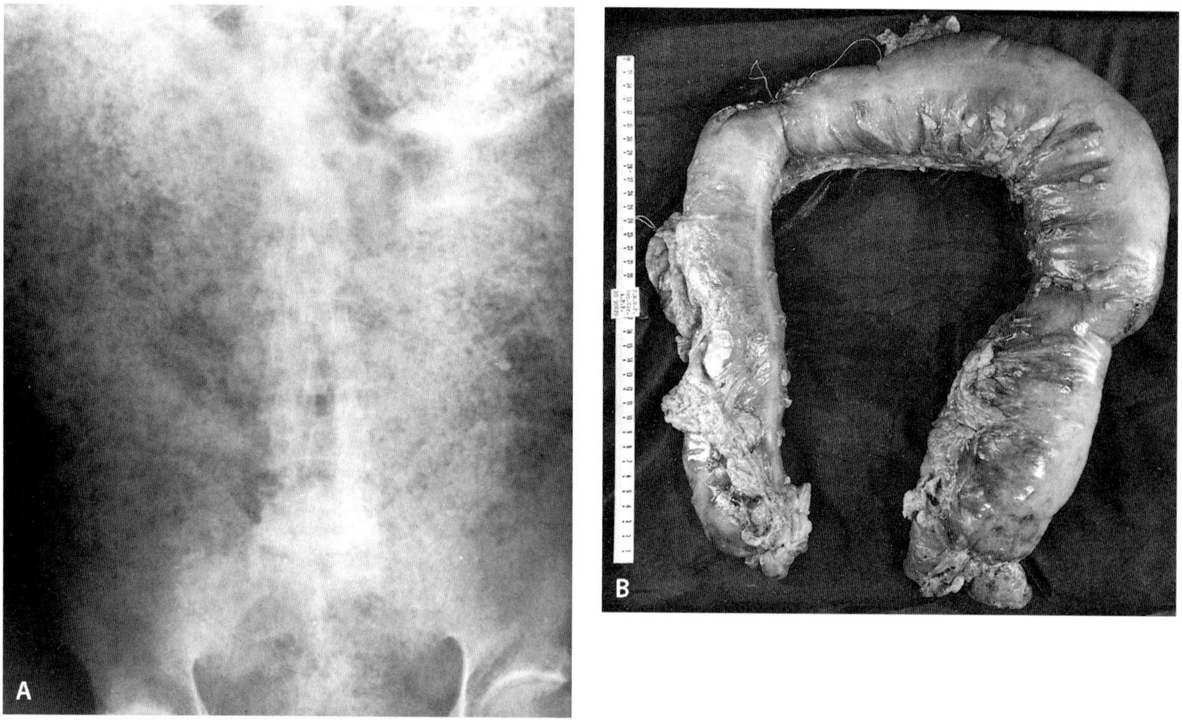

Fig. 4.17. A Chronic Chagas' megacolon with massive retained feces throughout a grossly dilated colon opacifying virtually the entire abdomen. This 51-year-old Brazilian man had progressive constipation for more than 14 years despite two previous partial resections of the colon. Following this examination, the entire colon was removed after it was emptied of fecaliths. The colon measured 10 cm in diameter and contained numerous small mucosal ulcers and secondary inflammation. (Courtesy of Dr. Clovis Simao, Sao Paulo) **B** The wall was not thickened uniformly, being thin in some places and thick in others. AFIP 69-2962

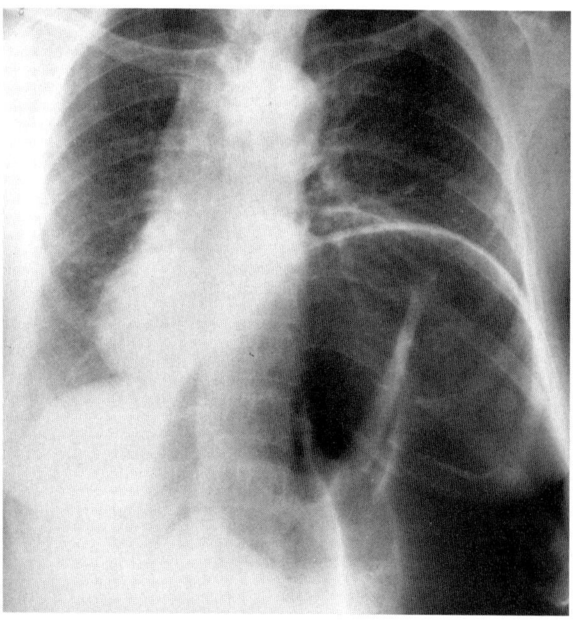

Fig. 4.18. Chagas' megacolon in an adult Brazilian woman showing a grossly distended splenic flexure beneath a markedly elevated left hemidiaphragm. In Brazil and adjacent countries of South America, this appearance is often due to Chagas' disease rather than an obstructing carcinoma of the distal colon, splenic flexure syndrome, or toxic megacolon. (Courtesy of Dr. Clovis Simao, Sao Paulo)

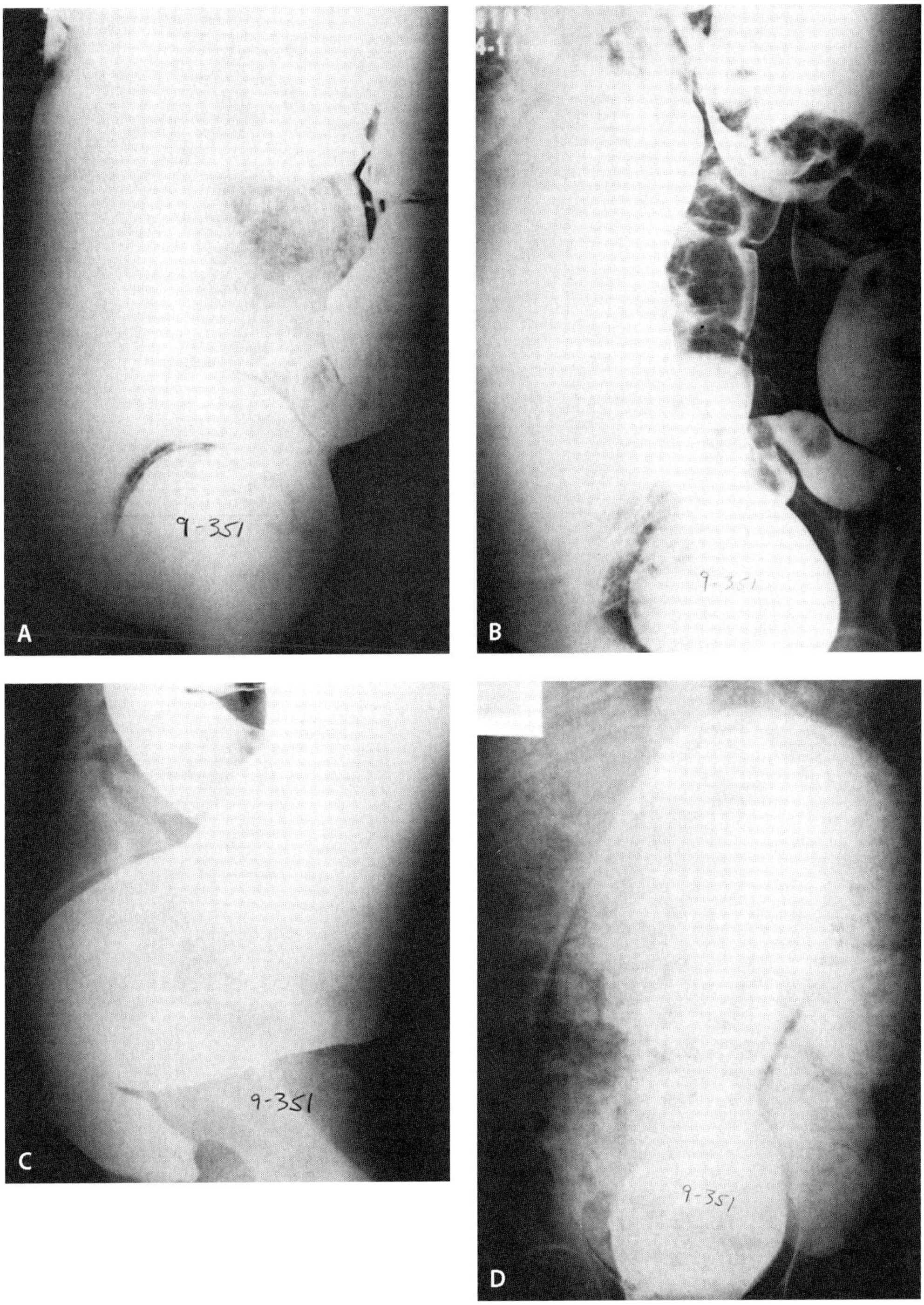

Fig. 4.19 A–D. Chagas' megacolon in a 56-year-old Brazilian woman with chronic obstipation. The AP (**A**), oblique (**B**) and lateral (**C**) views from a barium enema show massive dilatation of the entire rectosigmoid colon. Note the large fecaliths within the colon. The distal rectum is not dilated to the same degree as the sigmoid and descending colon because of the action of the pelvic musculature. A follow-up plain film of the abdomen taken 47 days later showed marked retention of barium from this examination (**D**). The patient had only a scanty bowel movement in the interval. (Courtesy of Dr. Clovis Simao, Sao Paulo)

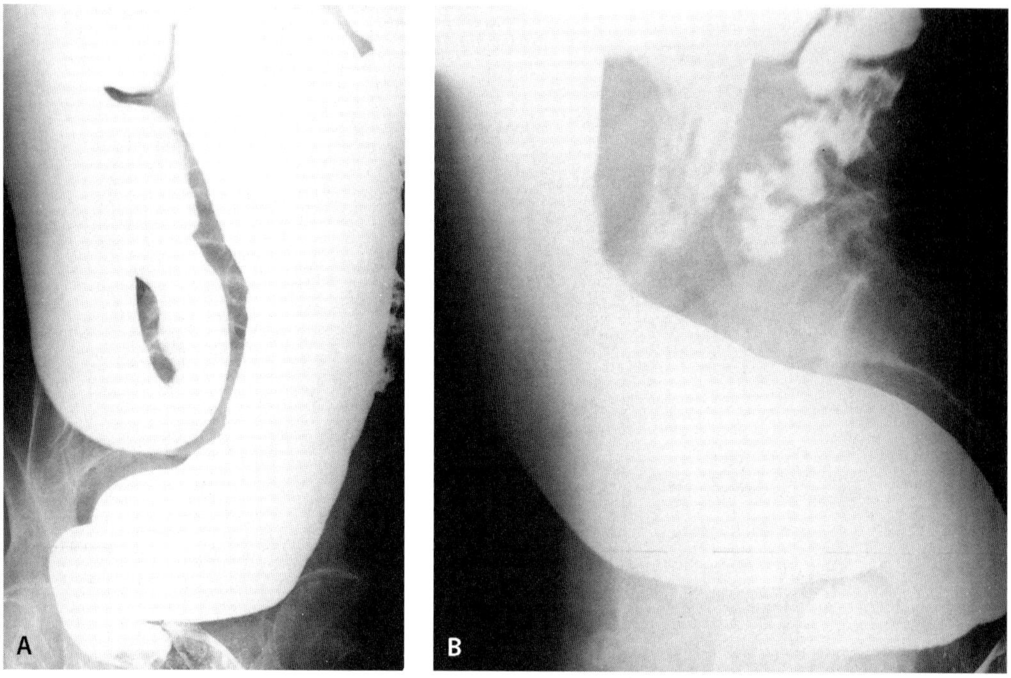

Fig. 4.20 A, B. Chronic Chagas' disease with megacolon in a Brazilian man. Oblique (**A**) and lateral (**B**) views show marked dilatation of most of the colon, especially the sigmoid colon, which is also somewhat elongated and redundant. The lower rectum is not dilated to the same degree as the sigmoid and descending colon because of the rigidity of the musculature of the pelvic floor. Loss of tone throughout the involved colon could be seen fluoroscopically. The patient had intestinal constipation beginning 5 years previously with bowel movements every 2–3 days. At the time of this barium enema he was defecating every 12 days but had no colic. His feces were dry and he needed a laxative for intestinal function. His Chagas' serology was positive. (Courtesy of Dr. Clovis Simao, Sao Paulo)

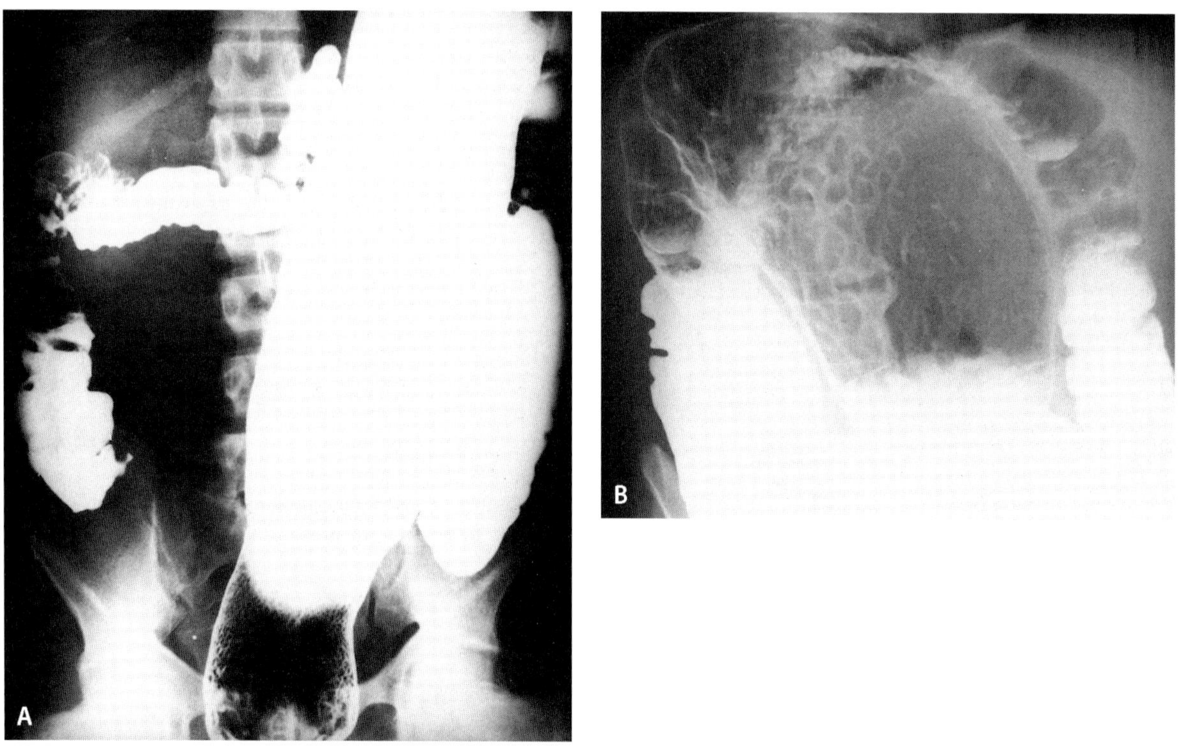

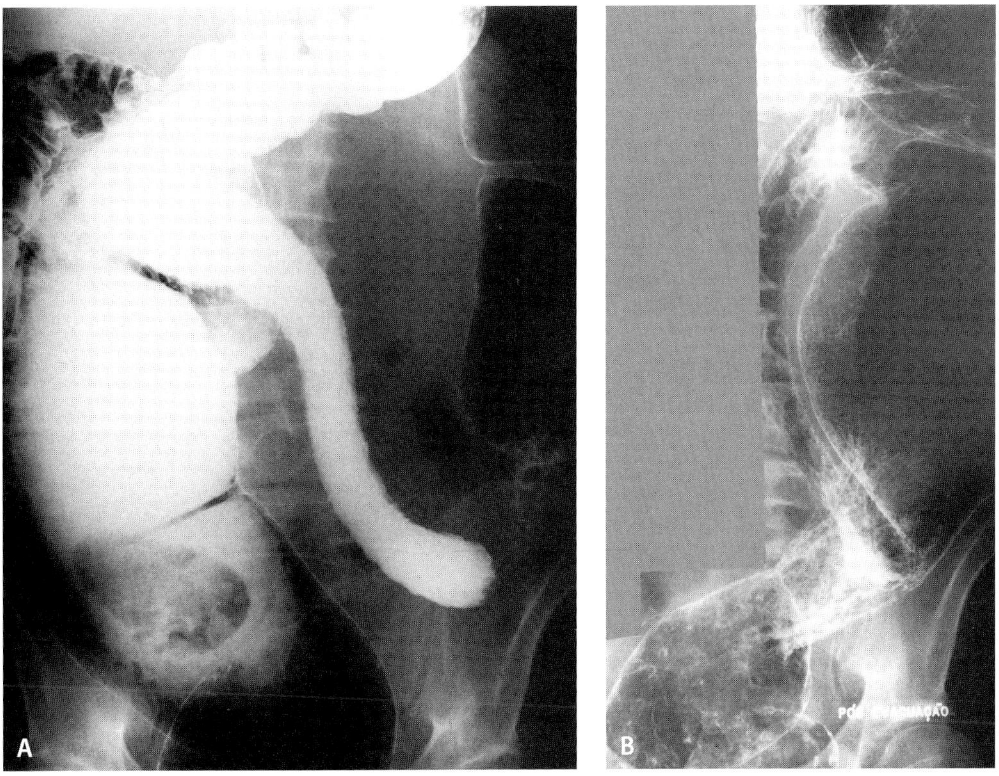

Fig. 4.22 A, B. Chagas' megacolon in a Brazilian adult showing numerous superficial ulcers throughout a somewhat narrowed proximal sigmoid colon. There is a tubular appearance to this portion of the sigmoid and loss of all haustral markings. The distal sigmoid and rectum are grossly distended. **A** AP view of barium enema taken after filling of the colon with barium and air. **B** Postevacuation film from the air contrast barium enema shows a hive-like mucosal pattern in the rectosigmoid colon and diffuse superficial ulceration. Some cases of megacolon show diffuse inflammatory changes and ulceration within the involved segment of bowel, primarily as a result of prolonged fecal stasis and impactions

◀ **Fig. 4.21 A, B.** Chagas' megacolon with hive-like appearance of the mucosa in two Brazilian men. **A** There is severe distention and elongation of the rectum and sigmoid and descending colon with normal caliber of the proximal colon. The hive-like mucosal pattern in the rectum is possibly secondary to chronic obstipation with fecal impactions and stasis ulcerations, but the pattern is similar to that seen with intestinal hives and could represent a hypersensitivity or autoimmune phenomenon. The grossly dilated sigmoid colon extends to the level of the left hemidiaphragm, and plain film examination of the chest showed marked distention of the colon, elevating the left hemidiaphragm and simulating the splenic flexure syndrome. **B** A similar hive-like pattern is seen in a grossly dilated and redundant sigmoid colon of another Brazilian, a 61-year-old black man, who had had constipation for 10 years. During that time, he had bowel movements every 2–3 days, and more recently, every 5–7 days with the use of laxatives. (Courtesy of Dr. Clovis Simao, Sao Paulo)

Occasionally, the dilatation of the colon is not uniform throughout, and one or more less distended short segments may be seen, presumably where ganglial destruction has not been as total as elsewhere in the bowel (Fig. 4.23). These segments may serve as a focus for volvulus in some patients, almost always involving the markedly distended and redundant sigmoid colon (Figs. 4.24–4.26). Air-fluid levels may be seen in the remarkably dilated, obstructed sigmoid colon proximal to the twist (Figs. 4.25, 4.26). In patients with megaesophagus, surgical resection with a colon transplant replacing the esophagus has proven effective in Brazil. In patients with megacolon, the most distended distal segments of the colon are surgically excised and an end-to-end anastomosis performed between the relatively normal caliber proximal colon and rectum (Fig. 4.25).

(Text continues on p. 378)

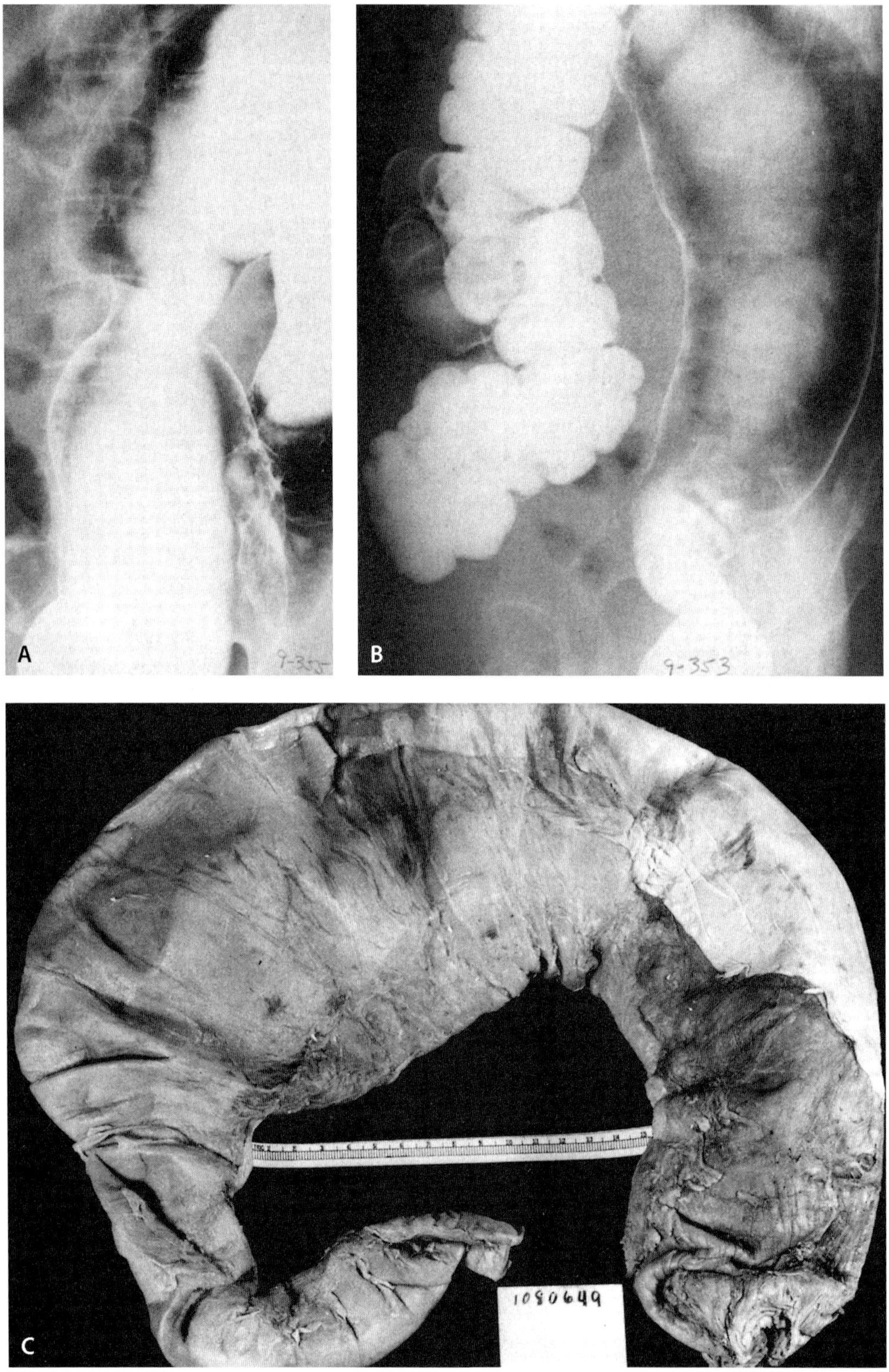

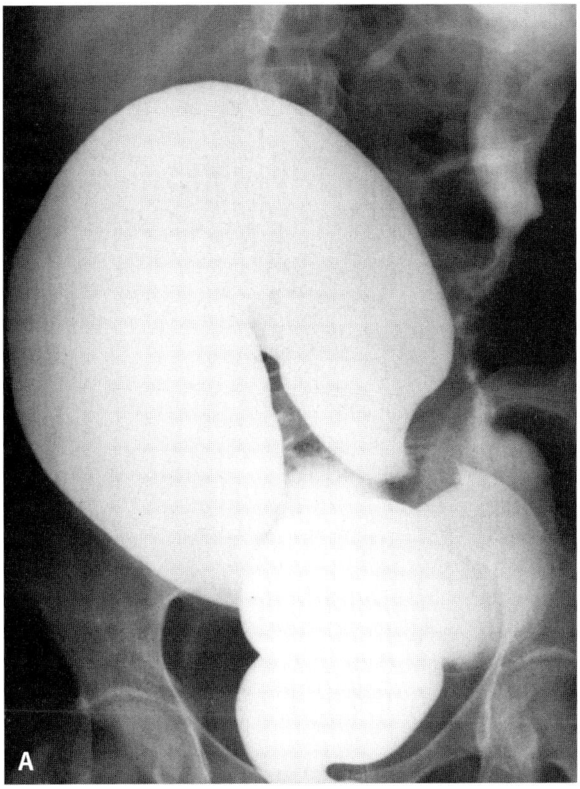

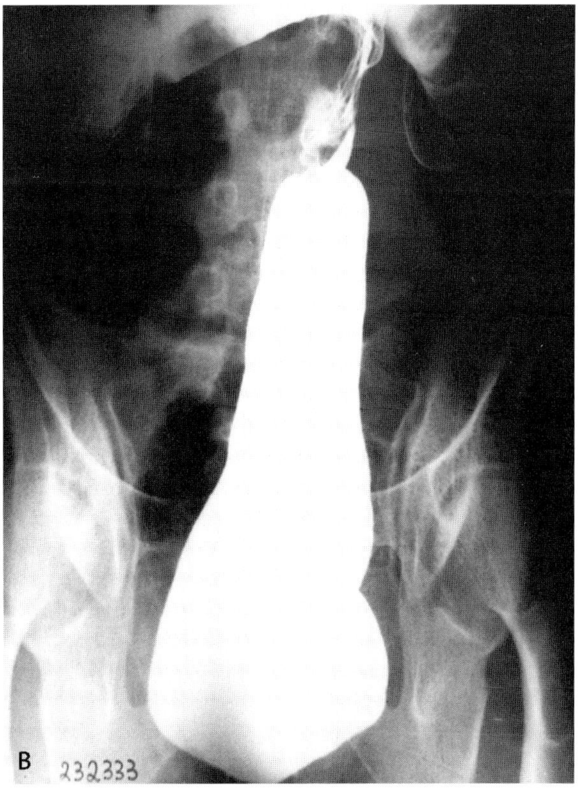

▲ **Fig. 4.24 A–C.** Sigmoid volvulus in two different Brazilian patients with Chagas' megacolon. In patient **A** there is the typical beak-like appearance of the barium column as it reaches the point of volvulus in the proximal sigmoid colon. In the second patient (**B, C**), the classical twisted appearance of the sigmoid is well seen, with a slight amount of barium passing beyond the area of volvulus in the mid-sigmoid colon. Note the considerable distention of the entire large bowel due to underlying Chagasic aganglionosis. Volvulus occurs in up to 10% of patients with Chagas' megacolon, almost always involving the distended and redundant sigmoid colon. (Courtesy of Dr. Clovis Simao, Sao Paulo)

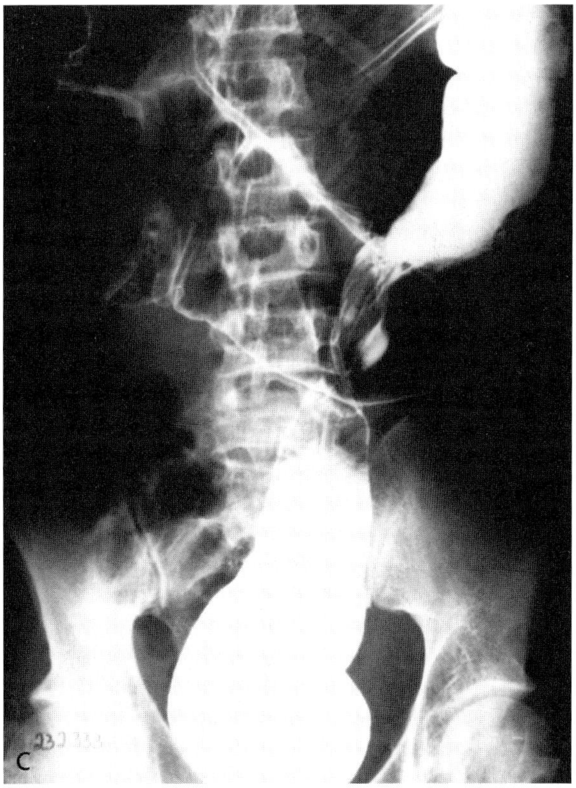

◀ **Fig. 4.23 A–C.** Chagas' megacolon in two different Brazilians showing localized nondistended segments in the sigmoid colon, presumably where destruction of ganglion cells has not been as complete as elsewhere in the adjacent bowel. These segments may serve as focal points for volvulus in such patients. Patient **A** was a 48-year-old Caucasian man with constipation for 18 years, requiring laxatives to promote bowel movements. The frequency of passage of feces, which was once every 3–5 days, was now every 18–20 days. He also complained of heart palpitations and dysphagia for dry foods. A systolic murmur was heard in the mitral area. Serological test for Chagas' disease was positive. Radiographic examination revealed typical megacolon and megaesophagus. Patient **B** was a 35-year-old Brazilian woman with constipation for several years. (Courtesy of Dr. Clovis Simao, Sao Paulo) **C** Grossly distended distal colon in another patient with Chagas' megacolon. Note the lack of distention of a localized segment (*bottom left*): such an area may cause volvulus. AFIP 67-5314

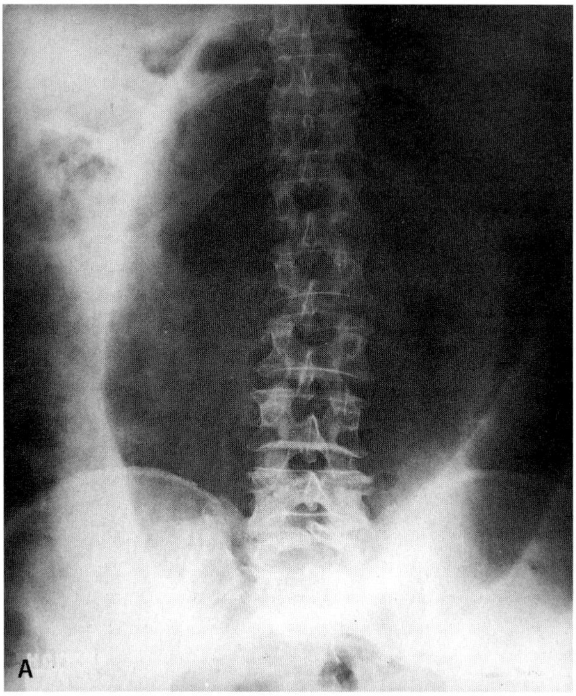

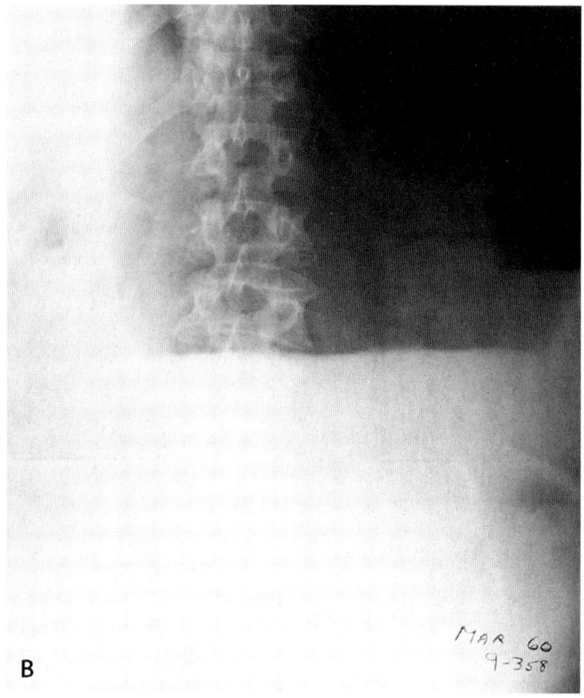

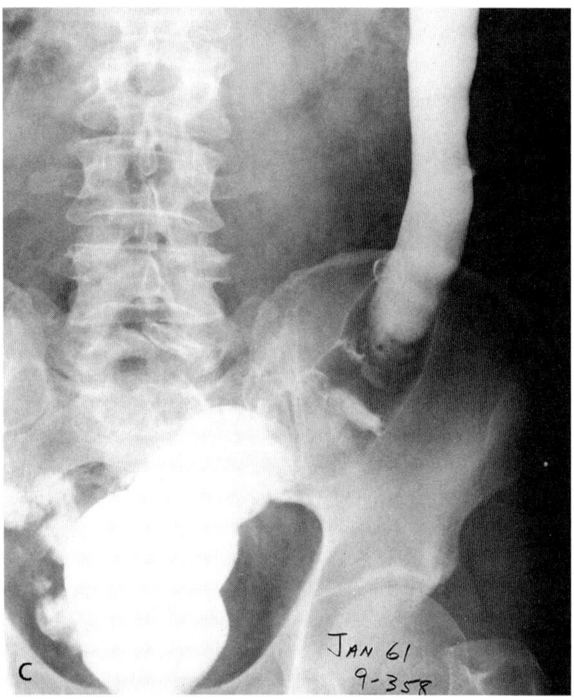

Fig. 4.25 A–C. Chagas' megacolon with volvulus of the sigmoid colon in a 59-year-old white Brazilian man who had severe abdominal colic and distention with no passage of stool or flatus for 15 days. He had a globus abdomen with asymmetrical distention of the left side which was painful to palpation. At operation, there was a 180° torsion of the mesosigmoid with considerable thickening and fibrosis of the mesosigmoid. Volvulus may often be the presenting manifestation in advanced cases of Chagas' disease. **A** Supine AP view of the abdomen showing marked distention of the twisted sigmoid colon which measures greater than 15 cm in diameter. **B** Erect AP view of the abdomen showing a prominent air-fluid level within the grossly dilated, twisted sigmoid loop. **C** A follow-up barium enema, performed 10 months after surgical resection of the dilated sigmoid colon and end-to-end anastomosis of the less involved descending colon with the rectum: there is only minimal distention of the remaining colon and a well-functioning anastomosis. For several decades this has been the surgical procedure of choice in patients with advanced megacolon, with or without volvulus. (Courtesy of Dr. Clovis Simao, Sao Paulo)

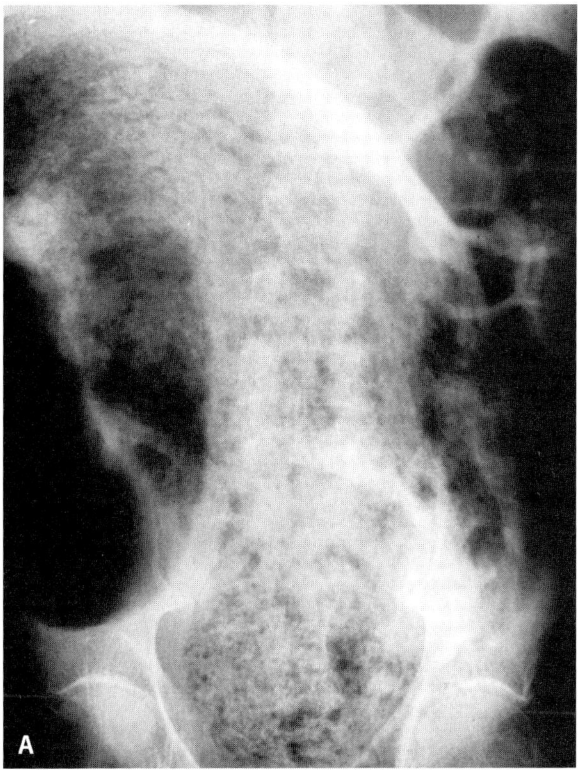

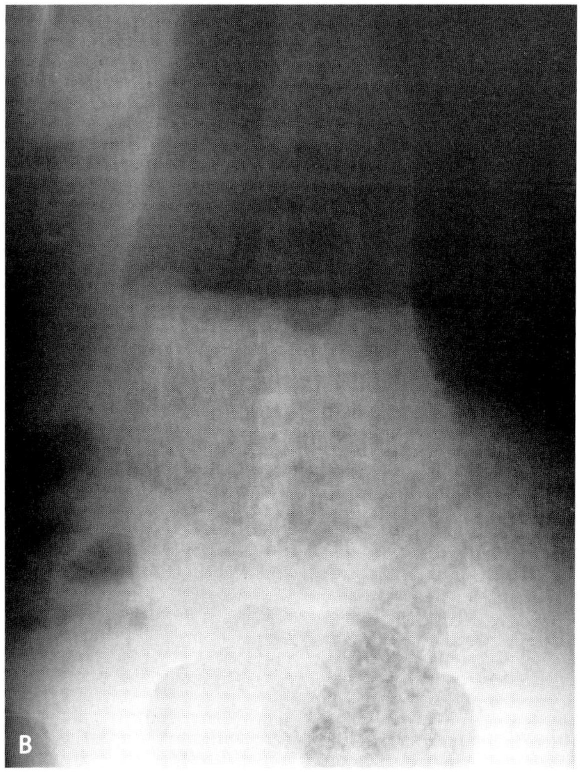

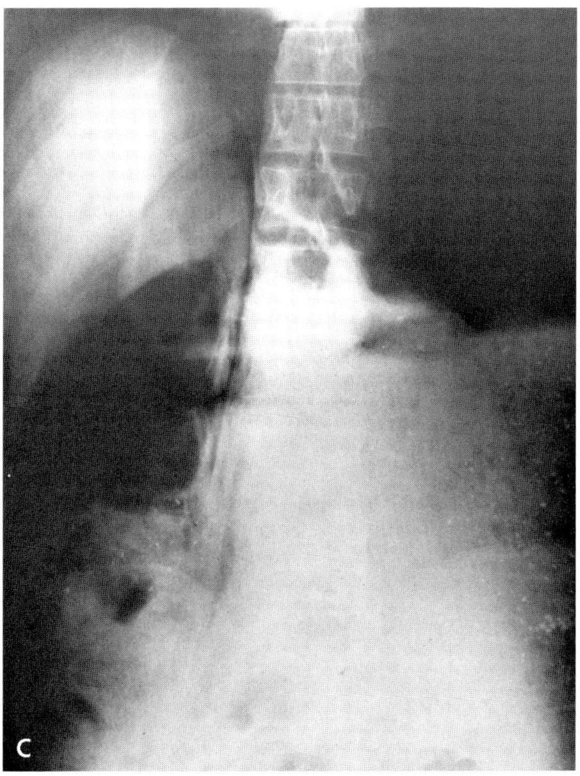

Fig. 4.26 A–C. Volvulus of the sigmoid colon with perforation in a Brazilian adult with Chagas' megacolon. **A** Supine AP view of the abdomen shows a massive amount of feces within a grossly dilated and twisted sigmoid colon. **B** Erect AP view shows a prominent air-fluid level within the distended, fecal-laden sigmoid colon. **C** An AP view of the abdomen taken later shows free air within the abdomen following perforation of the markedly distended sigmoid after an unsuccessful attempt at decompression and evacuation of feces. (Courtesy of Dr. Clovis Simao, Sao Paulo)

Chronic Chagas' Myocardiopathy (CCM)

Symptoms of acute Chagas' disease last only a few months in most patients, although about 15% of these seemingly recovered individuals will have an abnormal ECG. In any endemic area, the majority will be asymptomatic with latent or chronic trypanosomiasis.

Cardiac disease in these patients usually develops slowly over 10–20 years, during which time the patients remain asymptomatic. Over this period the number with an abnormal ECG will increase, until in some populations 50% will have myocardial damage. The majority (82%) will be 11–50 years of age, with the highest incidence in the third and fourth decades. There is a slight male predominance. These statistics vary in different parts of South America. In Argentina, for example, 2.5 million people are infected with *T. cruzi* and over 18% have chronic myocarditis; it is likely that 20% of these patients will die within 2 years of the diagnosis. In the rural areas of Venezuela in 1958, there were over half a million infected persons, of whom 50% had ECG abnormalities.

The pathogenesis of Chagas' cardiomegaly is controversial. It is generally accepted that the disease represents a chronic myocarditis caused by *T. cruzi*. However, for each myocardial fiber containing parasites there are thousands of damaged or destroyed fibers without amastigotes and this raises other hypotheses. The parasites may destroy myofibers indirectly by elaboration of a toxic substance or by an immunological mechanism; autoimmune destruction is suspected by many investigators since *T. cruzi* shares common antigens with cardiac myofibrils. However, a recent study by Tarleton et al. suggests that heart damage, and resulting sudden death, is due not to the body's immune response to heart tissue but rather to an immune reaction to the parasites within the heart itself despite the difficulty in finding *T. cruzi* there. They believe their data indicate the parasite load should be reduced in patients to prevent chronic disease progression, whereas currently victims of Chagas' disease usually are not treated for parasite eradication after the acute phase, chiefly because physicians believe the body's alleged autoimmune response would be difficult or impossible to treat. Despite millions of people infected or at risk, there is presently no vaccine development in progress, principally because of the engrained concept of an autoimmune origin of the disease. Tarleton believes that "even if autoimmunity is a component of the disease, we cannot treat this as an autoimmune disease. We must treat it as a parasitic disease. We must develop protocols to clear the parasites. If we do that, we can get rid of the disease."

Köberle and others believed that the cardiomegaly is caused by the same basic disturbance of intrinsic innervation as has been demonstrated in the alimentary tract. Most pathologists agree there is a marked reduction in identifiable ganglion cells in the heart. Microscopically, there is a diffuse inflammation of the myocardium involving the walls of all chambers, including the septum, and sometimes extending into the endocardium and epicardium. The valves and coronary arteries are not affected. Endomyocardial fibrosis and thinning occur, particularly at the apex of the left ventricle, where aneurysmal dilatation may develop in over 50%, and in some reports as many as 86%, of patients who come to autopsy (Fig. 4.27). Possible mechanisms for development of these apical aneurysms include ischemia, inflammation, herniation through the apical spiral bundles, and autonomic imbalance. There are frequently mural thrombi in the aneurysm or the apex of the ventricles or attached elsewhere to the endocardium of the atria or ventricles. The involvement of the right ventricle, as well as the left, with fibrotic areas and the presence of the apical aneurysms help to differentiate CCM from other cardiomyopathies.

Grossly, the cardiac chambers are all dilated and the muscles are flaccid. The dilatation widens the tricuspid and mitral annuli and leads to incompetence of those valves with functional tricuspid and mitral regurgitation. There is hypertrophy of the myocardium. The heart weight increases, in some cases up to 800 g.

Clinical Characteristics

The clinical findings in CCM depend on the severity and number of myocardial lesions, and the development of heart failure and various arrhythmias. In varying reports, 10%–50% of chronically infected patients will develop congestive failure and 50% of these individuals will be dead within 2 years. The immunological tests will be positive in over 90% of

Fig. 4.27 A–D. Chronic Chagas' myocardiopathy. **A** Chronic myocarditis with interstitial edema, fibrosis, and mild inflammatory cell infiltrate. H&E, ×80; AFIP 62-6106. **B** Necropsy specimen of an enlarged heart in a 36-year-old black Brazilian woman with CCM. The myocardium is pale and there is generalized dilatation of the cardiac chambers. Note the aneurysm at the apex of the left ventricle and notched appearance of the apical aspect of the interventricular septum. AFIP 69-2961-1. **C** Posterior half of the same heart showing generalized dilatation of the atria and ventricles and the aneurysm at the apex of the left ventricle. Continued on p. 379

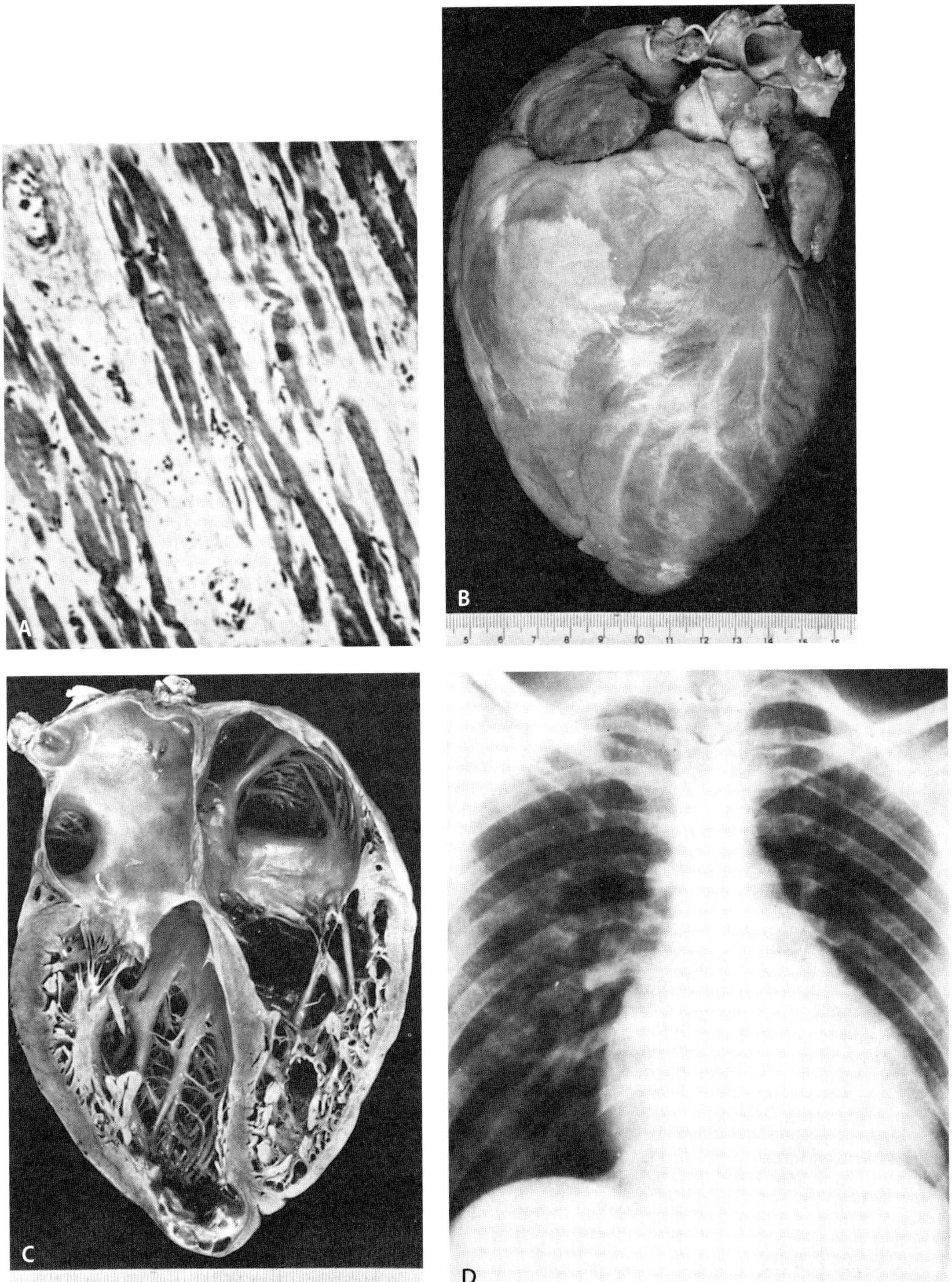

Fig. 4.27 (*continued*). The interventricular septum and ventricular walls are thin, as is the complexity of trabeculae near the insertion of the papillary muscles. AFIP 69-2961-2. **D** Moderate generalized cardiac enlargement is shown on the PA view of the chest of the same patient. Fluoroscopically, the cardiac pulsations were diminished. Note the clear lung fields with no pulmonary vascular congestion or pleural fluid. Clinically the patient had shortness of breath, cardiac palpitations, precordial pain, and pitting edema in the legs for 15 days prior to admission. The ECG showed supraventricular tachycardia and evidence of anteroseptal necrosis, with extension to the diaphragmatic area. Chagas' serology was positive. The patient progressively deteriorated and at autopsy the heart weighed 420 g and showed generalized enlargement with apical aneurysm. (Courtesy of Dr. Clovis Simao, Sao Paulo)

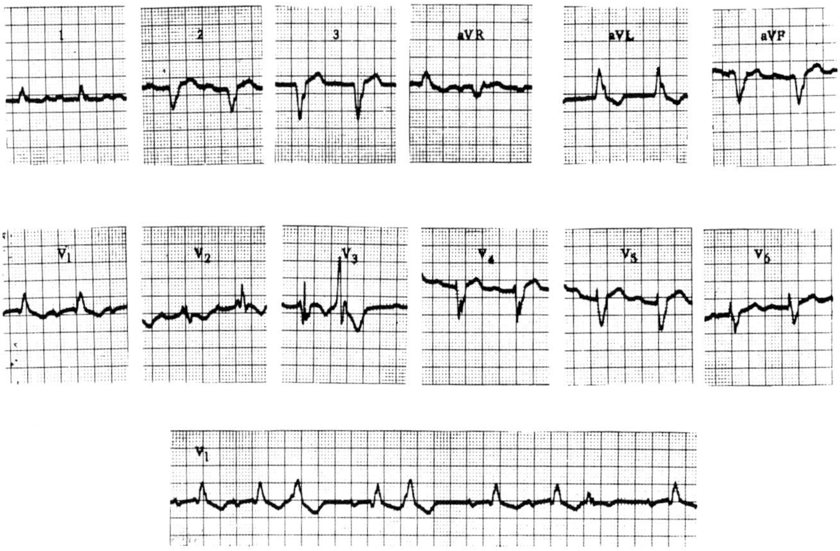

Fig. 4.28. ECG in CCM is often diagnostic, showing various conduction disturbances, principally right bundle branch block and left anterior hemiblock. Negative T waves of the primary type and alterations indicative of apical myocardial necrosis are also common. Frequent and multifocal ventricular extrasystoles are characteristic, as is a sinus bradycardia or an abnormally fixed sinus rhythm associated with heart failure. AFIP 69-4025

patients at this stage. On physical examination, there may be cardiac enlargement, irregularities of rhythm due to premature ventricular contractions or atrioventricular block, gallop rhythm, sinus bradycardia, diminished heart sounds, a widely split second pulmonary sound, and systolic murmurs from functional mitral or tricuspid regurgitation. There may also be an increase in systemic venous pressure and hepatomegaly. The systolic blood pressure is usually normal to moderately lowered, as is the pulse pressure.

The ECG in CCM is often diagnostic (Fig. 4.28). The panmyocarditis almost always causes conduction disturbances, principally right bundle branch block (seen in 30%–60% of patients) and left anterior hemiblock. Negative coronary T waves of the primary type and alterations indicative of apical myocardial necrosis are common. Apical aneurysms diagnosed by ECG or echocardiography are more frequent in enlarged hearts, but about 26% of patients with a normal radiographic cardiac series have ECG evidence of apical lesions. Frequent and multifocal ventricular extrasystoles are characteristic of CCM; a sinus bradycardia or abnormally fixed sinus rhythm associated with heart failure is highly specific and probably a consequence of partial or complete block of the autonomic nervous system or damage to the sinus node itself. This may produce a dysautonomic syndrome of postural hypotension, dizziness, and arrhythmias. A recent report of symptomatic patients with chronic Chagas' disease in Venezuela showed that almost 40% had a conduction abnormality, over 75% had ventricular arrhythmias, and nearly 33% had abnormal ST segment and T wave inversion.

The prognosis in patients with clinical CCM is grave. Embolic phenomena, particularly cerebral embolism, are a not uncommon way for patients to present and are the most common cause of stroke in young adults in endemic geographic regions. Many patients have syncope and may die suddenly from the effects of the disease on the conduction system, particularly ventricular fibrillation, while others develop progressive cardiac failure. Most patients with chronic Chagasic cardiopathy die between the ages of 20 and 40 years. Unfortunately, there is as yet no specific drug which is entirely effective against *T. cruzi*, especially in the chronic stage, when the morphological alterations of cardiopathy, megaesophagus and megacolon are organized and irreversible.

Imaging Diagnosis

In 20% of patients with severe CCM, the cardiac size is normal or only slightly enlarged. Equally, some patients who have severe heart disease clinically with cardiomegaly and advanced atrioventricular block have few or no symptoms. There is good correlation between the intensity of the microscopic changes and the degree of cardiac enlargement. The size of the heart depends on the severity and location of myocardial lesions and varies from normal to enormous dilatation and hypertrophy.

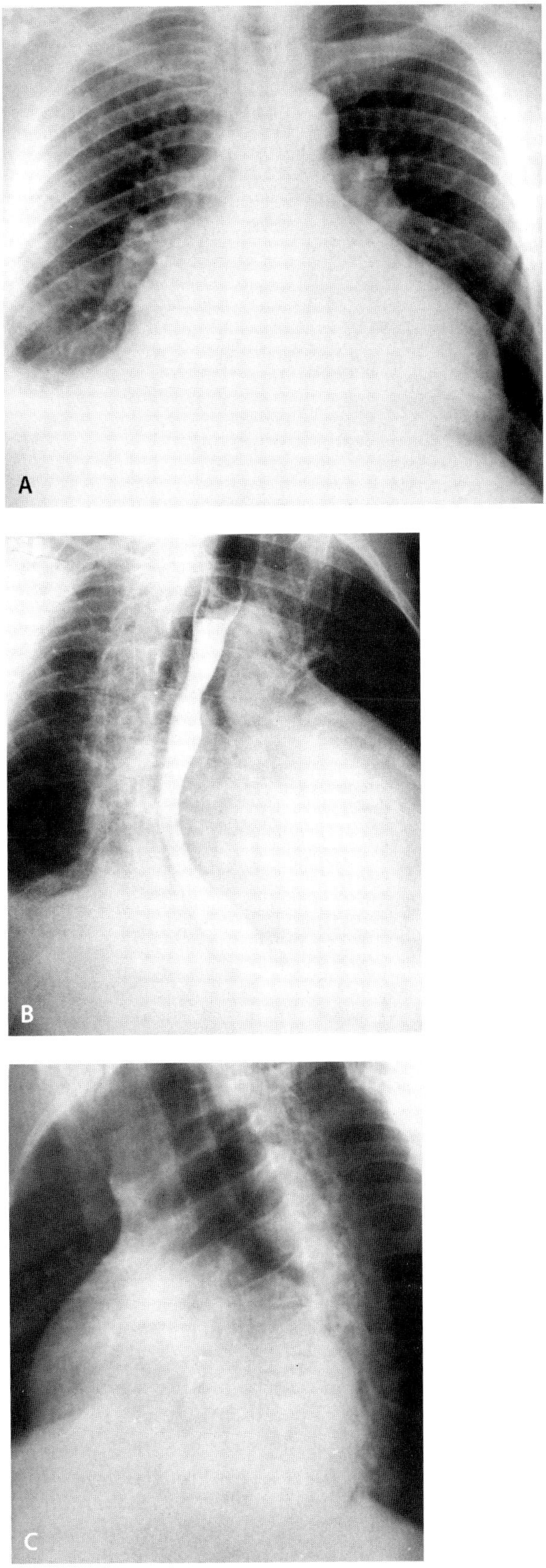

Fig. 4.29 A–C. Chronic Chagas' myocardiopathy in a 55-year-old black Brazilian man. PA (**A**), RAO with barium in the esophagus (**B**), and LAO (**C**) views of the chest show marked generalized cardiac enlargement with prominence especially of the left ventricle and left atrium. The latter causes a prominent indentation upon the barium-filled esophagus in the RAO view, and also elevation of the left main stem bronchus and straightening of the left heart border on the PA view. There is minimal pulmonary vascular congestion with some cephalization of venous blood flow. There is also dilatation of the superior vena cava and a small right pleural effusion. In such patients, loss of distensibility of the left ventricular wall from fibrosis may cause functional mitral valve incompetence and restricted diastolic filling of the left ventricle, with resultant pulmonary venous congestion. The cardiac silhouette, pulmonary vasculature, and hilar areas may resemble the radiographic appearance of mitral and/or aortic valvular disease rather than a myocardiopathy. Clinically, this patient had had shortness of breath, easy fatiguability, an enlarged liver, and weight gain for the past year. The heart sounds were weak, with a few premature beats. No murmurs were heard. ECG showed slight sinus tachycardia, complete right bundle branch block, left ventricular hypertrophy, a wide QT interval, and isolated premature ventricular contractions. Serological reaction for Chagas' disease (Machado-Guerreiro test) was positive. Necropsy showed Chagas' cardiopathy with a heart weight of 650 g, generalized cardiac enlargement, right ventricular infarction, chronic passive congestion of the viscera, hydrothorax and ascites, and partial denervation of the esophagus and Auerbach plexi of the sigmoid colon. (Courtesy of Dr. Clovis Simao, Sao Paulo) ▶

In the early stages of heart failure, isolated dilatation of the left ventricle may be present, since damage there is usually more severe than in other chambers and the left ventricle has a heavier work load. Loss of distensibility of the left ventricular wall due to marked fibrosis may cause annular dilatation and functional incompetence of the mitral valve, and restricted diastolic filling of the left ventricle with resultant pulmonary venous congestion. Dyspnea is then more marked and on chest radiographs the cardiac contour, lung fields, and hila resemble the radiographic appearance of mitral and aortic valvular disease rather than a myocardiopathy (Fig. 4.29). At times, the left atrium may be quite prominent and an apical systolic murmur may be present, imitating mitral insufficiency.

In the usual case of simultaneous left- and right-sided failure, signs of pronounced systemic venous hypertension overshadow those of pulmonary venous congestion. Dyspnea and orthopnea are not severe even in advanced disease. The chest radiograph typically shows prominent generalized cardiomegaly, but clear pulmonary fields without congestion and small to normal hila even when there is severe cardiac failure (Figs. 4.27, 4.30). The main pulmonary artery segment and peripheral vasculature are usually normal, probably because of the failure of the right ventricle to overload the lungs. In many pa-

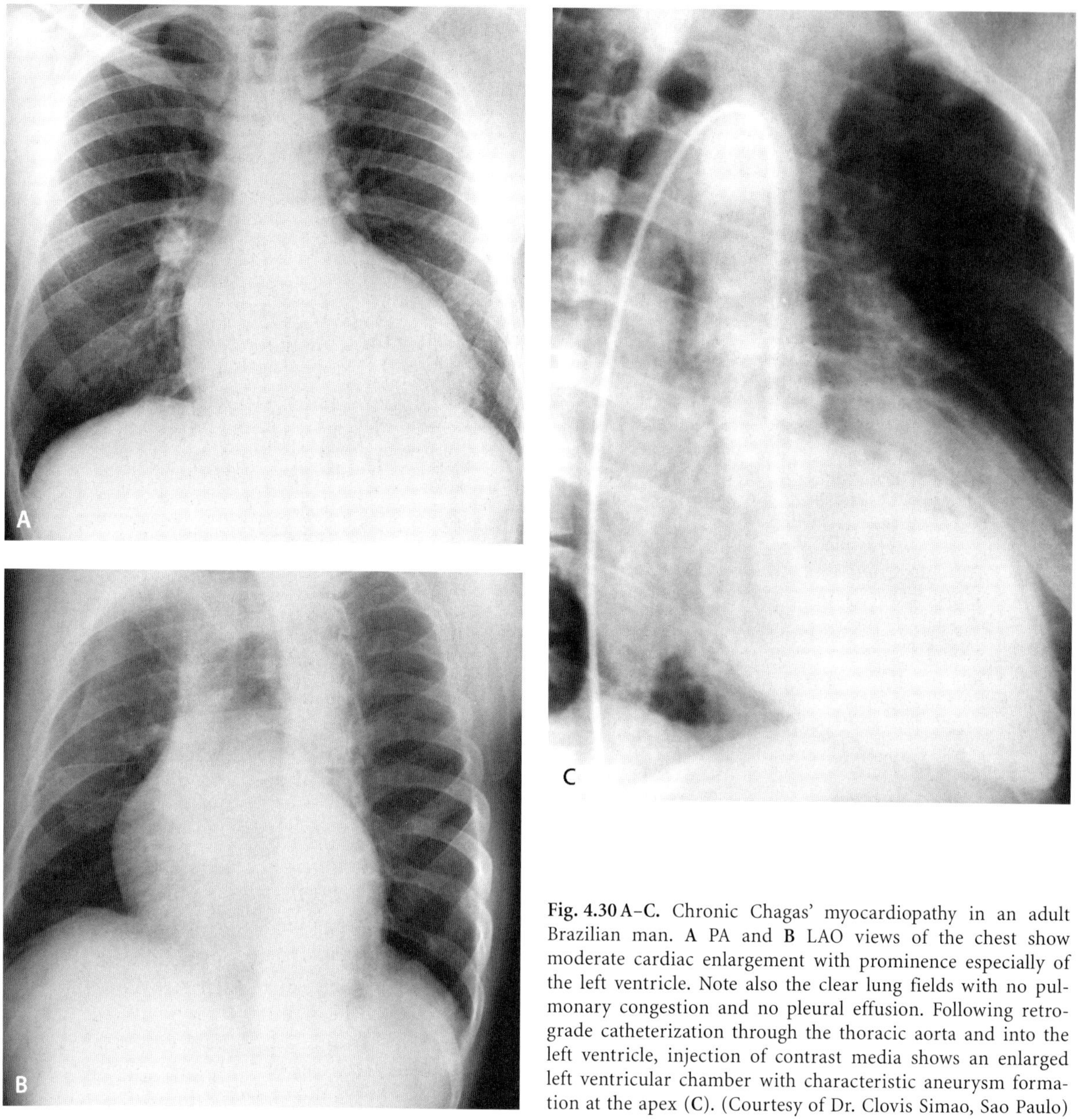

Fig. 4.30 A–C. Chronic Chagas' myocardiopathy in an adult Brazilian man. **A** PA and **B** LAO views of the chest show moderate cardiac enlargement with prominence especially of the left ventricle. Note also the clear lung fields with no pulmonary congestion and no pleural effusion. Following retrograde catheterization through the thoracic aorta and into the left ventricle, injection of contrast media shows an enlarged left ventricular chamber with characteristic aneurysm formation at the apex (**C**). (Courtesy of Dr. Clovis Simao, Sao Paulo)

tients with advanced congestive failure (Fig. 4.31), predominant right-sided failure with functional tricuspid insufficiency may develop.

Most patients with CCM will complain of chest pain, the pathophysiology of which is unknown, although myocardial necrosis and fibrosis are often identified at autopsy and cardiac autonomic impairment is a feature of the disease. In a study by Marin-Neto et al. (1992) of 23 patients with CCM and chest pain, thallium-201 myocardial scintigraphy was performed after maximal effort and 4-hour redistribution. Regional wall motion was evaluated by radionuclide and contrast angiography. Only one patient developed chest pain and no ischemic ECG changes occurred in any patient during the stress test. Scintigraphic evaluation of seven segments per patient showed perfusion defects in at least one segment in all patients. Of 161 myocardial segments, 16 showed fixed, 10 reversible, and 22 paradoxical defects (reverse redistribution). Most of the fixed perfusion defects (75%) occurred in dyssynergic regions, whereas reversible defects occurred in normal or mildly hypokinetic areas and reverse redistribution predominated in regions with normal wall motion (82%). Marked impairment of parasympathetic cardiac control was present, but no significant coronary abnormalities were seen in the 16 patients also studied by angiography.

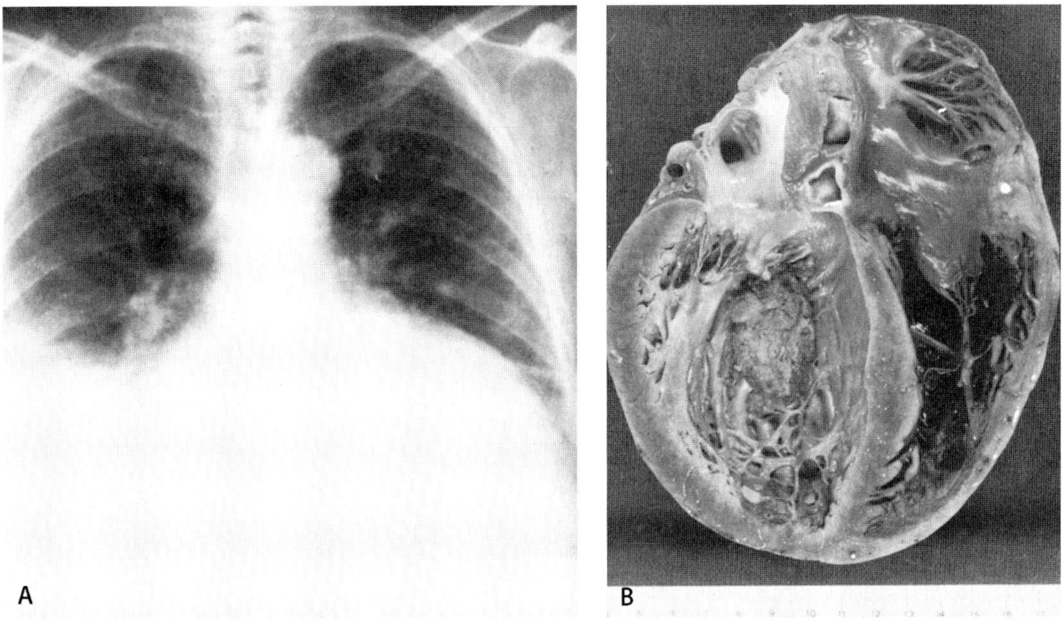

Fig. 4.31 A, B. Chronic Chagas' myocardiopathy in a 57-year-old white Brazilian woman with advanced biventricular failure. **A** PA view of the chest shows marked cardiac enlargement, predominantly left ventricular, with pulmonary vascular congestion and a large right pleural effusion. The patient complained of shortness of breath of 2 years' duration, progressively increasing in the past 2 months. She had two-pillow orthopnea, pitting edema of the lower extremities, and facial edema. Heart sounds were weak and there was an arrhythmia, but no murmurs. ECG showed left bundle branch block and multifocal ventricular extrasystoles. Chagas' serology was positive. At necropsy there was a generalized cardiac enlargement and hypertrophy with a heart weight of 550 g and mural thrombosis in the left ventricle (**B**). There was evidence of congestive heart failure with hydrothorax, chronic liver congestion, and lower leg edema. AFIP 69-2960. (Courtesy of Dr. Clovis Simao, Sao Paulo)

Carrasco et al. (1982) used cineangiography to identify left ventricular signs of myocardial damage and study the evolution of characteristic lesions in 126 chronic chagasic patients, divided into three groups. Group I patients had no clinical, ECG, or radiological evidence of heart disease; 41% of them showed apical or anterior apical asynergy, suggesting early subclinical myocardial damage. Group II patients had an abnormal ECG but no clinical signs of heart failure. Extensive asynergy, left ventricular dilatation, and decreased distensibility and contractility were present in 98% of these patients. Group III patients had congestive heart failure, a greatly dilated, hypokinetic left ventricle, and a 40% incidence of large apical aneurysms; 20% had thrombosis within the left ventricle. These investigators concluded that left cineventriculography enabled them to diagnose early myocardial damage and detect potentially resectable lesions such as ventricular aneurysms and apical thromboses. (Echocardiography and MRI would be equally accurate.)

Echocardiography is today the best imaging modality in the evaluation of CCM. The findings basically reflect cardiac dilatation and compromise of heart function. The abnormalities seen on 2 D echocardiography include: (1) dilatation and diffuse myocardial involvement, which characterize this myocardiopathy, with an increased volume/mass ratio; (2) increase in left ventricular systolic and diastolic volume; (3) septal and posteroinferior wall hypokinesis; (4) segmental hypokinesis of the posterior wall of the left ventricle; (5) diffuse hypokinetc pattern (observed in up to 25% of patients); and (6) decrease in ventricular function with reduced ejection.

Echocardiography can detect segmental or focal areas of myocardial involvement, including the apical aneurysms almost pathognomonic of this entity (Figs. 4.32–4.34). These aneurysms are caused by abrupt localized thinning of the myocardium, usually due to the myocarditis. The great majority of them (80%) are in the left ventricle, but they may occur less commonly in the right ventricle or both ventricles. Mural thrombi are often present in these aneurysms or even in patients without them (Fig. 4.35). Based on the study of these thrombi by ultrasonography (their location, shape, and echogenicity), their potential to cause emboli can be predicted, according to some investigators, thus aiding in therapeutic decisions such as the use of anticoag-

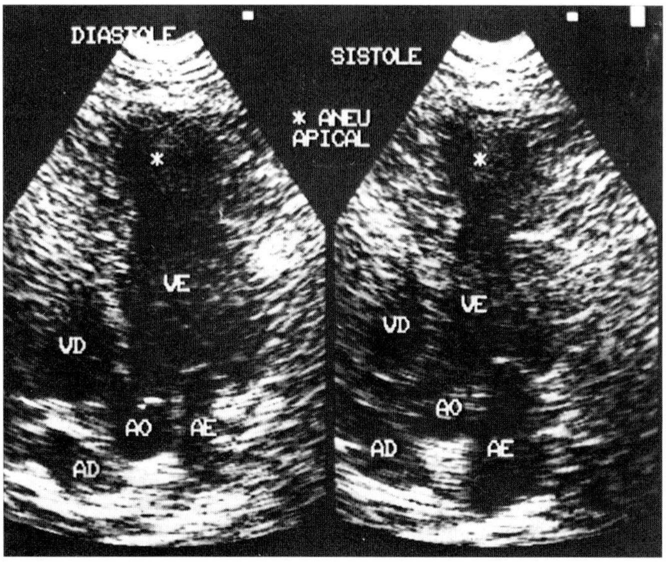

Fig. 4.32. An echocardiogram showing an aneurysm in the apical region of the left ventricle, with images obtained during systole and diastole. (Courtesy of Dr. Sergio Sales, Rio de Janeiro)

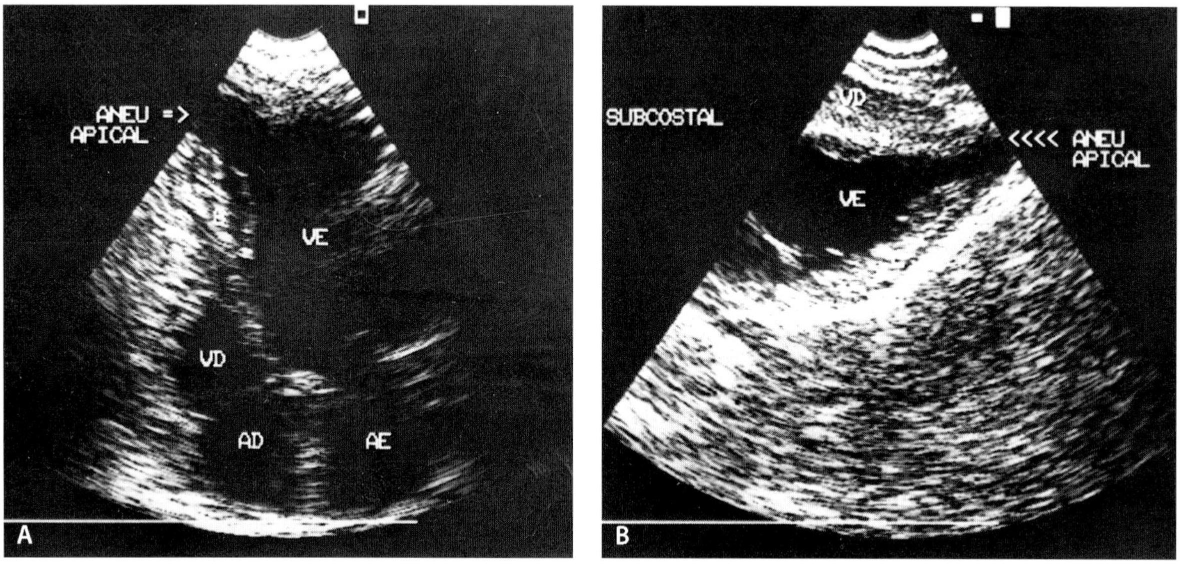

Fig. 4.33 A, B. An echocardiogram showing a "finger-shaped" aneurysm in the apical portion of the left ventricle in a patient with Chagas' myocardiopathy. (Courtesy of Dr. Sergio Sales, Rio de Janeiro)

ulants. Mural thrombi frequently embolize to the pulmonary and systemic circulation, causing infarcts that are most common in the lungs, brain, spleen, and kidneys. Ultrasonography or CT, MRI, scintigraphy, and angiography may be used as appropriate for the diagnosis and evaluation of the extent of these infarcts.

Doppler and color-Doppler echocardiography can detect mitral regurgitation due to left ventricular enlargement, papillary muscle dysfunction, valvular dilatation, and low ventricular flow, typical for this diffuse ventricular disease. Sometimes right ventricle dysfunction is difficult to evaluate by ultrasonography and, in these cases, radioisotopic ventriculography may be helpful.

Magnetic resonance imaging can also be used for imaging Chagas' myocardiopathy to show the heart changes in this disease, but is expensive and time consuming compared with ultrasonography. It is useful in differentiating between Chagasic cardiac insufficiency (caused by segmental cardiomyopathy) and idiopathic cardiac dilatation; it is useful also in detecting areas more severely affected with myocarditis, especially when biopsy of the heart is being considered for diagnosis. Areas of myocarditis may enhance with contrast agents (such as gadolinium)

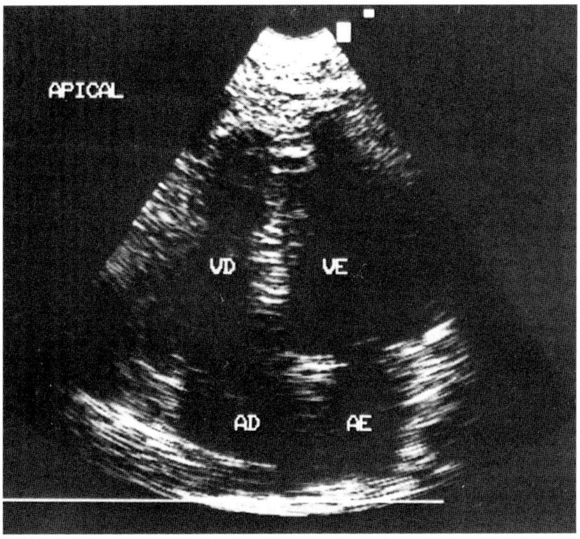

Fig. 4.34. An echocardiogram showing biventricular apical aneurysms (above *VD* and *VE*). (Courtesy of Dr. Sergio Sales, Rio de Janeiro)

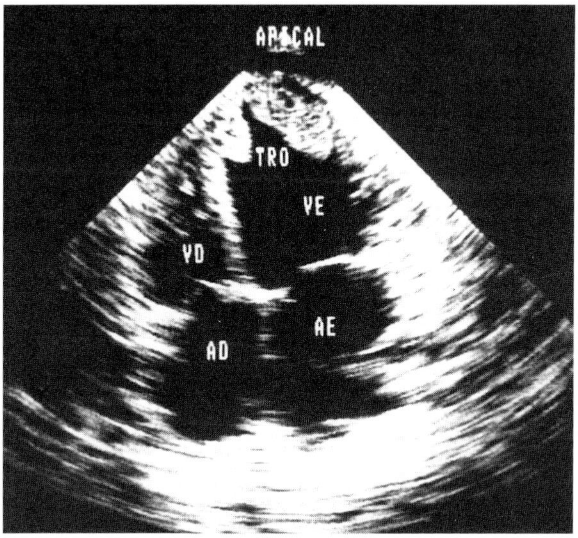

Fig. 4.35. An echocardiogram showing a large thrombus (*TRO*) in the apical region of the left ventricle in a patient with Chagas' myocardiopathy

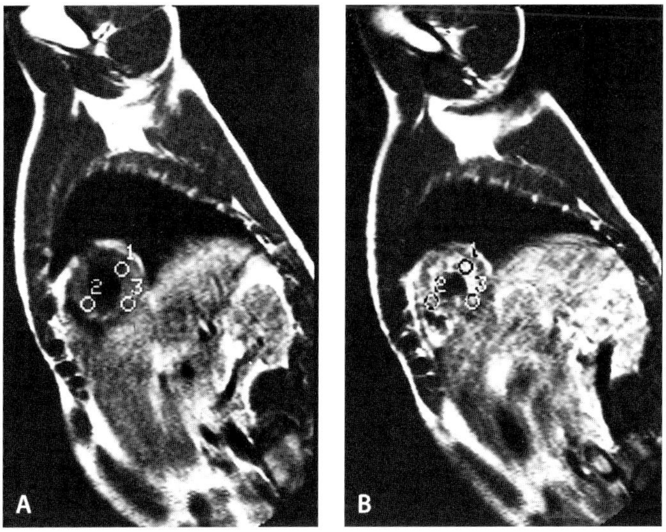

Fig. 4.36 A, B. An MRI study of the heart showing gadolinium enhancement of areas of myocarditis caused by Chagas' disease. A Precontrast; B post-contrast. (Courtesy of Dr. Giovani Guido Cerri, Sao Paulo)

on T1-weighted images (Fig. 4.36); ongoing work in this area is being done (1999) at the Heart Institute (INCOR) of Sao Paulo, Brazil. MRI can also demonstrate the presence of a mural thrombus (Fig. 4.37) or an apical ventricular aneurysm (Fig. 4.38).

As previously noted, in some endemic areas, chiefly Brazil, there is a high incidence of megaesophagus and megacolon and rarely dilatation and/or aperistalsis of other hollow viscera such as the stomach, duodenum, ureters, bladder, and bronchi. Certainly the combination of generalized cardiomegaly and megaesophagus or megacolon in a South American patient should suggest the diagnosis of chronic Chagas' disease (Fig. 4.39).

Neurological Symptoms in Chagas' Disease

Chagas' disease may cause neurological symptoms in both the acute and chronic phases.

In acute Chagas' infections, there may be clinically silent meningoencephalitis. There is perivascular inflammation, causing microglial proliferation, with lymphocytes, plasma cells, and parasitized cells. There is often leptomeningitis, with mononuclear cells. The inflammatory foci may destroy the ependymal epithelium and be subependymal. Similar inflammatory foci occur in the spinal cord.

In the chronic phase, the neurological abnormalities are probably the result of the meningeal thickening

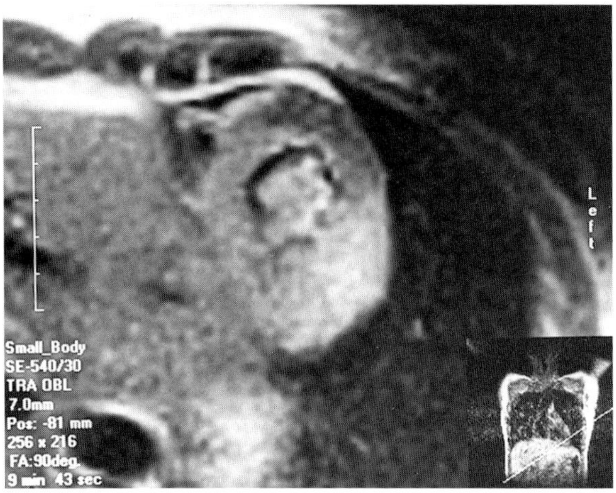

Fig. 4.37. An MRI study of the heart: axial section through the short axis of the apex of the left ventricle showing a high signal mural thrombus within the chamber

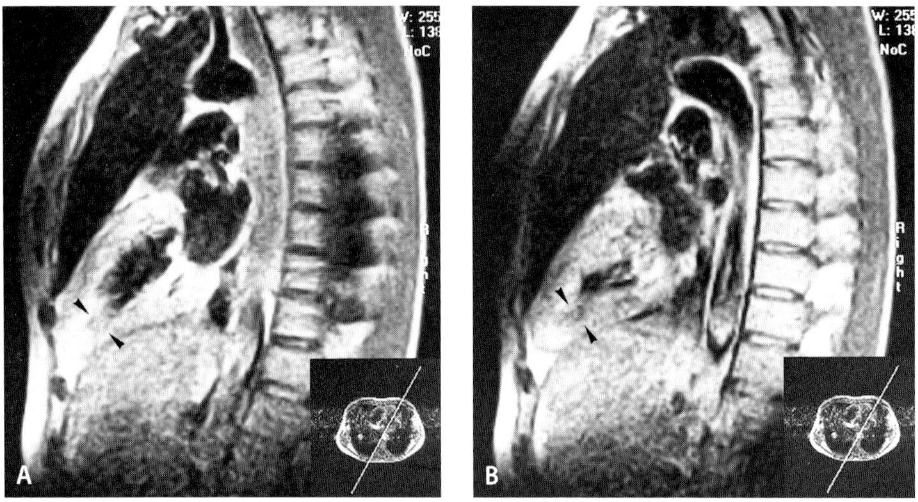

Fig. 4.38 A, B. An MRI study of the heart of a patient with Chagas' myocardiopathy. T1-weighted images obtained in a sagittal-oblique plane through the long axis of the left ventricle showing an apical aneurysm (*arrowheads*)

and gyral adhesions which follow the acute meningoencephalitis. However, in immunocompromised patients, reactivation of Chagas' disease may occur: the meningoencephalitis is then more severe and more diffuse, and can be fatal. There are more pseudocysts associated with necrotic, hemorrhagic foci. When the immunosuppression is due to AIDS, tumor-like lesions have developed; these are the result of wide areas of necrosis and hemorrhage, with an inflammatory reaction and parasitized glial cells (Fig. 4.40). (There may also be reactivation of the myocarditis.)

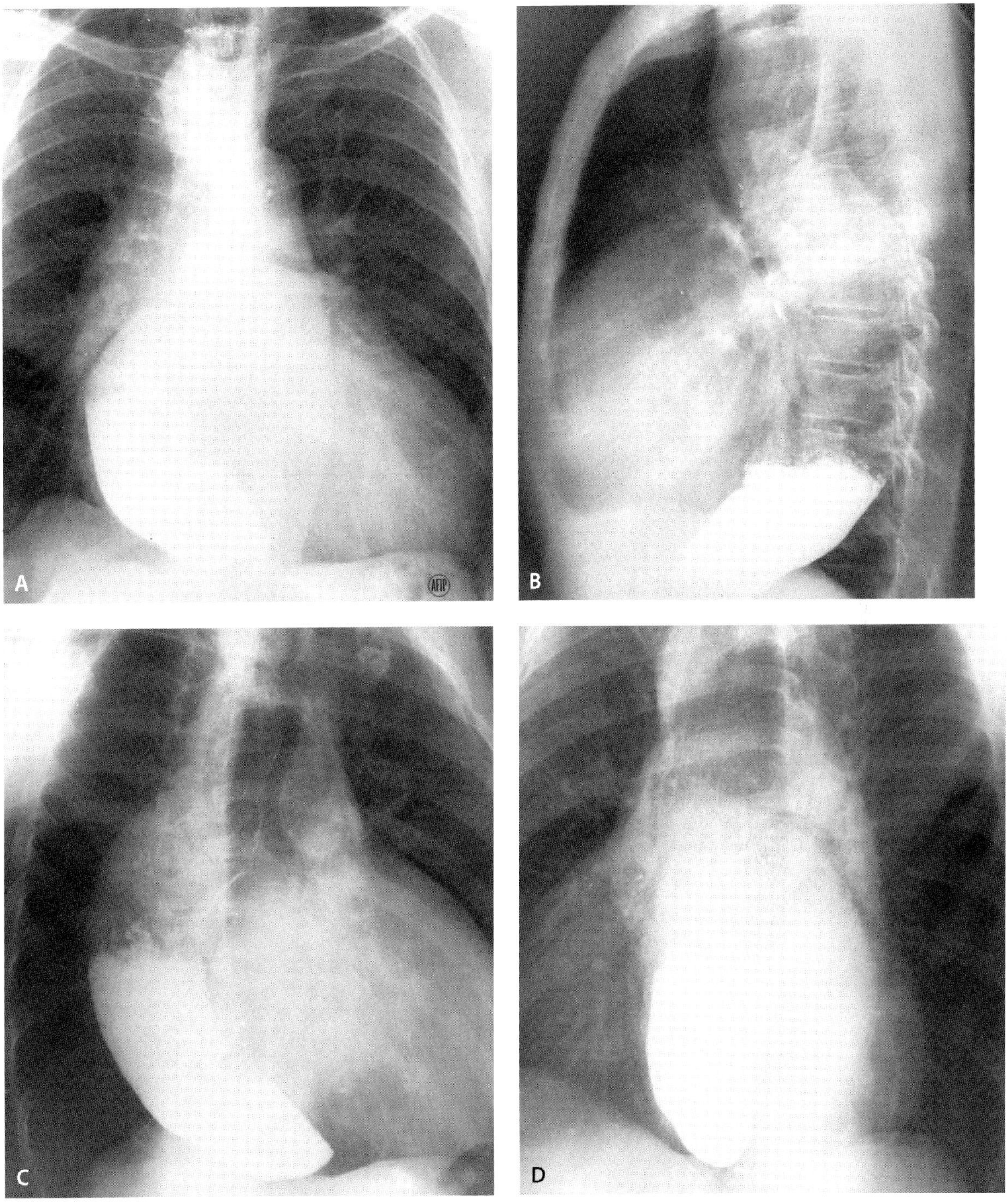

Fig. 4.39 A–D. Chronic Chagas' myocardiopathy and megaesophagus in a 58-year-old black Brazilian man. **A** PA view of the chest shows a prominent soft tissue density along the entire right mediastinal border, due to the greatly dilated esophagus partially filled with barium and fluid. The right and left cardiac convexities are prominent because of enlargement of both sides of the heart. The left atrial enlargement causes a bulge along the left upper cardiac border and upward displacement of the left main bronchus. There is no pulmonary vascular congestion or pleural fluid. The left lateral (**B**) and RAO (**C**) views show posterior displacement of the megaesophagus by the dilated left atrium. The grossly distended esophagus causes a wide area of increased soft tissue density from the apex to the diaphragm posterior to the trachea and heart outlines on the lateral view. **D** Gross cardiomegaly with enlargement of all chambers is seen on a left anterior oblique view. The markedly dilated left atrium elevates the left main bronchus, while the huge left ventricle protrudes well behind the vertebral column. Clinically, the patient had a 37-lb weight loss and dysphagia for both solid foods and fluids of 7 months' duration, with regurgitation of food several hours after eating. His heart rate was 36 beats per minute and arrhythmic, and a systolic murmur was heard in the mitral area. There was slight hepatomegaly. (Courtesy of Dr. Clovis Simao, Sao Paulo)

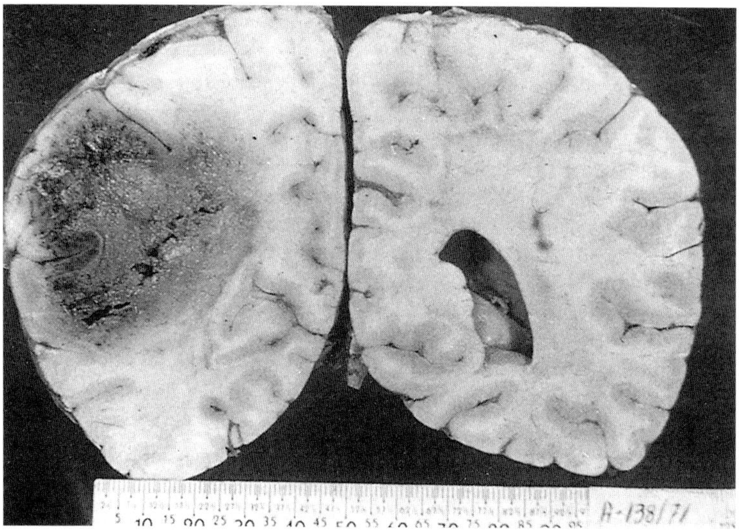

Fig. 4.40. Involvement of the CNS by Chagas' disease. A tumoral lesion is present in the brain of a 62-year-old patient who was in the indeterminate phase of the disease until the infection was reactivated in association with mycosis fungoides. A large hemorrhagic-necrotic mass is present in the left occipitoparietal region. (Courtesy of Prof. Aristides Cheto Queiroz, Bahia and Bittencourt and Ashworth 1995)

Bibliography

Abath GM, et al: Histopathology of skeletal muscle in Chagas' disease. *Am J Trop Med Hyg* 15:141–145, 1966

Acquatella H, Schiller NB: Echocardiographic recognition of Chagas' disease and endomyocardial fibrosis. *J Am Soc Echocardiogr* 1:60–68, 1988

Acquatella H, Schiller NB, Puigbo JJ, et al: M mode and two-dimensional echocardiography in chronic Chagas' heart disease. A clinical and pathological study. *Circulation* 62:787–789, 1980

Allain DS, et al: An evaluation of the direct agglutination test for Chagas' disease. *J Parasitol* 60:179–184, 1974

Anselmi A, et al: Myocardiopathy in Chagas' disease. 1 Comparative study of pathologic findings in chronic human and experimental Chagas' myocarditis. *Am Heart J* 72:469, 1966

Anselmi A, et al: Cardiovascular radiology in acute and chronic Chagas' myocardiopathy. Morphologic and dynamic study of the cardiac contour correlated with the histologic changes observed in myocardiopathies attributed to *Schizotrypanum cruzi*. *Am Heart J* 73:626, 1967

Arreaza N, Puigbo JJ, Acquatella H, et al: Radionuclide evaluation of left ventricular function in chronic Chagas' cardiomyopathy. *J Nucl Med* 24:563–567, 1993

Atias A, et al: Megaesophagus, megacolon, and Chagas' disease in Chile. *Gastroenterology* 44:433–437, 1963

Bittencourt AL, Ashworth TG: Trypanosomiasis. In: Doerr W, Seifert G: *Tropical pathology*, 2nd edn. Springer, Berlin Heidelberg, New York, 1995, pp 653–681

Bocchi EA, Kalil R, Rosenberg L, et al: Magnetic resonance imaging in Chagas' disease: correlation with endomyocardial biopsy. *Circulation* 84:1–266, 1992

Bocchi EA, Bellotti G, Uip D, et al: Long term follow-up after heart transplantation for Chagas' disease. *Transpl Proc* 25:1329–1330, 1993

Braile DM, Soares MJF, Rodrigues MCZ, et al: Cardiomyoplasty – clinical study of 26 patients: a six year follow-up. *Intercontinental Cardiology 2*. 631:71–78, 1993

Brasil A: Aperistalsis of the esophagus. *Rev Bras Gastroenterol* 7:21, 1955

Brasil A: Anatomical sino-atrial block: a new disturbance of the heart mechanism. *Arq Bras Cardiol* 8:159–221, 1955

Breniere SF, Carrasco R, Revollo S, et al: Chagas' disease in Bolivia: clinical and epidemiological features and zymodeme variability of *Trypanosoma cruzi* strains isolated from patients. *Am J Trop Med Hyg* 41:521–529, 1989

Byington CAB: Vectocardiografia em Doenca de Chagas. *Anaes do Congresso Internacional sobre a Doenca de Chagas. Vol 1.* Oficina Grafica da Universidade do Brasil, Rio de Janeiro, 1959, pp 357–374

Carrasco HA, Barbozo JS, Inglessis G, et al: Left ventricular cineangiography in Chagas' disease: detection of early myocardial damage. *Am Heart J* 104:595–602, 1982

Carvalhal S, et al: Alteracoes do complexo QRS nos derivacoes precordiais e seu substrato anatomico en pacientes portadores de miocardite chagasica cronica. *Rev Paul Med* 45:161, 1954

Chagas C: Nova especie morbida do homen, produzida por um Trypanosoma (*Trypanosoma cruzi*). Nota previa. *Bras Med* 23:161, 1909

Combellas I, Puigbo JJ, Acquatello H, et al: Echocardiographic features of impaired left ventricular diastolic function in Chagas' heart disease. *Br Heart J* 53:298–309, 1985

Cunha CLP, Urbanitz LAGT, Souza AM, et al: Evolutive Doppler echocardiographic changes in the indeterminate phase of Chagas' disease. *Eur Heart J* 14:135, 1993

De Freitas JLP: *Public health importance of Chagas' disease.* Pan American Health Organization, Washington, DC, WHO/Chagas' 4:1, 1960

Ferreira MS, et al: Acute, fatal *Trypanosoma cruzi* meningoencephalitis in a human immuno-deficiency-virus positive hemophiliac patient. *Am J Trop Med Hyg* 45:723–727, 1991

Ferreira-Santos R, Carril CF: Acquired megacolon in Chagas' disease. *Dis Colon Rectum* 7:353–364, 1964

Ferreira-Santos R: Aperistalsis of the esophagus and colon (megaesophagus and megacolon) etiologically related to Chagas' disease. *Am J Dig Dis* 6:700–726, 1961

Gluckstein D, et al: Chagas' disease. Another cause of a cerebral mass in the acquired immunodeficiency syndrome. *Am J Med* 92:429–432, 1992

Guerrero L, Carrasco H, Parada H, et al: Left ventricular mechanics in Chagas' disease and dilated cardiomyopathy: echocardiographic study [in Spanish]. *Arq Brasil Cardiol* 53:23–27, 1989

Hagar JM, Rahimtoda SH: Chagas' heart disease in the United States. *N Engl J Med* 325:763–768, 1991

Johnson CM: American trypanosomiasis. *Med Clin North Am* 27:822, 1943

Jung RC: Chagas' disease, a possible cause of megaesophagus and megacolon. *Am J Gastroenterol* 32:311–316, 1959

Kirchhoff LV, et al: American trypanosomiasis (Chagas' disease) in Central American immigrants. *Am J Med* 82:915–920, 1987

Kirchhoff LV: American trypanosomiasis (Chagas' disease) – a tropical disease now in the United States. *N Engl J Med* 329:639–643, 1993

Köberle F: Megaesophagus. *Gastroenterology* 34:460–466, 1958

Köberle F: Enteromegaly and cardiomegaly in Chagas' disease. *Gut* 4:399–405, 1963

Köberle F, et al: Patologia da molestia de Chagas. *Med Rev Fac Med Ribeirao Preto* 5:5–45, 1972

Lack EE, Filie A: American trypanosomiasis. In: Connor DH, Chandler FW: *Pathology of infectious diseases, vol 2.* Appleton & Lange, Stamford Conn., 1997, pp 1299–1304

Laranja FS, et al: Chagas' disease: a clinical, epidemiologic, and pathological study. *Circulation* 14:1035, 1956

Latin America's plague. *The Economist* May 5, 1990, p 105

Levin MJ, Mesri E, Benarous R, et al: Identification of major *Trypanosoma cruzi* antigenic determinants in chronic Chagas' heart disease. *Am J Trop Med Hyg* 41:530–538, 1989

Lorenzana R: Chronic Chagas myocarditis: report of a case. *Am J Clin Pathol* 48:39–43, 1967

Losavio A, Jones MC, Sanz OP, et al: A sequential study of the peripheral nervous system involvement in experimental Chagas' disease. *Am J Trop Med Hyg* 41:539–547, 1989

Marin-Neto JA, Marzullo P, Souza ACS, et al: Radionuclide angiographic evidence for early predominant right ventricular involvement in patients with Chagas' disease. *Can J Cardiol* 4:231–236, 1988

Marin-Neto JA, Marzullo P, Marcassa C, et al: Myocardial perfusion abnormalities in chronic Chagas' disease as detected by thallium-201 scintigraphy. *Am J Cardiol* 69:780–784, 1992

Marquez JS, et al: The electrocardiogram in Chagasic myocarditis. *Am Heart J* 59:321–322, 1960

Marsden PD: American trypanosomiasis. In: Cook GC (ed) *Manson's tropical diseases, 20th edn.* Saunders, London, 1996, pp 1197–1212

Massumi RA, Gooch A: Chagas' myocarditis. *Arch Intern Med* 116:531–536, 1965

Mattoso LF, Reeder MM: Radiological diagnosis of Chagas' disease (American trypanosomiasis). *Semin Roentgenol* 33:26–46, 1998

Mota E, Todd CW, Maguire JH, et al: Megaesophagus and seroreactivity to *Trypanosoma cruzi* in a rural community in northeast Brazil. *Am J Trop Med Hyg* 33:820–826, 1984

Mott KE, Hagstrom JWC: The pathologic lesions of the cardiac autonomic nervous system in chronic Chagas' myocarditis. *Circulation* 31:273–286, 1965

Neal RA: Epidemiology of Chagas' disease and methods of detecting *T. cruzi. Proc R Soc Med* 66:773–774, 1973

Ortiz J, Matsumoto AY, Monaco CAF: Echocardiography in Chagas' disease. *Echocardiography* 3:41, 1986

Puigbo JJ, et al: Clinical and epidemiological study of chronic heart involvement in Chagas' disease. *Bull World Health Organ* 34:655–669, 1969

Raia A, et al: Pathogenesis and treatment of acquired megaduodenum. *Am J Dig Dis* 6:757–771, 1961

Reeder MM, Hamilton LC: Tropical diseases of the colon. *Semin Roentgenol* 3:62–80, 1968

Reeder MM, Hamilton LC: Radiologic diagnosis of tropical diseases of the gastrointestinal tract. *Radiol Clin North Am* 7:57–81, 1969

Reeder MM, Simao C: Chagas' myocardiopathy. *Semin Roentgenol* 4:374–383, 1969

Reeder MM, Palmer PES: Infections and infestations. In: Freeny PC, Stevenson GW (eds) *Margulis and Burhenne's alimentary tract roentgenology, 5th edn.* Mosby, St. Louis, 1994, pp 1475–1542

Rezende JM, Moreira H: Chagasic megaesophagus and megacolon. Historical review and present concepts. *Arq Gastroenterol* 25 (special issue):32–43, 1988

Rosemberg S, et al: Fatal meningoencephalitis caused by reactivation of *Trypanosoma cruzi* infection in a patient with AIDS. *Neurology* 42:640–642, 1992

Rosenbaum MB: Chagasic myocardiopathy. *Prog Cardiovasc Dis* 7:199–225, 1964

Schiffler RJ, et al: Indigenous Chagas' disease (American trypanosomiasis) in California *JAMA* 251:2983–2984, 1984

Soubhie NV, Vichi RL: Acao de digitalicos na cardiopatia Chagasica cronica. *Rev Paul Med* 70:210, 1967

Szarfman A, et al: A simple method for the detection of human congenital Chagas' disease. *J Parasitol* 59:723, 1973

Tarleton R, Downs M, Zhang L: Chagas' disease: associated heart damage not due to autoimmune reactions. *Vaccine Weekly* Sept 22, 1997, pp 7–8

Troncon LE, Iazigi N: Scintigraphic study of the gastrointestinal transit of a liquid meal in patients with chronic Chagas' disease. *Braz J Med Biol Res* 25:145–148, 1992

Vichi FL, et al: Apical abnormalities in Chagas' cardiopathy. A radiological-electrocardiographic correlation. *Arq Bras Cardiol* 21:251–256, 1968

Winslow DJ, Chaffee EF: Preliminary investigations on Chagas' disease. *Milit Med* 130:826, 1965

Woody NC, Woody HB: American trypanosomiasis. First endogenous case in the United States. *JAMA* 159:676, 1955

Woody NC, Woody HB: American trypanosomiasis I. Clinical and epidemiological background of Chagas' disease in the United States. *J Pediatr* 58:568, 1961

World Health Organization: Chagas' disease: report of a study group. *WHO Tech Rep Ser* 202:1, 1960

World Health Organization: Control of Chagas' disease: report of a WHO expert committee. *WHO Tech Rep Ser* 811:1–91, 1991

5 Tuberculosis

With S.J. WAMBANI and PAUL REEVE

I see a lily on the brow
With anguish moist and fever dew
And on thy cheek a fading rose
Fast withereth too.

La Belle Dame San Merci
John Keats, 1795–1821

There was a time in the eighteenth and nineteenth centuries when tuberculosis was a fashionable affliction. All the best poets, musicians, and writers, not to mention politicians and heroines of operas, suffered from consumption and died either beautifully or in interesting ways. Of course, the unknown poor simply died, often unpleasantly, of the white plague. There were many names for this common disease, which has been recognized and described for centuries: the earliest definitive record is of pulmonary and spinal tuberculosis in the mummy of a 5-year-old Egyptian child of about 3400 B.C. A later mummy, of a young man dated at about 1000 B.C., had a psoas abscess as well as spinal lesions. In the Americas, a naturally mummified middle-aged Peruvian woman who died about 1000 years ago had primary pulmonary tuberculosis with calcified hilar lymph nodes. Tuberculosis was identified in this case because a unique DNA segment was identified in a lung lesion, using the polymerase chain reaction.

The word "tubercle" was first used in the seventeenth century by a Dutchman, Franciscus Silvius, of Leyden, to describe the lung lesions. Later (1839), Johann Schönlein called the disease "tuberculosis." It was not until 1882 that Robert Koch identified and described *Mycobacterium tuberculosis*. With this discovery much of the romance and many of the myths vanished.

If the source had been found, the cure had not, and tuberculosis continued as a major cause of death and no respecter of social rank: it was familiar and fatal to everyone. Probably more than 25% of the graves in the cemeteries of Europe and America were filled by people of all ages who had died of tuberculosis. There is a large and interesting literature on the disease and the remarkable ways in which it was treated. Most were in some way or other uncomfortable for the patient, and none were very successful. Then in 1943, Selman Waksman, a microbiologist at Rutgers University, fortuitously discovered streptomycin while investigating a peculiar fungus which was killing chickens. This discovery, together with the development of two other drugs in the next few years, led to the apparent conquest of tuberculosis.

But the bacillus which had undoubtedly affected history by killing so many in their youth may well have the same power once again. In 1993 the World Health Organization (WHO) declared that tuberculosis was a global emergency and estimated that it would kill 30 million people in the next decade. In 1996 it was the leading cause of deaths due to micro-organisms: there are eight million new cases every year. One-third of the world's population (1.7 billion) have been infected at some time and 20 million currently have active tuberculosis. (On average, about 10% of those infected go on to develop clinically active disease.) More than half of all those who have been infected live in Asia and Africa. WHO estimates (1995) that only 10% of tuberculous patients also have AIDS, but in the next decade there may be seven million with the combined infection, rising to 14 million by the year 2010. Almost every patient with both diseases will have active tuberculosis, because the AIDS virus destroys the cell which normally controls the micobacteria. (See Chap. 8, p. 681 for discussion of tuberculosis in AIDS.)

The global rise in population, the wars and disputes which have caused refugees and migration, and the decline in the level of public health services are also to blame for the recent reemergence of tuberculosis. WHO has shown (in Tanzania) that it is possible to find and cure over 80% of infectious cases and that 6–8 months of proper treatment will achieve this goal. The sputum bacterial counts fall rapidly and the sputum becomes negative for bacilli within 2 months of adequate treatment, resulting in control of the epidemic spread. In 1997, WHO was a little more optimistic that tuberculosis might be leveling off but warned that failure to treat the infection promptly would result in drug resistance, which is already at a level of at least 7% and rising and often takes the form of multidrug resistance.

Against this background it is important to add that "tropical" tuberculosis is not a product of the AIDS epidemic. This chapter in the first edition (1981) started by stating that "The causative organism of tuberculosis, Koch's bacillus, is morphologically and culturally the same in the tropics as in non-tropical countries. Yet the clinical disease "tuberculosis" appears in ways which may be unrecognizable to physicians trained in non-tropical countries. It is not a "chronic" disease in the majority of patients, but an acute and often fulminating infection whether it be in the chest, bones, joints or elsewhere. Moreover, it causes signs and symptoms and presents at sites which may be quite unexpected and contrary to the descriptions in many North American and European textbooks." To this it is now necessary to add, "unless those books refer to AIDS-related tuberculosis."

Both in the tropics and in HIV-positive patients, the difference lies in the immunological background, the state of nutrition, and the way of life; it is that mystical relationship between the bacillus and its host which changes the clinical course of the disease, aided by variations in the virulence of particular strains of bacilli. Tuberculosis in the tropics often mimics an infection in an immunosuppressed patient; it must be remembered as the possible etiology of almost any acute or unusual illness whether seen in the tropics or in a recent immigrant into nontropical countries, and this pattern of tuberculosis must not be assumed to be due to AIDS. There are many other common causes of immunosuppression. And in the same way, a person from a nontropical area moving into the tropics retains the nontropical pattern of disease; transplanting one's person does not immediately change one's nature. Only over several years may this phenomenon of "host-response" alter to the local pattern, unless a virus or other event intervenes.

Acute tuberculosis with unusual variations is not the monopoly of the tropics; the authors have seen cases following the severe "tropical" pattern in patients who do not have AIDS and who have spent their lives in North America or in Europe. Tuberculosis is a disease of infinite variation because it occurs in an infinite variety of people. The immunosuppression due to HIV infections has focused worldwide attention on the pattern of tuberculosis which has been the norm in the tropics, as it may well have been in the past wherever nutrition, hygiene, and living conditions were poor and parasites were plentiful.

Dr. Olive Shisana, Director General of the South African Department of Health and joint author of a 1996 WHO report, has summed up the situation: "Tuberculosis has become a disease more terrifying than AIDS or the Ebola virus." Worldwide, it is the principal cause of death amongst all adults. Referring to drug resistance, Dr. Donald Enarson, Director of the International Union Against Tuberculosis, based in Paris, has added, "This is the most frightening situation I have ever encountered. If we do not act now, we will have a situation that we cannot control."

Radiologists in the tropics or, indeed, anywhere else, should consider tuberculosis in almost every differential diagnosis: its manifestations, like its sufferers, are legion.

Synonyms

TB. Koch's disease. Pulmonary tuberculosis: Phthisis. Consumption. Tabes pulmonalis. Spinal tuberculosis: Pott's disease. Abdominal tuberculosis: Tabes mesenterica. Tuberculous cervical lymphadenitis: Scrofula. Struma. General tuberculosis: Hectic fever. Asthenia. *Ger*: Tuberkulose. Schwindsucht. *Sp*: Tisis, Tuberculosis. *Fr*: Phtisie.

Definition

Tuberculosis is an infection with the *Mycobacterium tuberculosis* or *Mycobacterium bovis*. Both are gram-positive, acid and alcohol fast, aerobic, non-spore forming rods, classified with the actinomycetes. *M. tuberculosis* is a facultative intracellular parasite, which, many believe, is capable also of extracellular growth and can remain dormant for years or even decades.

Geographic Distribution

Tuberculosis is a worldwide infection from which some three million people die annually, more than from any other single infectious disease. It is probable that, because of AIDS, drug resistance, and population stresses, the epidemic will increase in the future unless brought under control. The countries with the largest number of patients with tuberculosis are Bangladesh, Brazil, China, India, Indonesia, Nigeria, Pakistan, the Philippines, and Vietnam. The rate of disease is highest in sub-Saharan Africa. In some parts of the world, 80% of the population react positively to a tuberculin skin test by the age of 25 years and many react much earlier (unless they are HIV-positive). In developing countries tuberculosis accounts for 26% of avoidable deaths.

The reported incidence, however, may not be accurate: it is often a reflection of the efficiency and methods used to detect the disease rather than a true indication of its actual prevalence. Public health facilities vary greatly, but, for example, it was estimated East Africa (1971) that half a million persons were newly infected each year and that 75000 would develop clinical tuberculosis, of whom only 25000 would be diagnosed and 16000 treated. Such figures have improved in some countries, but not in all. A person, once infected, is likely to harbor the tubercle bacillus for the rest of his or her life and it may remain dormant unless there is a change in general health or immunity, as occurs with AIDS, diabetes, leukemia, or malnutrition. Much less commonly, there may be reinfection.

Epidemiology and Pathology

Tuberculosis affects everyone from infants to the very aged. It is spread by droplet infection or by contaminated foods, particularly milk from herds infected with *M. bovis*. In many countries bovine tuberculosis has been almost completely eliminated following the pasteurization of milk and the control of infected cattle. Unfortunately, there is a reservoir in wild species and it is known to have infected buffalo and rhinoceros in East and southern Africa, for example. Reinfection of domestic cattle is thus always possible.

The first infection is most commonly in the lungs, but can be in any part of the body. Both *M. tuberculosis* and *M. bovis* can directly infect the skin, presenting as a serpiginous ulcer, although this is uncommon. Lupus vulgaris is a secondary (immune) infection. Transplacental infection is possible but very rare: there are about 150 well-documented cases in the literature, but it may become more frequent in HIV-positive mothers.

Even if AIDS is not taken into account, tuberculosis is most prevalent in crowded cities, yet there is also a high incidence in rural areas. In the tropics it is a household infection and WHO has reported an incidence five to ten times higher in household contacts than among the general population. Living and sleeping in proximity to an infected person in a crowded house or hut is more risky than using public transport or working in ill-ventilated buildings.

The susceptibility of a person to tuberculosis is influenced by genetic and ethnic factors, malnutrition, the quantum of bacteria entering the body, and other illness, such as diabetes, pneumoconiosis, infection with multiple parasites, and anemia, as well as AIDS. There is an individual and herd variation in immunity. The Moslem community of southern India, the North American Indians and Eskimos, many Africans, and Malays have a high susceptibility and morbidity. Extensive campaigns by WHO utilizing mass radiographic surveys, BCG vaccination, and education were very successful, but now the disease is once again a major health problem throughout the tropics and is getting more common because of AIDS and drug resistance, as well as population movements.

Modern chemotherapy has made it possible for patients with active pulmonary tuberculosis to stay at home and have treatment without endangering other inhabitants of the house. As mentioned above, a bacillus-positive sputum will become negative after about 2 months of therapy. The real danger of spreading infection occurs before the disease is diagnosed. Ambulant treatment has encouraged many patients to accept the necessary regimen; previously, isolation or sanitarium treatment met with considerable resistance. Now the difficulty is to ensure that treatment is continuous and adequate.

There are also variations in the sensitivity of the organism to different drugs; for example, in southern India, where tuberculosis is common, the bacilli seem to be isoniazid-sensitive, whereas in the United Kingdom the response is not so good. *p*-Aminosalicylic acid is better tolerated by patients in the tropics. Thiacetezone is not tolerated by HIV-positive patients and may even be fatal. The atypical (nontuberculous) mycobacteria are also a cause of treatment failure, but the major therapeutic problem is the development of drug-resistant organisms, the frequency of which now varies from 7% to 20%. This is usually the result of inadequate and incomplete treatment: many patients do not feel the need to continue therapy for 6 or 8 months and abandon their pills as soon as they feel better. Poverty, the nonavailability of drugs in the regular market at normal cost, interference in the treatment by unqualified practitioners, and the side-effects of the drugs (e.g., tinnitus, deafness, neuropathies, hepatitis, gastroenteritis) all offer reasons for the failure of continuous treatment. Black market drugs at inadequate dosage add to the problem. Yet WHO reckons that 80% of patients can be cured with proper supervision and full treatment, and that even in the poorest countries a case reduction of 50% is possible.

A patient's resistance to tuberculosis is a very complex process, much of which is not yet fully understood. In very general terms, no two mycobacterial strains are genetically identical (as is the case with people), but if a person is infected with a virulent strain of tuberculosis, the outcome depends on the state of competence of the patient's cell-mediated immunity (CMI). With a competent CMI the body produces derivatives of the monocyte-macrophage cells that have the ability to kill and sequester mycobacteria. These derivatives are the activated macrophage, the epithelioid cells, and the Langhans giant cell. All these cells produce hydrogen peroxide and oxygen in forms which are toxic, such as hypochlorous acid and toxic enzymes: all of these kill mycobacteria. However, the effects are unfortunately not limited to the bacteria and these toxic products kill much more host tissue than mycobacteria, which is why the disease becomes chronic, resulting in persistent destruction as seen in fibrocaseous tuberculosis. This is known as hyperergic tuberculosis, a response which is characterized by the granulomatous reaction. It is the only effective defense and the only hope that the patient has of survival. A positive tuberculin skin test is an indication that CMI has developed, and there will be a sharp reduction in the number of mycobacteria and the development of a layer of palisaded epithelioid cells around the necrotic foci. Eventually there will be an outer layer of granulation tissue surrounding the necrotic foci and scars will form that contain any remaining mycobacteria.

When CMI is suppressed, becoming too weak or nonexistent, the mycobacteria can proliferate unchecked and destroy host tissues directly. This is anergic tuberculosis, which, unchanged, is progressive and soon fatal. It is characterized by broad areas of contiguous noncaseous necrosis, large numbers of bacilli, and very little or no granulomatous reaction. Caseous necrosis is flecked with mineral deposits, hence calcification, and retains for a short time a ghost outline of previously vital tissue. The necrosis of anergic tuberculosis does not have calcification or recognizable tissue. The suppression of CMI may occur for unexpected reasons, such as grief, trauma, exposure to cold, cytotoxic agents, x-radiation in large doses, and corticosteroids, as well as the more recognized causes such as malnutrition, alcoholism, diabetes, malignancy, and, of course, the AIDS virus. The problem with this oversimplified explanation is that it is difficult to confirm in the laboratory and there is no general explanation why patients who have apparently successfully overcome the infection should suffer a breakdown of this protective immunity, allowing the disease to surge again. One of the suggested explanations is the difference in the genetic background of the host, but this is also very controversial. For all these reasons, the terms "hypersensitivity," "immunity," and "acute" are used less often. Much remains to be clarified, especially about the cell envelope and the associated and secreted protein. It is not even clear how the effective immune response in 90% of people succeeds in killing tubercle bacilli. As so often happens in medicine, the natural history of the disease is fully understood, the explanation of why it happens is not. Research continues, and is particularly oriented toward the development of a vaccine against tuberculosis.

Laboratory Diagnosis

The only real proof of tuberculosis is the isolation on smear or culture of *M. tuberculosis* from the patient's sputum, other body fluids, or tissues. The histological mark is the epithelioid granuloma with mononuclear and Langhans giant cells, together with caseating necrosis. Clinically the tuberculin test is almost universally accepted as a fairly reliable way to detect a current or previous tuberculous infection, but there are sources of error: When the tests are properly applied and material is fresh and active, it is an effective screening method unless the individual is immunosuppressed. Another source of error, in which the test may be positive, is previous BCG vaccination. Sensitivity to tuberculin may also be related to unrecognized infection with similar micro-organisms which are not tuberculous. This "false" sensitivity is particularly common in the tropics and subtropics and has a variable geographic distribution both in Africa and in India; it is more common in low-altitude populations than in those who live on the mountains. The responsible organism has not yet been identified. Thus, when there is a weak reaction to low doses of tuberculin and a strong reaction to a high dose, it may indicate a nonspecific reaction rather than tuberculosis.

During severe and overwhelming generalized infections (including HIV) the skin tests may remain negative, as seen in very sick, undernourished children. A similar misleading result can occasionally occur in bone tuberculosis. It is not common, but is well documented. Thus, a negative skin test does not totally exclude tuberculosis, nor in the tropics does a positive test necessarily prove its presence. The new γ-interferon blood test, which is thought to be 98% specific and is without observer error, may solve many clinical problems.

Other laboratory tests do not differ in the tropics from those accepted elsewhere in the world, but unfortunately the host of parasitic infestations which are endemic in the tropics may confuse routine investigations. An elevated erythrocyte sedimentation rate (ESR), a raised eosinophil count, lymphocytosis, and anemia may all be due to the patient's "underlying normal" ill-health. Sputum or gastric aspirates remain the most reliable method of diagnosis, particularly in children. Under the age of 1 year, it is the lungs which are most commonly infected and positive recovery of the bacilli is possible in about 75% of cases. In older children, even when very ill, the recovery rate of bacilli may be only 40%. Examination of effusions in the pleura, peritoneum, or joints, or of the pus from a spinal or other abscess, may demonstrate the organism on smear or culture, but failure to recognize the bacillus does not exclude active tuberculosis. Unfortunately, culture is a slow process, expensive, and not always readily available. Apart from the classical histological findings, the polymerase chain reaction, a method amplifying specific DNA sequences, is successful in detecting mycobacterial DNA in clinical specimens, including fluids.

The cerebrospinal fluid (CSF) will only contain tubercle bacilli in about 10% of initial samples. More information can be obtained from the ELISA assay and the polymerase chain reaction. There is a latex particle agglutination assay which is inexpensive and suitable for use in developing countries. The spinal fluid will usually be under pressure and clear, with an increased protein content and reduced glucose level: there is often an increased CSF white blood cell count, with 90%–95% monocytes.

Examining urine for the bacillus was once suggested as a way of confirming generalized tuberculosis, but this is positive in less than 7% of samples (except when there is active genitourinary tuberculosis), and is too inaccurate to be used. General hematological examination is usually normal in tuberculosis, but can be confusing when there is acute tuberculous pneumonia because the white blood cell count may be increased. When there is bone marrow involvement, there may be leukopenia. A patient who has multiple parasites is also likely to have an abnormal hematological background.

In many patients in the tropics the disease is a severe, acute infection and no time can be wasted in waiting for laboratory results which may be of dubious value. Even when the skin reaction is negative, if the clinical suspicion of tuberculosis is high then therapy is often started and the patient reviewed, particularly as to the radiological findings after about 2 months of treatment. Hypercalcemia is an infrequently recognized complication of tuberculosis, particularly in small children and those with disseminated infection; it probably occurs because vitamin B_3 metabolites have a role in immunoregulation, and the level of these metabolites is regulated in granulomata by T-small cells.

Clinical Characteristics

Clinical tuberculosis is so well described in so many textbooks that there is little reason to repeat the findings. To the usual picture of malaise, tiredness, loss of weight, night sweats, and mild pyrexia must be added two important tropical variants: the acute form of the disease and the background of ill health which is so common in many of the tropical patients.

Ill health, anemia, malnutrition, pyrexia, and dysentery are so much a normal part of the low standard of living and hygiene of many tropical countries that these conditions cannot be used as an indication of possible tuberculosis. For example, in Egypt and elsewhere in Africa, many adults in rural areas normally have several varieties of parasites and this is equally true for much of India, Asia, and South America. This background of ill health makes the patient more susceptible to tuberculosis and the delicate balance of borderline ill health may have been upset by a recent tuberculous infection which has brought the patient to the physician.

In other patients, acute tuberculosis, whether in lungs or in joints or elsewhere in the body, may closely mimic an acute bacterial infection. The classical presentation of a low-grade illness is not the only way in which tuberculosis behaves. The history of the illness may be short, as when a child who has a temperature of 39.5 °C (103 °F) seems to have acute bacterial lobar pneumonia but actually has primary tuberculosis. Initial examination of the sputum (or gastric lavage) in such cases may be confusing because of secondary infection: the diagnosis of tuberculosis may not be made because the possibility is often forgotten. Similarly, acute osteomyelitis, septic arthritis, mastoiditis, and peritonitis may all be due to tuberculosis and not an "ordinary" pyogenic infection. There must be a high index of suspicion and clinical sixth sense, and tuberculosis should be included in almost every differential diagnosis.

Tuberculosis of the Respiratory Tract

Even before AIDS swept through the tropics, pulmonary tuberculosis had been one of the major causes of illness and death: it is not likely to relinquish this leading role for many years, even in the millions who are HIV-negative.

Tuberculosis of the Upper Respiratory Tract

The possibility of tuberculosis of the upper respiratory tract should always be considered in a patient from whom the sputum has been found to contain tubercle bacilli and yet the routine chest radiograph is normal. Clinically there will be excess sputum, hoarseness, and, usually, general symptoms of tuberculosis. Endoscopy, computed tomography (CT), and, in some cases, a contrast tracheogram will demonstrate the tuberculous ulceration and granulation tissue (when CT is not available, standard tomography can be helpful) (Figs. 5.1, 5.2). The trachea may be narrowed, the larynx swollen, and the cartilage eroded, all of which can be demonstrated on CT. Active tuberculosis is always much more extensive on CT scanning than it appears on endoscopy. Quite often the whole length of the trachea is thickened and it may extend into the major bronchi. The thickening is irregular, and where there is an intraluminal granulomatous mass, the degree of narrowing can be quite significant. The extent of the infection is most clearly seen on three-dimensional imaging, but actual images often show the relationship of the neighboring structures.

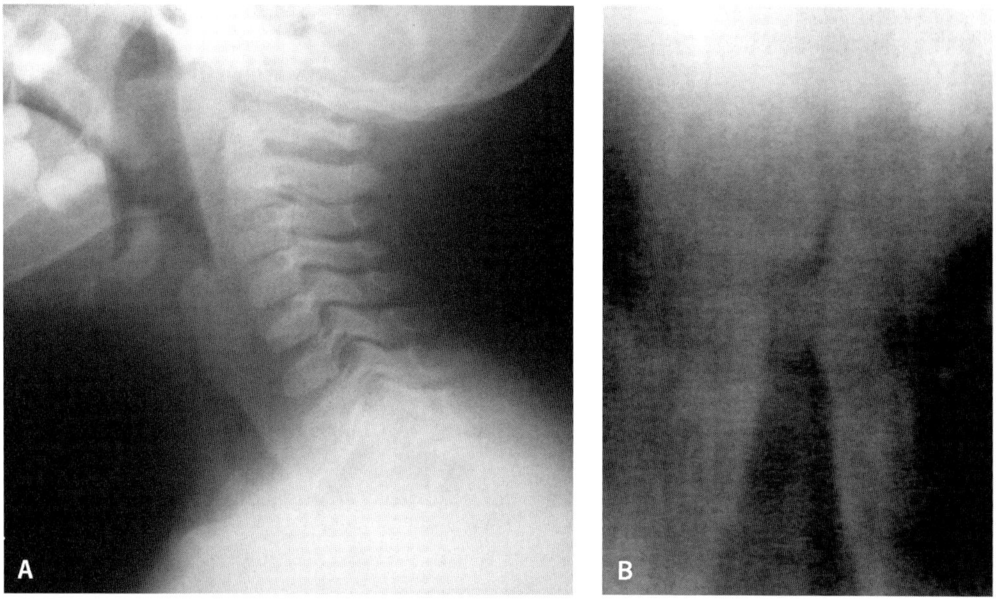

Fig. 5.1. **A** Laryngeal and subglottic tuberculosis in a 3-year-old girl from one of the Pacific Islands. There is narrowing and anterior displacement of the airway. The diagnosis was confirmed by bronchoscopy: both lungs showed miliary tuberculosis and there was tuberculous thickening of the ileocecal region also. Upper airway infection is usually part of generalized, hematogenous spread and this case was no exception. (Courtesy of Dr. Cheryl Sisler, Hawaii) **B** Linear tomograms of laryngeal tuberculosis which presented in an adolescent as upper airway obstruction. There was a granulomatous mass lesion in the larynx. (From Cremin and Jamieson 1995)

The fibrotic stage of tuberculosis usually results in smooth narrowing of the lumen and the thickening of the wall is less marked. When the disease spreads down to the main bronchi, the left main bronchus is often more involved.

Although pulmonary tuberculosis is common, laryngeal and tracheal infection are not, even as a complication in patients with heavily infected sputum. As an isolated infection, without pulmonary tuberculosis, laryngeal or tracheal tuberculosis is rare. While the granulomas can be imaged, there is no satisfactory radiological method to confirm that the etiology is tuberculosis.

Fig. 5.2 A–F. Tuberculosis of the trachea and major bronchi is best shown with multiplanar and three-dimensional reconstruction. **A** An irregular mass narrowing the trachea, with marked thickening of the whole length of the tracheal wall. **B** Three-dimensional CT scan of the same patient confirms the irregular and diffuse narrowing of the whole length of the trachea and the proximal main bronchi. **C** Thin-section CT, at the level of the thoracic inlet, clearly showing the marked thickening of the wall of the trachea and the narrow lumen. In the fibrotic stage, the distortion may be even more marked. **D** Three-dimensional CT scan of a 29-year-old woman shows marked irregular narrowing along the length of the left main bronchus. **E** A thin-section CT scan of the same patient, just below the carina, confirms the narrowing of the lumen and shows the marked thickening of the wall of the bronchus. **F** The coronal scan shows the full extent of the bronchial fibrosis. (Courtesy of Dr. Kyung Soo Lee, Seoul) ▶

Primary (Nonimmune) Tuberculosis

The prevalence of acute primary infection at any age, even without AIDS, is one of the major variations in tuberculosis in the tropics compared with other regions. In one series, more than 50% of the patients with the primary pattern of tuberculosis were over 18 years of age. Clinically patients may present with an acute illness which may be so severe that its true cause is not easily recognized. Other patients may seem to have a simple upper respiratory infection, perhaps one which does not improve clinically, and primary lung tuberculosis is an unexpected finding on a chest radiograph. There are five ways in which primary tuberculosis presents radiographically:

- Lobar pneumonia
- Bronchopneumonia
- Hilar and mediastinal adenopathy
- Pleural or pericardial effusion
- Miliary tuberculosis

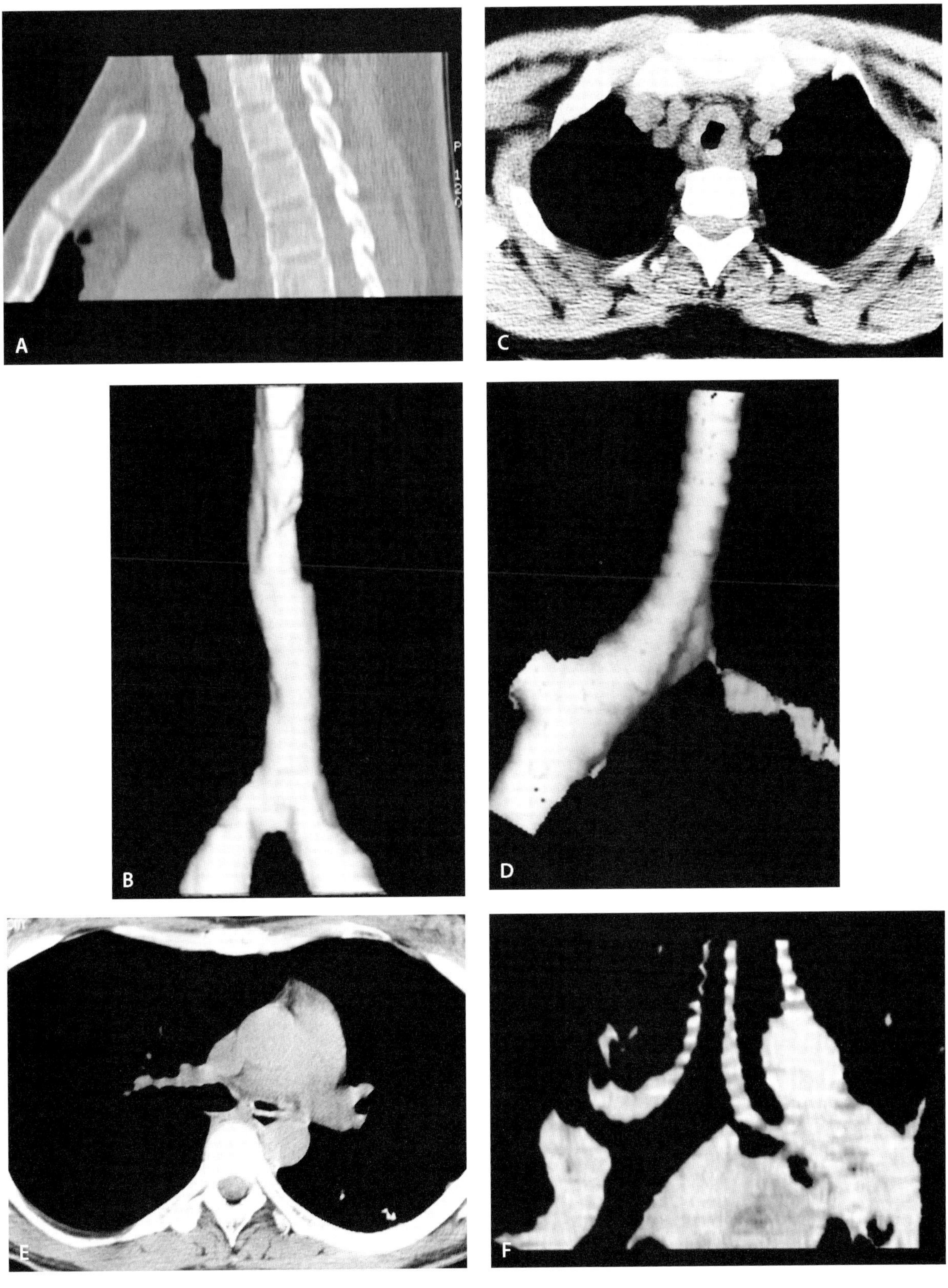
A
C
B
D
E
F

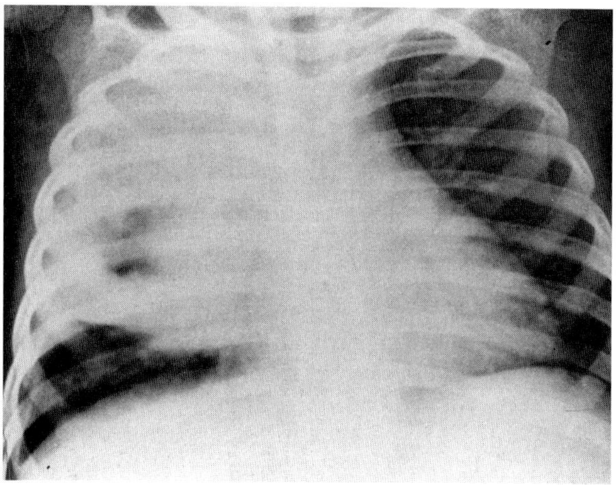

Fig. 5.3. Progressive primary tuberculosis. Right upper lobe tuberculous pneumonia has progressed, with central necrosis, and become a large tuberculous lung abscess. There is a small overlying pleural reaction. Shortly after this film was taken, the child developed an acute pneumothorax that required surgical decompression. (Courtesy of *Semin Roentgenol*, 1979)

Any of these patterns may appear on the first chest radiograph, separately or in any combination. In patients with poor immunity for any reason, the primary infection may never heal but continue on to severe cavitating, spreading pneumonia (Fig. 5.3). This is progressive primary tuberculosis (see also p. 403). The majority of primary infections, however, heal with little residual scarring; only a few will imperceptibly change to the secondary, or immune, pattern of tuberculosis with resulting fibrosis, distortion, and calcification. There is one particular end result, a "destroyed lung" or lobe. This outcome is common in the tropics; it is particularly frequent in Africa and India, but has also been seen in Asia, Australia, Hawaii, and South America. It occurs in children as well as in adults (see p. 409).

Lobar Pneumonia

The classical "primary" lobar pneumonia of nonimmune tuberculosis may affect any part of the lung, usually a whole lobe but sometimes only a segment (Fig. 5.4). It is probably a little more common in the upper lobes, but no part of the lung escapes and being influenced by the site of the lobar infection is not a safe way to exclude tuberculosis. Clinically the patient may present at any age, with a high temperature and the physical findings of lobar pneumonia. Quite contrary to this acute presentation, in other patients the lobar consolidation may be seen on a chest radiograph when there is little or no clinical ill health and the pneumonia is quite unsuspected. There is no atelectasis in the early stages, nor is there a pleural effusion associated with the lobar pneumonia (see p. 414).

There may be *M. tuberculosis* in the sputum or gastric lavage, but failure to find the bacillus does not invalidate the diagnosis. A tuberculin skin test may be negative or change to positive during the illness, usually in 2–3 weeks after the onset.

The lobar consolidation is definite but seldom dense, yet it is more opaque than the hazy and ill-defined consolidation which is usually seen in a viral infection. The distinctive feature of primary pulmonary tuberculosis is enlargement of the hilar and mediastinal lymph nodes, which is nearly constant in primary tuberculosis at any age; in adults, this lymphadenopathy can be seen on standard posteroanterior (PA), high kV, grid films of the chest. In children it may be necessary to obtain a lateral view as well as the frontal film to reliably identify the enlarged nodes: as always, full inspiratory radiographs are essential. Lymphadenopathy is a way to distinguish tuberculosis from pyogenic pneumonia, in which hilar adenopathy recognizable on standard radiographs is distinctly unusual (although it may be visible with CT). "If the nodes are enlarged and can be seen on standard radiograph in a case of lobar or segmental pneumonia, then suspect tuberculosis." This is a reliable dictum. It was the Viennese pathologist, Anton Ghon, who in 1912 first described the combination of a focal tuberculous lesion in the lung with regional lymphadenopathy. Radiologists have continued to recognize the Ghon complex as important evidence of a tuberculous infection.

Tuberculous consolidation resolves from the periphery towards the hilum, often with a well-defined edge (Fig. 5.5). When this occurs in a lung segment, such as the superior segment of the lower lobe, it may radiologically resemble a tumor, particularly if this is the appearance on the first chest radiograph (Fig. 5.6). In children this will be an unlikely diagnosis, and malignant disease of the lung (apart from metastases) is uncommon in many parts of the tropics at present.

Tuberculosis in one-third of babies may progress radiologically for as much as 3 months, even during intensive antibiotic therapy. In addition to extension of the lobar consolidation, there may also be increasing lymphadenopathy, thought to be the result of a high-sensitivity reaction during the first 2–10 weeks after infection. In most patients, the resolution of the radiographic changes of tuberculous pneumonia is slow: it often takes as long as 9 months even when adequate therapy has been given and when the clinical improvement has been dramatic (as is the case in many patients).

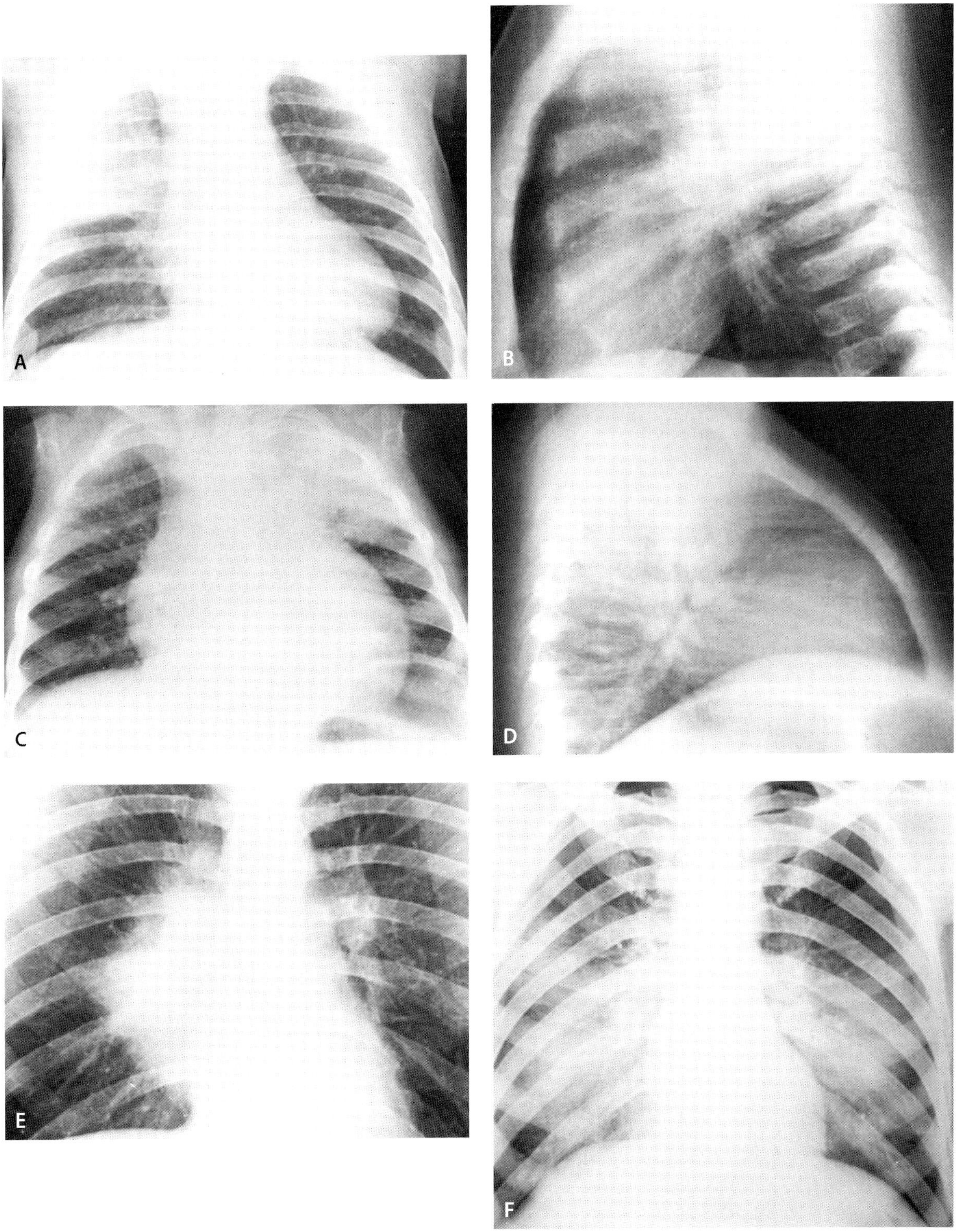

Fig. 5.4 A–F. Tuberculous primary lobar pneumonia can occur in any lobe or segment of lung. There is almost always hilar lymphadenopathy. **A, B** Primary pneumonia in the posterior segment of the right upper lobe, with right hilar lymphadenopathy. **C, D** Left upper lobe tuberculous pneumonia: the enlarged lymph nodes are only clearly seen in the lateral projection. There is also tuberculous infection in the lower thoracic spine. **E** Right lower lobar pneumonia. There is probably lymphadenopathy, partially obscured by the lung consolidation. **F** Bilateral primary pneumonia in the right middle lobe, the lingula, and the anterior segment of the right upper lobe. This child had had a mild but persistent cough and a low fever for 2 weeks. (**A, B, E, F** courtesy of *Semin Roentgenol*, 1979)

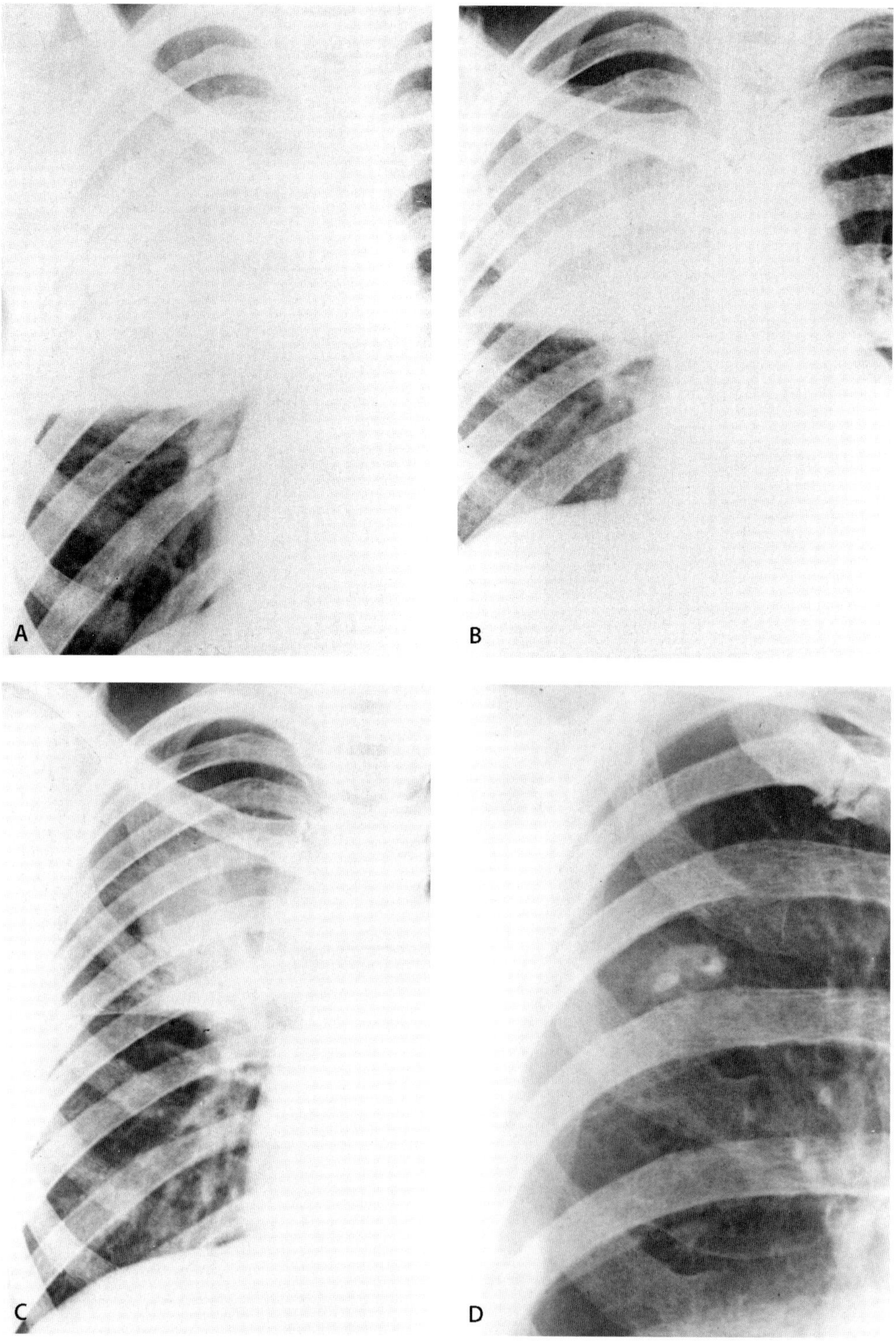

Fig. 5.5 A–D. The resolution of primary tuberculous pneumonia usually occurs from the periphery inwards towards the hilum. **A** Right upper lobe pneumonia, moderate pyrexia and cough, and a negative PPD. The patient was given penicillin, after which there was some clinical improvement but persisting pyrexia (December). **B** By January the PPD had converted and the lobar pneumonia had begun to resolve from the periphery towards the hilum. There were tubercle bacilli in the sputum and antituberculous therapy was started. **C** By March consolidation had decreased further towards the hilum. **D** One year later, after continuous treatment, there is calcification in the small residual granuloma. The patient had remained clinically fit. This pattern of healing can be seen in a patient of any age. (Courtesy of *Semin Roentgenol*, 1979)

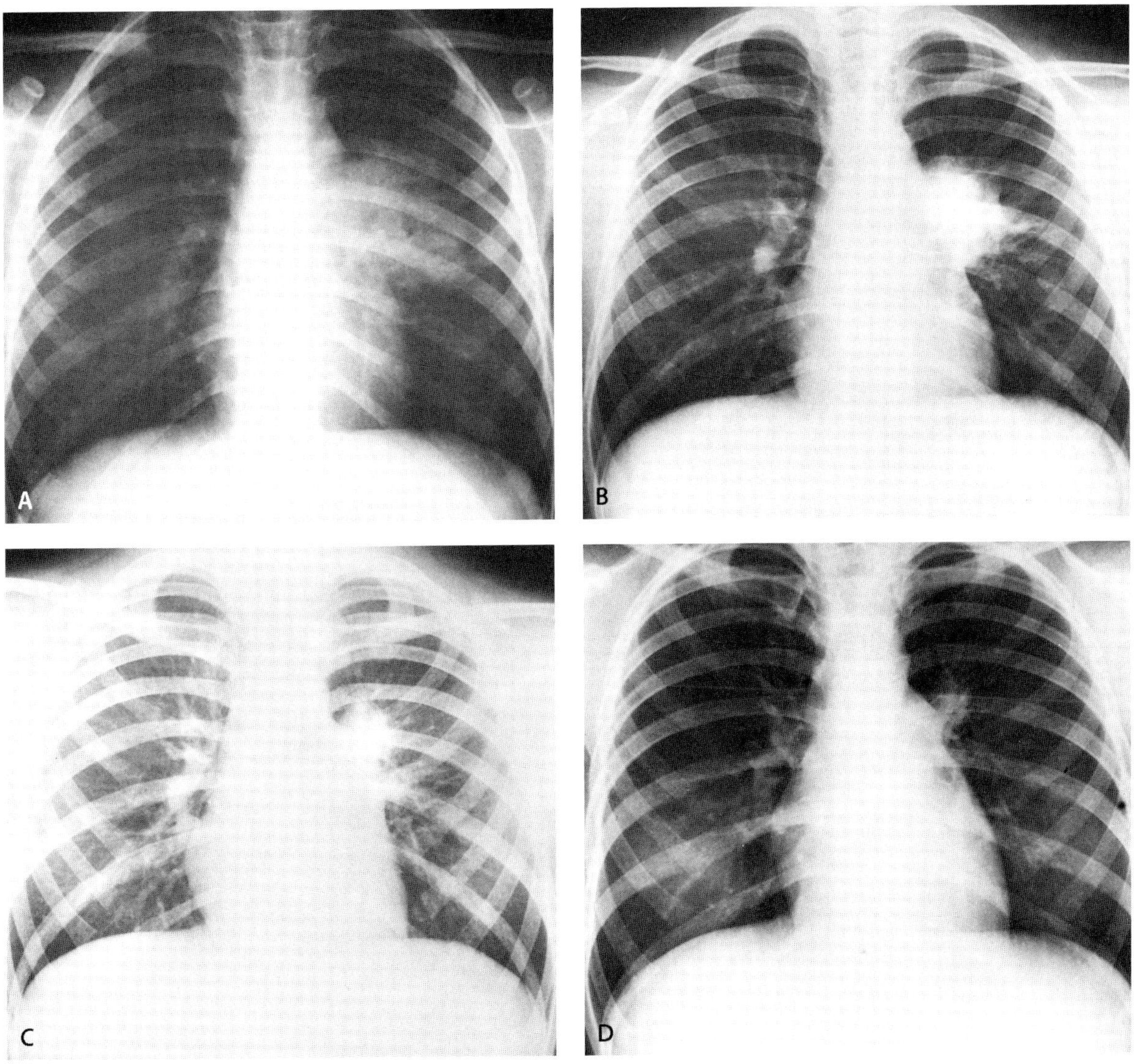

Fig. 5.6. A–D. The resolution of primary (nonimmune) tuberculosis in a young male adult. **A** July: Persistent loss of weight and cough due to a tuberculous infection in the superior segment of the left lower lobe, with perihilar lymphadenopathy. PPD was positive and there were *M. tuberculosis* in the patient's sputum. Treatment was started with three drugs. **B** Four months later consolidation is less pronounced but the lymph nodes are still enlarged and appear much more dense. **C** After a further 3 months' treatment the consolidation and nodes are again much smaller: shrinkage has continued from the periphery inwards. If the patient had been radiographed at this stage, or at the stage depicted in **B**, the "mass" could have been mistaken for a neoplasm. **D** After another 14 months of treatment there has been much improvement, but the lymph nodes are still slightly enlarged and the lung is a little more dense than normal

The considerable discrepancy between the x-ray appearance and the well-being of the patient may be useful confirmation of the diagnosis when there has been no other more positive proof of tuberculosis (see Figs. 5.5, 5.6). Any lobar pneumonia which disappears within 2 or 3 weeks, leaving a normal chest radiograph, is probably not tuberculous.

Radiologically visible calcification occurs quite early in tuberculosis, both in the peripheral focus in the lung and in the hilum. As the calcified lung focus shrinks, it may seem to be more dense; the end result is the calcified, healed primary complex (Fig. 5.7). In other patients, the peripheral granuloma will disappear altogether, leaving only residual calcification in the lymph nodes. Calcification seen radiologically is evidence that healing is occurring; unfortunately, it does not always mean that the infection has been conquered. It is possible for a partially calcified lymph node to rupture into a bronchus and cause inhalation bronchopneumonia. Because the lymph nodes, although starting to calcify, may still be large and soft, they may rupture

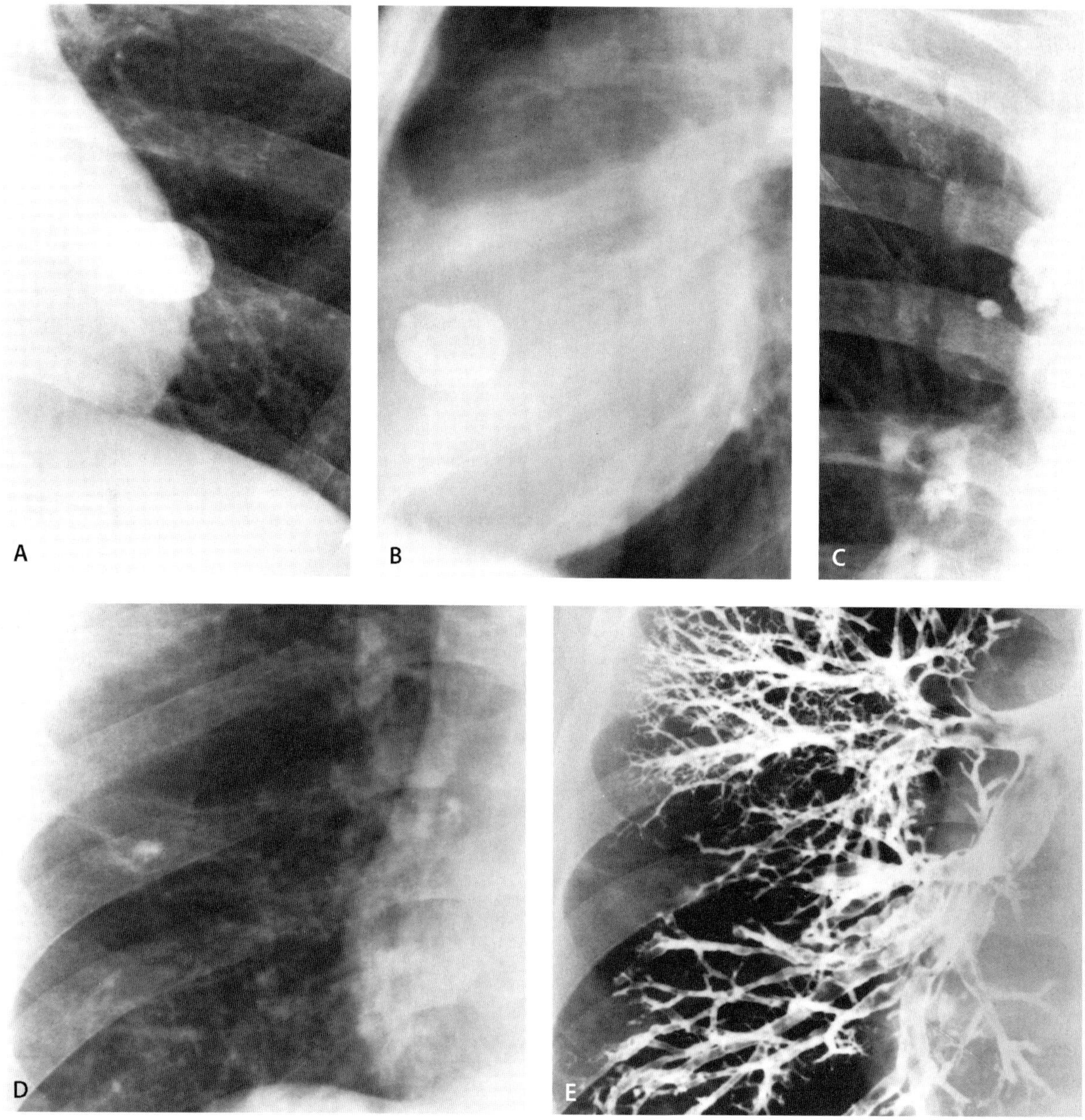

Fig. 5.7 A–E. In the majority of patients of any age, the end result of a primary tuberculous infection is a calcified granuloma: this is often a chance finding and seldom of clinical significance. **A, B** A well-defined, moderate sized calcified granuloma in the lingula of a physician, known to have been present for years. The PPD was positive and the patient was healthy. **C** Calcified hilar and right paratracheal lymph nodes. There is a very small calcified granuloma in the apical segment of the right lower lobe, seen alongside the paratracheal calcification. **D** Linear fibrosis can be seen around a small calcified peripheral granuloma. **E** Bronchography (performed for another reason) confirms the distortion of the bronchial pattern, localized emphysema, and some fibrosis, which is in a lower subsegmental branch of the right upper lobe. Such distortion is seldom of clinical significance, although occasionally it is the site of repeated infection. (Courtesy of *Semin Roentgenol*, 1979)

into a bronchus (Fig. 5-8 C–F) or cause external pressure resulting in peripheral atelectasis (see "The Destroyed Lung" p. 409).

The radiological differential diagnosis of primary lobar tuberculosis includes pyogenic or other lobar pneumonia, especially in those patients in whom the enlarged lymph nodes cannot be seen. Where there is consolidation in the lower lobe particularly, amebiasis will have to be excluded; both paragonimiasis and melioidosis can mimic tuberculosis, although usually at the later, cavitary stage of the disease.

Finally, it must be emphasized that because most tuberculous infections are airborne, a pulmonary lesion may subsequently develop wherever the tubercle bacilli happen to lodge in the lung. Thus, distribution is by chance. The majority of such contacts with bacilli leave no evidence or, at the most, microscopic foci which are not visible radiologically. Careful histopathology of many "normal" lungs has shown that most of these invisible lesions are in the lower lobes and seldom develop further. It is the minority of foci that cause the majority of radiological and clinical findings. Nevertheless, it is very important to recognize that no part of the lung is exempt from any pattern of tuberculosis and in the nonimmune patient there is usually a poor correlation between the radiological pattern and the clinical state of the patient.

Bronchopneumonia

Tuberculous bronchopneumonia presents radiologically as multiple, often bilateral, patchy, "cottonwool" densities. These occur when tubercle bacilli are forced or inhaled into multiple terminal bronchial segments during caughing, either when an open pulmonary lesion (cavity) communicates with a bronchus, or when an infected lymph node has ruptured into a bronchus (Fig. 5.8). In nontropical countries, this radiological pattern of bronchopneumonia usually suggests staphylococcal infection and the acute clinical presentation in the tropics may be very similar. The tuberculous patient, usually a young child or baby but sometimes an adult or elderly person, can be severely ill clinically. The sputum invariably contains many tubercle bacilli, but the tuberculin skin test is often negative, especially in the early stages or when the patient is HIV-positive.

Radiologically the infection is usually bilateral and widespread, but not always symmetrical. There may be multiple thin-walled cavities (lung abscesses), together with the fluffy ill-defined densities. The appearances change daily, and the thin-walled cavities may vary in size, be empty or contain fluid, expand, and develop a surrounding pulmonary reaction. This sequence depends not only on the severity of the infection and the resistance of the patient, but also on the accumulation of secretion in the cavity and how frequently and how well it is coughed out. In progressive primary tuberculous infections there will be marked bilateral adenopathy in almost every patient, the nodes being large and ill defined. (When a similar bronchogenic spread occurs during the secondary, or immune stage of tuberculosis, there is no adenopathy.) In this acute bronchopneumonic, cavitating pattern of tuberculosis, any of the peripheral tuberculous lung abscesses may rupture into the pleura or pericardium, resulting in a tuberculous empyema or pericarditis.

Histological examination at this stage shows that the lungs contain multiple thin-walled abscesses which are filled with caseous pus. This can be demonstrated by CT, particularly with high resolution and thin sections. It must be differentiated from bronchiectasis by the finding of relatively normal bronchi and the absence of atelectasis.

Calcification in this pattern of infection is uncommon, in either the lung foci or in the nodes. In some patients infection is so acute that it may cause death: if the patient recovers, the end result can be a remarkably normal chest radiograph or one showing only a little scarring.

The differential diagnosis includes staphylococcal pneumonia. Adenopathy is extremely rare in similar cavitating pyogenic infections, most of which are the result of septicemia with a visible source of infection, such as osteomyelitis or an infected skin ulcer. In both tuberculous and staphylococcal infections there can be hepatosplenomegaly.

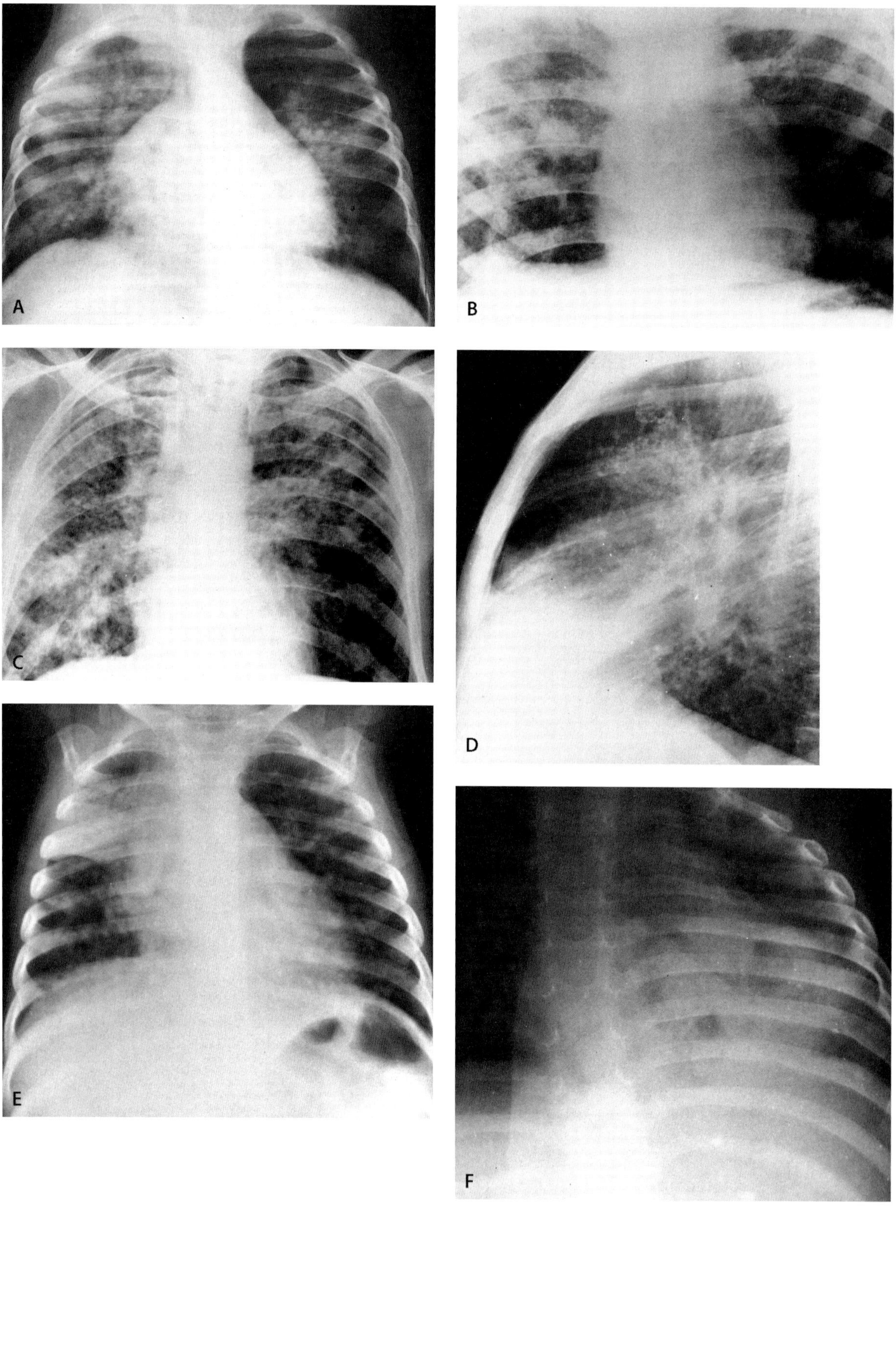
A
B
C
D
E
F

◀ **Fig. 5.8 A–F.** Complications of primary tuberculosis: the progressive primary infection. **A** An African infant from Kenya with bilateral bronchopneumonia and lymphadenopathy due to acute primary tuberculosis. **B** Bilateral "fluffy" bronchopneumonia in a young Indian adult. In the right lung some of the consolidation is cavitating. Clinically this was an acute illness resembling staphylococcal pneumonia, but the sputum contained many *M. tuberculosis*. **C, D** This adult has a 24-hour history of cough, sputum, headache, and feeling unwell. There is bilateral bronchopneumonia and hilar lymphadenopathy. The lateral view shows well-marked calcification in the paratracheal lymph nodes. There were many *M. tuberculosis* in the sputum. The response to antituberculous therapy was clinically dramatic, but much slower radiologically. Presumably this is a primary infection, unknown to the patient and healing satisfactorily as shown by the nodal calcification. One of the lymph nodes had ruptured into a bronchus and caused the acute bilateral inhalation bronchopneumonia and his acute illness. **E** This child was being treatment for primary tuberculosis and improving clinically. After 3 months treatment, she suffered an acute upper respiratory infection and became acutely ill, with a high temperature, severe cough, and obvious ill health. There is resolving right upper lobe pneumonia and enlarged right hilar and paratracheal lymph nodes complicated later (**F**) by bronchogenic spread throughout both lungs. The coarse and irregular pattern is unlike the fine and softer appearance of miliary tuberculosis. (C–E courtesy of *Semin Roentgenol*, 1979)

Hilar and Mediastinal Lymphadenopathy

The lungs may be normal but enlargement of the mediastinal lymph nodes may be the only presenting abnormality in tuberculosis, discovered on a radiograph of the chest taken because the patient is complaining of a cough, other pulmonary symptoms, tiredness, or weight loss (Fig. 5.9–5.12). Thoracic lymphadenopathy in tuberculosis occurs only in the primary (anergic nonimmune phase), and is not seen in the secondary (hyperergic immune) pattern (see p. 424).

The majority of patients with tuberculous hilar lymphadenopathy will have a positive tuberculin skin test; if it is negative it should be repeated after a short interval to exclude sarcoidosis, which is uncommon (although it does occur) in many parts of the tropics despite its frequency among Afro-Americans in the United States.

At any stage of the infection the nodes may enlarge sufficiently to rupture into a bronchus, causing an acute inhalation tuberculous bronchopneumonia. This may lead to severe clinical symptoms or, alternatively, may produce little clinical response. It should be suspected radiologically when fresh segments of patchy, consolidation appear unexpectedly during any primary tuberculous infection (see Fig. 5.8).

Enlarged mediastinal nodes can also rupture into the pericardium, causing acute tamponade or an acute tuberculous pericarditis. In some patients this causes sudden deterioration, but in others the clinical course is surprisingly benign (see p. 414).

Hilar and mediastinal lymphadenopathy may resolve completely, but this may take many months. There may be residual calcification, although the incidence of calcified nodes is variable in different parts of the tropics, possibly related to the state of nutrition. Statistically, in the tropics hilar calcification is more common in children than in adults, for which there are two possible explanations. Either calcification has occurred and subsequently been absorbed, or the background immunity and the state of nutrition of children and young adults is improving compared with their elder generation. AIDS may reverse this statistic, as it has many others.

The differential diagnosis of enlarged mediastinal and hilar lymph nodes is largely dependent on the local pattern of disease; in the tropics, tuberculosis usually will be the most likely etiology, especially when the more peripheral peribronchial and perihilar nodes are enlarged. Sarcoidosis occurs in the tropics, but not commonly and with considerable variation geographically; in sarcoidosis there is usually enlargement of the mediastinal and paratracheal nodes in particular, as well as bilateral symmetrical hilar node enlargement. Lymphoma, especially in children, may present with enlarged nodes in the chest and elsewhere, and is indistinguishable from tuberculosis. Similarly, Kaposi sarcoma in children in the tropics may present as an acute lymphadenopathy with very few of the characteristic pigmented skin nodules. (There is often lacrimal involvement.) But tuberculosis is also a common cause of peripheral lymphadenopathy in the tropics: for example, the majority of enlarged cervical nodes in Uganda in patients under the age of 50 years are tuberculous (see p. 524). In adults, malignant disease is often the initial diagnosis when mediastinal nodes are enlarged, but it must be remembered that even old people may have "primary" tuberculosis. When the patient is HIV-positive, intrathoracic lymphadenopathy is as likely to be tuberculous as malignant; for example, in West Africa over 80% of patients with combined TB and AIDS have mediastinal lymphadenopathy. At any age, biopsy and histopathology may be necessary to establish the correct diagnosis.

(Text continues on p. 409)

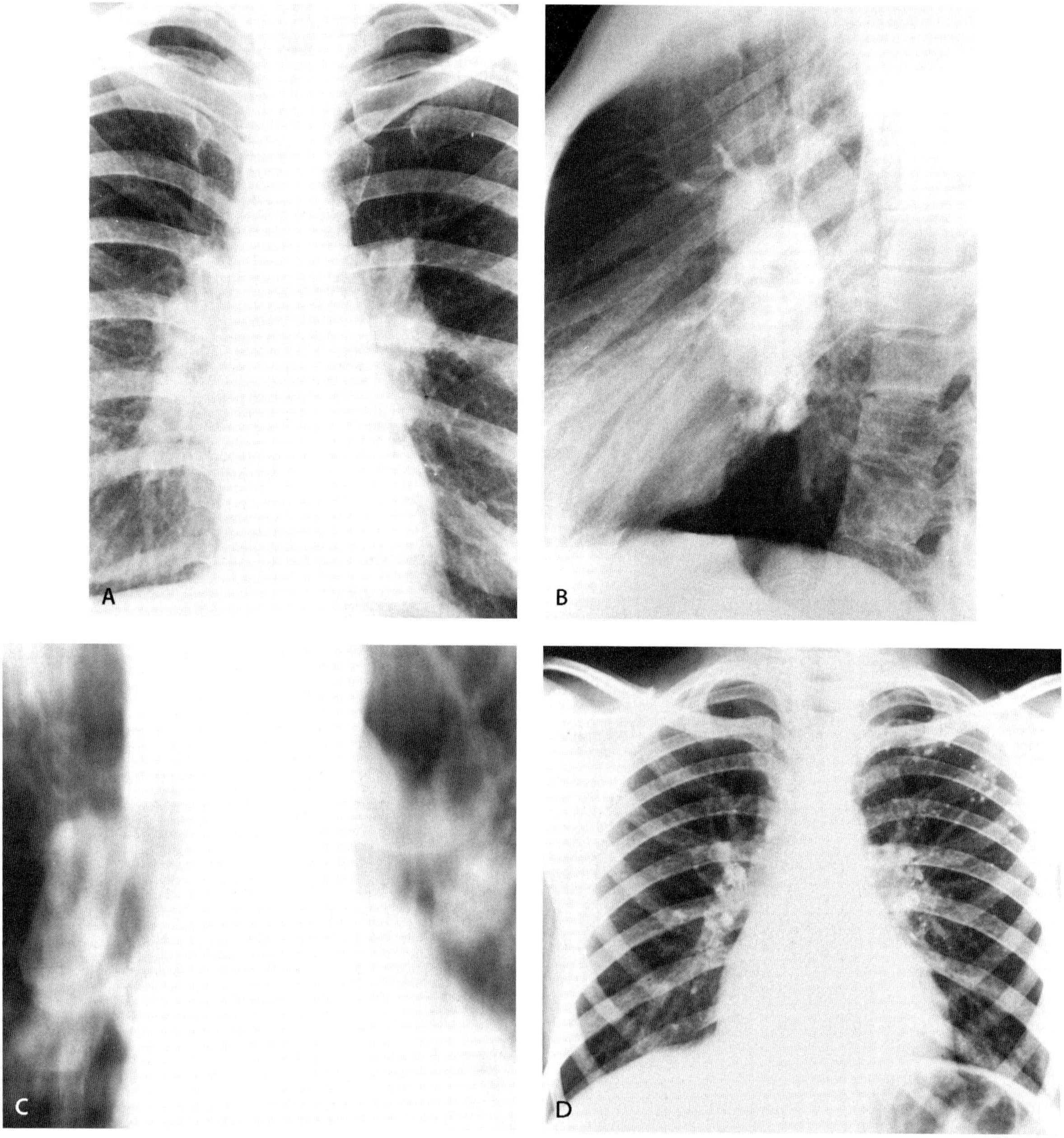

Fig. 5.9 A–D. Tuberculous lymphadenopathy. This is only found in the primary (anergic, nonimmune) phase. The pattern and density of the lymph nodes is very variable. **A** PA and **B** lateral radiographs of the a 32-year-old woman who had been "unwell" for some weeks, without specific complaints or cough. Her PPD was positive and she had a mild evening pyrexia. There is marked bilateral peribronchial and perihilar lymphadenopathy. **C** Standard tomography of a different patient shows large lymph nodes around the main branch of the major bronchi on both sides. **D** Multiple calcified granulomas in both hilar and right paratracheal lymph nodes. There is a calcified complex in the left upper lobe. (**D** courtesy of *Semin Roentgenol*, 1979)

Fig. 5.10 A–F. Tuberculous lymph nodes may enlarge and cause pressure on different parts of the bronchial tree. **A** Marked enlargement of the peritracheal nodes: no lung focus is visible. Only biopsy or therapeutic trial could differentiate between tuberculosis and lymphoma. **B** Standard tomography shows compression of the right main and the right upper lobe bronchi. There is also compression of the intermediate and right middle lobe bronchi, but a little less marked than that of the upper lobe. There is a large thick-walled cavity beyond the almost blocked upper lobe bronchus: the tuberculin test was positive, but the sputum did not contain *M. tuberculosis*. The adenopathy was tuberculous but the cavity was pyogenic, the result of the blocked upper lobe bronchus. **C, D** Partial atelectasis accompanying infection of the right middle lobe, with markedly enlarged hilar and mediastinal lymph nodes. **E, F** Enlarged mediastinal lymph nodes (best seen in **F**) which have caused obstructive emphysema, with over-expansion of the left lung and displacement of the mediastinum to the right. This was a young patient from the Pacific Isles. (**E, F** courtesy of Dr. Cheryl Sisler, Hawaii)

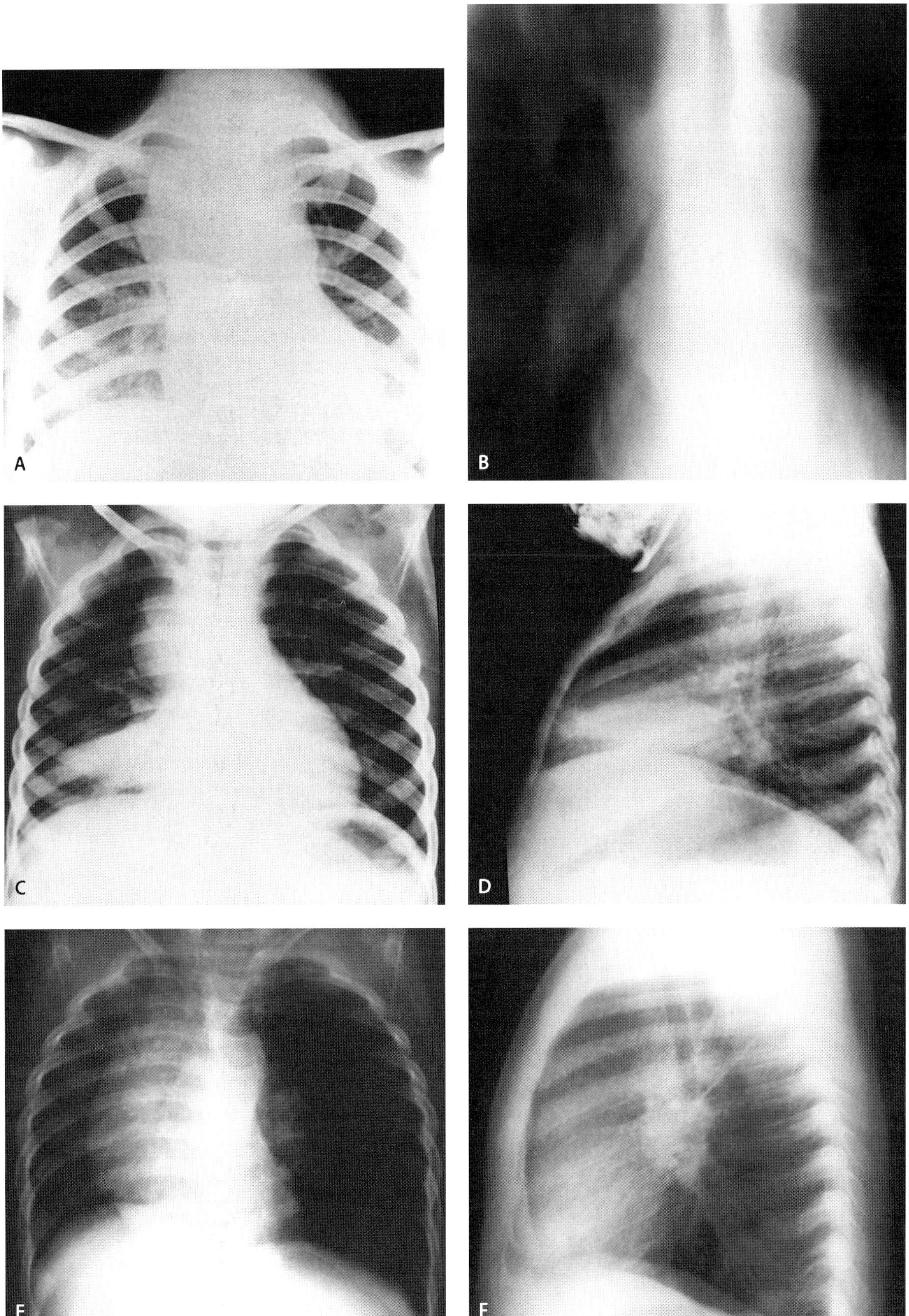
A
B
C
D
E
F

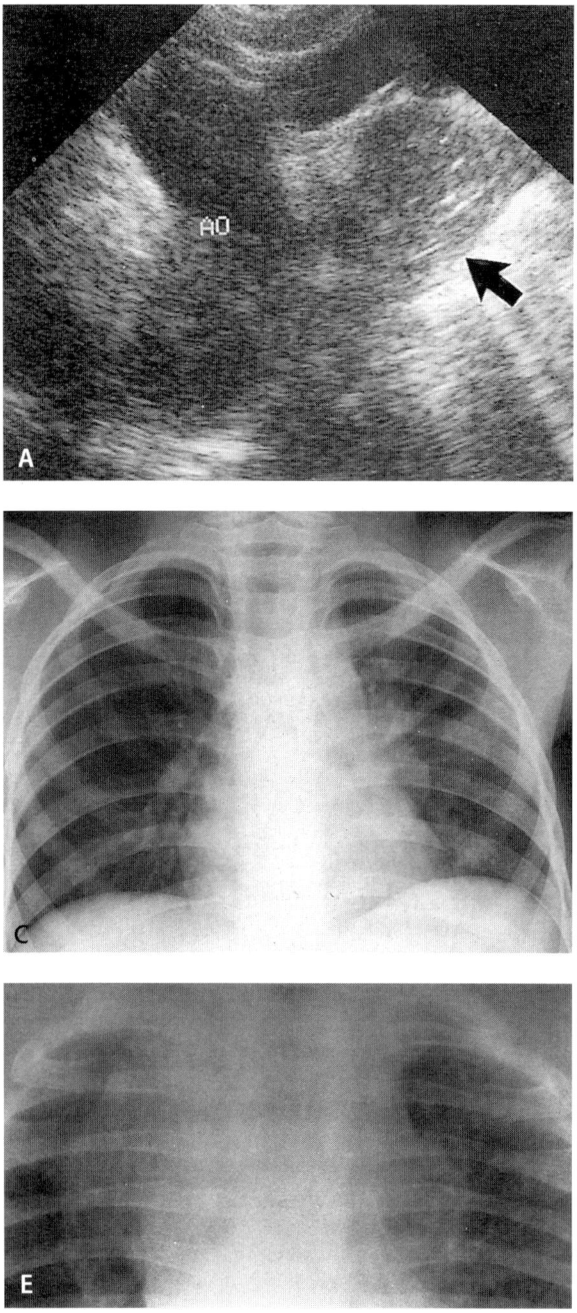

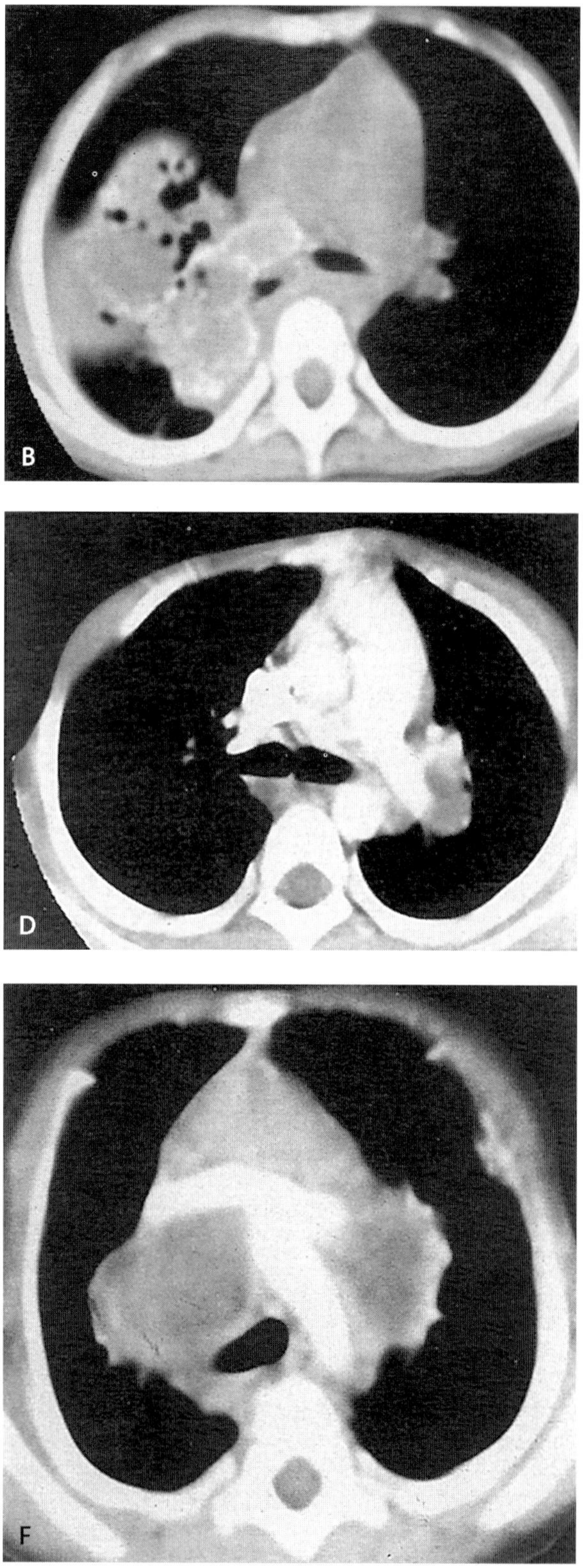

Fig. 5.11. **A** A left parasternal ultrasound scan shows a large lymph node adjacent to the aortic arch (*arrow*) below the left subclavian artery. **B** A CT scan shows calcification in the right lung parenchyma and mediastinal lymph nodes due to tuberculosis. **C, D** A frontal chest radiograph shows left hilar adenopathy; rim enhancement is seen on the contrast CT scan. **E, F** This child's chest radiograph shows a widened superior mediastinum which might be mistaken for the thymus; the contrast-enhanced CT scan shows large tuberculous lymph nodes, with rim enhancement. (From Cremin and Jamieson 1995)

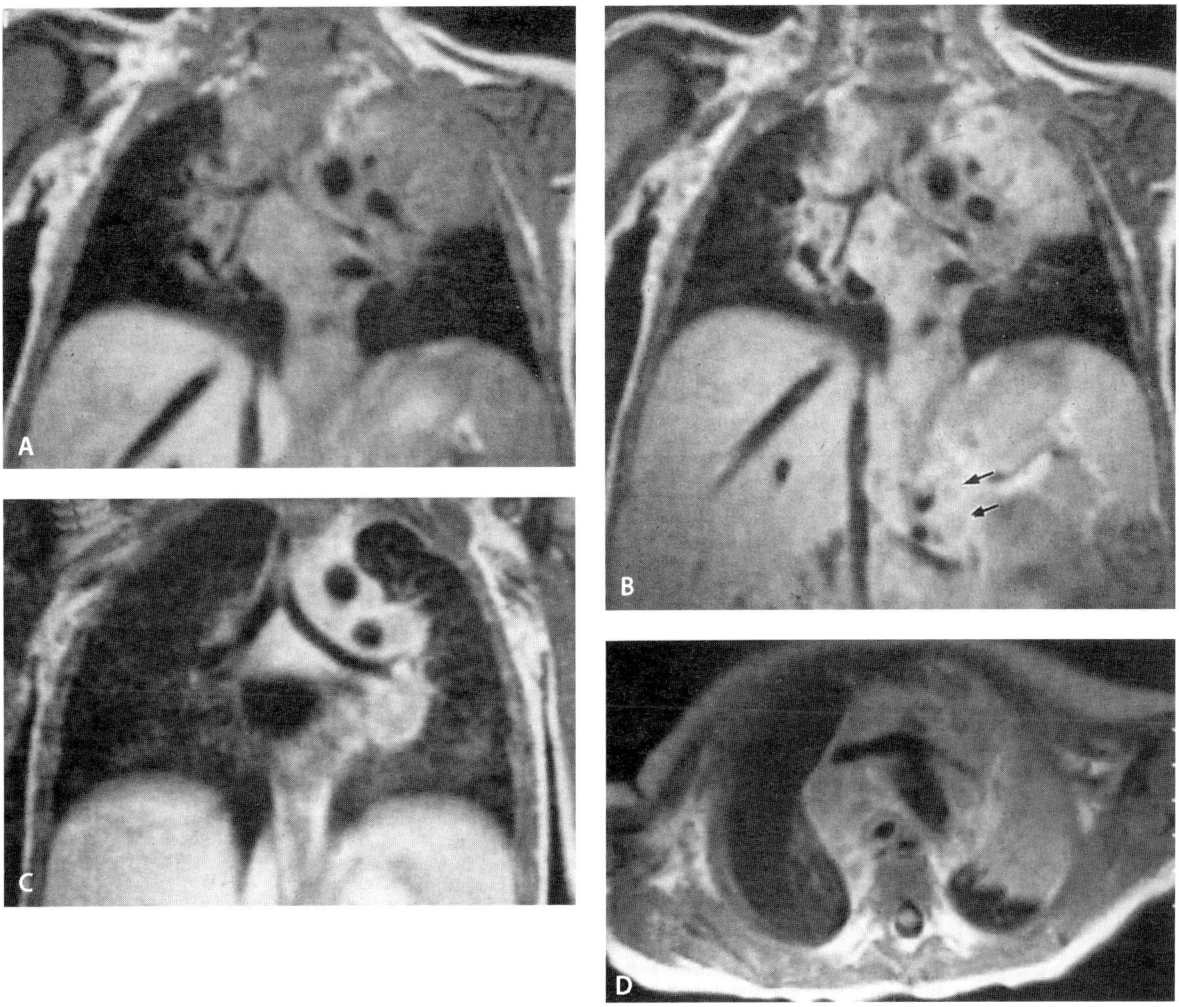

Fig. 5.12 A–D. MRI can also demonstrate both the pulmonary and nodal changes of tuberculosis. **A** The coronal T1-weighted and **B** coronal i.v. gadolinium-enhanced T1-weighted scans showing consolidation in the left upper lobe, which is enhanced, and nodal masses in the right superior mediastinum, right hilum, and below the carina, with rim-enhancement. There are also contrast-enhanced para-aortic nodes (*arrows*). **C** A coronal i.v. gadolinium-enhanced T1-weighted scan showing rim-enhancing nodal masses in the left hilum. **D** An axial T1-weighted scan showing superior mediastinal adenopathy and consolidation in the left upper lobe. (From Cremin and Jamieson 1995)

The Destroyed Lung

The "destroyed lung" describes the very characteristic radiographic appearance of a common end result of primary tuberculosis, or less often, of a nontuberculous mycobacterial infection, e.g., *M. avium-intracellulare* (Fig. 5.13).

The pathophysiology of the destroyed lung is easy to understand (Fig. 5.14). There are lymph nodes at the division of each major and segmental bronchus which are enlarged by a primary tuberculous infection. With such a close anatomical relationship, any swelling results in pressure on the bronchus, causing narrowing often to the extend of blockage. This may resolve as the nodes subside or the bronchial wall may be so involved and damaged that the cartilage is destroyed. If there is pressure or fibrosis sufficient to cause blockage of the bronchus, there may be collapse of the segment or even the lobe of the lung peripherally.

Enlarged tuberculous lymph nodes are the usual cause of the destroyed lobe or lung, which is a very common finding in Africa or India, but is also seen wherever tuberculosis is common (e.g., in the Australian aborigines). Statistically the left upper lobe is more frequently affected; in one extensive survey of admission chest x-rays in a large African hospital, left upper lobar pneumonia in young adults was more likely to be tuberculous. The right upper lobe is a little less often involved, and none of the other lobes escape. (The "right middle lobe syndrome" described in England results from similar lymph

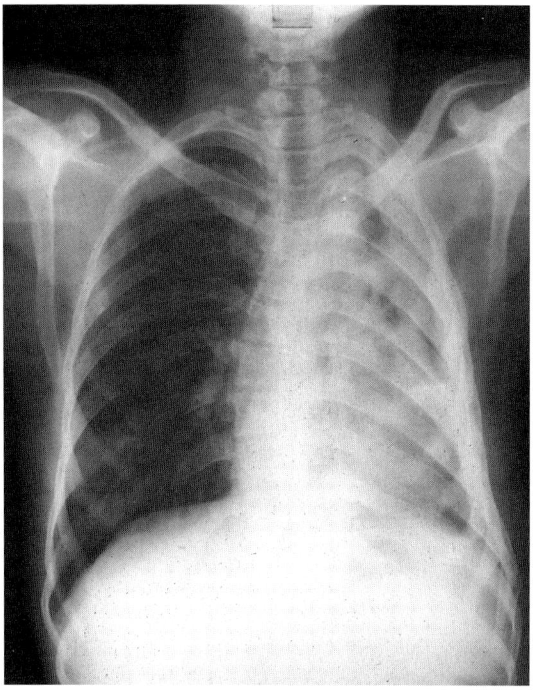

◀ **Fig. 5.13.** The characteristic radiograph of a "destroyed lung" in a patient from Malawi. There is flattening of the left chest wall, with displacement of the mediastinum to the left. There are cavities in the fibrotic left lung. Some pleural thickening is present on the left. The right lung is over-expanded, but otherwise normal. (The nodular shadow on the right lower lung field is the nipple.)

Fig. 5.14 A–F. The development of a "destroyed lung." **A** Primary left upper lobe tuberculous pneumonia. **B** Standard tomography shows the enlarged mediastinal and perihilar lymph nodes, compressing not only the apical posterior bronchus but also the other bronchi to the left lung. **C** Because of the compression and resulting obstruction, the left lung is shrinking and the mediastinum is moving to the left. The left chest wall is being flattened and there is some pleural reaction. **D** A bronchogram about a year later shows widespread bronchiectasis with overlying pleural thickening. There are adhesions along the diaphragm and widening of the lower half of the trachea. The right lung is over-expanded but is otherwise normal. **E** A similar destroyed lung, but on the right side. The mediastinum is shifted to the right and the right chest ist contracted. **F** The bronchogram shows the underlying shrunken right lung, with bronchiectasis, and the overlying pleural thickening ▶

node fibrosis.) The outcome of the fibrosis and bronchial constriction is often secondary pyogenic infection of the atelectatic segments. Bronchiectasis then develops, often being both tuberculous and pyogenic in origin (Fig. 5.15). Because of the underlying lung collapse and fibrosis, the chest wall flattens, particularly over upper lobe disease, and the mediastinum is pulled by the fibrotic lung towards the same side. The lung damage is slowly progressive, with recurrent infection and further fibrosis. There may be cavity formation, and as the disease heals it is very difficult to decide clinically or radiologically whether a fresh cavity is the result of recurrent tuberculous infection or secondary infection or whether there are fibrotic bullae only. Although no longer commonly performed where CT scanning is available, bronchography in these patients is dramatic and demonstrates the extent and pattern of lung damage. When the underlying sequence of lymphadenopathy, atelectasis, infection, bronchiectasis, fibrosis, contraction, and scarring is understood, it is so characteristic that it is possible to look at the plain chest radiograph and describe the bronchogram (or CT scan; Fig. 5.16) without actually performing it (which is much appreciated by the patient).

During the process of healing, local pleural effusions frequently occur over the destroyed area of lung, especially over the apex. Such fluid is usually trapped by adhesion over the upper lobe, so that the costophrenic angles frequently remain clear. Fluid does not have any prognostic significance but may resemble a mass: CT or ultrasonography may help to distinguish between pleural fluid (mobile) and pleural thickening.

Subsequently, the major clinical problem in patients who have a "destroyed lung" is recurrent infection. This may be tuberculous or pyogenic, or even both, and can be contaminated by a fungus or other saprophyte. Examination of the sputum is very misleading; it almost always contains a multiplicity of organisms and it is difficult to identify tuberculous bacilli. Management of these patients presents a problem; some control of the pyognic infection may be obtained by antibiotics, but such treatment is not always successful, the outcome depending on the extent of the fibrosis and on the drainage from the affected area. Surgery is sometimes attempted but can be extremely difficult because the pleura is thickened and adherent, and the underlying lung fibrotic and friable. The end result may be a disastrous tuberculous empyema. Localized thoracoplasty has helped to enhance the drainage in some patients, but masterly inactivity is another option.

In summary, a destroyed lung is easy to recognize and describe radiologically but there are no satisfactory criteria to distinguish the etiology of subsequent infections. Clinical recognition is equally straightforward, but treatment remains a recurring problem in some patients.

(Text continues on p. 414)

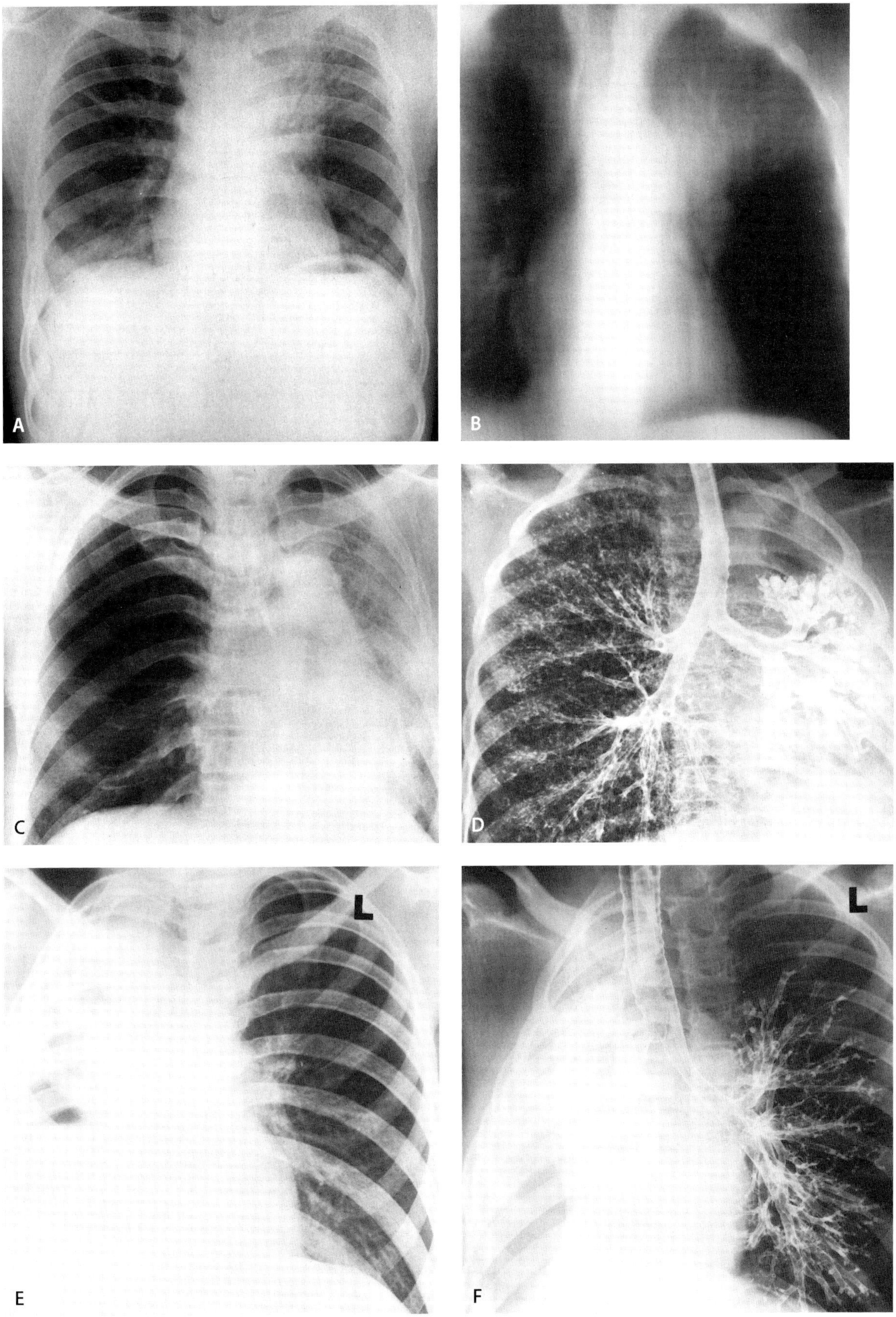
A
B
C
D
E
L
F
L

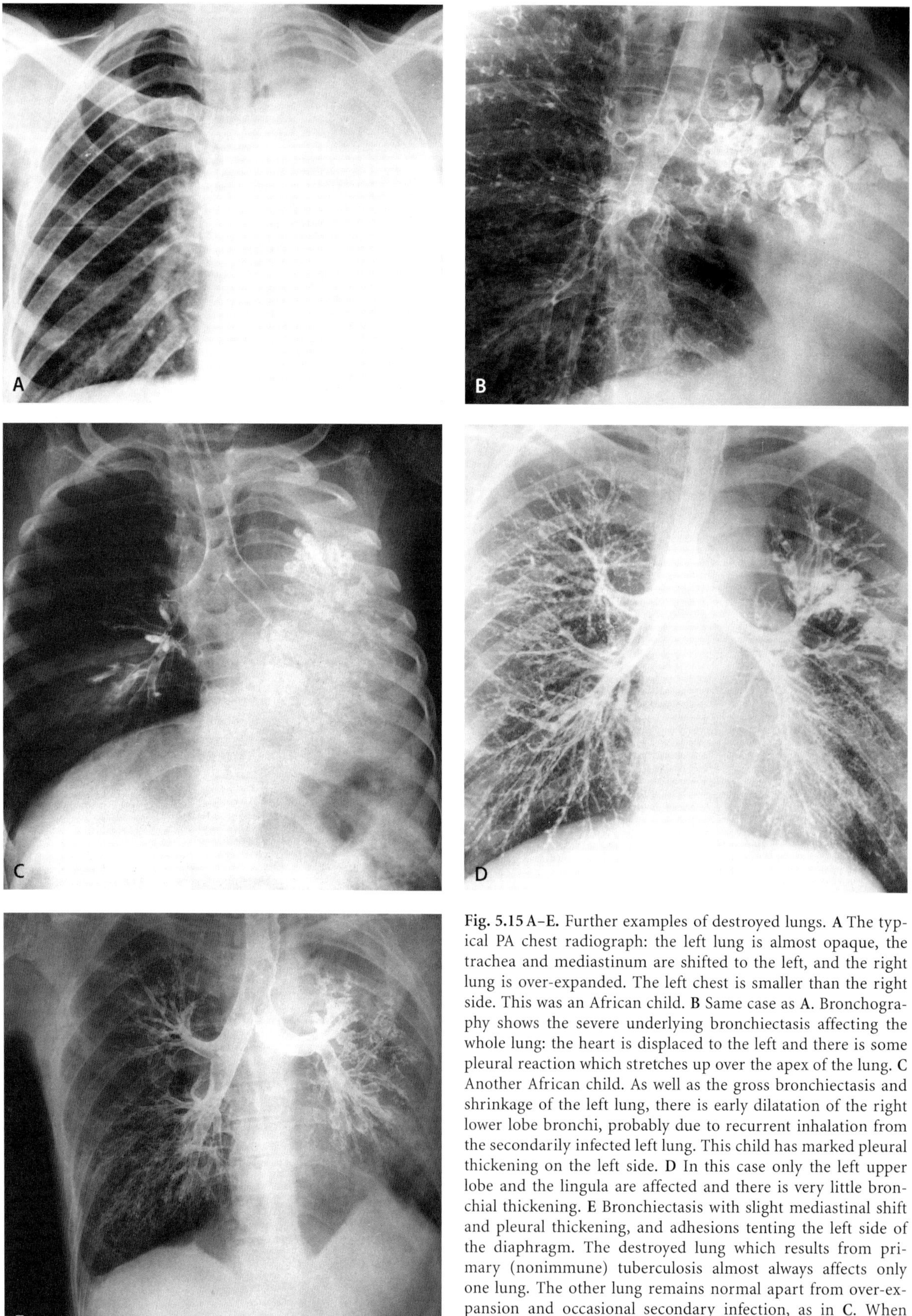

Fig. 5.15 A–E. Further examples of destroyed lungs. **A** The typical PA chest radiograph: the left lung is almost opaque, the trachea and mediastinum are shifted to the left, and the right lung is over-expanded. The left chest is smaller than the right side. This was an African child. **B** Same case as **A**. Bronchography shows the severe underlying bronchiectasis affecting the whole lung: the heart is displaced to the left and there is some pleural reaction which stretches up over the apex of the lung. **C** Another African child. As well as the gross bronchiectasis and shrinkage of the left lung, there is early dilatation of the right lower lobe bronchi, probably due to recurrent inhalation from the secondarily infected left lung. This child has marked pleural thickening on the left side. **D** In this case only the left upper lobe and the lingula are affected and there is very little bronchial thickening. **E** Bronchiectasis with slight mediastinal shift and pleural thickening, and adhesions tenting the left side of the diaphragm. The destroyed lung which results from primary (nonimmune) tuberculosis almost always affects only one lung. The other lung remains normal apart from over-expansion and occasional secondary infection, as in **C**. When bronchiectasis follows secondary (immune) tuberculosis, it is nearly always bilateral

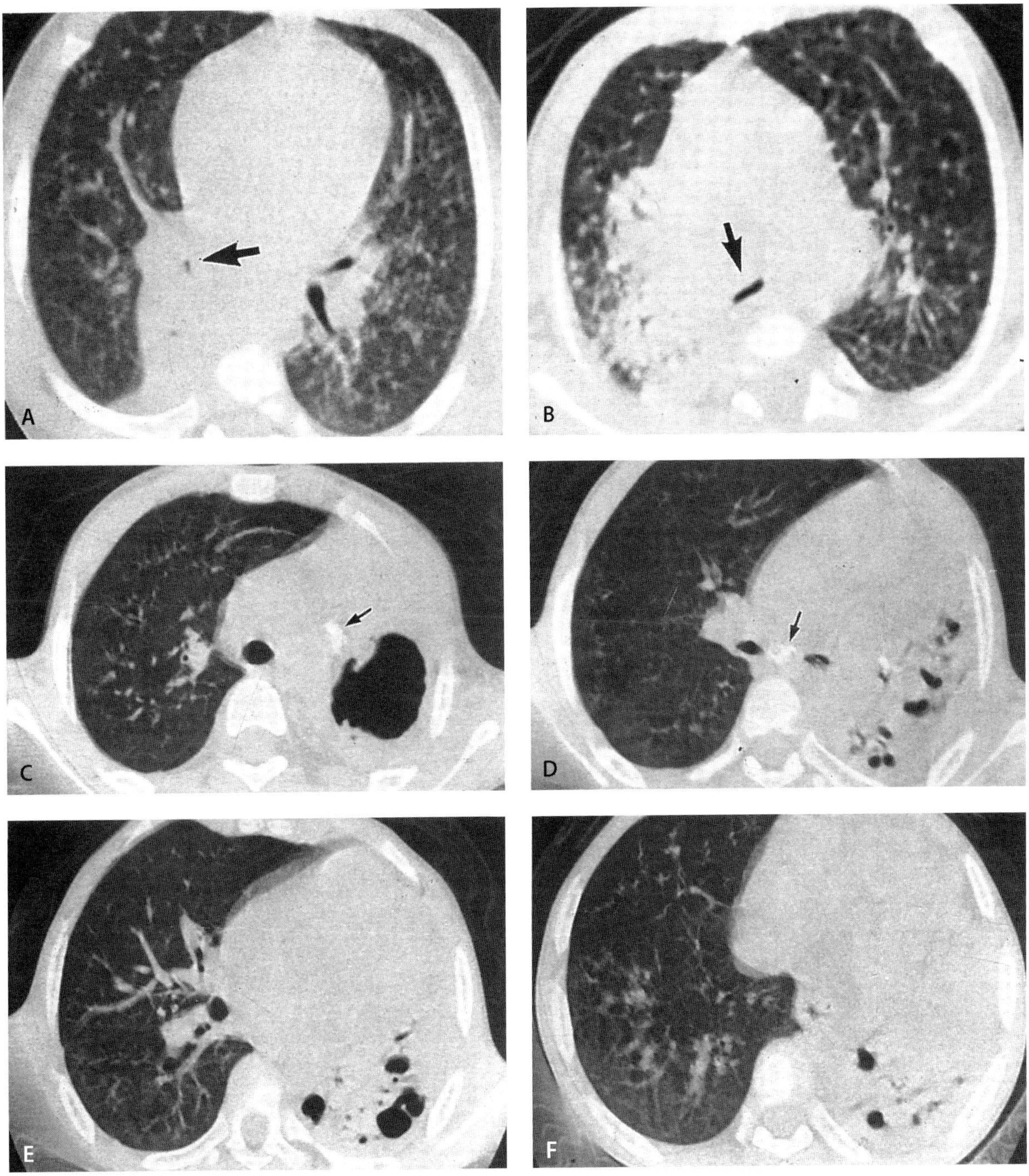

Fig. 5.16 A–F. CT of the destroyed lung. **A** Marked compression of the right lower lobe bronchus (*arrow*) by enlarged nodes. There is segmental consolidation and compensatory emphysema in the remainder of the right lung. **B** Severe compression of the trachea (*arrow*) due to mediastinal lymphadenopathy: there is right upper lobe consolidation. **C–F** Scans at different levels in the same patient showing destruction of the left lung, with volume loss, cavitation, and consolidation. There is early calcification in some of the left hilar and subcarinal nodes (**C, D** *arrows*). There is no gross pathology in the right lung. The patient eventually had a left pneumonectomy. (From Cremin and Jamieson 1995)

Pleural and Pericardial Effusions

Tuberculous pleural effusions at any age are usually a manifestation of primary, anergic (nonimmune) tuberculosis. The fluid may be serous, proteinaceous, bloody, or occasionally purulent (Fig. 5.17). Pleural biopsy and DNA fingerprinting are reliable methods of establishing the diagnosis. Mediastinal lymphadenopathy often can be demonstrated by CT or tomography, even when there is no radiologically visible pulmonary parenchymal lesion. The majority of tuberculous effusions will be unilateral, but bilateral effusions are not uncommon in tuberculosis in the tropics. (Whenever there is a bilateral effusion, a tuberculous infection of the thoracic spine should also be excluded.) Ultrasonography is an excellent way to localize fluid (Fig. 5.18) and exclude a subphrenic cause, such as an hepatic amebic abscess or ascites.

Tuberculous effusions may loculate anywhere, including over the upper zones of the lung or in the pleural fissures. The radiological appearance may then suggest local consolidation or a tumor, and decubitus radiographs and lordotic views may be necessary for differentiation. Ultrasonography will demonstrate the septate adhesions and pleural thickening.

Removal of a large amount of pleural fluid in a malnourished patient may cause sudden clinical deterioration. Aspiration should be controlled and guided by ultrasonography, so that only sufficient fluid is removed to permit a functioning lung volume; if the fluid is purulent, total and continuous drainage will be required. If this is not adequate, pleural thickening and lung encasement will follow. Most tuberculous pleural effusions respond well to appropriate drug therapy.

Pleural calcification may be the sequel to a tuberculous pleuritis (Fig. 5.19). The calcification may have a feathery or lacy pattern, or be linear around an encysted effusion. Calcification is not evidence of cure, and decalcification may occur, particularly if the infection becomes active again. Calcification in the diaphragm is almost always due to asbestosis, and not to tuberculosis. It must be distinguished from calcification of the diaphragmatic pleura; but this also is uncommon following tuberculosis and is much more likely to be due to asbestosis. Of course, asbestosis and tuberculosis may coexist, and in some parts of the world frequently do.

Tuberculous pericarditis (Fig. 5.20) may be a primary anergic tuberculous infection or may follow rupture of adjacent mediastinal lymph nodes into the pericardium. The posterior aspect of the pericardium is in close apposition to the mediastinal lymph nodes beneath the carina. Rupture of these nodes may cause an acute clinical crisis, with tamponade, or may be a subclinical event. Subsequent healing can be complete, leading to an apparently normal pericardium, or may result in severe thickening and calcification. Because both layers of the pericardium are involved, adhesions are frequent and may be extensive; the epicardium may be involved. When there is restrictive (constrictive) pericarditis there may be a need for surgical decompression; this procedure can be hazardous because the cardiac muscle and small epicardial coronary arteries can be damaged. Careful ultrasonography may delineate the extent of the fibrosis before surgery.

Constrictive pericarditis may exist without any radiologically visible calcification, and may be better recognized with CT, magnetic resonance imaging (MRI), or ultrasonography (Fig. 5.21). When the constriction is severe, it may present as cor pulmonale with a radiographically normal heart size. In many patients extensive pericardial calcification has little physiological effect on the heart, while in others, minimal calcification seen on a plain radiograph may be the only sign of extensive pericardial fibrosis.

A solitary pericardial tuberculoma has been reported, forming a small mass along the left heart border. It is not easy by any method to distinguish a pericardial tumor from pericardial thickening.

Cardiac tuberculosis see Chap. 25.

Fig. 5.17 A–F. Tuberculous primary (nonimmune) pleural effusion. **A** A young African man with a right-sided pleural effusion and right hilar adenopathy. With antituberculous treatment, the fluid resolved more rapidly than the lymph nodes, which eventually calcified. **B** A teenage girl with a left-sided pleural effusion which extends up into the interlobar fissure. There is probably left hilar adenopathy, partially obscured by the fluid. **C** Localized pleural effusion on the right side which has been present for years. No pleural effusion is "safe". This type of effusion may become reactivated quite unexpectedly. **D** An encapsulated effusion along the right chest wall. The central density over the right chest is due to pleural thickening and fluid lying posteriorly. There was no change over many years and the patient remained quite healthy. **E** Bilateral pleural effusions in a young African girl. The lateral views clearly showed mediastinal lymphadenopathy; tuberculosis was confirmed by pleural biopsy. **F** A large pleural effusion almost filling the left side of the chest and partially collapsing the underlying lung. Although this resembles a destroyed lung, the mediastinum is shifted away from the density and the left side of the chest has not collapsed significantly. The main left bronchi can be seen clearly and are not obstructed. (**A, B, D** courtesy of *Semin Roentgenol*, 1979) ▶

(Text continues on p. 420)

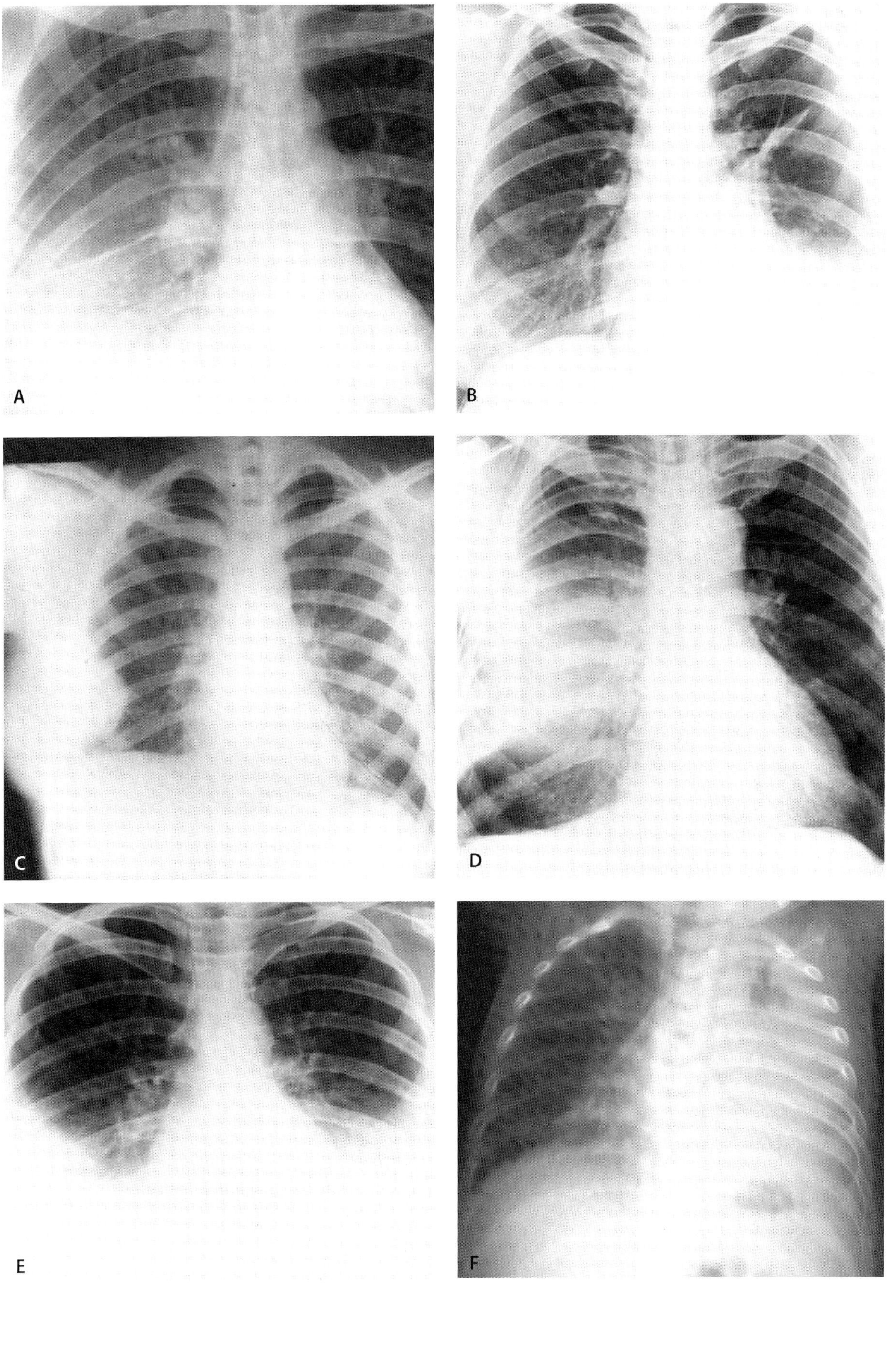
A
B
C
D
E
F

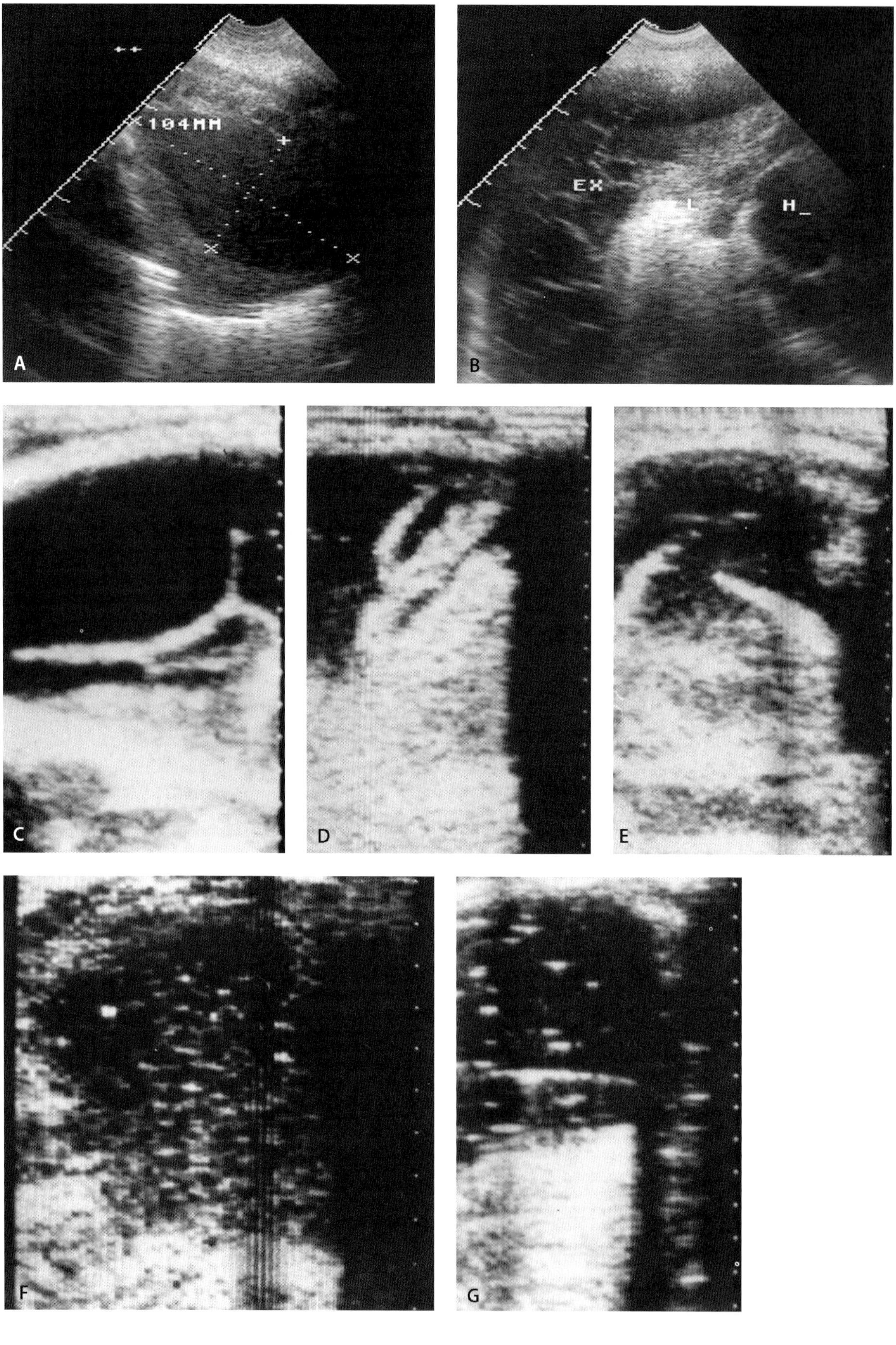
104MM
EX
L
H
A
B
C
D
E
F
G

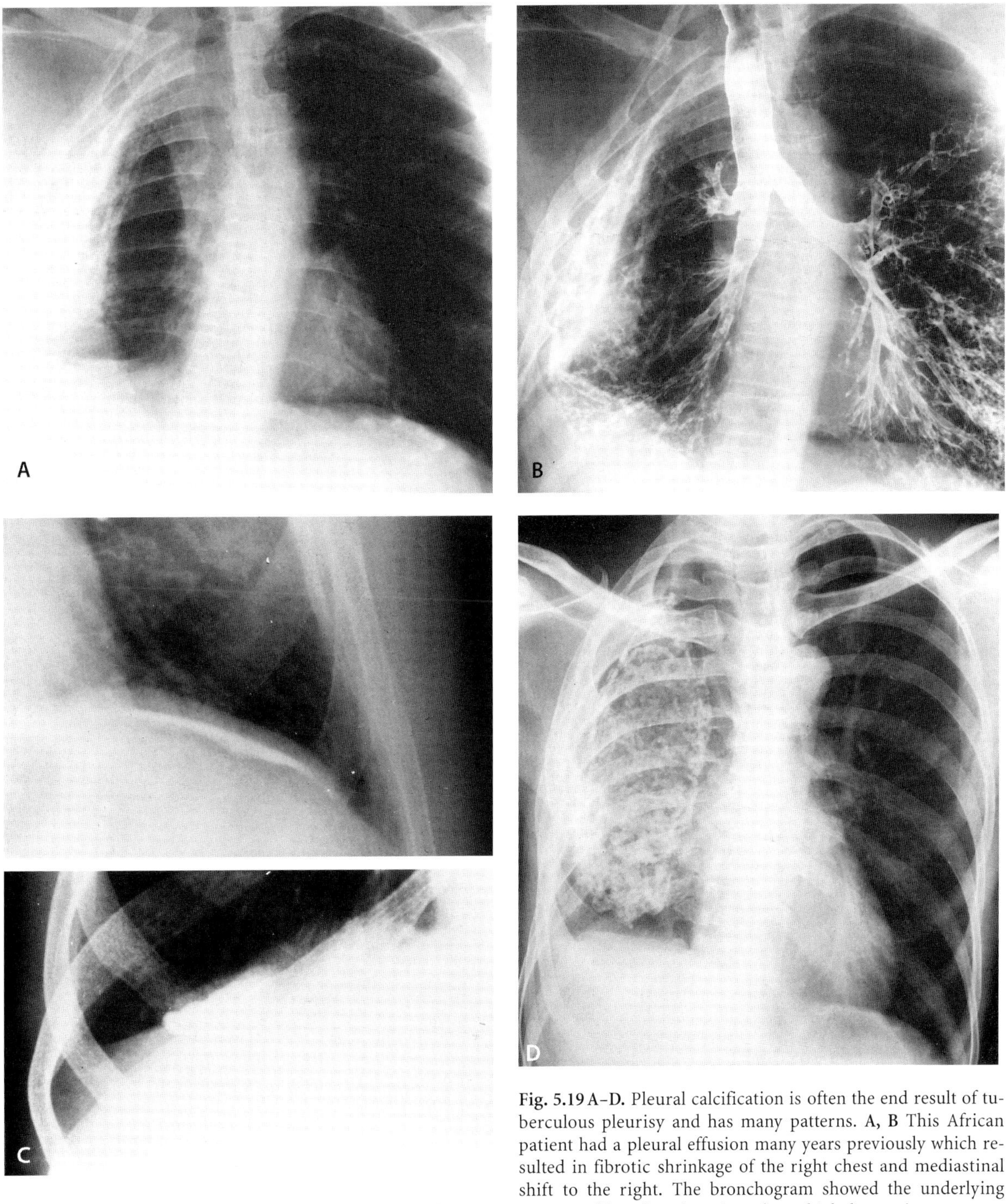

Fig. 5.18 A–G. Ultrasonography in tuberculous pleural effusions. A Fluid in the left chest; this could be tuberculous or pyogenic. Aspiration and biopsy would be necessary to discover the etiology. B A multiseptate right-sided pleural exudate due to tuberculosis. A and B are patients from Zimbabwe. (Courtesy of Dr. Sam Mindel) C–E Three different patients with septate tuberculous pleural effusions: the serous bands are adherent to both the visceral and parietal pleura. F, G Many tuberculous pleural effusions will have multiple internal linear echoes, which move freely when the patients changes position. This is a characteristic of tuberculosis. These patients are from Uganda. [Courtesy of Dr. L. Belli, Turin, and *Radiol Med* (*Torino*), 1992]

Fig. 5.19 A–D. Pleural calcification is often the end result of tuberculous pleurisy and has many patterns. A, B This African patient had a pleural effusion many years previously which resulted in fibrotic shrinkage of the right chest and mediastinal shift to the right. The bronchogram showed the underlying contracted lung but there is no bronchial obstruction or saccular bronchiectasis as is found in a destroyed lung. The pleural fibrosis has caused the right side of the chest to contract. The left lung is emphysematous but otherwise normal. C Typical diaphragmatic calcification due to asbestosis, seen in a patient who has never had tuberculosis. This can be bilateral or unilateral, and is seldom symmetrical. Both costo-phrenic angles are clear; had the calcification been the result of a tuberculous effusion there would have been pleural thickening. D This Indian had a right pleural effusion which healed, leaving pleural thickening laterally and calcification posteriorly. Although the right chest is a little contracted, there is no mediastinal shift

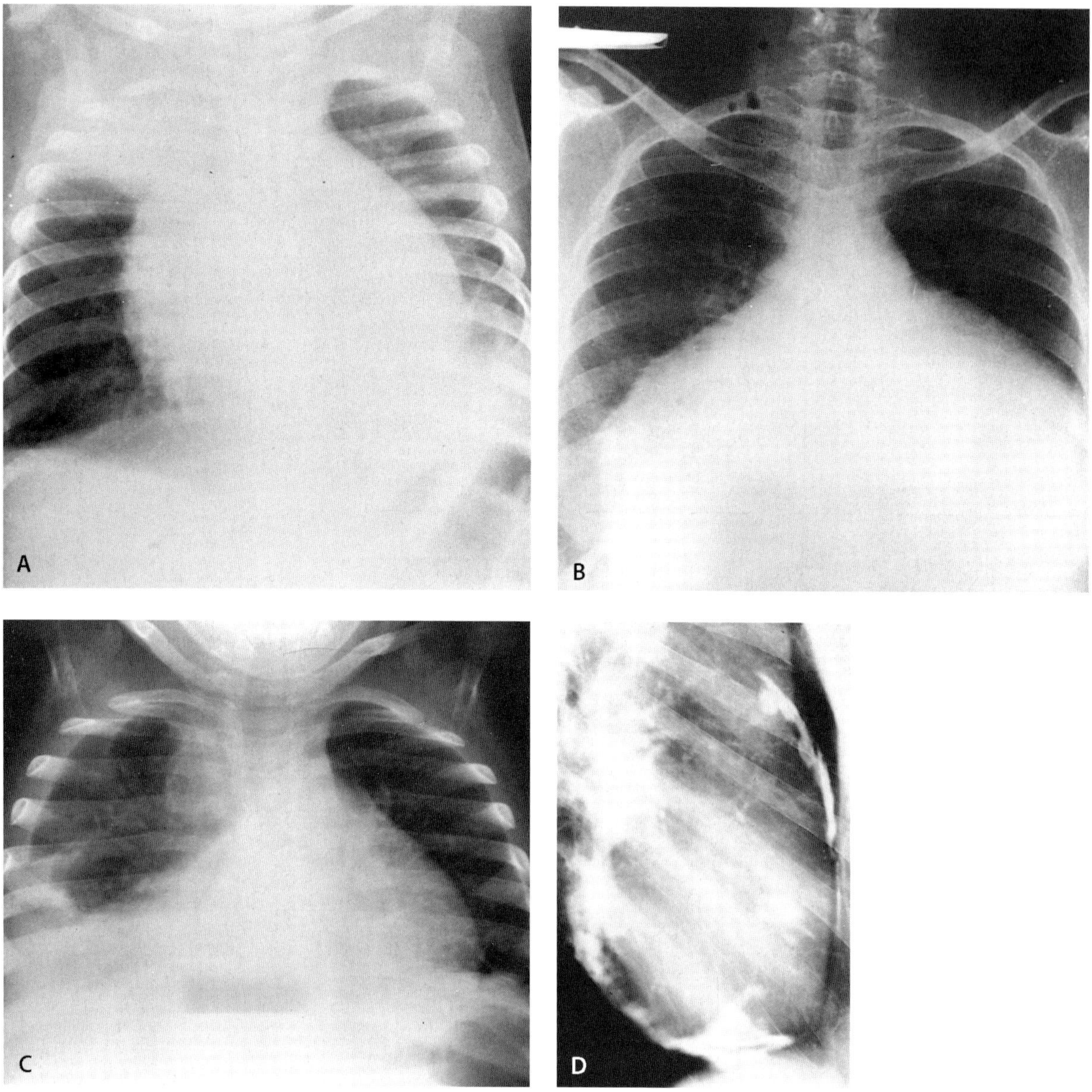

Fig. 5.20 A–D. Tuberculous pericarditis may be a primary tuberculous infection of follow rupture of an adjacent lymph node. **A** This African child had a right upper lobe primary tuberculous pneumonia and marked lymphadenopathy; she then developed a pericardial effusion and a left pleural effusion. **B** A huge cardiac outline which results from a large pericardial effusion. There is no evidence of cardiac failure or pleural fluid at this stage. **C** An African child from Zimbabwe with a large right pleural effusion and right lower lobe pneumonia. The right paramediastinal shadow is caused partly by pleural fluid and partly by enlarged lymph nodes. Other enlarged lymph nodes can be seen through the heart shadow around the left hilum. She had a pericardial effusion which needed to be removed, but which did not contain *M. tuberculosis*. However, the bacilli were present in her sputa. **D** Extensive calcification of the pericardium seen in a lateral view of the heart. The amount of pericardial calcification does not indicate the degree of pericardial constriction. This patient did not suffer from constrictive pericarditis. (**A**, **C** courtesy of *Semin Roentgenol*, 1979)

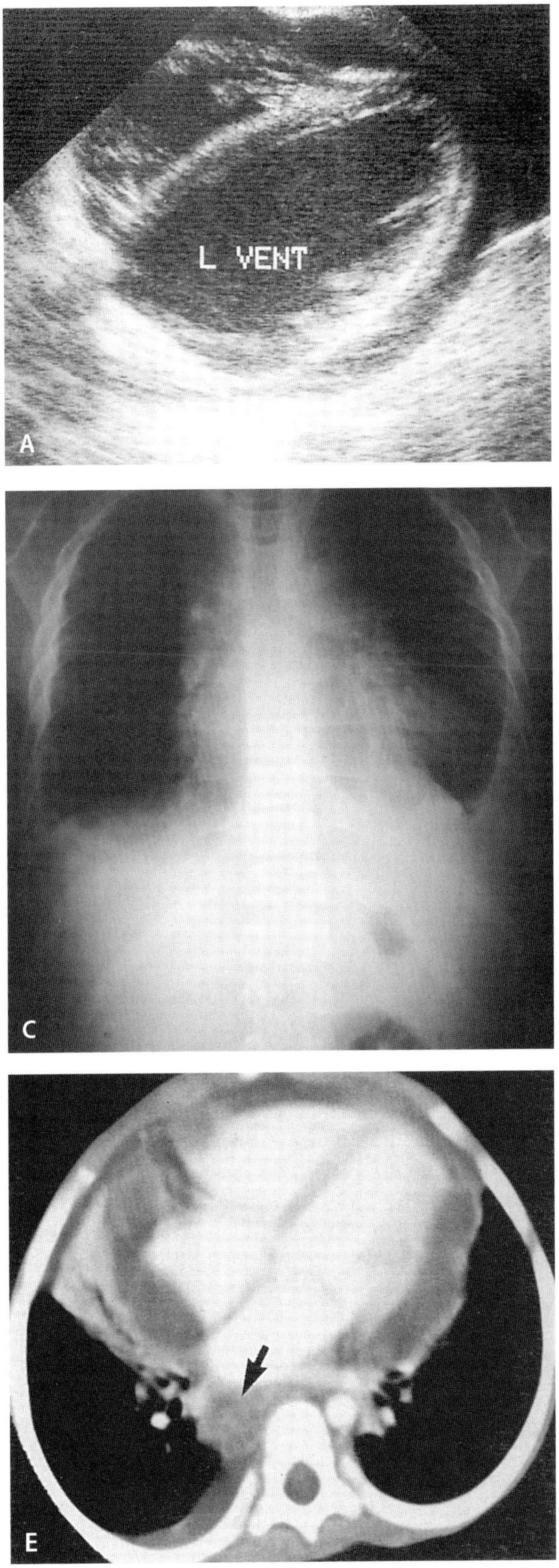

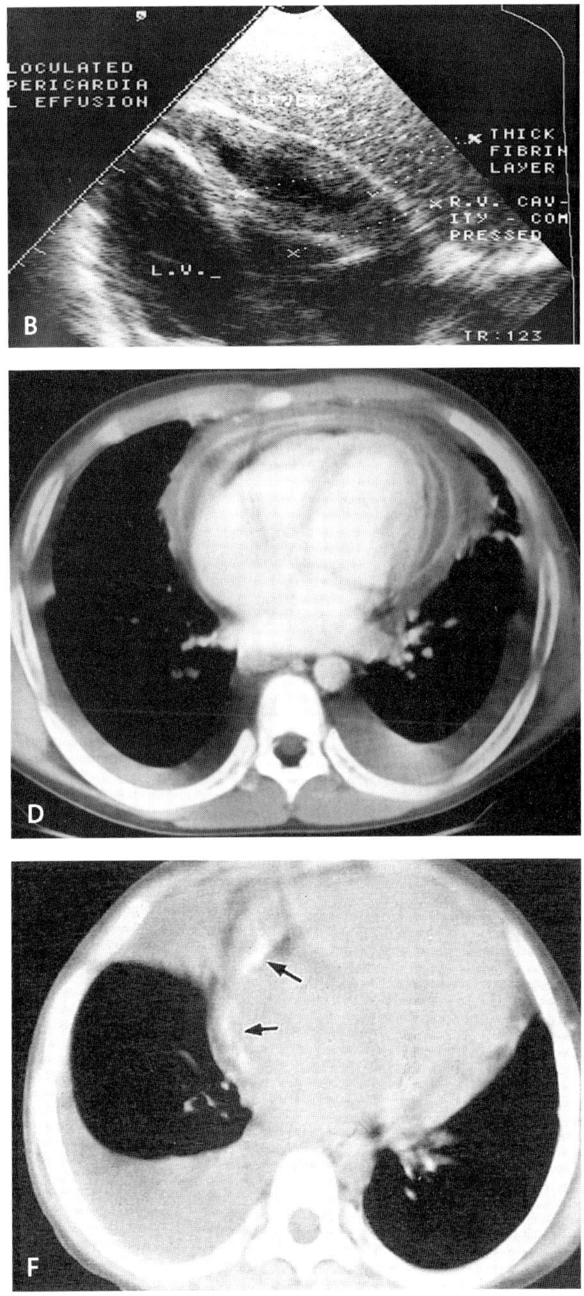

Fig. 5.21. **A** Ultrasonography is an excellent way to identify pericardial fluid, as in this child from southern Africa. **B** A loculated pericardial effusion with fibrous septa and marked thickening of the pericardium. There is some compression of the right ventricle (R.V.). This was an African from Zimbabwe with known tuberculosis. **C** A 13-year-old Polynesian boy with a pericardial effusion and bilateral pleural effusions. There is mediastinal lymphadenopathy. **D** The CT scan of the same patient, confirming the pericardial fluid, bilateral pleural effusions, and moderate lymphadenopathy. **E** A large tuberculous pericardial effusion in a child from South Africa, shown by contrast-enhanced CT: there is a large tuberculous lymph node (*arrow*) and consolidation in the right middle lobe. **F** Pericardial calcification seen on a CT scan (*arrows*). There is a right pleural effusion and right middle lobe consolidation. **G–I** see p. 420

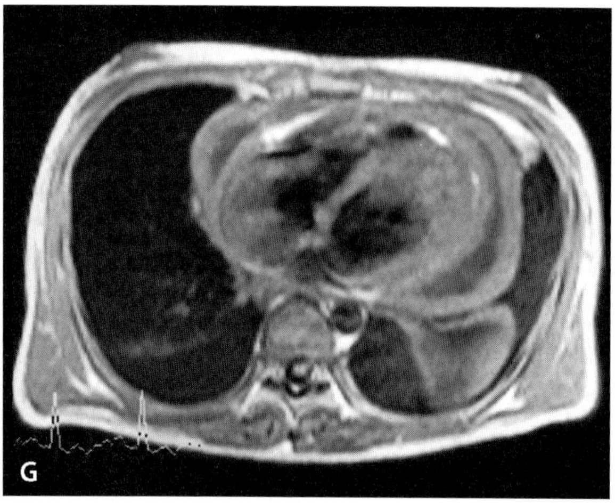

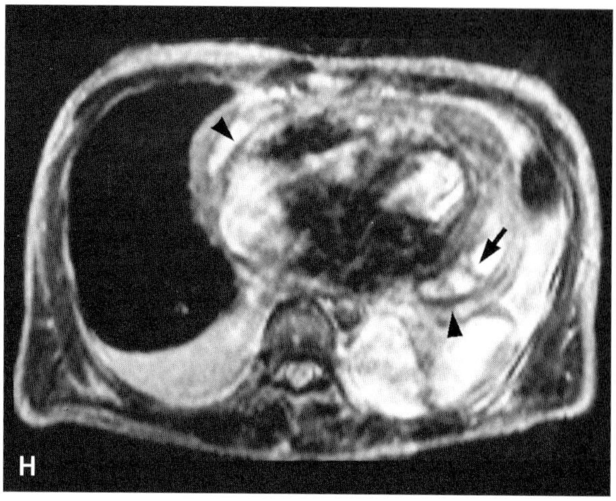

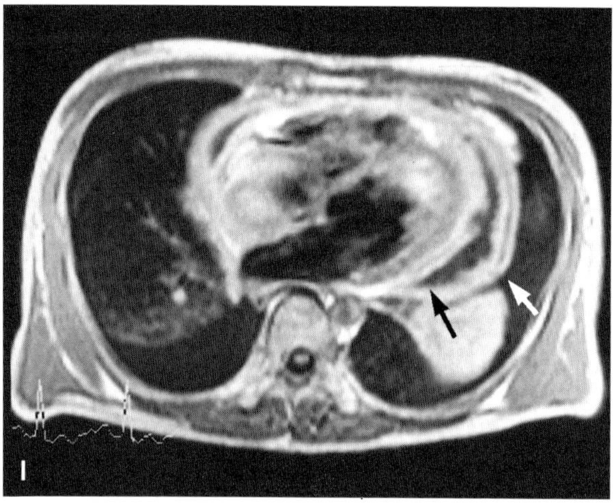

Fig. 5.21 (*continued*). **G–I.** MRI of tuberculous pericarditis shows marked percardial thickening. **G** T1-weighted image showing the pericardium with the same signal intensity as the myocardium. **H** T2-weighted image demonstrating low signal intensity on the inner surface of the thickened pericardium (*arrowhead*). The pericardial effusion also shows a low signal (*arrow*). – The lower scan is gadolinium enhanced, showing enhancement of thickened parietal and visceral pericardium (*arrow*). (**A, E, F** from Cremin and Jamieson 1995; **B** by courtesy of Dr. Sam Mindel; **C, D** courtesy of Dr. Cheryl Sister, Hawaii; **G–I** courtesy of H. Hayashi and *Br J Radiol*, 1998)

Miliary Tuberculosis

Miliary tuberculosis is an acute disseminated infection, the result of hematogenous spread; the primary focus may not be recognizable and may be extrapulmonary (Fig. 5.22). In other patients, miliary spread occurs during active pulmonary tuberculosis when there is rupture of a caseating lymph node or a cavity into a blood vessel. Even with good treatment there is a mortality of 13%–50%. Only about 30% of patients with miliary tuberculosis will have the bacillus in their sputum; up to 60% may have negative skin tests. Miliary tuberculosis is always evidence of a life-threatening infection. While it is usually easy to recognize the miliary pattern on a chest radiograph of a patient of any age, there is no correlation between the number or size of miliary nodules and the clinical health of the patient. Often those who are very ill show fewer nodules. The patient's general health and state of nutrition are very important factors.

Clinical correlation is essential to differentiate miliary tuberculosis from other causes of miliary nodulation, many of which may be found during the investigation of any debilitating illness. The initial chest radiograph may be normal, and reexamination of the chest should be requested "if symptoms persist," because miliary tuberculosis may only become apparent radiologically up to 10 days or more after the clinical illness has started; it may be recognized earlier, however, with high-resolution CT. There is also considerable variation in the "miliary" pattern radiologically, again with little correlation with the patient's clinical status. In some patients, at first there is only interlobular septal thickening, which can be very difficult to recongize, particularly on the chest x-ray of a small child: high-resolution CT is more reliable. The traditional miliary (millet seed) nodules are tiny, discrete, and all about the same size, less than 2 mm. These nodules may coalesce into patchy and more irregular opacities, and high-resolution CT will show even more variation (Fig. 5.23). The distribution of the nodules is not symmetrical and there are differences in size and density, which may represent different episodes. High-resolution CT may also show cavitation which

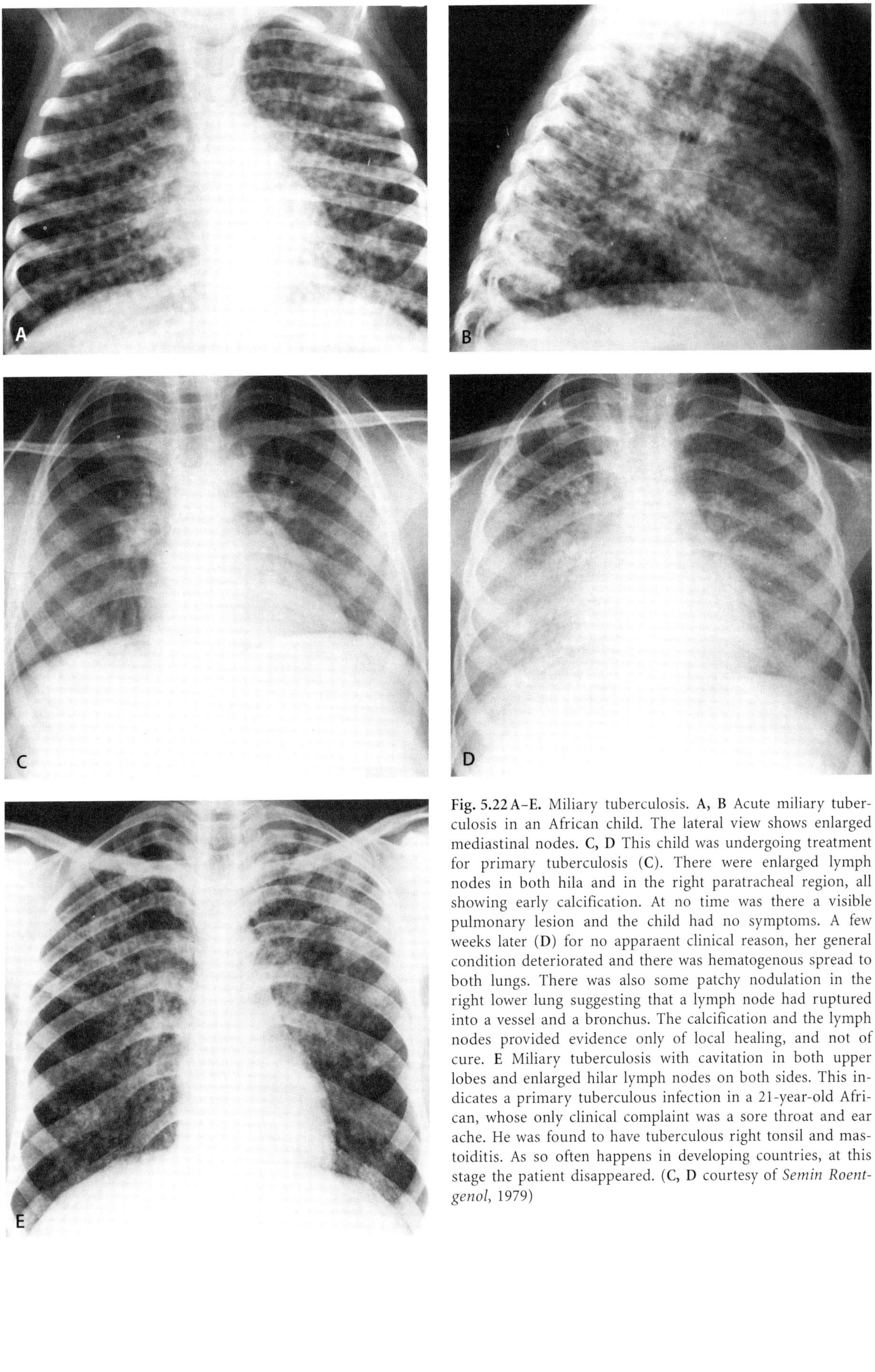

Fig. 5.22 A–E. Miliary tuberculosis. A, B Acute miliary tuberculosis in an African child. The lateral view shows enlarged mediastinal nodes. C, D This child was undergoing treatment for primary tuberculosis (C). There were enlarged lymph nodes in both hila and in the right paratracheal region, all showing early calcification. At no time was there a visible pulmonary lesion and the child had no symptoms. A few weeks later (D) for no apparaent clinical reason, her general condition deteriorated and there was hematogenous spread to both lungs. There was also some patchy nodulation in the right lower lung suggesting that a lymph node had ruptured into a vessel and a bronchus. The calcification and the lymph nodes provided evidence only of local healing, and not of cure. E Miliary tuberculosis with cavitation in both upper lobes and enlarged hilar lymph nodes on both sides. This indicates a primary tuberculous infection in a 21-year-old African, whose only clinical complaint was a sore throat and ear ache. He was found to have tuberculous right tonsil and mastoiditis. As so often happens in developing countries, at this stage the patient disappeared. (C, D courtesy of *Semin Roentgenol*, 1979)

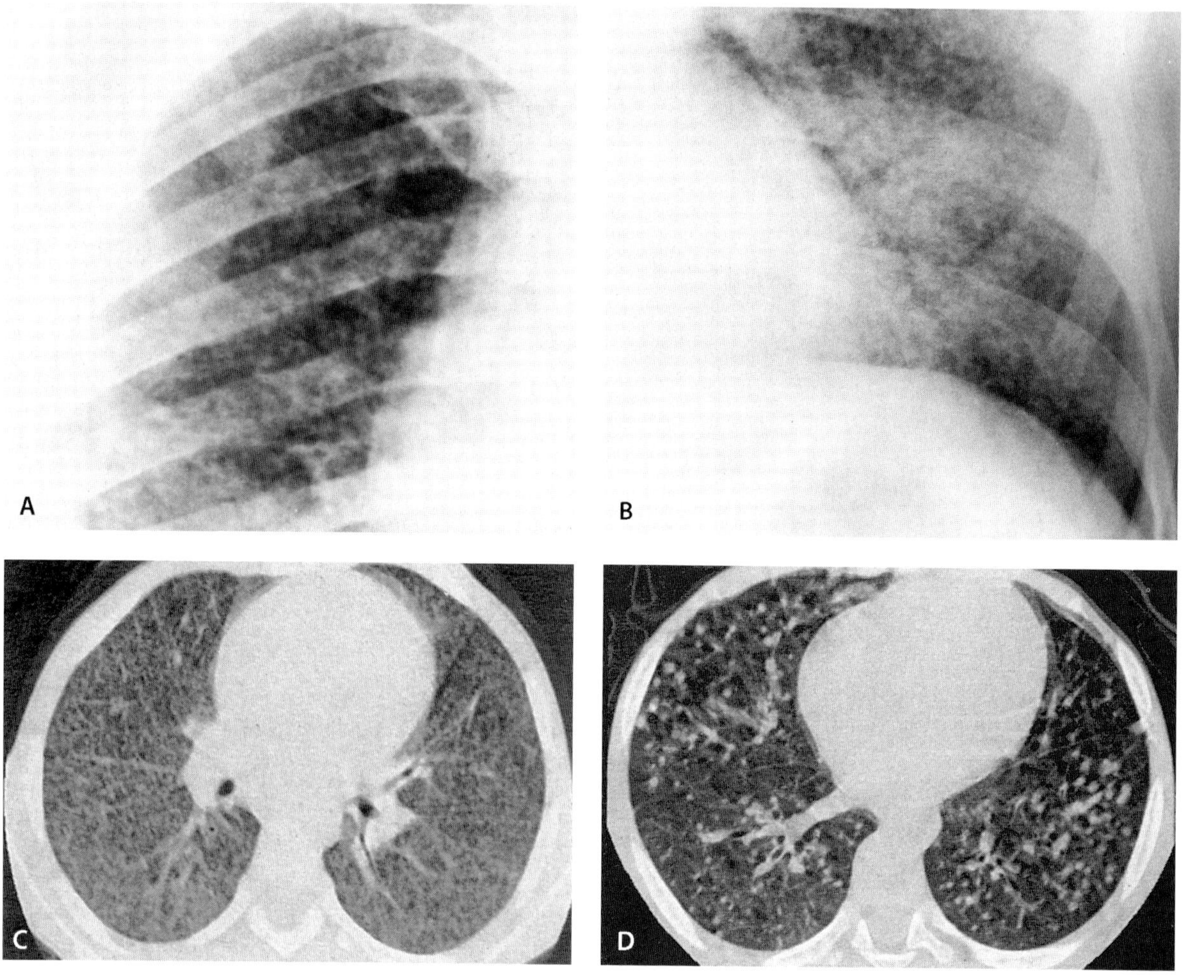

Fig. 5.23 A–D. Miliary tuberculosis. The miliary nodules vary considerably. **A** Fine nodulation in the right upper lobe, evenly distributed but with some nodules beginning to coalesce. **B** The left lower lobe of another patient with more numerous nodules varying a little in size. In this patient the nodules did not coalesce. **C** High-resolution CT showing small widespread nodules with interlobular septal and interstitial thickening. **D** High-resolution CT in another child from South Africa, with multiple nodules of two sizes, suggesting two episodes of hematogenous dissemination. Early diagnosis of hematogenous spread is important to reduce the high mortality. (**C, D** from Cremin and Jamieson 1995)

has not been suspected on the chest radiographs. In some patients there may be hilar lymphadenopathy, but in others the miliary disease is so acute that the lymph nodes are normal.

Hepatosplenomegaly often occurs in association with miliary infection, and on ultrasonography is seen as a granular echoic appearance in the liver or spleen. In some patients there may be multiple small hypoechoic nodules, some of which have central echogenic necrosis. On CT the small nodules are of low density and usually do not enhance with contrast, except occasionally around the rim of the nodule. These granulomas may become confluent, appearing as hypoechogenic or echogenic masses up to 2 cm in size. Both hepatic and splenic nodules may calcify (see p. 461).

Miliary tuberculosis in the tropics may occur at any age, including in the elderly, even when the patients are HIV-negative. But patients who have altered immunity (e.g., from AIDS, malnutrition, recurrent infection, diabetes, leukemia, lymphoma or other malignancy) are at risk when exposed to tuberculosis and are particularly liable to develop miliary spread. The differential diagnosis includes the miliary pattern caused by the passage of larvae of various parasites through the lungs, during which there will in most cases be a peripheral blood eosinophilia; unfortunately, this can be misleading, because miliary tuberculosis may be superimposed on the parasitic background of the patients, and is not excluded by eosinophilia. Fortunately, in the majority of parasitic infections the radiological appearances

change rapidly, whereas in miliary tuberculosis the nodules may become more apparent but the overall pattern does not fluctuate within a short period. Miliary tuberculosis may take 2 or 3 months to fade, even with adequate therapy. Only rarely does it result in miliary calcification.
There are many miners (for coal, tin, gold, etc.) throughout the tropical world in whom silicosis and silicotuberculosis must be considered in the differential diagnosis of miliary patterns in the lungs. Silicotuberculosis also occurs in women (see below).

Silicosis

Any pneumoconiosis, but silicosis in particular, carries an increased risk of tuberculosis. Routine chest radiography is required by law in many countries before anyone may work underground and is repeated every year. The increased risk of tuberculosis is such that many countries provide a pension, not only for silicosis but whenever a miner develops tuberculosis while at work or within 1 year of leaving the mines or high-risk occupation. The radiological differential diagnosis between silicosis and miliary tuberculosis can be extremely difficult, and depends on the distribution of the miliary nodules in the lung. In silicosis the nodules are almost invariably first recognized in the intraclavicular, upper midzone of the frontal chest film; over a period of months they become visible in the apices and the lower lung sequentially, and the original nodules become more prominent. Miliary tuberculosis has no such differential distribution and may occur everywhere (both lungs) at the same time. If both diseases occur together (silicotuberculosis) the radiologist is quite often unable to recognize the underlying pathological process and must resort to careful study of the preceding films and a sound clinical knowledge of the patient. High-resolution CT may help in the differential diagnosis. Lymphadenopathy can suggest tuberculosis, but also occurs in silicosis, developing a significant and almost unique "eggshell" pattern (sarcoidosis is the only other likely cause of this calcification). The development of a large, irregular, fibrotic "conglomerate mass" (massive fibrosis) in an upper zone is indicative of silicosis, but some authorities believe that there must also be infection before this occurs.
Silicosis can occur in unexpected places and persons, and not only in those who work in high-risk occupations, e.g., miners, quarriers, stone workers, and even sculptors in stone. In the Transkei in the Republic of South Africa, approximately half a million women developed silicosis because, from childhood onwards, the girls and women ground corn between two stones which had a high silica content

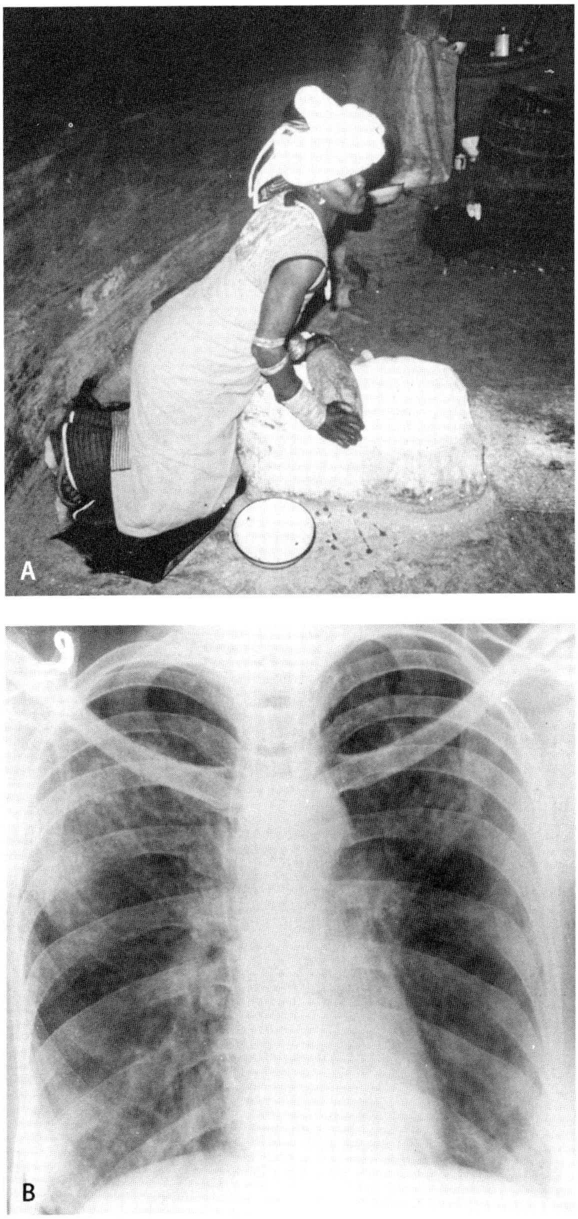

Fig. 5.24 A, B. Nor every miliary pattern on a chest radiograph is due to tuberculosis. This African woman had been grinding corn between stones since she was 9 years old. She was under treatment for miliary tuberculosis until it was realized that the distribution of the miliary nodules within her chest was not compatible with this diagnosis, and there had been no response to antituberculous therapy. The sputum did not contain *M. tuberculosis* nor did her clinical condition suggest active miliary tuberculosis. She had silicosis and was lucky, because many of the women who ground corn in this was developed silicotuberculosis. The possibility of some alternative diagnosis must always be considered when the patient's clinical condition does not match the radiographic appearance. (Courtesy of *S Afr Med J*, 1967)

(Fig. 5.24). The stones slowly disintegrated and as the women leaned over to add pressure to powder the corn finely, they inhaled large quantities of the silica-containing dust. Their children, strapped to their backs or running around the huts, were exposed to silica in the same way. The dust in these huts became full of silica of the correct particle size and characteristics to cause silicosis; as a result many of the young girls and women not only developed silicosis but there was an increased incidence of tuberculosis (more accurately, silicotuberculosis). This had a strange collateral effect; their husbands, many of whom worked underground in the gold mines of the Transvaal but under good health surveillance, went home and then returned to the mines from the rural areas with a higher incidence of tuberculosis than their fellow miners whose wives made flour by more modern methods! The whole population became at risk because of this domestic occupation. Moreover, even those who produced the grindstones were likely to suffer from silicosis as, for example, in a village north of Kano in Nigeria, West Africa, where sandstone is quarried in pits from which grindstones are hewn and then widely used throughout Nigeria for grinding guinea corn. A total of 126 workers were examined and 49 had silicosis, 17 of them in an advanced stage of massive fibrosis. Among these, seven also had pulmonary tuberculosis. No doubt similar hazards exist elsewhere in the tropical world for equally unexpected reasons (and elderly American Indian women have been shown to have faced the same hazards from grinding corn).

Summary

Primary, anergic or nonimmune tuberculosis occurs in any combination of the patterns described. This is significant in establishing the differential diagnosis; for example, it is unusual to see both lobar pneumonia and bronchopneumonia on the same chest radiograph in a pyogenic infection. Similarly, patchy bronchopneumonia with a small pleural effusion, or lobar pneumonia with pericarditis, is more likely to be tuberculous than pyogenic. Lobar pneumonia which does not clear in a few weeks is probably not pyogenic. Any chest infection at any age which does not respond appropriately to antibiotic therapy may be tuberculous, unless, particularly in adults, it is secondary to bronchiectasis or underlying neoplasm. Multiple cavities in young children may be tuberculous or staphylococcal. Enlarged hilar and mediastinal lymph nodes with any form of pneumonia, abscesses, or pleural or pericardial fluid should always suggest tuberculosis. Pleural effusions in young teenage patients, especially if bilateral and with no cardiac or renal disease, are probably tuberculous. Miliary lung disease, especially when accompanied by lymphadenopathy and effusions, also suggests tuberculosis.

It is very important to recognize that the lung changes in primary (nonimmune) tuberculosis go through a progressive spectrum, and that the first radiograph may be taken at any stage in the sequence. In some there may be lobar pneumonia and/or hilar lymphadenopathy, while in others there may be a healing peripheral focus or bronchogenic spread or pleural effusions; furthermore, there may be a combination of any of these events. Primary tuberculosis is not a static process, and the progress shown radiographically may provide the diagnosis when it is not clear on the initial film. Unlike a pyogenic infection, tuberculosis seldom simply fades away. The rate at which these changes develop and heal depends on what is called, in broad terms, the "resistance" of the individual patient, together with the success of any treatment. It is this whole repertoire of change which may allow the correct diagnosis, hopefully before it is too late for the patient.

Immune Tuberculosis (Also known as Secondary, Hyperergic, Reactivation, or Adult Tuberculosis)

The term "adult" tuberculosis is misleading because this pattern of disease can occur in any patient at almost any age beyond infancy. The majority of cases of "adult" pattern tuberculosis develop as a separate illness, or as a complication of other ill health, e.g., AIDS, diabetes, or malnutrition. There are a few patients whose immunity alters during the course of a primary tuberculous infection and an "adult" pattern develops without an interval. Whatever the sequence, the radiologist must not, therefore, hesitate to diagnose "adult" tuberculosis in a child, particularly one who has received BCG vaccination.

Secondary or immune tuberculosis is usually bilateral. In one survey only 4% of patients had unilateral disease. Cavitation is the rule rather than the exception, particularly during the active stage of the disease. When there is bilateral infection in the upper lobes, it is almost certainly due to tuberculosis; if it is bilateral and in the lower lobes, it may well be pyogenic bronchiectasis, following pertussis (whooping cough) or chronic sinus infection. If the infection involves one upper lobe and the opposite lower lobe, it is likely to be tuberculous. In Asia, all these appearances may also be due to paragonimiasis or to melioidosis.

Clinical Characteristics

The clinical symptoms of patients in the tropics are similar to those of patients in nontropical areas, but may be more severe. Hemoptysis, cough, fever, night sweats, and general debility are common. Many patients have clinical evidence of lung fibrosis, which causes asymmetrical flattening of the chest wall and shift of the trachea (mediastinum): there are often associated physical signs of cavitation. Clinically the differential diagnosis must include pyogenic pneumonia, chronic lung abscess, bronchiectasis, fungal infections, paragonimiasis or melioidosis (where appropriate), amebic infection of the lung (usually but not invariably associated with a large liver), and malignant disease.

Imaging Diagnosis

In the majority of patients the radiological diagnosis of hyperergic secondary (immune) tuberculosis is not difficult. Tuberculosis is a necrotizing infection in which cavitation and fibrosis can occur together or separately; both are usually bilateral in the upper lobes, especially tending to involve the apical and posterior segments. The superior segment of a lower lobe is another common site, but no lung segments escapes. Any multilobar infection with fibrosis and cavitation is likely to be reinfection tuberculosis, or an atypical mycobacterial infection. If the fibrosis is sufficient to shift the mediastinum, tuberculosis is even more likely. The mediastinal and hilar lymph nodes are not usually enlarged and may or may not be calcified. Sometimes it is possible to identify a primary parenchymal granuloma (such granulomas are usually calcified), but failure to do so does not exclude tuberculosis. There will often be pleural thickening, particularly in the costophrenic angle or over the lung apices. The rate of progress is very variable, but is usually slow and insidious, except when tuberculosis complicates some other severe illness, such as AIDS.

The initial lesion of reactivation tuberculosis is usually an alveolar haze with a few small pulmonary nodules, from which there may be some interstitial lines, often radiating to the hilum (Fig. 5.25). Further ill-defined opacities develop, with commencing distortion of the interstitial pattern due to fibrosis. At this stage the appearances often change if the patient is radiographed each month, with further distortion of the normal vascular and interstitial patterns. Contraction can progress until the interlobar fissure and hilum are displaced, usually upwards until one or both hila are much higher than normal.

Even without treatment, the infection may be arrested at any stage. This leaves residual scarring but in many cases the healing process is complicated by endobronchial involvement and there is stenosis or kinking of one or more peripheral bronchi. This results in secondary pyogenic infection and bronchiectasis, superimposed on the contracted fibrotic lung. In some patients this destructive process progresses to such an extent that it resembles the destroyed lung of primary infections (see p. 409). Unfortunately, at any stage the infection may be reactivated, sometimes after many years. Reactivation has been recorded from 35 to 51 years after the initial diagnosis. It is therefore not possible to describe any patient as being "cured." It may be better to report "probably old tuberculosis" or "apparently well healed." Unfortunately, clinicians are not much better at judging the future course of the disease.

Contrary to what is often taught, cavitation (Fig. 5.26) has diagnostic significance but no prognostic value, because necrosis and liquefaction are the normal course of tuberculosis. Cavities appear in 37%–75% of all cases of active secondary tuberculosis. They may be thick walled or thin walled and may be surrounded by a parenchymal reaction or appear to cause no local disturbance. They are more common in the upper lobes and the superior segments of the lower lobes than elsewhere, but may occur in any part of either lung. Cavities fluctuate considerably during treatment; radiographically, they may increase or decrease in size, may contain fluid, and may show a fluid level or apparently be empty, depending on the reabsorption, expectoration, or bronchial spread of the contents.

When there is obvious cavitation on standard radiographs, the sputum will be positive for bacilli in 80% of patients, but not always at the first examination; a negative sputum does not therefore exclude tuberculosis or indicate cure. Cavities may not disappear: 7%–10% of all cavities become bacteriologically sterile under treatment but remain patent. If, following surgery, cavities are examined histologically, part of the cavity wall may show healing while in another part there is active infection. Histopathologically, tuberculous cavities are abscesses and the wall of the cavity is lined with necrotic tissue. The only slight help which may be obtained in identifying active infection is when the inner wall of the cavity becomes radiographically ill-defined and the outer wall becomes less distinct. Unfortunately, a secondary infection, particularly fungal, can have exactly the same effect. Each and every radiological characteristic of the cavities can alter month by month, while the clinical condition of the patients may improve or worsen without any relationship to any radiological change in the cavities.

(Text continues on p. 429)

Unfortunately, space does not permit the illustration of all the vagaries of pulmonary tuberculosis in the tropics: the most important differences (between nontropical and tropical patients) are the rapidity with which tuberculosis may change or progress in the tropics, and how slowly it may heal even during adequate treatment. Equally important is the often acute and unexpected pattern of the infection, which may make it difficult to accept that it may be due to tuberculosis, whether in the primary (nonimmune) or in the secondary, reactivation (immune) phase.

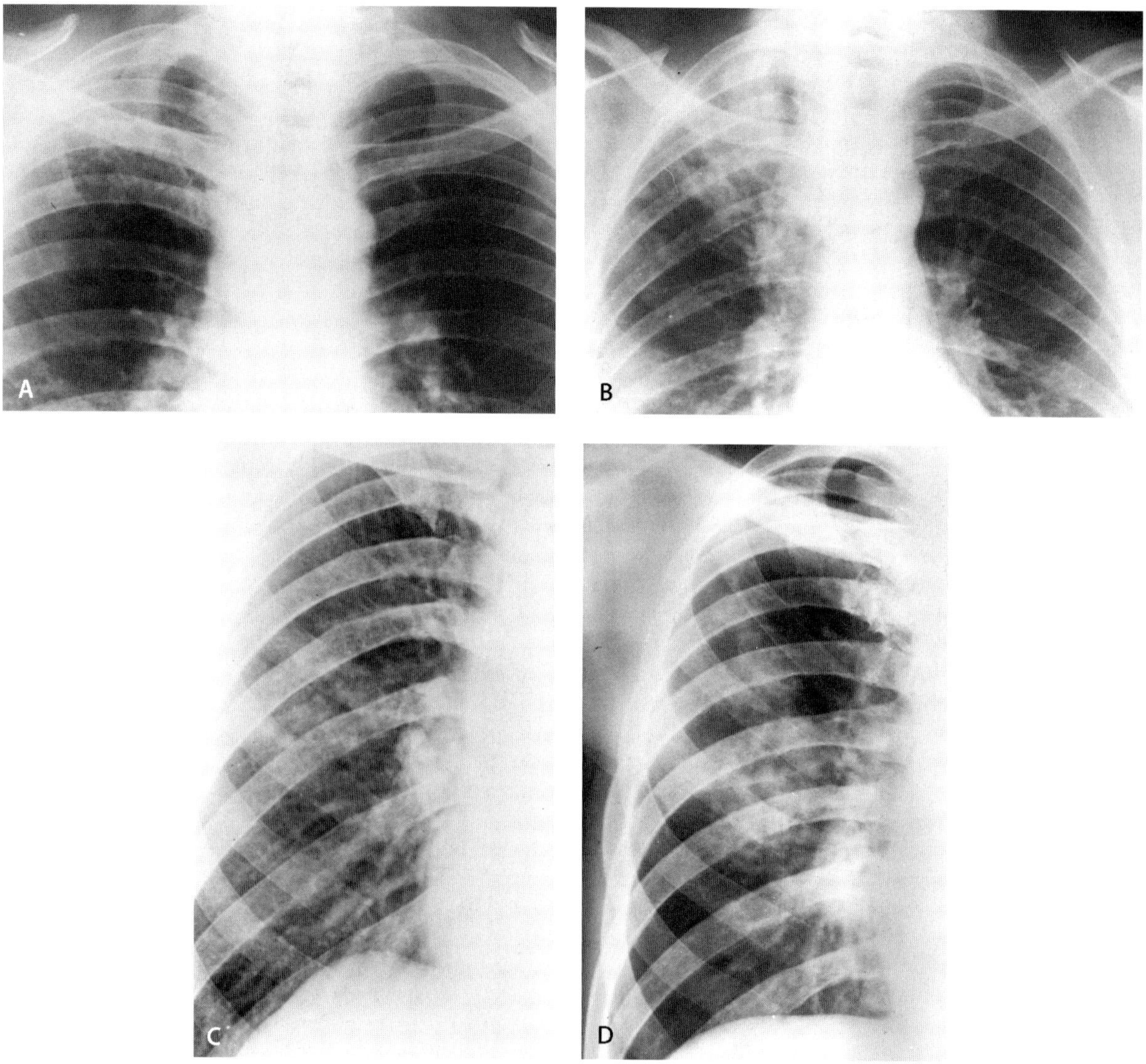

Fig. 5.25 A–D. The earliest evidence of immune (reactivation) tuberculosis is a soft alveolar haze, usually in the apex or upper lobe. This African man worked in a hospital and had routine chest radiograph which was normal 3 weeks before he became ill, with a cough, sputum, and minimal hemoptysis. His next radiograph (**A**) showed the clouding in the right apex with a few small tubercles. There were *M. tuberculosis* in the sputum. Although treatment was started, 12 weeks later (**B**) the infection had spread and was beginning to cavitate. The patient was found to be diabetic. **C** Another patient, who had lost weight and was unwell. There is a soft alveolar haze with small nodules in the periphery of the lung, probably in the anterior segment of the right upper lobe. The sputum contained *M. tuberculosis* and treatment was started: the patient improved clinically but after 7 months (**D**) the radiographic appearances seemed to have deteriorated

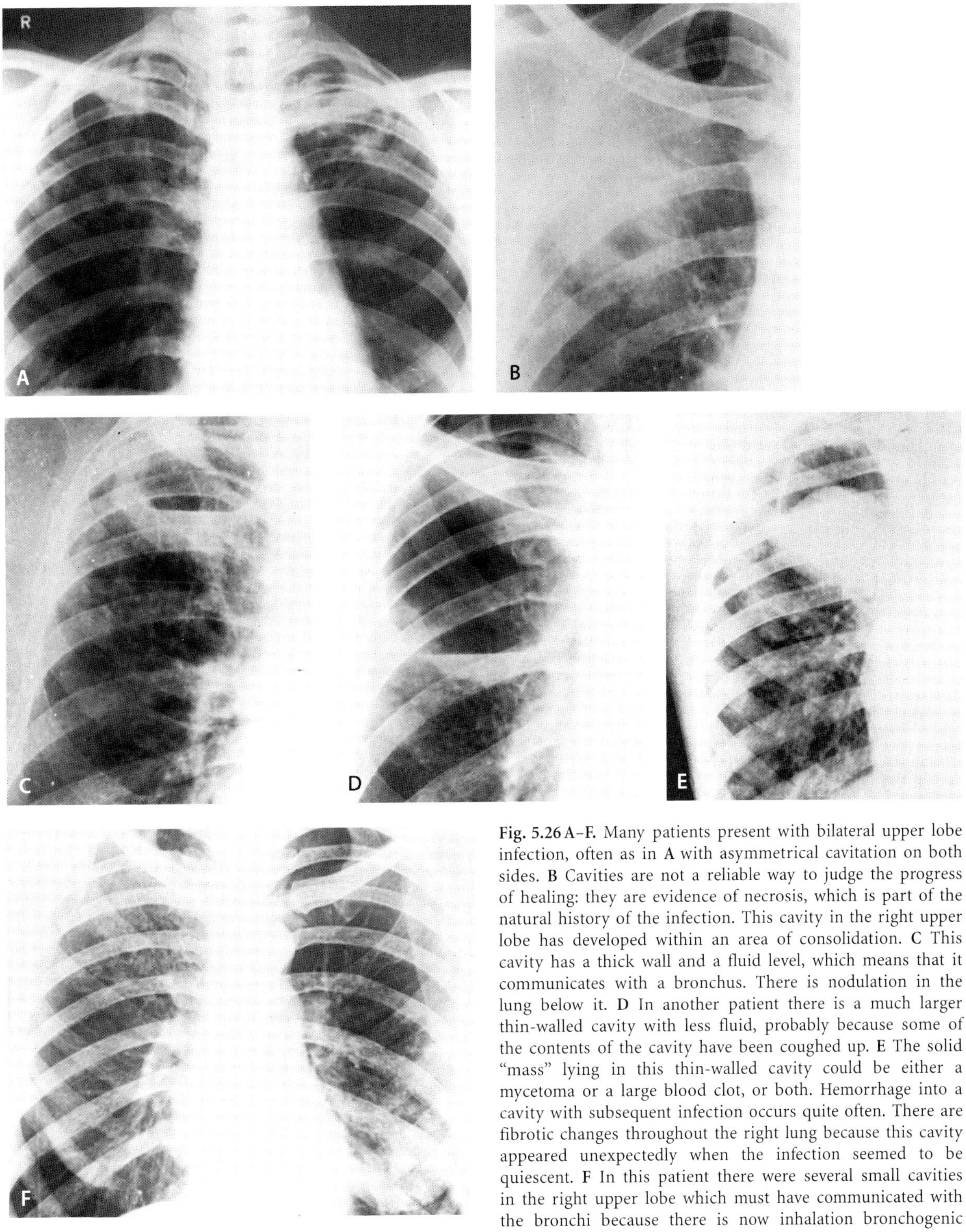

Fig. 5.26 A–F. Many patients present with bilateral upper lobe infection, often as in **A** with asymmetrical cavitation on both sides. **B** Cavities are not a reliable way to judge the progress of healing: they are evidence of necrosis, which is part of the natural history of the infection. This cavity in the right upper lobe has developed within an area of consolidation. **C** This cavity has a thick wall and a fluid level, which means that it communicates with a bronchus. There is nodulation in the lung below it. **D** In another patient there is a much larger thin-walled cavity with less fluid, probably because some of the contents of the cavity have been coughed up. **E** The solid "mass" lying in this thin-walled cavity could be either a mycetoma or a large blood clot, or both. Hemorrhage into a cavity with subsequent infection occurs quite often. There are fibrotic changes throughout the right lung because this cavity appeared unexpectedly when the infection seemed to be quiescent. **F** In this patient there were several small cavities in the right upper lobe which must have communicated with the bronchi because there is now inhalation bronchogenic spread into the left lower lobe. This pattern, with infection of an upper and a lower lobe, is very common

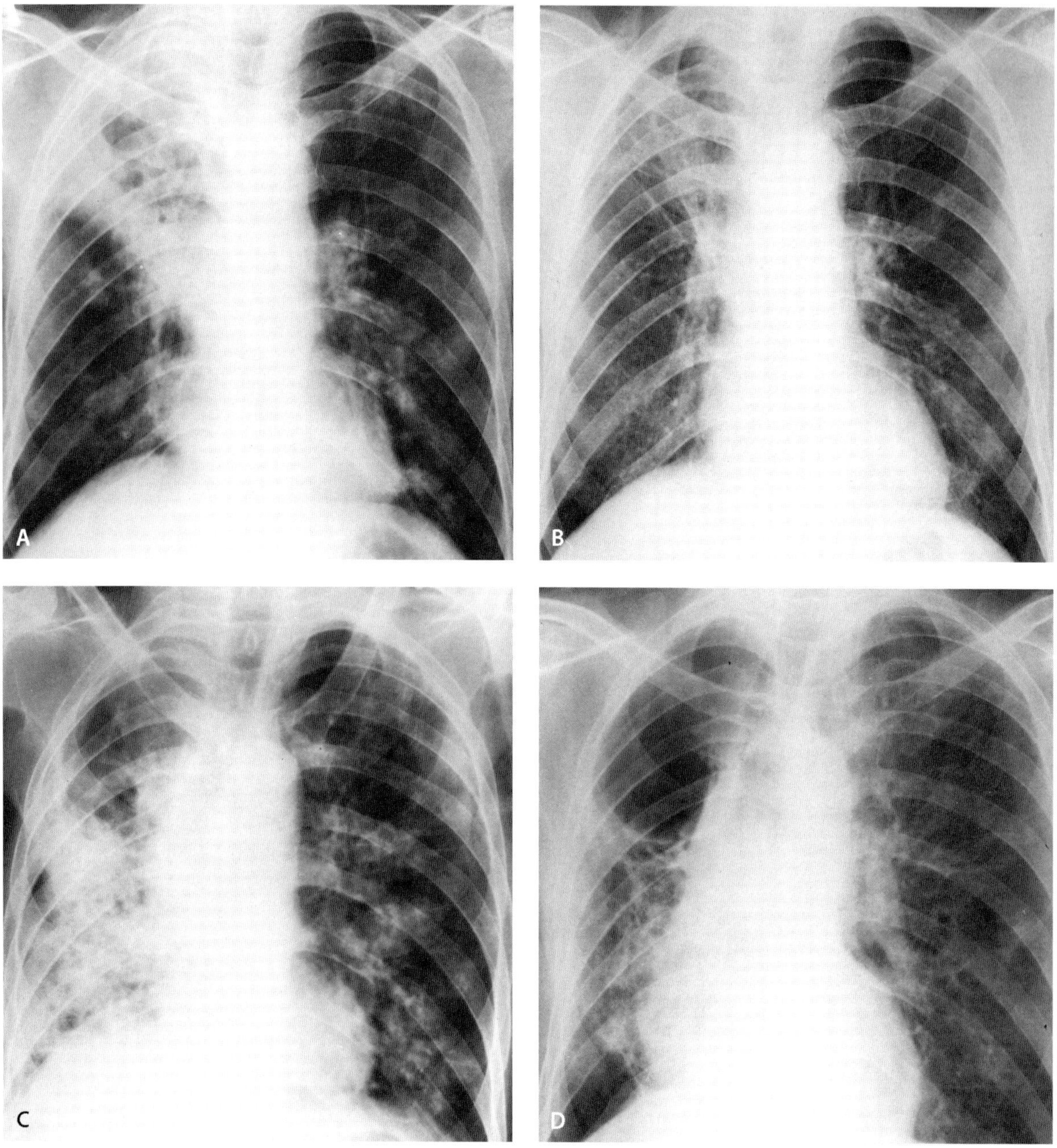

Fig. 5.27 A–D. The success, and failure, of treatment for tuberculosis. This African patient had started treatment in November for active tuberculosis. **A** Two months later the sputum was still positive for tuberculosis. Cavitation and consolidation are still present in the right upper lobe, with some overlying apical fluid. Some shrinkage of the upper part of the right lung has occurred, with slight mediastinal shift to the right. Infection is present in the left lung, particularly in the lower lobe but also in the apex. **B** By June, after 7 months' treatment there has been remarkable improvement. The right upper lobe has contracted and become fibrotic. The cavity has disappeared and the fluid over the apex of the lung has been absorbed. The left lung has also improved, leaving some minimal fibrosis only. The sputum was now negative. **C** Unfortunately, 1 year later there has been a severe relapse; a tuberculous focus has probably ruptured into a bronchus, with resulting widespread bronchopneumonia in both lungs. There is now consolidation in the right lung and a huge cavity in the right upper lobe. There is active disease and cavitation in the left lung. The mediastinum is still shifted a little to the right because of the underlying fibrosis and the right side of the chest is smaller than the left. Treatment was continued with slow improvement until (**D**) (4 years after the original radiographs. A large emphysematous bulla is present in the right upper lobe and the right lower lobe is also emphysematous. The middle lobe is severely contracted. This lung is also fibrotic and shows some small bullae. The sputum had been negative for about a year, but the fibrotic contraction and formation of bullae had continued until the right lung was virtually destroyed. Though fibrotic, the left lung is the only functioning remainder. The right lung is bronchiectatic and will often be secondarily infected. From this stage onwards it will be very difficult to decide whether any clinical illness is evidence of further reactivation of the tuberculosis

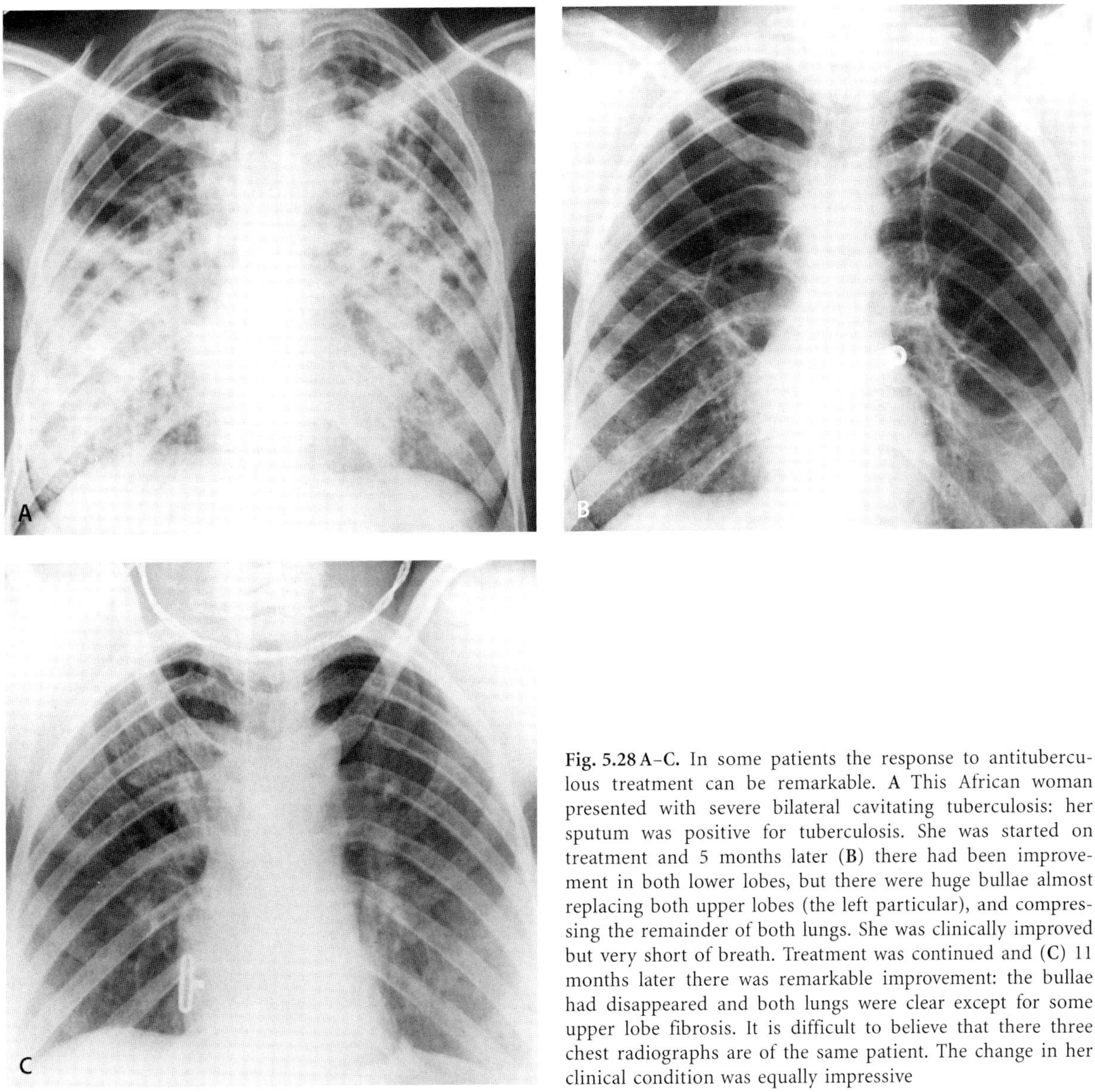

Fig. 5.28 A–C. In some patients the response to antituberculous treatment can be remarkable. **A** This African woman presented with severe bilateral cavitating tuberculosis: her sputum was positive for tuberculosis. She was started on treatment and 5 months later (**B**) there had been improvement in both lower lobes, but there were huge bullae almost replacing both upper lobes (the left particular), and compressing the remainder of both lungs. She was clinically improved but very short of breath. Treatment was continued and (**C**) 11 months later there was remarkable improvement: the bullae had disappeared and both lungs were clear except for some upper lobe fibrosis. It is difficult to believe that there three chest radiographs are of the same patient. The change in her clinical condition was equally impressive

The significance of cavitation has been overemphasized; it is but one event in the natural history of the disease. It is not even unique to human tuberculosis, air-fluid levels having been reported in the lungs of a tuberculous cockatoo!

When there is hemoptysis, the hemorrhage may come either from the lining of a cavity or from endobronchial disease, as when bronchoscopy shows that the blood comes from a lung segment in which there is no radiologically visible cavity. In tuberculosis, arteriography has not been a very satisfactory method of diagnosing or treating the source of the hemorrhage, probably because there is almost always a great deal of associated fibrosis and scarring. A clot in a tuberculous cavity can mimic a mycetoma or become infected by a fungus. It is only the reabsorption of the clot after a relatively short period, 1 or 2 weeks, which can exclude a fungus ball. Most cavities heal by obliteration, leaving a scar, but some remain as thin-walled bullae.

Fibrosis is equally unrewarding prognostically (Figs. 5.27–5.29). Change is almost always slow, so that comparison with a radiograph taken a few weeks previously may show no alteration. It is essential always to compare findings with the very earliest film available. It is never possible to judge the status of the infection from one radiograph; even extensive pulmonary fibrosis may include active disease. The radiological assessment of activity is very unreliable (Fig. 5.30), and is often made more difficult by a secondary pyogenic infection in the fibrotic lung: clinically it may be some other

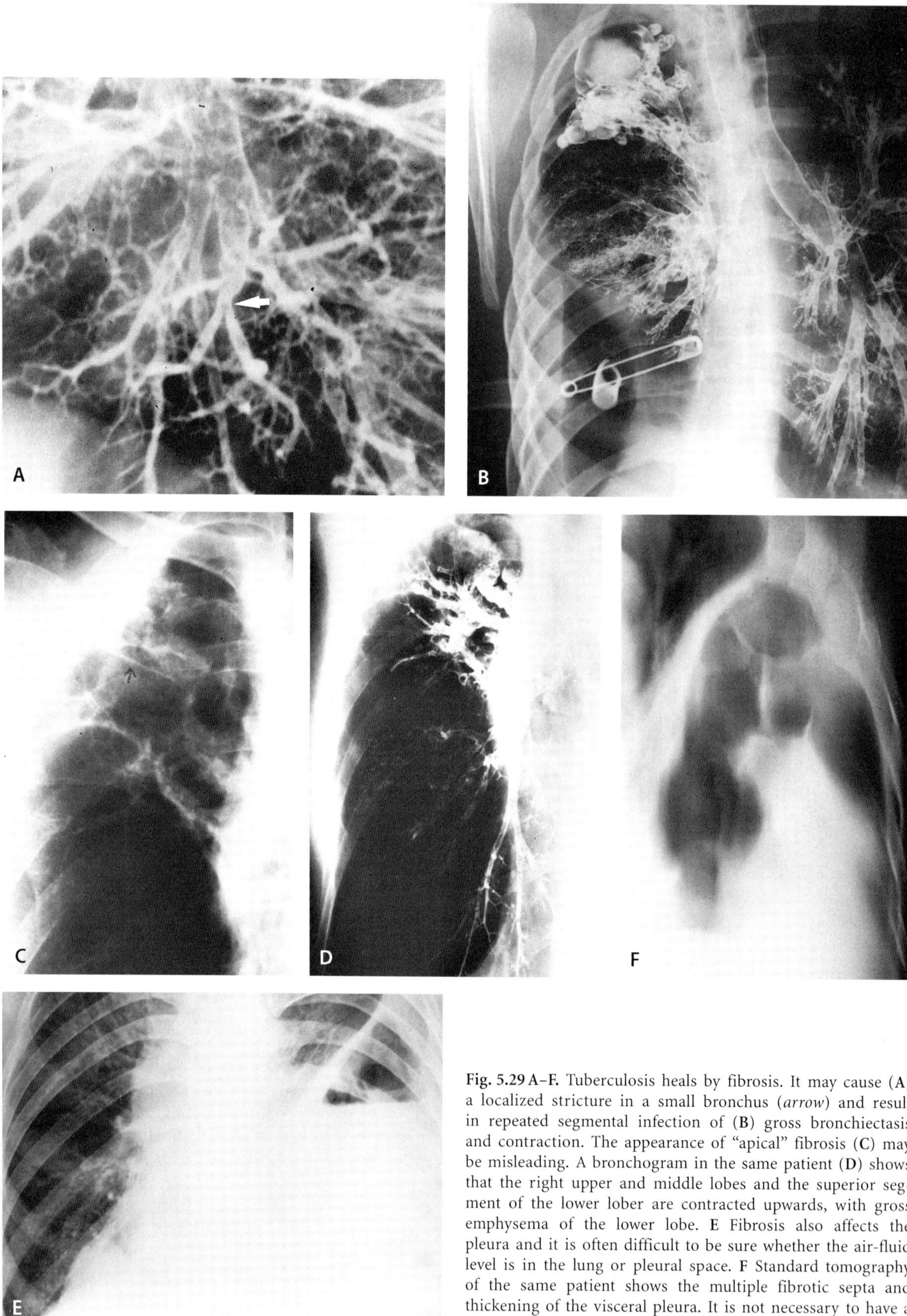

Fig. 5.29 A–F. Tuberculosis heals by fibrosis. It may cause (**A**) a localized stricture in a small bronchus (*arrow*) and result in repeated segmental infection of (**B**) gross bronchiectasis and contraction. The appearance of "apical" fibrosis (**C**) may be misleading. A bronchogram in the same patient (**D**) shows that the right upper and middle lobes and the superior segment of the lower lober are contracted upwards, with gross emphysema of the lower lobe. **E** Fibrosis also affects the pleura and it is often difficult to be sure whether the air-fluid level is in the lung or pleural space. **F** Standard tomography of the same patient shows the multiple fibrotic septa and thickening of the visceral pleura. It is not necessary to have a secondary pyogenic infection to produce this result

concomitant illness, such as amebiasis or dysentery, which has led to deterioration in the patient's general health. When there is lung fibrosis it is impossible by any imaging technique to differentiate pyogenic infection from recurrent tuberculosis, or to exclude contamination by a saprophytic fungus (Fig. 5.31). The diagnosis has to be made clinically with the help of the bacteriologist; unfortunately, relapsing secondary infections are common.

However, to end this section on a more positive note, the majority of patients eventually heal or fibrose their tuberculosis into a state of inactivity provided they continue with adequate treatment.

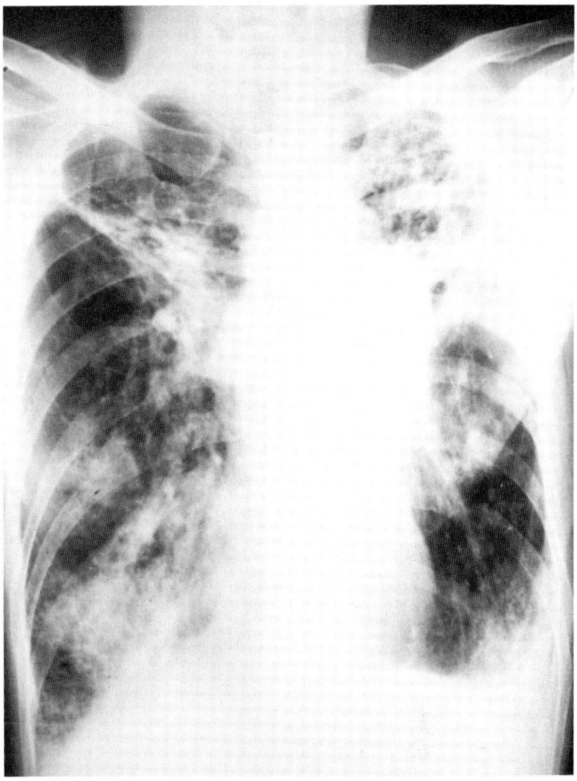

▶

Fig. 5.30. Severe bilateral chronic tuberculosis will remain unchanged radiographically for many years. In this 70-year-old patient no part of the lung has escaped. He occasionally produced sputum which contained a few *M. tuberculosis* bacilli and so remained a danger to his family, with whom he lived. Surgery was obviously impossible, but the success of continuing antituberculous therapy is doubtful

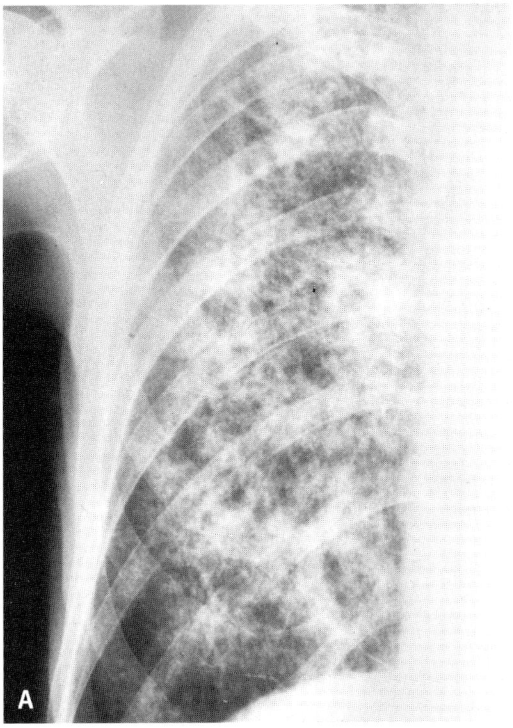

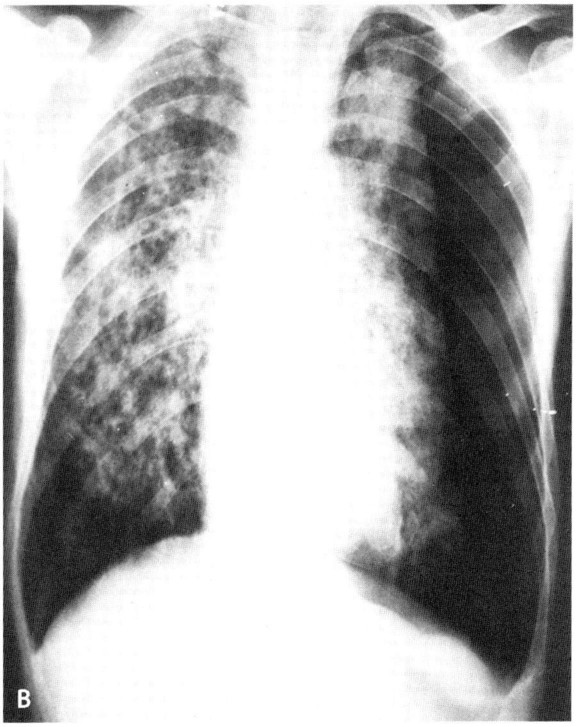

Fig. 5.31 A, B. Reactivation tuberculosis must be included among the many causes of interstitial fibrosis, particularly in middle-aged patients. The clinical complaint is usually of dyspnea and generall ill health. **A** Both lungs of this 50-year-old man showed severe interstitial fibrosis and honeycombing. The sputum was consistently negative for *M. tuberculosis* and the diagnosis was established by surgical biopsy. There was no radiographic change after 12 months of antituberculous therapy. **B** Lungs with interstitial fibrosis are fragile. An acute pneumothorax can develop after paroxysmal coughing, in this case bilaterally but much more severely on the left

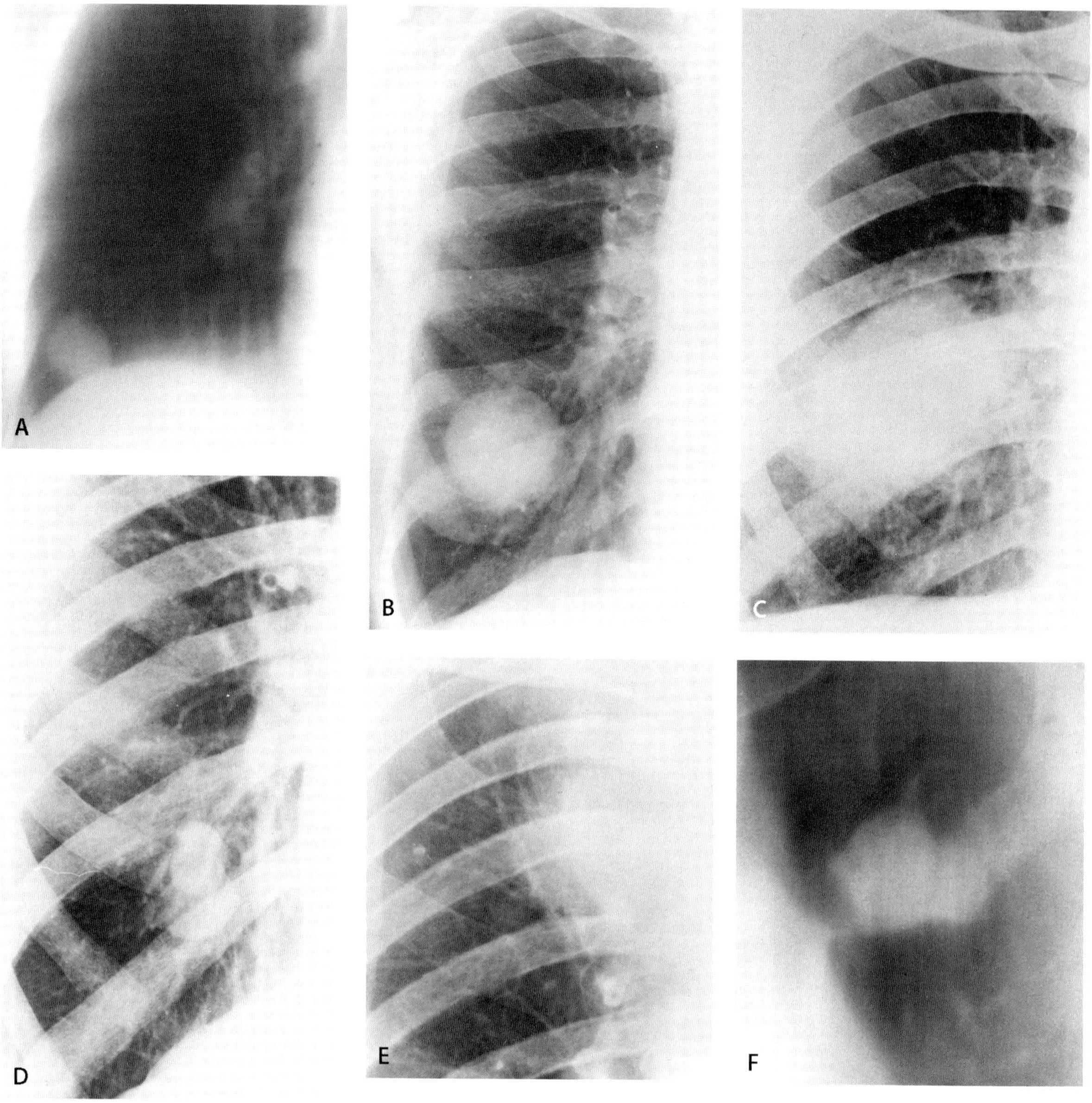

Fig. 5.32 A–J. Tuberculomas may appear in any part of the lung, at any age; they may be single or multiple and are of varying size. The sputum is almost always negative for *M. tuberculosis*. **A** Standard tomography of a small tuberculoma in the right lower lobe just above the diaphragm. **B** A larger smooth round tuberculoma in the right lower chest of a young woman. This did not change in spite of treatment over a period of many months. **C** A large ill-defined tuberculoma in the right lower lobe of an elderly patient. The initial diagnosis was carcinoma of the lung, but fortunately the sputum was positive for tuberculosis. **D** Some tuberculomas are lobulated or multiple. These two in the right middle lobe are well defined and could be mistaken for metastases. **E** A paramediastinal tuberculoma, clinically and radiologically suspected of being malignant. The diagnosis was made after surgical removal. **F** Standard tomograms of a lobulated tuberculoma in the left upper lobe, which was removed surgically. Even if tomography (including CT) demonstrates calcification, it is seldom possible to completely exclude malignancy by imaging. G–J see p. 433

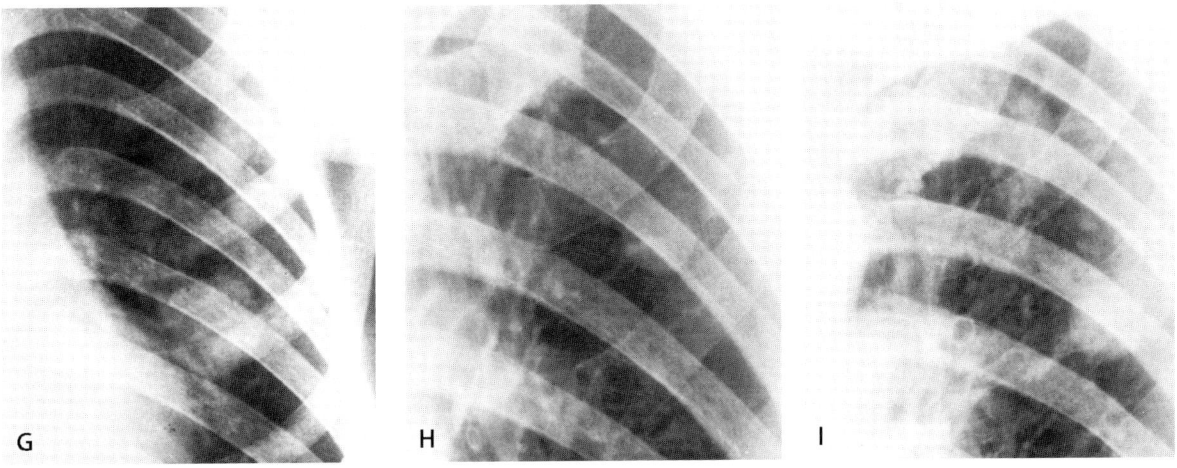

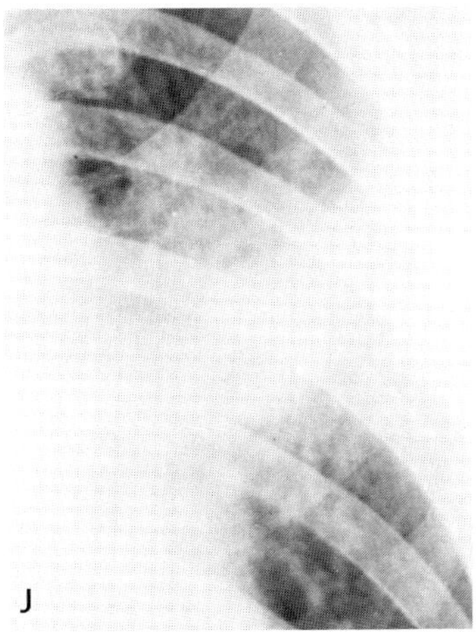

Fig. 5.32 (*continued*). **G** Multiple well-defined tuberculomas in the left mid-lung. These closely resemble metastases, but in this young African patient there was no known primary. **H** Tuberculomas are not always quiescent and harmless. There is a small tuberculoma with satellite nodules in the left upper lobe: it had not changed over 4 months. The patient refused surgery because he was clinically well. **I** Six months later the outline had become indistinct and further nodules had spread throughout the upper lobe. He remained clinically well but antituberculous therapy was started. **J** Unfortunately in spite of treatment, the infection continued to spread and coalesced into a caviating area of pneumonia which eventually led to further bronchogenic spread into the left lower lobe

Tuberculoma

Histopathologically, a tuberculoma is a focus of caseating pneumonia, although this is an oversimplified definition using a controversial explanation. Radiologically, a tuberculoma is a nodular, usually circular opacity in the lung, from 1 to 10 cm in diameter. Tuberculomas may be dense or hazy: while most are well defined, a few are more irregular in outline. CT or careful radiography may demonstrate small satellite tubercles. About ten percent of tuberculomas have central cavitation (necrosis). Tuberculomas are usually solitary but may be multiple; sometimes several occur in one lung segment. They may be found in any part of the lung, most often towards the periphery. Calcification, if present, can be central or eccentric, granular or in the form of small scattered flecks best seen with CT. The majority of tuberculomas show no calcification, even on CT or tomography, and there is no hilar lymphadenopathy; there is seldom hilar calcification. Most tuberculomas do not have any surrounding parenchymal reaction, although occasionally there will be haziness of part of their outline, apparently due to some increased vascularity or lymphatic thickening directed toward the hilum; this may result from continued activity or reactivation.

A tuberculoma may be found in a patient of any age, sometimes by chance on a radiograph taken for some other reason. Other patients present with cough and loss of weight. The appearance of the tuberculoma may remain unchanged for weeks or months, or it may unexpectedly break down as the result of some alteration in the patient's immune status. This can cause bronchogenic infection, or local spread becoming an area of pneumonia. No tuberculoma is "safe," even when unchanged for a long period.

The differential diagnostic problems are considerable: many tuberculomas are only diagnosed after surgical removal because a tumor has been suspected. If the patient is young, malignancy is unlikely and in the tropics, tuberculosis will be the most common etiology. A mycotic infection, such as histoplasmosis or coccidiomycosis, is possible; an early pyogenic or amebic lung abscess must be ex-

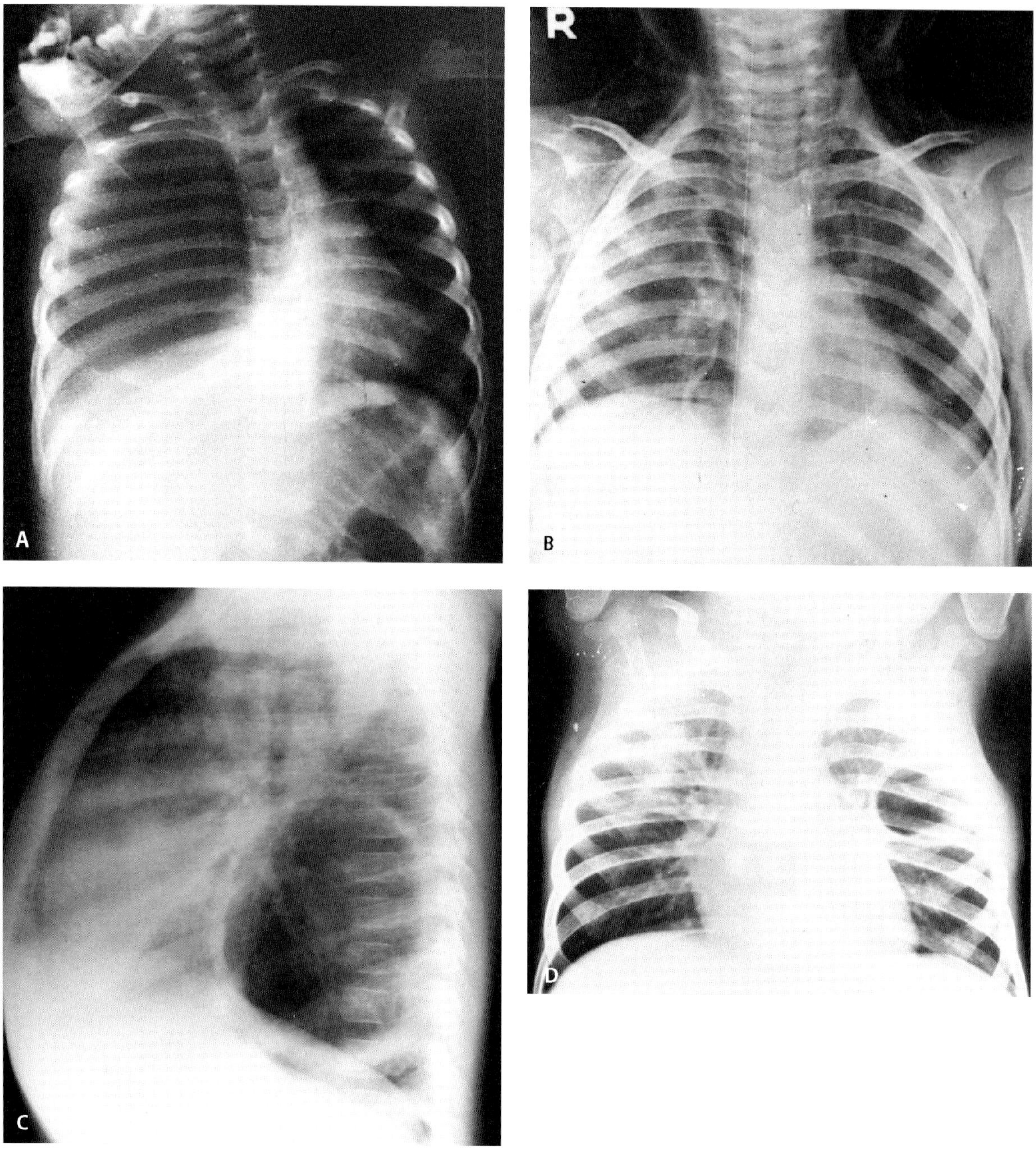

Fig. 5.33 A–D. Large emphysematous bullae can develop in children and adults, and can occur spontaneously or in association with isoniazed therapy. **A** A large thin-walled air-containing cyst in the right lung, displacing the mediastinum to the left. It is very easy to mistake this for a pneumothorax and attempt to decompress it. This may result in a bronchopleural fistula, but in some patients the pressure is so severe that the risk has to be taken. **B** Spontaneous rupture of a similar cyst has caused subcutaneous emphysema and a pneumomediastinum. If the pressure increases, this may be fatal. **C** The lateral radiograph showing a similar large cyst in a child. This is quite thick walled, and there is tuberculous lymphadenopathy. However, this is not a tuberculous cavity. **D** Another child with a large bulla in the left mid-lung. The patients illustrated in **C** and **D** were both being treated with isoniazid

cluded. Unlike the majority of tuberculomas, lung abscesses are progressive and seldom remain unchanged. The tuberculin skin test will usually be positive, but this may not be a helpful differentiating feature. A hydatid cyst will have to be excluded, but this is usually not too difficult (see Chap. 3). In adults, primary carcinoma of the lung must be considered, although it is still uncommon in many parts of the tropics. For the solitary nodule which strongly resembles primary or metastatic lung carcinoma radiographically, and which is too small or inaccessible for CT-guided biopsy, surgical excision may be the only way to establish the diagnosis, but if tuberculosis is considered possible, it is a wise precaution to give the patient adequate antituberculous therapy prior to biopsy or surgery.

Isoniazid Cysts

Isoniazid is used in chemoprophylaxis, particularly to prevent development of tuberculosis in infected persons or those who have been in contact with patients who have sputum which is positive for tuberculous bacilli. It is also used for treatment, together with antibiotics. Prolonged therapy with isoniazid, apart from risking liver damage and peripheral neuropathy, may result in the development of thin-walled cysts (Fig. 5.33). Such cysts may regress or develop ball-valve obstruction due to blockage of the segmental bronchi. They may enlarge to resemble a single emphysematous bulla and may burst, causing an acute pneumothorax or pneumomediastinum. This can happen in children or in adults.

Chronic Pleural Disease

A pleural effusion during the reactivation stage of tuberculosis almost always means direct spread of the infection into the pleural cavity and is really an empyema. It is a different process to the primary pleural effusion which occurs in the nonimmune patient. If there is a spontaneous air-fluid level in the pleura, then a bronchopleural fistula has developed. Tuberculosis often causes adhesions between the parietal and visceral pleura, causing loculation of the pleural fluid, and, following aspiration, there may be loculated air-fluid levels within thick-walled pleural cavities. On a standard chest radiograph it can be very difficult to differentiate this from pulmonary cavitation; ultrasonography, CT, or standard tomography may be helpful, but intrapleural contrast examinations may be necessary to show the cavity and the connections if decortication is considered. Eventually, many, but not all, tuberculous effusions and pleuritis result in pleural calcification (see p. 417) which may be extreme in some individuals, extending over half or more of the involved hemithorax.

Chest Wall

Direct spread of tuberculosis from the lung or pleura to any part of the chest wall does occur, but is extremely uncommon. It is a little more frequent in atypical mycobacterial infections. When there is a tuberculous empyema the ribs can be directly involved (Fig. 5.34). Infection of the sternum, ribs or spine occurs in children, particularly during the progressive primary type of infection. Hematogenous dissemination accounts for other cases with skeletal involvement (see Fig. 5.89, p. 511).

In many cases of spinal tuberculosis, there is no pulmonary infection (see p. 475), but an abscess from infected vertebrae can track around the intercostal space and surface alongside the sternum (see p. 506). The vertebral lesion may not be obvious radiologically and radioisotope bone scans or CT or MR may be advisable, or standard tomography where scanning is not available.

Tuberculosis of the ribs or sternum follows the same pattern as skeletal tuberculosis elsewhere (see p. 507).

Congenital Tuberculosis

Infection of an infant within the uterus or during parturition is rare. However, many infants become infected from their mother within a few days after birth. There are about 150 recorded cases of undoubted congenital tuberculosis. The skin reaction to tuberculin is not always positive and the diagnosis can be difficult. About half these children will die wihin 3 or 4 weeks. It is not known whether this pattern or frequency of congenital infection will change in mothers who are HIV-positive. A chest radiograph of the infant will show a pattern of either miliary disease or primary tuberculosis, and progressive tuberculosis may develop. Some may be born with or develop primary skin tuberculosis. It is possible that the mother will have no radiological and little clinical evidence of tuberculosis.

Immunization with BCG

Many countries with a high incidence of tuberculosis recommend BCG vaccination (bacille Calmette-Guérin, an attenuated but live strain of *M. tuberculosis*), often during the first few days of life. The protection privided varies in different countries: it

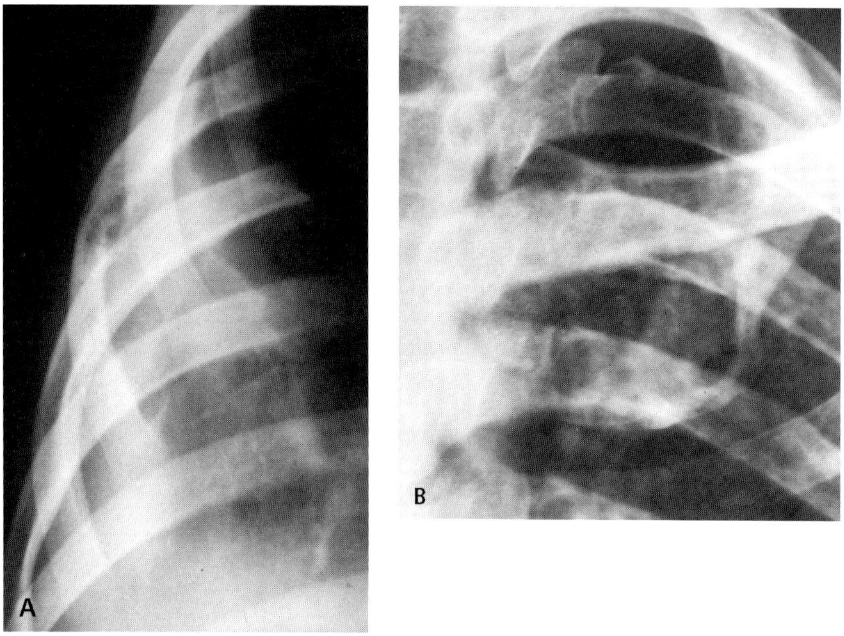

Fig. 5.34 A, B. Tuberculosis of the chest wall is uncommon. **A** This patient had a tuberculous empyema and the fifth right rib became infected directly from the empyema. There is also some periosteal reaction along the underside of the sixth right rib. **B** There is a lytic lesion in the anterior end of the first left rib which was found on biopsy to be tuberculous. The lung was not infected and no other source of tuberculosis was found. (See also Fig. 5.85 on p. 507.)

has been excellent in Haiti, but less successful in parts of India and Puerto Rico. The difference in results is not easily explained; sometimes it is due to technical problems with the vaccine and its administration. Another theory suggests that where environmental mycobacteria are common (see p. 394), people are already protected. However, where successful, the main benefit has been to reduce the risk of tuberculous meningitis and acute disseminated infections.

Protection following BCG immunization can last from 10 to 20 years; there are a few complications. Between 3 and 6 months after vaccination, children occasionally develop axillary (or inguinal) lymphadenitis on the same side (Fig. 5.35). This is probably no more than a classical primary complex, but in some children the nodal swelling is considerable and a very few nodes may suppurate: other children may be generally unwell and pyrexial, but the chest x-ray is almost invariably normal and remains so. Some countries use a more potent BCG vaccine when immunizing neonates, and this has been inadvertently used for older children. Although there was an increased skin reaction, which took longer to heal, there were no other complications and after 6 months the resulting scar was much the same as if the correct strength has been used.

The response to BCG vaccination is very dependent on the state of health and nutrition of the individual. When healthy, a positive reaction will be obtained in 85% of those vaccinated. The BCG response is grossly impaired in children and young adults with kwashiorkor (severe protein deficiency) and very depressed also when the patients are marasmic with kwashiorkor (combined protein and calorie deficiency). However, if the individual is marasmic only (calorie deficient) the successful vaccination rate is the same as in healthy patients. This is important, because the pattern of tuberculosis which may develop in those who have been vaccinated is very dependent on the success or otherwise of the vaccination. After successful BCG vaccination the tuberculin skin reaction should be positive and, if active tuberculosis does develops some years later, it will follow the hyperergic (secondary immune) pattern.

Although BCG osteomyelitis has been recorded, it is rare. The lesion is usually eccentric in the metaphysis of a long bone, breaking the cortex but seldom causing a periosteal reaction. Generalized BCG tuberculosis and tuberculous meningitis are even more rare; these complications may have an increased incidence in HIV+ patients. Intravesical BCG has been used successfully in the treatment of bladder carcinoma: subsequent miliary tuberculosis (recognized on a chest radiograph) has been recorded in two patients. The response to appropriate antituberculous therapy has been good.

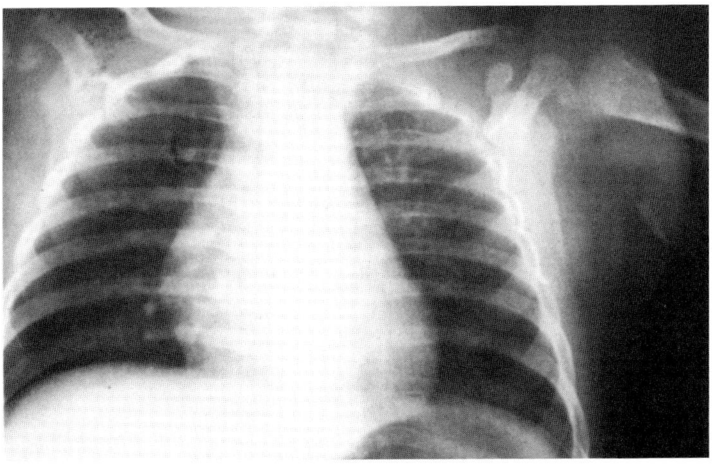

Fig. 5.35. The chest radiograph of a child who had had BCG vaccination 4 months previously. The chest is normal but the left axillary lymph nodes are considerably enlarged. It is very unusual for there to be any pulmonary abnormality following BCG vaccination

PPD Conversion

When an individual known to have a negative tuberculin skin test (PPD, Heaf or Mantoux) converts "spontaneously" to a positive reaction it is presumptive evidence of a tuberculous infection, although the site of the focus may never be found. A year of isoniazid or other therapy is often recommended. Several large series have shown that routine chest x-rays during this treatment are unnecessary, provided the patient takes the prescribed drugs correctly and continuously for at least 9 of the required 12 months. Only if treatment is discontinued or is inadequate should chest radiographs be taken regularly. Not all authorities agree with this regimen, and in the tropics the conversion may be due not to tuberculosis but to other mycobacteria (see p. 394). There is also some health risk from the chemotherapy, statistically about the same as for an otherwise healthy individual developing active tuberculosis after the tuberculin skin reaction has become positive. The risks of isoniazid-induced hepatitis are age dependent, and many authorities do not recommend its use in patients older than 40 years. Even if patients are not given active prophylaxis, repeated chest radiographs should not be routine but be taken only when indicated by the clinical condition of the individual.

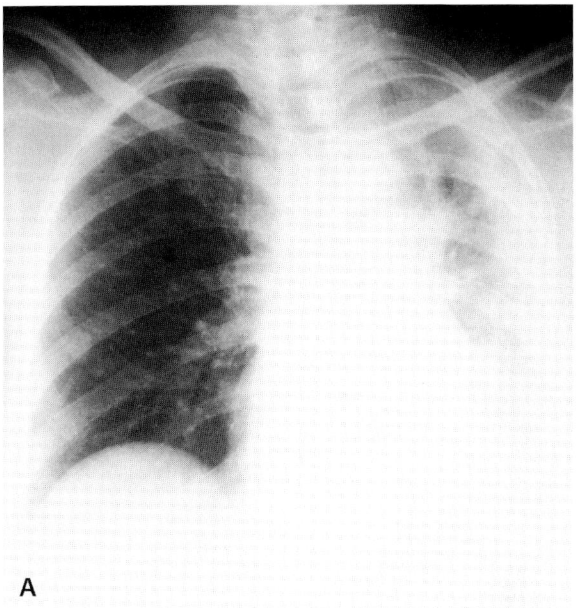

A

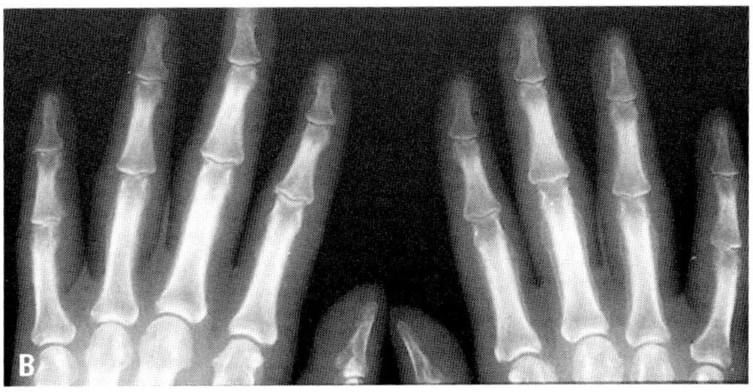

B

Fig. 5.36 A, B. Clubbing is much less common in patients with pulmonary tuberculosis than in the past. **A** This middle-aged patient with chronic tuberculosis, which has caused fibrosis of his left lung and pleura with flattening of the left chest wall, has (**B**) well-marked hypertrophic pulmonary osteoarthropathy. There is some apical fibrosis in his right lung, but he was not more dyspneic than would be expected, and there was no other reason for his clubbing. (There was no evidence of any bone foci.)

Clubbing

Hypertrophic pulmonary osteoarthropathy, "clubbing," is not now usually associated with pulmonary tuberculosis (Fig. 5.36). It used to be more common and was a frequent finding in America and elsewhere before antituberculuous therapy was available. However, it may still occur in up to one-third of African men with debilitating pulmonary tuberculosis. It seems to be more common in those who are undernourished but cannot be correlated with the extent of the findings on the chest x-ray or any other likely cause. Whether clubbing is increasing again in pulmonary tuberculosis in other regions is not yet recorded. It is important as a possible explanation for periosteal reaction on the clavicles, femora, digits, or elsewhere.

The Other Mycobacterioses

Nontuberculous mycobacterial infections (MOTT or "mycobacteria other than tuberculosis") cannot be distinguished clinically, radiologically, or pathologically from tuberculosis in the lungs or any other organ system, including bones. Some authorities state that there are about 40 different species; others recognize over 60 species. All agree that about half are potentially able to cause disease in humans. The distinction between *M. tuberculosis* and nontuberculous mycobacteria can only be made in the laboratory and requires selective culture, biochemical, DNA/polymerase chain reactions, and RNA sequencing, as well as serology. Differential skin testing is unreliable and cross-sensitivity occurs; almost all MOTT produce hypersensitivity to tuberculin and confuse the validity of the standard tuberculin skin tests (PPD, Heaf, or Mantoux reactions).

These nontuberculous mycobacteria are all common in the environment and all are acid-fast. The commonest human pathogens are:

- *Mycobacterium leprae* (with reservoirs in man, armadillos, and perhaps some species of monkeys)
- *M. ulcerans* (skin and subcutaneous tissue)
- *M. kansasii* (lungs, bones; can disseminate)
- *M. marinum* (*M. balnei*) (skin granuloma)
- *M. avium-intracellulare* (lungs), *M. scrofulaceum* (lymph nodes) complex: the MAIS complex, formerly the Battey bacillus, can disseminate (see also discussion of *M. paratuberculosis* below)
- *M. xenopi*
- *M. fortuitum* complex (can disseminate rapidly)
- *M. chelonei* (can disseminate rapidly)
- *M. simiae* and *M. szulgai* (both of which are very rare)
- *M. malmoense* (rare: mainly in northern Europe)

Apart from *M. ulcerans*, all have low virulence and poor infectivity and seem to lack person-to-person transmission, but there is evidence that this may be altered by immunosuppression, since all the nontuberculous mycobacterial infections are being seen much more frequently because of the AIDS epidemic. The majority are resistant to most antituberculous drugs, but may be treated by multidrug regimens, often aided by surgery.

The frequency of MOTT in Europe and North America is 1%–3% of all new cases of tuberculosis. In Western Australia the frequency has increased to 16%. The prevalence of tuberculosis is not affected by other mycobacteria, nor do the MOTT bacilli give any protection against tuberculosis. Repeated isolation of the same mycobacterium is required before suggesting that this is the causal organism for any illness. If *M. tuberculosis* is also present, then this is likely to be the dominant organism. Although the incidence of MOTT disease is now showing a marked increase due to the AIDS epidemic, it has in the past been uncommon in most developing countries except when patients had preceding lung damage; for example, MOTT were cultured twice as often in African gold miners who had silicosis compared with those who did not. Despite AIDS, MOTT is still less common in the tropics than elsewhere. The MOTT bacteria may be more important as subliminal infections.

Many MOTT are low-grade pathogens and others exist as saprophytes. The known precipitating factors in infections are chronic lung damage, such as emphysema and bronchitis, industrial lung disease (both mining and agricultural), urban air pollution, and immunosuppression. All MOTT (except *M. ulcerans*) can rarely cause pulmonary lesions. *M. scrofulaceum* may cause cervical lymphadenitits in children under 12 years old. *M. kansasii* and *M. avium-intracellulare* often affect males over the age of 45. *M. ulcerans* infects mainly the panniculus; *M. marinum* (balnei) also affects the skin, as do *M. fortuitum* and *M. chelonei*.

There have been many descriptions of the radiological appearances of different MOTT pulmonary infections, and there are some small differences, but as already noted, it is not possible to distinguish radiologically between the mycobacteria. When an otherwise healthy patient with an apparently straightforward tuberculous infection fails to respond to adequate therapy, the commonest cause is drug resistance and the alternative is infection with a nontuberculous mycobacterium.

Mycobacterium paratuberculosis (Johne's bacillus). Within the *M. avium-intracellulare* complex is *M. paratuberculosis*, which is very common in the intestine of many animals, including cattle, sheep, and primates. It has been cultured from humans with chronic intestinal inflammation, resembling Crohn's disease. It is very difficult to recognize by culture and in some instances cannot be cultured at all. It is very resistant to most antituberculous drugs.

Its incidence in the tropics is not documented, but it has caused cervical lymphadenitis and chronic granulomas of the small intestine, closely resembling those found in the animal infection. Radiologically, a cobblestone appearance of the mucosa, with segmental narrowing of the terminal ileum, has been reported. Human infection is acquired from drinking infected milk from animals which may be apparently well and are subclinically infected. The AIDS epidemic, lowering the human immunity, opens the way to more widespread infection by this bacillus.

Tuberculosis of the Alimentary Tract

Despite the overall prevalence of tuberculosis in many parts of the tropics, there is no part of the world where tuberculosis commonly affects the gastrointestinal system. In the past, before drug therapy became available and patients died of advanced tuberculosis, about 80% were found to have abdominal tuberculosis at autopsy; the more advanced the pulmonary tuberculosis, the more likely there was to be bowel infection. However, now that treatment has become possible, the correlation of pulmonary tuberculosis with abdominal tuberculosis has altered, and less than 50% (in some series 25%) of patients with abdominal tuberculosis have pulmonary tuberculosis also. This ratio may again alter significantly with AIDS; for example, already in Haiti patients with AIDS are 3.5 times more likely to have extrapulmonary tuberculosis than patients who are HIV-negative.

Tuberculosis in the bowel starts as a localized inflammation of the lymphoid tissue and progresses to necrosis. The reaction can be ulcerating or hypertrophic or both. Tuberculous ulcers in the bowel are often transverse and linear, rather than round. Throughout the alimentary tract, tuberculosis forms granulomas which may be demonstrated as a mass, as distortion due to fibrosis, or as a stricture. When the infection has healed, there may be a residual scar, adhesions, or an ulcer on the damaged tissue.

Except in tuberculous peritonitis (p. 457) there are no clinical or laboratory criteria which are of any significance other than the histology. Stool culture for tuberculosis is unreliable. The symptomatology is vague and cannot be related satisfactorily to the abdominal lesions in the majority of patients. Ill health, vomiting, diarrhea (30%), and constipation (20%) are all generalized symptoms. Malabsorption is not uncommon. Analysis of the blood is normal except for anemia, which is very common in tropical countries and is more likely to indicate the presence of parasites rather than tuberculous bowel. There is no close relationship between pulmonary and alimentary tuberculosis. Many patients will have active lung disease, but a normal chest x-ray does not exclude tuberculosis in the alimentary tract.

The development of imaging by scanning (ultrasonography, CT, or MRI) has provided a better understanding of the pathophysiology and clinical pattern of tuberculosis in the abdomen. The diagnostic index of suspicion for tuberculosis has been raised, but unfortunately this is all that imaging can do; there are no specific changes for any form of intra-abdominal tuberculosis. Nevertheless, all current methods of imaging provide very useful guidance and are invaluable in follow-up during or after treatment.

The two most common alimentary forms are peritoneal and cecal tuberculosis; other sites are less frequently affected. But again, it is probable that the incidence and pattern will change in AIDS patients, particularly late in their disease, adding to the already difficult problem of differential diagnosis.

Tuberculosis of the Esophagus

There are three ways in which tuberculosis may present in the esophagus: (1) as a long stricture; (2) as gross dilatation above a narrow stricture, and (3) as ulceration, with or without a diverticulum. A tuberculous granuloma presenting as a mass in the esophagus does not appear to have been reported, but is a theoretical possibility.

The common site of infection is in the upper half of the esophagus (Fig. 5.37). The patient may present with difficulty in swallowing or with sudden impaction of food and acute dysphagia. Intrinsic tuberculosis of the upper third of the esophagus must be differentiated from the traction and fusiform pseudodiverticula which may be caused by fibrotic tuberculosis in the lung apices. In these patients the trachea is always deviated. Many texts state that traction diverticula in the mid-third of the esophagus are the result of adhesions from tuberculous mediastinal lymphadenopathy. None of the authors of this book, who together have considerable tropical and tuberculous experience, have ever seen this occur; it may happen, but it is not the cause of most esophageal diverticula. There are many thousands of patients with tuberculous mediastinal lymphadenopathy and very few with esophageal diverticula.

Tuberculosis may cause a hard nodular swelling in the thyroid, which often grows quite rapidly; it is only later in the disease that an abscess develops, either in the neck or, rarely, behind the sternum. A mediastinal tuberculous abscess spreading from nodal or vertebral infection also may cause pressure displacement of the esophagus but a pyogenic abscess or an intrathoracic goiter must also be considered. Tuberculous infection of the esophagus has been known to cause both bronchoesophageal fistu-

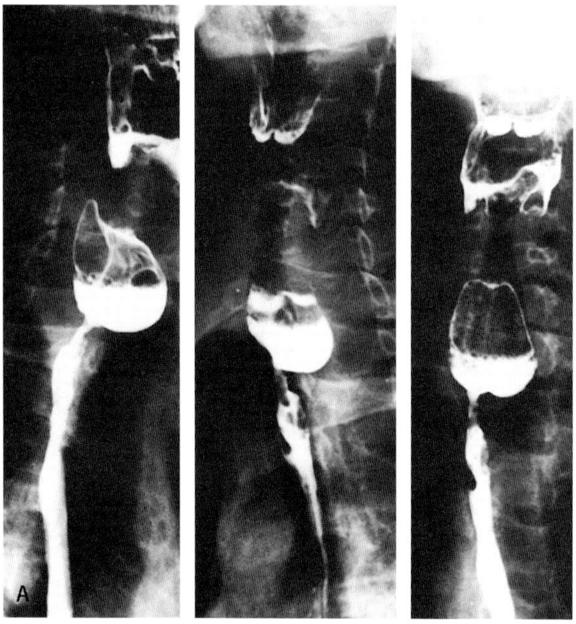

Fig. 5.37. A Tuberculosis of the esophagus. A stricture in the upper third of the esophagus which has all the characteristics of a carcinoma: only the histology can provide the diagnosis. (Courtesy of Dr. Jack Farman, Great Neck) B Mucosal edema and ulceration in the upper third of the esophagus of an Indian: he suffered from pain and dysphagia. This type of tuberculosis may eventually perforate (C) into the mediastinum but will still heal satisfactorily with the correct treatment. D A similar infection which has formed a pseudodiverticulum posteriorly in the lower third of the esophagus

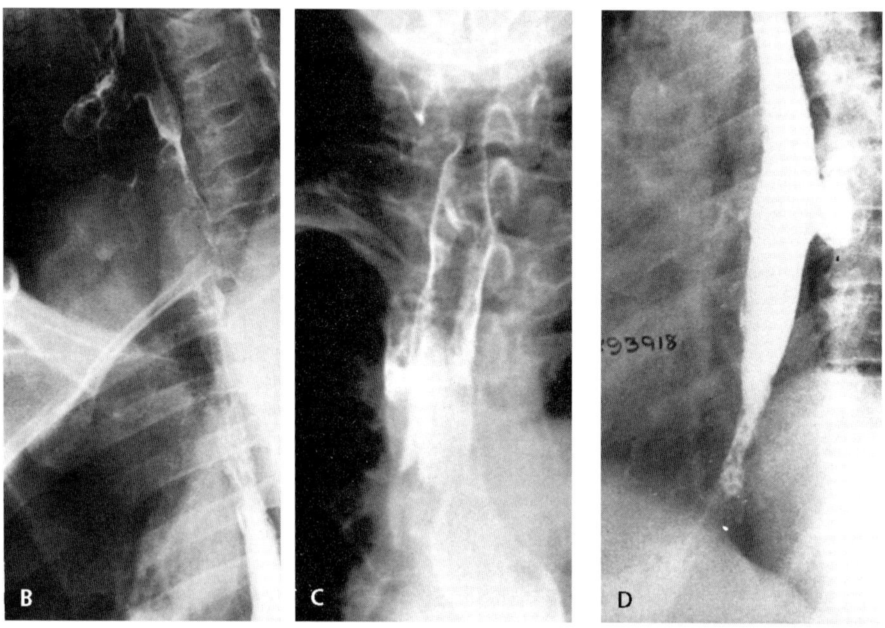

lae and erosion into an aortic aneurysm. These complications may become more common with AIDS.

Long-segment esophageal strictures with irregular granulations on the surface have to be differentiated from caustic burns, inflammatory or fungal esophagitis, and malignancy (Fig. 5.38). Carcinoma of the esophagus in the tropics may be multifocal and extend over 15 cm (6 inches) or more. Short-segment tuberculous strictures involving the lower third of the esophagus have to be differentiated from achalasia, peptic esophagitis and neoplasm; tuberculosis is a rare cause, and such differentiation is often impossible radiologically.

Tuberculosis of the Stomach

Tuberculosis of the Stomach is a very uncommon form of tuberculosis, although it may become more frequent in AIDS patients. However, it is unlikely to become easier to diagnose either clinically or radiologically. The clinical history and the imaging appearance may suggest simple peptic ulceration, other granulomatous diseases, lymphoma, or carcinoma of the stomach. Even at surgery the macroscopic appearances can resemble malignancy and the differential diagnosis may only be made histologically.

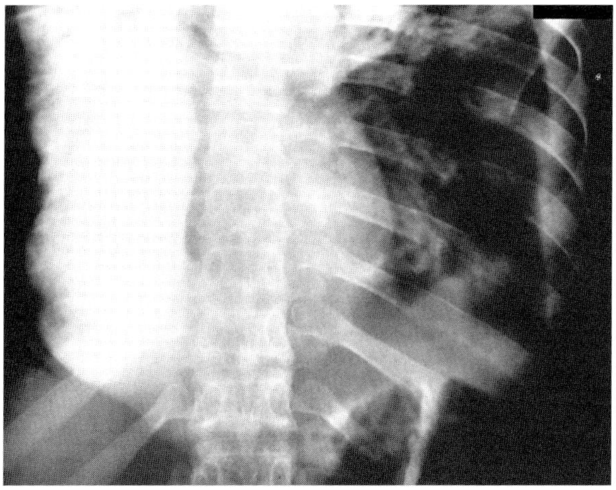

Fig. 5.38. Tuberculosis of the lower end of the esophagus causing a stricture just above the cardia. The huge dilated esophagus lies on the right side of the mediastinum and closely resembles the esophagus in achalasia or Chagas' disease. The patient had active pulmonary tuberculosis and a left pleural effusion, but histological examination of the esophagus provided the correct diagnosis. (Courtesy of Ms. A. A. Whitemore, Harare)

Radiologically, tuberculosis of the stomach may present as shallow ulceration, (which can be extensive), a granulomatous mass or as fibrosis (Fig. 5.39). The most common of these is ulceration at the pylorus, which causes gastric outlet obstruction. It resembles and often cannot be distinguished from fibrosis following peptic ulceration or from malignancy. Tuberculosis is yet another cause of gastric dilatation, but is sufficiently rare as to be a surprise to both the radiologist and the surgeon when histology is obtained. Tuberculous gastric ulceration has been reported on both the greater and lesser curvatures off the stomach, usually surrounded by induration and therefore reducing peristalsis.

These ulcers are usually shallow but can be quite large. The likely mistaken radiological diagnosis will be lymphoma or carcinoma.

The tuberculous granulomatous mass in the stomach is the least common presentation of this uncommon form of tuberculosis. With such a mass, there is always associated mucosal ulceration and surrounding fibrosis. The ulcers are chronic and will be mistaken for malignancy.

The shape of the stomach (and duodenum) can be distorted by extrinsic pressure from enlarged tuberculous lymph nodes (Fig. 5.40, 5.41). These usually compress on the distal third of the stomach and in some cases are adherent. In one such patient there was a very large gastroesophageal mass at the cardia causing distortion, with an overlying gastric ulcer. Although ultrasonography, CT or MRI can demonstrate the lymphadenopathy, the correct diagnosis is not likely to be achieved by imaging.

Fibrotic tuberculosis can mimic linitis plastica, scirrhous carcinoma, infiltrating lymphoma, or even syphilis. To this differential diagnosis must be added Crohn's disease, which is rare in the tropics.

Tuberculosis of the Duodenum and Small Intestine (Fig. 5.41, 5.42)

The clinical presentation in most cases is of upper small bowel obstruction, but occasionally the obstruction is lower, in the ileum. There is usually a history of intermittent attacks of abdominal pain, with nausea and sometimes vomiting; when the small bowel is involved, malabsorption and malnutrition occur more frequently. Eventually the obstruction becomes persistent.

Abdominal radiographs in the supine and erect positions will show dilated loops of small bowel and fluid levels. In one series from India, there were dilated loops of bowel in 54% of patients with abdominal tuberculosis and, in over half of them, there were fluid levels on the erect radiographs. Tuberculosis causes different patterns of small bowel disease. Infiltrating tuberculous granulomas around the duodenum result in loss of normal mucosal pattern, rigidity, and narrow strictures; a stricture of the third part of the duodenum (particularly in India) should raise the suspicion of tuberculosis. In the ileum, the Peyer's patches are affected and transverse ulcers develop with typical undermined edges. In the early stages, when there is minimal dilatation of the ileal loops with excess fluid in the lumen and no significant stricture, the barium forms bubbles with ill-defined edges; later as the strictures become well established, the barium column is trapped proximal to the stricture, and outlines the stricture and dilated lumen. The dilated ileum can reach mammoth proportions. It may be necessary to introduce a peroral small intestinal tube for a selective small-bowel enema to demonstrate the stricture. These strictures are most common in the ileum but may be seen in the jejunum and even in the duodenum. Tuberculous strictures are not as long as those of regional enteritis, and in addition, as noted earlier, Crohn's disease is extremely rare in India and many other tropical countries. Occasionally in tuberculosis there are fistulae in addition to the strictures, and the differential diagnosis then becomes impossible without histological examination. Calcified enteroliths are commonly seen within dilated loops of small bowel proximal to tuberculous strictures, but are uncommon in any other chronic enteritis (see Fig. 5.42 F and p. 457).

(Text continues on p. 448)

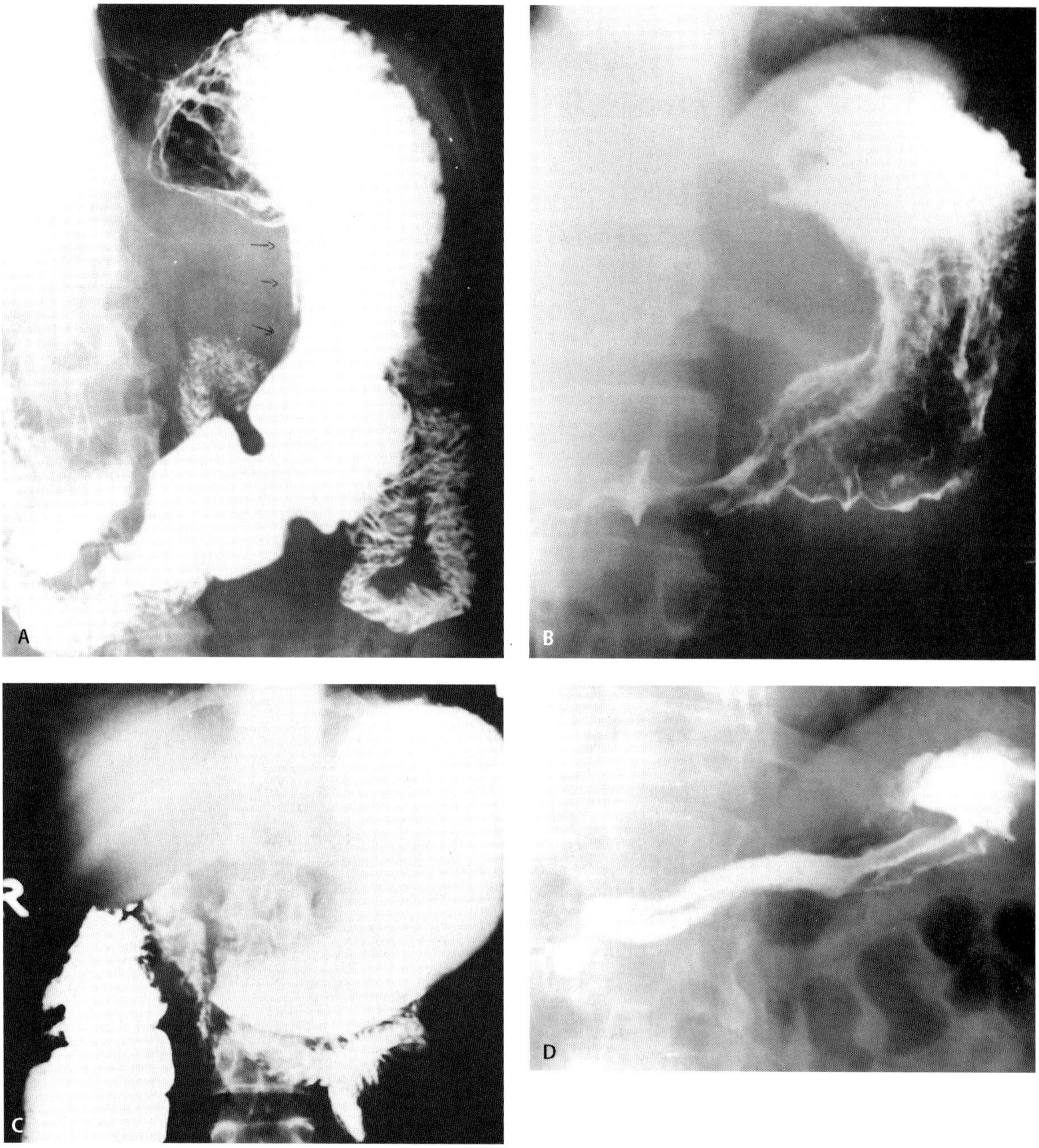

▲ **Fig. 5.39 A–D.** Tuberculosis of the stomach. **A** Mucosal ulceration and edema along the lesser curvature of the stomach of a patient from India. **B** Tuberculous gastritis causing thickening of the wall of the stomach and narrowing of the pyloric antrum of an African patient. **C** Granulomatous tuberculosis thickening and immobilizing the lesser curvature of the stomach from below the cardia down to the pylorus. In each of these patients the radiological diagnosis is likely to be carcinoma or lymphoma because tuberculosis of the stomach is rare. **D** Tuberculosis of the stomach resembling linitis plastica. The stomach would not distend beyond this size and peristalsis was absent. The radiological diagnosis was malignancy: it may be impossible even at surgery to distinguish tuberculosis without histological confirmation

Fig. 5.40 A–F. Pressure on the stomach and duodenum from tuberculous lymphadenopathy. **A** Displacement of the second part of the duodenum downwards and the third portion upwards. An African patient. **B** Distortion of both the lesser and greater curvature of the stomach and the pyloric antrum, with stretching of the pylorus and partial obstruction of the second and third parts of the duodenum. **C** Persistent pressure on the great curvature of the stomach which was thought to be due to carcinoma of the pancreas. The patient complained of abdominal swelling and pain. At surgery there was a large inoperative "tumor" which was found on histology to be due to active tuberculosis. Where it had originated remained undecided, but the patient responded to appropriate treatment. (Courtesy of the University of Capetown, Radiology Library) Continued on p. 443

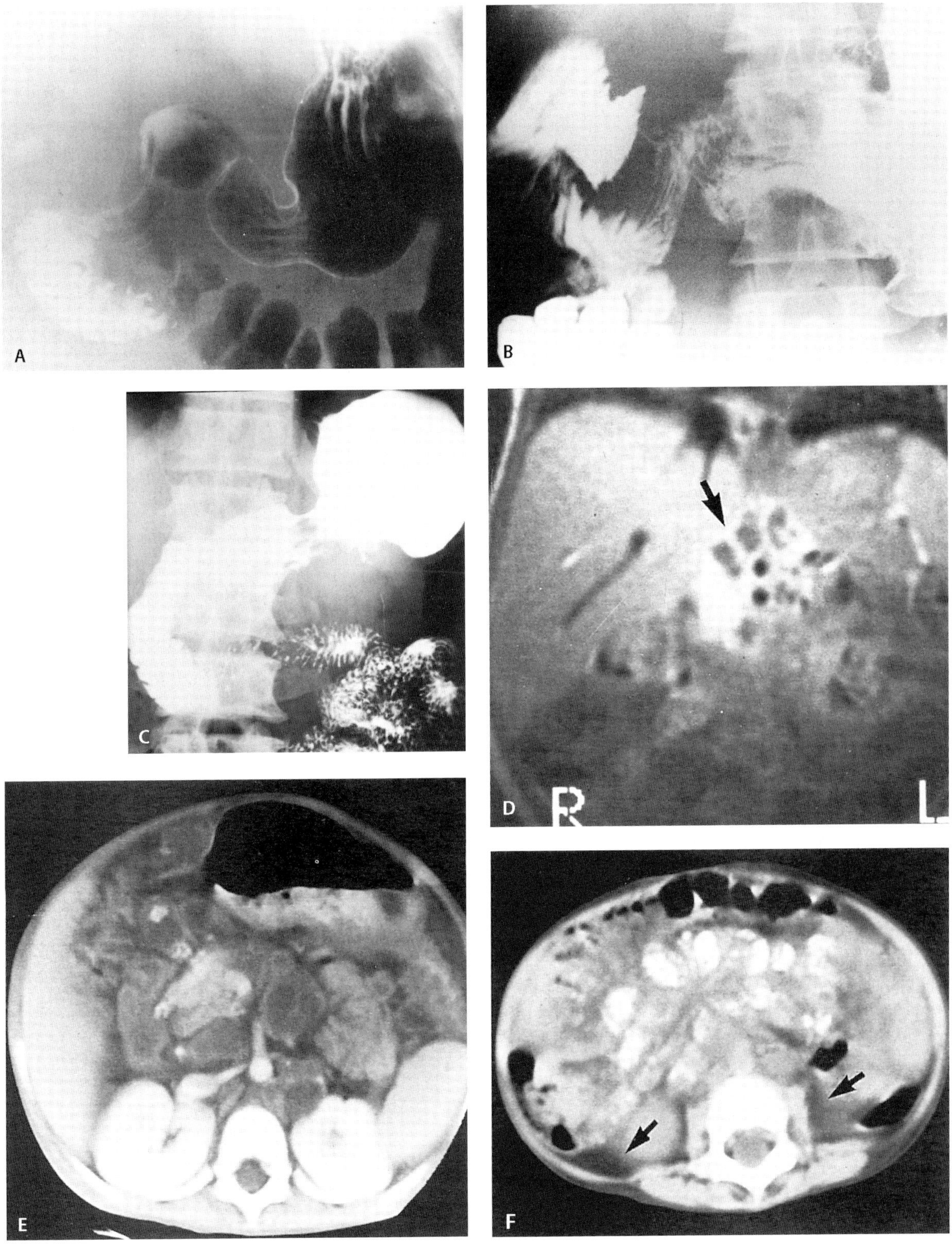

Fig. 5.40 (*continued*). **D** Intravenous gadolinium-enhanced T1-weighted MR scan showing an enhanced nodal inflammatory mass (*arrow*) with areas of nonenhancing necrosis. **E** A contrast-enhanced CT scan showing multiple rim-enhancing nodes in the periaortic region. **F** A CT scan of a child from South Africa shows diffuse calcification in enlarged mesenteric lymph nodes. There is also some ascites (*arrows*). (**D–F** from Cremin and Jamieson 1995)

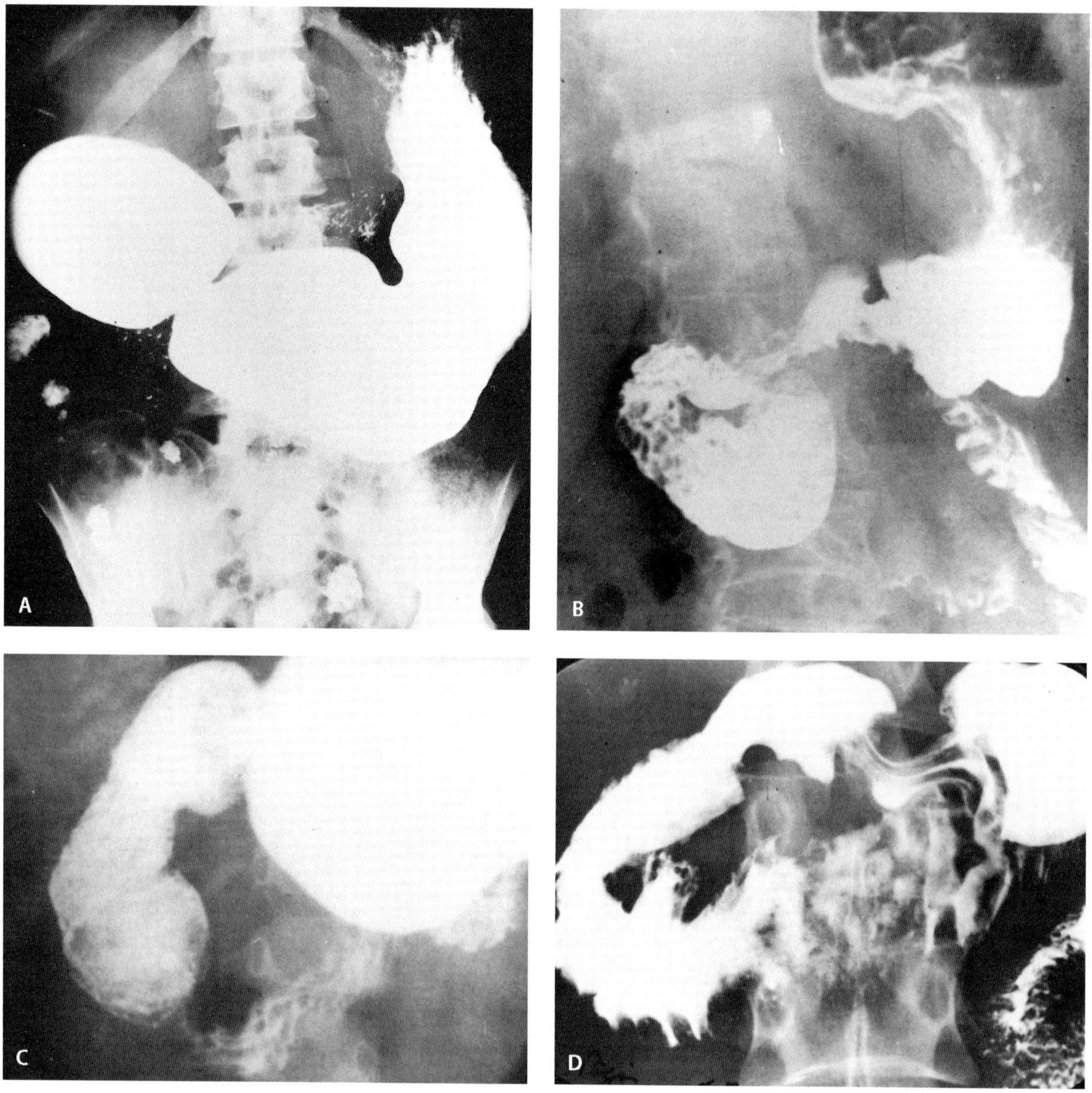

Fig. 5.41 A–H. The pressure from tuberculous lymph nodes may eventually cause obstruction in the duodenum. **A** A large duodenal bulb due to obstruction of the second part of the duodenum, caused by fibrosis following tuberculous lymphadenitis. **B** A stricture at the junction of the second and third parts of the duodenum of a 6-year-old child from India, which caused partial obstruction. This was the result of adhesions from previous tuberculous lymphadenitis. Both A and B could be misdiagnosed as the result of congenital bands (Ladd's syndrome). **C** Pressure on the second part of the duodenum and obstruction at the junction of the third and fourth parts by enlarged lymph nodes and tuberculous duodenitis. **D** Tuberculous mucosal ulceration and edema of the second, third, and fourth parts of the duodenum. This could be mistaken for lymphoma or even a severe parasitic infection. With proper treatment this condition may heal completely, or result in strictures. **E–H** see p. 445

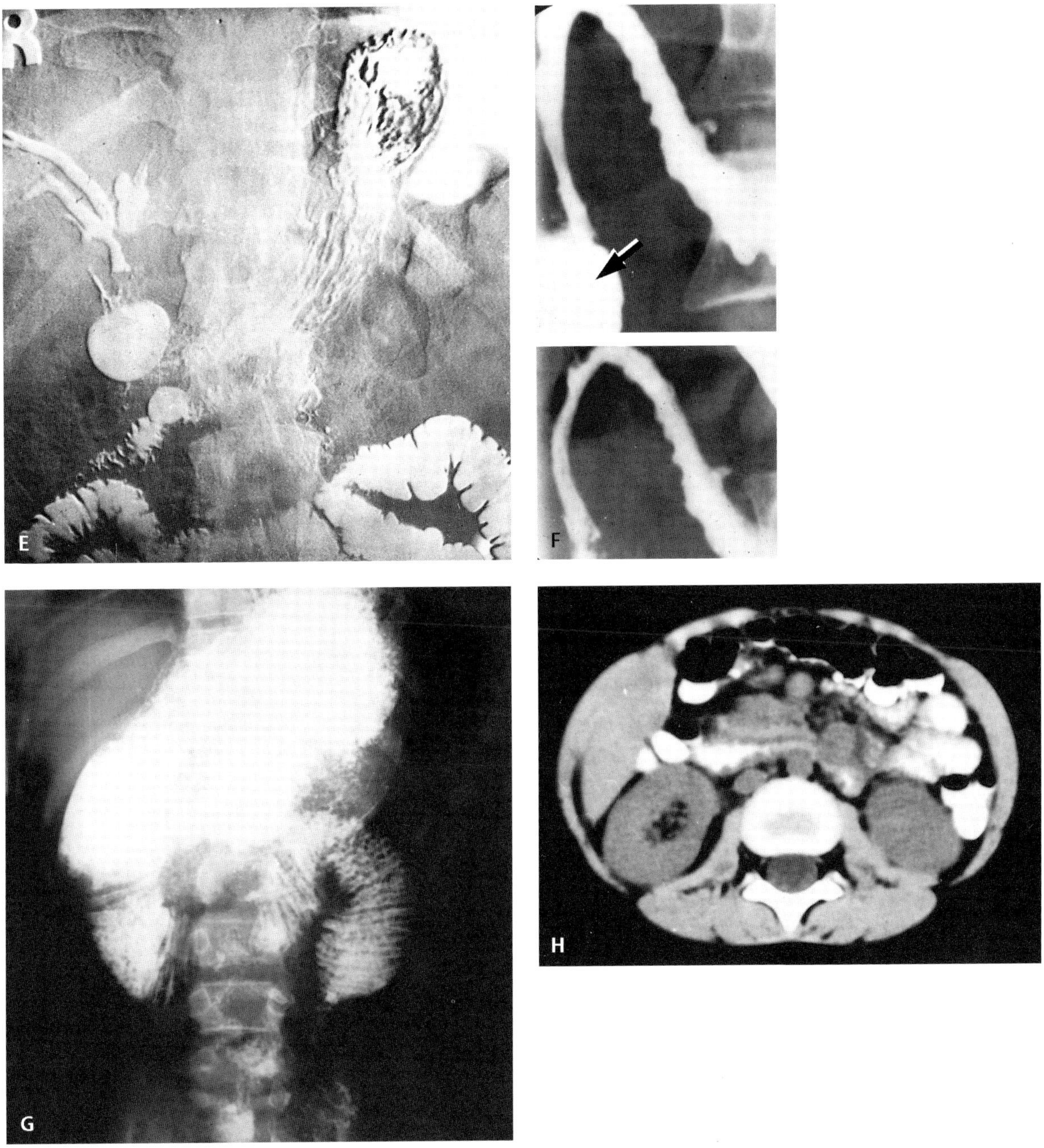

Fig. 5.41 (*continued*). **E** Perforation of a tuberculous ulcer of the second part of the duodenum into the biliary tract, with reflux of bile. (There are two incidental duodenal diverticula.) **F** Intense spasm due to tuberculous ulceration of the first and second parts of the duodenum of an Arab patient. Tuberculosis was confirmed histologically. (The *arrow* points to an artefact.) **G** A funnel-shaped stricture in the proximal jejunum of a 12-year-old Arab female. **H** A CT scan shows pressure on the transverse duodenum from lymphadenopathy. There was also an ileal stricture which is not demonstrated

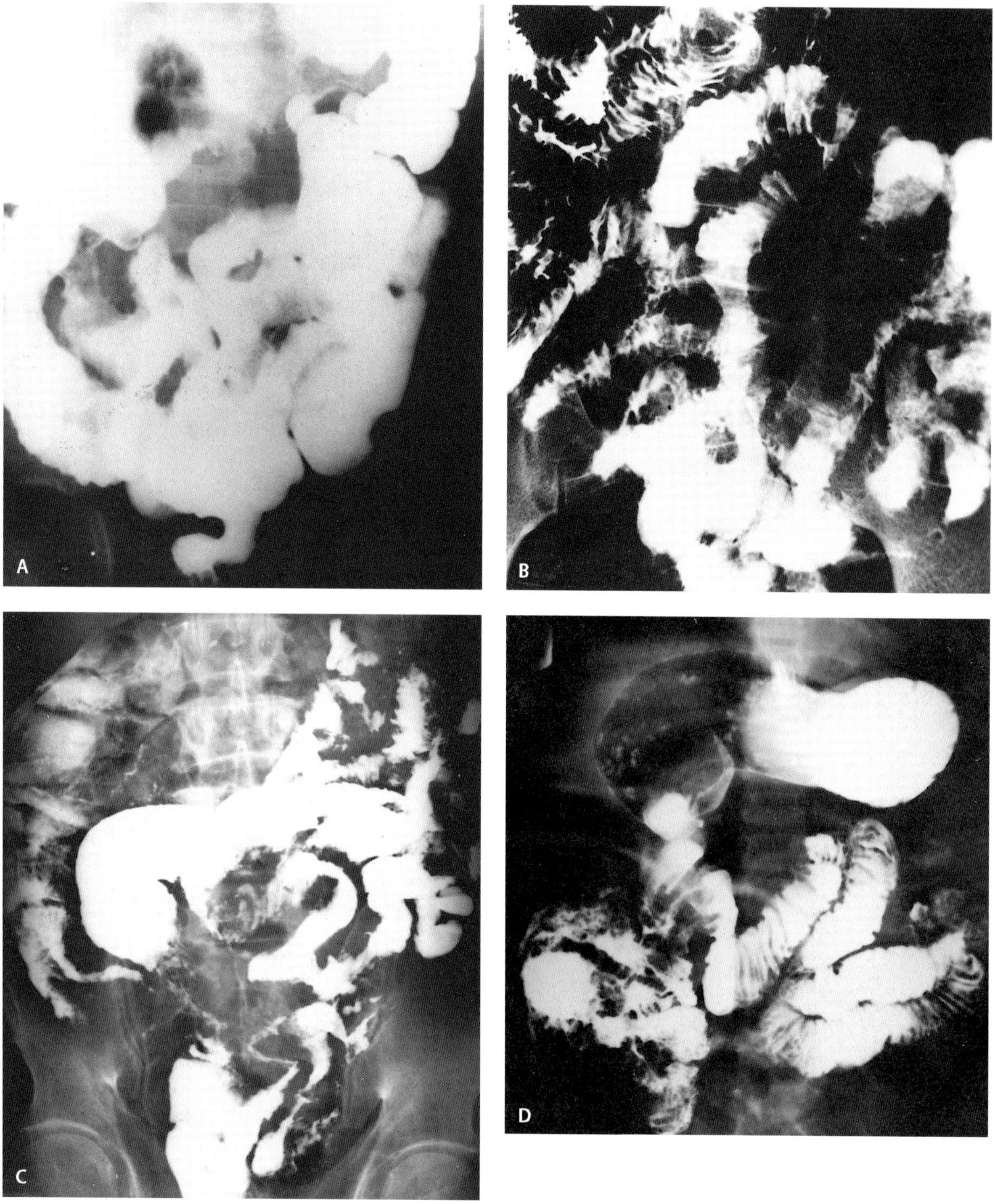

Fig. 5.42 A–H. Tuberculosis of the small intestine. **A** The acute phase with loss of normal bowel pattern, excess fluid within the gut, and rapid transit of barium. **B** Multiple granulomatous strictures and dilated lengths of bowel. **C** Multiple lengths of dilatation and strictures with fistula formation, indistinguishable from regional enteritis except by histology. **D** A tuberculous duodenal-colic fistula in a 7-year-old child with malabsorption (incidental stomach rotation). **E–H** see p. 447

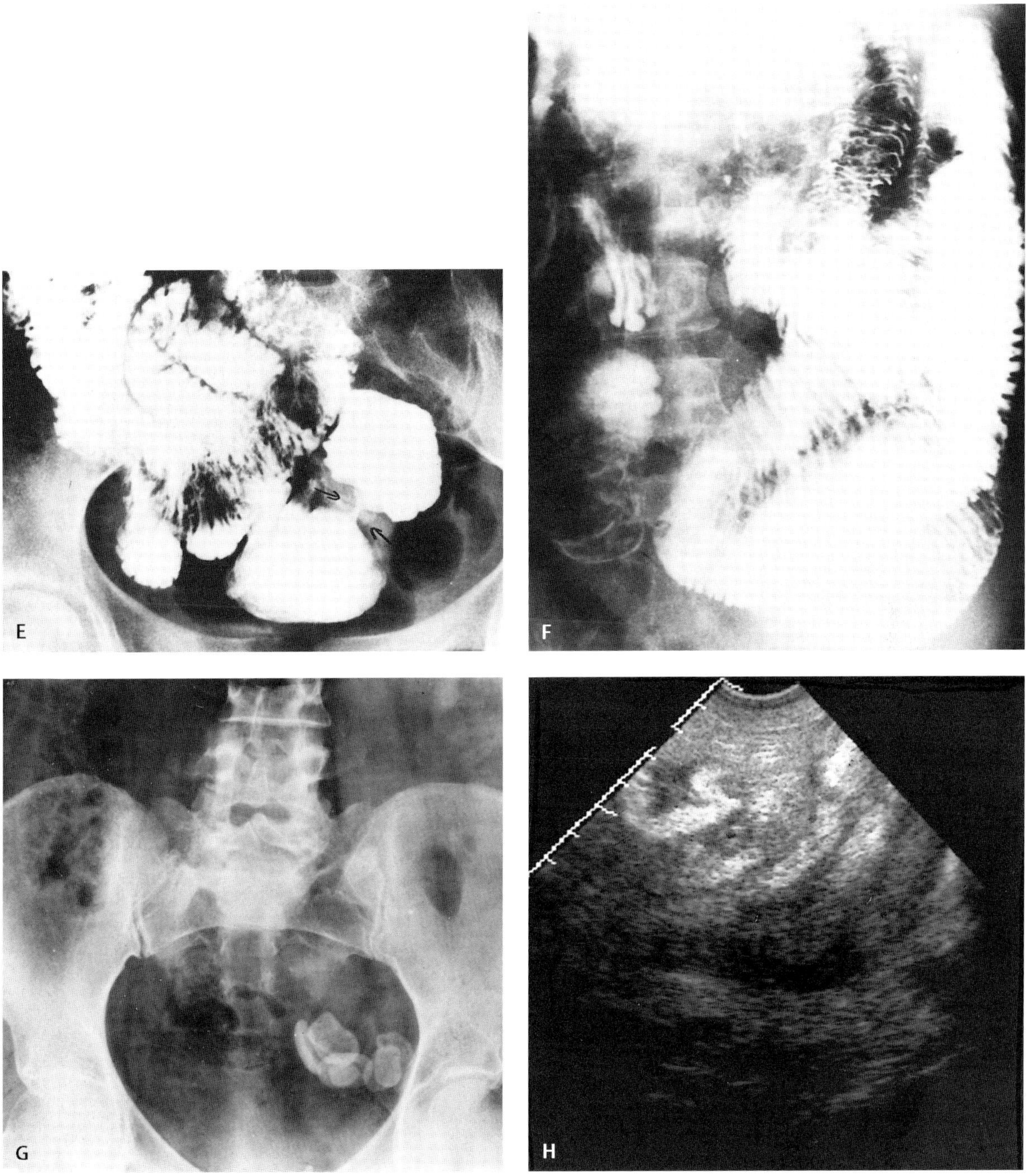

Fig. 5.42 (*continued*). **E** A narrow "apple core" stricture in the ileum (*arrows*). **F** Partial obstruction of the mid-ileum due to tuberculous granulation tissue. **G** Enteroliths in the small bowel of a patient from India, with multiple strictures in the small bowel from tuberculosis. **H** Ultrasonography can be used to show the thick wall of tuberculous small bowel and will often demonstrate that the bowel loops are adherent of clumped together. This patient was an African male, aged 43 years, from Zimbabwe. (**B** courtesy of the University of Capetown Radiology Library; **C** AFIP 229499; **D** courtesy of Dr. D. Makanjuola and *Eur J Radiol*, 1998; **H** courtesy of Dr. Sam Mindel)

When scanned by ultrasonography, CT, or MRI, the bowel lesions demonstrate the same imaging pattern. There is concentric bowel wall thickening, often with ulceration; this may be seen in any region of the small bowel or even into the colon. There is also narrowing of the lumen, which can be correlated with barium studies. It is not always easy to demonstrate such strictures by scanning. The bowel loops become matted together and adhesions, exudates, inter-loop fluid, or abscess may form complex masses. A "sandwich" appearance has been described when fluid collects close to the bowel wall and there is focal ascites; this results in alternating echogenic and echo-free layers through the wall of the bowel, showing the serosa, the fluid, and then the pattern of the adjacent bowel wall. Omental thickening (described as "caking") can also be demonstrated; a tuberculoma of the omentum has been recorded. Some loops of bowel will be dilated, others more normal or narrowed. Bowel wall thickness of more than 5 mm during contraction and 3 mm during distention is said to be abnormal, but whether this also applies in patients who have malabsorption or added parasitic infection is not known. In abdominal tuberculosis there is likely to be concomitant lymphadenopathy (p. 457), and any part of the small bowel, but especially the duodenum and jejunum, can be distorted and displaced by enlarged tuberculous lymph nodes. Adhesions are frequent and the mucosal folds may be stretched over the nodes. It is unusual for complete obstruction to result from this type of extrinsic lesion.

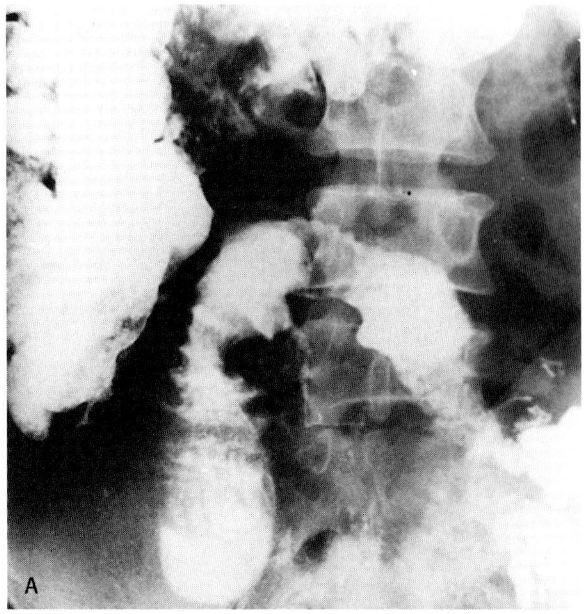

A

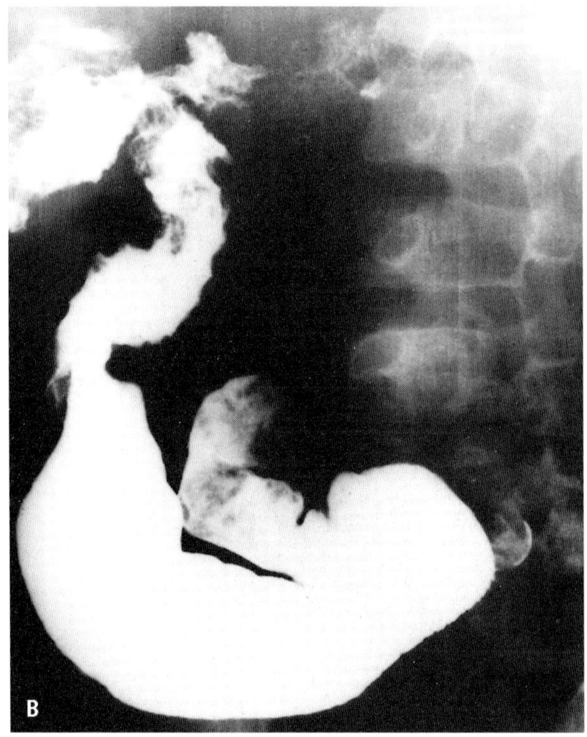

B

Fig. 5.43 A–E. Tuberculosis of the terminal ileum and cecum. A Dilatation, edema, and ulceration of the terminal ileum. B The contracted cecum which is the result of tuberculosis in a five-year-old child from India. There is marked adynamic dilatation of the terminal ileum, mucosal ulceration, and loss of the normal ileal pattern. C–E see p. 449

Tuberculosis of the Cecum (Hyperplastic Tuberculosis of the GI Tract)

Tuberculosis of the cecum is one of the most common types of intra-abdominal tuberculosis, and in some series it accounts for up to 60% of all tuberculous bowel infections. (The other common sites are the peritoneum and lymph nodes.) The clinical symptoms are vague. There may be alternating diarrhea and constipation, changes in bowel habit, a palpable mass and vague crampy pain in the right iliac fossa, general ill health, and anemia, but all are nonspecific. When tuberculosis affects the cecum and distal ileum (Fig. 5.43), initially there will be intense ileocecal spasm seen on barium studies or small bowel examination (Stierlin's sign). Later, the lumen and size of the cecum are compromised as the granulomas form into a mass and undergo fibrosis. The mesocolon of the cecum contracts; the cecum is pulled up out of the right iliac fossa and shrinks (Figs. 5.44, 5.45), often drastically, culminating in the classical conical, pyramidal, or at times, pear-shaped configuration. The associated fibrosis

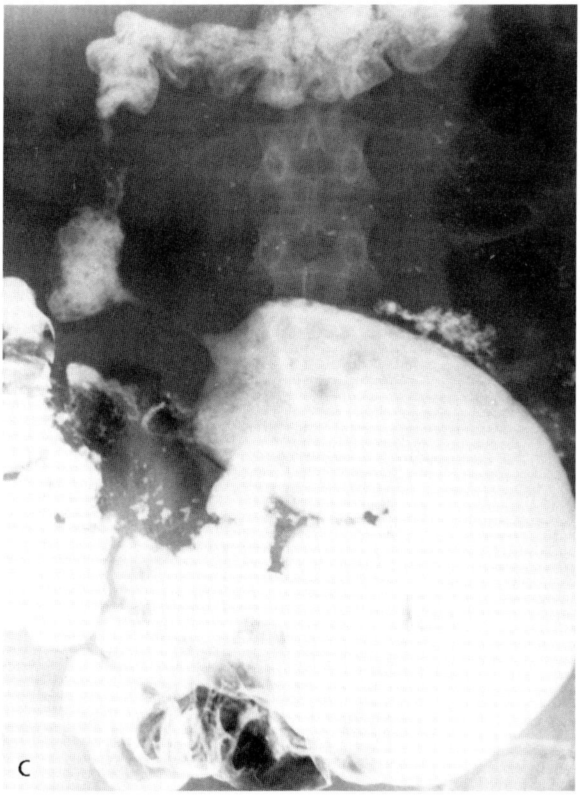

causes a partial stricture at the ileocecal region and the dilated terminal ileum appears to be suspended from the cecum like a pendulum. There is restricted movement of the cecum on palpation, not only transversely but also in the craniocaudal axis. Sinus formation is uncommon unless there has been inadequate surgical interference; sinus formation and osteomyelitis of the ilium suggest a mycotic infection, usually actinomycosis, not tuberculosis.

Scanning by any method, but particularly ultrasonography will show thickening of the bowel wall in the ileocecal region and in the ascending colon (Fig. 5.46, p. 452). In many patients the right iliac fossa may be comparatively empty because the cecum has been drawn up by fibrosis. When thickening occurs, it is nearly always concentric but may be distorted by the peritoneal adhesions. Ulceration in the ileocecal area is always associated with bowel wall thickening and may be superficial or deep. The correlation between scanning and barium studies is good, but the typical appearance as shown by barium enema may be more diagnostically accurate. The irregular pattern of spicules and progressive narrowing, together with displacement of the cecum, is likely to be more marked than in amebiasis.

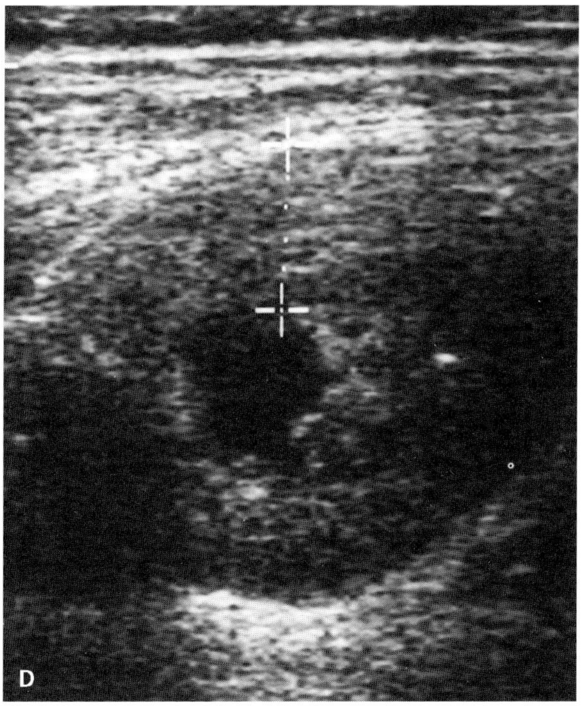

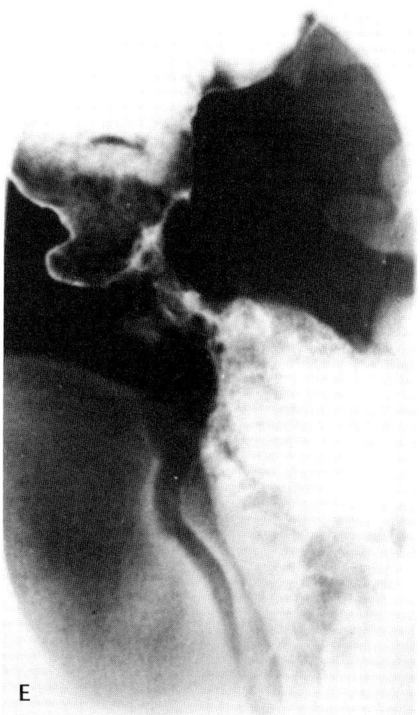

Fig. 5.43 (*continued*). **C** Gross dilatation of the terminal ileum above a long stricture proximal to a contracted tuberculous cecum. **D** The sonogram of the thickened cecum of a child from the Pacific Islands with ileocecal tuberculosis. **E** A tuberculous ulcer at the ileocecal junction, causing marked constriction and distortion, with resulting obstruction and dilatation of the ileum above it. (**D** courtesy of Dr. Cheryl Sisler, Hawaii)

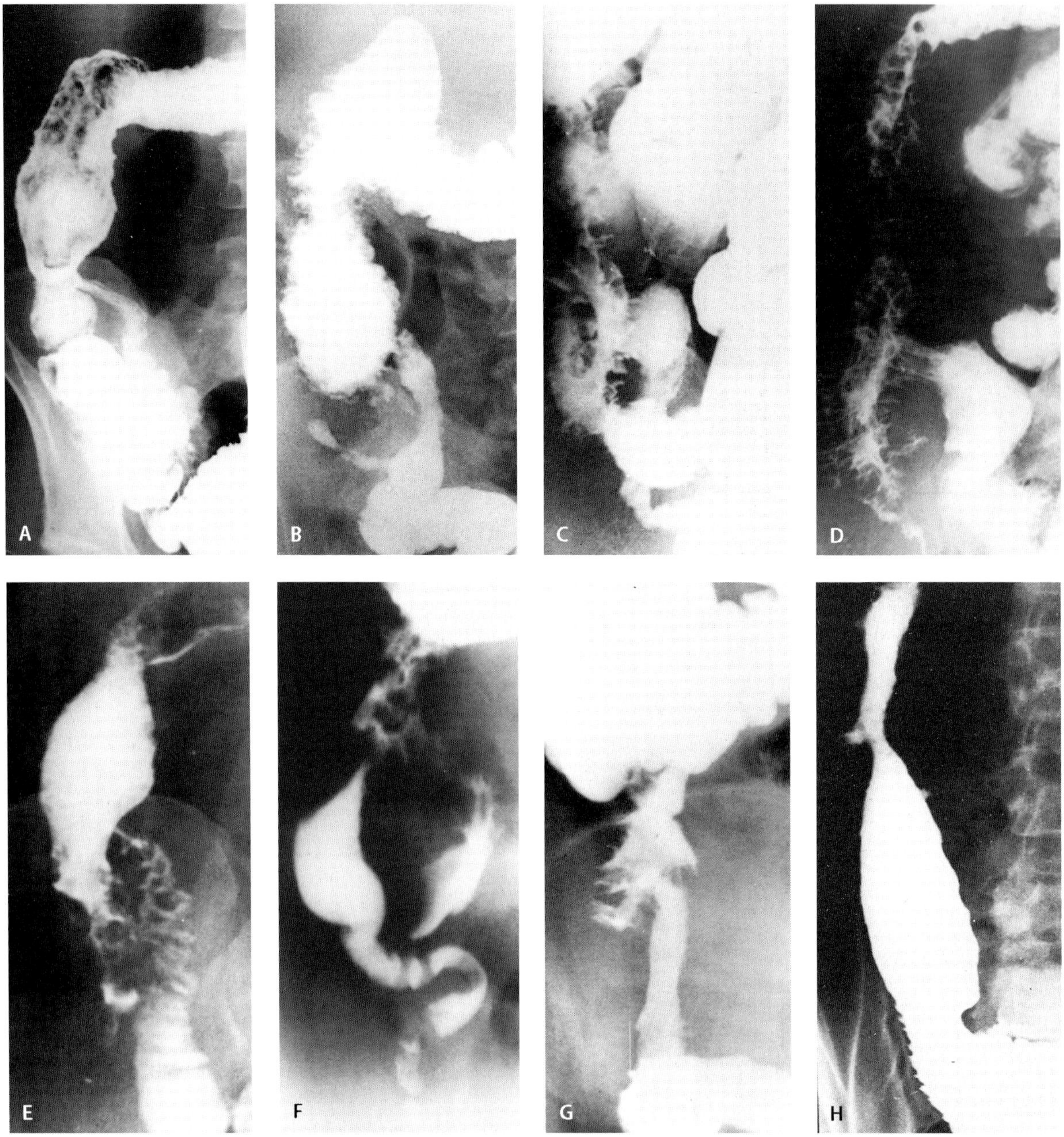

Fig. 5.44 A–H. Tuberculosis affects the cecum in different ways, but the end result is almost always contraction and considerable distortion. These figures illustrate eight different cases from different parts of the world. **A** Early mucosal ulceration and edema, with shrinkage. The infection has caused ulceration of the proximal half of the transverse colon. **B** Mucosal edema and ulceration of the right side of the colon and of the terminal ileum, which is beginning to dilate. The appendix is also infected. **C** The cecum is contracted, grossly edematous, and ulcerated, and the terminal ileum is dilated. **D** Gross and extensive mucosal edema with nodulation and spiculation of the cecum and ascending colon. The ileocecal valve is patent and the terminal ileum is also edematous and nodular. **E–H** Four different examples of shrinkage of the tuberculous cecum. In **E** and **F** the terminal ileum is not affected or even obstructed, but the cecum is much reduced in size. In **G** there is some ulceration of the terminal ileum, but only minimal obstruction and mild dilatation. In **H** the cecum is very small, and the ileum is dilated and almost seems to hang from the small narrow cecum

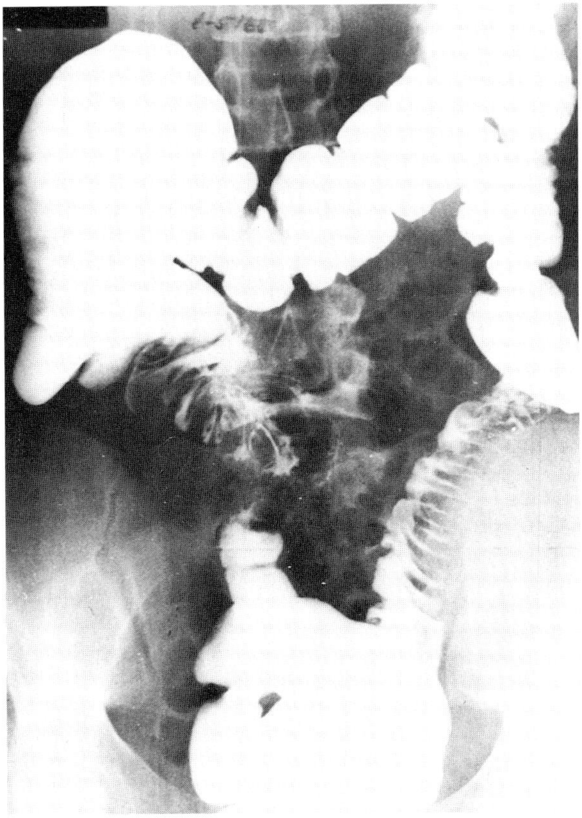

Fig. 5.45. Tuberculosis often affects more than one part of the bowel. This patient had a palpable mass in the right iliac fossa which clinically suggested malignancy. The barium enema showed that the cecum was displaced upwards and both the cecum and terminal ileum had edematous, swollen mucosa. However, there were marked mucosal changes in the sigmoid colon also, which led to the alternative diagnosis of amebiasis. Tuberculosis was not considered but the combination of fixation of the ileocecal junction, the contracted cecum, and small bowel adhesions is typical of tuberculosis. The palpable mass was due to enlarged lymph nodes

In children in particular, the ileocecal valve may be so thick that it mimics a mass in the cecum; it remains patent because of the fibrosis. Oral contrast is helpful with CT scanning to show the thickness of the bowel wall and narrowing of the lumen. However, in many cases only histology will provide the correct diagnosis.

The differential diagnosis includes an appendiceal abscess, amebiasis, actinomycosis, granulomatous colitis, and malignancy. Tenderness on palpation is maximal with appendiceal abscess, tethering of the cecum is maximal in tuberculosis, and sinus formation and adjacent osteomyelitis are most common in actinomycosis. Reflux into the ileum due to loss of ileocecal sphincter action is easily demonstrated in amebiasis and malignancy, in spite of the tumor; reflux is less common in tuberculosis in the early stages because of spasm, and later because of fibrosis. Amebic infection can present as granulomatous disease also, but the fibrosis accompanying tuberculosis is more severe than that seen in amebiasis. Multiple granulomas and strictures may also occur in amebic infection, but in over 90% of patients with amebiasis only the last 6 inches of small bowel are involved, whereas in tuberculosis and Crohn's disease the terminal ileum is involved in 45%–50% or more of patients with cecal disease. Lymphoma will have to be considered, but carcinoma, granulomatous colitis, and ischemic colitis are all rare in most tropical countries.

Tuberculosis of the Large Intestine

When tuberculosis affects the large bowel, the clinical symptoms vary from constipation to diarrhea. The presentation may be incomplete obstruction; there is seldom pain, but the majority of patients are in general ill health (though a small number are surprisingly well).

Radiologically and endoscopically, tuberculous granulomas present in the colon either as colitis or stricture; both can be multifocal. In the early stages the mucosa may be ulcerated (Fig. 5.47). There may be aphthoid ulcers (with central flecks of barium, some surrounded by a translucent halo on a normal mucosa). Short lengths are most commonly affected; tuberculosis does not involve the colon extensively, but in some cases it is associated with small bowel infection.

The radiological differential diagnosis can be very difficult and tuberculous colitis cannot be distinguished from amebiasis (Fig. 5.48); however, aphthoid ulcers are more commonly associated with Crohn's disease or amebiasis. Tuberculous granulomas cause strictures quite indistinguishable from an ameboma and both tuberculosis and amebiasis can also mimic the apple-core stricture of carcinoma of the colon, producing the same chronic, progressive obstruction. Radiological differentiation may be impossible; only histology can be accurate. Fortunately, malignant disease of the large bowel is uncommon in much of the tropics.

(Text continues on p. 455)

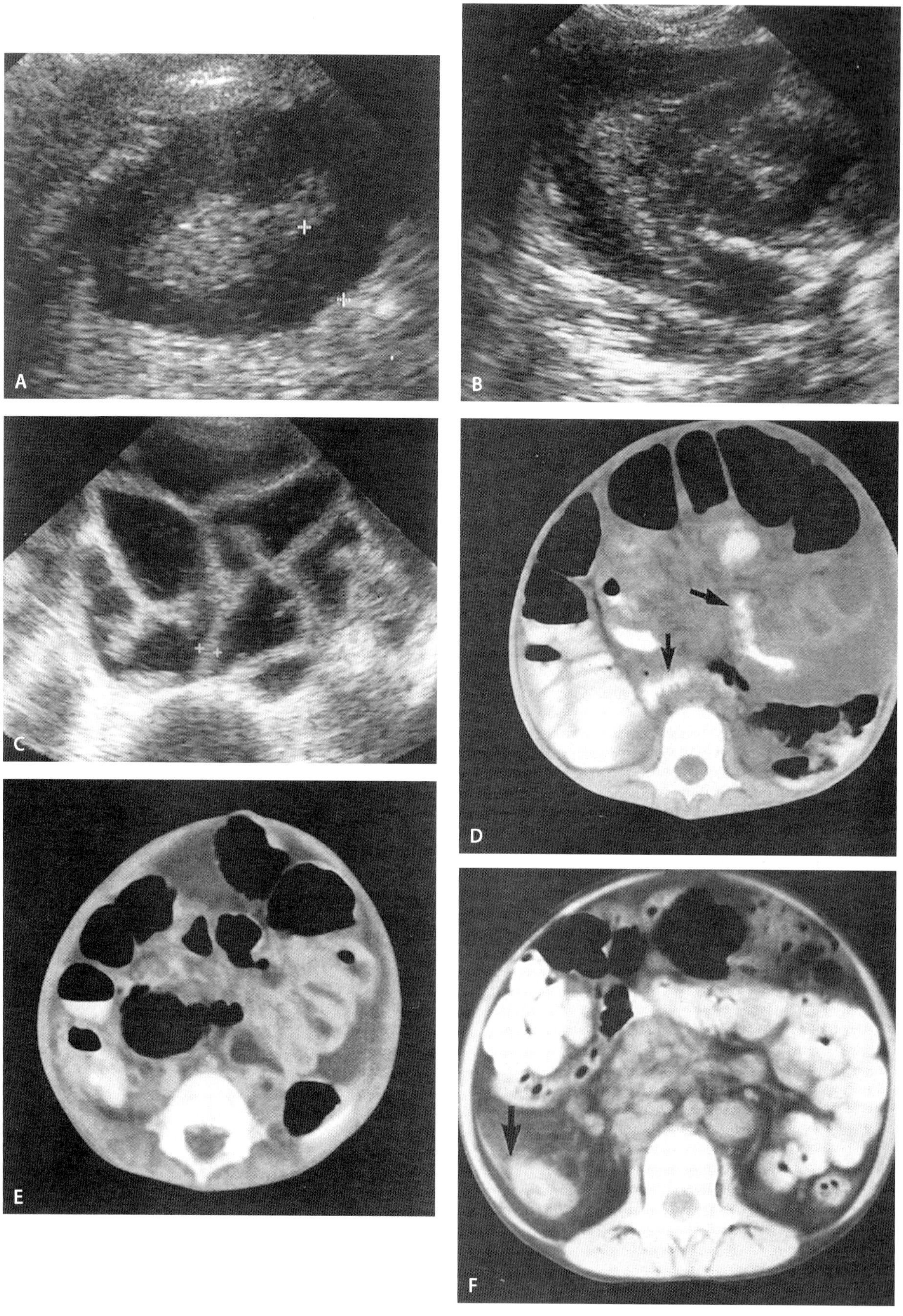
A
B
C
D
E
F

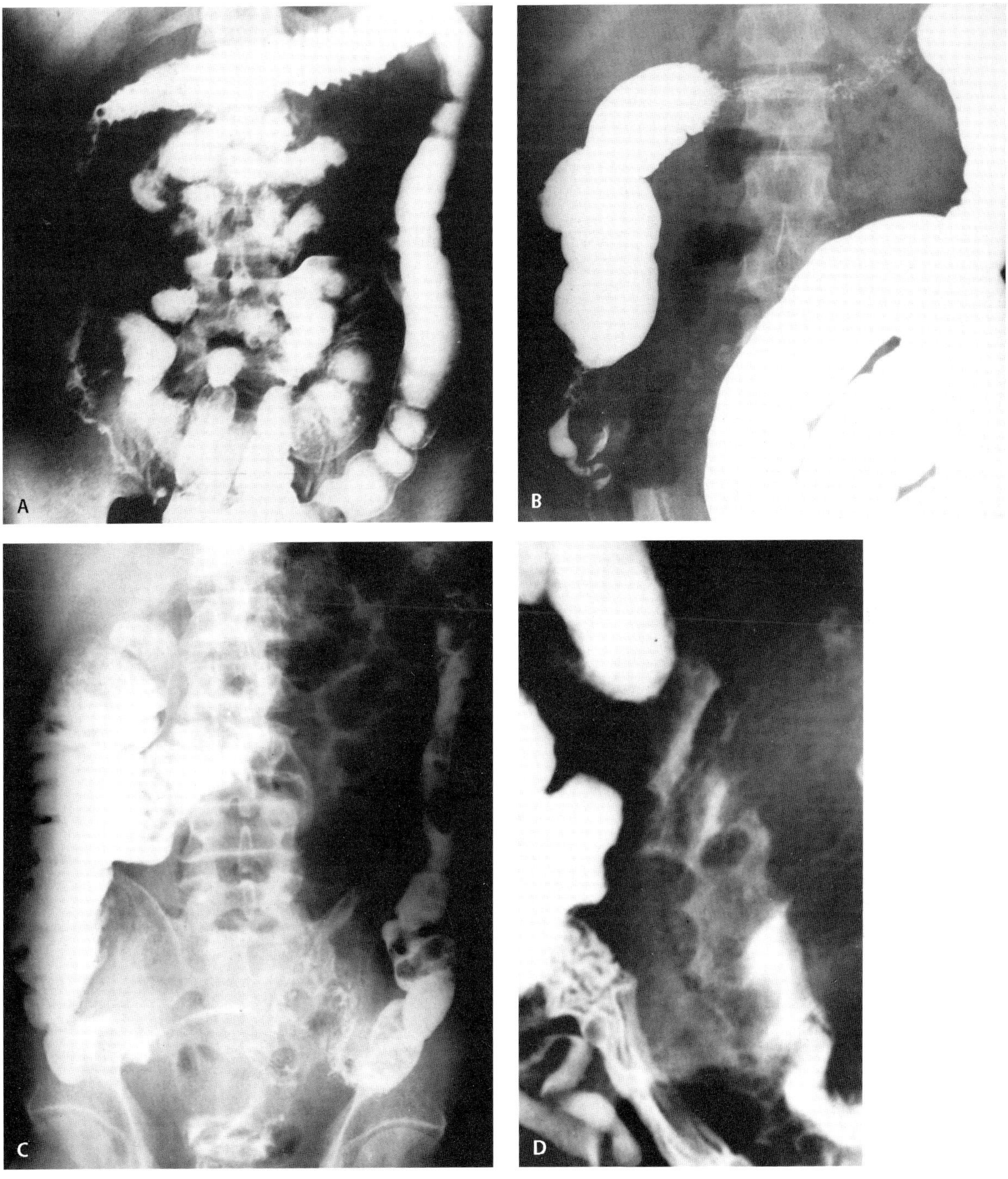

Fig. 5.46 A–F. Scanning, both ultrasonography and CT, can demonstrate the type of mass shown in Fig. 5.45 but can also be used to show thickening of the bowel wall and ascites. **A–C** Sonograms showing thick-walled bowel, groups of thick-walled bowel matted together, and distended small bowel with echogenic walls and ascites. **D–F** scans of children showing the thick walls of ileum (*arrows*) filled with contrast, contrast-enhanced mural thickening, and a thickened irregular contrast-filled cecum (*arrow*). The patients shown in **D–F** all had ascites. (From Cremin and Jamieson 1995)

Fig. 5.47 A–H. Tuberculous colitis can affect any part of the large bowel. **A** Tuberculosis affecting the cecum, ascending colon and much of the transverse colon. **B** Tuberculosis affecting the cecum, apparently sparing the ascending colon but involving the transverse colon. **C** Tuberculosis affecting the left half of the colon. In each of these patients there is spasm, saw-tooth distortion of the bowel wall, mucusal ulceration, and edema. In **A** and **C** there is excess mucus which is better seen in **B**, in which the edema is so acute that there is thumbprinting. This patient had active pulmonary tuberculosis. **D** Mucosal ulceration in the sigmoid colon of a child: the lower part of the colon is straight because of the peritoneal thickening. It would be difficult by any imaging method to distinguish any of these cases from amebiasis. E–H see p. 454

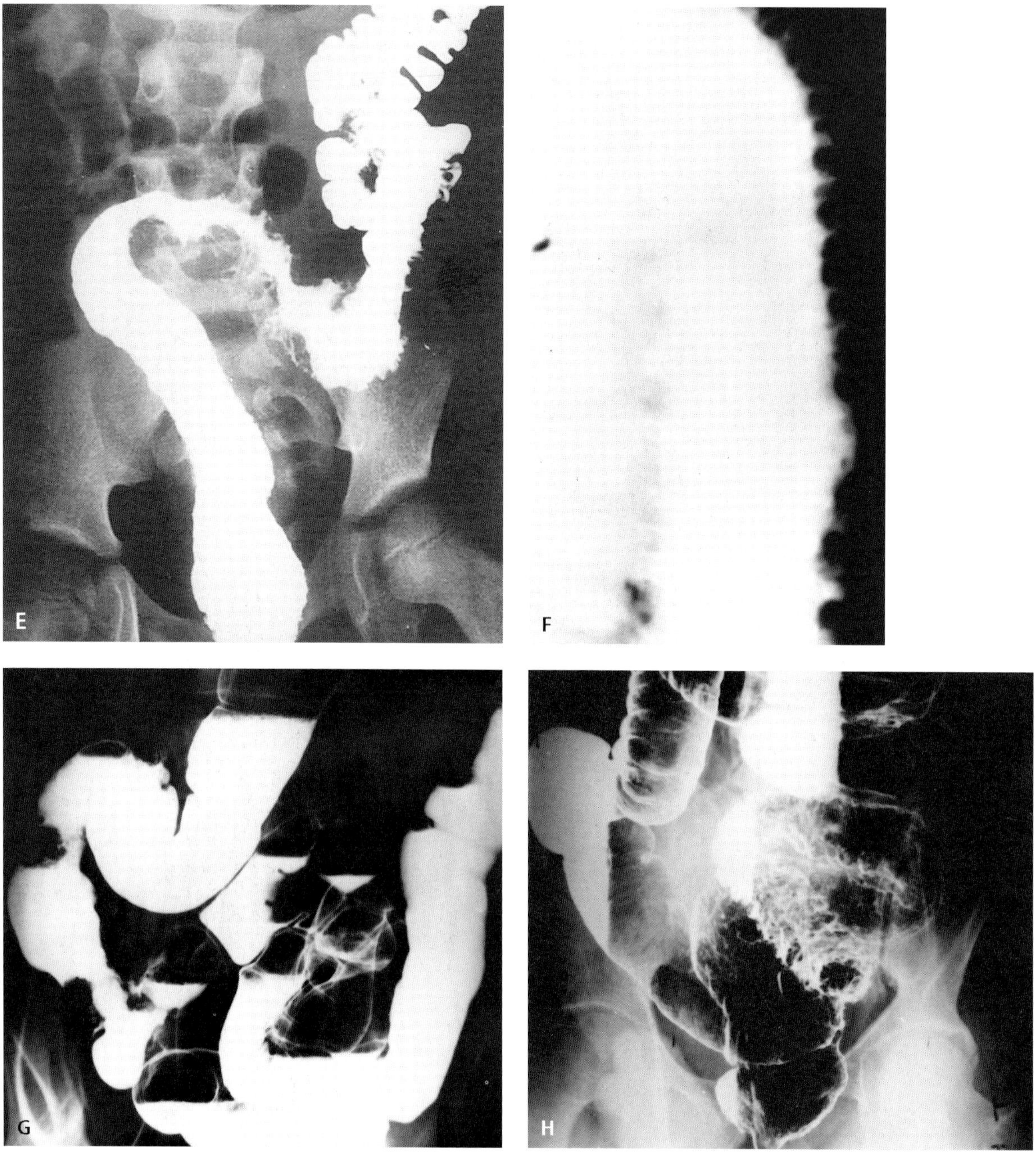

Fig. 5.47 (*continued*). **E** The irregular saw-tooth appearance of tuberculous mucosal ulceration (descending colon). **F** Spasm and mucosal edema affecting the whole of the descending and proximal sigmoid colon of a 53-year-old African patient. The cecum and ascending colon were also affected, but could not be filled with the barium enema because of the spasm and discomfort. **G** Skip ulcers encircling and constricting the ascending colon of a 42-year-old Arab female. **H** Extensive transverse ulceration without any narrowing in the sigmoid colon of a 38-year-old Arab female. (C AFIP 229499; E from Cremin and Jamieson 1995)

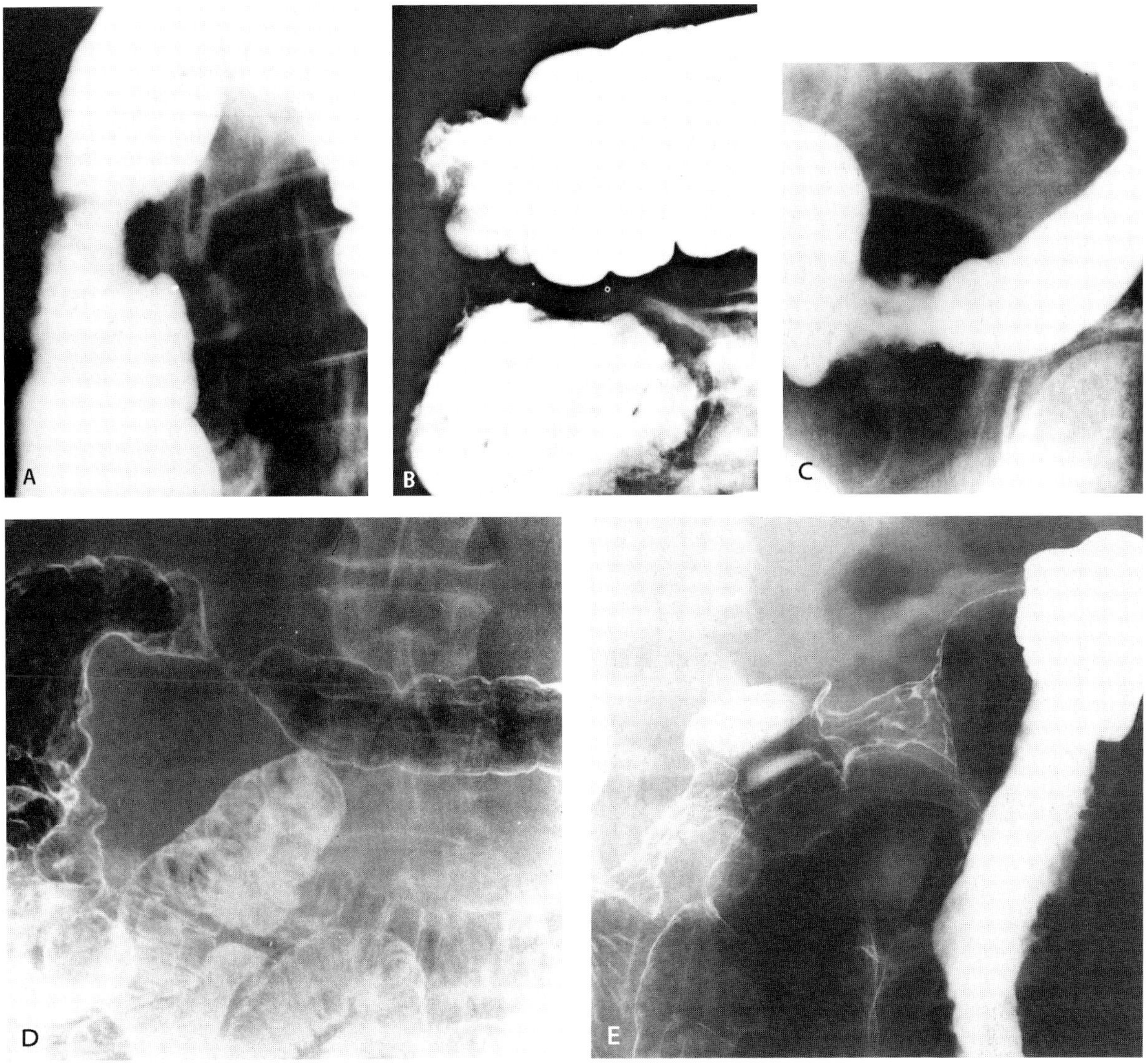

Fig. 5.48 A–E. Tuberculosis can cause local narrowing in any part of the bowel at any age. The differential diagnosis is then very difficult. **A** Stricture in the ascending colon of a 40 year old man. **B** A very tight stricture just proximal to the hepatic flexure in a young woman. **C** A constriction with ulceration in the sigmoid colon of a middle-aged man; these tuberculous strictures resmble localized amebomas, and carcinoma would have to be considered, although it is rare in some parts of the tropics. **D** A tight stricture in the proximal transverse colon. **E** Two elongated strictures in the transverse colon of a child: there is also ulceration and thickening of the descending colon. These patients come from three different continents: all had normal chest radiographs and in each the diagnosis of tuberculosis was confirmed histologically. (**E** from Cremin and Jamieson 1995)

Tuberculosis of the Rectum

The rectum is the least common site for tuberculosis in the gastrointestinal tract. There may be ulcerating procitis, fistulas and even stricture (Fig. 5.49). Any chronic ischiorectal abscess in the tropics should raise the possibility of underlying tuberculosis. A chest x-ray is often requested in patients who have a perianal or ischiorectal abscess but who are otherwise in good health. The majority of these will be negative. Imaging with barium, ultrasonography, or CT may demonstrate the abscess but it can be very difficult to demonstrate any fistula or connection between the abscess and deeper tissues. The differential diagnosis will include lymphogranuloma venereum, schistosomiasis, amebiasis, and rarely, actinomycosis or Crohn's disease.

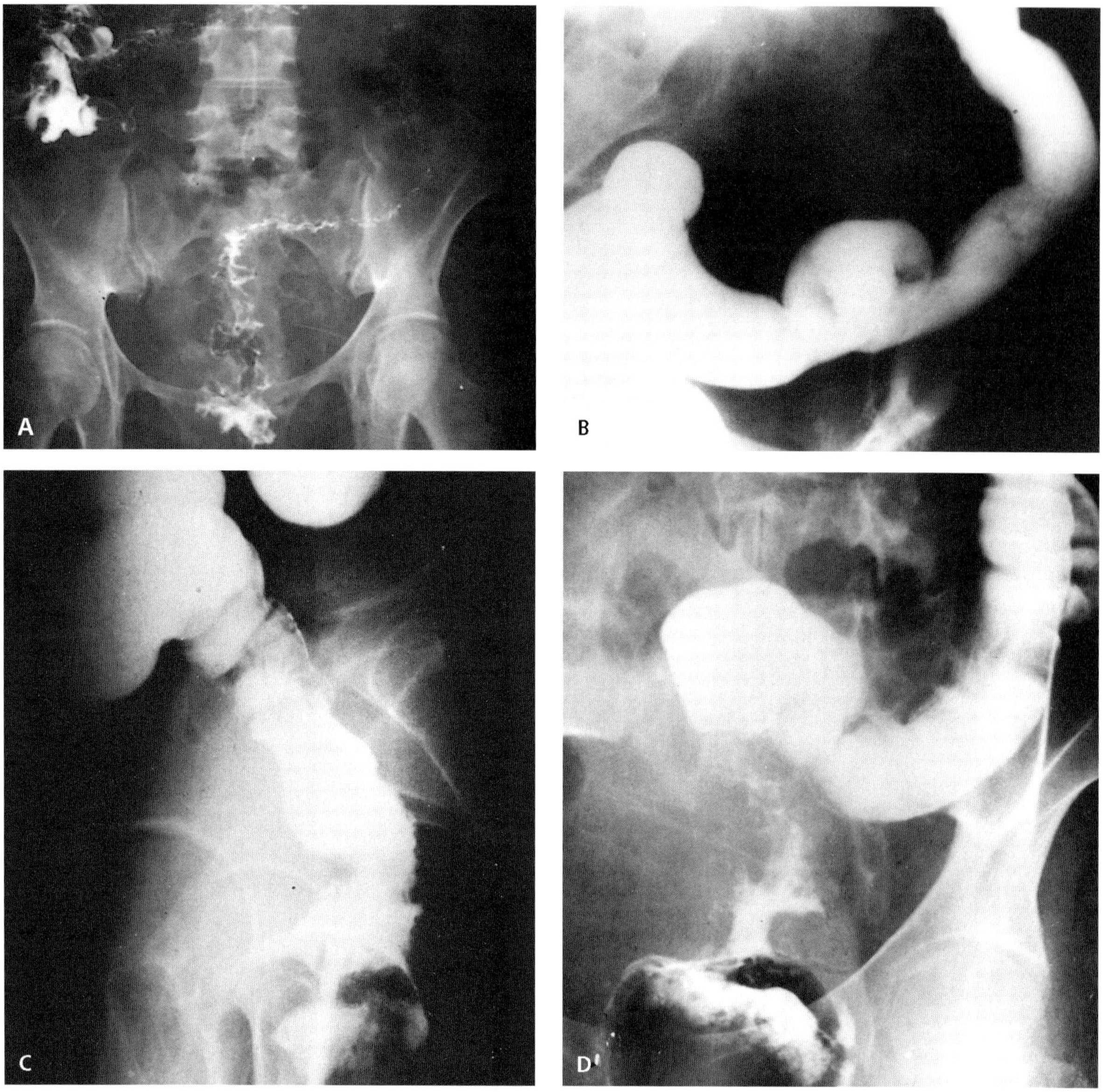

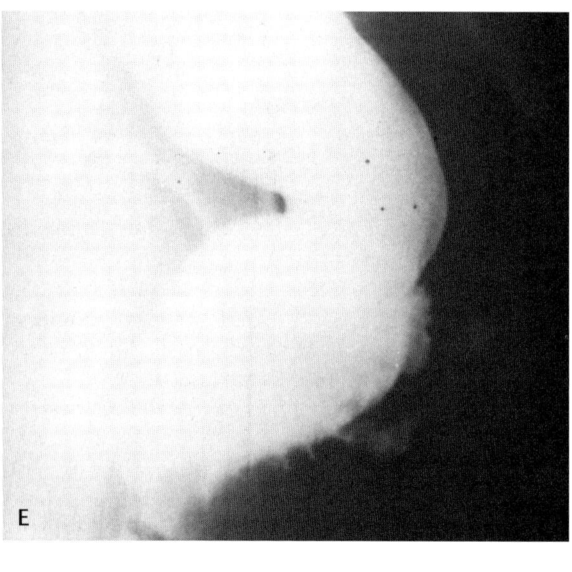

Fig. 5.49 A–E. Sigmoid and rectal tuberculosis. **A** Sigmoid colitis extending into the upper part of the rectum, with edema, ulceration, and mural thickening. **B** The possible end result: the sigmoid is smooth, lacking normal haustration or mucosal pattern. In both the acute and chronic stages, tuberculosis resembles amebiasis or any other ulcerating colitis. **C, D** The rectum is narrowed, ulcerating, and thickened. There is minimal obstruction at this stage, but if untreated the rectum will narrow and the sigmoid will dilate. **E** A different lateral projection of the same patient shows two fistulae which may connect with the skin in the perineum. Only biopsy will differentiate tuberculosis from lymphogranuloma venereum or amebiasis. Schistosomiasis can cause the same mucosal changes but fistulae are much less common. (**A** AFIP 68-2419-4; **B** AFIP 29499-185)

Enteroliths

Intestinal calculi are not seen very frequently, but may occur above any chronic bowel stricture. They seem to be more common in India than elsewhere, but isolated cases have been noted from many countries where tuberculosis is common. When the stricture is high within the small bowel, the enteroliths are composed of choleic acid and are usually radiographically nonopaque but may be seen as a dense mass on ultrasonography or CT. In the lower bowel, where there is a greater alkaline content and a higher concentration of calcium salts, enteroliths often become radiographically opaque (see Fig. 5.42 G, p. 447). Some are completely opacified, but others have translucent centers with a ring of calcification. These calcified enteroliths may be found in the lower ileum or colon in up to 3%–4% of cases of intestinal tuberculosis. They vary from multiple small stones to a single large laminated calculus. Massive nontuberculous enterolithiasis has been associated with ileal dysgenesis: the enteroliths were located in the distal ileum and there was an ileo-transverse-colonic fistula. Enteroliths must also be differentiated from calcified granulomatous lymph nodes, renal stones, gallstones, or less commonly, vesical stones. Cross-sectional imaging with ultrasonography or CT is an ideal way to localize them accurately. Barium studies may not always be successful because of the bowel stricture which is the underlying cause.

Tuberculosis of the Peritoneum and Abdominal Lymph Nodes

Tuberculous peritonitis occurs at any age and in both sexes, and in some series accounts for 30% of all nonpulmonary tuberculosis and for at least 20% of all cases of ascites. In most countries about half the cases of abdominal tuberculosis will be due to peritoneal infection, but in children and young adults the frequency is even higher. In almost every case there is associated abdominal lymphadenopathy; the infection may originate from a primary intestinal or gynecological source, or be blood borne; it is seldom possible to locate the primary focus.
The major clinical symptoms are abdominal distention and abdominal pain, vomiting and diarrhea are less common, occurring in under 30% of patients. Nonspecific findings, such as weight loss and tiredness, are difficult to evaluate in the tropics, but occur consistently in tuberculous peritonitis.
Clinical examination shows that 30% of the patients are afebrile, but almost all have ascites, which is clinically detectable in only about one-third. The tuberculin skin reaction varies geographically, but is often negative (Nigeria 70%, Ethiopia 23%), and the chest radiograph is often normal (India 60%, Ethiopia 50%, Iran 40%). Over 30% of the patients will have lymphadenopathy elsewhere, most commonly cervical. On palpation the abdomen has an ill-defined "doughy" feeling, and in 15% or more of patients there will be palpable abdominal masses. The liver and spleen are often enlarged. There is a very reliable laboratory test for tuberculous peritonitis. If the fluid is examined and the adenosine deaminase (ADA) level is over 32.3 µ/l, there is a 98% sensitivity and 95% specificity for tuberculosis.
Laparoscopy is one way to obtain a tissue biopsy because even culture of the ascitic fluid may be negative. It is useful to exclude other causes of ascites, such as carcinomatosis, lymphoma, or even worms. However, laparoscopy is not without risk, and in tuberculous patients carries a mortality of 3%–12%.
The course of the disease may be relatively benign (except in AIDS patients), and the response to antituberculous therapy quite rapid. The ascites may persist, even when the patient is improving clinically. Histological examination shows that the majority of the infected abdominal lymph nodes will be caseating and necrotic. These nodes may rupture into the peritoneum, disseminating small tubercles all over the peritoneal cavity and occasionally causing an acute clinical reaction and hemorrhagic exudate. When this happens, the protein content of the ascitic fluid will be high (over 45 g/l) and the fluid/blood glucose ratio will be below 0.96, with marked lymphocytosis. The tubercle bacilli can be seen on direct staining of the fluid or subsequently on culture. Another initially rare complication is intestinal obstruction, which increases in frequency as the fluid is absorbed and adhesions form. At autopsy, cecal or ileal ulceration may occasionally be found.

Tuberculous Peritonitis

Ultrasonography is the method of choice for imaging tuberculous peritonitis. There are three imaging patterns. There may be ascites (the "wet" form), there may be multiple caseous nodules and adhesions (the plastic or "dry" form), or there may be a combination in which loops of bowel, omentum, or mesentery have clumped together, often becoming palpable and associated with ascites.
When there is ascites, it can be free, localized or loculated (Figs. 5.50, 5.51). When free, it is either clear fluid or contains multiple thin strands, septa, or floating debris. These strands may be mobile and quite delicate or relatively thick so that adhesions occur. Fluid may be trapped between the thickened loops of bowel, producing alternating echoic and echo-free bands (the "sandwich" appearance). Both on ultrasonography and CT the density of tubercu-

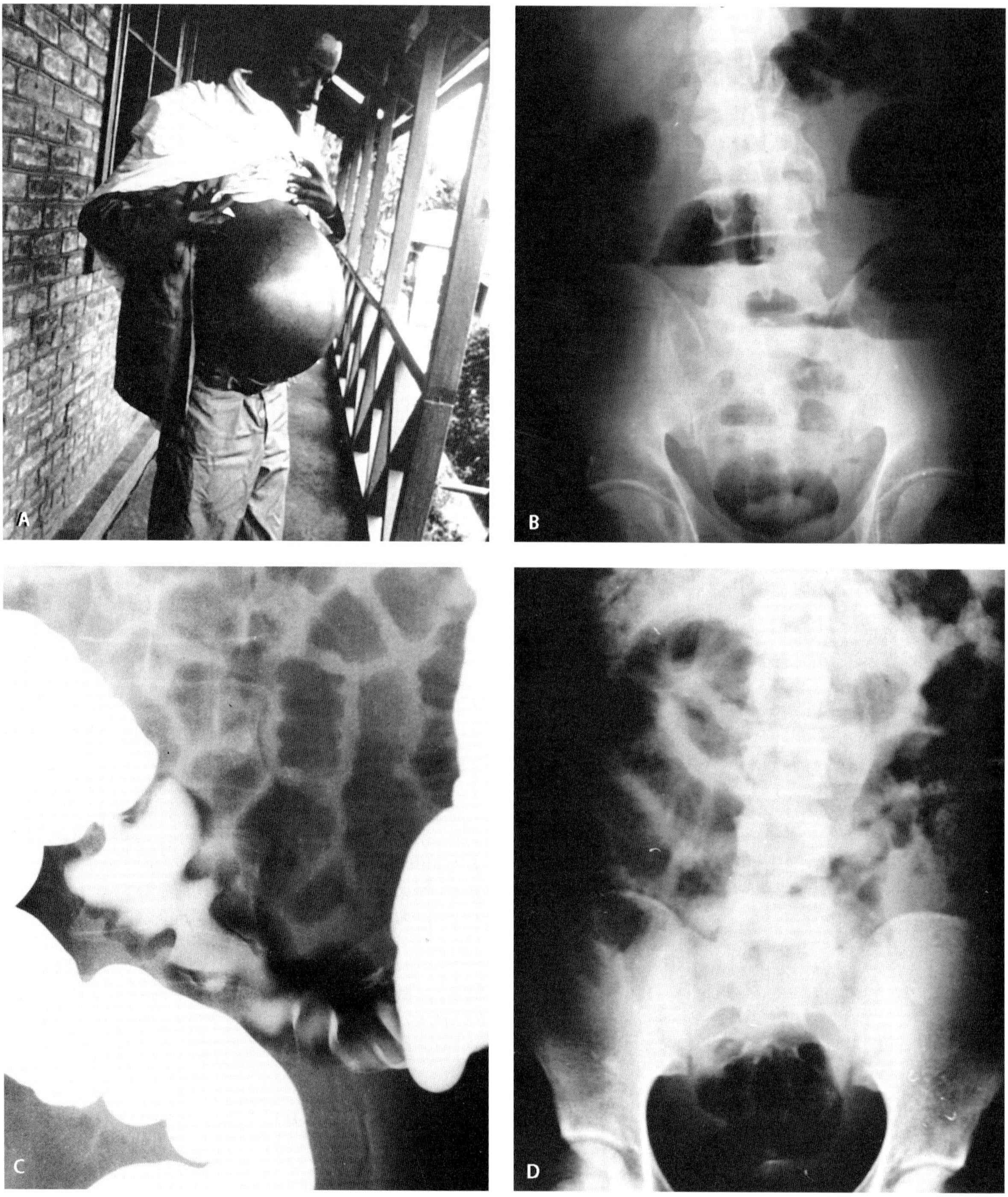

Fig. 5.50 A–F. Tuberculous peritonitis **A** An Ethiopian patient with tense ascites. (Courtesy of Dr. Richter) **B** Multiple loops of dilated bowel, with fluid levels, floating in ascites. It can be very difficult to decide whether this is due to obstruction or ileus. **C, D** Dilated loops of small bowel with thick edematous walls. This is still an ileus, but obstruction may develop later because of adhesions. **C** is an African and **D** a patient from India. **E, F** see p. 459

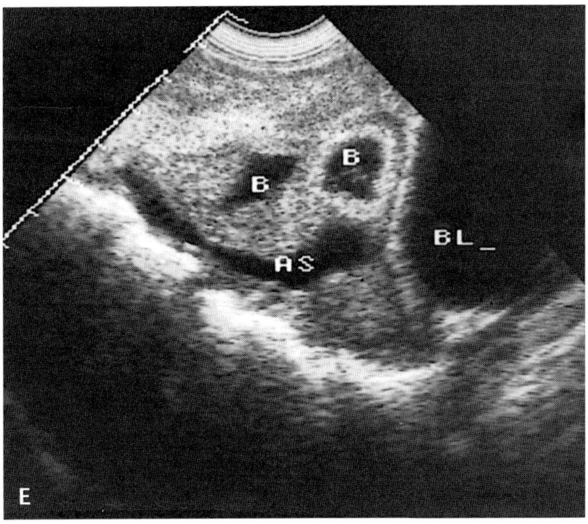

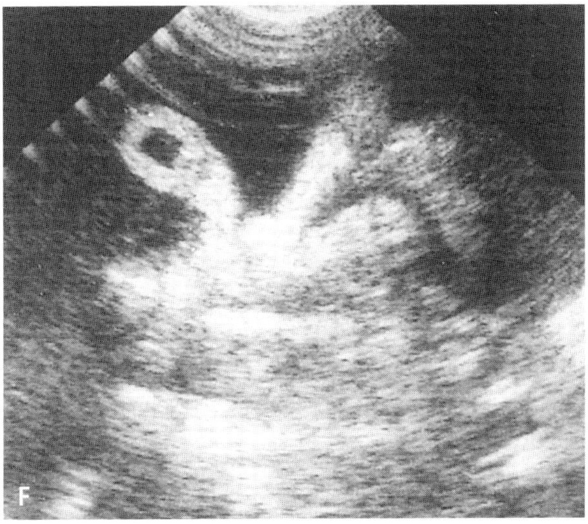

Fig. 5.50 (*continued*). **E** A sonogram showing thickened bowel walls and ascites due to tuberculosis in a 44-year-old African from Zimbabwe. *B* bowel; *AS* ascites; *BL* urinary bladder. (Courtesy of Dr. Sam Mindel) **F** A sonogram of a South African child showing echogenic bowel loops radiating from the mesenteric root, with ascites. (From Cremin and Jamieson 1995)

lous ascites is variable; when clear, it is a transudate in the early stage and becomes thickened later. There may be progression to an abscess, seen on ultrasonography as well-defined localized fluid collections, septate and with internal echoes. Aspiration of this thick fluid can be difficult or even impossible due to its consistency and the multiple septate divisions. But even at this stage, there can be good response to antituberculous therapy.

Computed tomography can demonstrate the ascites and the plastic changes, but preliminary oral contrast should be used within the bowel so that the thickening of the bowel wall, the omentum, and the lymph nodes can be differentiated. CT may be better than ultrasonography for the anatomical localization of the fluids and to show where it is loculated or has been walled off into a thick abscess. In patients with AIDS the progress is similar but exaggerated.

In the dry form of peritonitis, ultrasonography will demonstrate irregular echo-free or echo-poor, nodular or laminar thickening of the peritoneum. The nodules are poorly echogenic and occur almost anywhere on the peritoneal surface. Histologically they are caseating granulomas. The mesenteric thickening may lead to fixation of the bowel and, when there is fluid, these loops of bowel and mesentery have been described as "radiating from the mesenteric root in a stellate configuration." This is more clearly seen with CT. On MRI performed with gadolinium enhancement, lymphadenopathy can be demonstrated. However, there is seldom any great advantage in using either CT or MRI compared with ultrasonography.

Routine supine and erect radiographs of the abdomen will show free fluid and multiple distended loops of small bowel, often with thickened intestinal walls. There may be scattered fluid levels in the erect position, but the findings are those of an ileus rather than obstruction. The amount of fluid in the abdomen may make the details of the bowel somewhat hazy. The proximal colon may be involved and also dilated to the same extent.

As healing occurs, the degree of dilatation lessens and the wall of the gut is less thickened. Adhesions may form and there may be subacute obstruction with fluid levels. At this stage, barium contrast gastrointestinal studies may be helpful and careful fluoroscopy with palpation will make it possible to decide whether the loops of bowel are fixed or mobile. However, apart from adhesions, the majority of cases will have a normal radiological examination of the small intestine without any obvious bowel involvement.

Tuberculous Abdominal Lymph Nodes

At least one-third of patients with tuberculous peritonitis will have lymphadenopathy, and in some countries, e.g., India, the frequency of lymph node involvement may be as high as 70%. Lymphadenopathy may occur without detectable bowel involvement. All groups of nodes within the abdomen can be infected, particularly those around the pancreas, portal region, aorta, and vena cava. On ultrasonography the enlarged nodes are usually hypoechoic (Fig. 5.51 A, B), and some display central echogenic areas where caseation has started. Some nodes will be discrete, while others adhere together into large

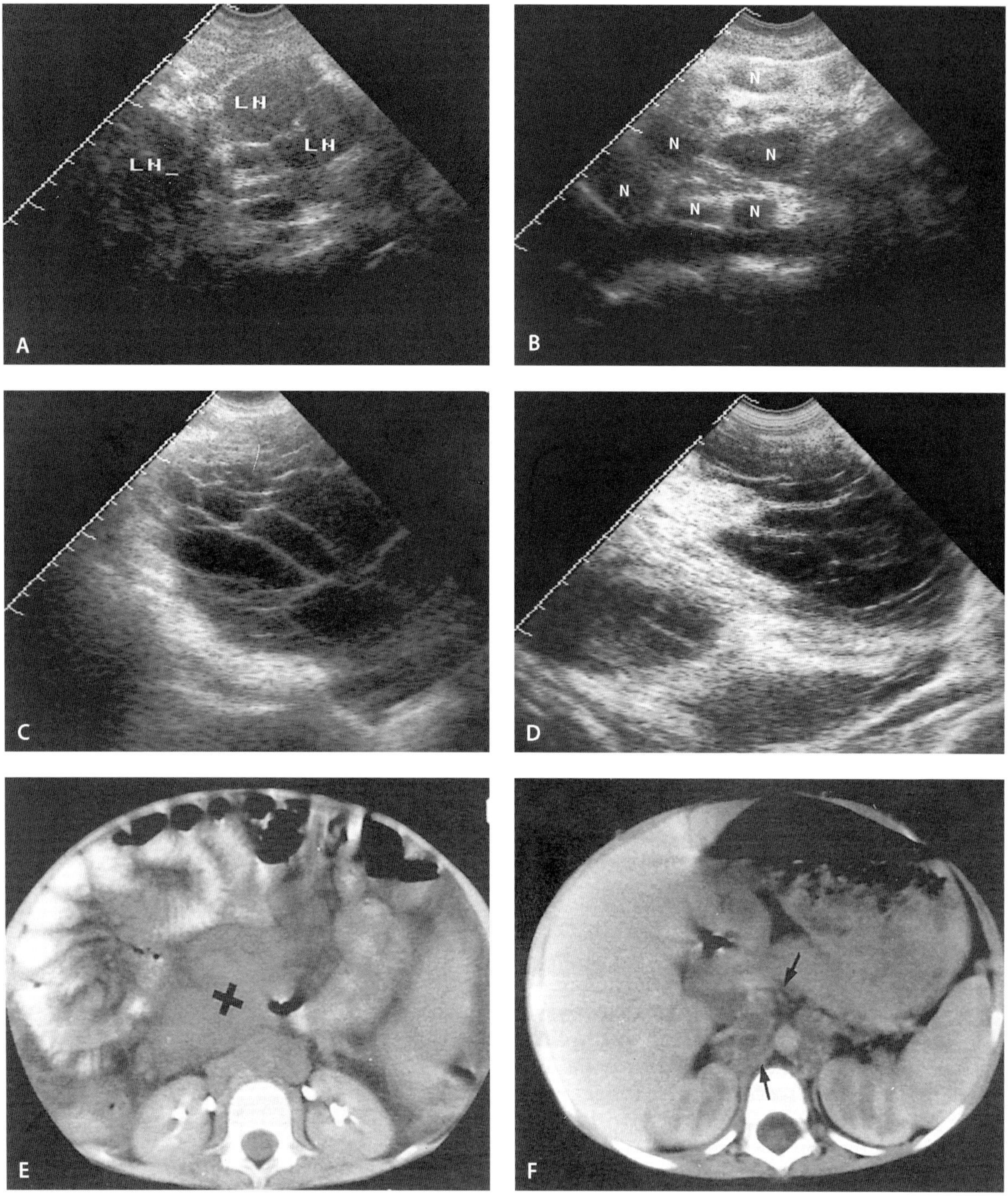

Fig. 5.51 A–F. With scanning it is possible to identify lymphadenopathy and peritoneal fluid: it is not always possible to be sure of the etiology. **A, B** Ultrasonography shows multile enlarged tuberculous lymph nodes (*LN/N*) and ascites. **C, D** Loculated peritoneal fluid, a very common finding in tuberculous peritonitis. (A–D are all patients from Zimbabwe, courtesy of Dr. Sam Mindel) **E** A contrast-enhanced CT scan (with contrast also in the bowel) shows the thickened intestinal loops and a large omental mass (*X*). There is loculated low-density ascites. **F** Contrast-enhanced CT showing rim-enhancing para-aortic lymph nodes (*arrows*). (**E, F** are children from South Africa, from Cremin and Jamieson 1995)

masses. Both CT and ultrasonography can demonstrate nodal calcification before it can be seen on a plain radiograph. On CT, most nodes are of low density with some peripheral rim enhancement (Fig. 5.51 F). It is probable that some of the abscesses (cold abscesses) within the peritoneum result from extensive caseation of lymph nodes; they have a very variable ultrasound and CT appearance depending on the degree of caseation, central necrosis, and septation.

Enlargement of the abdominal lymph nodes may cause direct pressure on various parts of the gut; there may be distortion of the pyloric antrum, duodenal loop, and upper jejunum in particular (see pp. 442–444). If the nodes are very large and swollen, the bowel may become adherent to them and involved in the tuberculous process. This results in a spiky irregular outline of the intestinal mucosa, localized edema, and ileus. Rupture of enlarged nodes into the intestine has been reported, but only happens when this adhesive process has occurred. It can present as a communicating diverticulum.

Calcification of the mesenteric nodes may be seen on healing, but is not as common as might be expected. It will be detected earlier by CT scanning (see p. 443). Although the presence of caseation and calcification suggest tuberculosis, metastatic malignancy and histoplasmosis can occasionally also calcify. When healing, tuberculous calcification may be seen as discrete lines on both CT and ultrasonography. Radiographically visible abdominal nodal calcification due to tuberculosis is uncommon in Africa and many parts of the tropics despite the frequency of the infection. (However, calcification in nodes elsewhere, such as the neck, mediastinum, and inguinal region, is quite common.)

Lymphangiography has been used for the evaluation of lymph nodes in abdominal tuberculosis, using pedal injections. Sharply outlined central filling defects, extending in some cases to the periphery, have been described as a feature of tuberculous lymphadenitis. As would be expected, the bunching of the lymph nodes together in an adherent mass can also be seen. The central filling defects are probably tuberculous caseation. In some lymph channels there is obstruction to the flow. Most of the changes described on lymphangiography can also be seen in lymphoma and metastatic disease. Ultrasonography and CT scanning have replaced lymphangiography for diagnosis in most countries (which is probably appreciated by the patient).

A rare tuberculous involvement of a large giant cystic lymphangioma has occurred in an Ethiopian male immigrant to Israel. His father had tuberculosis. The patient had a draining right axillary sinus, a large fluctuating abdominal mass, and an equally large reducible right inguinal hernia. There was no palpable lymphadenopathy. Imaging showed this to be one cystic mass extending from the posterior mediastinum into the pelvis, and aspiration of the fluid was positive for *M. tuberculosis*. The mass responded to antituberculous therapy and fluid aspiration. Two similar infections have been reported in cystic hygromas of the hand.

Tuberculosis of the Liver, Spleen, and Pancreas

Hematogenous, disseminated tuberculosis can result in small (miliary) tuberculous nodules in any organ. Clinically, generalised hepatomegaly and less often splenomegaly may be palpated when there is abdominal tuberculosis. Isolated tuberculomas of the spleen have also been reported.

There may be multiple small tuberculous granulomas (tubercles) in the liver (Fig. 5.52 A–F) or spleen (Fig. 5.53) which on ultrasonography have a granular echoic or hypoechoic appearance. The granulomas can become macronodular, depending on the stage of development. Some will have central, more echogenic areas. If a tuberculous abscess develops, the hypoechoic center will be surrounded by a hyperechoic rim. One or more areas of caseous necrosis may develop. This is less common in the spleen. In some tuberculous granulomas there will be calcification, seen on plain radiographs or causing acoustic shadowing on ultrasonography.

Large tuberculous masses are unusual, but have been reported. One such mass was 3.5×5.5 cm, and situated in the left lobe of the liver (Fig. 5.52 G–I). On CT the mass was hypodense and showed peripheral enhancement with contrast. Celiac arteriography in this case showed stretched hepatic vessels and some neovascularity, which suggested that the mass was inflammatory rather than neoplastic in origin.

Only very rarely will a solitary hepatic, splenic, or pancreatic abscess or tuberculoma be the presenting evidence of tuberculosis. Almost always there will be marked tuberculous lymphadenopathy within the abdomen, and often in peripheral nodes also.

Pancreatic tuberculosis may be nodular or (less commonly) form an abscess, usually of complex echogenicity but with less surrounding pancreatitis than a pyogenic abscess. The nodular pattern is less easily recongized. Pancreatic lesions are unlikely to be seen in children. In adults they are probably going to become more common in patients with AIDS.

All tuberculous granulomas may calcify and then be demonstrated by any method of imaging (Fig. 5.53 A, B). Many cases of splenic or, less often, hepatic calcified tuberculous granulomas are chance findings.

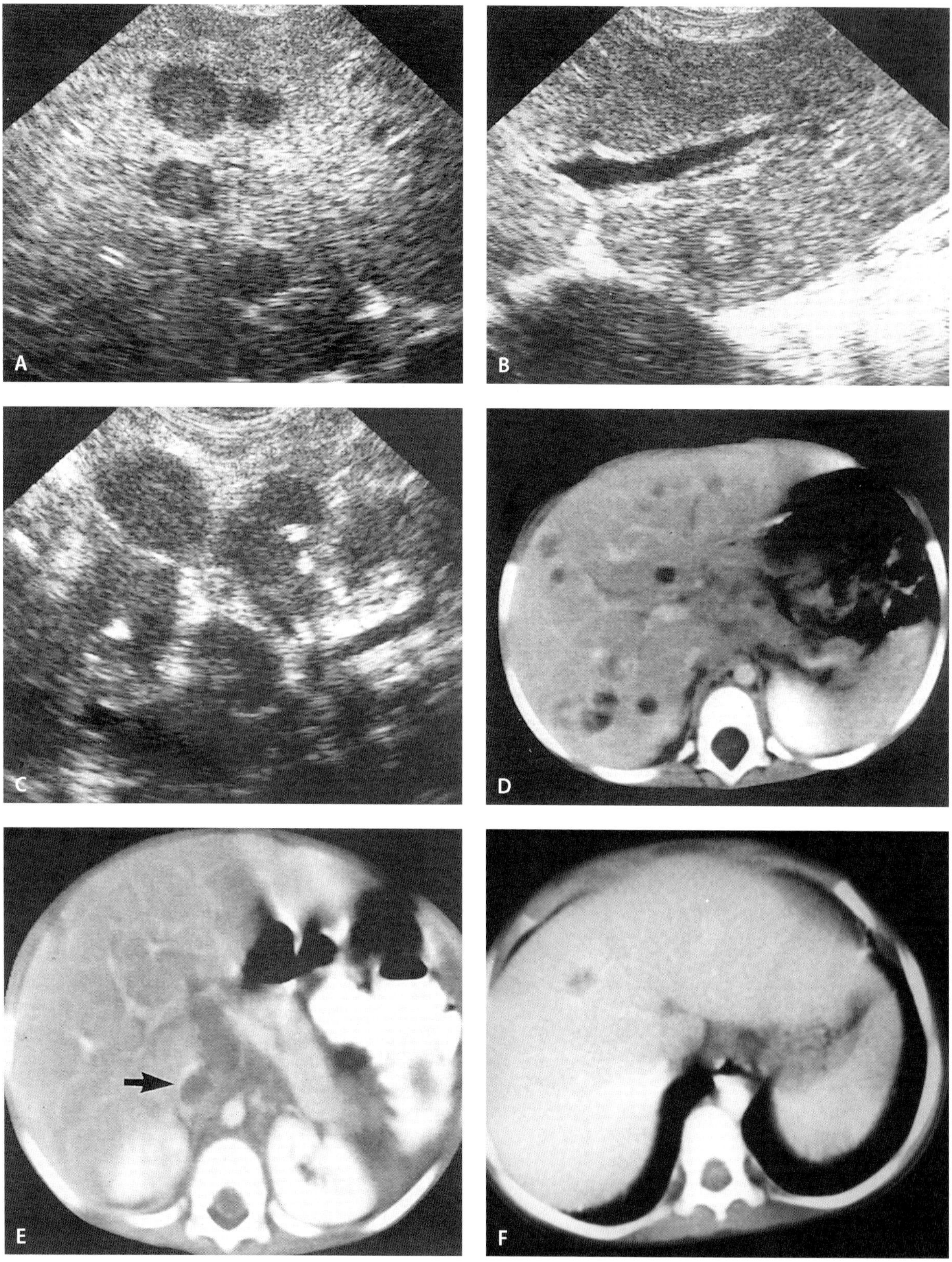

Fig. 5.52 A–I. Tuberculosis of the liver. **A, B** Ultrasonography showing hypoechoic granulomas and a granuloma with an echogenic center in the livers of two children. **C** In another child there are hypoechoic lymph nodes with echoic calcification at the porta hepatis. **D** A contrast-enhanced CT shows multiple nonenhancing granulomas in a child's liver. **E** In a different child there are rim-enhancing nodes (*arrow*) at the porta hepatis. **F** A child from a Pacific Island has a similar granuloma in the liver. **G–I** see p. 463

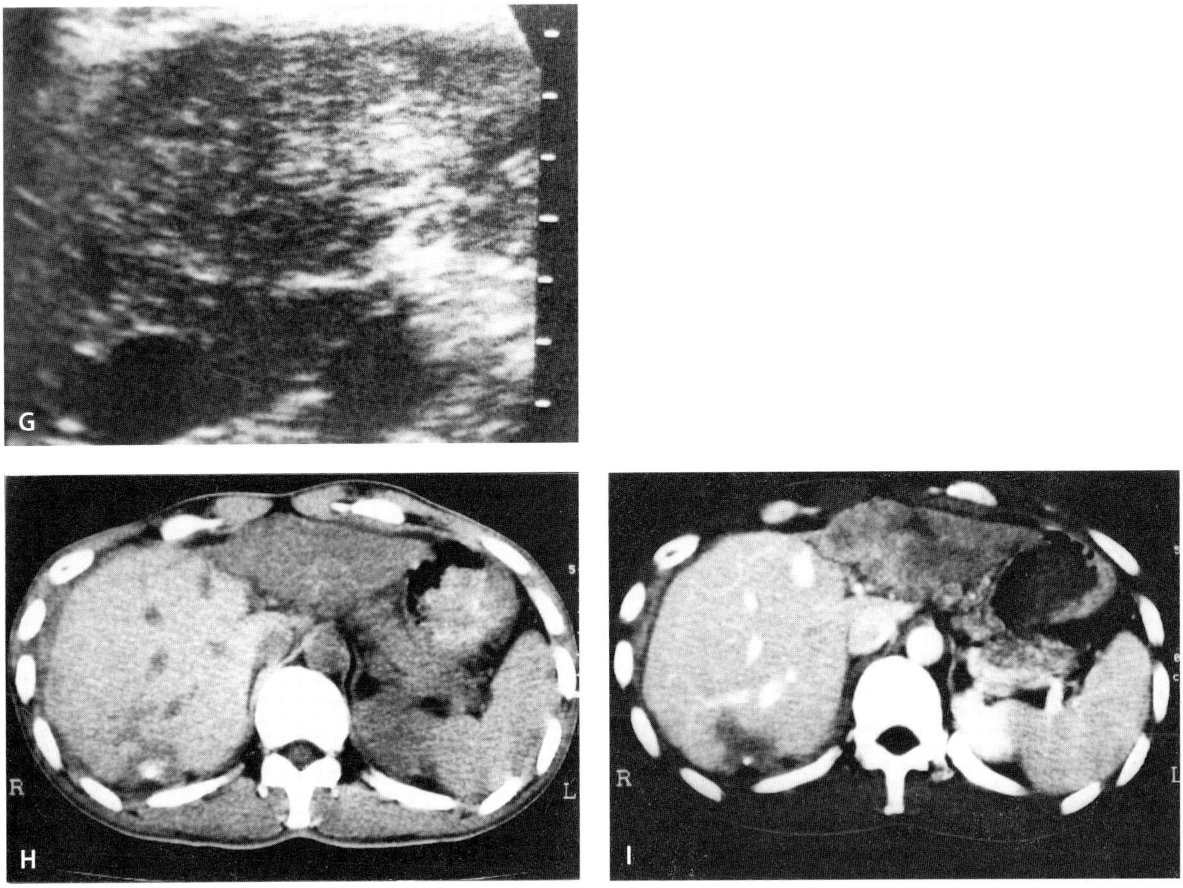

Fig. 5.52 (*continued*). **G** Tuberculoma of the liver: A 3.5×5.5 cm hyperechoic mass in the lateral segment of the left lobe (sonogram). An isolated hyperechoic nodule with calcification was also found in the right lobe. **H, I** CT scans of the same patient show a large hypodense lesion almost filling the lateral segment of the left lobe of the liver. The other nodule in the right lobe, is hypodense with a central hyperdense focus. **I** After intravenous contrast, the lesion in the left lobe shows peripheral enhancement and central hypodensity; the nodule in the right lobe remains hyperdense. The patient was a 30-year-old male, a known hepatitis B carrier, complaining of right upper quadrant abdominal pain. His chest radiograph showed diffuse reticulonodulation and pleural thickening due to pulmonary tuberculosis and pleurisy. Ultrasound-guided liver biopsy showed acid-fast bacilli. After 9 months of antituberculous treatment the tuberculoma had almost disappeared. (**A–E** from Cremin and Jamieson 1995; **F** courtesy of Dr. Cheryl Sisler, Hawaii; **G–I** courtesy of Dr. T. C. F. Tan et al. and *Br J Radiol*, 1997)

The differential diagnosis can be difficult because of the rarity of active infection in the liver, pancreas, or spleen. A chest x-ray may be normal, but the tuberculin skin test is usually positive. Most of these tuberculous lesions in solid organs will be nonenhancing, although there may be rim enhancement at some stage. If noncalcified, they can be mistaken for hydatid disease, amebic abscesses, or, more commonly, malignancy. Image-guided aspiration can be used to make the diagnosis and, in some cases, for instillation of drugs. When lesions are calcified their etiology can be more difficult to identify, since they may resemble a collapsed hydatid cyst, an old pyogenic or mycotic infection, or even a calcified hematoma following trauma (especially in the spleen). For noncalcified, active granulomas or abscesses, imaging can be used to follow treatment, and prolonged follow-up is advisable because recurrence of tuberculosis from these isolated abscesses has been recorded.

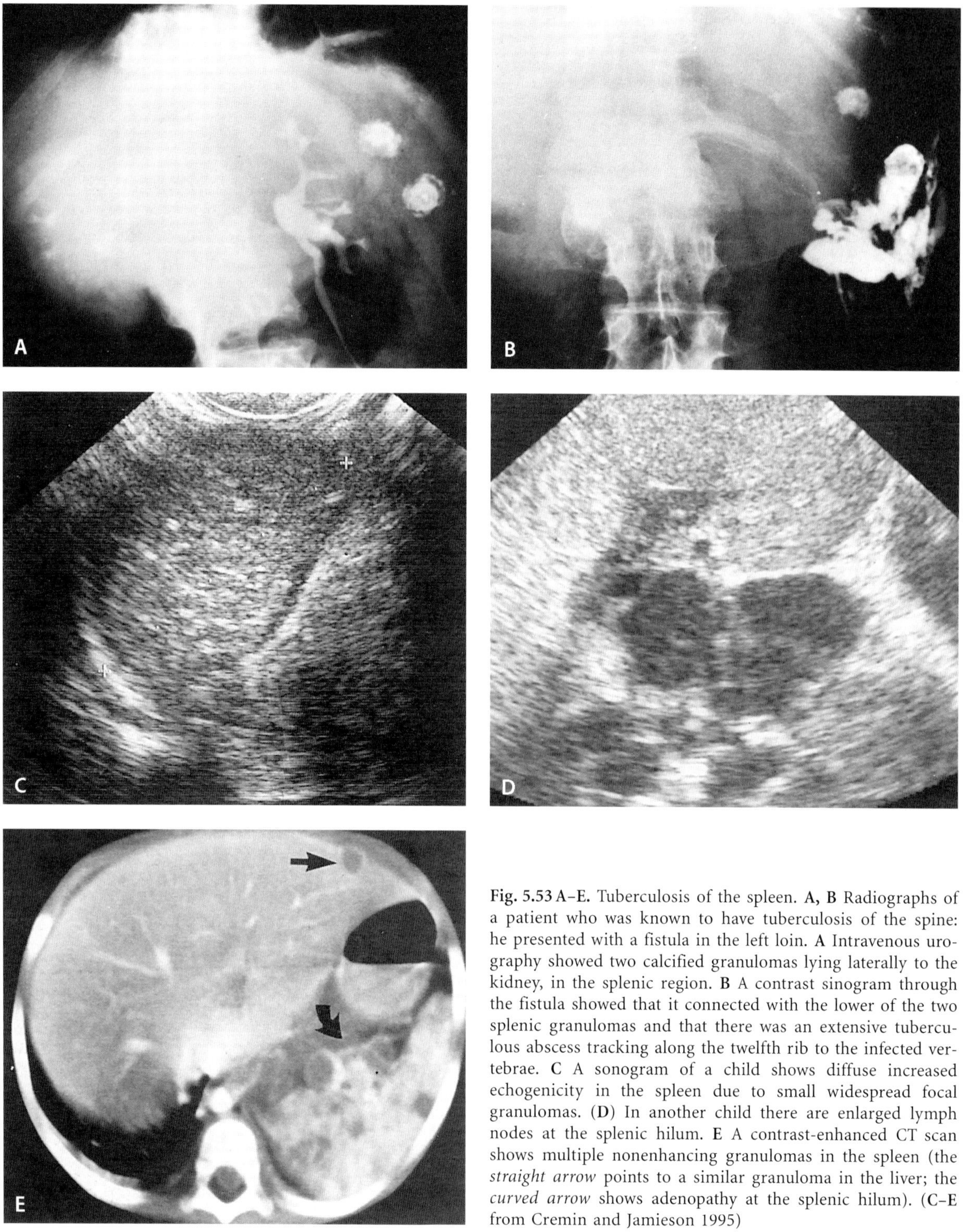

Fig. 5.53 A–E. Tuberculosis of the spleen. **A, B** Radiographs of a patient who was known to have tuberculosis of the spine: he presented with a fistula in the left loin. **A** Intravenous urography showed two calcified granulomas lying laterally to the kidney, in the splenic region. **B** A contrast sinogram through the fistula showed that it connected with the lower of the two splenic granulomas and that there was an extensive tuberculous abscess tracking along the twelfth rib to the infected vertebrae. **C** A sonogram of a child shows diffuse increased echogenicity in the spleen due to small widespread focal granulomas. (**D**) In another child there are enlarged lymph nodes at the splenic hilum. **E** A contrast-enhanced CT scan shows multiple nonenhancing granulomas in the spleen (the *straight arrow* points to a similar granuloma in the liver; the *curved arrow* shows adenopathy at the splenic hilum). (C–E from Cremin and Jamieson 1995)

Tuberculosis of the Urinary Tract

Kidneys and Ureters

The incidence of tuberculosis of the kidney varies throughout the tropics; wherever it occurs, it is more common in the higher socioeconomic groups, repeating the pattern of the disease in Europe. It is uncommon in tropical Africa, despite the fact that tuberculosis is prevalent in most other tissues. It occurs frequently in much of Asia and India, particularly in association with diabetes. There are often tuberculous foci in the chest and skeleton also.

Renal tuberculosis in the tropics is probably almost always bilateral, although it may be first identified on one side only, especially if contrast urography is used to make the diagnosis. It usually starts as a localized caseating lesion, most commonly in the upper pole of either kidney, although it may arise anywhere. Such foci are caused by hematogenous spread. Alternatively, it may present as pyelonephritis as the result of reflux from an infected bladder.

The nidus of infection in the renal parenchyma enlarges and ruptures into a neighboring calyx, discharging necrotic caseous material and distorting the calyx (Fig. 5.54). This can be demonstrated by intravenous or retrograde urography, ultrasonography, CT, or MRI. If there is a communication into the tuberculous cavity, it may fill during an intervenous contrast examination; the affected calyx becomes an ulcerated cavernous lesion. The infection spreads to involve the draining calyceal infundibulum, which may then develop a stricture and seal off the infected calyx. If the ulcer and stricture are located in the renal pelvis, there will be obstruction to the outflow of urine and the calyces will become clubbed. Later, a stricture of the renal pelvis can seal off the kidney, and fibrosis and calcification may follow. This may result in autoamputation of the kidney. If there is direct extension of the tuberculous infection into the rest of the kidney, the entire kidney becomes a bag of caseous necrotic pus.

Ultrasonography is a very satisfactory way to image each step of this pathological process (Fig. 5.55). Although it is possible to demonstrate the irregular and dilated calyces and the connecting cavities by urography, ultrasonography gives a better image of the renal parenchyma and will show increased echogenicity and mixed echogenicity around the calyceal lesions. Focal parenchymal granulomas which cannot be seen radiographically may be identified by ultrasonography. (Scanning should always include both kidneys even when there is an obvious lesion on one side only. On ultrasonography a tuberculous abscess will appear as an echogenic, irregular mass, often containing debris. Local or general hydronephrosis can be imaged and in the end stage the kidney will become irregular in outline, with varying thickness of the cortex. Eventually there may be calcification in the granulomas or abscess, showing as bright areas on an ultrasound scan (Fig. 5.56). Punctute calcification of the upper pole and curvilinear calcification outlining the entire kidney are the two extremes of renal involvement. CT and MRI are alternative ways to scan.

Autoamputation, the end result of advanced tuberculosis, can cause remarkably little clinical disturbance, especially in patients who are malnourished and in ill health for other reasons. There can be complete nonfunction on contrast urography or scintigraphy, a finding noted in half the patients in one pediatric series. On ultrasonography or CT, the distorted renal mass can be accurately demonstrated, showing the ultrasonically echogenic fibrosis and contraction and the bright echoes of calcification.

In tuberculosis, the ureters are dilated proximally, with irregular granulomas which result in one or more strictures and which ultimately lead to hydronephrosis (Fig. 5.57). Eventually, spotty ureteric calcification develops; in extreme cases this may merge into extensive pipe calcification along the length of the ureters. Intravenous, or even better, retrograde pyelography is the most accurate way to delineate the full length of the ureters to demonstrate strictures or calcification. Although the echogenic irregularity and granulomatous masses, as well as the dilatation of the ureters, can be demonstrated by ultrasonography, it is not so easy to assess the peristalsis. CT and MRI are less reliable (and MRI particularly is not a good way to demonstrate calcification) and are both a more costly way of evaluating the ureters.

Differentiation from schistosomiasis is usually fairly reliable. In schistosomiasis calcification is first seen in the lower end of the ureters and the bladder and then extends up the ureters; it is most unusual to see much ureteric calcification without bladder calcification, and the nodular irregularity of the ureters as seen on contrast studies will be useful in making the differentiation. In tuberculosis, the calcification extends down the ureter and the bladder is very seldom calcified to the same extend as in schistosomiasis. The multiple strictures and nodules of ureteritis cystica are rare in the pattern of urinary tuberculosis in the tropics. Transitional cell carcinoma of the ureter is rare in much of the tropics but does produce irregular strictures with mucosal destruction and nodular masses, often with the characteristic goblet or champagne glass appearance.

(Text continues on p. 471)

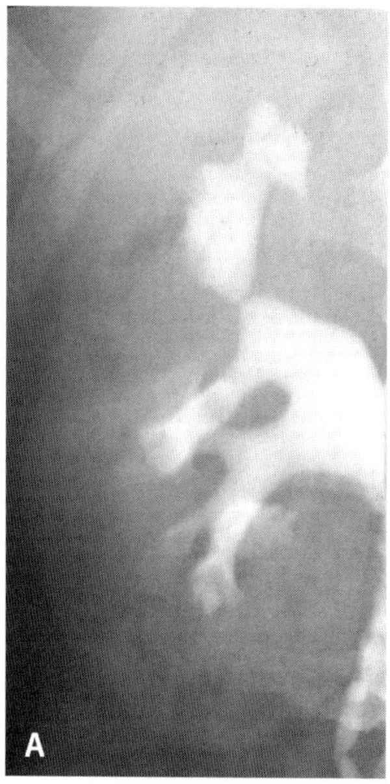

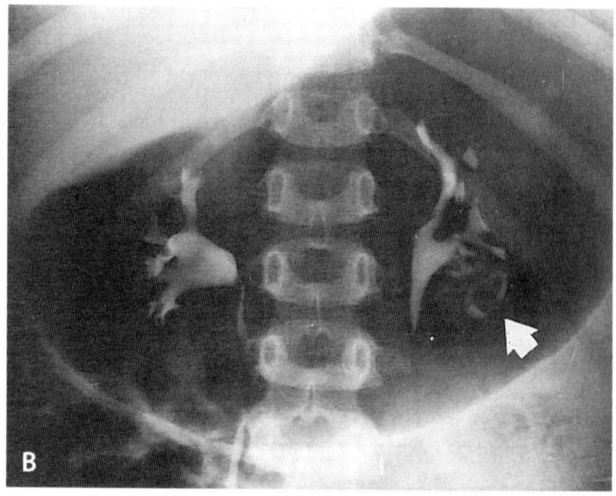

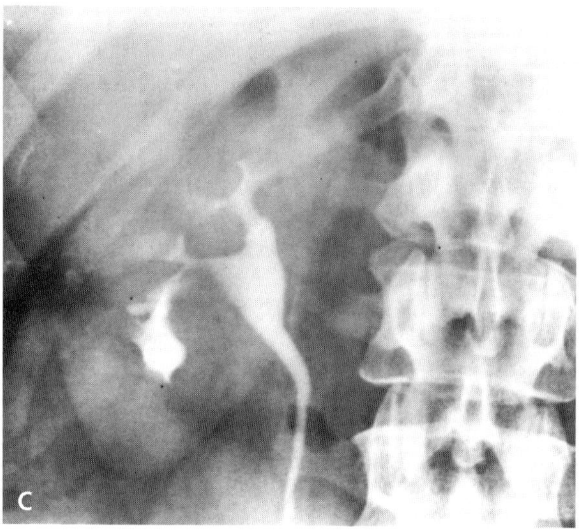

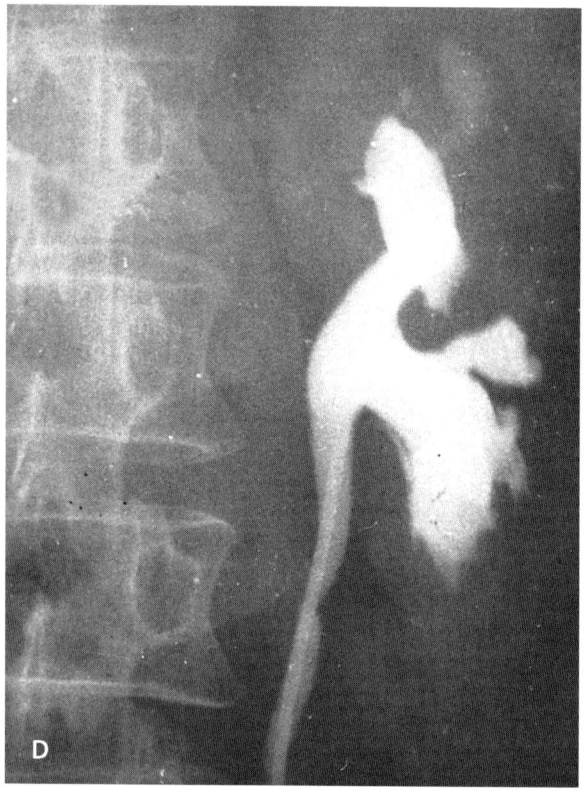

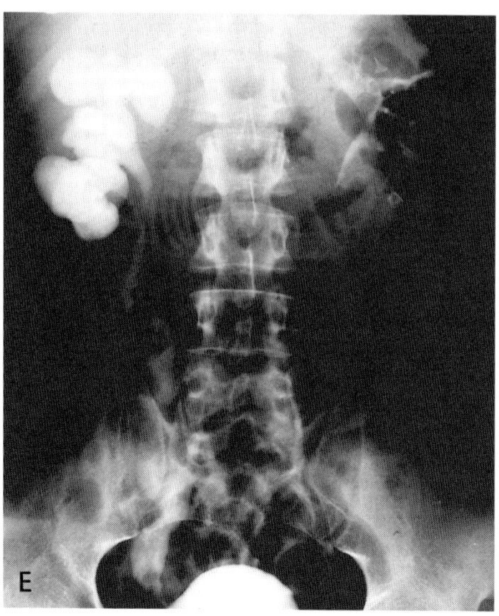

Fig. 5.54 A–F. Tuberculosis of the kidney; appearance on excretory urograms. **A** Widening and distortion of the upper calyces of the right kidney, with a stricture just above the renal pelvis. **B** Destruction of the lower calyces in the left kidney (*arrow*) with the formation of crescents outlining the edges fo the tuberculous abscess (cavity) **C** A tuberculous cavity in the lower pole of the kidney. **D** All the calyces in this left kidney are clubbed and distorted, and there is an abscess in the upper pole. **E** A more advanced infection in the right kidney with hydronephrosis and dilatation of the lower half of the right ureter. The left kidney and ureter are normal so far

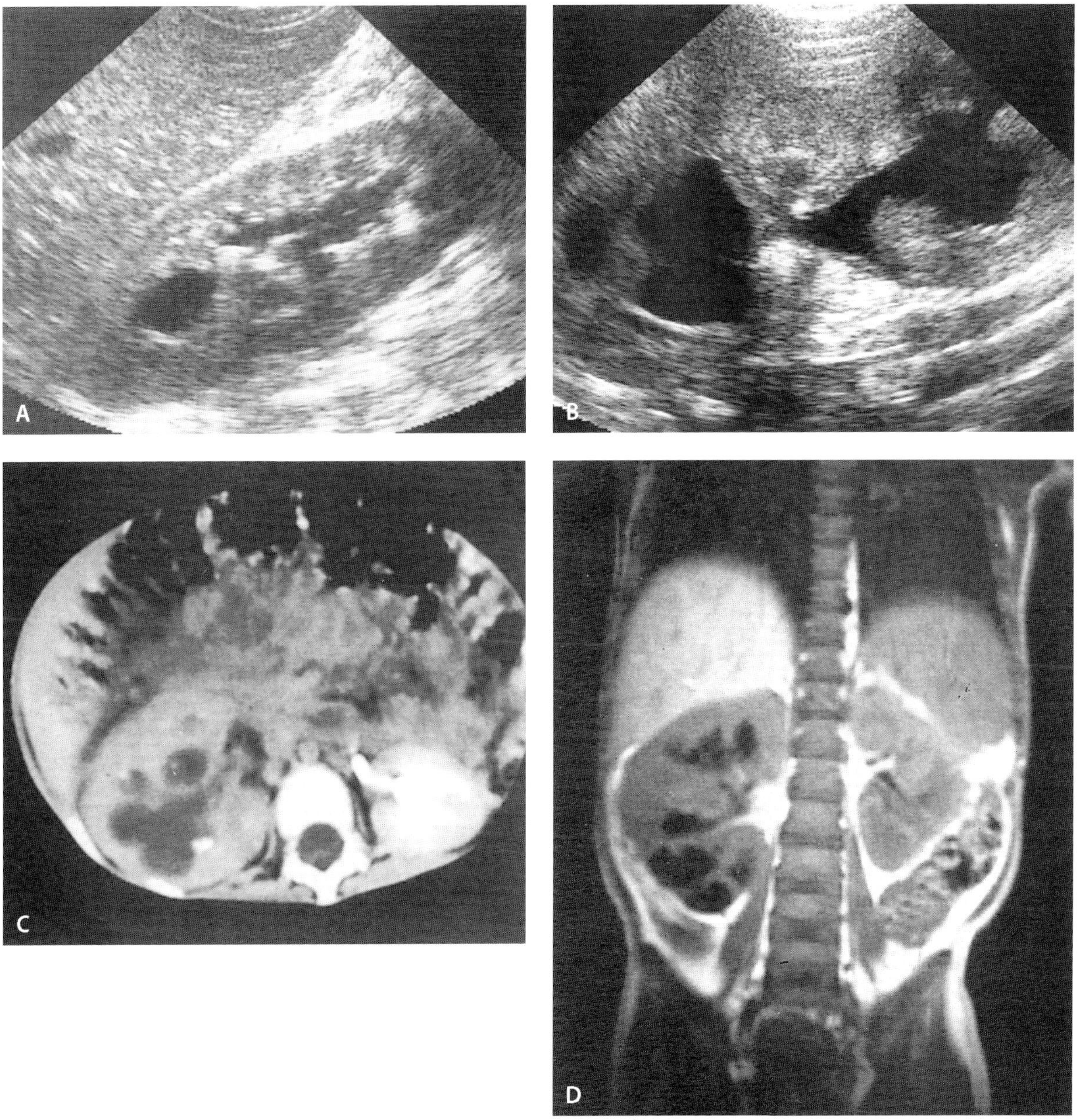

Fig. 5.55 A–F. Scanning can show parenchymal tuberculosis and its progress more accurately than urography. A, B Ultrasonography shows echogenic foci in the renal parenchyma as well as irregular caliectasis. C More advanced destruction of the calyceal system in the right kidney, with some parenchymal foci. D A coronal T1-weighed MR scan of the same patient showing the extent of the renal infection. E, F see p. 468

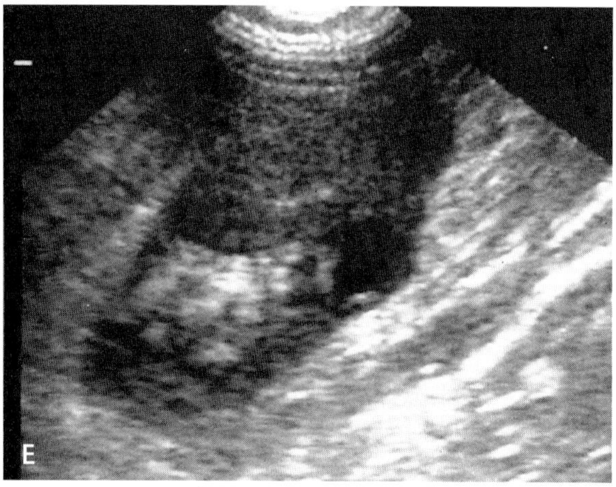

Fig. 5.55 (*continued*). **E** Ultrasonography of a different patient showing an abscess in the right kidney. **F** Angiography is useful in the differential diagnosis between a tumor and infection. The extent of the renal tuberculosis is well shown in this right renal series. (**A–D** from Cremin and Jamieson 1995; **E** courtesy of WHO: *The manual of diagnostic ultrasound*, Geneva, WHO, 1995; **F** courtesy of the University of Capetown Radiology Library)

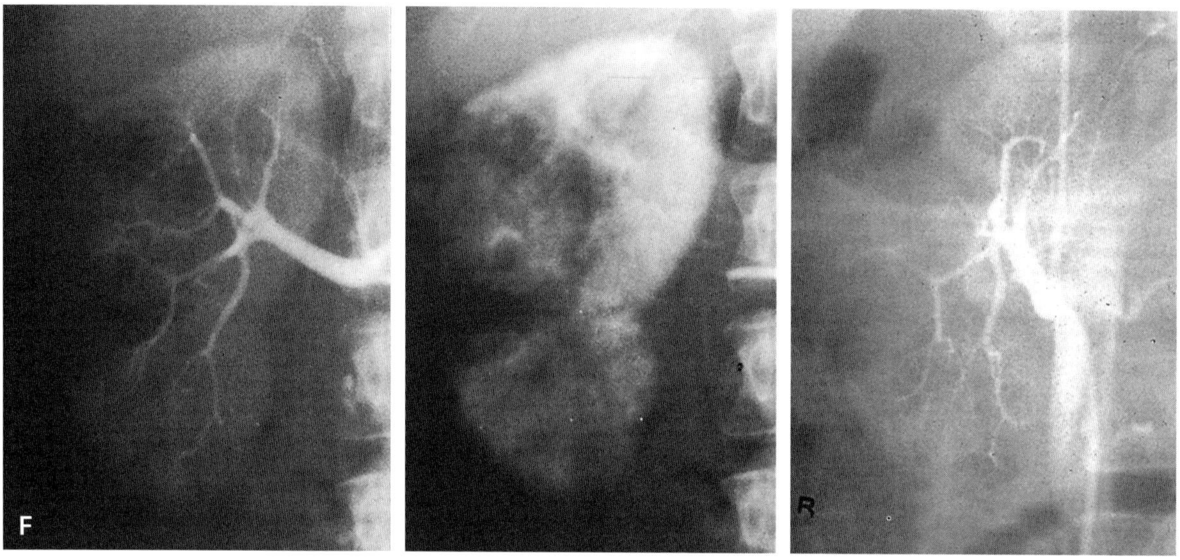

Fig. 5.56 A–E. When renal tuberculosis heals, it usually calcifies. **A** A large parenchymal granuloma in the lower pole of the left kidney. **B** Fine scattered calcification in the upper pole of the left kidney and the lower pole of the right kidney with scarring and shrinkage of the renal parenchyma. **C** Almost complete calcification of the right kidney. (There is no contrast medium.) An African from Kenya. This is the end result of renal tuberculosis. As well as heavy calcification within the right kidney, linear calcification can be seen in the right ureter, but not in the bladder. The ureteric calcification is unlike the intermittent, spotty calcification seen in schistosomiasis and, if that were the cause, there would almost certainly by bladder calcification also and a comparatively normal kidney. **D, E** Auto-amputation shown by ultrasonography (**D**) and by contrast CT (**E**). In **D** there is also echogenic material blocking the renal pelvis. (**C** courtesy of Dr. S. Malik, Nairobi; **D, E** from Cremin and Jamieson 1995) ▶

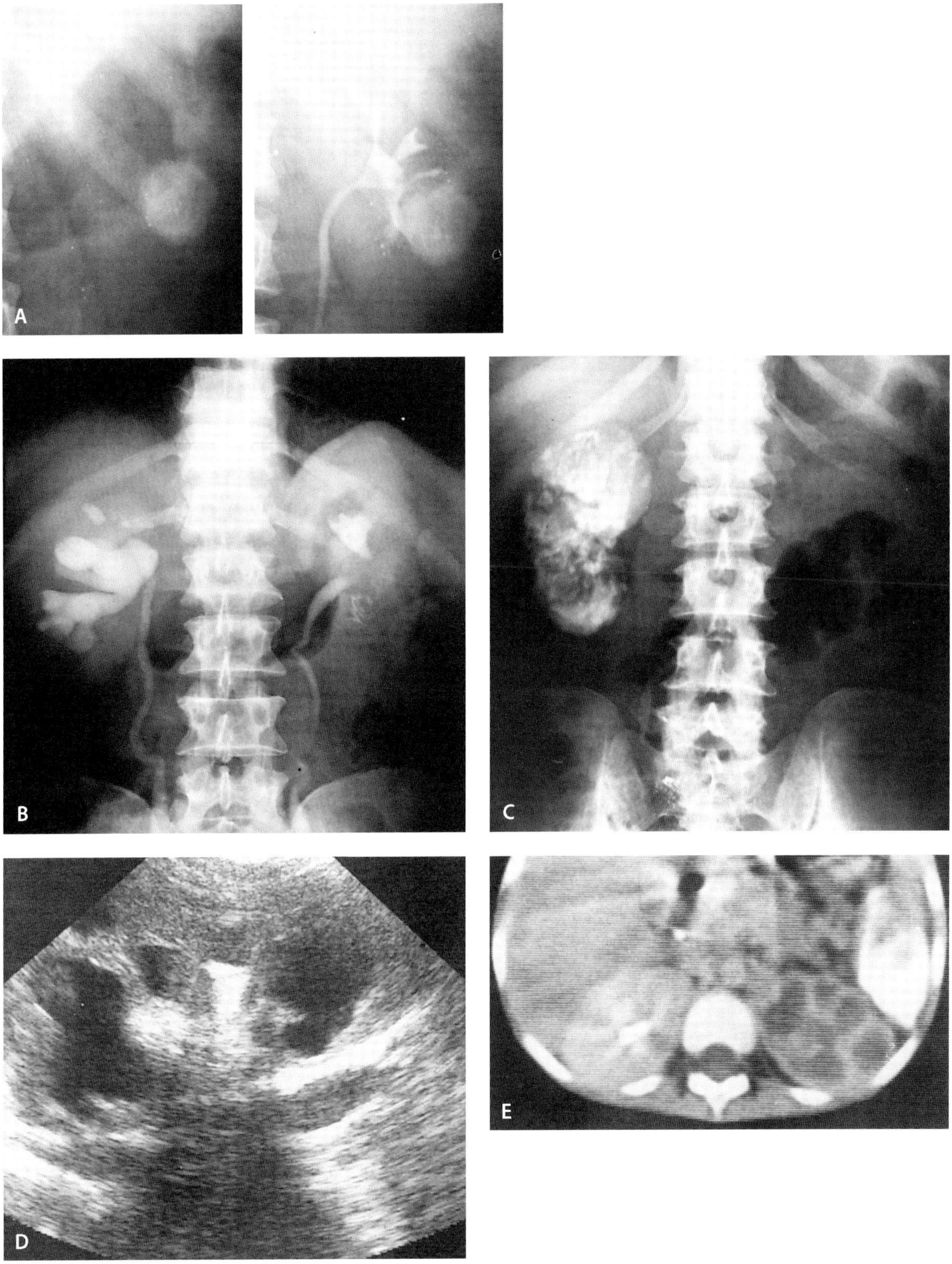
A
B
C
D
E

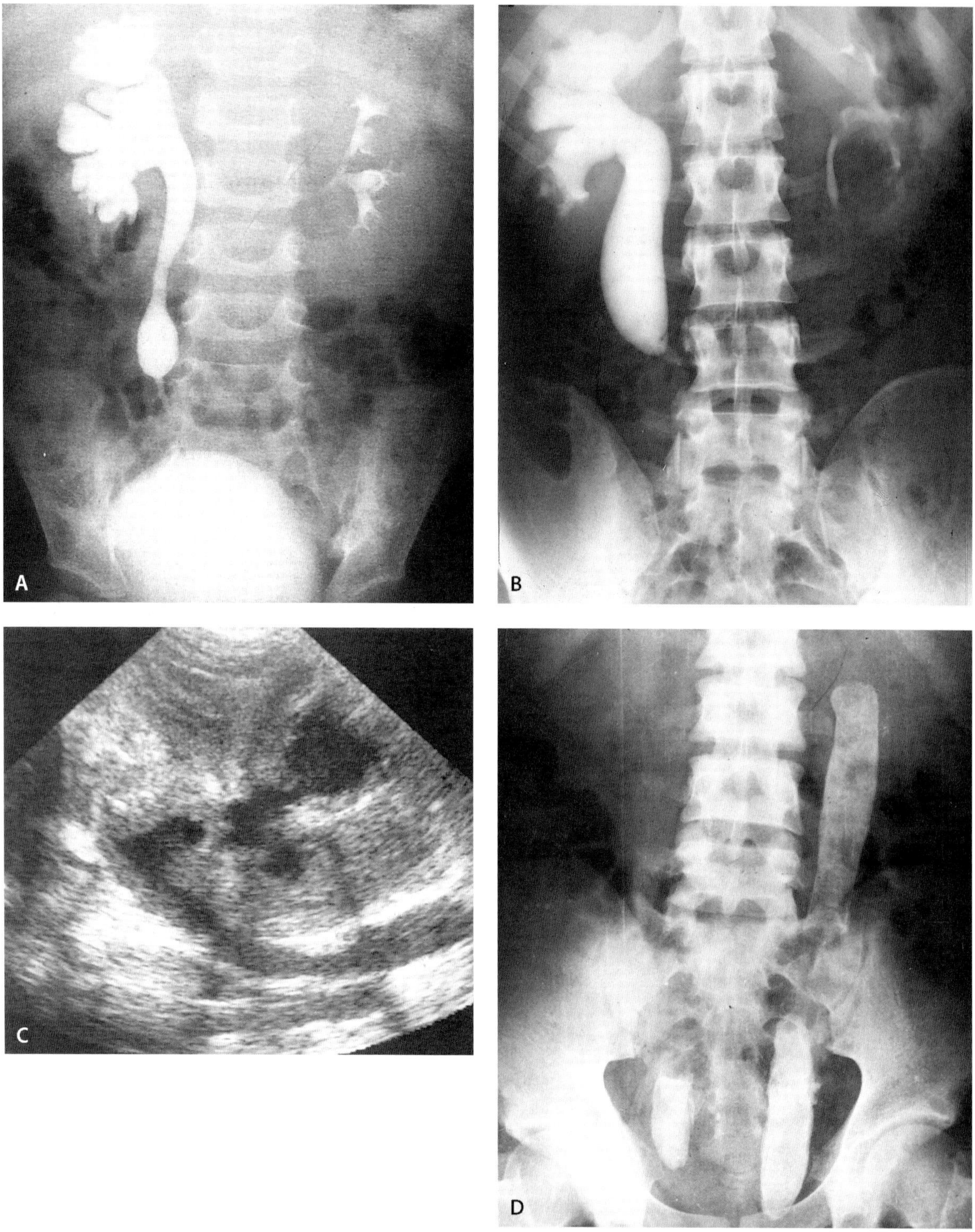

Fig. 5.57 A–D. Tuberculosis of the ureters. Strictures and dilatation can occur at almost any level along the ureter. **A** Hydronephrosis of the right kidney resulting from a stricture of the distal ureter in a child from South Africa. **B** A similar almost complete ureteric obstruction in an adult Kenyan African. It is difficult to know whether the kidney is also infected, or only obstructed. **C** Ultrasonography showing dilatation of the upper ureter and thickening of the ureteric epithelium, as well as parenchymal cavitation. **D** Advanced bilateral ureteric calcification. Unlike schistosomiasis, the bladder is not calcified. (**A**, **C** from Cremin and Jamieson 1995)

Bladder

When tuberculosis affects the bladder there is gradual and usually localized thickening of the bladder wall, with increasing diminution of the bladder volume. Trabeculation of the mucosa may develop. The vesicoureteric orifices are affected by this progressive fibrosis and there will then be bilateral, often asymmetrical hydroureter and hydronephrosis. Both CT and ultrasonography will demonstrate the irregular and thick bladder wall caused by the tuberculous granulomas (Fig. 5.58). To show this clearly, the bladder must be full which, in some patients with tuberculosis, may cause considerable discomfort because chronic contraction is usual. Contrast radiography or cystography is likely to demonstrate reflux up to the dilated ureters because the orifices will usually be rigid and held open. Bladder calcification due to tuberculosis is very uncommon and, when it occurs, is patchy. Calcification in small granulomas may be seen more easily on ultrasonography or CT. When bladder calcification is seen on a radiograph, schistosomiasis is the diagnosis until proven otherwise. Spontaneous tumor calcification can occur in bladder neoplasm (particularly in India), and needs to be differentiated from tuberculosis (but only after schistosomiasis has been excluded).

Adrenal Tuberculosis

Ultrasonography and CT (and MRI) have shown that adrenal tuberculosis is a little more common than previously suspected. It is usually bilateral, which is important in the differential diagnosis from adrenal hemorrhage in adults or from tumors (although metastases, especially from a lung primary, can also be bilateral).

Both ultrasonography and CT will shown enlargement of the adrenal glands: if it is easy to see the adrenals with ultrasonography they are probably enlarged (except in infants). On CT, there can be enhancement after contrast injection. When healing occurs, there will be calcification in the tuberculous granuloma and it can be diffuse, localized, or punctate: it is not always easy to recognize on plain radiograph. Tuberculous abscesses in the adrenal are initially well defined but later become complex.

The differential diagnosis is not difficult, particularly when there is calcification. Adrenal hemorrhage is not uncommon bilaterally during infancy but usually occurs on one side only in adults. Tuberculosis often causes bilateral enlargement and the enlargement may decrease but still persist after healing and calcification.

Genital Tuberculosis

Tuberculosis can infect any part of the genital tract but most commonly it is the fallopian tubes which are affected (Fig. 5.59 B–E). Hydrosalpinx and pyosalpinx are fairly common and may be large. There may be calcification of the pyosalpinx.

Hysterosalpingography shows flask-shaped dilatation of the fallopian tubes due to obstruction at the fimbriae. Sometimes, the block is at the uterine opening, and then the tubes are not visualized. Tuberculous endometritis and cervicitis may show as synechiae, irregular uterine mucosal lining, or an elongated cervix with loss of differentiation at the uterocervical junction. Surprisingly, tuberculous endometritis is not a significant cause of sterility (2% or less), whereas fallopian tube blockage will be, whatever the cause. Both ultrasonography and CT can demonstrate these changes and show the anatomical relationship clearly. However, the overall picture provided by hysterosalpingography has some advantages, particularly in the investigation of sterility.

Tuberculous masses within the pelvis can be the result of tuberculous peritonitis (see p. 457), with matting of the omentum, mesentery, and bowel, or they can be due to tuberculous tubo-ovarian abscesses. Both types of mass can be large and have been mistaken for carcinoma of the ovary or, in males, for the large nodal mass of lymphoma. On ultrasonography, such masses will have mixed echogenicity and there will be mixed density on CT because almost all will have both solid and cystic components. At least one tuberculous abscess has involved the bladder and vagina. Tuberculous tubo-ovarian abscesses may calcify and be seen in either side of the pelvis (together or singly) as well-defined homogeneous circular masses, sometimes with areas of increased density, probably due to the granuloma. Serpiginous or linear calcification can occur in the fallopian tubes.

Tuberculosis can affect the testes, presenting clinically as a swollen testes with a hydrocele. Ultrasonography will show a mass of mixed echogenicity, often with a central cavity containing debris (Fig. 5.59 A). It can be very difficult to differentiate tuberculosis from a tumor or other infection. Ultrasonography can also demonstrate the thickening due to edema caused by tuberculosis of the epididymis and vas deferens, both of which may eventually calcify and be seen on radiographs of the male pelvis. This must be differentiated from schistosomiasis and diabetes. Contrast studies of the vas and spermatic cord have not proven useful.

(Text continues on p. 474)

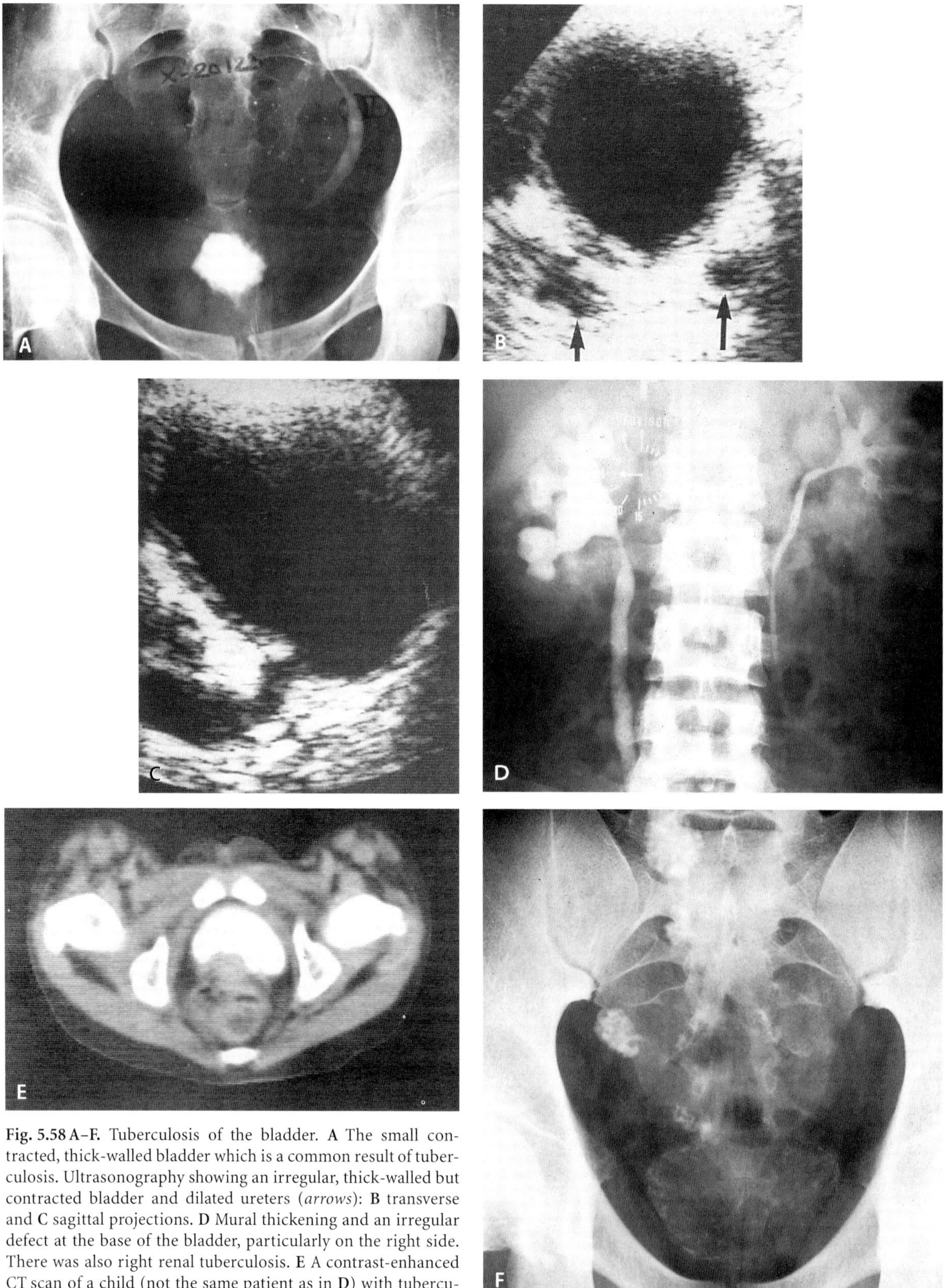

Fig. 5.58 A–F. Tuberculosis of the bladder. **A** The small contracted, thick-walled bladder which is a common result of tuberculosis. Ultrasonography showing an irregular, thick-walled but contracted bladder and dilated ureters (*arrows*): **B** transverse and **C** sagittal projections. **D** Mural thickening and an irregular defect at the base of the bladder, particularly on the right side. There was also right renal tuberculosis. **E** A contrast-enhanced CT scan of a child (not the same patient as in **D**) with tuberculous thickening at the base of the bladder. **F** Speckled calcification throughout the bladder and the lower left ureter. There are calcified granulomas in the lymph nodes in front of the sacrum on the right. It is unusual for tuberculous calcification to be so extensive: it is more commonly present in one bladder segment only. This was proven to be tuberculosis, without any evidence of schistosomiasis. (**B, C, E** from Cremin and Jamieson 1995)

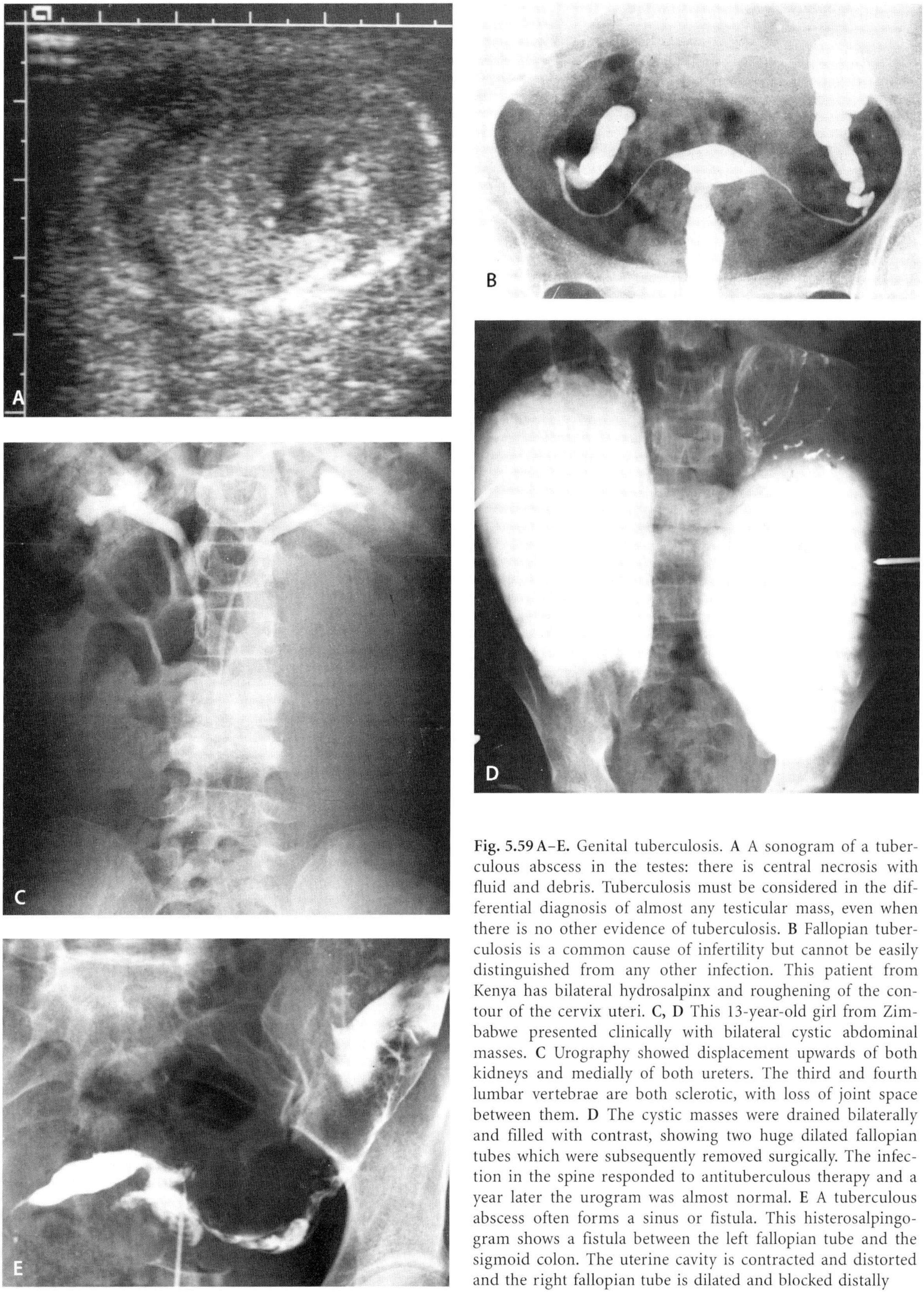

Fig. 5.59 A–E. Genital tuberculosis. A A sonogram of a tuberculous abscess in the testes: there is central necrosis with fluid and debris. Tuberculosis must be considered in the differential diagnosis of almost any testicular mass, even when there is no other evidence of tuberculosis. B Fallopian tuberculosis is a common cause of infertility but cannot be easily distinguished from any other infection. This patient from Kenya has bilateral hydrosalpinx and roughening of the contour of the cervix uteri. C, D This 13-year-old girl from Zimbabwe presented clinically with bilateral cystic abdominal masses. C Urography showed displacement upwards of both kidneys and medially of both ureters. The third and fourth lumbar vertebrae are both sclerotic, with loss of joint space between them. D The cystic masses were drained bilaterally and filled with contrast, showing two huge dilated fallopian tubes which were subsequently removed surgically. The infection in the spine responded to antituberculous therapy and a year later the urogram was almost normal. E A tuberculous abscess often forms a sinus or fistula. This histerosalpingogram shows a fistula between the left fallopian tube and the sigmoid colon. The uterine cavity is contracted and distorted and the right fallopian tube is dilated and blocked distally

Tuberculosis of Bone

There are three important characteristics of bone and joint tuberculosis in the tropics which differ from the non-AIDS cases in North America and Europe: it is often an acute osteomyelitis or arthritis, it is often a destructive condition which can affect any and every bone in the skeleton, and it is frequently multifocal.

Bone and joint tuberculosis is extremely common in tropical countries; there is a tendency to focus on pulmonary tuberculosis as the major public health problem, but skeletal infection is a neglected and serious disease for which there are few accurate statistics. It is common in India, Asia, much of tropical Africa, and South America. It is fueled by malnutrition, inadequate housing, poor medical services, and, perhaps most importantly, lack of health education; to this list must now be added AIDS. Many patients report to the doctor only when the disease is advanced and when they are paraplegic, crippled, or deformed. The majority of cases are not due to bovine tuberculosis; they arise from hematogenous spread, but in many patients the original site of infection will not be identified. There are no accurate figures on the relationship of bone tuberculosis to diagnosed pulmonary tuberculosis. A normal chest radiograph does not exclude a tuberculous etiology for a bone or joint infection, but neither does pulmonary tuberculosis mandate the same etiology for any osteomyelitis or arthritis; pyogenic infections are as common as tuberculosis. Whatever the state of the lungs, when there is a skeletal infection in the tropics tuberculosis should be considered in the differential diagnosis, whether the patient is HIV negative or positive.

No age is exempt. Skeletal tuberculosis may occur in babies from 6 months upwards and become an advanced disease; the elderly are similarly affected. It is most common in children and young adults, but is not rare in any age group. It occurs most frequently in the spine; the hip is the most common joint affected, followed by the knee, ankle, elbow, wrist, and shoulder in decreasing frequency. Tuberculous osteomyelitis can affect the skull, mandible, pelvis, ribs, and scapula. No bone escapes. Next to trauma it is the commonest cause of crippling and deformity and is such a common disease that it is cared for in general hospitals all over the tropical world. Drug therapy is usually effective, often dramatically so, but the late stage at which the patients appear necessitates skilled orthopedic correction which is not always available. Although the clinical presentation may be acute, the radiological findings often indicate that the infection has been present for a considerable time.

The majority of patients with skeletal tuberculosis (if they do not have AIDS) will be positive tuberuclin reactors, but a small percentage, perhaps less that 2%, will have negative skin tests. This can cause difficulty in diagnosis. Equally, because so many of the population will be positive reactors anyway, the finding of a positive tuberculin test in a patient with bone or joint infection is only really significant in infancy and the first few years of life. The diagnosis must be suggested by a high clinical index of suspicion, and confirmed by biopsy and culture. Unfortunately, not all biopsies will yield positive results; it may be necessary to treat the disease because of the clinical and radiological findings, despite a negative culture. A "sterile" culture is most likely to be tuberculosis and is useful in that it helps to exclude a pyogenic and typhoid etiology.

Because of poor host immunity, tuberculosis (even in those without AIDS) often behaves as an acute disease and must be treated in the same way. Surgical biopsy, even aspiration, is not a benign procedure and may result in widespread hematogenous dissemination and septicemia. A potentially tuberculous bone or joint should be treated with the same caution as a pyogenic dental abscess and surgery should be carried out under a therapeutic "umbrella" of antituberculous drugs; this rule should be violated only in cases of paraplegia due to an abscess or some similar acute emergency. The clinical and radiological diagnosis is surprisingly accurate in the majority of patients; biopsy will be confirmatory and provide a culture for the sensitivity of the organism, rather than being an immediate necessity. In the spine, removing the "pus" may be therapeutic also.

Tuberculous osteomyelitis and arthritis are often associated with marked peripheral lymphadenopathy (also tuberculous). This combination is particularly found in spinal tuberculosis and conversely, when children have gross lymphatic involvement, concomitant bone or joint disease should be carefully excluded. In one reported series from the Philippines, 7 out of 39 children with lymphatic tuberculosis were found, on radiological examination, to have spinal tuberculosis which had been clinically unsuspected. This combination occurs throughout the tropics, particulary in India and Africa; skeletal involvement can be remarkably silent in its early stages and may only become obvious because of a complication. In AIDS, skeletal tuberculosis becomes yet another part of the onslaught of infections.

The best way to image any part of the skeleton will depend very much on the site involved, but because tuberculous bone infections are so often multifocal and may be present in different parts of the skeleton and yet be clinically silent, scintigraphy is a very valuable early investigation. However, when such a scan shows multiple active sites in the patient who is clinically ill and has lost weight, the possibility of malignancy will also have to considered. To make the differential diagnosis more difficult, the tumormarker CA 125 may be positive in destructive skeletal tuberculosis and even in tuberculous peritonitis.

Tuberculosis of the Spine

Synonyms

Caries. Pott's disease. Pott's paraplegia. *Ger*: Pott-paraplegie. *Fr*: paraplégie de Pott.

Clinical Characteristics

The description and statistics in this section refer to HIV-negative patients. For those with AIDS, the clinical and imaging findings are similar, but often more advanced, and the site incidence may be different. Tuberculosis in AIDS is "tropical tuberculosis," but more progressive and often more advanced. In most tropical countries tuberculosis of the spine accounts for more than 50% of all cases of skeletal tuberculosis. Clinically, paraplegia is the commonest presenting symptom. It may be complete and acute, with bladder paralysis and inability to walk; depending on the level of the infection, it may present as quadriplegia. In other patients the symptomatology may be less severe, but neurological involvement occurs in half of those who have tuberculous spines. The remainder complain of the deformity, of pain, or of general weakness and ill health which bring them to the physician. Some will complain of a mass in the groin, which may be a hernia, but the possibility of a psoas abscess should be remembered in every such case. Whatever the presentation, a careful examination will reveal some neurological deficit (often unsuspected) in the majority of patients when first seen; yet they may have very gross spinal deformity but still be ambulatory.

Clinico-pathological-radiological Correlation: Spinal Tuberculosis

If the radiological findings in tuberculosis of the spine are to be understood, it is important to have a clear idea of the underlying pathological changes. These were beautifully described in 1936 by Compere and Garrison, working at the University of Chicago. They made longitudinal whole-body sections of tuberculous spines and correlated these with radiological findings and the histological examination. Their autopsy research has since been confirmed at surgery by Hodgson and others in Hong Kong (1969). Now, in recent years, CT and especially MRI have imaged the pathophysiology, and provided three-dimensional confirmation. There are two basic premises: (a) cartilage resists destruction by tuberculosis and (b) there is no blood supply to the intervertebral disc, although there is a rich blood supply to the vertebrae. The vertebral blood supply does not cross the articular surface; the disc obtains its nutrition from lymphatics.

The intervertebral disc is a fibrocartilaginous ring, the annulus, blended with hyaline cartilage plates above and below and enclosing the nucleus pulposus. The nucleus is an interlacing matrix of fibrous tissue and fibrocartilage, with semigelatinous substance within the mesh; because this is liquid it is incompressible, and therefore narrowing of the disc can only take place when there is extrusion or destruction of the nucleus or, alternatively, dehydration. Tuberculosis commonly starts by hematogenous implant and more rarely by direct extension from infected lymph nodes. It is essentially a bone-destroying infection, with little evidence of repair in the early stages. When it occurs beneath cartilage, the cartilage is eventually destroyed but the annulus and nucleus tend to survive much longer. It is only when there is fissuring of the annulus that the infection can involve the disc proper. Even when the vertebral body has become caseous, wedged, and destroyed, careful histological search will nearly always show the nucleus, either intact or in part, having prolapsed into the softened bone or debris. Primary tuberculous invasion of the annulus has not been demonstrated. Narrowing of the disc space occurs when the annulus eventually becomes infected and fluid escapes, or when the nucleus is extruded. At this stage there will be loss of the disc space when imaged.

Compere and Garrison also showed very clearly the spread of tuberculous abscesses under the anterior or, more rarely, the posterior spinal longitudinal ligaments. When this occurs the infection involves the vertebral bodies and the disc remain intact for a considerable time. They illustrated pathologically what may be demonstrated by imaging, i.e., that multiple vertebrae can be involved above and below the original focus and yet the disc and the dura may remain intact. The cartilaginous plate of the vertebra is a barrier, more effective in children than in adults because it is thicker during childhood.

The studies of Compere and Garrison showed pressure on the spinal cord is likely to be from an epidural or subdural abscess, and sometimes from a prolapsed disc. Direct pressure from a collapsed vertebra is rare. Paraplegia thus results from the ab-

scess, from the prolapsed disc or tuberculous debris, or occasionally from edema of the cord due the neighboring infection.
The same authors also pointed out that tuberculous peritonitis from direct spread of a spinal abscess is uncommon and that most cases of tuberculous spinal meningitis are hematogenous in origin.
Compere and Garrison showed that in pyogenic infections, invasion of the intervertebral disc occurs more rapidly, is seen earlier, and is more common. This is because the cartilaginous plate is destroyed by proteolytic enzymes and the nuclear substance is extruded more rapidly, with dissolution of the annulus. This occurs in all pyogenic infections, but particularly in brucellosis. The ability of the intervertebral disc to survive a tuberculous infection during the early stages is important in the differential diagnosis. It is particularly well illustrated in Figs. 5.60 B, C and E, 5.61 A, and 5.66. The anterior spread of an abscess is well illustrated in Fig. 5.71 B.

Imaging of Spinal Tuberculosis

There are important general principles which guide the imaging of spinal tuberculosis:

1. Plain skeletal radiography provides a great deal of information, but it does not show the extent of the very important intradural abscess or of its paravertebral extension. It does not always demonstrate every locus of bone infection, nor does it show the nucleus palposus.
2. Because spinal tuberculosis is often multifocal, bone scintigraphy is a very valuable early examination; not only will other vertebral foci be seen, but early infection elsewhere in the skeleton may be discovered.
3. Ultrasonography is useful in demonstrating the paravertebral abscess and any associated lymphadenopathy. Beyond this, it does not provide useful information in most cases.
4. CT is excellent for demonstrating the exact extent of the skeletal disease, the deformity, and the size and position of the abscess (if any). It does not demonstrate intramedullary foci.
5. MRI provides very accurate information about both the soft tissue and bone involvement. It is accurate in the demonstration of bone lesions and is the only way to image focal myelitis in the cord. It is a poor method of imaging calcification as it occurs during healing.

Vertebral Body

Although the destructive process of spinal tuberculosis is best imaged by CT or MRI, plain radiography and standard tomography can provide useful information, particularly if the underlying pathological process is understood.
The original tuberculous focus may be marginal, central, or subperiosteal and is usually in the vertebral body (Fig. 5.60). Infection starting in a pedicle is not all that uncommon, and can be bilateral. In nontropical countries destruction of the pedicle suggests malignancy, either metastatic or lymphomatous, but in the tropics it may be tuberculous. It is not very uncommon for only the neural arch to be affected, the vertebral body remaining intact.
This can be difficult to detect with plain radiography, but is well seen by CT. The transverse processes are rarely involved except as part of the spread of infection; the spinous process is occasionally affected, but causes little deformity.
Many tuberculous spinal infections are multifocal: when suspected in any vertebra, the whole spine should be radiographed (if there has not been previous scintigraphy). Infection may be centered in one, two, three, or four contiguous vertebrae, or there may be normal vertebrae between other sites of infection, above or below that originally discovered. In some patients there will be more than two involved areas, each separated by normal vertebrae.

Fig. 5.60 A–I. Tuberculosis can affect any part of the vertebral body or neural arch. In the early stages, the intervertebral disc space may remain normal. **A** Destruction in the center of the vertebral without any change in shape. A patient from Tanzania. **B** This vertebral body has also maintained its shape but there is more advanced central destruction and the upper border will probably collapse. **C** The upper border of this vertebra is beginning to collapse and there is minimal lose of disc space. The central focus of infection was clearly visible only on tomography. **D** Similar infection in the lower half of the body. On the routine films, the loss of the cortical margin was visible but not the central destruction. **E** Central destruction of the lower half of the vertebral body, only seen on the anteroposterior view. The disc space is slightly narrowed. **F** Destruction of the right side of the vertebral body and the neural arch, with the remainder of the body maintaining its shape. The lower disc space is narrowed on the right side; the upper space is almost normal. A small lytic defect is present on the right side of the body below, and there is a small paravertebral abscess. The extent of the bony destruction is usually underestimated by plain radiography and is better seen by CT or MRI (see also Figs. 5.68–5.70). **G, H** Tuberculosis affecting the spinous process only. This is very unusual. **I** A CT scan of a child from South Africa, showing destruction of the neural arch on both sides, as well as of the vertebral body. *Arrows*, anterior spinal abscess. (**A** courtesy of Dr. Harold G. Jacobson; **I** from Cremin and Jamieson 1995)

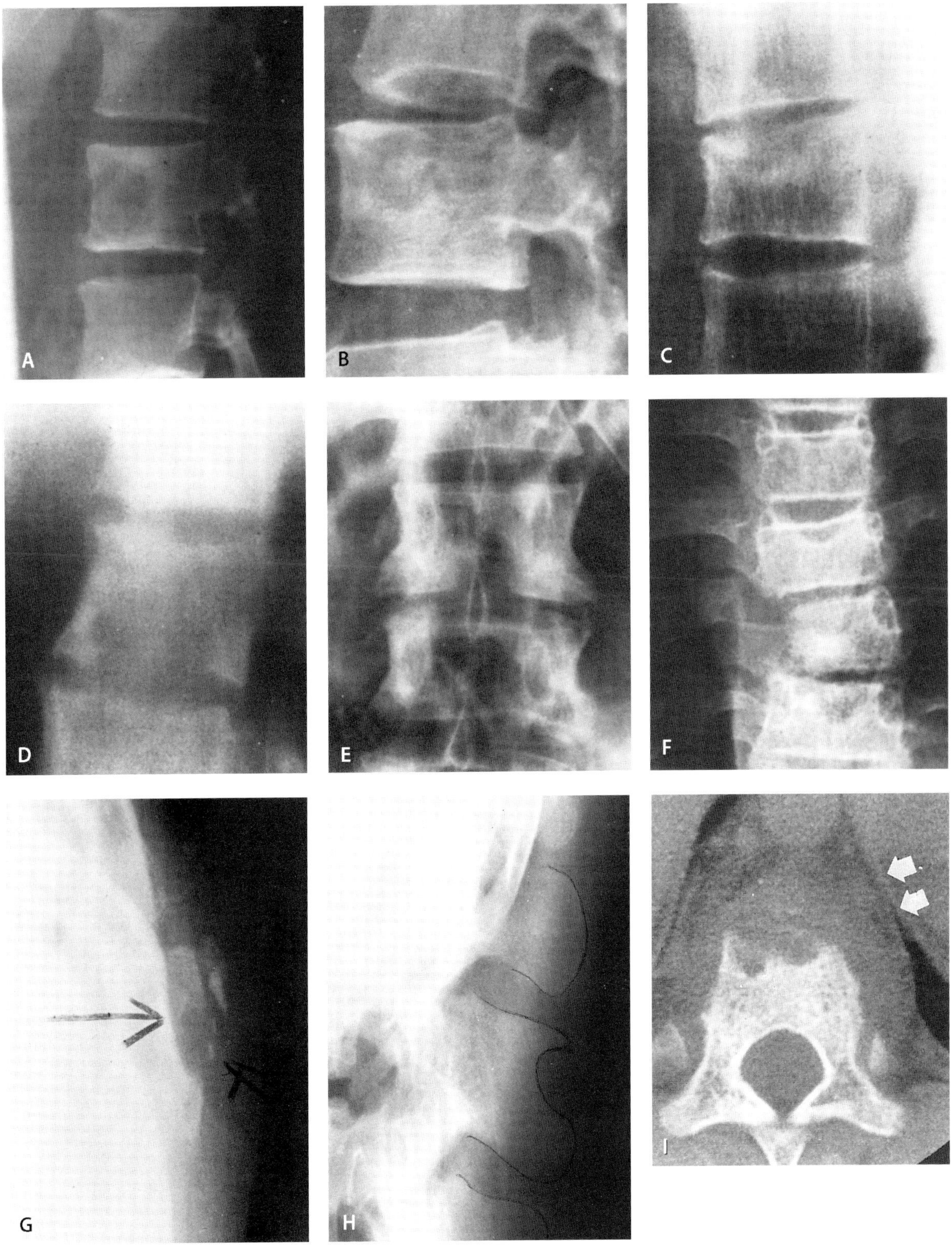
A
B
C
D
E
F
G
H
I

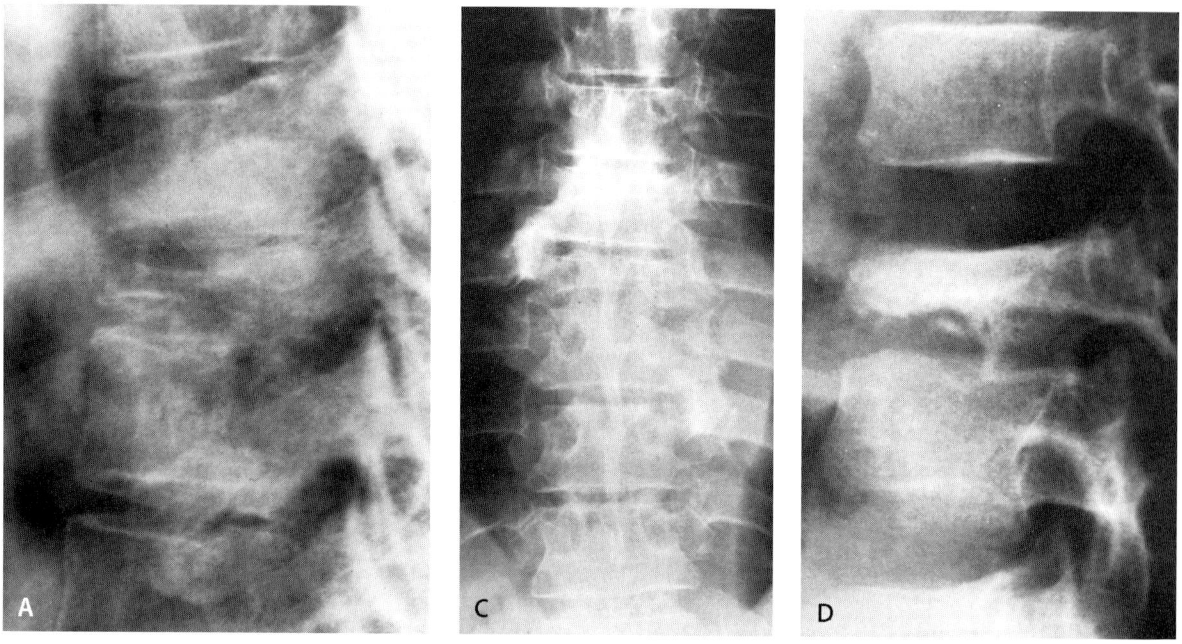

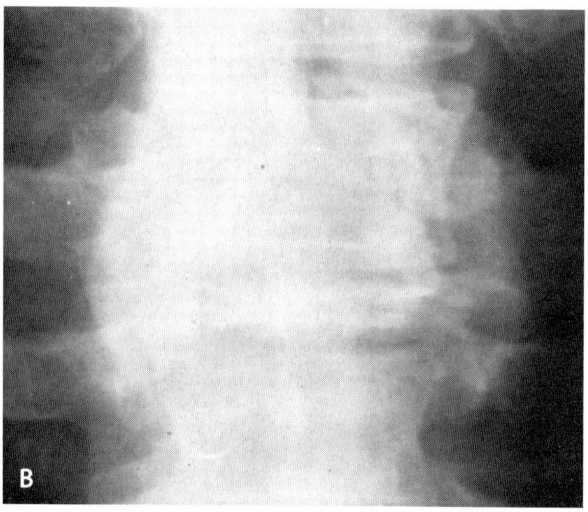

Fig. 5.61 A–D. Vertebra plana. Four different patients. **A** The vertebra has collapsed and yet the upper and lower margins remain intact and the disc spaces are clear. **B** More extensive collapse with small bilateral paravertebral abscesses. **C** This mid-thoracic vertebra has collapsed in the same way, with intact upper and lower margins, and clear disc spaces. However, there is some new bone on either side and there is some destruction of the left upper border of the vertebra below. There is a left paravertebral abscess, but none is visible on the right. **D** A pseudo-vertebra plana: the top half of the body is intact and becoming sclerotic. The disc space above is clear, but the anterior half of the lower margin has been destroyed although the posterior edge remains normal. These four patients were all Africans from Zimbabwe

The degree of bone destruction when the patient is first radiographed is infinitely variable. There may be an area of increased lucency, occasionally localized by low-grade clinical pain and perhaps identified after radionuclide scanning. Standard tomography, CT, or MRI, may be necessary to find the defect within the vertebral body. Unfortunately, this is the least common presentation; most patients are first seen when the vertebral lesions are easily visible on routine films.

Because of the bone destruction the extent of the change in the vertebral shape is variable. The vertebra may be intact, with no change in its outline or there may be one or more peripheral defects; this can occur in any part of the vertebral body. Alternatively, collapse may be so complete that there is a "vertebra plana" (Fig. 5.61). In nontropical countries it is a diagnostic "rule" that vertebra plana is never tuberculous, but we have a personal series of more than 40 such cases, all of them proven tuberculosis, and many other radiologists in the tropics have seen similar cases. Tuberculosis in the tropics does not follow European and North American rules.

Wedge formation is the commonest finding and is a complex process with many variants. The majority of vertebrae collapse anteriorly; some demonstrate lateral collapse and only in a minority will the collapse first occur posteriorly. (This is said to be more common in pyogenic infections, but it can happen in tuberculosis.) The wedge may be formed of only one vertebral body which has collapsed on itself, either with both the upper and lower borders falling inwards towards the center, or with one or other border remaining intact and the wedging occurring onto it (Figs. 5.62, 5.63). However, the radiological appearance of a wedge can be misleading and what at first seems to be one vertebra may be a wedge formed of two or even more. The disc space may seem to be totally obliterated. In such cases, the upper border of the top vertebral body and the lower border of the one beneath remain intact but are no longer parallel, and the central parts of both vertebrae merge to become the wedge. The angulation can vary so that the wedge is around either the upper or lower vertebra, or both. The same destructive process can extend to involve three vertebrae or, rarely, four. When this happens the middle vertebral body disappears. It is thus essential to identify each pedicle when assessing tuberculous wedging, and if possible also to localize the vertebral ends of the ribs to be sure of the number of vertebrae involved. A seemingly severely wedged small vertebral body may be all that is left of three or, at the most, four vertebrae. Fusion may be complete, the cortical margins may be reestablished, and there may be no trace of the original anatomy. The resulting spinal deformity is equally variable. There may be little clinical abnormality, even when there is marked vertebral destruction; alternatively, there may be severe kyphosis (Fig. 5.64), and if two regions of the spine are infected, the curvature is often bizarre and myelography (see later) becomes a major problem. In the majority of patients the spinal cord manages to adapt to amazing curves, and paraplegia is seldom due to the bony deformity; it usually results from the abscess within the spinal canal. When paraplegia occurs without pus, it is due to vascular or toxic changes, or, as MRI has demonstrated, the intramedullary lesion; very rarely paraplegia is due to vertebral disc displacement. The disc is involved late in tuberculosis, and is more often displaced into the vertebral body than posteriorly into the cord. Even when most of the rest of the disc has disappeared, very late in the infection, MRI can often show the fluid in the nucleus.

Healing of a tuberculous infection in the spine occurs in many different ways. The vertebral body may return to normal and be reconstituted with apparently normal margins and only slight increase in trabecular density to indicate the previous infection. When two vertebral bodies have fused, the resulting bone may also look almost normal, apart from the wedge shape. In other cases vertebrae sclerosis occurs, so that all or part of the vertebral body is increased in density (Fig. 5.65); this is evenly distributed and is seldom patchy. In temperate climates it is commonly said that tuberculosis does not cause sclerosis, but this is not applicable in the more acute pattern of the disease in the tropics. However, sclerosis does not always follow the expected distribution of the bone necrosis; it may be seen radio-

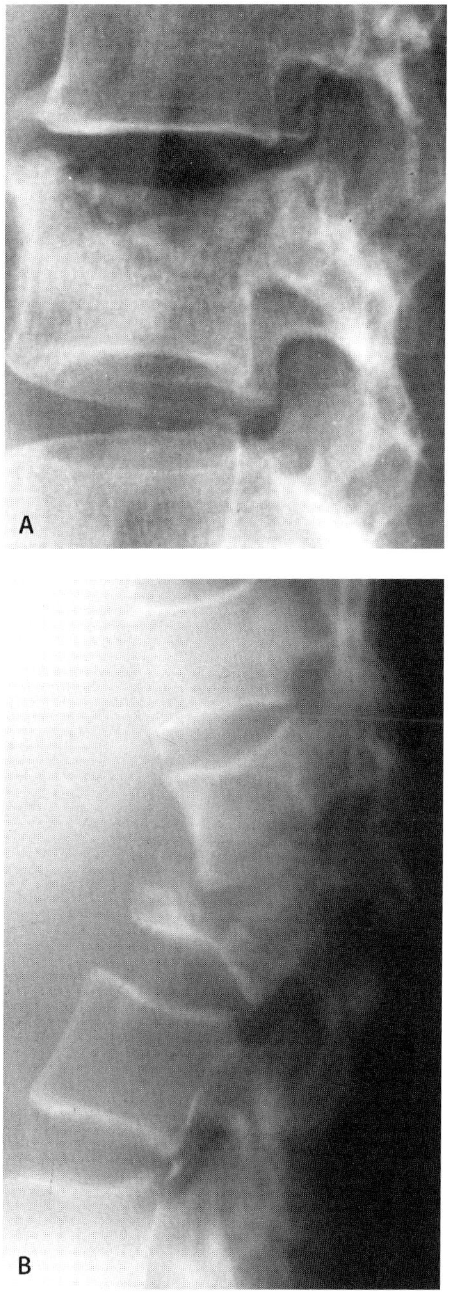

Fig. 5.62 A, B. In early spinal tuberculosis, the commonest finding is decrease in the disc space and some destruction of the vertebral body. **A** Most of the upper part of the vertebral body has given way and the intervertebral disc has probably sunken into the necrotic bone. The vertebra above is intact, but the disc space is narrowed. **B** This vertebra has given away even more, so that the disc and the vertebra above have caused it to split. Yet the disc spaces above and below are normal and no other infected vertebrae are visible on this radiograph. (Though there is the possibility of other foci of infection above or below and these should be sought and excluded. Increasing kyphosis and, eventually, spinal cord damage are inevitable unless this is treated.)

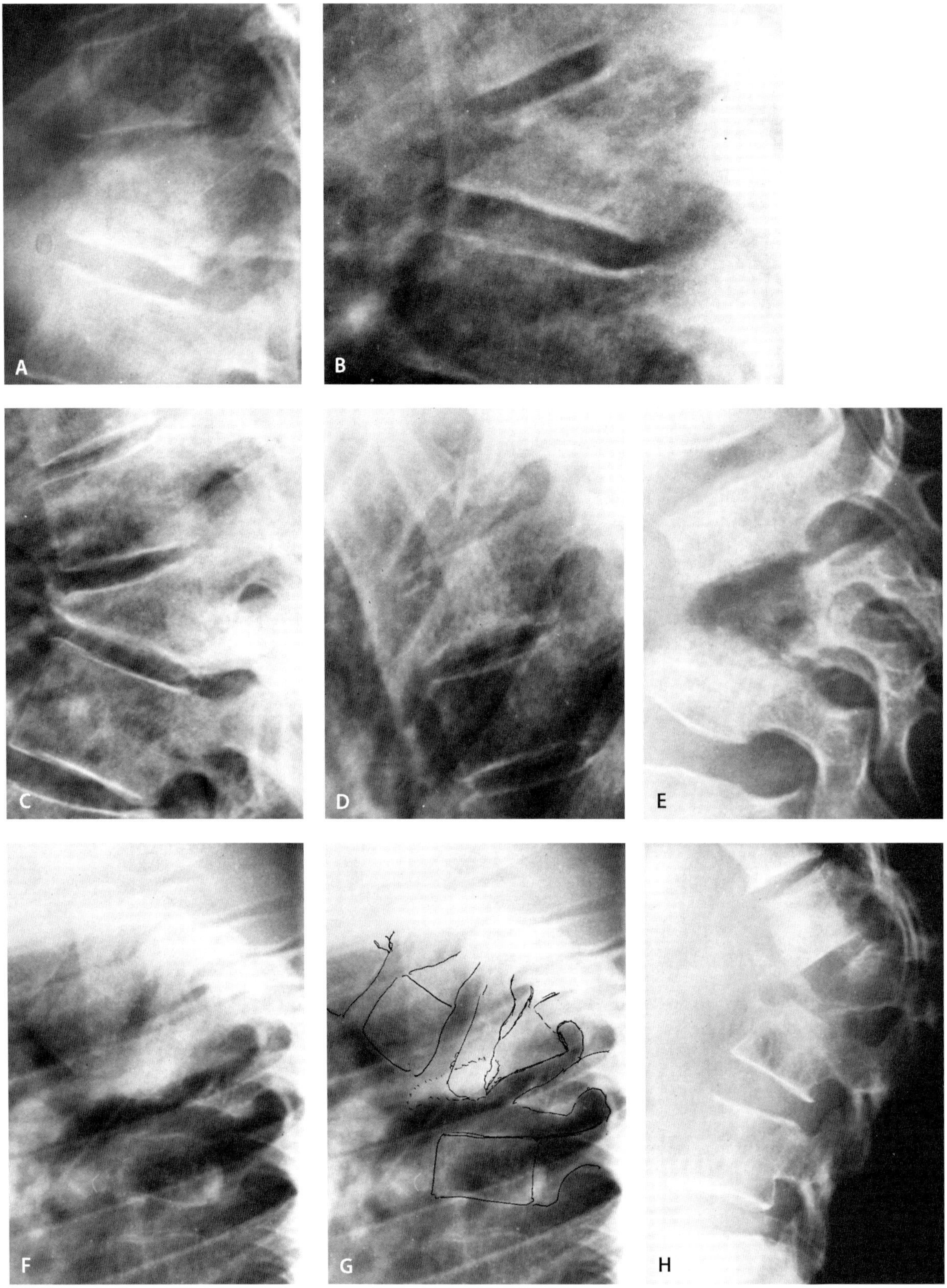
A
B
C
D
E
F
G
H

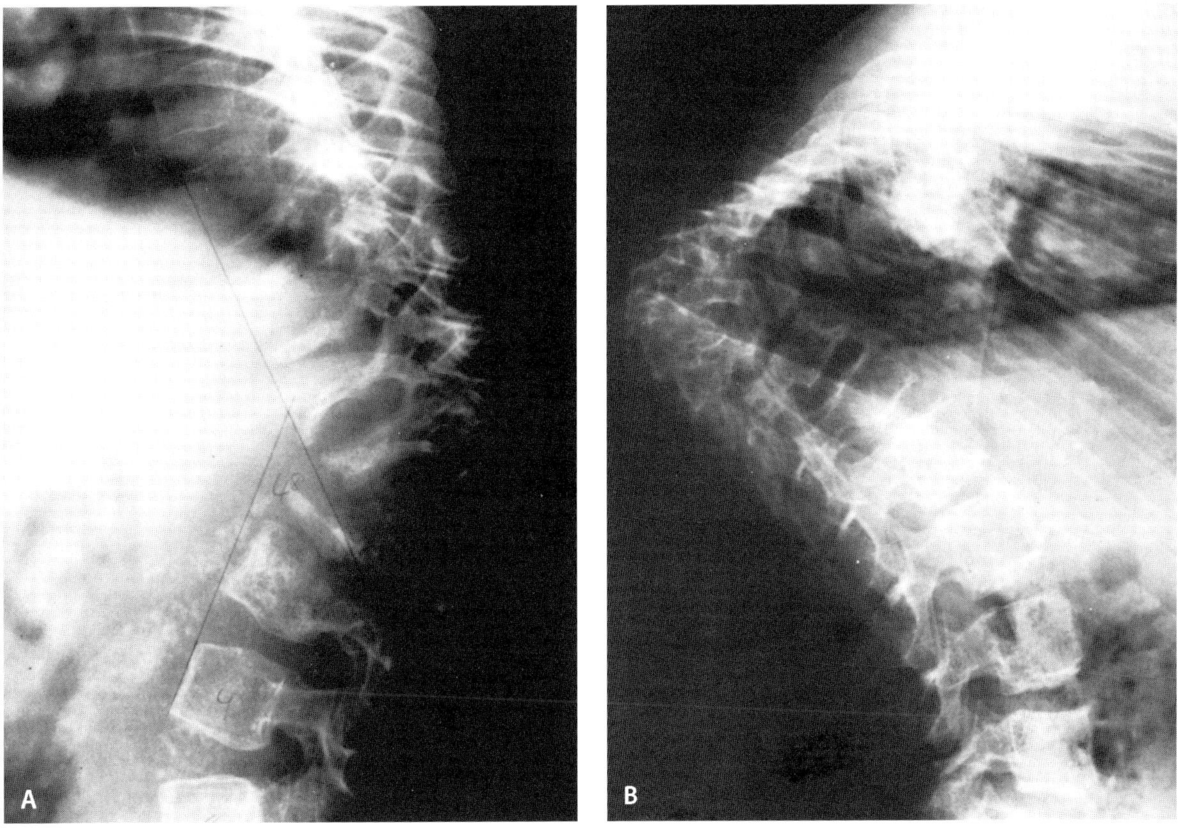

Fig. 5.64 A, B. Tuberculous kyphosis. Two African patients with severe kyphosis and infection of multiple vertebrae. **A** Eight vertebrae are infected. Three have become individual vertebrae plana. The wedge in the center is formed from the 12th thoracic and the first lumbar vertebrae combined. There is a large calcified psoas abscess extending anteriorly down into the pelvis. **B** Similar mid-thoracic infection involving multiple vertebrae which are now healed. There is a calcified abscess anteriorly. There is no vertebral rotation and the anteroposterior view showed there was very little scoliosis

◀ **Fig. 5.63 A–H.** The way in which wedge formation in tuberculosis occurs depends on the number of vertebrae involved. **A** Opposing surfaces of two thoracic vertebrale have been infected, and the disc space is no longer visible. **B** Twelve months later (with treatment) the bones are healing and fusing into one. **C** Thirty-one months after film **A**, there is a solid wedge made from two vertebral bodies, with well-defined edges. The disc spaces above and below the wedge are normal: there will probably be no further change until degenerative arthritis develops. Wedge formation can be more complicated. **D** One complete vertebral body has collapsed into a wedge, but with normal vertebrae above and below. **E** Two vertebrae have become wedged and the opposing surfaces of the vertebrae above and below are also infected. **F, G** There are three vertebrae at the center of this kyphosis and they will probably fuse into one solid wedge. If there is no abscess, this degree of curvature does not immediately cause neurological symptoms in children, but as their growth alters from age 12–13 years onward, there may be pressure on the cord. The end results may resemble **H**. This healed wedge formed from two vertebrae and fused with the vertebral body immediately below

logically in parts of the vertebra which have up to then been considered normal. CT, MRI, or standard tomography of a tuberculous spinal infection usually demonstrates considerably more bone destruction than can be appreciated on routine films, and during healing the sclerosis may follow this distribution. (Except when affecting the upper thoracic vertebrae, the indication to scan or tomograph tuberculous vertebrae, particularly when the diagnosis has been firmly established, should be based more on the neurological examination than the radiographic appearances.) Bone sclerosis does not necessarily indicate secondary infection; it can occur as a result of tuberculosis without any complications.

Spinal tuberculosis in the tropics often heals with marked anterior and lateral bony bridging, to such an extent that it may resemble ankylosing spondylitis (Figs. 5.66, 5.67). It may be surprisingly symmetrical, but the normal sacroiliac joints in this pattern of tuberculosis may help to establish the correct diagnosis.

(Text continues on p. 484)

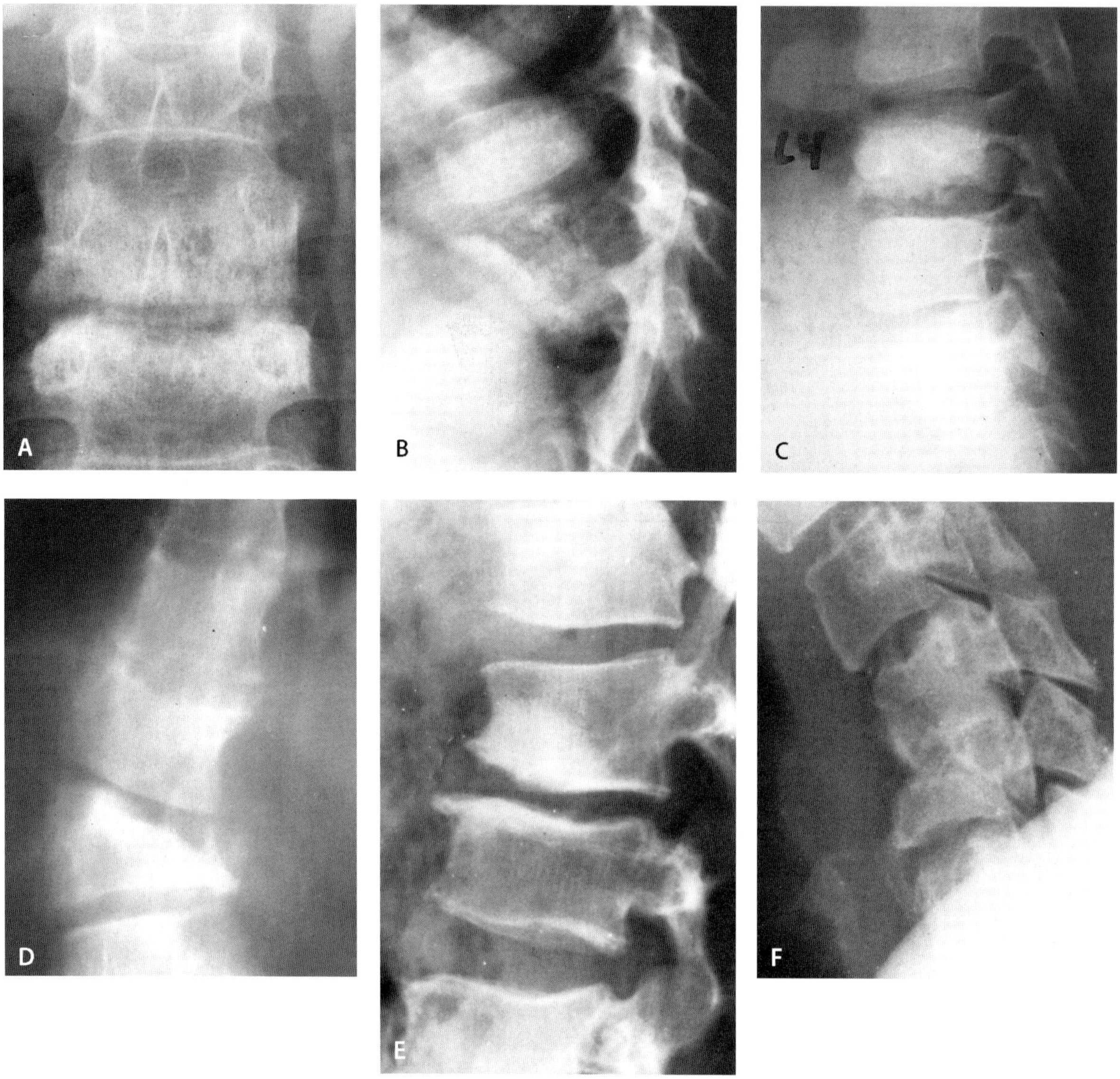

Fig. 5.65 A–F. The healing of spinal tuberculosis. Sclerosis represents initial evidence of repair but it does not reliably indicate that the infection has healed completely. **A** Increased trabecular density occurring about 3 months after starting antituberculous treatment. **B** Increasing density in the lower part of a wedge of vertebrae. **C** Increased density of a whole vertebral body, which is irregular in outline and smaller than the two normal vertebrae above and below it. The disc spaces are surprisingly clear. **D** The lateral aspect of this vertebra had collapsed and the bone is increasing in density and will probably not wedge any further. The upper margins of the two vertebrae above are also slightly increased in density, suggesting that they were previously infected. **E** A well-healed sclerotic tuberculous focus in the lower anterior portion of a vertebral body, with decrease in disc space and some reactive sclerosis in the vertebra below. This was a young African man who had been treated for more than 2 years to reach this stage. **F** Healing can take place without increased bone density, but will then involve a lot of fibrosis. This could be mistaken for the result of trauma, but was proven tuberculosis. (C courtesy of Dr. Harold G. Jacobson)

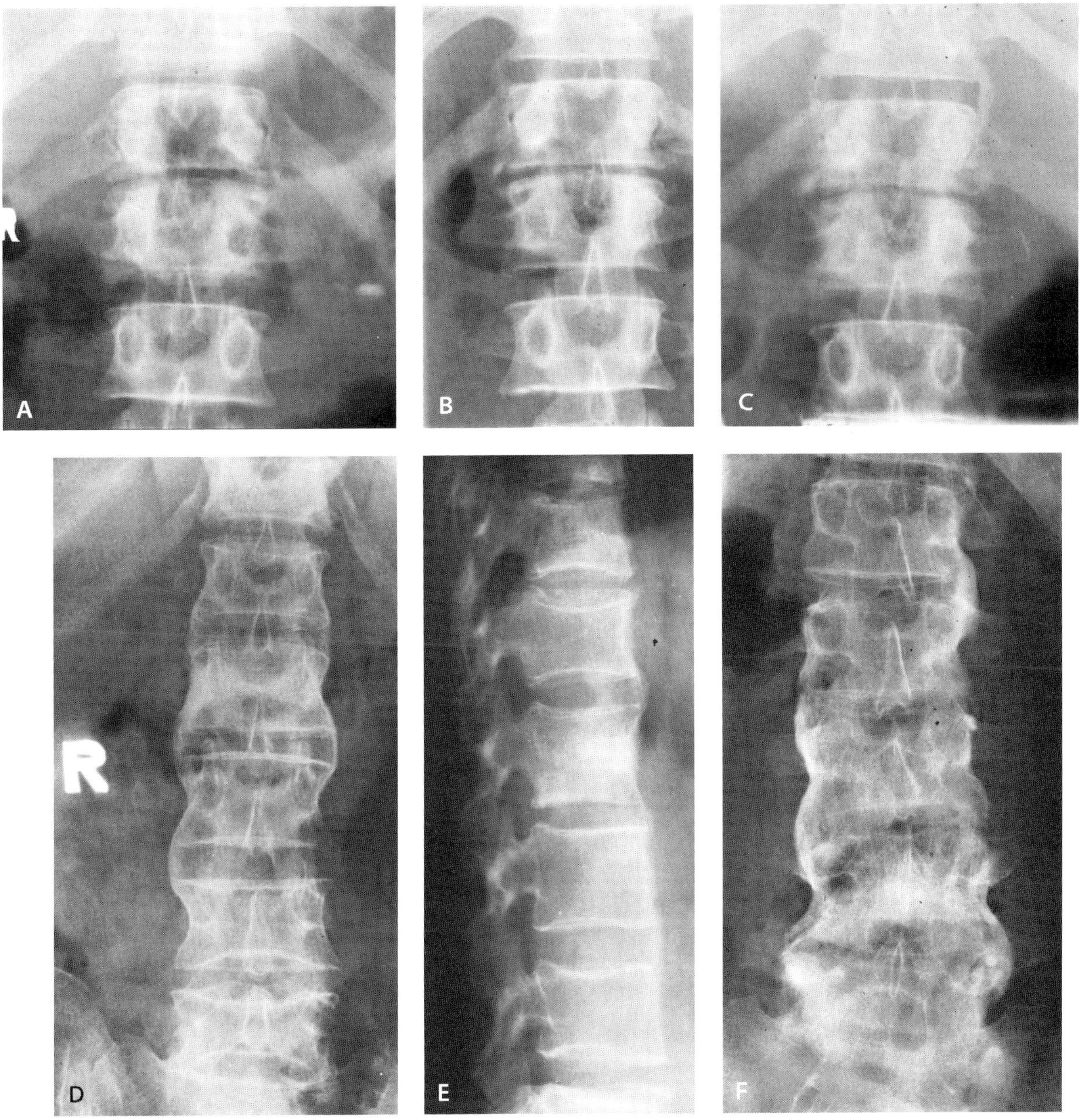

Fig. 5.66 A–E. Spinal tuberculosis heals with "bridge" formation between vertebrae until, in some patients, it may resemble the bamboo spine of ankylosing spondylitis. The bridges form surprisingly quickly. **A** Loss of joint space between the 12th thoracic and the first lumbar vertebrae. There is little other change except for some slight irregularity of the opposing surfaces. **B** Six weeks later there is new bone forming a bridge between the two vertebrae on the right side and, more surprisingly there are bridges on both sides of the normal space between the 11th and 12th thoracic vertebrae. **C** Three months later there is firm bridging between the 11th and 12th thoracic vertebrae and some increase in thickening of the partial bridges between the 12th thoracic and first lumbar vertebrae. There is now a faint bridge forming on the left side at this level and bridging has started between the first and second lumbar vertebrae, although that disc space is also normal. **D, E** The end result of healing. The sclerosis in the center of the body of the second lumbar vertebra and (in the lateral view) the healed focus of infection on the anterior edge of the 12th thoracic vertebrae show that this is post-tuberculosis. The sacroiliac joints are normal. This African from Zimbabwe has been under treatment for spinal tuberculosis for 3 years. **F** It is difficult to recognize this as the end result of tuberculosis, but this African has also been treated and observed for more than 3 years. Although these patients (**D–F**) show bridging between most of their lumbar vertebrae, the process may be limited to only two or three and occur at any level (see Fig. 5.67)

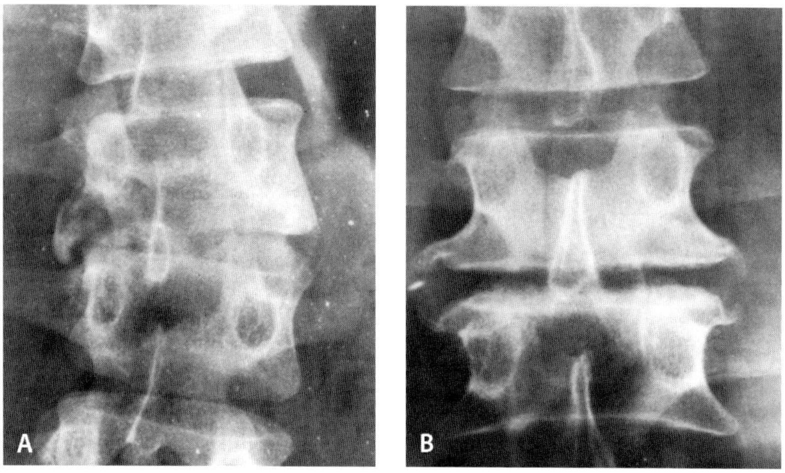

Fig. 5.67 **A** Unilateral bridging around a focus of infection in the lower corner of one vertebral body. **B** Small bilateral bridges across a narrow disc space, with marked sclerosis of the vertebral bodies. There is considerable variation in the frequency of bridging and in some countries sclerosis may be less common

Bone formation and bridging can be unexpectedly rapid or may occur slowly; it can be localized between one or two vertebrae, may be extensive at one side of the spine and not the other, may occur anteriorly and not laterally, or may occur in any combination. Many of the bony bridges are arched, leaving a clear space between the vertebrae. In many cases there is no vertebral collapse, which is a distinguishing feature from previous trauma. In others there is marked destruction.

There is some geographic variation in the pattern of tuberculosis of the spine and its healing. In most of Africa, bony bridging is relatively common; in Asia the process is much more destructive and there is much more rarefaction; this heals with either normal bone replacement or some increase in the trabecular density superimposed on the deformity.

One of the most difficult radiological problems is to assess the degree of healing; this can only be done after review of serial radiographs, preferably at 2–3 months intervals, to assess progress. Lack of further change may be the first sign of healing. The difficult surgical decisions are when to operate, to decompress, to use a bone graft, or only to immobilize. The "correct" treatment of spinal tuberculosis is still controversial. It was shown by Konstam in West Africa that a short preliminary period of drug therapy in hospitals could be followed by ambulatory care with a spinal cast. The results were excellent even when there was considerable neurological and urological deficit when the patient entered the hospital. His research was confirmed that the most important factor in the effective treatment of spinal tuberculosis is drug therapy. This must be continued, of course, for an adequate time and patients must be reviewed regularly. If the patient is in a cast, surgeons must be persuaded to change it at a review visit, so that the progress of the spine may be properly assessed radiologically; attempts at review when radiographs have been taken through the cast are highly unreliable. A more surgical approach was used by Roper in Zimbabwe, Kircaldy-Willis in East Africa, and Hodgson in Hong Kong, combining surgery, cast, and drug therapy. The results are usually excellent, but whether every case needs surgery is very much a matter of opinion. Ambulatory care is successful and thus of great importance in developing countries, where hospital beds and skilled nursing are in short supply.

Paravertebral Abscess

Not every vertebra infected with tuberculosis will have a paraspinal abscess. Tuberculous abscesses present in many different ways:

1. There may be an abscess but no bone lesion (or a bone lesion but no abscess).
2. The abscess may be unilateral or bilateral.
3. The abscess may be lateral, or anterior, or both.
4. The abscess may appear below, or occasionally above, the obvious bone focus.
5. There may be a large abscess with no clinical symptoms or a small abscess with paraplegia.
6. Abscesses may surface almost anywhere on the skin but particularly in the inguinal region, in the thighs, in the loin, near the sternum, or in the neck. A retropharyngeal abscess may cause difficulty in swallowing. A psoas abscess may connect with any part of the intestine and present as a fecal fistula.

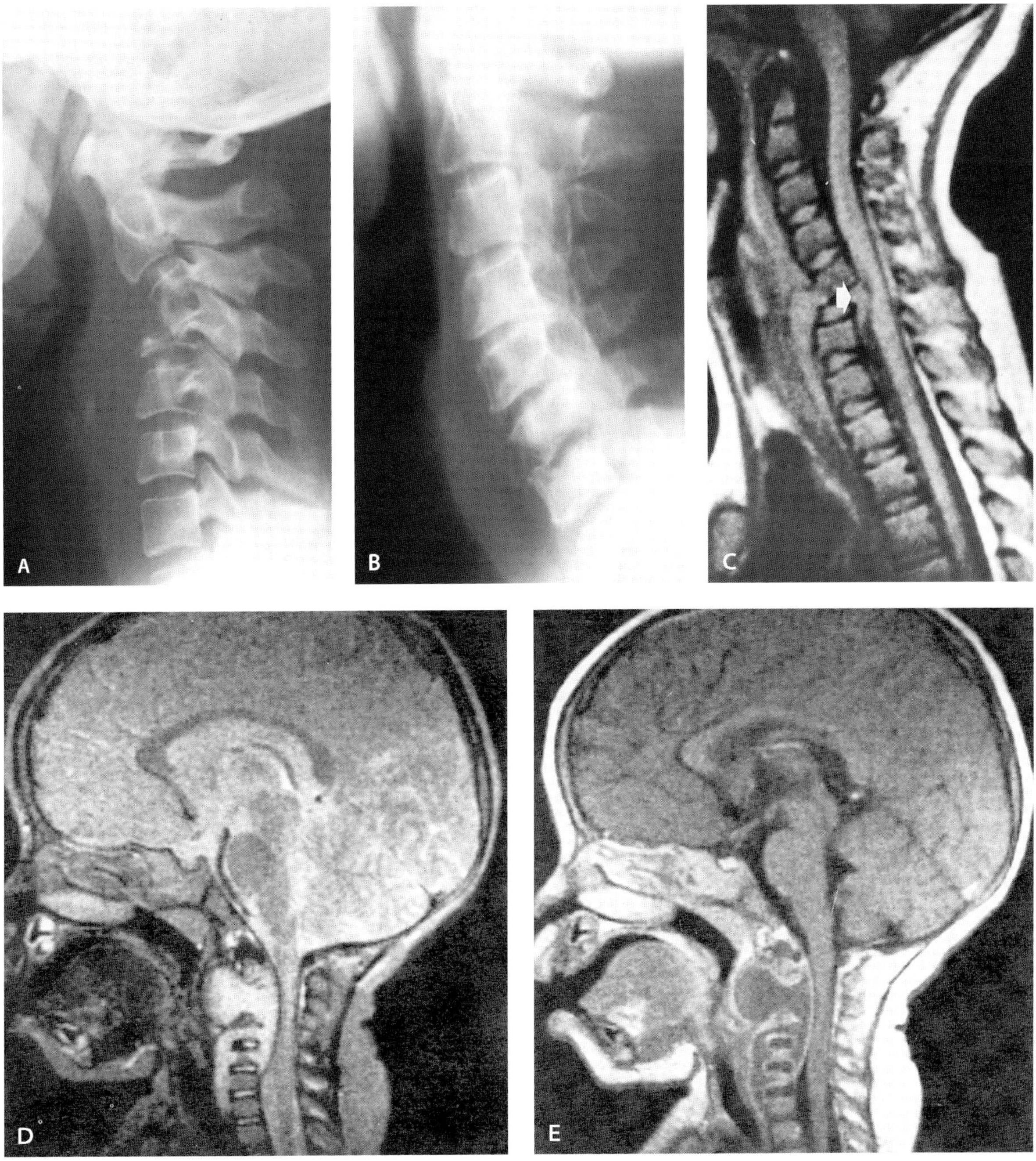

Fig. 5.68 A–F. Tuberculous abscesses. The best way to image an abscess around a tuberculous spinal infection is by scanning, particularly with CT and MRT. However, when these modalities are not available, abscesses can be seen with plain radiography or, occasionally, with contrast media. They are usually much larger than the plain radiographs suggest. **A** There is a large abscess in front of the cervical spine, displacing the trachea and esophagus anteriorly. **B** Another patient with a similar abscess a little lower in the cervical spine. Both these abscesses could have been demonstrated by ultrasonography, but radiography gives a better image of the spine as well. **C** This 5-year-old child was quadriparetic because of the anterior cord compression from a tuberculous abscess at the level of C5 (*arrow*) shown by T1-weighted MRI. **D** T2-weighted MR-scan in another child shows destruction of C2–4 with anterior and posterior abscesses. **E** with intravenous gadolinium there is peripheral enhancement but the necrotic content of the abscess does not enhance. (**D, E** from Cremin and Jamieson 1995)

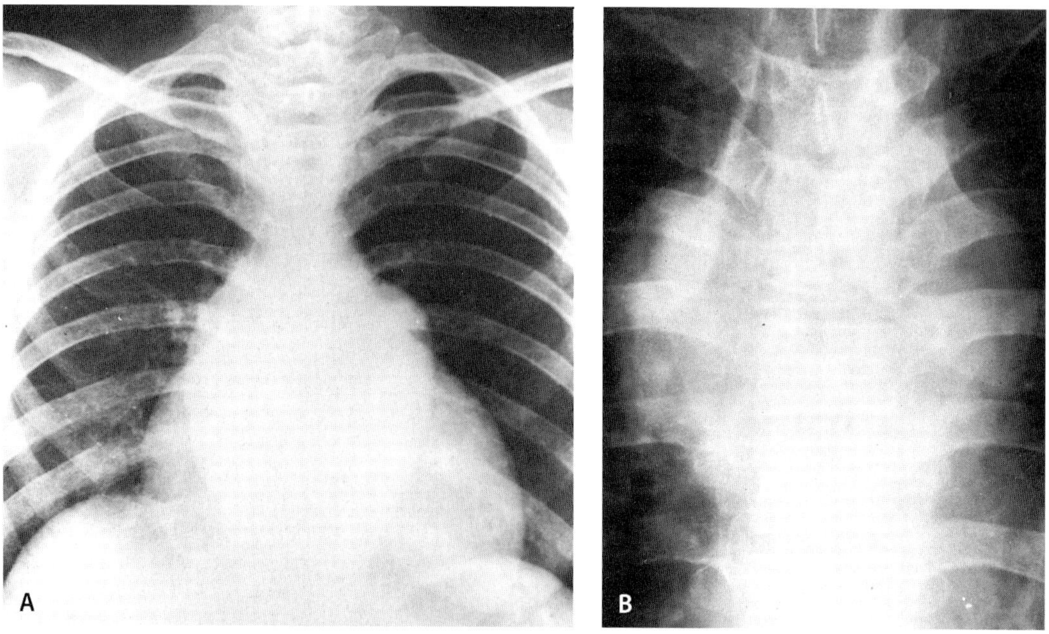

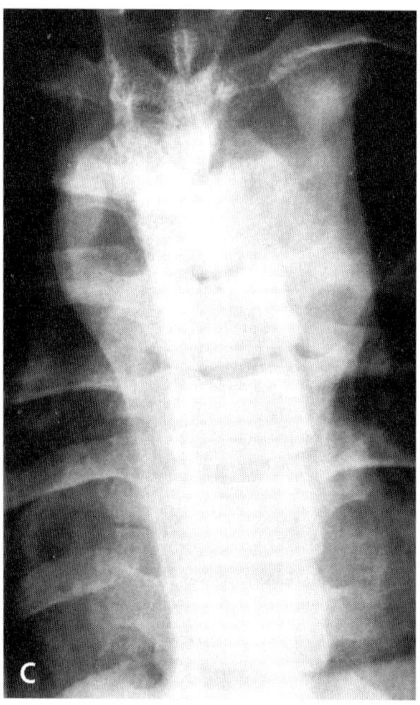

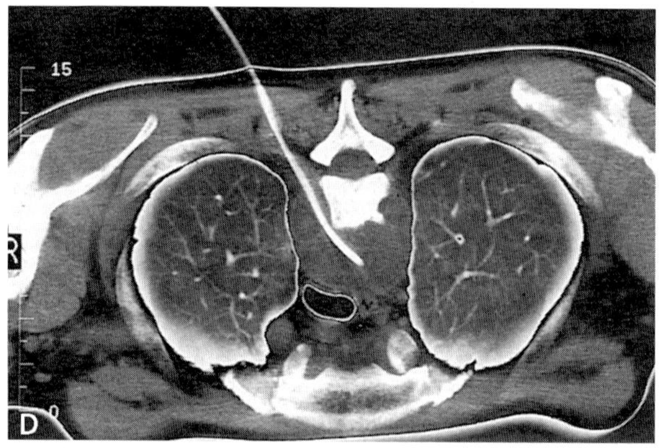

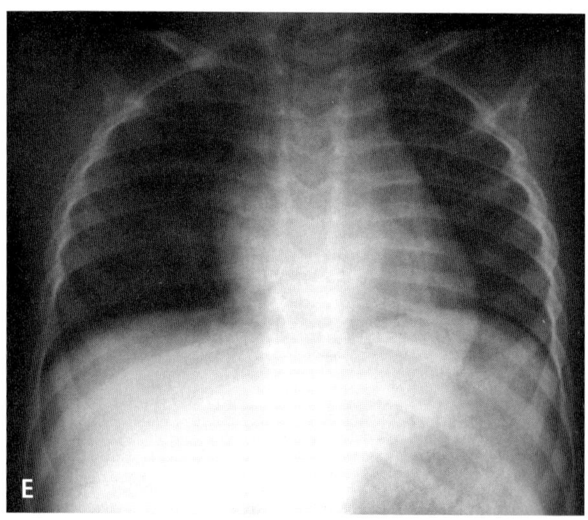

Fig. 5.69 A–I. Tuberculosis of the thoracic spine. **A–C** These three different patients each had a large bilateral paravertebral abscess, seen through the mediastinum. Such abscesses can be large enough to compress the trachea, particularly in children. **D** CT-guided drainage of an anterior paravertebral abscess with the patient supine; there is destruction of the thoracic vertebral body. These are all African patients. **E** Similar mid-thoracic abscess in a child from the Pacific Islands. **F, G** The CT scan shows left upper cavitating pneumonia (**F**) and, at a lower level, destruction of the vertebrae with fluid on both sides (**G**). **H** The MR scan confirms the pneumonia and shows the size of the abscess and the destruction of the vertebrae. **I** The lateral MR scan shows the cord compression. F–I see p. 487

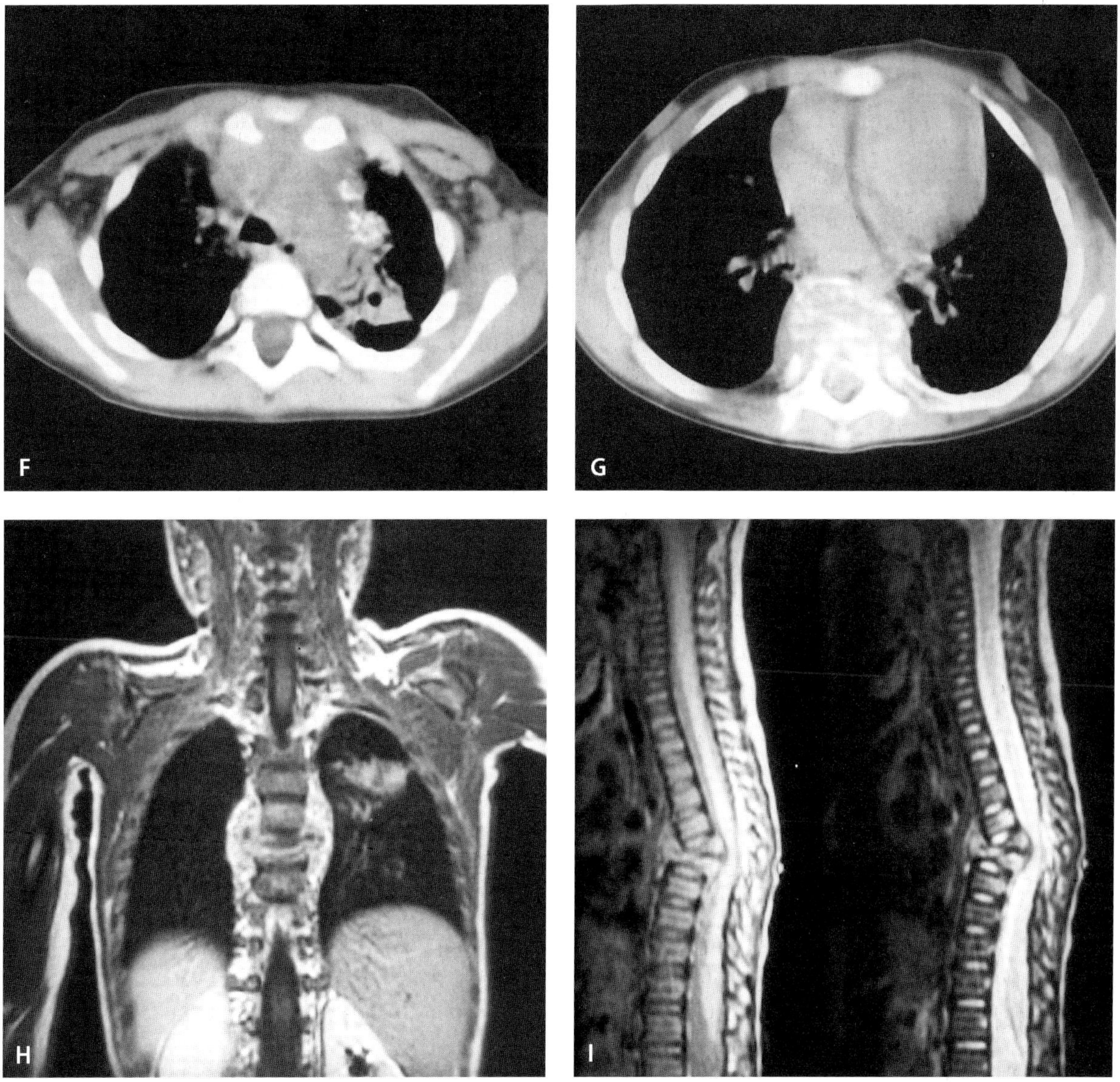

Fig. 5.69 F–I. Legend see p. 486

CT and MRI have radically altered our knowledge of these tuberculous abscesses by showing them, and bone foci, where they cannot be imaged on plain radiographs (Figs. 5.68–5.70). In particular, the full extent and position of any fluid can be demonstrated by CT or MRI.

Wherever the abscess presents, there should be careful imaging of the whole spine, starting preferably with isotope scintigraphy. Paravertebral abscesses occur at all levels and may be present on one side only, on both sides symmetrically or asymmetrically, or only in front of the spine without any lateral extension. Some may be dumb-bell in shape, protruding wherever space permits. They vary considerably in size and shape. When there is an anterior spinal abscess, underneath the spinal ligaments, the anterior edge of the vertebral bodies may become concave because of the transmitted aortic pulsation. The vertebral cartilages are not affected and the pressure absorption of the body may be minimal or considerable, so that it resembles the concavity caused by an aortic aneurysm. MRI is the best way to demonstrate what is actually happening, and CT is also suitable for this purpose.

A psoas abscess may connect with any part of the bowel, may be extensive and surround the kidney or the liver, or may burst through the skin onto the surface almost anywhere (see Fig. 5.71). In many cases sinography is required, but careful technique is essential. The examination should be carried out

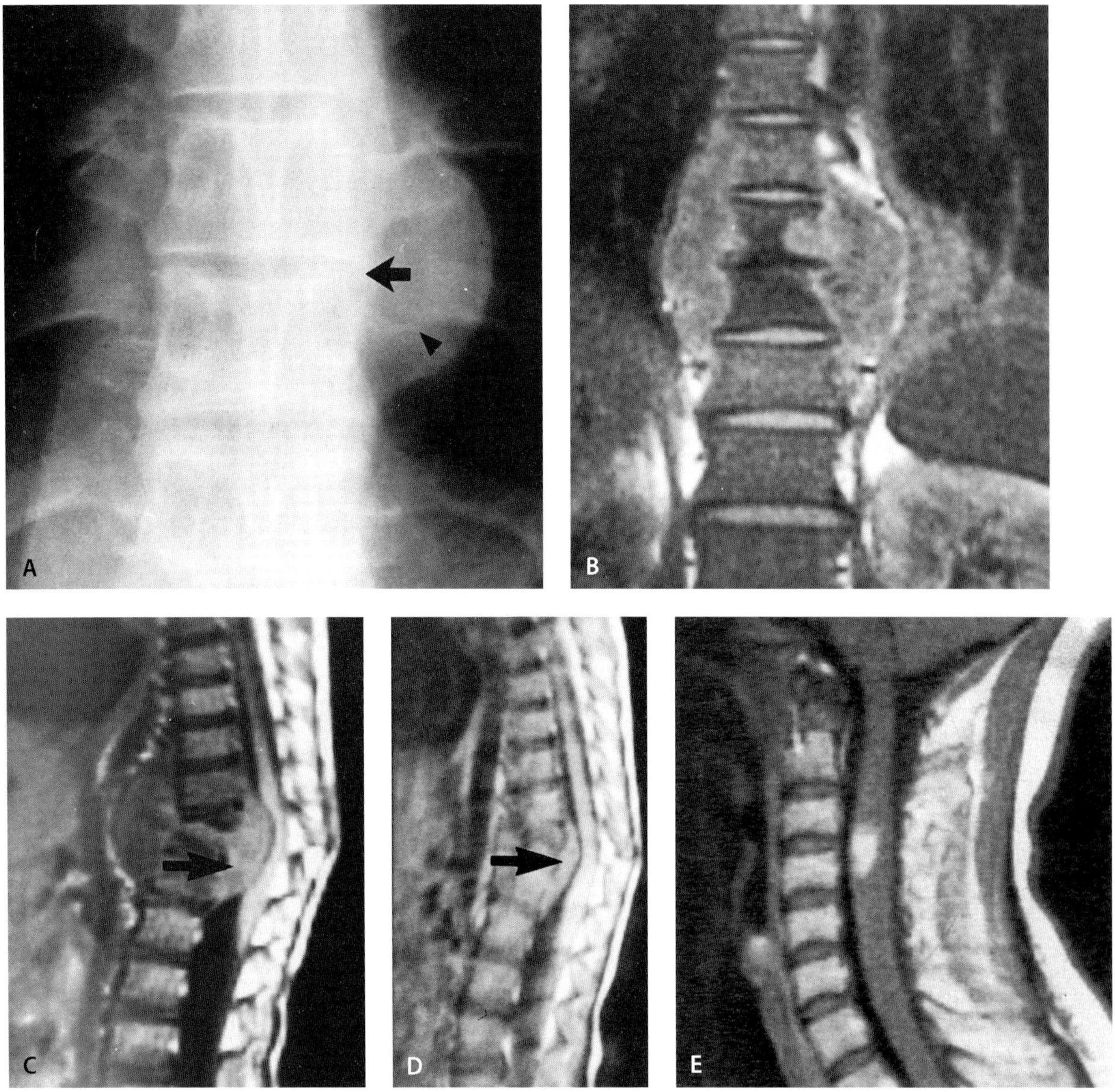

Fig. 5.70. A A 25-year-old African complained of backache ans was found to have a left paravertebral abscess and erosion of the medial end of left tenth rib (*arrowhead*). **B** A T1-weighted coronal MR scan showed bilateral abscesses and low-intensity signals from the marrow of T8 and T9. **C** The T1-weighted sagittal MR scan showed the large abscess anteriorly and posteriorly, with destruction of the vertebral bodies and compression of the cord (*arrow*). **D** After 6 weeks of antituberculous treatment the abscess is much smaller and the cord is less compressed (*arrow*). It was realized more than 30 years ago (Konstam) that many of the neurological signs are caused by the abscesses rather than the spinal deformity. CT and MRI have confirmed this dramatically. (Courtesy of Dr. Peter Corr, Durban) **E** Apart from pressure on the cord from an abscess, there may be a tuberculoma, as shown at the level of C4 in a different patient, a child. This is an intravenous gadolinium-enhanced T1-weighted MR scan. (From Cremin and Jamieson 1995)

under aseptic conditions and under fluoroscopic control. The sinus should be blocked by using the largest catheter that can be inserted; a balloon catheter will often help in achieving a tight connection. Pus should be aspirated, if possible, and pressure on the surrounding tissue or the suspected site of the abscess may help this drainage. Contrast material should then be injected and considerable pressure may be required if the full extent of the abscess is to be visualized. The case illustrated in Fig. 5.71 A and B was a patient who presented with a sinus in the left side of the lower abdomen, without any obvious etiology. The only organism cultured from it was *E. coli*. A barium enema and an upper gastrointestinal series with a follow-through examination did not show any connection to any part of the bowel.

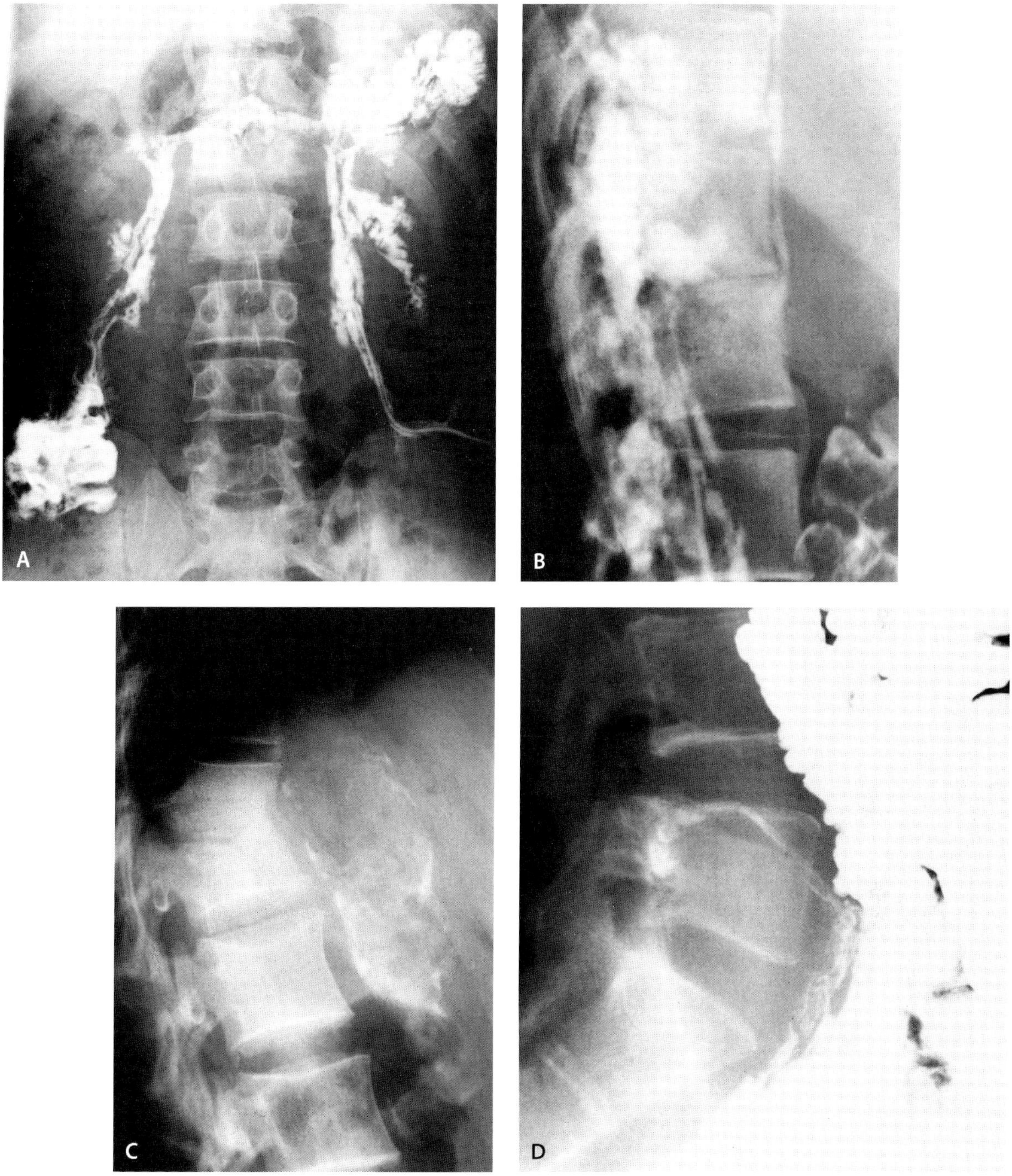

Fig. 5.71 A–D. Psoas abscesses can be very extensive and have unexpected connections. This young African has a persistent left flank sinus contaminated with *E. coli.* **A** The sinogram from the left lower flank, close to the iliac crest, showed that the fistula was connected to an enlarged left perirenal tuberculous abscess, which had started in a tuberculous infection between the 12th thoracic and first lumbar vertebrae. The abscess had also drained down in the right psoas and connected with the cecum, which was the source of the *E. coli* infection. **B** The lateral view of the same patient shows contrast running in front of the vertebrae, above and below the infection. This demonstrates how anterior abscesses can transmit aortic pulsation and also the etiology of the anterior bone bridging which occurs when the periosteum and anterior spinal ligaments are lifted. The aortic pulsation can bow the front of the vertebrae, as is shown in **C** in a much older patient with advanced aortic athromatous calcification. A previous tuberculous infection has resulted in fusion and increased density of the two lower thoracic vertebrae. **D** Another African patient with a fistula connecting the terminal ileum with a paraspinal abscess, which originated in lower thoracic tuberculosis. It is not always possible to demonstrate these fistulae with a barium gastrointestinal series. *E. coli* contamination is usually sufficient proof, even if the actual fistula cannot be imaged. (C courtesy of Dr. Harold G. Jacobson)

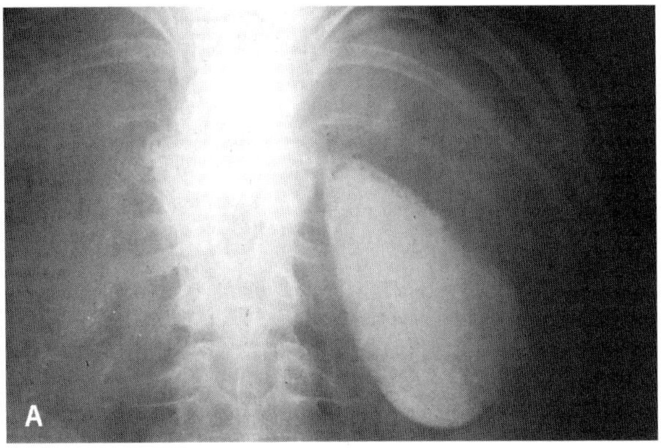

Fig. 5.72 A–E. Tuberculous abscesses of the lower spine. Thoracic and lumbar abscesses track along the psoas and can present at the inguinal region. When they heal, they often calcify. **A** Well-defined, heavily calcified abscess starting at the lower thoracic region in a patient with severe kyphosis. **B** Bilateral loculated and less densely calcified psoas abscesses. **C** A unilateral calcified psoas abscess in the lumbar region. There is bridging between the upper lumbar vertebrae, well above the visible abscess. **D, E** Sonograms of a right psoas abscess, displacing the kidney, in an African patient from Zimbabwe. *RK* right kidney. (**A** courtesy of Dr. Harold G. Jacobson; **D, E** courtesy of Dr. Sam Mindel)

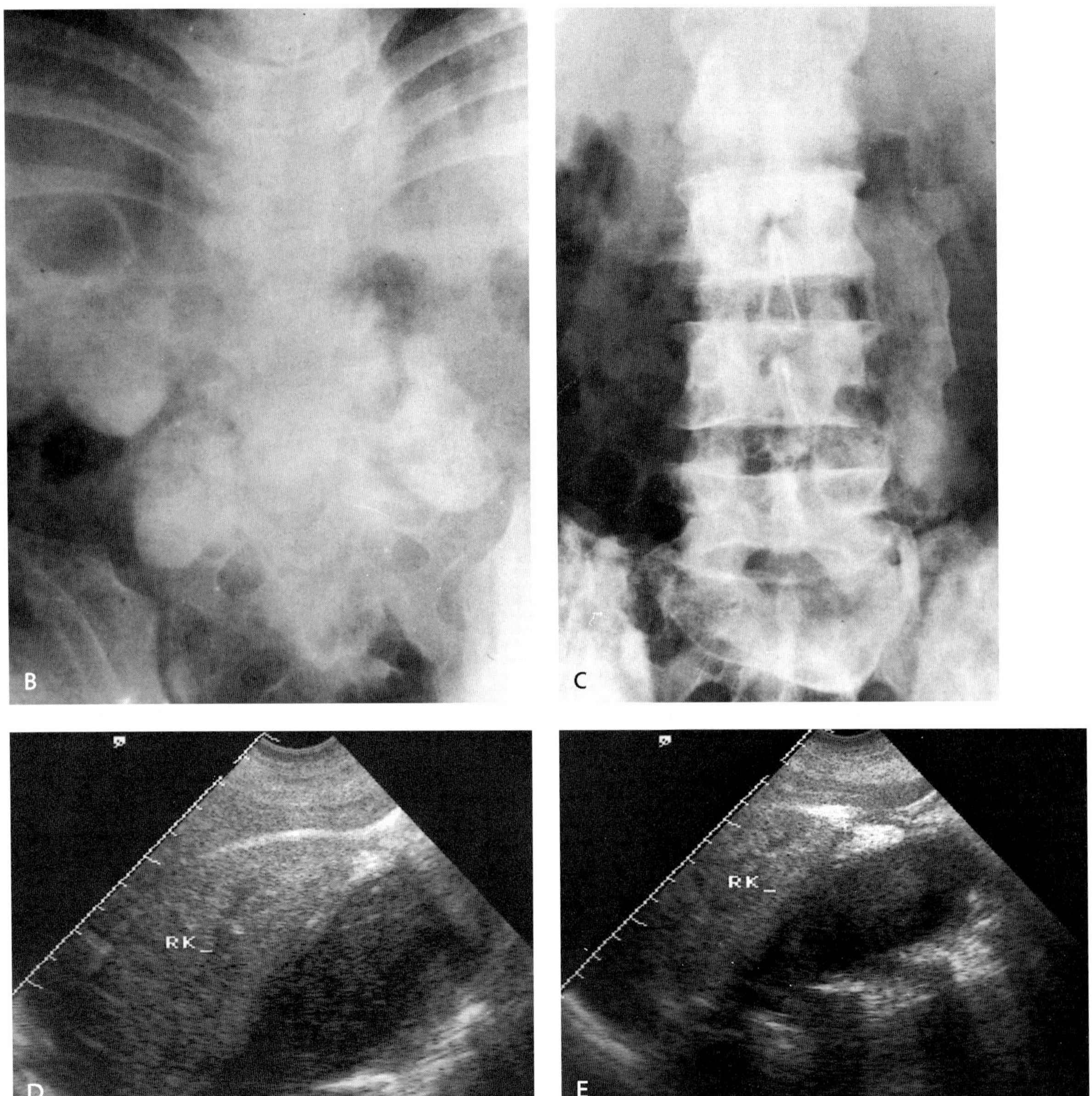

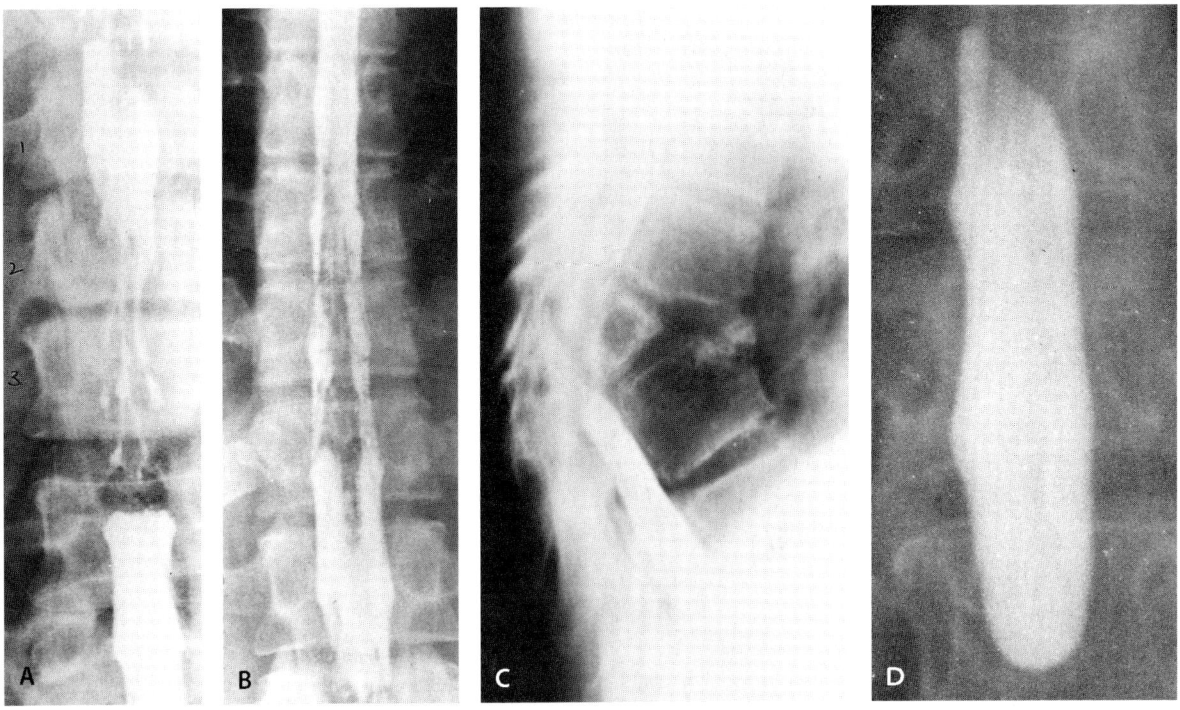

Fig. 5.73 A–D. Myelography in tuberculous paraplegia. Where scanning is not available, there is no contraindication to myelography under fluoroscopic control. **A** There is narrowing of the disc space between the second and third lumbar vertebrae, but the myelogram shows distortion not only at this level, but also one space above. **B** A patient with thoracic paraplegia. Myelography shows long irregular defects, between the tenth and 12th thoracic vertebrae. **C** Myelography in a kyphotic patient can be difficult. In spite of the angle, in this patient there was no obstruction on myelography: it can be difficult to retain the contrast at the level of the curve when it flows freely in either direction. **D** The myelogram may show complete block. (**D** courtesy of Dr. Harold G. Jacobson)

Two limited sinograms were performed before the patient was referred to the author, who blocked the sinus and, using considerable pressure, showed the abscess extending up the left psoas and surrounding the left kidney, across the midline between T12 and L1, and then coursing down the right psoas to connect posteriorly with the cecum. This was, therefore, a sinus draining from the left lower abdomen and yet connected with the cecum on the opposite side through a tuberculous abscess of the spine. (A very similar case has been seen in an American who has never been near the tropics!)

Paravertebral tuberculous abscesses shrink and often show calcification as they heal and fibrose (Fig. 5.72). Unfortunately, calcification does not always indicate sterility. There may be active caseous material contained within the fibrotic bag.

Scanning, Paraplegia, and Myelography

As already mentioned, MRI is the ideal way to examine a patient with a tuberculous spine. A T1-weighted scan shows tuberculous spondylitis as an area of low signal intensity where there is normally a higher intensity from the bone marrow, adjacent to the end plate of the vertebra. On a T2 weighted scan these lesions have a high intensity. Liquid pus also yields a high-intensity signal on a T2-weighted scan. MRI gives an accurate image of the spinal cord compression associated with intraspinal abscesses. At surgery, almost all patients with paraplegia will have at least a small abscess; even if it has not been visualized on plain radiography, it will probably be clearly seen on MRI (Fig. 5.73). Paraplegia indicates that there is about 50%–60% extradural compression above the conus, provided there is no vertebral instability. Peripheral nerves below the cauda or extraspinal nerves are not likely to be affected by compression. In some cases of paraplegia, the cord will appear to be intact, in which case there is likely to be a vascular deficit, a toxic reaction, or, as MRI can demonstrate (by showing a

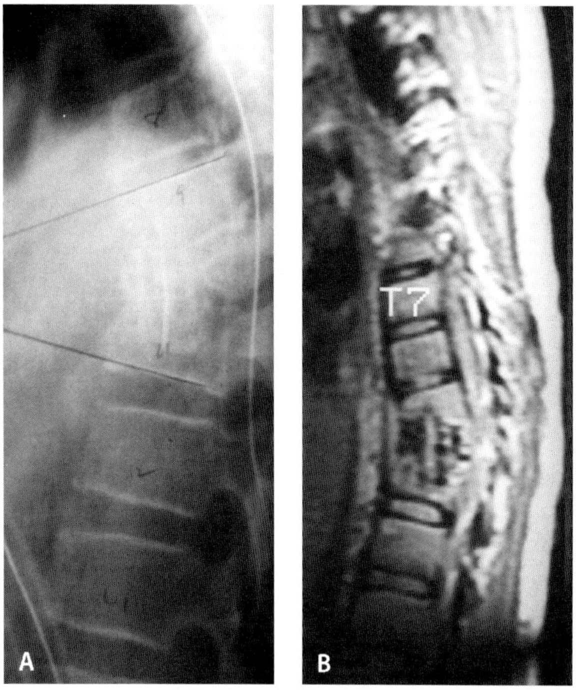

Fig. 5.74 A, B. Postoperative spinal tuberculosis. It is very difficult to assess healing, which may take years. These are the postoperative images of a 2-year-old girl from the Pacific Islands. **A** The lateral radiograph shows the graft across the infected and wedged thoracic vertebrae (T9–11). **B** T2-weighted MRI shows the residual abscess and granulation tissue and the exact extent of the bone destruction. (Courtesy of Dr. Cheryl Sisler, Hawaii)

Fig. 5.75 A–H. The case history of spinal tuberculosis. A young man from Saudi Arabia had been complaining of pain between his shoulder blades for some months before he came to hospital one weekend, with rapidly developing paraplegia. Plain radiography (**A**) showed wedging of two upper thoracic vertebrae. Myelography (**B**) showed almost complete block at this level and CT scan (**C**) showed destruction of the vertebra, particularly on the right side, and of the medial end of the rib at the same level. Fluid was present in the right side of the chest. **D–G** Pre- (**D**) and postgadolinium (**E–G**) MR scans show the full extent of the paraspinal abscess, and of the epidural granulomatous tissue. The findings on the CT scan are confirmed but shown more clearly. Subsequent surgical decompression revealed both caseation and granulomatous tissue with *M. tuberculosis* on direct smear microscopy. The patient made a good recovery. (Courtesy of Dr. Frank McGuiness, Ryadh) ▶

high-intensity focus on a T2-weighted scan), damage to the cord, probably due to prolonged compression. This focal myelitis has a poor prognosis and the paraplegia is likely to be irreversible. However, as Konstam demonstrated, rest and drug therapy may relieve paraplegia which is of short duration, and simple decompression, either by needle aspiration or surgery, may be all that is needed in the early stages. Whenever any intervention is planned, it is a wise precaution to have the patient already on antituberculous therapy to obviate the risk of tuberculous septicemia.

Whatever method of imaging is used, it is essential that the whole cord or spinal canal is examined because the obstruction may not occur at the site of the obvious bone lesion, but rather be above or below it, depending on the extent of the fluid, necrotic tissue displacement, or granulation tissue.

If MRI is not available, myelography, with or without CT, is a very useful investigation and should be performed as early as possible and always before surgery to localize the exact site of any obstructions (Fig. 5.74). There are no contraindications to myelography although in some patients the kyphosis may make it extremely difficult. Where there is a double curve, careful manipulation of the patient (especially in the lateral decubitus position) may permit the column of contrast material to travel throughout the length of the spinal canal. Sometimes this is technically impossible, even when there is no blockage, because of severe spinal angulation. Fortunately, paraplegia is less often due to kyphosis or bony deformity than to an abscess or soft tissue pressure. The decision as to whether myelography needs to be repeated during treatment should be based on the clinical examination.

Following surgery in patients with spinal tuberculosis it is very difficult to assess healing, which may take years. Again, MRI is the best method for this purpose (Fig. 5.75).

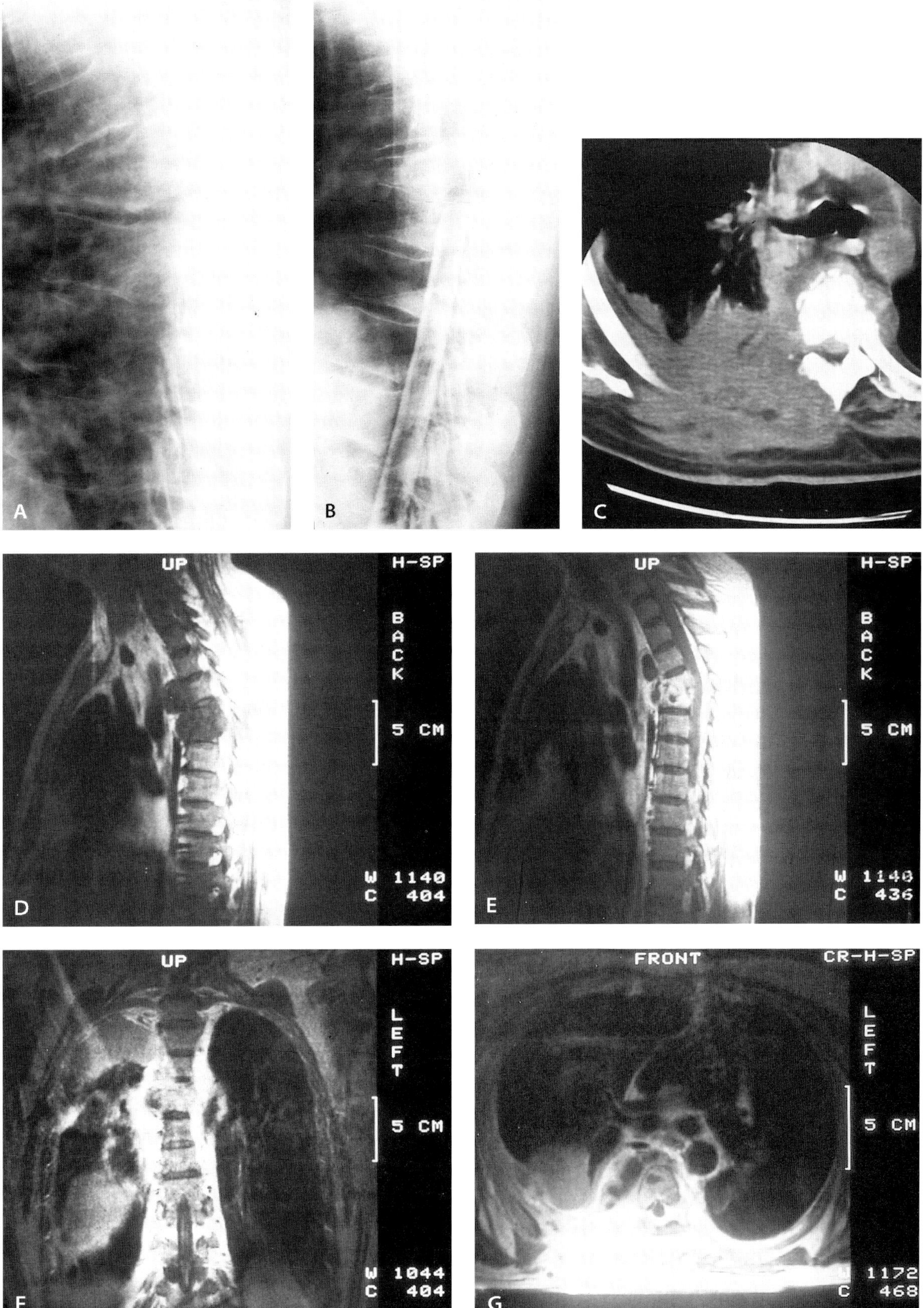
A
B
C
UP
H-SP
BACK
5 CM
W 1140
C 404
D
UP
H-SP
BACK
5 CM
W 1140
C 436
E
UP
H-SP
LEFT
5 CM
W 1044
C 404
F
FRONT
CR-H-SP
LEFT
5 CM
1172
C 468
G

Differential Diagnosis

Theoretically any type of bone infection may cause a paravertebral abscess. In practice, the majority of spinal abscesses in the tropics are tuberculous; if there is active pulmonary tuberculosis, the possibility of spinal infection also being tuberculous is enhanced. It is unusual for a pyogenic or typhoid infection to cause a large paravertebral abscess, and even less often do such abscesses point to the surface as occurs with tuberculosis. On MRI, pyogenic disc infection usually has a high intensity on T2-weighted scans, but in tuberculosis less than one-third show this. However, pyomyositis (tropical myositis) can present in this way, usually without any osseous lesion (see Chap. 30). Brucellosis may also produce a paravertebral abscess (see Chap. 32). There may be paravertebral thickening in lymphoma (particularly in Burkitt's lymphoma) which may resemble an abscess, and the bony destruction may also be very confusing because Burkitt's lymphoma may involve a vertebral body or a pedicle (see Chap. 41). Sometimes the differential diagnosis is impossible with any method of imaging, but in the majority of cases there will be other evidence of Burkitt's or other lymphoma to establish the correct diagnosis (see Chap. 41). Wedging, particularly wedging and fusion of two or three vertebrae, is very uncommon in any infection other than tuberculosis.

Because tuberculous osteomyelitis in the tropics (even in patients without AIDS) is often an acute disease, it is difficult to differentiate from other infections and the clinical condition of the patient may be very important when giving a radiological opinion. Nontuberculous spinal infections usually cause more severe clinical symptomatology than tuberculosis, with more systemic reaction, a higher pyrexia, and a raised white cell count, but none of these criteria are absolute and biopsy or aspiration and culture are essential.

The differential diagnosis of tuberculosis from acute trauma is seldom difficult, if only because of the clinical history. Trauma does not cause as much bone loss and destruction as tuberculosis. Long-standing cases need serial review, both clinical and radiological. In the majority of such problem patients the etiology is of no immediate clinical significance, permitting a more cautious approach. Scintigraphy or other imaging survey of the rest of the spine may show other involved vertebrae and allow the differentiation between trauma and infection.

In all patients, the possibility of malignancy will have to be excluded, particularly when the bone destruction involves the pedicles. Many malignant tumors cause paravertebral swelling resembling an abscess; obtaining a tissue specimen, either through needle aspiration or biopsy, becomes essential. Most errors are made because the possibility of tuberculosis is overlooked in the elderly or in the very young.

Tuberculosis of Bones and Joints (Nonspinal)

Tuberculous Arthritis

A tuberculous infection of a joint can occur at any stage, but is more common in the younger age groups. Even babies from 6 months onwards may present with quite severe skeletal infection. The joints most affected in order of frequency are the hips, knees, ankles elbows, wrists, sacroiliac joints, and shoulders (Fig. 5.76, 5.77). In 98% of HIV-negative patients the tuberculin skin test will be positive. The way in which tuberculosis affects a joint depends on whether the original focus is in the synovium or in the adjacent bone. Spread of the infection from bone into a joint is more common and has a poorer prognosis.

Nontuberculous mycobacteria may cause arthritis and bone infection. This is uncommon, but may become more frequent in patients with AIDS. *Mycobacterium kansasii* has been known to infect knee joints, and *M. intracellulare* has infected the shoulder, the spine, and, in one patient, both wrists. The differential diagnosis will only be made by joint aspiration or synovial tissue culture.

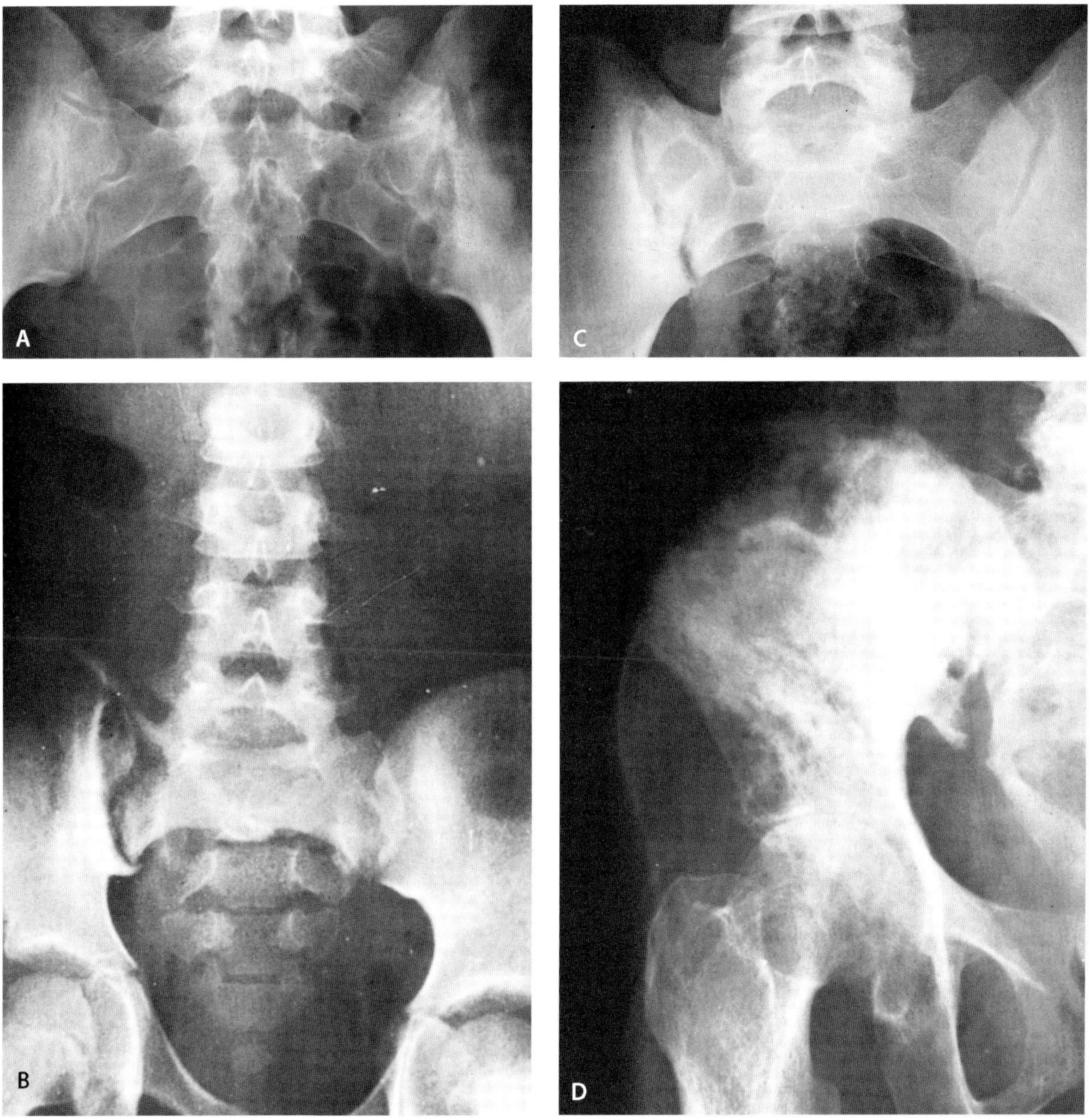

Fig. 5.76 A–D. Skeletal tuberculosis. The pelvis. Infection of the sacroiliac joints can be destructive and then, as healing occurs, become sclerotic and fused. **A** Widening and irregularity of the left sacroiliac joint. **B** Sclerosis on the iliac side of the right sacroiliac joints. **C** In another patient there is infection on both sides of the sacroiliac joint, particularly the sacrum. **D** Extensive destruction of a right sacroiliac joint in a different African patient. The infection must have spread through the right ilium, which is becoming sclerotic. The joint is widened throughout its length. The right hip joint is narrowed and probably also infected. (**A**, **C** courtesy of Dr. Harold G. Jacobson)

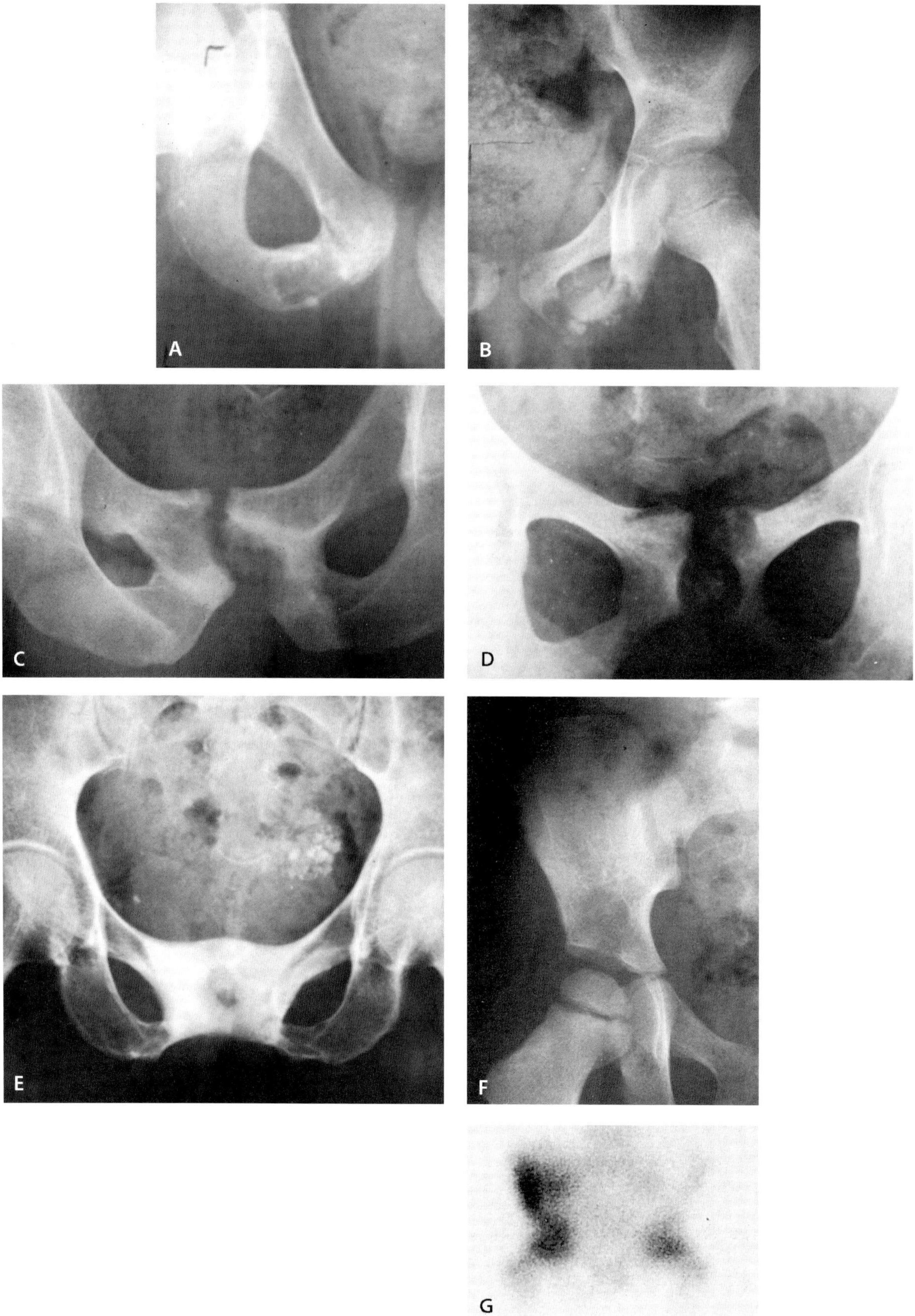
A
B
C
D
E
F
G

◀ **Fig. 5.77 A–G.** Tuberculosis of the ischium and symphysis pubis. In the early stages most tuberculous lesion in the ischium are ill-defined lucent areas; they later become sclerotic. **A** A lucent focus of infection in the left ischium, with some early surrounding sclerosis. **B** A more destructive lesion closer to the hip in another patient, with some loose bone fragments. **C** There are foci on both sides on the symphysis and in the left ischium. **D** Both sides of this symphysis have been infected, the joint is widened, and there is a central sequestrum. An African from Zimbabwe. **E** A different patient from the same country in which a similar infection has healed causing sclerotic fusion across the symphysis. **F** There is a lytic area of infection above the acetabulum in this child from South Africa, but the hip joint remains normal. **G** An isotope scan of the same patient shows that the iliac infection is more extensive than seen on the radiograph. Tuberculosis is the proven cause in all these cases. (**A–C** courtesy of Dr. Harold G. Jacobson; **F, G** from Cremin and Jamieson 1995)

Synovial Tuberculosis

Patients will first complain of either slight pain or stiffness in the affected joint, and of limitation of movement. In the early stages pain is minimal and it is only as the joint swells that it becomes significant. In many cases there will be a dull, ill-defined ache, often worse at night, but in developing countries such discomfort is often ignored, and it is not until the disease has progressed further that the patient seeks help.

In the beginning, it will be difficult to detect any clinical abnormality to account for the symptoms. Later there will be edema and swelling around the joint, with some limitation of passive movement and increase in local temperature; an effusion often develops early and aspiration of the fluid usually shows it to be clear or straw-colored with few cells; it is sterile on culture. The diagnosis may have to be presumptive, because it may not be possible to find any positive proof of tuberculosis. At this stage, scintigraphy is a reliable way of excluding bone infection; ultrasonography and MRI, and to a lesser extent CT, can be useful in demonstrating the soft tissue changes. Radiographically the joints may be entirely normal in the early stages, and it may take 2–6 weeks before there are positive radiological findings (Fig. 5.78).

The earliest change is loss of clarity of the bones forming the joint; their margins become hazy and difficult to define. There is a mild generalized osteoporosis but not localized bone destruction. The joint space may be widened because of the effusion. Progress of the infection is slow, but a little more rapid once the radiological changes have developed. The osteoporosis becomes more pronounced and there will be soft tissue swelling around the joint. It may be difficult to define any bone erosion because of the osteoporosis and the variable change in bone density. Eventually foci of bone destruction become more definite as the cartilage is destroyed. At this stage the radiological appearance is "ghost-like," particularly when compared with the opposite normal side. If only the synovium is involved, and if treatment is adequate, the disease shows no further progress but slowly heals with a return of the joint towards normality. In the majority of cases, however, there is permanent damage to the cartilage and occasionally to the underlying bone which may lead to degenerative arthritis. When the synovial involvement has been severe, the joint may eventually ankylose.

Osteoarticular Tuberculosis

Scintigraphy is a very useful way of locating tuberculous bone infection and ensuring that it is not multifocal. In the majority of patients, tuberculous infection of a joint is due to spread from a focus within an adjacent bone. An effusion is evidence of this spread but may also occur before actual cartilage destruction has taken place. The bony focus may be close to the articular surface, a few milimeters away from it, or in the metaphysis. The very early bone focus (as well as the soft tissue involvement) can be shown by MRI, and the extent of marrow replacement can be assessed. Gadoliniumenhanced T1-weighted images show differential rim enhancement. Such foci can be single or multiple, and although they are usually opposite one another on opposing sides of the joint, they need to be so closely related. On plain radiographs or CT, the lesion within the bone appears as an area of decalcification, without any definite edge and of no particular shape. This slowly spreads up the shaft, but also across the epiphysis into the joint. At this stage clinical symptoms will be minimal. Some patients may complain of a dull ache or "spasm" in the joint or occasionally some swelling. Careful clinical examination may show some restriction of movement, but this may be so slight that there is little suspicion of an underlying osteomyelitis.

As the infection bursts into the joint, there will be a considerable reaction, with fluid and tuberculous debris in the joint space. The sacroiliac joints can be the most difficult to assess on plain radiography. Scintigraphy can be helpful but the uptake ratio between the sacroiliac joint and the os sacrum can vary with age. In any joint, CT and MRI provide more definite evidence of bone destruction on either side of the joint, and of subsequent joint involvement. Clinically, at this stage, there is no doubt that a limb joint is abnormal. It will be painful, swollen, and immobile.

(Text continues on p. 500)

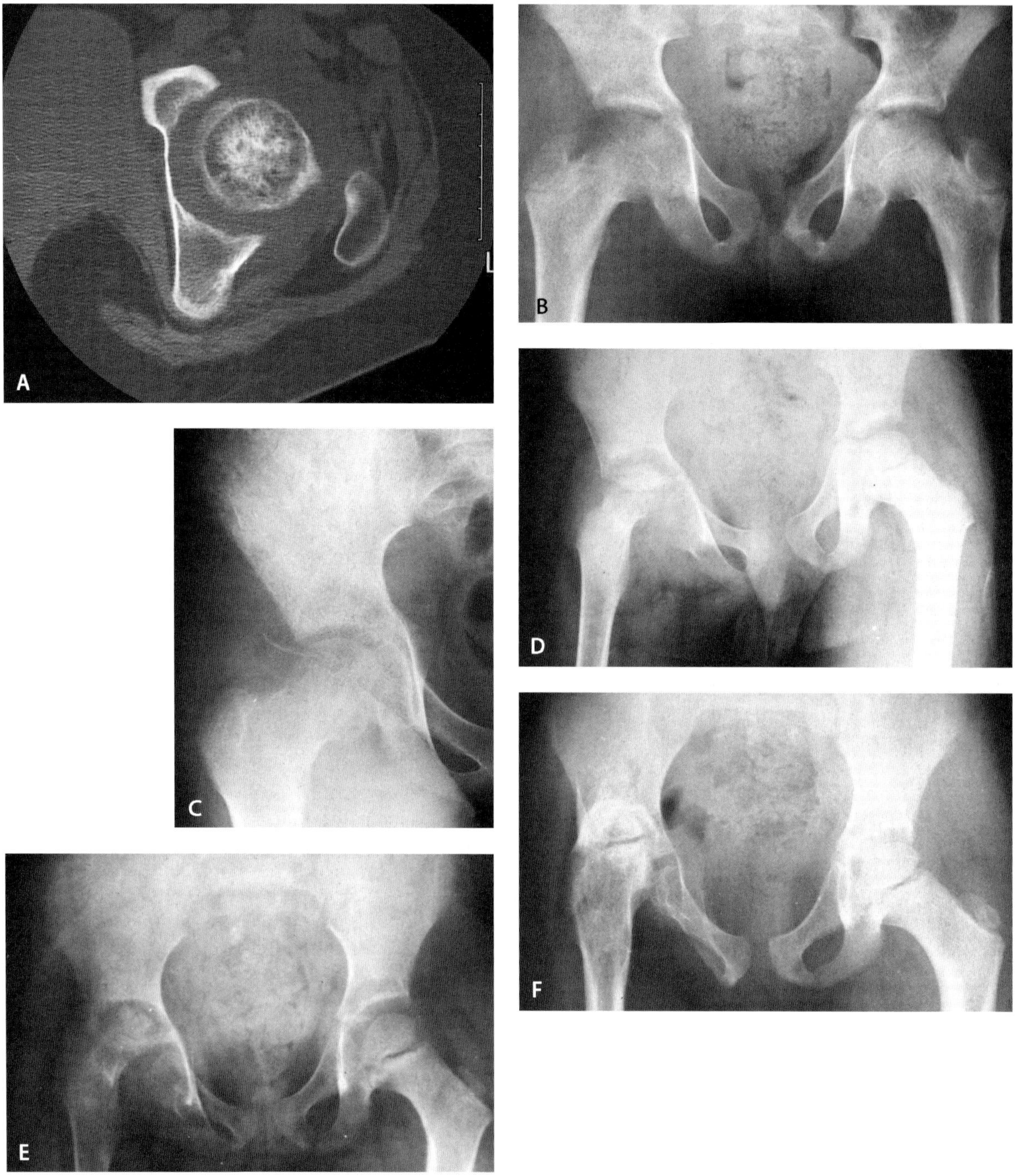

Fig. 5.78 A–F. Tuberculosis of the hip. The earliest evidence of infection may be an effusion into the joint. **A** The CT scan did not show any bone lesion but there were *M. tuberculosis* in the effusion. **B** In other patients there may be soft tissue swelling, osteoporosis, and loss of bone definition, as can be seen by comparison with the normal left hip. **C** A different but similar infected hip in which the ill-defined, hazy appearance of the joint and the soft tissue swelling around the acetabulum, particularly medially, are clearly shown. **D–F** The same patient (an African from Zimbabwe) over a period of 3 years. **D** There is soft tissue swelling and an effusion in the hip joint with destruction of the acetabulum and femoral head. **E** Six months later there is less fluid and the bone density is improving: in spite of the bone destruction, there are no sequestra. **F** Two years later the joint has fused: there will be shortening of the limb and there is significant deformity of the right side of the pelvis. (**A** courtesy of Dr. Cheryl Sisler, Hawaii)

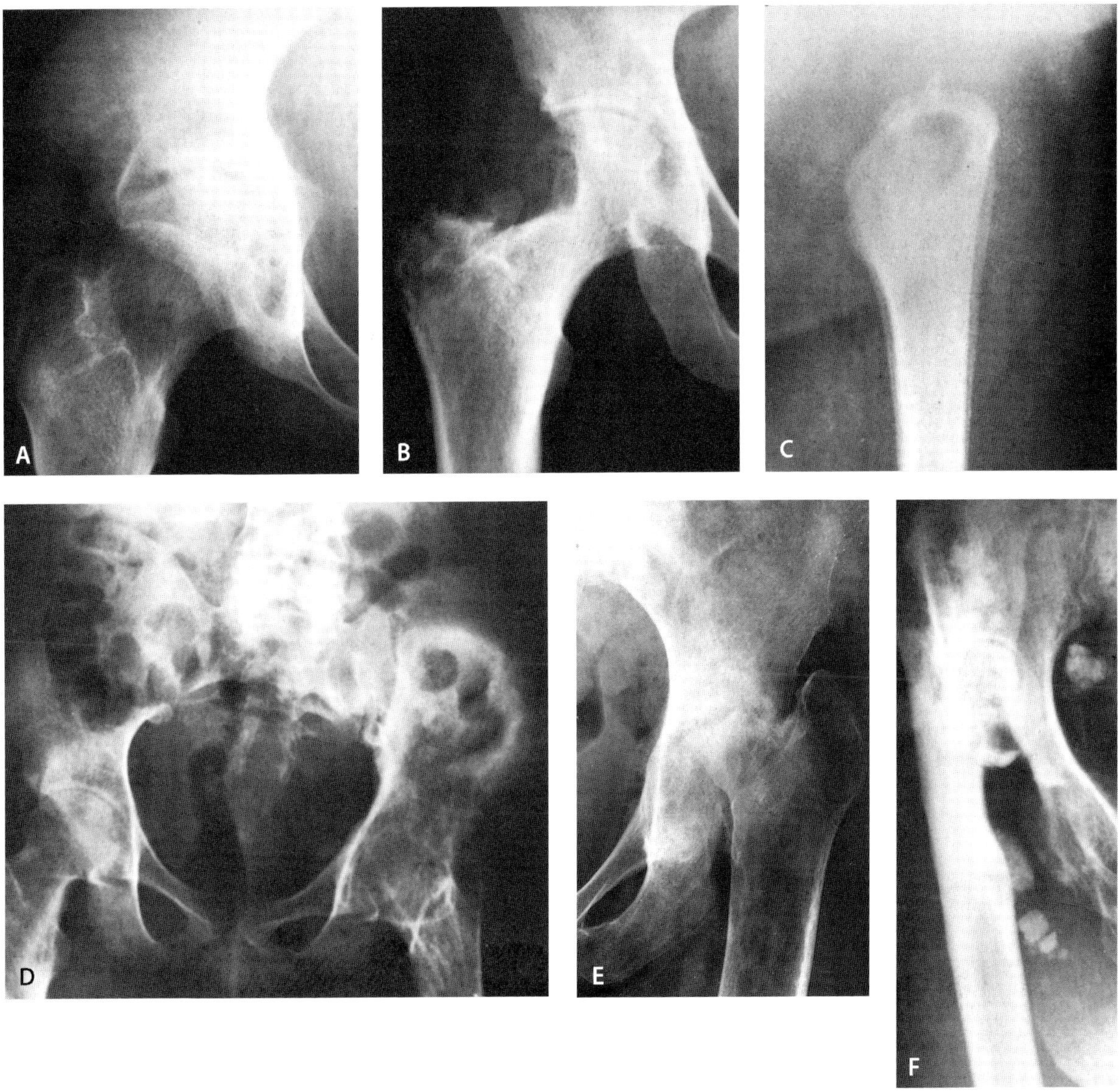

Fig. 5.79 A–F. Tuberculosis of the hip. In some patients the femoral head remains surprisingly intact, while in others it is eventually destroyed. **A** A cystic lesion in the acetabulum of a young African male: the hip joint is narrowed and irregular. There was also infection in the inferior pubic ramus. **B** There is destruction of the greater trochanter in this adult African and a cystic lesion in the neck of the femur, spreading into the femoral head. The joint space is not affected. **C** In this child there is central destruction of the upper end of the left femur, with a periosteal reaction along the shaft. The joint is infected and the femoral head has been dislocated and will never develop properly. **D** Advanced tuberculosis of the left hip and the left part of the pelvis. The hip joint is fused and there is dense sclerotic bone around the three lytic foci in the left iliac bone. This could be mistaken for a pyogenic infection. **E** The femoral head has disappeared, the acetabulum is irregular and sclerotic, and there are cystic changes both in the femoral neck and around the joint. The end result will be fusion, and there may be fixed fibrosis already. **F** The joint has been completely destroyed and dislocated and is surrounded by calcified debris. There will be marked shortening of the right leg and the hip is fixed. (Courtesy of the University of Capetown Radiology Library)

The disease progresses with further destruction and disorganization; the soft tissues, already swollen, become involved with the tuberculous process, best shown by MRI or CT. The joint may subluxate. In weight-bearing joints such as the hip (one of the most commonly affected: Figs. 5.78, 5.79), involvement of the acetabulum may lead to rupture of the femoral head into the pelvis, particularly where treatment has been delayed and weight bearing has been continued. CT and MRI, and occasionally ultrasonography, can show a soft tissue mass within the pelvis when this occurs. There will usually be multiple, very small sequestra within the mass. The margin of the infected lesion in the bone will probably show reactive sclerosis. Angiography has been used to show the soft tissue mass, which is usually vascular, but it is unlikely that this will provide much useful information.

As healing occurs, the joint space usually narrows; the bones increase in density but do not remodel and the deformity persists. Ankylosis is almost inevitable and may in fact be beneficial because it often permits limited use of the limb. The entire process may take months, even with adequate drug therapy, and the principal imaging problem is to assess the progress of healing, because the changes occur slowly and are often minimal. Ankylosis may become complete, but because of fibrous tissue rather than bony fusion. In such cases the infection may be quiescent but not fully healed. As with all other types of tuberculosis, experience must be combined with careful clinical judgment and continuous observation of the patient to obtain the best end result.

This process, either synovial or osteoarticular, may occur in any tuberculous joint and the same pattern will be followed. Variations occur depending on the type and location of the joint, whether or not it is weight bearing, and how much it is used. For example, when foci oppose each other on either side of a joint [usually the knee (Fig. 5.80), but also the elbow, shoulder, and hip], dense areas of bone may be seen ("kissing sequestra"). There is some individual variation depending on the host resistance, but this is more in terms of the time taken for the changes to be complete rather than in the pattern of the disease.

Fig. 5.80 A–H. Tuberculosis of the knee. **A** The earliest signs of infection may be a large joint effusion and mild generalized osteoporosis, without any visible bone defect. **B, C** Another African patient from Zimbabwe. The soft tissue swelling and effusion are marked but there is a lytic bone focus in the lower end of the femur and periosteal elevation around the full diameter of the femoral shaft. There is accentuated growth of both the femoral and tibial epiphyses. The lytic bone focus is important in the differential diagnosis, because nonarticular rheumatoid arthritis and hemophilia can both give similar appearances before there is any bone destruction. **D** Another patient with a lytic bone focus medially in the lower end of the femur, but also in the femoral epiphysis with a slight sclerotic margin. There is a joint effusion. **E** A tuberculous infection of the patella with a suprapatellar effusion. **F, G** The end stages of a tuberculous joint infection. In **F** there were foci on both sides of the joint; the lateral femoral and tibial condyles had been partially absorbed and destroyed. New bone is present on the lateral aspect of the joint with some fragmentation. There is angulation which may progress. The joint will probably fuse, with either fibrous tissue or bony anyklosis, but in some patients it may remain a lax unstable joint. **H** A healed but badly damaged joint, with partial destruction of the upper end of the tibia, and a lot of new bone and loose fragments. There is calcified debris in the supra-patellar bursa

Tuberculosis of Bones

Osteomyelitis due to the tubercle bacillus is a common condition and need not always involve a joint; in fact it can occur in virtually any bone in the skeleton (Figs. 5.81–5.85). It is most common in childhood but no age is immune; it is frequently multifocal. Scintigraphy is very helpful in identifying the possible multiple sites.

As with pyogenic organisms, the infection most commonly begins in the metaphysis. Its effect on the adjacent joint has already been described. Away from the joint the early changes, localized areas of osteoporosis without any surrounding bone reaction, are often more easily seen than delineated. They have no particular shape, but follow the contour of the bone; in the skull they may be large and apparently spreading. The initial lesion may be seen in the diaphysis, but this is rare. Multiple bones may be infected or the same bone may have foci in different places, not initially connected.

If there is a lesion close to the cortex, expansion is common and cortical thinning occurs. There will be an associated periosteal reaction with a fine lamellar pattern, spreading proximally and distally from the original focus. Ultrasound can identify the edema and the periosteal reaction and be used to guide aspiration biopsy to establish the diagnosis. Both CT and MRI can image the infection, but are unlikely to add much to the accuracy of the diagnosis. This type of reaction is most common in the smaller bones, such as the phalanges (tuberculous dactylitis) and is most frequently seen in children (Figs. 5.86, 5.87). The changes are more marked at this age because the cortex is relatively soft and expansion occurs more easily. The old descriptive term "spina ventosa" (spina = short bone; ventosa = inflated with air) is thus especially appropriate (see Fig. 5.86 A).

(Text continues on p. 504)

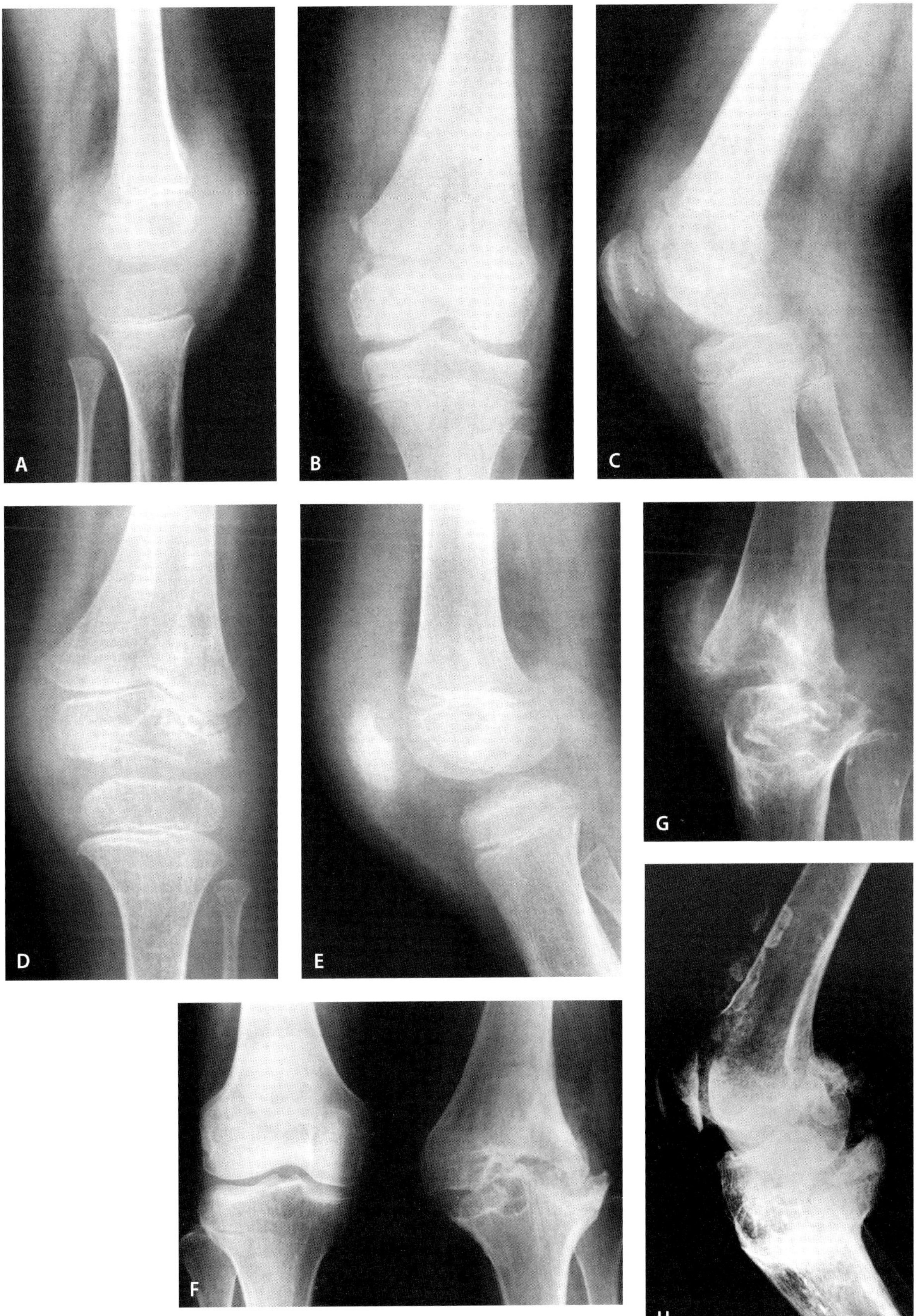
A
B
C
D
E
G
F
H

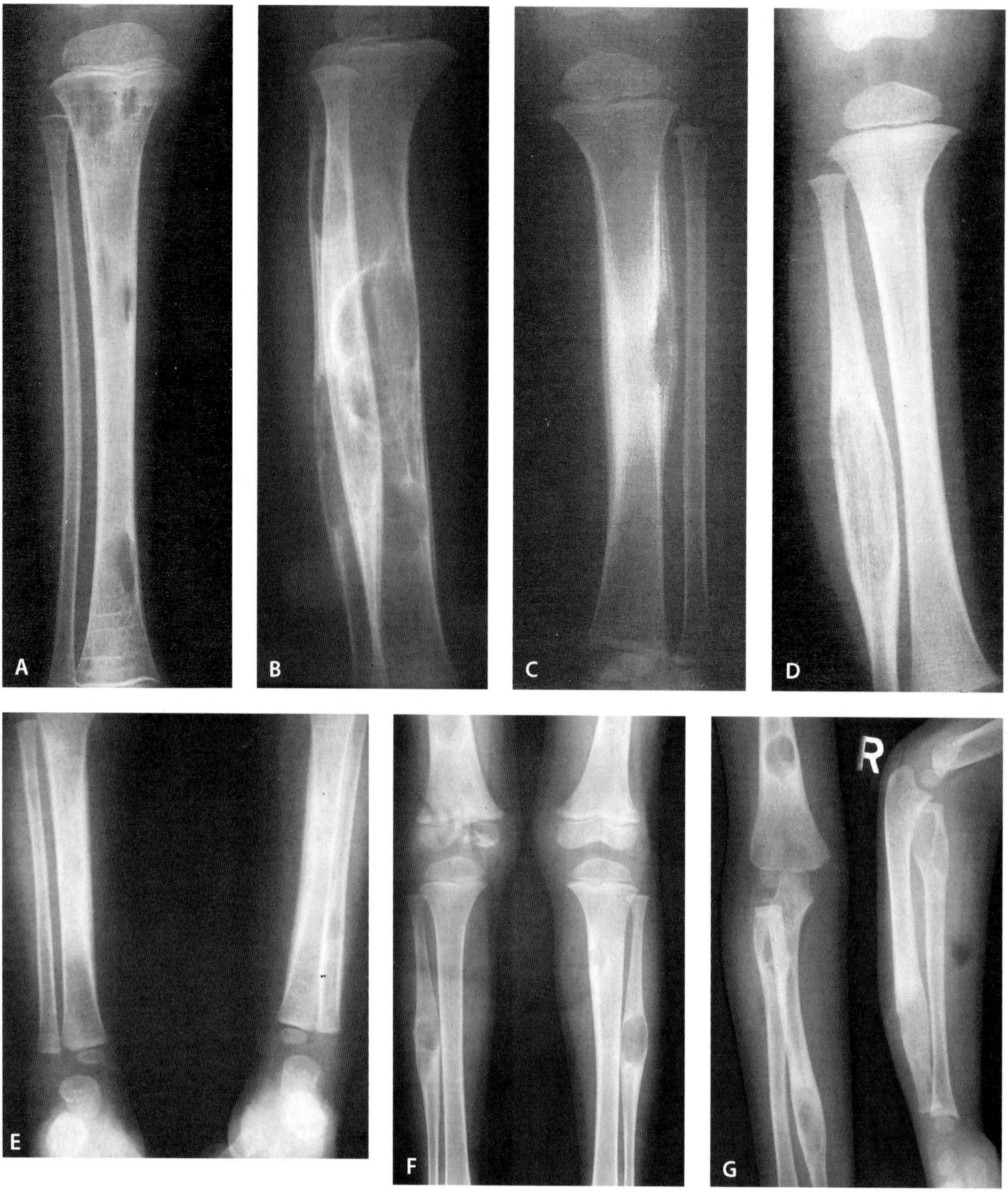

Fig. 5.81 A–G. Tuberculosis in the lower leg. Many tuberculous foci in the long bones are cystic and are often multiple. There is nearly always periosteal reaction. **A** Multiple cystic foci in the tibia and lower femur. There is minimal periosteal reaction along the upper half of the tibia laterally. **B** Multiple similar cysts in the tibia and fibula of another patient, with a periosteal reaction in the fibula particularly. Some of the cystic foci have minimal sclerotic but incomplete borders. **C** A focus of infection in the center of the tibia with a layered periosteal reaction. **D** An expansile lesion in the fibula, with the ghost of the original shaft running through it. **E** Tuberculous foci may appear in more than one limb. In this African there is a periosteal reaction around the shafts of tibiae and the left fibula, with several faint foci of infection. **G** An African child from Kenya with tuberculous foci in both fibulae, the left tibia, and the lower ends of both femora. He also had similar foci in the right humerus, radius, and ulna. This type of tuberculous bone infection usually responds quite well to appropriate treatment (see Fig. 5.88). (**B** courtesy of Dr. Harold G. Jacobson ; **A, C, D** from Cremin and Jamieson 1995)

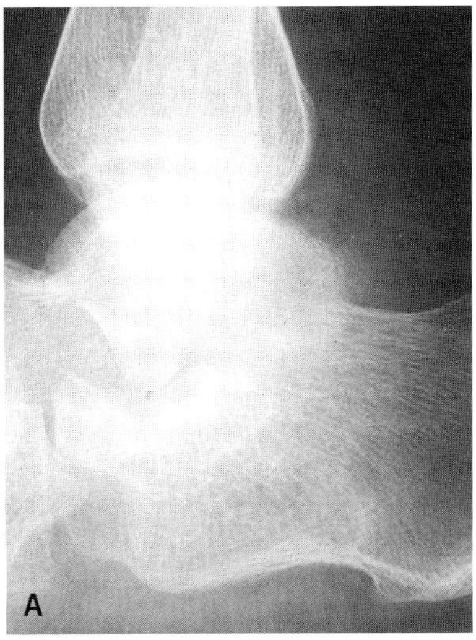

Fig. 5.82 A–F. Tuberculosis around the ankle joint. **A** Very early infection. There is synovial thickening and a small effusion, as well as a minimal bone defect in the cortex of the upper surface of the talus posteriorly. **B** Infection of the lower end of the tibia, with an effusion into the ankle joint. There is marked soft tissue swelling. **C** A large defect medially and posteriorly in the lower end of the tibia with generalized osteoporosis and a small focus in the fibula. The ankle joint is decreased and a focus of infection is seen in the talus posteriorly. There is marked soft tissue swelling, and a joint effusion. **D** Collapse and destruction of the os calcis with marked soft tissue swelling and generalized osteoporosis. The infection is in the os calcis, but the whole joint will eventually be destroyed. **E** Cystic and sclerotic tuberculous infection in the posterior two-thirds of the os calcis, only affecting the cortex in one small area of the upper margin, near the tendo Achillis. **F** A more localized infection of the os calcis, with a sequestrum and extensive disruption of the upper surface. In **D–F** the differential diagnosis would include pyogenic and mycotic infections. (Courtesy of the University of Capetown Radiology Library)

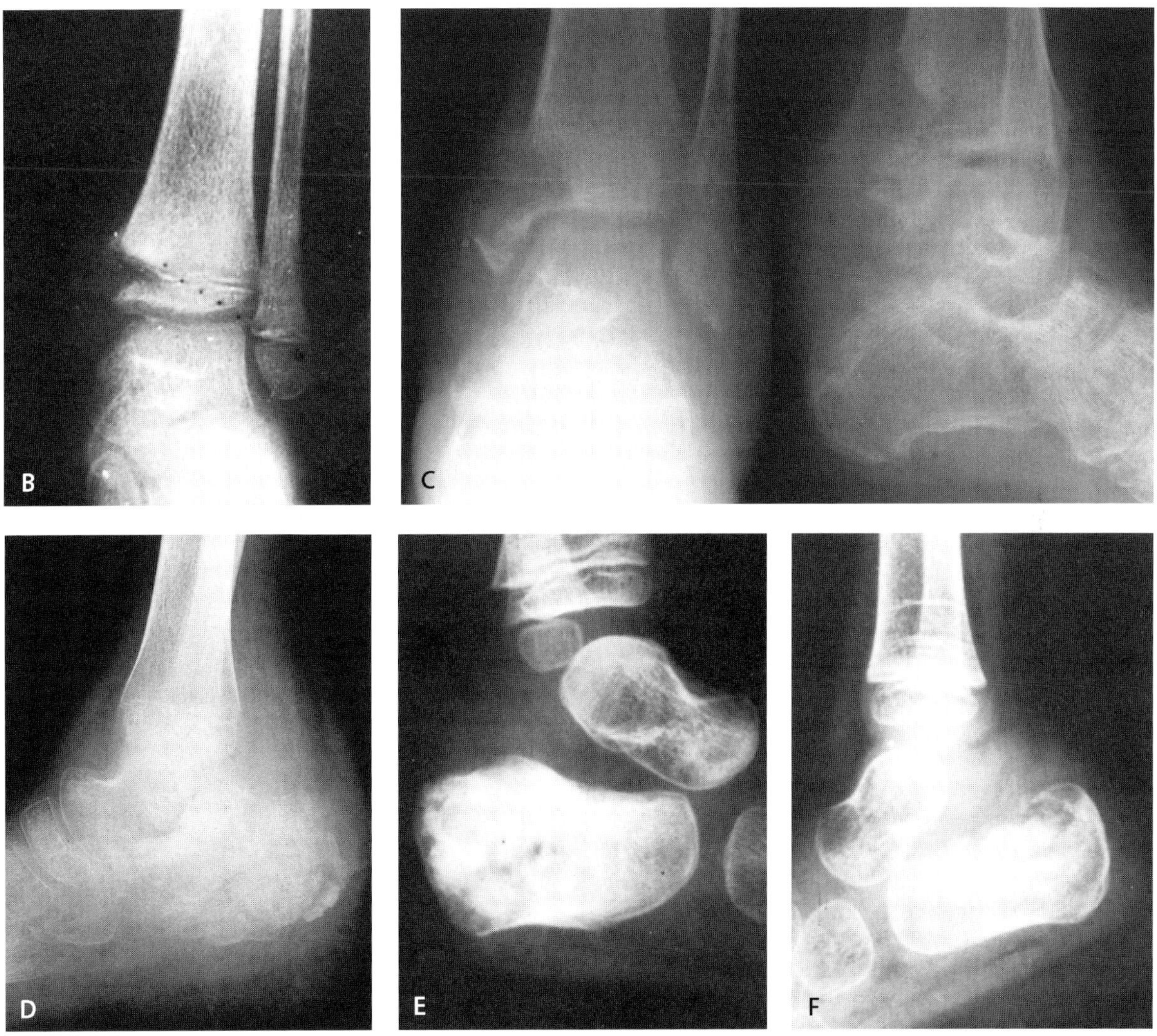

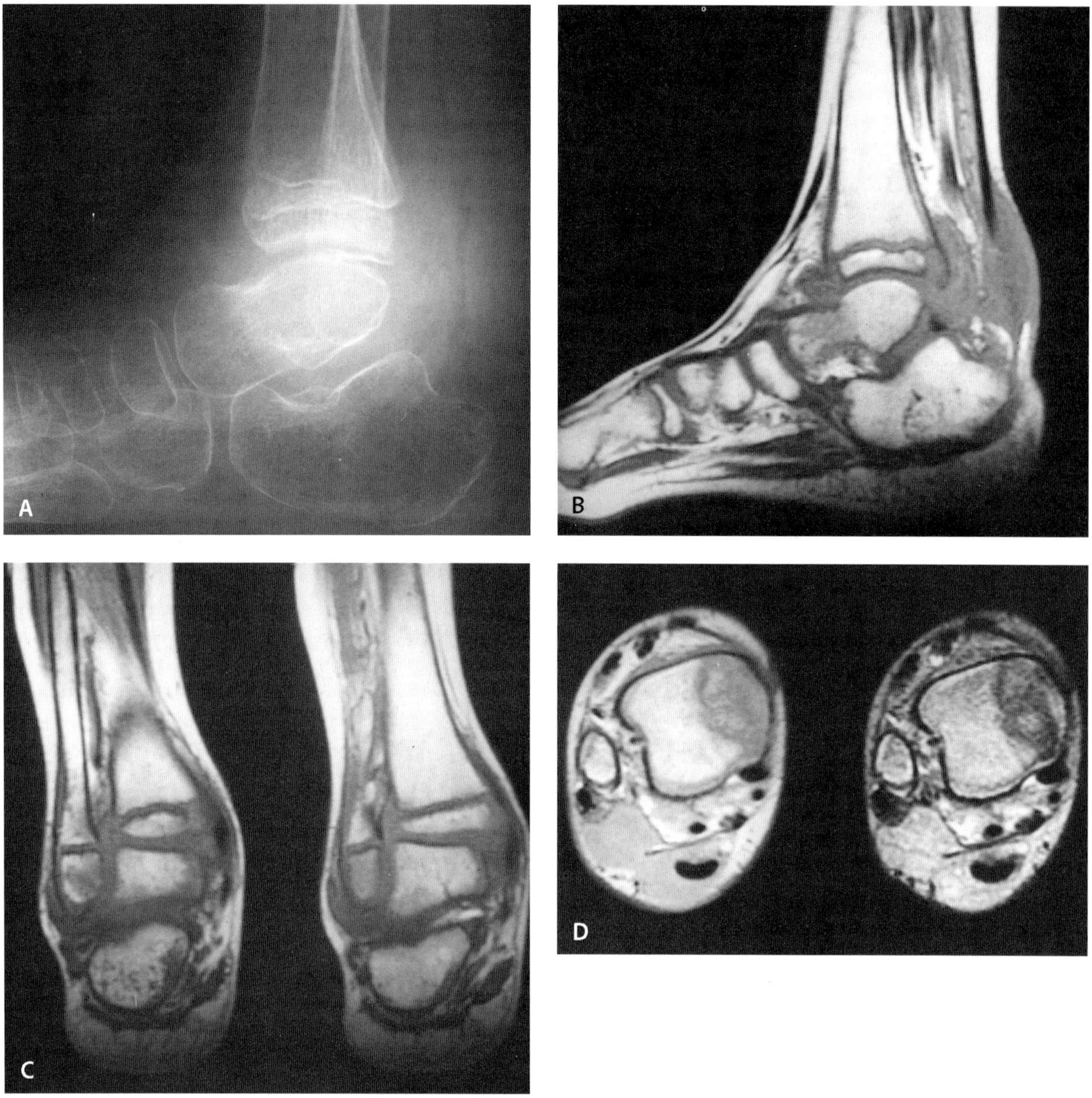

Fig. 5.83 A–D. The swollen ankle of a 7-year-old boy from the Pacific Islands. **A** There is generalized osteoporosis, but it is difficult to be sure that there is any bone focus. **B–D** MR scans show the joint effusion, and destruction of both the talus and the posterior part of the tibial epiphysis. The unfortunate child had tuberculous meningitis and miliary tuberculosis

The radiolucent areas are filled with tuberculous granulation tissue, which causes the expansion. As the cortex expands and thins, subperiosteal new bone is laid down on the outer aspect; this new bone may be layered, quite thick and dense, and sclerotic. Because there is the appearance of an involucrum, the possibility of a pyogenic infection should be considered. The differential diagnosis then depends largely on the patient's clinical condition. In tuberculosis the pain is not marked, pyrexia is minimal, and the whole condition is relatively benign. A pyogenic osteomyelitis causing such a reaction would be acutely painful, swollen, and inflamed, with a generalized systemic reaction which is often absent in the tuberculous variety.

Radiographically detectable sequestration does not often occur in tuberculosis because the blood supply has not been affected, but there are exceptions and tuberculous sequestra do occur without any other associated infection (cf. Fig. 5.82 F). CT may detect very small sequestra when a bone lesion has spread rapidly into the soft tissues, e.g., in the pelvis.

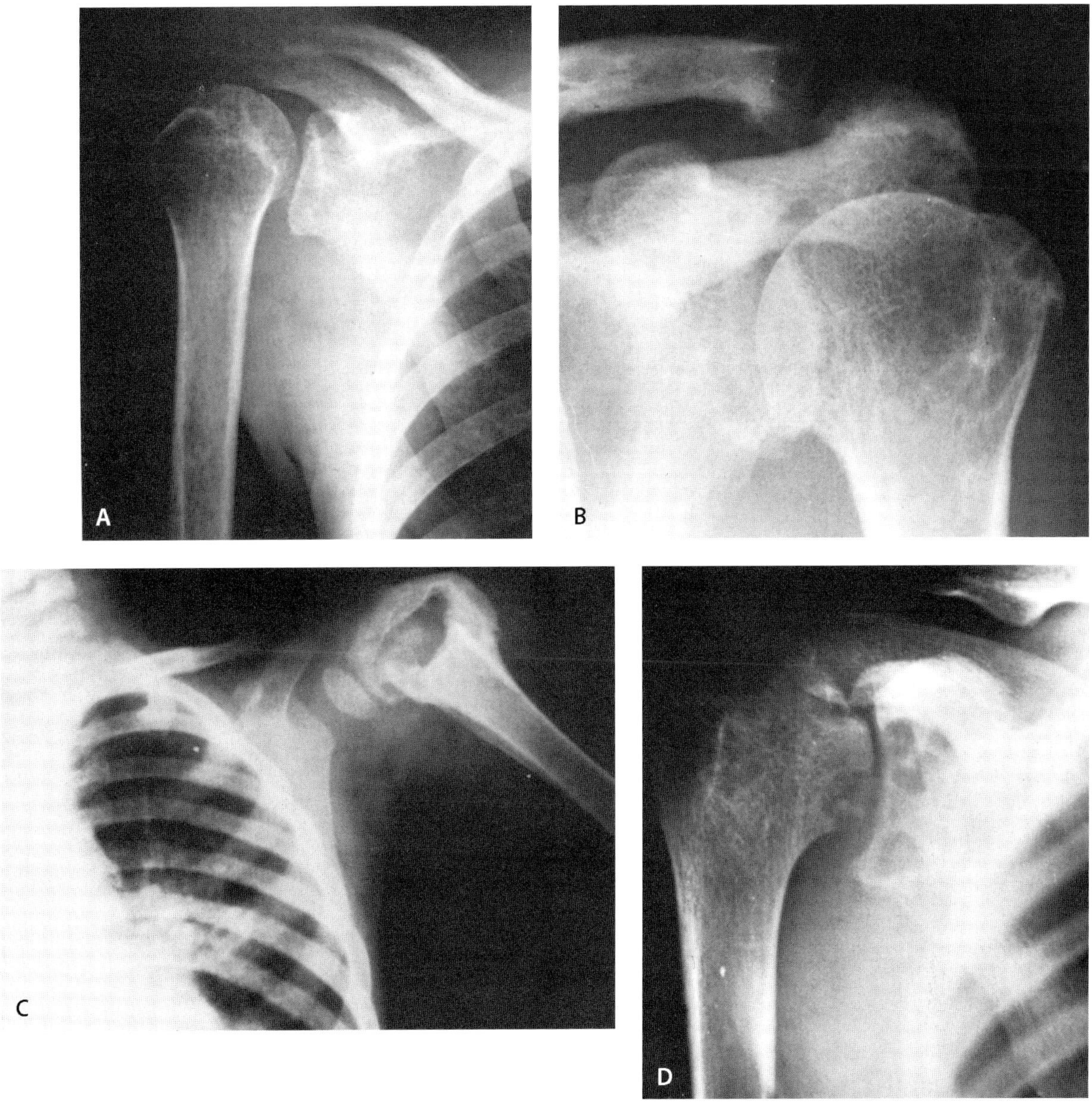

Fig. 5.84 A–H. Tuberculosis of the shoulder. **A** Acute tuberculosis with marked osteoporosis of all the bones around the shoulder. There is minimal periosteal elevation along the clavicle, but there is no bony defect. **B** A more chronic infection with multiple lytic areas in the head of the humerus, the clavicle, and the acromion process. The acromioclavicular joint is disrupted, but the shoulder joint is still relatively intact. **C** Considerable destruction of the head of the humerus in a child. There is left hilar lymphadenopathy. **D** Cystic tuberculosis in the right shoulder of a middle-aged African. The glenoid is almost destroyed, and filled with multiple cystic lesions. Next to it, the head of the humerus shows similar defects and there is destruction of the articular surface. The joint space is narrowed. The acromion was also affected. **E–H** see p. 506

In Europe and North America, the same multifocal lytic lesions can occur, but they are better demarcated and cyst-like. They are most common in the long bones of children and young adults; sometimes they are symmetrical. Probably the difference between the tropical and nontropical pattern is related to immunity or more prompt treatment. The "tropical" pattern will be seen in AIDS anywhere and will often be more destructive and spread more rapidly.

In the skull, scapula, and ribs, as well as the long bones, there may be similar lytic foci without any bone response. In the skull this results in quite large, destructive lesions. Solitary skull foci also occur, sometimes with a reactive edge and a central "button" sequestrum. Because these solitary tuberculous foci are associated with a fluctant "cold" abscess they were named "a puffy tumor" by Sir Percival Pott in the eighteenth century.

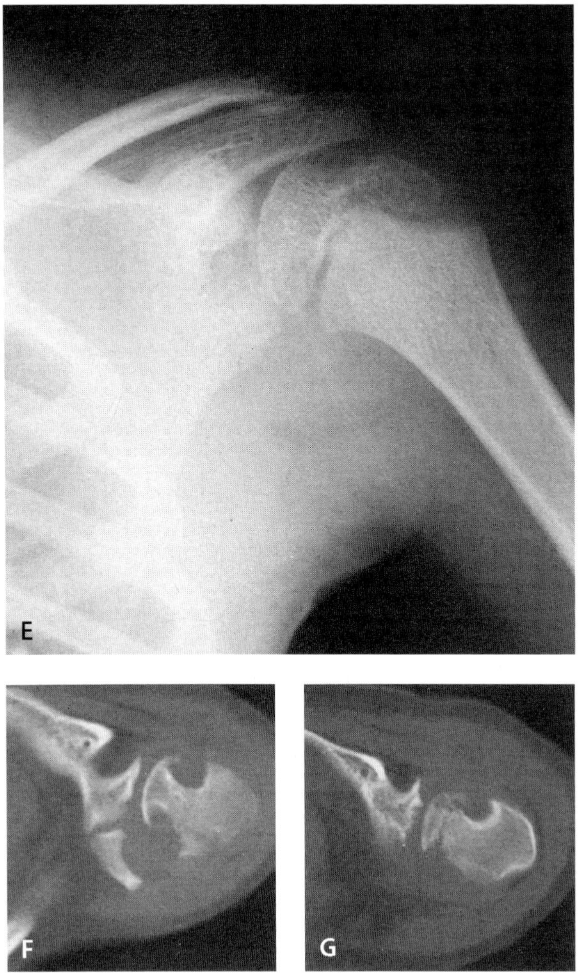

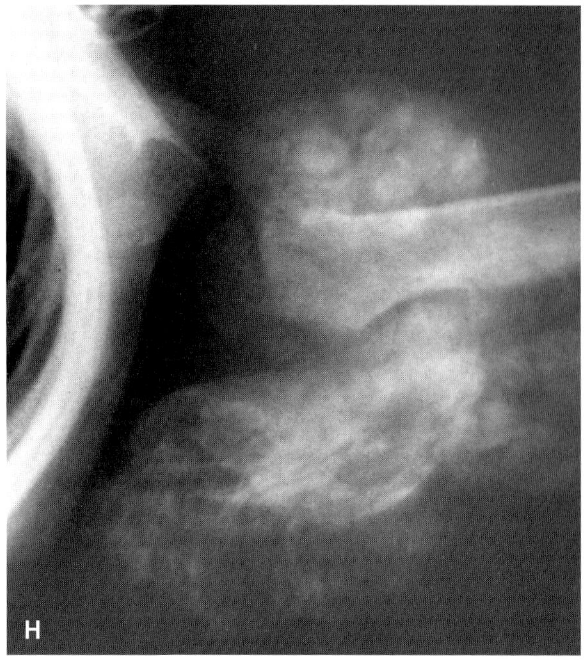

Fig. 5.84 (*continued*). **E** Erosion of the glenoid and humeral head in a child. **F, G** two CT scans in the same patient showing the defect in the humeral head and the partial destruction of the glenoid (**G**). **H** The late stage of tuberculosis; there is calcified debris all around the joint, with partial destruction of the end of the clavicle. The acromion was also involved. The humeral epiphysis is very decalcified. The calcified masses could be mistaken for tumoral calcinosis, but the destruction of the clavicle and acromion provide evidence of infection. (**E–G** from Cremin and Jamieson 1995)

In the ribs there may be quite a marked periosteal reaction and localized swelling (Fig. 5.85 E, F). Some care has to be taken to differentiate tuberculous osteomyelitis of a rib from a tuberculous abscess tracking around the intercostal space from its origin in the thoracic spine. Such as abscess will also cause swelling, and there may be some local periosteal reaction on adjacent ribs. Ultrasonography (or CT/MRI) may help to track the abscess more accurately and, like scintigraphy, will locate any intrinsic bone focus. Radiographically, in slender bones such as ribs it may not be easy to see the destructive areas within the bone itself, particularly when the periosteal reaction is marked; an exactly similar process can occur in the long bones. Periosteal new bone is not the "hallmark" of pyogenic infection; it can also be seen in tuberculosis.

In the tropics this type of "cystic" and periosteal tuberculous bone infection (cf. Fig. 5.81) may be relatively slow and benign, or can be progressive, depending on the host resistance and the rapidity with which treatment is commenced. In young children the imaging changes may appear worse than the clinical condition. When tuberculous osteomyelitis occurs in adolescence and adults, it takes longer to heal and may be more significant. In the skull vault the infection usually spreads outwards; only rarely does it involve the meninges, leading to an intracerebral tuberculous abscess (see Fig. 5.95).

Healing follows the same slow pattern already described (Fig. 5.88). The bone density returns; the defect may be filled in with new bone, or may persist for some time. The bone may be sclerotic, heavily trabeculated, or relatively normal. Some areas may be dense, resembling sequestra; the dense sclerosis in some bones, especially in the diaphysis, may mimic a chronic pyogenic (Brodie's) abscess. Healing is more rapid in the long bones and digits than in the flat bones and tends to leave less deformity except when the epiphyseal place has been involved, which commonly results in shortening. Almost all diaphyseal lesions respond well to therapy.

(Text continues on p. 510)

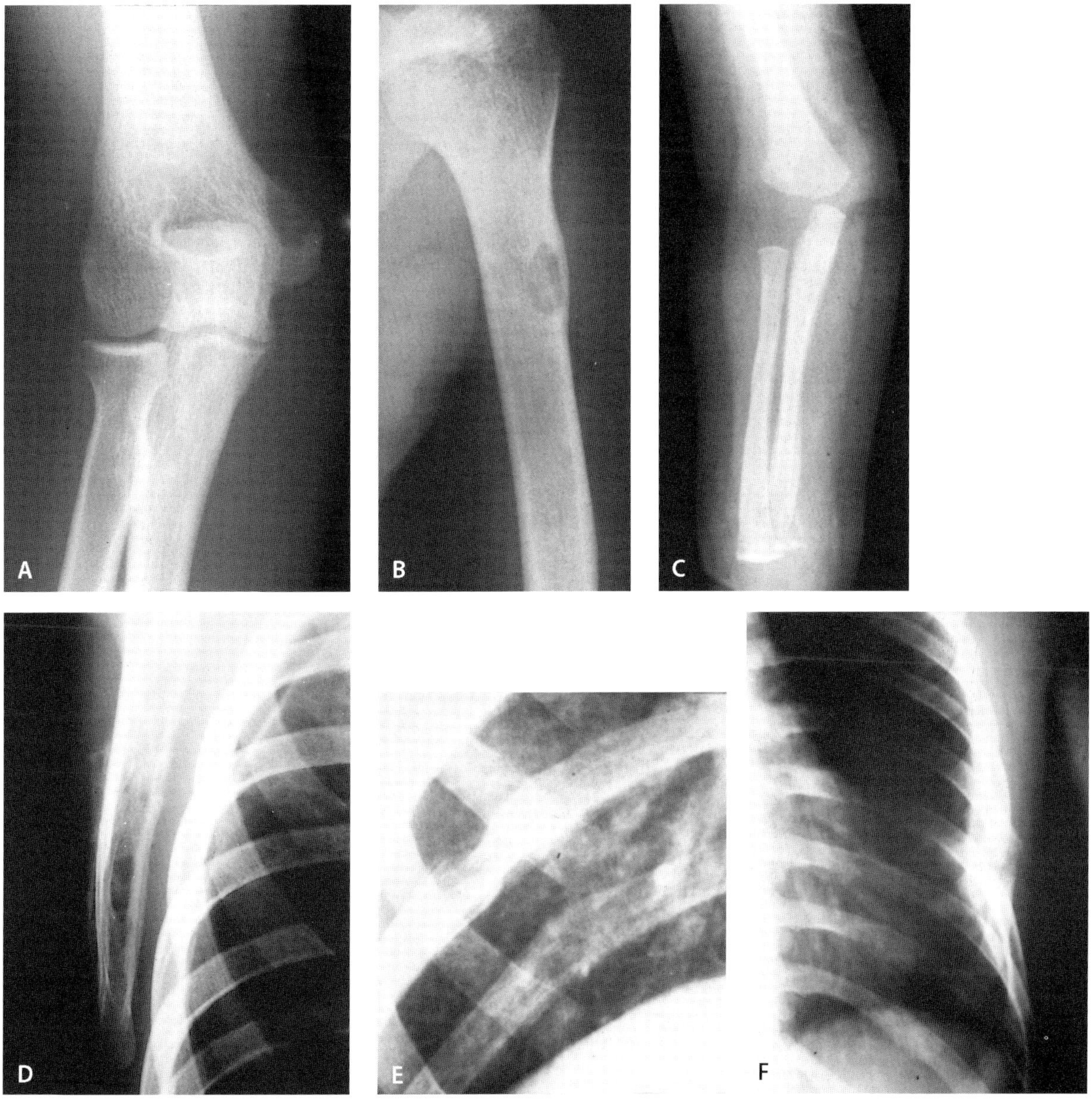

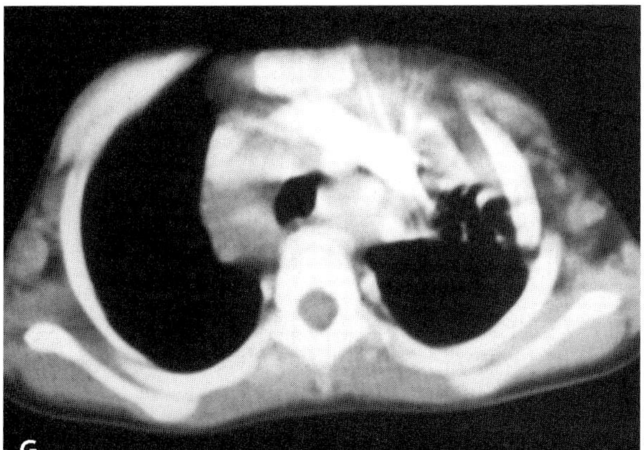

Fig. 5.85 A–G. Tuberculosis in the arm, scapula, and chest wall. **A** A lytic defect in the lower end of the humerus, will ill-defined edges, destruction of the cortex, and a minimal periosteal reaction. A similar but earlier lesion is suspected in the head of the radius. **B** A well-defined lytic focus in the upper end of the humerus, with a smaller, less clear focus in the middle of the shaft. **C** Periosteal reaction along the radius and ulna, with disruption of the lower end and widening of the upper end of the ulna and some lytic foci in the lower end of the radius. **D** Lytic destruction and minimal periosteal reaction in the lower part of the scapula. **E, F** Tuberculosis of the ribs. In **E** there is cortical destruction and periosteal reaction, and in **F** the infection is a little more advanced. There is also a pleural reaction. **G** A CT scan showing tuberculous infection of the left upper chest wall of a 4-year-old child from the Pacific Islands. He had widespread adenopathy, left upper lobe tuberculous infection, and tuberculous foci in the liver. (A progressive primary infection.) (**D–F** courtesy of Dr. Harold G. Jacobson; **G** courtesy of Dr. Cheryl Sisler, Hawaii)

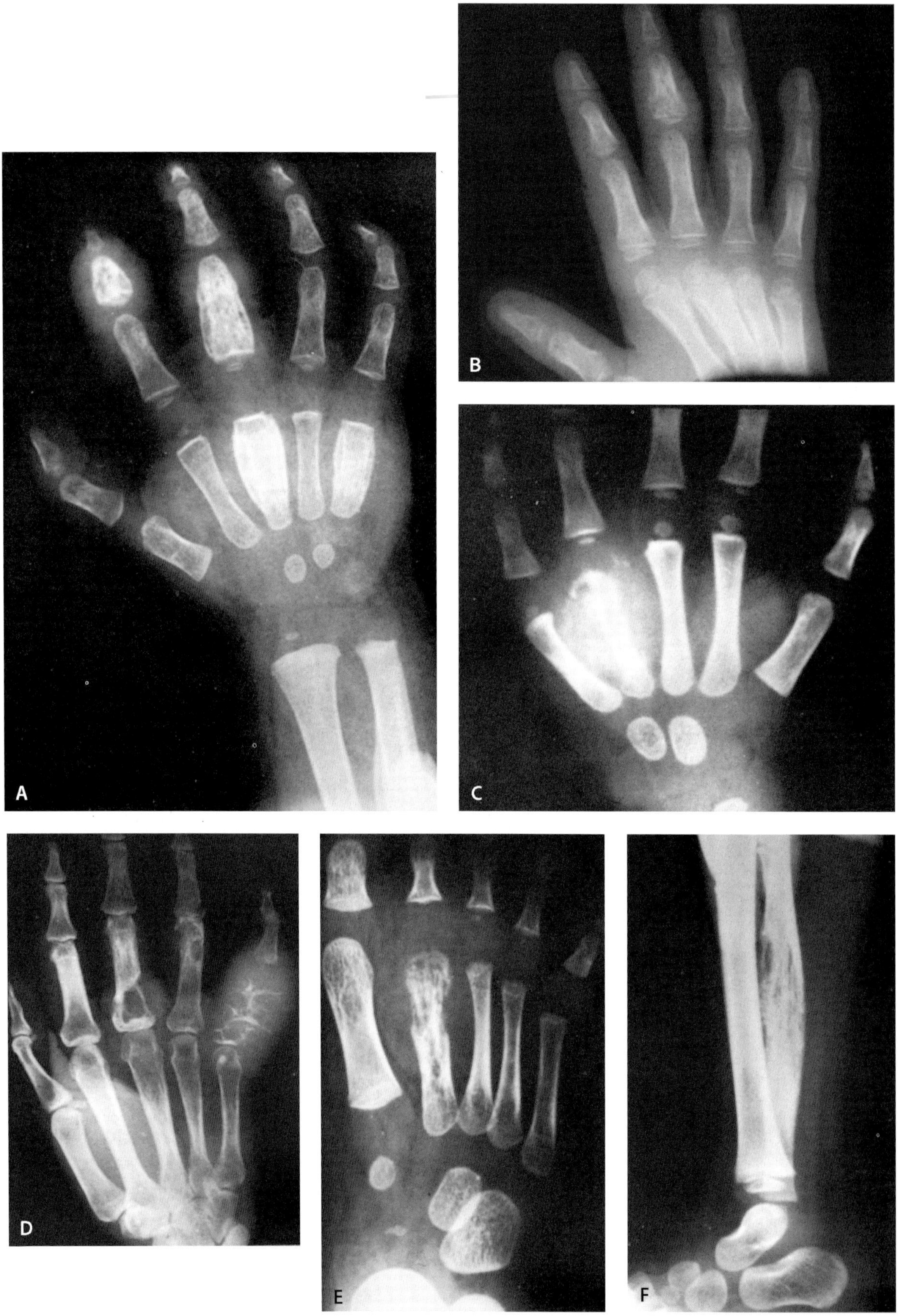
A
B
C
D
E
F

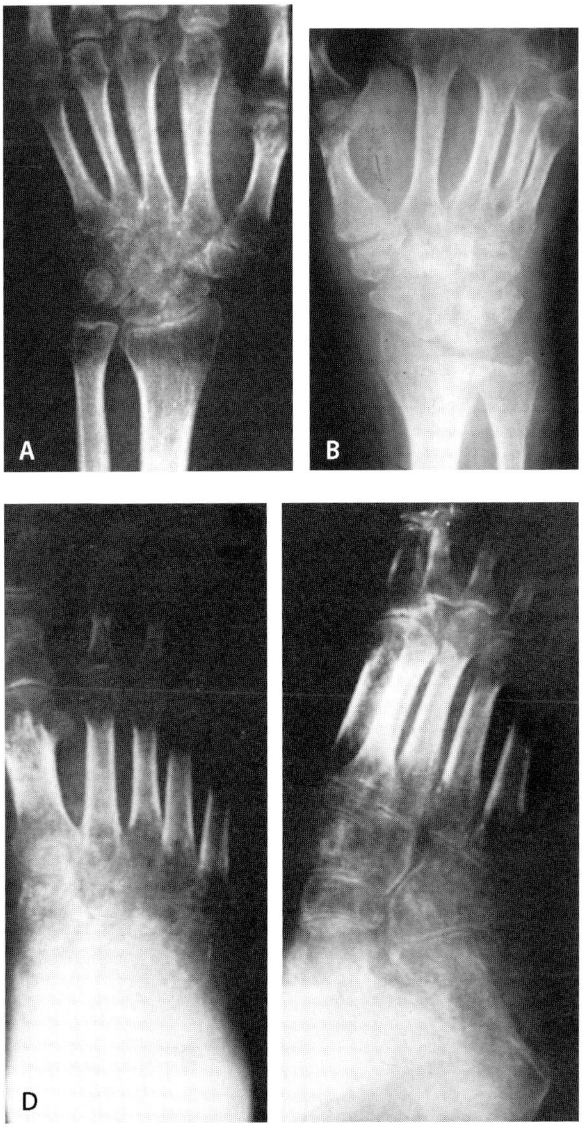

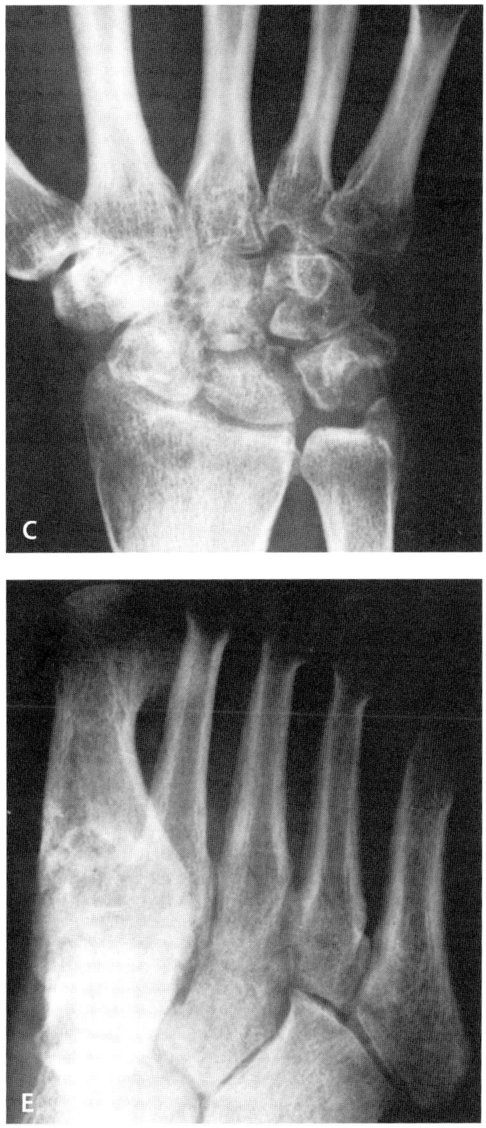

◀ **Fig. 5.86 A–F.** Tuberculosis of the extremities. Infections of the hands and feet produce similar images. **A** The hand of an infact showing marked periosteal elevation and multiple lytic areas of bone destruction. There is a periosteal reaction along the ulna also. Lytic defects are present without periosteal reaction in some of the digits. **B** In this child there is also some epiphyseal damage and less periosteal reaction. The infection was by atypical mycobacteria, but this could not be recognized by looking at the images. **C** Destructive tuberculous osteomyelitis affecting the fourth left metacarpal. **D** The hand of an older patient with more advanced tuberculosis; the proximal phalanx of the fifth finger has been almost entirely replaced by granulation tissue and there are also multiple lytic foci in the phalanges of the third and fourth fingers. This is an unusual form of tuberculosis and it could be mistaken for multiple enchondromas or even metastases. **E** Osteomyelitis of the second right metatarsal and **F** the fibula of the same patient, a young African girl; her hand is shown in **C**. Her chest x-ray was normal and there were no other bone foci. (**A** courtesy of Dr. Harold G. Jacobson; **C, E, F** courtesy of the University of Capetown Radiology Library)

▲ **Fig. 5.87 A–E.** Tuberculosis of the carpal and tarsal bones in different patients. All show generalized osteoporosis, particularly at the ends of the digits and around the carpal and tarsal joints. No bone foci are visible because the disease is mainly synovial. Bone destruction is likely to occur eventually and fusion will be the end result. **A** Osteoporosis is well marked. **B** The wrist of another patient in which bone destruction has started, involving the radius and ulna as well as the metacarpals. The carpus is collapsing. **C** In this patient the cystic and destructive tuberculous infection could be mistaken for rheumatoid arthritis or even severe gout. **D** Similar changes in the tarsus: generalized osteoporosis particularly around the joints. There are a few bone foci in the metatarsals. **E** A more chronic infection at the proximal end of the right first metatarsal and the medial side of the tarsus. The cystic lesions are becoming sclerotic and the joints are fused. There is a periosteal reaction along the shaft of all the metatarsals, but this may be due to the soft tissue reaction rather than local bone infection. This African patient was treated for many months but there was no significant change in his foot. (**B** courtesy of Dr. Harold G. Jacobson)

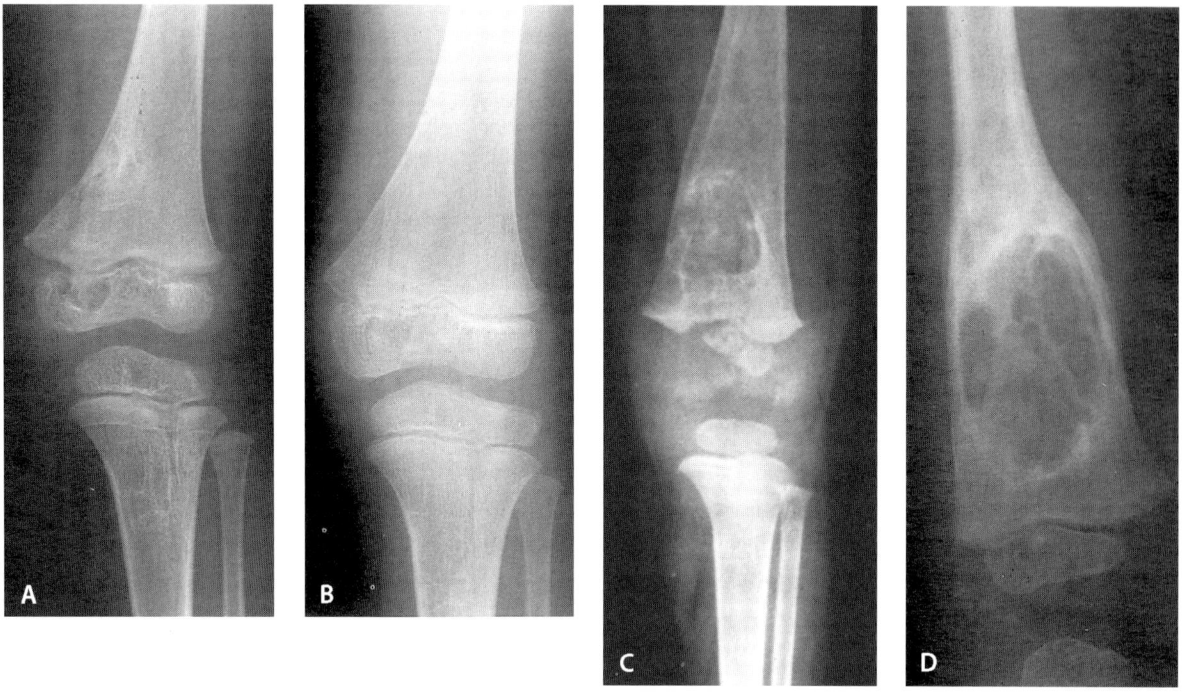

Fig. 5.88 A–D. The healing of tuberculous bone foci. **A** Cystic changes in the lower end of the femur and the upper end of the tibia, including their epiphyses. Eighteen months following the completion of 6 months of antituberculous treatment, the changes have responded well. They will probably leave only small dense foci. **C** This young African child had been on treatment for 3 months and the large cystic focus was healing with sclerosis. The periosteal reaction along the medial aspect of the femur has also thickened. Unfortunately, there is considerable disruption of the normal growth pattern of the femoral epiphysis. **D** A longstanding lesion in the lower end of the femur of another child with a multicystic appearance, periosteal thickening, and widening of the lower end of the femur. In this case the epiphysis is small but otherwise appears normal

Differential Diagnosis

The differential diagnosis of tuberculous bony lesions can be very difficult, particularly if this possible etiology is not considered early. The patient's clinical condition may help to differentiate tuberculosis from acute pyogenic infections, but even this may not ensure accuracy. The mycotic infections, such as North American blastomycosis, can simulate tuberculosis, particularly in their early stages. The multifocal destructive lesions of histoplasmosis duboisii (see Chap. 6) may resemble the aggressiv form of tuberculosis.

In the early stage osteoporosis is more marked in tuberculosis compared with pyogenic infections, but tropical (or AIDS) tuberculosis (unlike tuberculosis in Europe or North America) may behave quite acutely and change can be rapid. Sequestration is not common in tuberculosis, but can occur. Spread of infection across an epiphyseal plate is uncommon in pyogenic infections, but is frequent in tuberculosis. Eosinophilic granuloma may mimic tuberculosis (or vice versa) and infections associated with sickle cell disease, such as typhoid osteomyelitis, may closely resemble tuberculosis in their early stages in the bones of the skull vault or in the spine. Later there tends to be more periosteal reaction and the clinical condition is more acute in nontuberculous infections. The frontoparietal lytic lesions of tuberculosis are usually ill defined, compared with the clearly beveled edge of histiocytosis. Syphilis can produce very similar osteolytic lesions.

Particularly in children it is important to differentiate early rheumatoid arthritis, especially the monarticular variety. Cystic lesions could be mistaken for hydatid disease of bone, but this is uncommon in the midshaft of long bones.

The pattern of tuberculosis is the same in the bones of the skull, and may be found in the sphenoid, mastoid, zygoma, as well as the calvarium (Figs. 5.89–5.95). The maxilla and the mandible can also be involved and the differential diagnosis can be extremely difficult.

Tropical tuberculosis affects the skeleton in many ways, and this possible etiology must be remembered when any bone infection, "acute" or "chronic", is being reviewed.

(Text continues on p. 515)

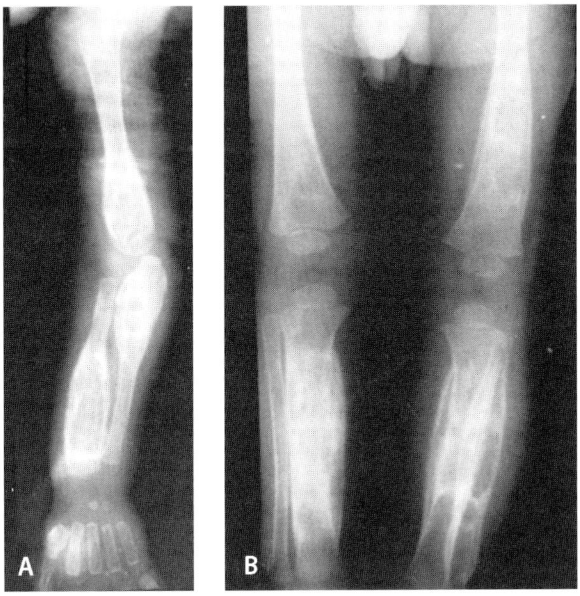

◀ **Fig. 5.89 A, B.** Tuberculosis is very frequently multifocal, particularly in patients who have a depressed immune system for any reason. Although multifocal infection is seen most commonly in children as part of the progressive primary tuberculosis, it may also appear in adults, even in old age if the infection is reawakened. **A** This 10-month-old African baby had widespread skeletal tuberculosis. There are cystic lesions with marked periosteal reaction in almost all the long bones. In the right arm, the lower end of the humerus, the upper end of the radius, and the lower half of the ulna are affected. There is dactylitis of the fifth right metacarpal. There were similar lesions in the left arm. **B** There cystic lesions in both lower limbs, in each femur; the left is more severely affected and shows a greater periosteal reaction. In the lower legs only the right fibula seems to have escaped. Whenever there is multifocal disease, a radioisotope bone study may reveal unexpected foci. The only reason that this child was brought to a hospital was because of swelling of the left lower leg. (Courtesy of the University of Capetown Radiology Library)

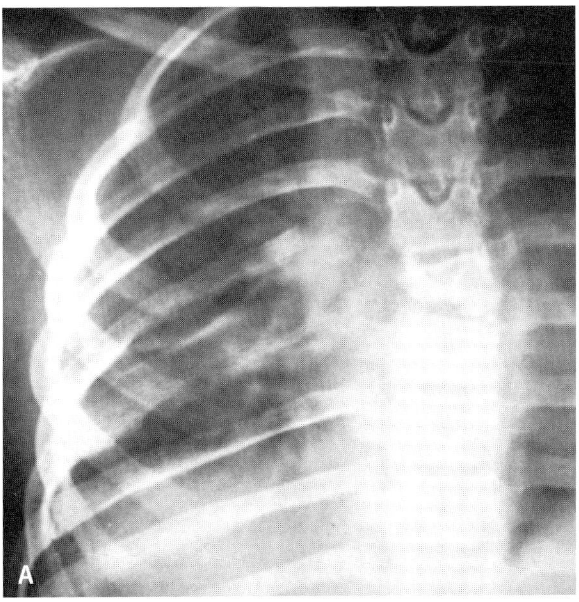

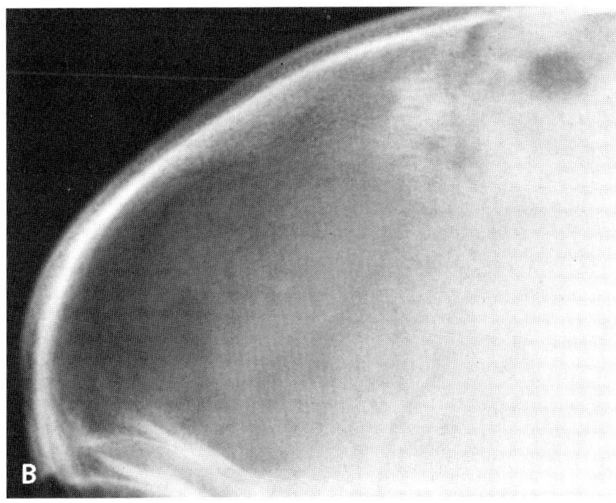

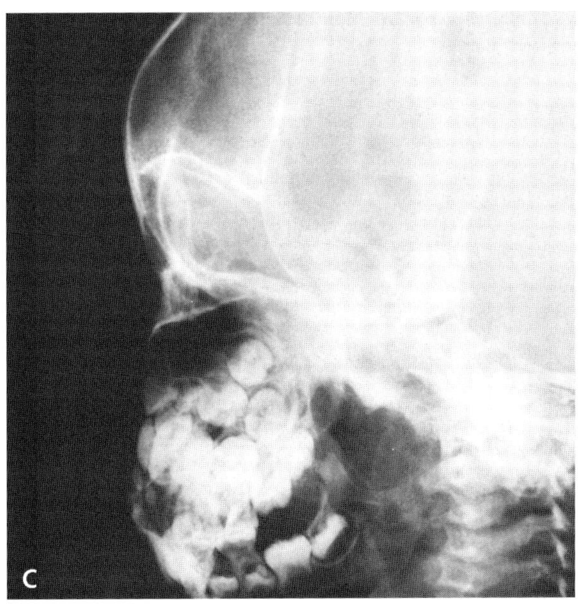

Fig. 5.90 A–C. Tuberculosis in the spine may be the clinical reason why a patient comes to hospital, but there are often foci of infection elsewhere. **A** In this small African child there is destruction of the inner ends of the sixth and seventh ribs and the infection has spread along the seventh right rib. The right side of the sixth thoracic vertebra has collapsed, although so far the disc space has remained relatively intact. There is a large right paravertebral abscess and a smaller one on the left. It is probable that the rib became infected from the spinal foci, because there is a periosteal reaction along to the anterior ends of both the sixth and seventh right ribs. The child also had two tuberculous foci in the vault of the skull (**B**) and destruction of the condyle of the mandible (**C**)

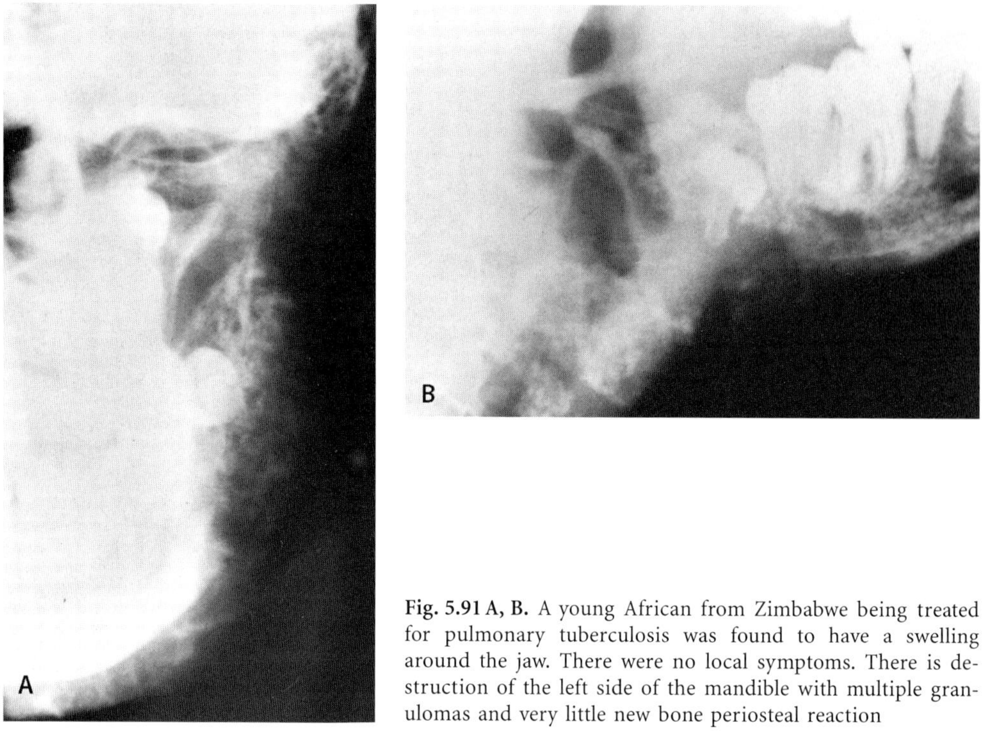

Fig. 5.91 A, B. A young African from Zimbabwe being treated for pulmonary tuberculosis was found to have a swelling around the jaw. There were no local symptoms. There is destruction of the left side of the mandible with multiple granulomas and very little new bone periosteal reaction

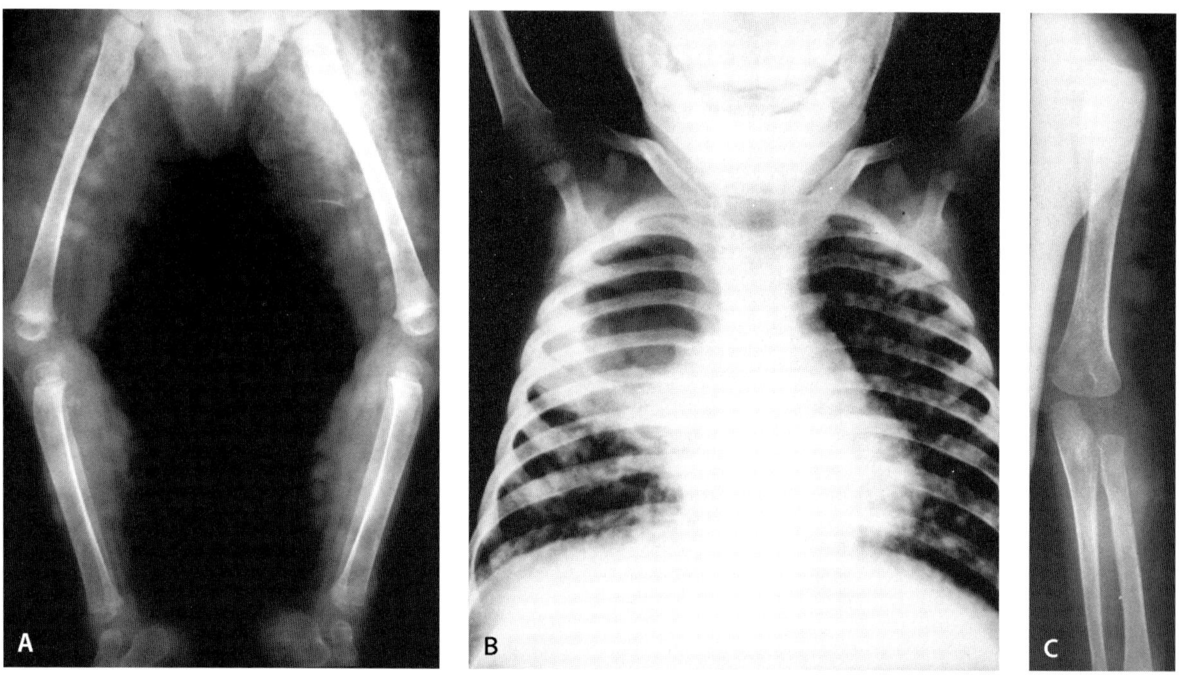

Fig. 5.92 A–C. This young African child had an overwhelming tuberculous infection and presented (**A**) with multiple cutaneous lesions covering the whole body. The only bone focus was in the upper end of the left humerus (**B**), seen on the chest radiograph. There was a large cavity almost replacing the right upper lobe, pneumonia, and multiple tuberculous foci throughout both lungs. Young children with lowered immunity may suffer from hematogenous miliary spread and present with papules, erythematous macules, or purpuric lesions over most of the body. The tuberculin skin test is usually negative and the prognosis is often poor, but this child improved after 2 months of treatment (**C**). The skin lesions are regressing, and there is a thick periosteal reaction around the upper end of the humerus, seen through the shadow of the shoulder

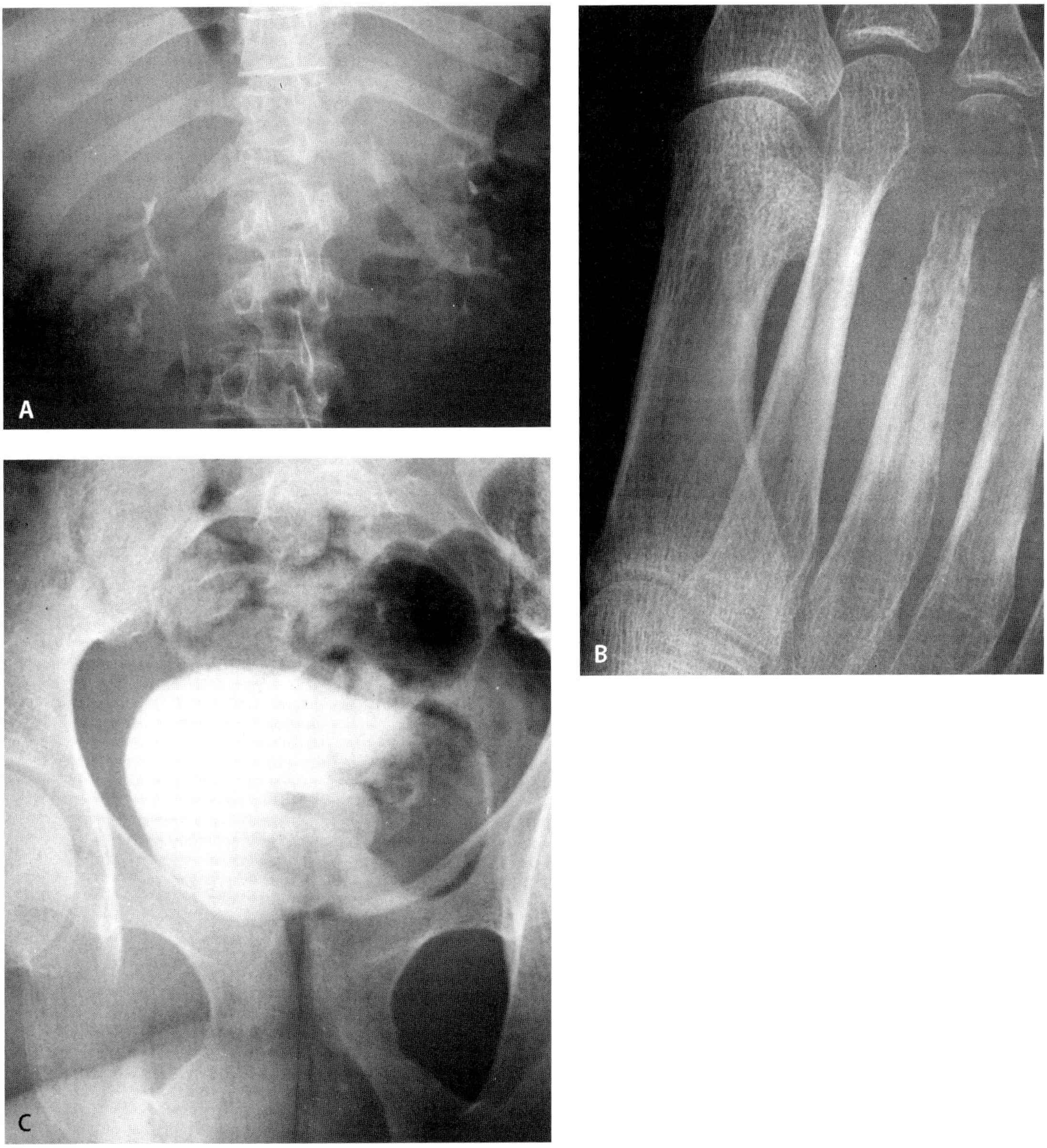

Fig. 5.93 A–C. This African patient came to hospital with a complaint of frequency of micturition. An intravenous urogram showed that he had a tuberculous infection of the spine (A) with almost complete destruction of the 12th thoracic vertebra. There was a large left paravertebral abscess, and destruction and subluxation of the 12th left rib. A large lytic defect was present in the right 10th rib. The patient was started on antituberculous therapy but later complained of a pain in his foot where there was a similar destructive lesion in the third metatarsal (**B**). The urogram had also shown tuberculous swelling of the left side of the bladder (**C**) and another incidental finding was almost complete destruction of the right lower pubic ramus. Despite all these lesions, the patient's main complaint was still urinary!

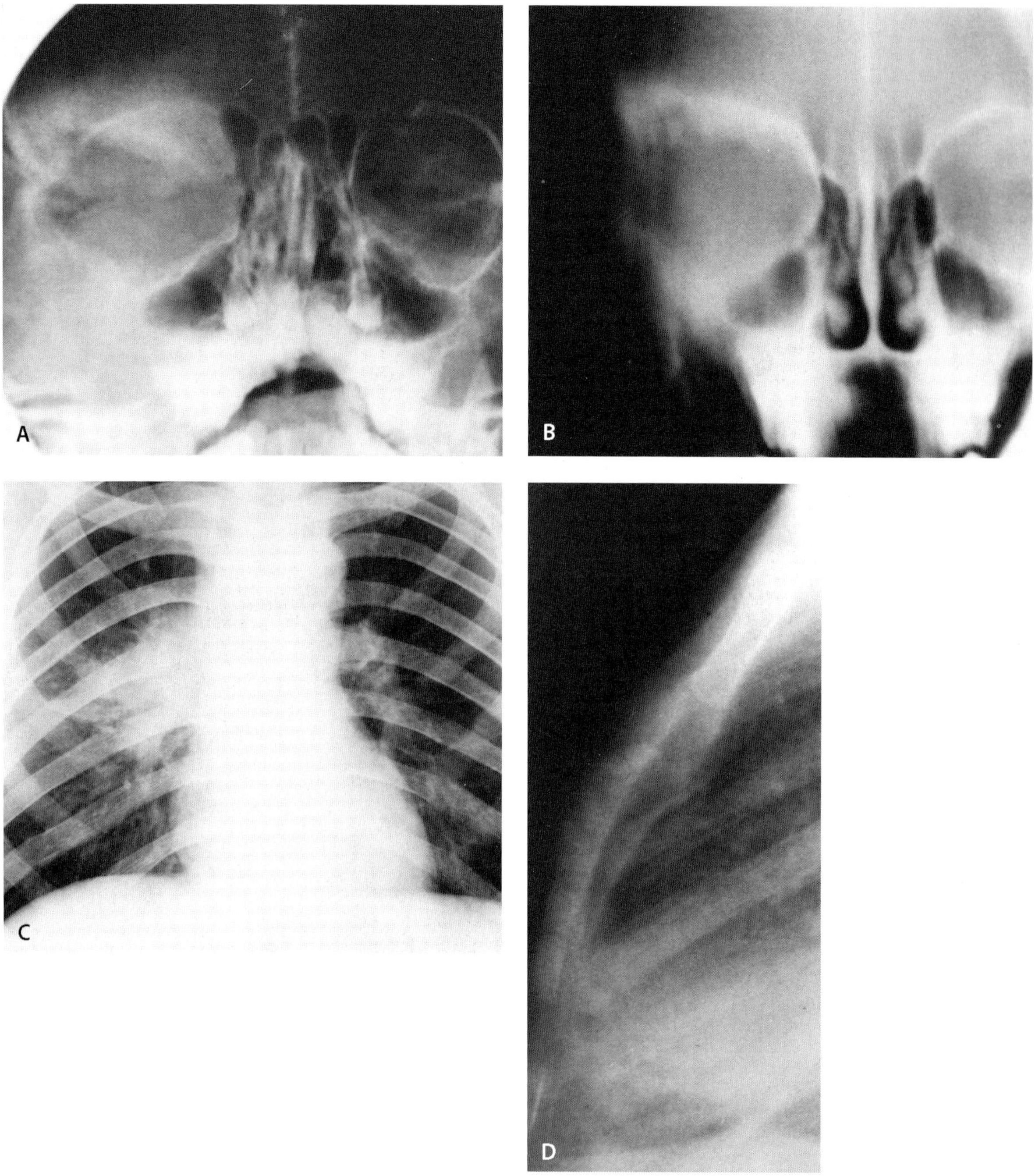

Fig. 5.94 A–D. When the infection is tuberculosis, patients may only complain of part of the infection. This teenage African came to hospital with swollen right orbit (**A, B**) and was found to have a destructive bone infection of the right orbital margin. Standard tomography (**B**) showed not only the sclerotic thickening, but a sequestrum within a lytic area above the eye. His chest radiograph (**C**) showed a primary tuberculous infection, with lymphadenopathy and the lateral radiograph (**D**) showed that he also had a tuberculous sternum.

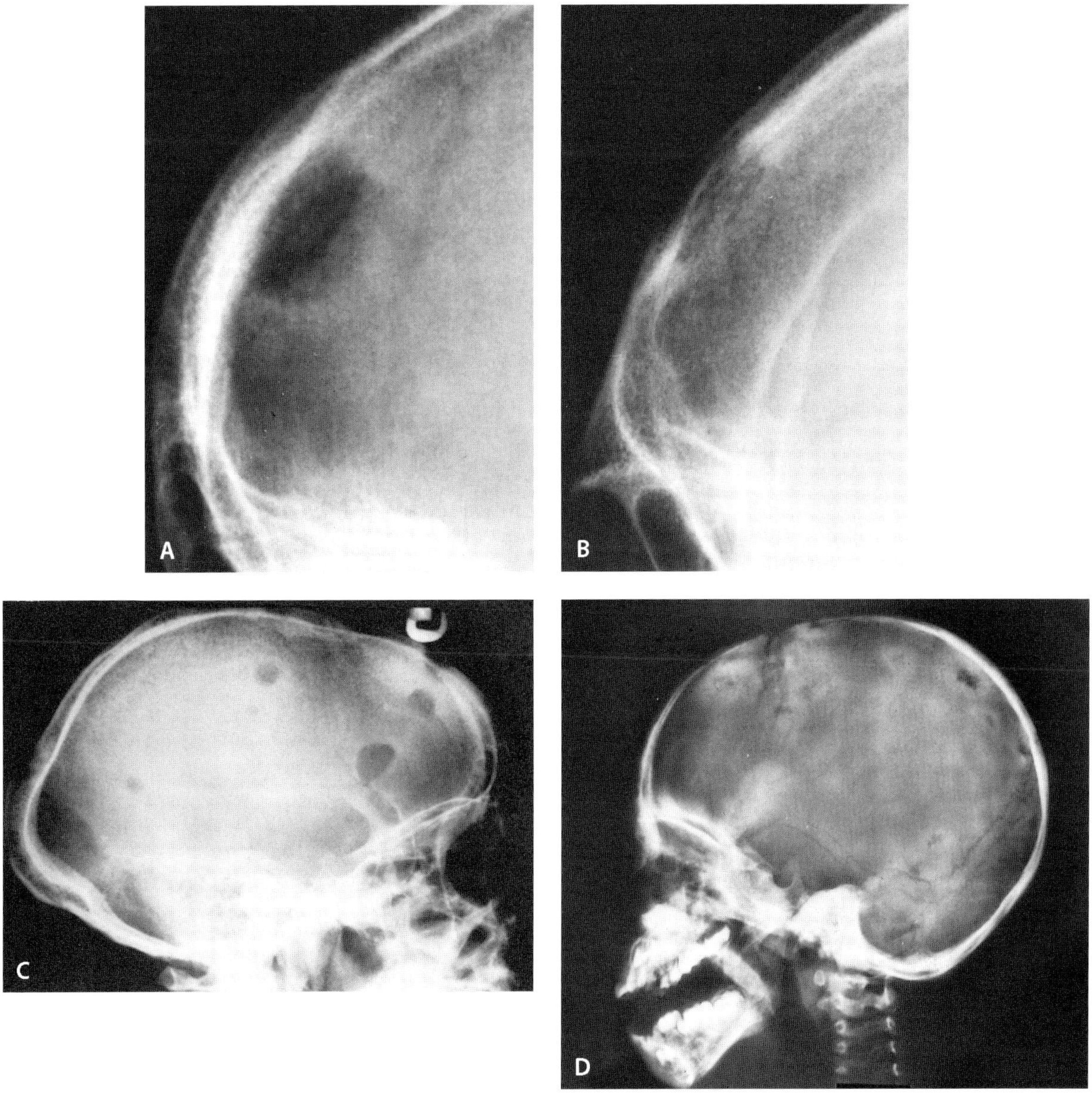

Fig. 5.95 A–D. Tuberculosis may affect any part of the skull. **A, B** Two different views of a lytic area in the frontal bone. **C** Multiple lytic areas across the skull vault. **D** Similar foci with surrounding bone reaction suggesting healing or a more chronic infection

Tuberculosis of the Central Nervous System

CT and MRI have changed our knowledge of the incidence and significance of tuberculosis of the central nervous system (CNS). It was not possible previously to image satisfactorily the different lesions caused by tuberculosis: plain radiography seldom gives much information or allows an accurate diagnosis (Fig. 5.96), and many foci that cannot be demonstrated with plain radiography are recognized on CT or MRI.

Tuberculomas of the brain probably have a variable geographic distribution, seemingly being more common in India and southern Africa. But this may also reflect the availability of imaging facilities and, particularly with the AIDS epidemic, CNS tuberculosis is likely to become more common. Tuberculosis involves the CNS by hematogenous spread, except in a few cases which result from rupture of cranial osteitis, e.g., from the mastoid or frontal bones. The tubercle bacilli may be seeded anywhere but are most common superficially over cerebral and cerebellar hemispheres and the ventricular system.

(Text continues on p. 518)

Tuberculosis of the central nervous system affects the meninges (which is probably the most important, because it carries a poor prognosis but if treated early may respond) and causes granulomatous masses (tuberculomas) which vary considerably in size and significance. Tuberculous abscesses are probably the result of central necrosis in a tuberculoma. Most tuberculomas respond to treatment, some may resolve spontaneously and the minority calcify. Plain radiography seldom gives much information or allows an accurate diagnosis. CT and MRI are the important imaging methods

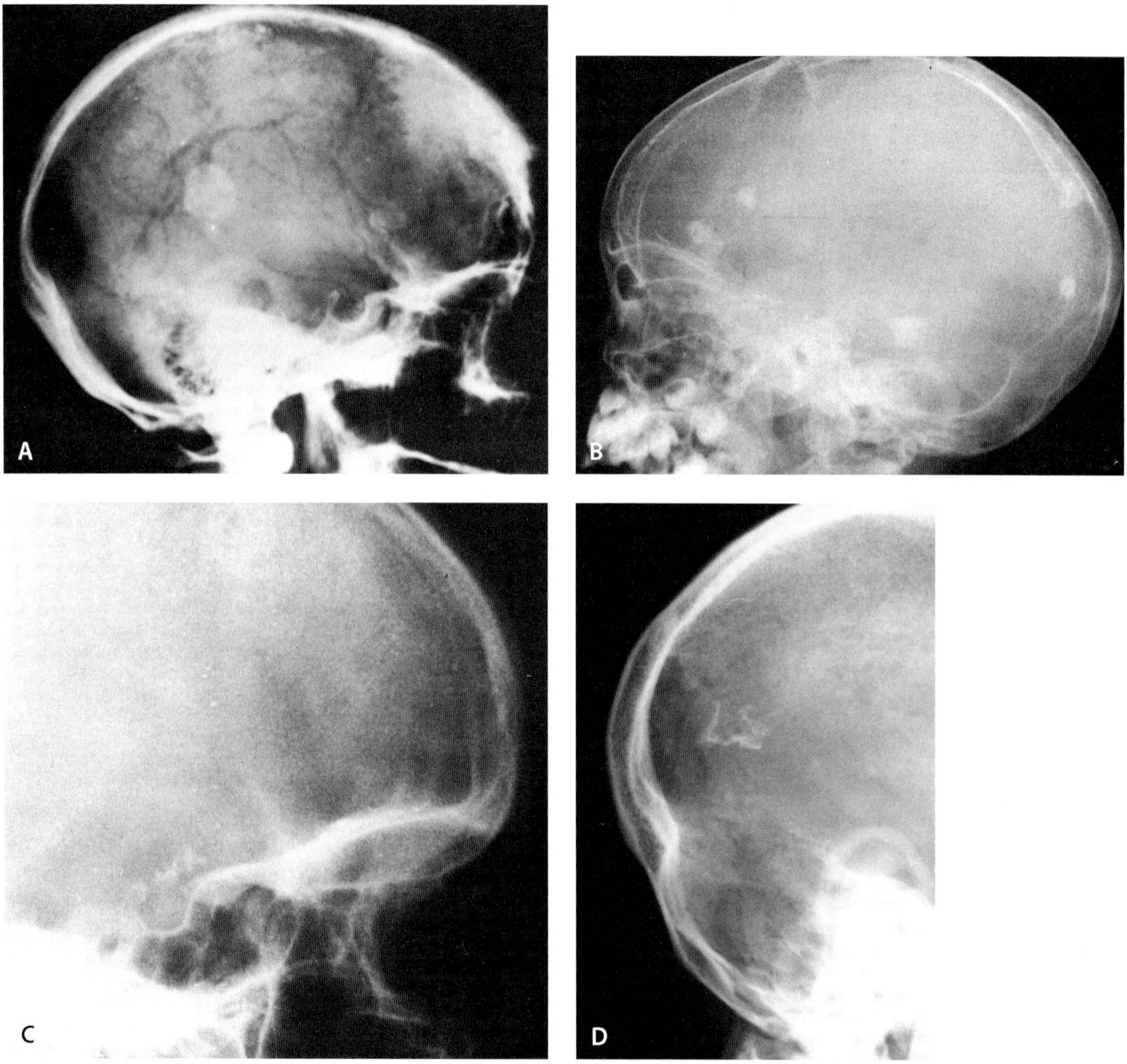

Fig. 5.96 A–H. Plain radiography of the skull may show calcification in tuberculomas or basal meninges. A normal skull radiograph does not, of course, exclude tuberculosis. **A** Multiple calcified tuberculomas with calcification of the meninges, probably also tuberculous. **B** Multiple calcified tuberculomas in a child. **C** Calcification of the basal meninges. **D** Curvilinear calcification in a tuberculoma in the left occipital region. **E–H** see p. 517

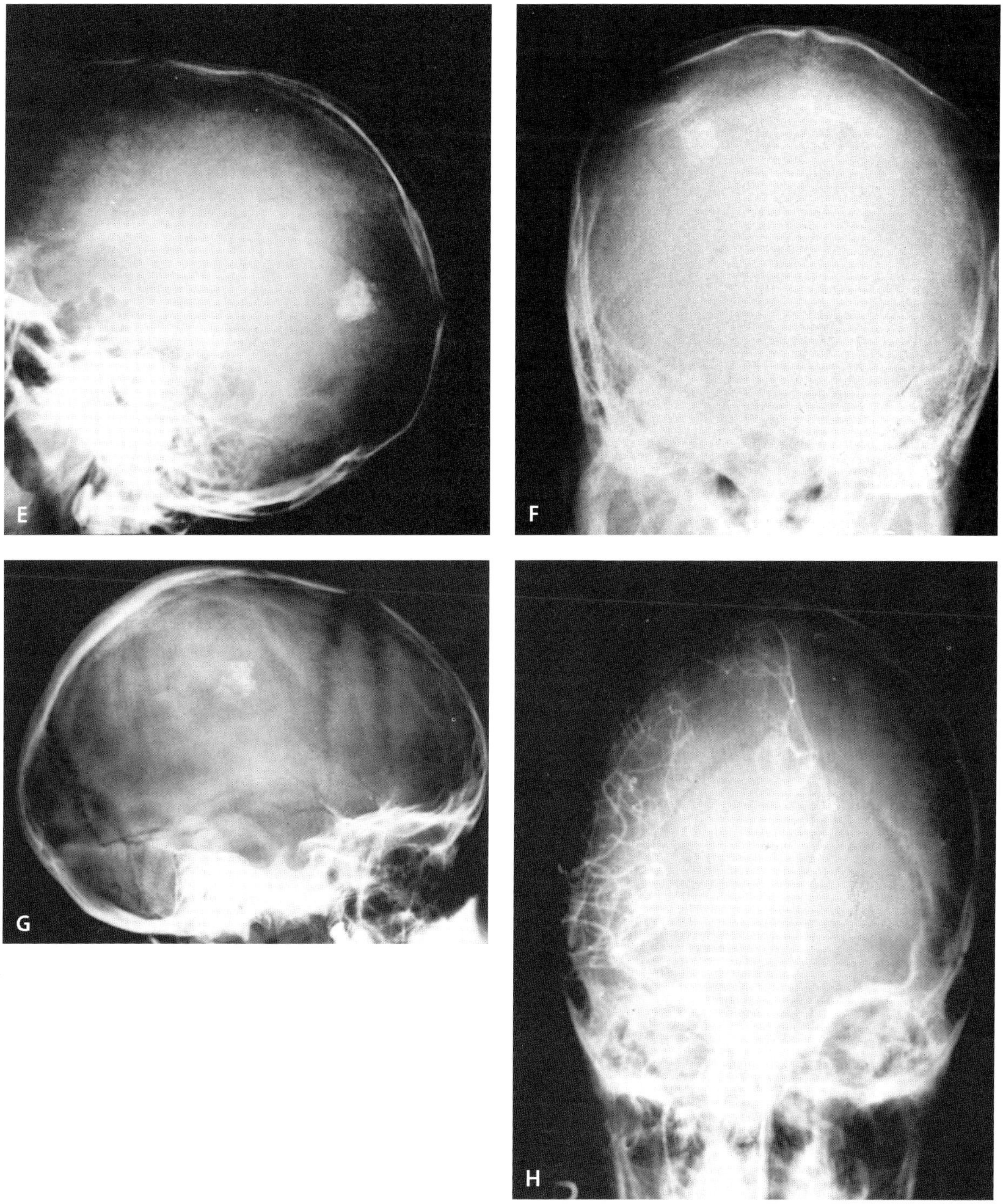

Fig. 5.96 (*continued*). **E, F** A calcified tuberculoma which was a chance finding in a patient who suffered a head injury. The depressed fracture had to be elevated and the tuberculoma was removed to confirm the histology. **G, H** Angiography is not usually helpful in making the diagnosis. However, it may indicate the size of the mass, if scanning is not available. A lateral radiograph (**G**) shows suture diastasis and a calcified mass. Arteriography (**H**) shows that this is a avascular and indicates that the size of the tuberculoma is much larger than the calcification would suggest. (**G, H** courtesy of Dr. L. Handler, Capetown) None of these radiographs would permit an accurate diagnosis of tuberculoma

As tuberculosis develops and caseates, involving the meninges, the infection can spread to the subarachnoid space. The most extensive reaction is at the base of the brain, where a thick exudate develops and surrounds the cranial nerves, compressing blood vessels and blocking the foramina of the fourth ventricle. The general inflammatory response also causes raised intracranial pressure.
Two main patterns of CNS tuberculosis develop:

1. Tuberculous meningitis
2. Parenchymal or meningeal mass lesions, tuberculoma

In some patients both varieties develop together, becoming a very complex infection.

Tuberculous meningitis

Tuberculous meningitis as a presenting illness is most common in children and carries a significant mortality and complication rate if not treated early. It is often associated with progressive primary tuberculosis and will also be seen in immunosuppressed patients. Cranial nerve damage may occur and ischemic infarction can occur in any part of the brain: these are the two most common causes of long-term complications. The incidence of infarction is high, perhaps 40%–60%. As the blood vessels become involved with the proliferative arachnoiditis, spasm and occlusion may result in infarction.
Plain radiography has little part to play in the imaging of tuberculous meningitis. Small infants may have suture diastasis as intracranial pressure rises, but this is a nonspecific finding. In babies and if the diastasis is sufficient, ultrasonography can be used to demonstrate the basal meningeal changes and the ventricular dilatation. Most children are too old for ultrasonography to be really useful.
Where available, CT and MRI are the most important imaging modalities (Figs. 5.97, 5.98). Following infarction, CT will show ill-defined hypodense areas, which may enhance with contrast. MRI is more accurate and a contrast enhanced T2-weighted scan can demonstrate a mass effect and hyperintense areas. These may progress to show cavitation. On T1-weighted scans these areas are well defined and hypointense.
Hydrocephalus develops in most cases of tuberculous meningitis unless treatment is started very promptly (Fig. 5.99). The obstruction is usually in the basal cisterns or the aqueduct. Immediate surgical shunting may be necessary. The end results, even with treatment, may be fibrosis and continued basal obstruction. Healing may be recognized by lack of contrast enhancement on CT but the end stage is difficult to judge. A small number of cases will resolve completely.
Cerebral arteriography during the active phase of meningitis may show vascular irregularity of the larger vessels basally, probably due to arteritis because of the surrounding inflammation. Sometimes complete obstruction of the vessel can be demonstrated. These findings correlate well with the CT images and it is doubtful whether arteriography is indicated during tuberculous meningitis. Occasionally tuberculous meningitis may form plaques or clusters of thickening around major cerebral vessels, demonstrated by CT. These have not been reported commonly from tropical patients, but this may represent infrequency of scanning rather than absence of the pathology.
It is important to note that the incidence of intracranial tuberculomas complicating tuberculous meningitis is 4%–28%: at least one such case has developed during adequate antituberculous treatment. The presence of an intracranial tuberculoma may be indicated by clinical deterioration and may be thought to be due to a resistant organism. When a clinical change occurs, MRI or CT scanning is indicated.

Tuberculomas

Any granuloma may develop into a tuberculoma, forming a mass anywhere on or within the meninges. A tuberculoma can be single and nodular, or there may be more than one (Fig. 5.100). Provided they are treated, almost all will resolve without residual imaging abnormality; untreated many will continue to become calcified granulomas (Figs. 5.96, 5.100 A, B). A few, during development, may become tuberculous cerebral abscesses. These have thin walls and are smooth but can be multiloculated. They are indistinguishable from pyogenic abscesses except histologically. Many have surrounding edema which can be demonstrated by CT (hypodense) and T2-weighted MRI (hyperintense) (Fig. 5.101).
The tuberculoma without central necrosis is hypodense on CT and hyperintense on T1-weighted MR scans. T2-weighted scans show hypointensity. On both CT and MRI there is contrast enhancement. If there is central necrosis, this does not enhance and there will be a ring mass (Fig. 5.101 C, D). The central necrosis of tuberculoma may have two origins. The granulation tissue may undergo necrosis or it may result from cellular components which can be caseous or quite liquefied, more like pus. Both types of necrosis may be present in the same abscess and will react differently on CT and MRI. When due to a granuloma, the necrotic area does not enhance, is hyperdense on CT, and is hypointense on T2-weighted MRI. When liquid, it is hypodense on CT and hyperintense on T2-weighted MRI (Fig. 5.102).

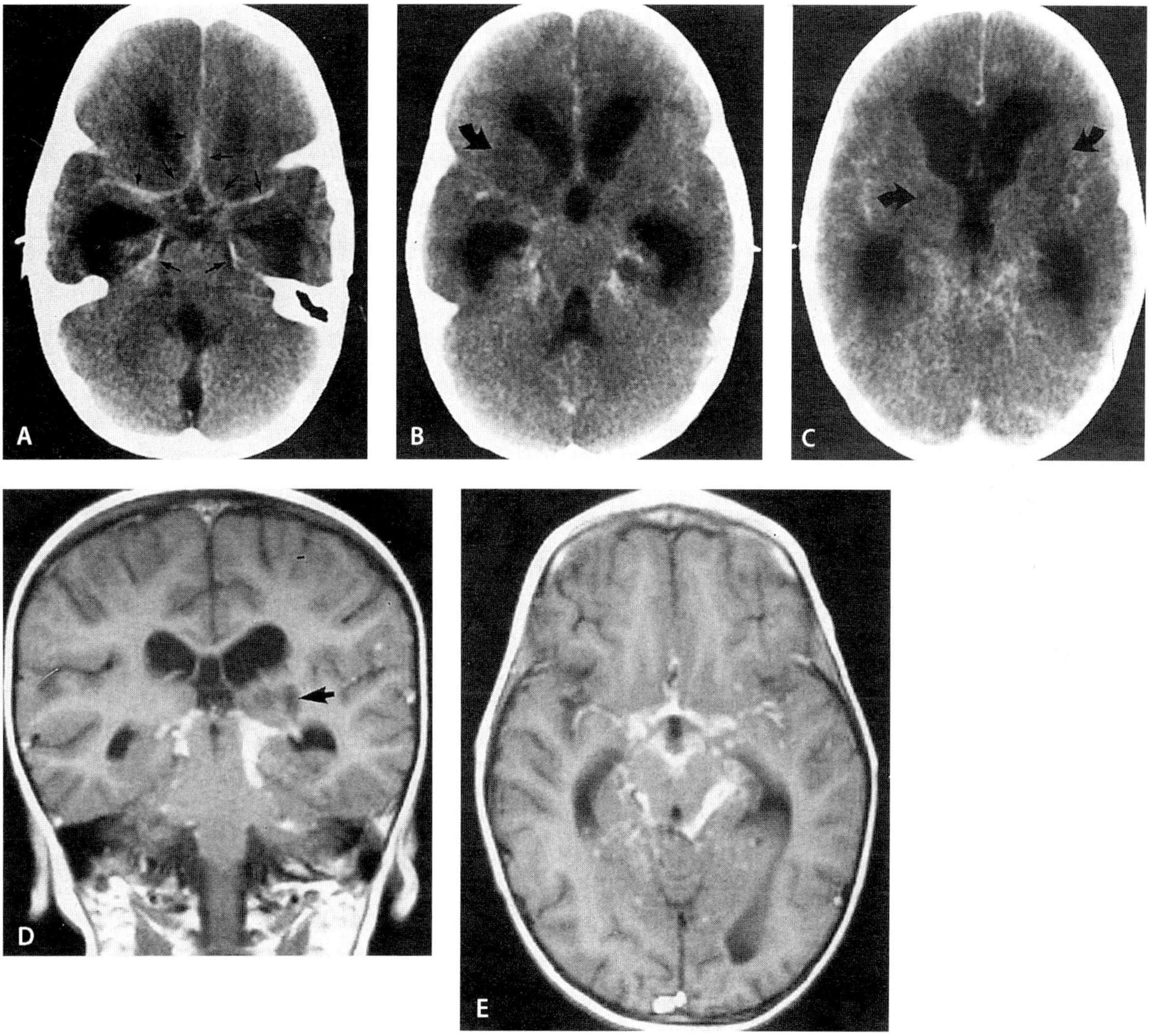

Fig. 5.97. A–C. Three important findings on CT scanning of tuberculous meningitis: **A** basal leptomeningeal enhancement (*small arrows*); **B, C** infarction in the basal ganglia (*curved arrow*) and hydrocephalus. **D, E** MRI with gadolinium enhancement in another child showing basal leptomeningeal enhancement, as well as a cavitated infarct deep in the left gray matter (*arrow*) and hydrocephalus. (From Cremin and Jamieson 1995)

Some tuberculomas under treatment may resolve in 3 or 4 months, but others may take over a year. Of those which are treated, about 5% probably calcify; this is a surprisingly small figure, because CT and MRI scans undertaken for other reasons have shown granulomas in patients with no previous history or knowledge of a CNS tuberculous infection: natural resistance must result in calcification more often than occurs with therapy.

Cerebral arteriography can demonstrate the mass lesion of a tuberculoma, depending on its size and situation. They are almost all avascular, but a small minority have a ring blush.

The differential diagnosis for tuberculous meningitis in the early stages includes any pyogenic infection. Tuberculomas can be mistaken for an intracranial neoplasm, or almost any other disease process causing mass lesions in the brain (such as subacute trauma, hemorrhage, pyogenic abscesses, or hydatid disease).

Careful clinical history, the clinical examination, and a high index of suspicion are very important. Mycotic infections can give rise to identical clinical and imaging findings (see Chap. 7, p. 641).

Tuberculosis of the skull vault results in multifocal, lytic, and well-circumscribed fluctuant swellings (Fig. 5.95). The majority are symptom free, and they almost always occur under the age of 20 years. A few may discharge to the surface and then become secondarily infected. Internal extension is very common.

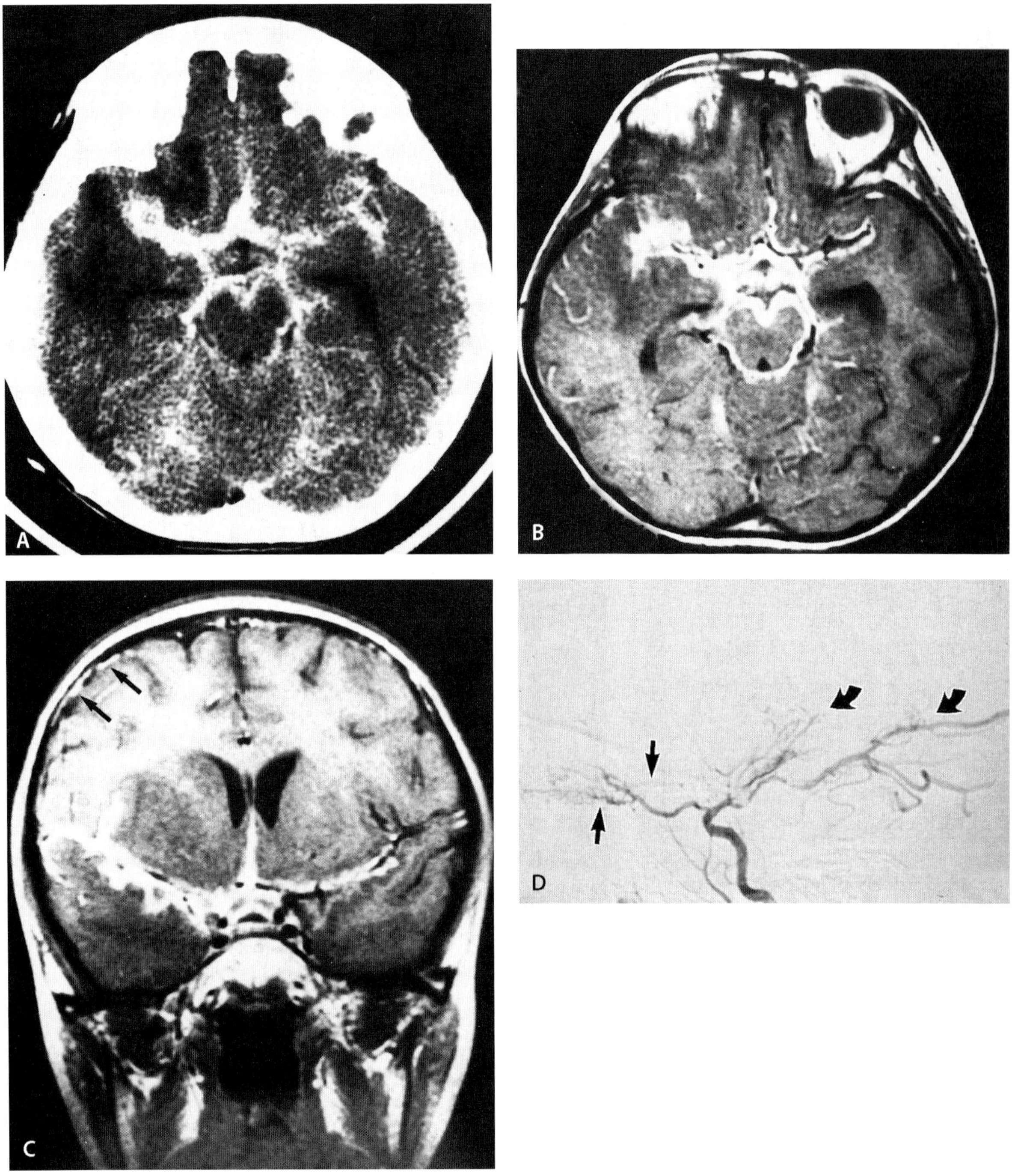

Fig. 5.98 A–D. A 9-year-old girl from the Pacific Islands with tuberculous meningitis. **A** Contrast-enhanced CT scan shows edema in the right temporal lobe and inflammatory reaction in the basal cisterns and sylvian fissures, with has enhanced. **B, C** T1-weighted MR images with contrast show similar enhancement of the basilar cisterns and the sylvian fissures, encasing the middle cerebral arteries. **D** Another child; a right carotid angiogram shows nearly complete occlusion of the artery as it traverses the meninges. An alternative collateral supply has been derived from the middle meningeal artery (*long arrows*), the ophthalmic artery (*short arrows*), and the posterior system (*curved arrows*). (**A–C** courtesy of Dr. Cheryl Sisler, Hawaii; **D** from Cremin and Jamieson 1995)

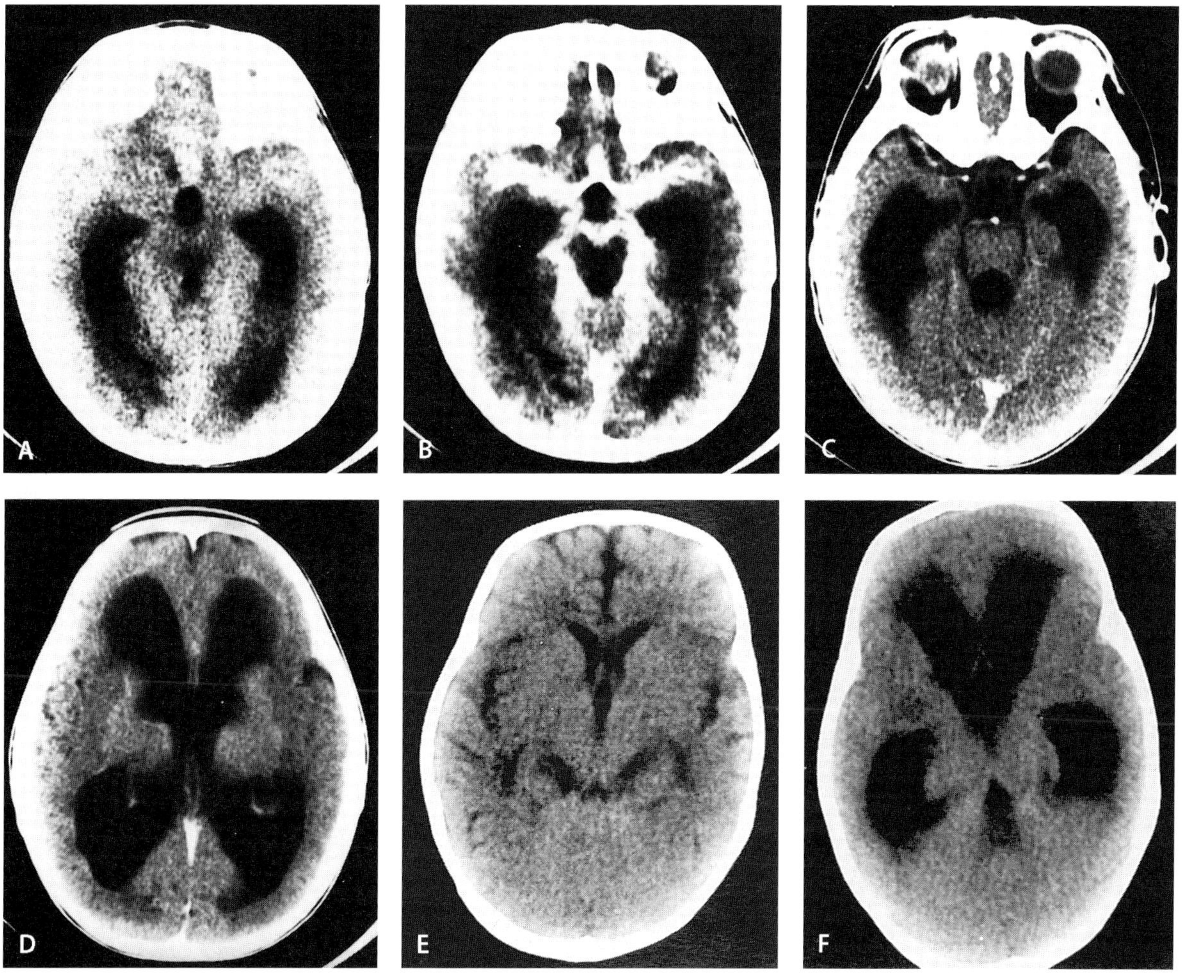

Fig. 5.99 A–F. Ventricular dilatation is common with tuberculous meningitis, but is not always permanent. **A** A 14-month-old boy from the Pacific Islands with tuberculous meningitis and positive CSF culture for *M. tuberculosis*; a nonenhanced CT shows ventricular enlargement. **B** With contrast there is enhancement of the basilar cisterns and sylvian fissures. **C** A 23-month-old girl, also from the Pacific Islands, was treated successfully for tuberculous meningitis when she was 6 months old. The enhanced CT scan shows persistent ventricular enlargement, but there is no enhancement of the basal cisterns. **D** The lateral, third and fourth ventricles, also enlarged, showing that there is communicating hydrocephalus. **E** This is the admission CT scan of another child with active tuberculous meningitis, already on treatment. **F** A repeat scan of the same child 1 month later. Another scan after 3 months did not show any significant change. (**E, F** from Cremin and Jamieson 1995)

These are the "puffy tumours" described by Sir Percival Pott. The soft tissue swelling can be quite significant. They can be imaged with ultrasonography, CT, or MRI. It is important to distinguish them from histiocytosis or a low-grade pyogenic infection. These and other tuberculous lesions within the bones of the skull have been described on pp. 505, 515.

(Text continues on p. 524)

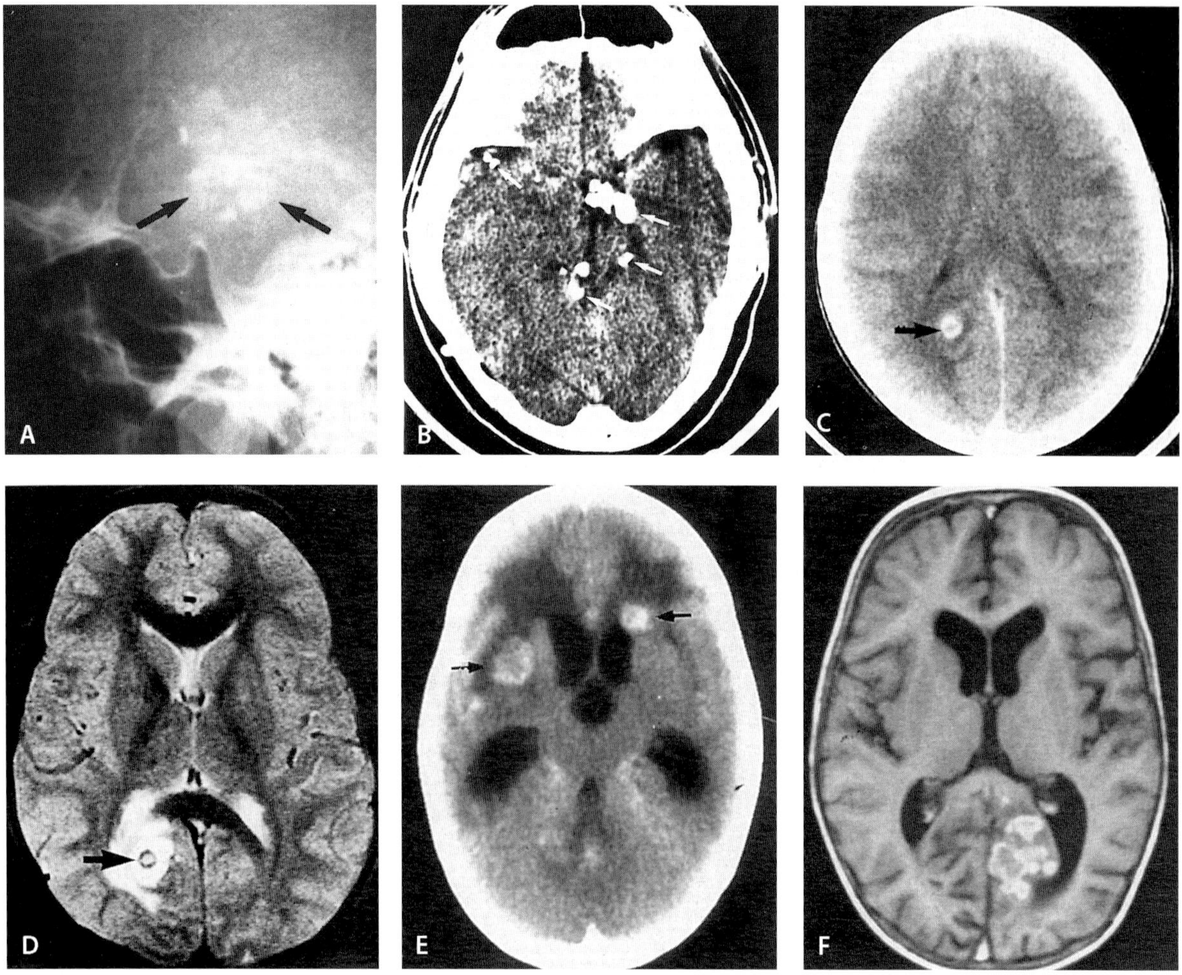

Fig. 5.100 A–F. Tuberculous granulomas. **A** The lateral radiograph of the skull of a 35-year-old man from the Pacific Islands who had tuberculous meningitis when he was 19 year old. There is a group of calcified granulomas (*arrows*) which are better seen on the nonenhanced CT (**B**: *arrows*). There are more than would be expected from the plain radiograph. **C** The contrast-enhanced CT scan of another child from South Africa showing that the granuloma has a hypodense center and surrounding edema (*arrow*). **D** T2-weighted MR scan of the same patient shows that the caseous necrotic center is T2 hyperintense, the rim of the granuloma is hypointense (*arrow*), and the edema is T2 hyperintense. **E** Several granulomas (*arrows*) are shown on a contrast-enhanced CT of another patient. There is also basal enhancement and hydrocephalus. **F** A gadolinium-enhanced T1-weighted MR scan of another patient shows a cluster of granulomas in the left occipital lobe. (**A, B** courtesy of Dr. Cheryl Sisler, Hawaii; **C–F** from Cremin and Jamieson 1995)

Fig. 5.102 A–C. Tuberculous abscesses do not image in the same way as tuberculomas. **A** A contrast-enhanced CT scan shows rim enhancement with a hypodense center. There is also a group of enhancing granulomas posterior to the abscess. **B** A T2-weighted MR scan without enhancement shows that the abscess has a hypointense rim and a hyperintense center. **C** A T1-weighted MR scan of the same patient, with gadolinium enhancement, shows that the center of the abscess is hypointense and the wall of the abscess enhances. (From Cremin and Jamieson)

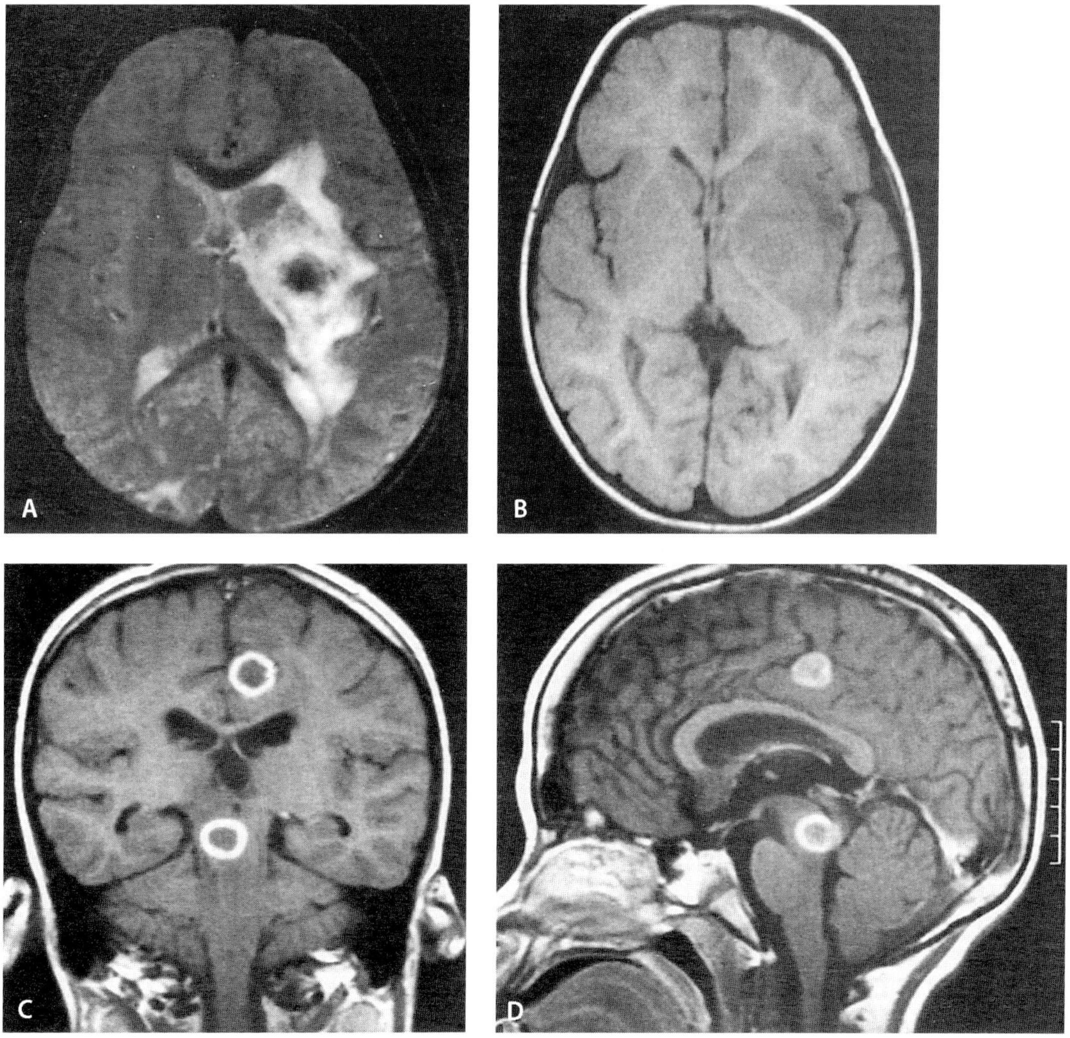

Fig. 5.101 A–D. Some tuberculomas have been described as "gummatous" and become quite large. **A** T2-weighted MR scan of a large tuberculoma. There is hyperintense edema surrounding a predominantly hypointense granuloma. **B** On a T1-weighted MR scan, the tuberculoma is isointense. **C, D** Gadolinium-enhanced MR scans of another patient show that the central necrosis is hypointense but there is strong rim enhancement. Both tuberculomas imaged in the same way. (From Cremin and Jamieson 1995)

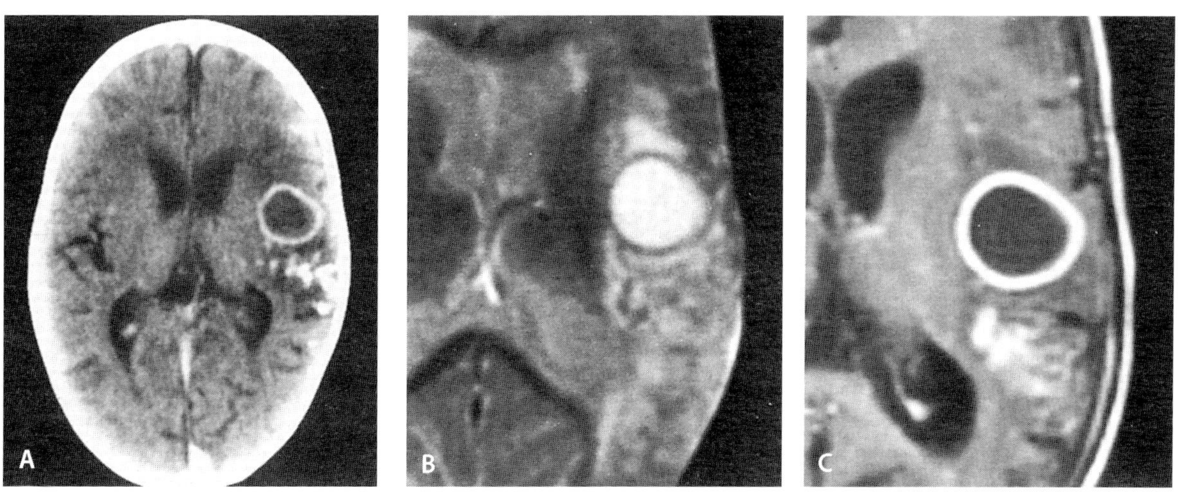

Tuberculosis Involving Other Sites

Tuberculous Lymphadenopathy

Abdominal tuberculosis (see p. 459)

Tuberculous lymphadenitis (scrofula) is by no means rare in many parts of the tropics; one study in Uganda showed that 41% of all enlarged cervical nodes were tuberculous. While tuberculosis is the most common cause of lymphadenopathy under the age of 30 years (unless the patient has Burkitt's lymphoma) there will also be a significant number of elderly patients in whom cervical lymphadenopathy is tuberculous in origin. Ultrasonography can accurately demonstrate the lymphadenopathy (as can CT or MRI), but cannot establish the etiology. Most lymph nodes will appear as hypoechoic masses with a regular outline; often multiple enlarged nodes are present. Ultrasonography is most useful for the accurate follow-up of resolution during treatment. During the acute stage there are no changes of radiological significance; when the infection has healed, calcification frequently follows. Calcified lymph nodes may be seen not only in the neck, but in the axilla, around the shoulder, in the inguinal region, in the popliteal fossa, and elsewhere (Fig. 5.103). All must be differentiated from other causes of soft tissue calcification, e.g., parasites, or, in the limbs, from tumoral calcinosis. This is usually possible because calcified tuberculous granulomas are irregular in size and shape but, more importantly, their anatomical situation may suggest the diagnosis.

Calcified tuberculomas may be seen in the liver and spleen, but have little clinical and no radiological significance (see p. 461). A tuberculous granuloma can calcify anywhere and only histological examination will differentiate its nature. Even this may be difficult because of the fibrosis.

Tuberculosis of the Breast

Although not common anywhere, tuberculosis of the breast is not rare in the tropics and significant series have been reported. The most common presentation is a mass in the breast of a 30- to 40-year-old woman. It is usually painful, but if there is a sinus tract leading from the "mass" (which is the tuberculous breast abscess) to the skin (Fig. 5.104), the surface ulceration is often painless unless secondarily infected. Many tuberculous breast lesions are quite chronic and have been felt by the patient for some months; a few may be more acute, with a history of only a few days, and such rapid onset occurs particularly in the lactating breast. The clinical diagnosis is usually of a carcinoma or, in the more acute cases, a pyogenic breast abscess.

Mammography shows the palpable mass as a diffuse density, which, when there is fluid, may change in shape and density on the two standard mammographic projections. There may be one or more sinus tracts connecting the mass to the thickened, overlying skin. In some patients the skin bulges (Fig. 5.104 C), probably at the stage before the sinus tract has formed. The underlying breast stroma is coarse, and may be reticulated. There is almost always nipple retraction. The breast size is often reduced. Ultrasonography can be used to confirm the fluid, but does not give much further information.

In some patients there will be minimal regional lymphadenopathy, but in others the lymph nodes are normal. The usual mammographic diagnosis is "chronic breast inflammation or breast abscess," but many of the masses will suggest malignancy. Recognition of the sinus tract and the skin thickening should suggest tuberculosis, particularly when there is little surface pain clinically. Unfortunately, many sinus tracts become secondarily infected and there is then a pyogenic breast abscess: only histology will show the underlying tuberculosis. (The differential diagnosis, apart from malignancy and pyogenic abscess, will include, in the painless lesion, syphilis, mycotic infections, and parasites such as guinea worm.)

Tuberculosis of the Parotid Gland

Tuberculosis of the parotid gland is uncommon, but can be the presenting symptom of tuberculosis. There may be associated tuberculous cervical lymph nodes, but in the majority of patients there is no systemic symptom of tuberculosis and the chest radiographs are normal. Clinically, parotid tuberculosis resembles a tumor, and biopsy to establish the diagnosis is usually necessary. However, CT scanning may show characteristic thick-walled, smooth, round, rim-enhancing lesions, usually with central lucency. The clinical mass will be shown on scanning to be multiloculated; the thick enhancing rim surrounding the low-density central tissue is often corrugated and irregular. If the enhanced rim is thin, biopsy becomes essential. Contrast sialography does not add significant information and may be contraindicated because in some cases it has exacerbated the inflammatory reaction.

There may be similar lesions in the lymph nodes, and there may be lymph node tissue within the parotid glands.

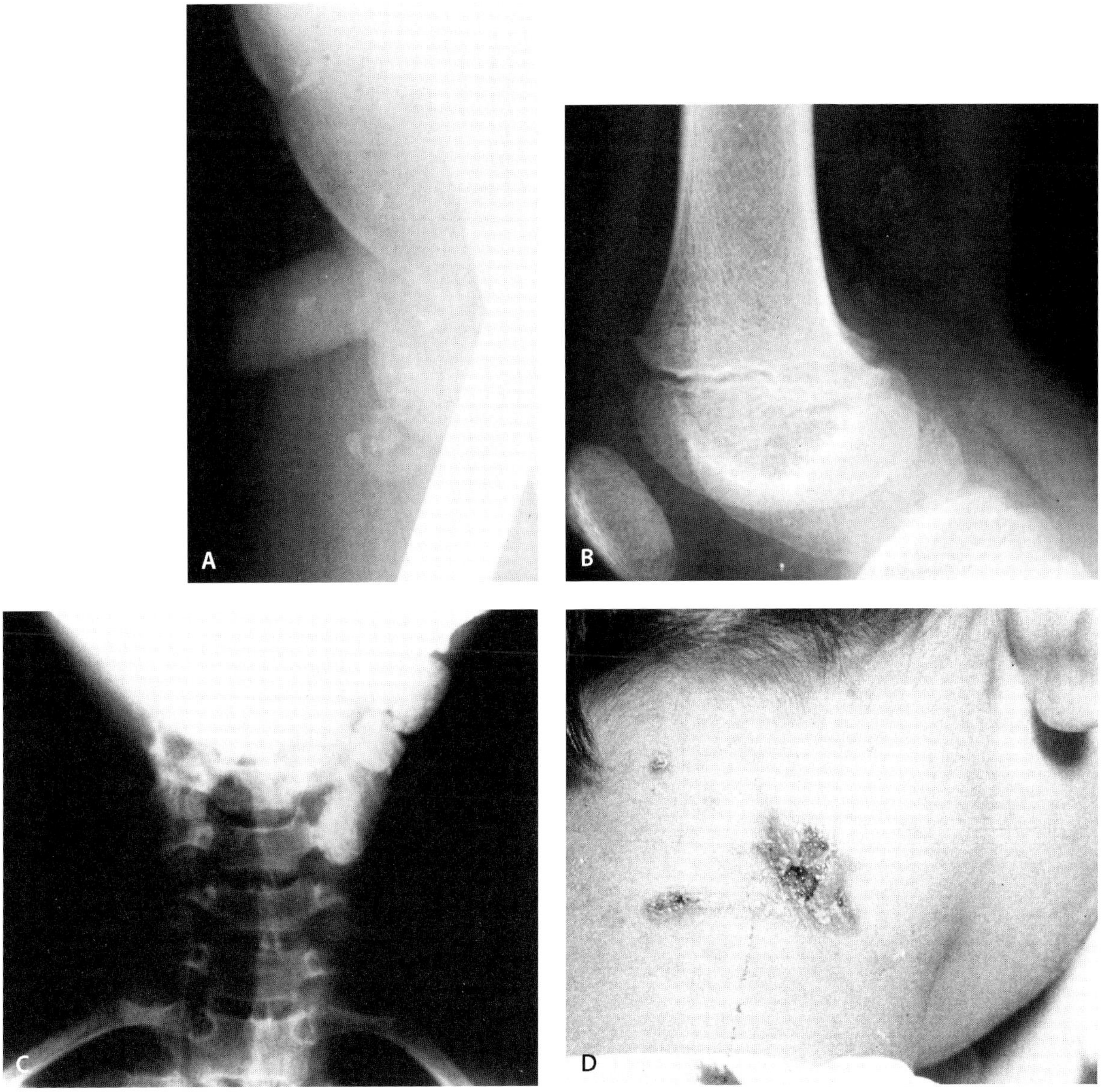

Fig. 5.103 A–D. Calcification in tuberculous lymphadenitis is not difficult to recognize in the chest or abdomen, but may occur unexpectedly wherever there are lymph nodes. **A** Calcified lymph nodes in the groin of a child and **B** in another patient, behind the knee. These small calcifications must be differentiated from parasites and early tumoral calcinosis. There is seldom a clinical history of significance. **C** Heavily calcified lymph nodes in the neck of a child from the Pacific Islands with a discharging sinus (**D**). This is the scrofula well known for centuries and in this child was, in fact, caused by *M. scrofulaceum*

Ocular Tuberculosis

Ocular tuberculosis is rare and usually associated with pulmonary or skeletal infection. Scleral tuberculosis has been reported but has no imaging significance.

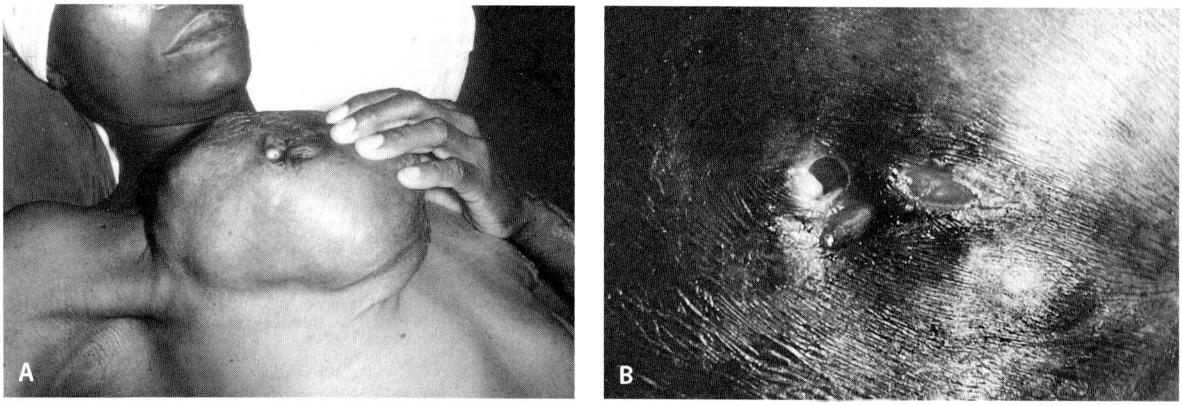

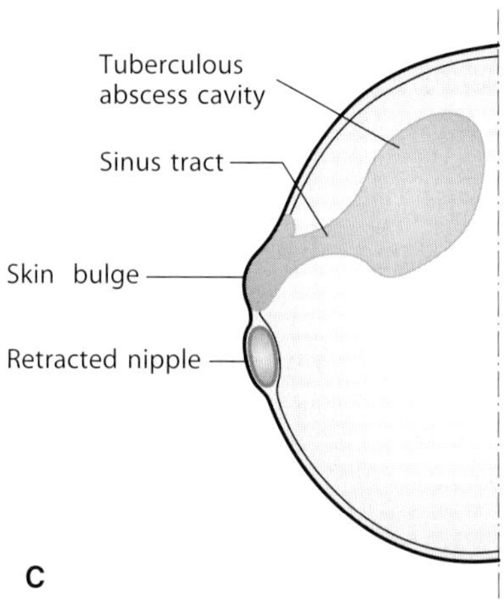

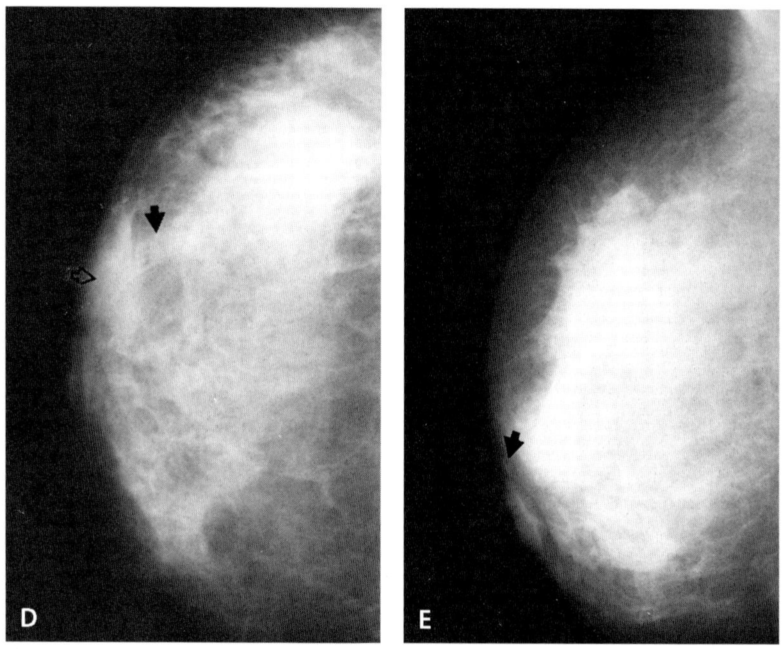

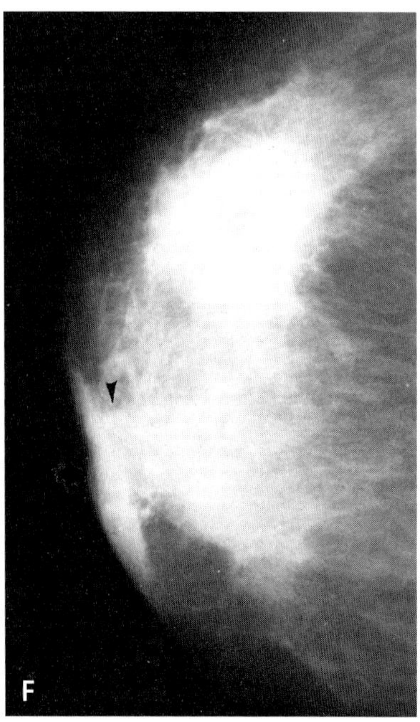

Fig. 5.104 A–F. Tuberculosis of the breast. It can be very difficult clinically to distinguish between a breast abscess, tumor, and tuberculosis. If there is a discharging sinus, tuberculosis is more likely. **A** A large lobulated mass in the right side of the breast of this African patient was firm and painless. The sinus (**B**) was flat with little surrounding reaction. The ulcer had been present for some months and was initially painless, but is now probably secondarily infected. **C** The sinus tract between the tuberculous abscess and the skin shows clinically as a bulge in the skin, often close to the nipple. This is an important feature of the mammograms. **D** Craniocaudal mammogram of the left breast shows an ill-defined density in the upper outer quadrant connected by the dense linear tract (*solid arrow*) to localized skin thickening (*open arrow*) and a bulge above it (*arrow head*). **E** An oblique mediolateral mammogram showing the skin thickening and the change in the outline of the breast mass. **F** The craniocaudal mammogram of a different patient with a smaller breast but showing a similar change in outline and the dense masses. The sinus tract is clearly seen (*arrowhead*) and there is localized skin thickening close to the nipple (*arrow*). Ultrasonography can also be used to show a fluid collection and sometimes the sinus tract also. (**C–F** courtesy of Dr. D. Makanjuola and *Clin Radiol*, 1996)

Bibliography

Abdelwhab IF, et al: Atypical skeletal tuberculosis mimicking neoplasm. *Br J Radiol* 64:551–555, 1991

Abrams IS, Holden WD: Tuberculosis of the gastrointestinal tract. *Arch Surg* 89:282–288, 1964

Adams WM, Fitzgerald R: Abdominal tuberculosis: unusual findings on CT. *Clin Radiol* 50:734–735, 1995

Aderle WI: Radiological patterns of pulmonary tuberculosis in Nigerian children. *Tuberculosis* 61:157–163, 1980

Ahmed FB, et al: Tuberculous enteritis. *BMJ* 313:215–217, 1996

Aldossary J, Grant CS: Abdominal tuberculosis: a frequent diagnostic challenge. *Ann Trop Med Parasitol* 79:163–167, 1985

Allen CM, Craze J, Grundy A: case report: tuberculous broncho-oesophageal fistula in the acquired immuno-deficiency syndrome. *Clin Radiol* 43:60–62, 1991

Anderson DH, et al: Pulmonary lesions due to opportunistic myobacteria. *Clin Radiol* 26:461–471, 1975

Anscombe AR, Keddie NC, Schofield PF: Caecal tuberculosis. *Gut* 8:337–341, 1967

Apps MCP, Harrison NK, Blanth EIA: Tuberculosis of the breast. *BMJ* 288:1874–1875, 1984

Aston NO, DeCosta AM: Tuberculous perforation of the small bowel. *Postgrad Med J* 61:251–252, 1985

Avery GR, Chippendale AJ: Case of the month: a single diagnosis. that is the question. *Br J Radiol* 68:665–666, 1995

Bahdur P, et al: Tuberculosis of the mammary gland. *J Indian Med Assoc* 80:8–12, 1983

Bailey IC: The Pattern and presentation of cerebral tumours in Uganda. *East Afr Med J* 48:565–575, 1971

Baker RD: Endocardial tuberculosis. *Arch Pathol* 19:611–635, 1935

Ball PAJ: Abdominal tuberculosis. In: Davey WW (ed) *Companion to surgery in Africa*. E & S Livingstone, Edinburgh, 1968, pp 267–270

Balthazar EJ, Gordon R, Mulnick D: Ileocecal tuberculosis: CT and radiologic evaluation. *Am J Roentgenol* 154:499–503, 1990

Bankier AA, et al: Update: abdominal tuberculosis. Unusual findings on CT. *Clin Radiol* 50:223–228, 1995

Barnes P, et al: An unusual case of tuberculous peritonitis in a man with AIDS. *West J Med* 144:467–469, 1986

Barson AJ, Kirk RS: Colonic tuberculosis with carcinoma. *J Pathol Bacteriol* 101:289–292, 1970

Bastani B, et al: Tuberculous peritonitis. Report of 30 cases and review of the literature. *Q J Med* 56:549–557, 1985

Bateson EM, Woo-Ming M: Destroyed lung: a report of cases in West Indians and Australian aborigines. *Clin Radiol* 27:223–226, 1976

Bell GM, de Klerk JN: Tuberculose van die penis (corpora cavernosa). *S Afr Med J* 50:1489–1490, 1976

Belli L: Studio ecografico dei versamenti tuberculori. *Radiol Med (Torino)* 83:659–661, 1992

Betoulieres P: The lymphangiographic appearances of lymph node tuberculosis. *J Radiol Elec* 49:1–5, 1968

Bevans M, Wilkins SA: Tuberculous endocarditis. *Am Med J* 24:843–849, 1942

Bhansali SK: Abdominal tuberculosis. Experiences with 300 cases. *Am J Gastroenterol* 67:324–337, 1977

Bhargave S, et al: Case report: tuberculosis of the parotid gland – diagnosis by CT. *Br J Radiol* 69:1181–1183, 1996

Black GA, Carsky EW: Duodenal tuberculosis: *AJR* 131:329–330, 1978

Bohrer SP: Tuberculous synovitis with widening of the intercondylar notch of the distal femur. *Br J Radiol* 42:703–704, 1969

Bolton JM, Snelling MR: Review of tuberculosis among the Orang Asli (Aborigines) in West Malaysia. *Med J Malaysia* 30:10–29, 1975

Brauner M, et al: Sonography and computed tomography of macroscopic tuberculosis of the liver. *J Clin Ultrasound* 17:563–568, 1989

Brenner SM, Annes G, Parker JG: Tuberculous colitis simulating nonspecific granulomatous disease of the colon. *Am J Dig Dis* 15:85, 1970

Brody JM, et al: Gastric tuberculosis: a manifestation of the acquired immuno-deficiency syndrome. *Radiology* 159: 347–348, 1986

Brombart M, Massion J: Radiological differences between ileocecal tuberculosis and Crohn's disease. *Am J Dig Dis* 6:589–603, 1961

Burack WR, Hollister RM: Tuberculous peritonitis: a study of forty-seven proved cases encountered by a general medical unit in twenty-five years. *Am J Med* 28:510–521, 1960

Burke GJ, Zafar SA: Problems in distinguishing tuberculosis of bowel from Crohn's disease in Asians. *BMJ* 4:395–397, 1975

Calder JF, Norredam K: Chylous ascites due to tuberculosis. *East Afr Med J* 49:684–686, 1972

Camiel MR: Ileocecal tuberculosis. *Radiology* 44:344–351, 1945

Carazo-Martinez O, et al: Realtime ultrasound evaluation of tubercular pleural effusions. *J Clin Ultrasound* 17:407–410, 1989

Cardocio SA, Locker GY: Elevated serum CA 125 secondary to tuberculous peritonitis. *Cancer* 72:2016–2018, 1993

Cardozo LJ, et al: Tuberculous meningitis in adult Africans; problems of diagnosis and management. *East Afr Med J* 53:136–142, 1976

Carroll SR, Newsom SWB, Jenner JR: Treatment of septic arthritis due to *Mycobacterium kansasii*. *BMJ* 289:591–592, 1984

Casselman ES, et al: CT of meningitis in infants and children. *J Comput Assist Tomogr* 4:211–216, 1980

Chan HS, Pang J: Isolated giant tuberculomata of the liver detected by computed tomography. *GI Radiol* 14:305–307, 1989

Chandracharoensin C, Viranuvalti V: Tuberculous abscess of the retrosternal thyroid gland. *Diagn Imaging (Netherlands)* 50:29–31, 1981

Charatan FB: Quoted in the Proceedings of the National Academy of Science (March, 1994). "Peruvian mummy shows that TB preceded Columbus." *BMJ* 308:808, 1994

Chatfield WR, et al: The investigation and management of infertility in East Africa (a study of 200 cases). *East Afr Med J* 47:212–216, 1970

Chatterji DN: Tuberculosis in children (pattern of intrathoracic lesions in hospitalised patient). *J Indian Med Assoc* 67:217–223, 1976

Chanuhry UR, Ghani MU: Diagnosis of tuberculous basal meningitis by CT scan and transcranial Doppler (TCD) studies. Proc. 19th Int. Cong. Radiol., PP 1.2 Beijing, 1996

Chazan BI, Aichison JD: Gastric tuberculosis. BMJ 2:1288–1290, 1960

Choe KO, Jeon P: Reexpansibility of the lung after decortication in tuberculous empyema. Proc. 19th Int. Cong. Radiol, SS 3.16. Beijing, 1996

Citron KM: BCQ – vaccination against tuberculosis: international perspectives. *BMJ* 306:222–223, 1993

Clark RA, et al: Hematogenous dissemination of *Mycobacterium tuberculosis* in patients with AIDS. *Rev Infect Dis* 13:1089–1092, 1991

Cohen C: Tuberculous mastitis: *S Afr Med J* 52:12–16, 1977

Collins CM, Yates MD, Grange JM: Names for mycobacteria. *BMJ* 288:463–464, 1984

Compere EL, Garrison M: The correlation of pathologic and roentgenologic findings in tuberculous and pyogenic infection of the vertebrae. The fate of the intervertebral disc. *Ann Surg* 104:1038–1067, 1936

Cook SM, Frank TS: Detection and characterization of atypical mycobacteria by the polymerase chain reaction. *Mod Pathol* 6:104 A, 1993

Cope AP, Heber M, Wilkins EGL: Valvular tuberculous endocarditis: a case report and review of the literature. *J Infect* 21:293–296, 1990

Corr P: MRI of tuberculous spondylitis. *Imaging S Afr Mag* 17–20, 1990

Corr P, Handler L, Davey H: Pott's paraplegia and tuberculous spondylitis. Evaluation by magnetic resonance. *Neuroradiology* 33 (Suppl):109–110, 1991

Cremin BJ: Radiological imaging of urogenital tuberculosis in children, with emphasis on ultrasound. *Pediatr Radiol* 17:34–38, 1987

Cremin BJ: CT in tuberculous spondylitis. *Clin Radiol* 49:433–435, 1994

Cremin BJ, Jamieson DM, Hoffman EB: CT and MRI in the management of advanced spinal tuberculosis. *Pediatr Radiol* 23:298–300, 1993

Cremin BJ, Jamieson DM: *Childhood tuberculosis*. Springer, Berlin Heidelberg New York, 1995

Cremin BJ, Levinsohn MW: Multiple bone tuberculosis in the young. *Br J Radiol* 43:638–645, 1970

Dahlene DH, et al: Abdominal tuberculosis: CT findings. *J Comput Assist Tomogr* 8:443–445, 1984

Damrongsak C, et al: Functional hepatogram and coeliac arteriogram in tuberculosis of the liver. *J Med Assoc Thai* 60:285–288, 1977

Danziger J, et al: Cranial and intracranial tuberculosis. *S Afr Med J* 50:1403–1405, 1976

DaRoche-Afodu JT: Tuberculous thyroiditis. *West Afr Med J* 23:159–161, 1975

Das MK, Indudhara R, Vaidyanalthan S: Sonographic features of genitourinary tuberculosis. *Am J Roentgenol* 158:327–329, 1991

Dastur HM, Shah MD: Intramedullary tuberculoma of the spinal cord. *Indian Pediatr* 5:468–471, 1968

Davey WW: Tuberculous pericarditis. In: Davey WW (ed) Companion to surgery in Africa. E & S Livingstone, Edinburgh, 1968, pp 310–312

De Labarthe B, et al: Acute, lethal miliary tuberculosis due to *Mycobacterium bovis. Poumon Coeur* 34:139–142, 1978

Denath FM: Abdominal tuberculosis in children. CT findings. *Gastrointest Radiol* 15:303–306, 1990

Dent DM, Webber BL: Tuberculosis of the breast. *S Afr Med J* 51:611–614, 1977

Denton T, Hossain J: A radiological study of abdominal tuberculosis in a Saudi population. *Clin Radiol* 47:409–414, 1993

Dineen P, Homan WP, Grafe WR: Tuberculous peritonitis: 43 years of experience in diagnosis and treatment. *Ann Surg* 184:717–722, 1976

Dixon JM: Breast diseases. *Br Med J* 309:947–949, 1994

Dong-Ho-Lee, et al: Sonographic findings of intestinal tuberculosis. *J Ultrasound Med* 12:537–540, 1993

Dorff GJ, et al: Musculoskeletal infections due to *Mycobacterium kansasii. Clin Orthop* 136:244–246, 1978

Downey DB, Nakielny RA: Aphthoid ulcers in colonic tuberculosis. *Br J Radiol* 58:561–562, 1985

Doy RW: Tuberculosis presenting as an acute surgical emergency. *Cent Afr J Med* 18:91–93, 1972

Ehlers MRW: The biology of *mycobacterium tuberculosis* and the host-pathogen relationship. In: Cremin BJ, Jamieson DM (eds) Childhood tuberculosis. Springer, London Berlin Heidelberg New York, 1995, pp 7–17

El Masri SH, et al: Abdominal tuberculosis in Sudanese patients. *East Afr Med J* 54:319–326, 1977

Er-hu J, et al: CT diagnosis of tracheobronchial tuberculosis. Proc. 19th Int. Cong. Radiol. 33. 3.15. Beijing, 1996

Fisher D, Hiller N: Case report: giant tuberculous cystic lymphangioma of posterior mediastinum, retroperitoneum and groin. *Clin Radiol* 49:215–216, 1994

Foster DR: Miliary tuberculosis following intravesical BCG treatment (letter). *Br J Radiol* 70:429–431, 1997

Fowler WC: A preliminary report on the treatment of tuberculosis with turtle vaccine. *Tubercle* 12:12–17, 1930

Fox E: Tuberculosis. In: Strickland GT (ed) Hunter's tropical medicine, 7th edn. Saunders, Philadelphia, 1991, pp 458–483

Gaines W, Steinbach HL, Lowenhaupt E: Tuberculosis of the stomach. Radiology 58:808, 1952

Ganguli PK: *The radiology of bone and joint tuberculosis with special reference to tropical countries.* Asia Publishing House, London, 1963

Garber EK, Bluestone R: Tuberculous arthritis of the knee with a cold abscess communicating with the knee joint. *Skeletal Radiol* 6:76, 1981

Gawne-Cain ML, Hansell DUR: The pattern and distribution of calcified mediastinal lymph nodes in sarcoidosis and tuberculosis: a CT study. *Clin Radiol* 51:263–267, 1996

Gerritsen J, Knol K: Hypercalcaemia in a child with miliary tuberculosis. *Eur J Pediatr* 148:650–651, 1989

Gershon-Cohen J, Kremens V: X-ray studies of the ileocecal valve in ileocecal tuberculosis. *Radiology* 62:251–254, 1954

Gilinsky NH, et al: Abdominal tuberculosis: a 10 year review. *S Afr Med J* 64:849–857, 1983

Godfrey-Fausset P, et al: Evidence of transmission of tuberculosis by SNA finger printing. *Br Med J* 305:221–223, 1992

Goldblatt M, Cremin BJ: Osteo-articular tuberculosis: its prevention in coloured races. *Clin Radiol* 29:669–677, 1978

Granet E: Intestinal tuberculosis: a clinical, roentgenological and pathological study of 2086 patients affected with pulmonary tuberculosis. *Am J Dig Dis* 2:209, 1935

Grassi R, et al: Case report: massive enterolithiasis associated with ileal dysgenesis. *Br J Radiol* 70:207–209, 1997

Graybill JR, Geiger J: Naturally acquired tuberculin hypersensitivity in Ethiopia. *East Afr Med J* 49:597–603, 1972

Greenberg SD, et al: Active pulmonary tuberculosis in patients with AIDS: spectrum of radiographic findings (including a normal appearance). *Radiology* 193:115–119, 1994

Gulati P, et al: Impact of MRI in the management of spinal tuberculosis. Proc. 18th Int. Congr. Radiol. Singapore, S410.186, 1994

Gupta RK, et al: MR Imaging of intracranial tuberculomas. *J Comput Assist Tomogr* 12:280–285, 1988

Halleran WJ, Martin NL: Non-tuberculous mycobacterial arthritis. Kans Med Soc J 83:284–286, 1982

Hancock SM: Hyperplastic tuberculosis of the distal colon. *Br J Surg* 46:63–68, 1958

Hanson J: CT of tuberculous peritonitis. *Am J Roentgenol* 144:931–933, 1985

Hayashi H, et al: Case report: tuberculous pericarditis. *Br J Radiol* 71:680–682, 1998

Herlinger H: Angiography in the diagnosis of ileocecal tuberculosis. *Gastrointest Radiol* 2:371–376, 1978

Hermon-Taylor J, et al: *Mycobacterium paratuberculosis* cervical lymphadenitis, followed five years later by terminal ileitis similar to Crohn's disease. *Br Med J* 316:449–453, 1998

Hersch C: Tuberculosis of the liver: a study of 200 cases. *S Afr Med J* 38:857–863, 1964

Hodgson G, et al: the x-ray appearances of tuberculosis of the spine. The intervertebral disc. Charles C. Thomas, Springfield, Ill. 1969, pp 34–40

Hoffman EG, Crosier JH, Cremin BJ: Imaging in children with spinal tuberculosis. *J Bone Jt Surg [Br]* 75:233–239, 1993

Hollins FR: Tuberculosis in the African community in the city of Salisbury (Rhodesia). *Cent Afr J Med* 22:25–28, 1976

Hoon JR, Dockerty MG, Pemberton JdeJ: Collective review: ileocecal tuberculosis including comparison of this disease with nonspecific regional enterocolitis and noncaseous tuberculous enterocolitis. *Int Abstr Surg* 91:417, 1950

Hossain J, Kiniroms M, Lewis RR: Laparoscopy does have a role in tuberculous peritonitis (letter). *Br Med J* 313:1145–1146, 1996

Hsu LCS, Leong JCY: Tuberculosis of the lower cervical spine (C2 to C7) – a report of 40 cases. *J Bone Jt Surg [Br]* 66:1–5, 1984

Hughes HJ, Carr DT, Geraci JE: Tuberculous peritonitis: a review of 34 cases with emphasis on the diagnostic aspects. *Dis Chest* 38:42–50, 1960

Hulnick DH, et al: Abdominal tuberculosis: CT evaluation. *Radiology* 157:199–204, 1985

Jain R, et al: Sonographic diagnosis of early abdominal tuberculosis. Proc. 18th Int. Congr. Radiology. Singapore, S 213.184. 1994

Jain SK, et al: A clinico-radiological study of secondary mycoses in pulmonary tuberculosis. *Indian J Med Sci* 45:81–84, 1991

Jain VK, et al: The far cry of a TB brain. Report of a case of tuberculous meningitis, multiple tuberculomas and tubercular abscess. *Clin Neurol Neurosurg* 91:171–176, 1989

Jamieson DH, Cremin BJ: High resolution CT of the lungs in acute disseminated tuberculosis, and a pediatric radiology perspective of the term miliary. *Pediatr Radiol* 23:380–383, 1993

Jena A, et al: Demonstration of intramedullary tuberculomas by magnetic resonance imaging: a report of 2 cases. *Br J Radiol* 64:555–557, 1991

Jinkins JR: Computed tomography of intracranial tuberculosis. *Neuroradiology* 33:126–153, 1991

Kapoor R, et al: Ultrasound detection of tuberculomas of the spleen. *Clin Radiol* 43:128–129, 1991

Kawamori Y, et al: Macronodular tuberculoma of the liver: CT and MR findings. *Am J Rad* 158:311–313, 1992

Kedar RP, et al: Sonographic findings in gastrointestinal and peritoneal tuberculosis. *Clin Radiol* 49:24–29, 1994

Kent PW: The pattern of tuberculosis in East Africa. *East Afr Med J* 48:450–455, 1971

Kipps A, et al: Negative tuberculin tests. *S Afr Med J* 40:108–114, 1966

Klimach OE, Ormerod LP: Gastrointestinal tuberculosis: a retrospective review of 109 cases in a district general hospital. *Q J Med* 56:569–578, 1988

Kolawale TM, Lewis EA: Radiologic study of tuberculosis of the abdomen. *Am J Roentgenol* 123:348–358, 1975

Konstam PG, Bleskovsky A: The ambulant treatment of spinal tuberculosis. *Br J Surg* 50:26–38, 1962

Kool HES: HIV seropositively and tuberculosis in a large general hospital in Malawi. *Trop Geogr Med* 42:128–132, 1990

Kulholma P, et al: Tuberculous peritonitis simulating peritoneal carcinomatosis. *Acta Obstet Gynaecol Scand* 61:491–494, 1982

Kurpiewska-Radzimska D, Makuchowa K: Multifocal pseudocystic bone tuberculosis in children. *Chir Narzadow Ruchu Ortop Pol* 42:293–298, 1977

Lachman E, Moodley J, Pitsoes B: Peritoneal tuberculosis imitating ovarian carcinoma. "Special category". *Acta Obstet Gynecol Scand* 64:677–679, 1985

Lagundoye SB, Singh SP: Tuberculosis of the mastoid masquerading as a glomus jugulare tumour: a case report. *Niger Med J* 8:161–163, 1978

Lawn SD, et al: Pulmonary tuberculosis: radiological features in West Africans co-infected with HIV. *Br J Radiol* 72:339–344, 1999

Le CT, Yoiung LW: Radiological case of the month. Non-tuberculous mycobacterial infection. *Am J Dis Child* 139:608–608, 1985

Leader M, Revell P, Clark G: Synovial infection with *M. kansasii. Am Rheum Dis* 43:80–82, 1984

Lee KS, et al: The evaluation of tracheo-bronchial disease with helical CT, with multiplanar and three dimensional reconstruction: correlation with bronchoscopy. *Radiographics* 17:555–567, 1997

Lennard-Jones JE: Clues to the elucidation of Crohn's disease. *Trans Coll Med S Afr* 40:34–41, 1996

Lesar MS, et al: Pericardial tuberculoma. *Radiology* 136:309–310, 1981

Lester FT, Tsega E: Tuberculous peritonitis in Ethiopian patients. *Trop Geogr Med* 28:169–174, 1976

Levine C: Primary macro-nodular hepatic tuberculosis. US and CT appearances. *Gastrointest Radiol* 15:307–309, 1990

Levine R, et al: Tuberculous abscess of the pancreas. Case report and review of the literature. *Am J Dig Dis* 377:1141–1144, 1992

Lewis EA, Kolawole TM: Tuberculous ileocolitis in Ibadan: a clinico-radiological review. *Gut* 13:644–653, 1972

Lobo PI: The first reported case of sarcoidosis in an East African. *East Afr Med J* 49:45–48, 1972

Locke EA: Secondary hypertrophic osteoarthropathy and it's relation to simple club fingers. *Arch Intern Med* 15:659–713, 1915

Ly HM, et al: Skin test responsiveness to a series of new tuberculins of children living in three Vietnamese cities. *Tubercle* 70:27–36, 1989

Mahendra KK, et al: Lymphangiography in the tubercular abdomen. *Indian J Radiol* 26:287–289, 1972

Makanjuola D, et al: Mammographic features of breast tuberculosis: the skin bulge and sinus tract sign. *Clin Radiol* 51:354–358, 1996

Makanjuola D, et al: Radiological evaluation of complications of intestinal tuberculosis. *Eur J Radiol* 26:261–268, 1998

Malone JL, et al: Intracranial tuberculoma developing during therapy for tuberculous meningitis. *West J Med* 152:188–190, 1990

Manni JJ: Tuberculous laryngitis. *Trop Geogr Med* 34:109–112, 1982.l

Marsot-Dupuch K, et al: Tuberculosis of the ear; contribution of radiology. *Ann Radiol (Paris)* 26:473–476, 1983

McDonal Jb, Middleton PJ: Tuberculosis of the colon simulating carcinoma. *Radiology* 118:293, 1976

Medical Research Council (UK): Controlled trial of short course regimens of chemotherapy in the circulatory treatment of spinal tuberculosis. *J Bone Jt Surg [Br]* 75:240–248, 1993

Mehta JB: Abdominal tuberculosis mimicking neoplasia on computerized tomography. *South Med J* 78:1385–1386, 1985

Menzies IM, Fitzgerald JM, Mulpeter K: Laparoscopic diagnosis of ascites in Lesotho. *Br Med J* 291:473–475, 1985

Metcalf C: A history of tuberculosis. In: Cooradia HM, Benctar SR (eds) *A century of tuberculosis.* Oxford University Press, Cape Town, 1991, pp 1–31

Miles MM, Shaw RJ: The effect of inadvertent intradermal administration of high dose percutaneous BCG vaccine. *Br Med J* 312:1205, 1996

Milika-Cabanne N, et al: Radiographic abnormalities in tuberculosis and risk of co-existing human immuno-deficiency virus infection. Methods and preliminary results from Bujumbura, Burundi. *Am J Resp Crit Care Med* 152: 794–799, 1995

Milika-Cabanne N, et al: Radiographic abnormalities in tuberculosis and risk of co-existing human immuno-deficiency virus infection. Results from Dar es Salamm. Tanzania. *Am J Resp Crit Care Med* 152:786–793, 1995

Miller WT. Spectrum of pulmonary non-tuberculous mycobacterial infection. *Radiology* 191:343–350, 1994

Mitchell RS, Bristol LJ: Intestinal tuberculosis: an analysis of 346 cases diagnosed by routine intestinal radiography on 5529 admissions for pulmonary tuberculosis, 1924–1949. *Am J Med Sci* 227:241–249, 1954

Moore EH: Atypical mycobacterial infections in the lung: CT appearances. *Radiology* 187:777–782, 1993

Morgan M: Breast tuberculosis. *Surg Gynecol Obstet* 52:593–603, 1931

Morse D, Brothwell DR, Ucko PJ: Tuberculosis in Ancient Egypt. *Am Rev Respir Dis* 90:525–535, 1964

Mortenson W, et al: Radiologic aspects of BCG-osteomyelitis in infants and children. *Radiology* 124:858, 1977

Moskovic E: Macronodular hepatic tuberculosis in a child: computed tomographic appearances. *Br J Radiol* 63:656–658, 1990

Naim-Ur-Rahman J: Atypical forms of spinal tuberculosis. *J Bone Joint Surg [Br]* 62:162–165, 1980

N'Dhatz M, et al: Les aspects de la radiographie thoracique chez les tubercleux infectes par le VIH en Cote d'lvoire. *Rev Pneumol Clin* 50:317–322, 1994

Obisesan AA, et al: Radiological features of tuberculosis of the spine in Ibadan, Nigeria. *Afr J Med Sci* 6:55–67, 1977

Okoro EO, Komolafe OF: Gastric tuberculosis: unusual presentations in two patients. *Clin Radiol* 54:257–259, 1999

Onuora VA: Nonthyroid neck masses in tropical Africans. *Trop Geogr Med* 39:256–259, 1987

Palmer PES: Pulmonary tuberculosis. In: Middlemiss H (ed) *Tropical Radiology.* Heinemann, London, 1961, pp 191–200

Palmer PES: Pulmonary tuberculosis-usual and unusual radiographic presentations. *Semin Roentgenol* 14:204–243, 1979

Palmer PES, Daynes G: Transkei silicosis. *S Afr Med J* 41:1182–1188, 1967

Palmer PES, Rothman WT: The incidence and pattern of chest disease in an African hospital. *Clin Radiol* 15:211–218, 1963

Paterson DE: Tuberculosis of the upper alimentary tract. In: Middlemiss H (ed) *Tropical radiology.* William Heinemann Medical Books, London, 1961, pp 223–224

Pathria MN: Septic arthritis. Proc. 18th. Int. Congr. Radiol. Singapore, 203–204, 1994

Perneger TV, et al: Does the onset of tuberculosis in AIDS predict shorter survival? Results of a cohort study in 17 European countries over 13 years. *Br Med J* 311:1468–1471, 1995

Phemister DB, Hatcher CH: Correlation of the pathological and roentgenological findings in the diagnosis of tuberculous arthritis. *Am J Roentgenol Radium Ther Nucl Med* 29:736–740, 1993

Pinto RS, Zausner J, Bernbaum ER: Gastric tuberculosis. Report of a case with discussion of angiographic findings. *Am J Roentgenol* 110:808, 1970

Pomerance A: Tuberculoma of the intraventricular septum. *Br Heart J* 25:412–414, 1963

Premkumar A, Lattimer J, Newhouse JH: CT and sonography of advanced renal tract tuberculosis. *Am J Roentgenol* 148:65–69, 1987

Primack L, et al: Pulmonary tuberculosis and *mycobacterium avium-intra cellulare*: a comparison of CT findings. *Radiology* 194:413–417, 1995

Puliyel JM, et al: Adverse local reaction from accidental BCG overdose in infants. *Br Med J* 313:528–529, 1996

Raffa H, Mosieri J. Constrictive percicarditis in Saudi Arabia. *East Afric Med J* 67:609–613, 1990

Rajshekhar V, et al: Differentiating solitary small cysticercus granulomas and tuberculomas in patients with epilepsy. Clinical and computerized tomography criteria. *J Neurosurg* 78:402–407, 1993

Ramages LJ, Gertler R: Aural tuberculosis. A series of 25 patients. *J Laryngol* 99:1073–1076, 1985

Rathakrishan V: Osteoarticular tuberculosis. A radiological study in a Malaysian hospital. *Skeletal Radiol* 18:267–272, 1989

Reed DH, Nash AF, Valabhji R: Radiological diagnosis and management of a solitary tuberculous hepatic abscess. *Br J Radiol* 63:902–904, 1990

Reede DL, Bergeron RT: Cervical tuberculosis adenitis. CT manifestations. *Radiology* 154:701–704, 1985

Reeve PA et al: Clubbing in African patients with pulmonary tuberculosis. *Thorax* 42:986–987, 1987

Richter C, et al: Clinical features of HIV seropositive and HIV seronegative patients with tuberculous pleural effusion in Dar-es-Salaam, Tanzania. *Chest* 106:1471–1475, 1994

Richter C, et al: Chest radiography and beta-2-microglobulin levels in HIV-seronegative and HIV-seropositive African patients with pulmonary tuberculosis. *Trop Geogr Med* 46:283–287, 1994

Rochat T: Tuberculose 1992: Nouveaux aspects clinique, epidemiologiques et diagnostiques. *Schweiz Med Wochenschr* 123:140–147, 1993

Rosenzweig DT, Stead WW: The role of tuberculosis in the pathogenesis of bronchiectasis. *Am Rev Respir Dis* 93:769–785, 1966

Saini JS et al: Scleral tuberculosis. *Trop Geogr Med* 40:350–352, 1988

Saunders NA: State of the art: typing *Mycobacterium tuberculosis. J Hosp Infect* 29:169–176, 1995

Schaffer R, Becker JA, Goodman J: Sonography of the tuberculous kidney. *Urology* 22:209–211, 1983
Schatz A, Bugie E, Waxman SA: Streptomycin, a substance exhibiting antibiotic activity against gram positive and gram negative bacteria. *Proc Soc Exp Biol Med* 55:66–69, 1944
Schofield PF: Abdominal tuberculosis. *Gut* 26:1275–1278, 1985
Schulze K, Warner HA, Murray O: Intestinal tuberculosis. *Am J Med* 63:735–745, 1977
Scott JW et al: Tuberculous false aneurysm of the abdominal aorta with rupture into the stomach: a case report with review of the literature. *Am Heart J* 37:820–827, 1949
Segal T: Intestinal tuberculosis; Crohn's disease and ulcerative colitis in an urban black population. *S Afr Med J* 65:37–44, 1984
Serrano-Heranz A, et al: Tuberculous cardiac tamponade and AIDS. *Eur Heart J* 16:430–432, 1995
Shanan DH, Kibel MA: Tuberculosis. In: Stanfied P, et al. (eds) *Diseases of children in the subtropics and tropics,* 4th edn. Edward Arnold, London, 1991, pp 519–552
Sharif HS et al: Role of CT and MR imaging in the management of tuberculous spondylitis. *Radiol Clin North Am* 33:787–804, 1995
Sharma N, Prescott S: BCG vaccine in superficial bladder cancer. *Br Med J* 308:801–802, 1984
Smith RL, et al: Factors affecting the yield of acid-fast sputum smears in patients with HIV and tuberculosis. *Chest* 106:684–686, 1994
Staples WG et al: Disseminated tuberculosis with bone marrow necrosis and lymphoma. *S Afr Med J* 52:680–683, 1977
Stassa G: Tuberculous Peritonitis. *Am J Roentgenol* 101:409–500, 1967
Stewart CA et al: Unusual pattern of lung uptake of technetium 99 m sulfur colloid seen on the liver scan of a patient with pulmonary tuberculosis. *Clin Nucl Med* 14:271–274, 1989
Stoker DJ: Spinal infection. Proc. 18th Int. Congr. Radiol. Singapore, 1994, pp 199–202
Suri S, et al: Computed tomography in abdominal tuberculosis: a pictorial revue. *Br J Radiol* 72:92–98, 1999.
Sutinen S: Evaluation of activity in tuberculous cavities of the lung. *Scand J Resp Dis Suppl* 67:5–78, 1968
Swensen SJ, Hartmann TE, Williams DE: Computerized tomography diagnosis of *Mycobacterium avium-intracellulare* complex in patients of *Mycobacterium avium-intracellulare* complex in patients with bronchiectasis. *Chest* 105:49–52, 1994
Tabar L, et al: Tuberculosis of the breast. *Radiology* 118:587–589, 1976
Takhtani D, et al: Radiology of pancreatic tuberculosis; a report of three cases. *Am J Gastroenterol* 91:1832–1834, 1996.
Tam PKH, Saing H, Lee JMH: Colonoscopy in the diagnosis of abdominal tuberculosis in children. *Aust Paediatr J* 22:143–144, 1986
Tan TCF, et al: Tuberculoma of the liver presenting as a hyperechoic mass on ultrasound. *Br J Radiol* 10:1293–1295, 1997
Tandon RK, et al: A clinico-radiological reappraisal of intestinal tuberculosis – changing profile. *Gastroenterol Jpn* 21:17–22, 1986
Templeton AC, Schmanz R: Cervical lymphadenopathy in Uganda. *East Afr Med J* 47:582–587, 1970
Thijn CJP, Steensma JT: *Tuberculosis of the skeleton: focus on radiology,* 1st edn. Springer, Berlin Heidelberg New York, 1990, p 12.l
Ting YM, et al: Lung carcinoma superimposed on pulmonary tuberculosis. *Radiology* 119:307, 1976
Umerah BC: Radiological patterns of spinal tuberculosis in the African. *East Afr Med J* 54:598–605, 1977
Vaidya MG, Sodhi JS: Gastrointestinal tract tuberculosis: a study of 102 cases including 55 hemicolectomies. *Clin Radiol* 29:189–195, 1970
Villoria MF, et al: MR imaging and CT of central nervous system tuberculosis in the patient with AIDS (review). *Radiol Clin North Am* 33:805–820, 1995
Vogel H, Rodrigues GHC: Peritonitis tuberculosa des Kleinkindes. *Roentgenol* 36:118–119, 1983
Voigt M, et al: Diagnostic value of ascites adenosine deaminase in tuberculous peritonitis. *Lancet* I:751–754, 1989
Wainwright J: Tuberculous endocarditis. A report of 2 cases. *S Afr Med J* 56:731–733, 1979
Walley J, Porter J: Chemoprophylaxis in tuberculosis and HIV infection. *Br Med J* 310:1621–1622, 1995
Weaver P, Lifeso RM: The radiological diagnosis of tuberculosis of the adult spine. *Skeletal Radiol* 12:178–186, 1984
Werbeloff L, et al: The radiology of tuberculosis of the gastrointestinal tract. Br J Radiol 46:329–336, 1973
Westall J: Tuberculosis leveling off worldwide. *Br Med J* 314:921, 1997
Wilms GE, et al: Computed tomographic findings in bilateral adrenal tuberculosis. *Radiology* 146:729–730, 1983
Witcombe JB, Cremin BJ: Tuberculosis erosion of the sphenoid bone. *Br J Radiol* 51:347–350, 1978
World Health Organisation: Tuberculosis, a global emergency. *World Health Forum* 14:438, 1993
World Health Organisation: Need for action against tuberculosis. *World Health Forum* 16:218, 1995
Yang PJ, et al: Brain abscess: an atypical CT appearance of CNS tuberculosis. *Am J Neuroradiol* 8:919–920, 1987
Yang SO: MR imaging diagnosis of musculoskeletal tuberculosis. Proc. 18th Int Congr Radiol Singapore C 19:222, 1994
Yang ZH, et al: DNA fingerprinting and phenotyping of *Mycobacterium tuberculosis* isolates from human immunodeficiency virus (HIV) – sero-positive and HIV-sero-negative patients in Tanzania. *J Clin Microbiol* 33:1064–1069, 1995
Yaniv E, Avedillo H: Parotid tumour as a presenting symptom of tuberculosis – a report of two cases. *S Afr Med J* 68:613–615, 1990
Young D: Gene deletion behind drug resistance: quoted in editorial. *Br Med J* 305:441, 1992
Zheng JW, Zhang QH: Tuberculosis on the parotid gland. A report of 12 cases. *J Oral Maxillofac Surg* 53:849–851, 1995
Zvetina JR, et al: *Mycobacterium intracellulare* infection of the shoulder and spine. *Skeletal Radiol* 8:111–113, 1982

6 The Mycoses

Diseases Caused by Fungi and Filamentous Bacteria

There are endless varieties and uncountable species of fungi, with estimates varying from 100 000 to 600 000. There is a vast worldwide literature describing the many diseases caused by fungi and the clinical problems of millions of sufferers. Yet, in reality, and fortunately, relatively few, perhaps 150 fungi, are pathogenic to humans and only about 30 are common causes of infection. Of these, about 12 cause serious illness. This chapter is a brief summary of the more clinically and radiologically important varieties and emphasizes those which are common in the tropics and subtropics. Some, such as coccidioidomycosis, are equally or more common in temperate climates. No attempt has been made to provide more than a general description of each entity.

Mycology has been a somewhat neglected subject in radiology, partly because many of the pathogenic fungi have a very provincial geographic distribution ("endemic mycoses"). Examples are *Blastomyces dermatitidis, Coccidioides immitis, Histoplasma duboisii*, and *Paracoccidioides brasiliensis*. However, fungi have flourished and become more widespread in the last few years because of mass migration, increased tourism, and the evolution of AIDS, together with the use of immunosuppressive drugs and antibiotics that wipe out preexisting bacterial flora. Previously localized fungi have appeared in patients in geographic regions where they have been unknown. Those who are immunosuppressed may be killed by normally non-aggressive saprophytic fungi, such as *Cryptococcus neoformans*.

The main responsibility for the diagnosis of mycotic infections lies with the physician caring for the patient, who must include fungal etiologies in almost any differential diagnosis. However, laboratory support is essential; the pathologist who sees the organism in the context of an inflammatory reaction and the mycologist who identifies the culture must decide on cause and effect. The mycologist must try to identify the species and, for certain organisms, determine sensitivity to antifungal agents. Good mycology laboratories are expensive to operate and there are not enough of them, but because of the increasing population of immunosuppressed patients, general diagnostic laboratories are becoming more familiar with the more common pathogenic fungi. Mycology is a very specialized subject and considerable experience is required to identify the many species found in tissue sections, aspirates, and cultures. In most tropical countries, where the necessary laboratory facilities are not always available, imaging can be a very useful initial screening tool leading to more accurate diagnosis and treatment. Imaging can also show the extent and distribution of fungal lesions in soft tissues, and determine whether the infection is superficial or deeply invasive. Imaging allows early recognition of skeletal infection and in both soft tissues and bone can help select the site for biopsy. It is sometimes possible to differentiate mycotic from nonmycotic infections and even to diagnose the actual species of fungus. Furthermore, imaging is a good way to assess the effectiveness of treatment and help in the selection of those patients who may need surgery. Equally important, radiologists must be aware of the specific imaging patterns of fungal infections, because such awareness may not only help to establish the correct diagnosis but also, when the laboratory results and the imaging diagnosis are incompatible, lead to review of all the available information.

True and False Fungi

Included in this chapter are diseases caused by filamentous bacteria which bear a superficial resemblance to fungi and which have traditionally been described in medical mycology. They clinically and radiologically closely resemble true fungi: they form grains in the tissues and cause swelling and draining sinus tracts. These bacteria are *prokaryotic*, with cells and other properties which are very different from those of the true fungi: they include members of the genera *Actinomyces, Nocardia*, and *Streptomyces*.

True fungi are eukaryotic organisms which have no chlorophyll, but their cells resemble those of eukaryotes, including those of mammals which may be infected by fungi. When they invade body tissues,

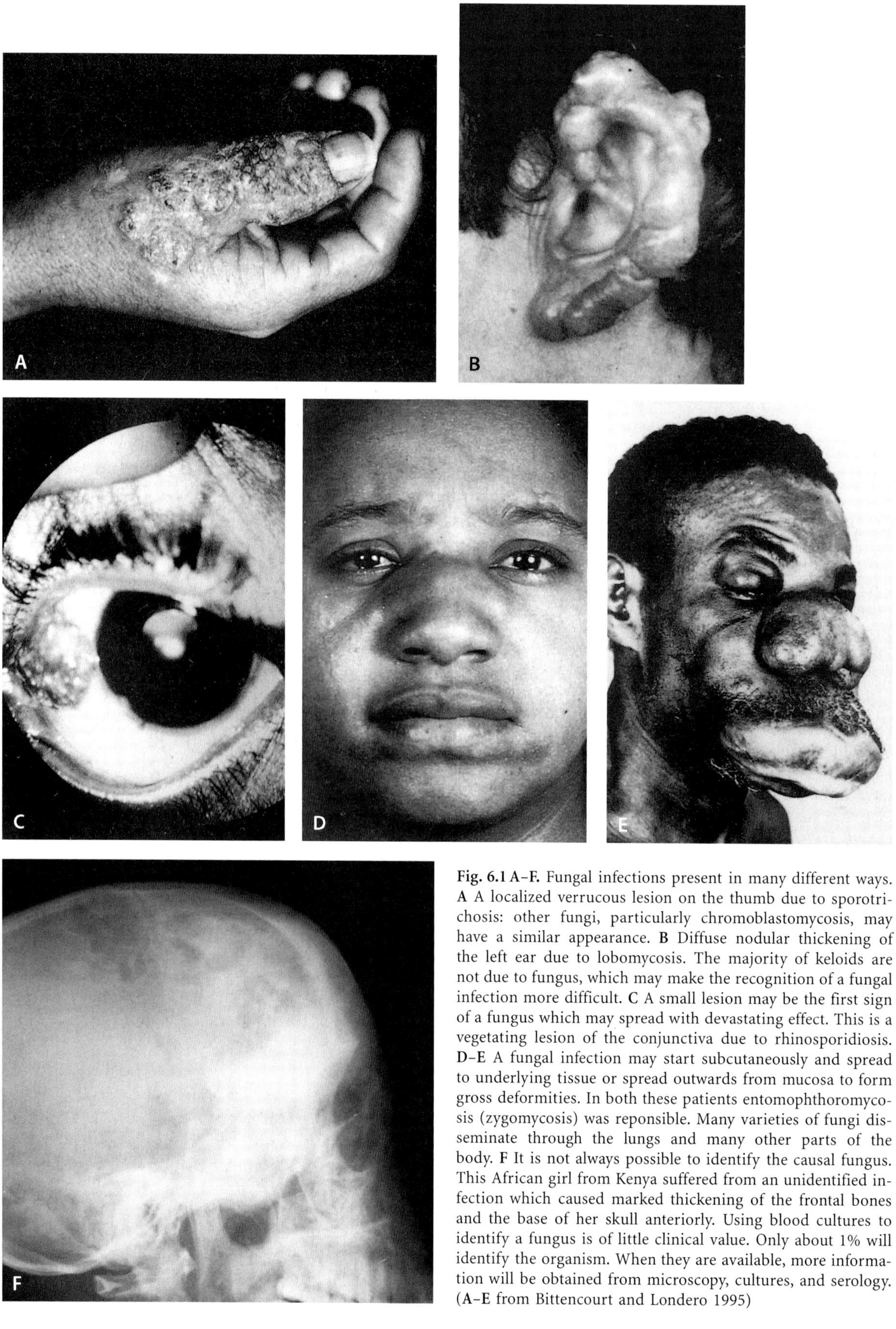

Fig. 6.1 A–F. Fungal infections present in many different ways. **A** A localized verrucous lesion on the thumb due to sporotrichosis: other fungi, particularly chromoblastomycosis, may have a similar appearance. **B** Diffuse nodular thickening of the left ear due to lobomycosis. The majority of keloids are not due to fungus, which may make the recognition of a fungal infection more difficult. **C** A small lesion may be the first sign of a fungus which may spread with devastating effect. This is a vegetating lesion of the conjunctiva due to rhinosporidiosis. **D–E** A fungal infection may start subcutaneously and spread to underlying tissue or spread outwards from mucosa to form gross deformities. In both these patients entomophthoromycosis (zygomycosis) was reponsible. Many varieties of fungi disseminate through the lungs and many other parts of the body. **F** It is not always possible to identify the causal fungus. This African girl from Kenya suffered from an unidentified infection which caused marked thickening of the frontal bones and the base of her skull anteriorly. Using blood cultures to identify a fungus is of little clinical value. Only about 1% will identify the organism. When they are available, more information will be obtained from microscopy, cultures, and serology. (A–E from Bittencourt and Londero 1995)

they grow as budding, round, or oval cells, or as filaments, hyphae, or mycelia (molds). Many of the medically important fungi are Fungi Imperfecti, meaning that their sexual phase has not been recognized. Others are "perfect fungi", i.e., they have a specific sexual phase which classifies them as Ascomycetes, Basidiomycetes, or Zygomycetes: they can reproduce by forming sexual spores of asexual conidia. In nature they are biodegraders and make an essential contribution to the natural balance. They require an exogenous carbon source (heterotrophic). In vivo they can release enzymes to break down tissues to obtain their nourishment.

There are two distinct clinical types of fungal infection: (1) the superficial mycoses, in which the fungi live in nonliving keratin-containing parts of skin, hair, or nails and (2) the intermediate and deep mycoses, where fungi invade deep tissues from the skin. The superficial mycoses, including the so-called dermatophytes, will not be discussed in detail. Only the more significant fungi that cause deep and systemic, often life-threatening disease in humans, are described in this chapter. Each can only be summarized, because there is immense variety and no two are alike (Fig. 6.1). There are many very complex alternatives, for example, the vegetative phase may last a few days or several decades, but always precedes the reproductive phase. Some invade human tissues as hyphae (filaments), some as yeast forms, and some as both; these are called biphasic fungi and sometimes the two phases are morphologically identical. Most fungi that cause disease are saprophytic, degrading vegetation in soil and water, and only appear to infect humans and other animal species accidentally. The reproductive structures are disseminated by movement of air and only infrequently are the fungi spread from one animal directly to another. Two pathogenic species, *Histoplasma capsulatum* and *Cryptococcus neoformans*, are found in bird droppings or on soil which the droppings have contaminated.

Fungi can be grouped as *primary pathogens*, which can establish an infection in the immuno-normal host, usually by inhalation or by implantation of their spores, or as *opportunistic*, fungi which can cause disease when the natural defenses of the host are lowered or absent. This division is not absolute, as some of the fungi which are primary pathogens may also affect immunodeficient hosts. The pathogenic fungi can adapt to the higher temperature of tissues (thermotolerance) or the lower oxidation-reduction potential of tissue (Eh tolerance) and then overcome host defenses by a combination of increased multiplication and relative insensitivity to phagocytosis. Several systemic pathogens exhibit thermal dimorphism. The infectious conidia or spores of the mold (mycelial) phase invade human tissues when inhaled or implanted, and, under the influence of body temperature and other effects, change to the yeast phase. This dimorphism permits a morphological form to change to a yeast form and commonly takes place when tissue invasion occurs: the reverse can be seen during culture. At the same time other changes occur, including the composition of the cell wall. This process is also reversible. Histoplasmosis, blastomycosis, coccidioidomycosis, and paracoccidioidomycosis are diseases caused by fungi that exhibit dimorphism. Candidiasis is caused by yeasts which also can change their morphology although this is not really dimorphism. *Cryptococcus neoformans* is usually monomorphic, i.e., yeast-like, in the infected host and in culture.

The opportunistic fungi are probably the commonest cause of human infections and can result in both superficial and systemic disease. They are usually less virulent than viruses or bacteria, and may coexist peacefully in most people, causing no harm until there is a change in their immune status. Examples are *Aspergillus*, *Candida*, *Cryptococcus*, and the genera causing mucormycosis. These fungi cannot exhibit thermal dimorphism and thus remain either in a mycelial hyphae stage (e.g., *Aspergillus*) or in the yeast stage (e.g., *Cryptococcus neoformans*), invading tissues in hosts with an abnormal immune system.

Classification

A radiology text is not the proper place to classify the fungi!

Descriptions and classification of fungi can be controversial and experts admit that the terminology is sometimes ambiguous and changes frequently. If a detailed classification is required, reference should be made to one (or more) of the standard texts on clinical mycology. Sometimes reference to more than one text causes more confusion!

Laboratory Tests

Fungi can be recognized in cultures from biopsy specimens, exudates, or body fluids. Identification of the genus is often a challenge; deciding on the species is often even more difficult. Histopathology can provide the most rapid means of identification, but it is customary to set aside half of any tissue or fluid for culture to obtain in vitro morphological identification. Growth may be slow and may take several weeks before there are characteristic morphological forms. A recurring problem is in deciding whether the presence of an organism is of clinical significance. For example, *Actinomyces* may be present in the oral cavity in increased numbers when there are carious teeth, and *Candida albicans* may be found in the oral and respiratory mucosa without being invasive or pathogenic. Close correlation with clinical, imaging, and histopathological findings is required to determine the correct diagnosis and its relevance for any patient. Analysis of small aspiration biopsy specimens or sputum, pleural effusions, or bronchial washings is less reliable than excisional biopsy, because histopathology allows recognition of the tissue inflammatory response to the fungus. Unfortunately, negative tissue examination does not entirely exclude a fungal cause for infection, and culture may then be necessary.

The light microscope enables the identification of about 20 pathogenic fungi and the rapidly expanding fields of immunohistochemistry and electron microscopy have made histopathological diagnosis more accurate. However, the reaction to a fungus varies with the patient's immune status. When cell-mediated immunity is defective (in cryptococcosis and histoplasmosis, for instance), tissue response to the fungi is minimal and the organisms proliferate and disseminate, but when the immune status is good, there are fewer fungi and the reaction tends to be vigorous. The primary site of infection for airborne fungi is usually the lungs. If there is an acute inflammatory response, the alveoli fill with fibrin and neutrophils, showing on imaging as consolidation. Many primary lesions, including those caused by *Histoplasma capsulatum, Cryptococcus neoformans, Blastomyces dermatitidis*, and *Coccidioides immitis*, may heal in a few weeks without dissemination. When the patient is immunodeficient, however, the infection spreads widely by lymph and blood to multiple organs. Some fungi, such as *B. dermatitidis, P. brasiliensis*, and *C. immitis*, cause a mixed pyogranulomatous reaction.

Other pathogenic genera, e.g., *Aspergillus*, include almost 100 well-described species: they rarely can be speciated in tissue sections, but some species can be identified when the tissue is well fixed and special stains are expertly used.

Skin tests are generally useful in epidemiological studies, but less useful in the diagnosis in individual patients, unless conversion from negative to reactivity is demonstrated. Serological tests are useful for diagnosis and prognosis in coccidioidomycoses, cryptococcosis, histoplasmosis, and paracoccidioidomycosis. More specific descriptions of the tissue response will be summarized in each section.

Grain-Forming Filamentous Bacteria (Actinomycetes)

Table 6.1. Classification of the grain-forming filamentous bacteria

Anaerobic	Aerobic	
	Nocardia	*Streptomyces*
Actinomyces israelii	*N. asteroides*	*Actinomadura madurae*
A. bovis	*N. brasiliensis*	*S. somaliensis*
A. naeslundii	*N. farcinica*	*Actinomadura pelletieri*
Arachnia propionica	*N. otitidiscaviarum*	

Actinomycosis

Synonyms

Leptotrichosis. Lumpy jaw (also found in cattle). Streptotrichosis. Ray fungus. *Ger*: Aktinomycose (Strahlen Pilzkrankheit durch Actinomyces). *Fr*: Actinobacillose. *Sp*: Actinomicose. Actinomicosis

Definition

Actinomycosis is an infection with one of the *Actinomyces* species, most commonly *Actinomyces israelii*, causing a chronic pyogranulomatous reaction characterized by multiple nodular swellings, tissue destruction, and multiple discharging sinuses. These sinuses discharge puscontaining organisms, either as invisible filaments or in colony forms, the so-called grains or white or yellow "sulfur granules."

Geographic Distribution

The distribution of actinomycosis is worldwide.

Epidemiology and Pathology

These pathogenic, grain-forming, filamentous bacilli are anaerobic and are normal human flora. They frequently colonize the surface and spaces around teeth and the tonsillar crypts. They are possible involved in the formation of dental plaques. They are seldom found elsewhere unless there is an active infection, and then almost always on previously injured tissue. The characteristic grains or sulfur granules are a matrix of bacterial filaments and cellular debris. The filaments branch, are gram positive, are usually aligned at right angles, and have intermediary gram-negative segments. They may be associated with other anaero-

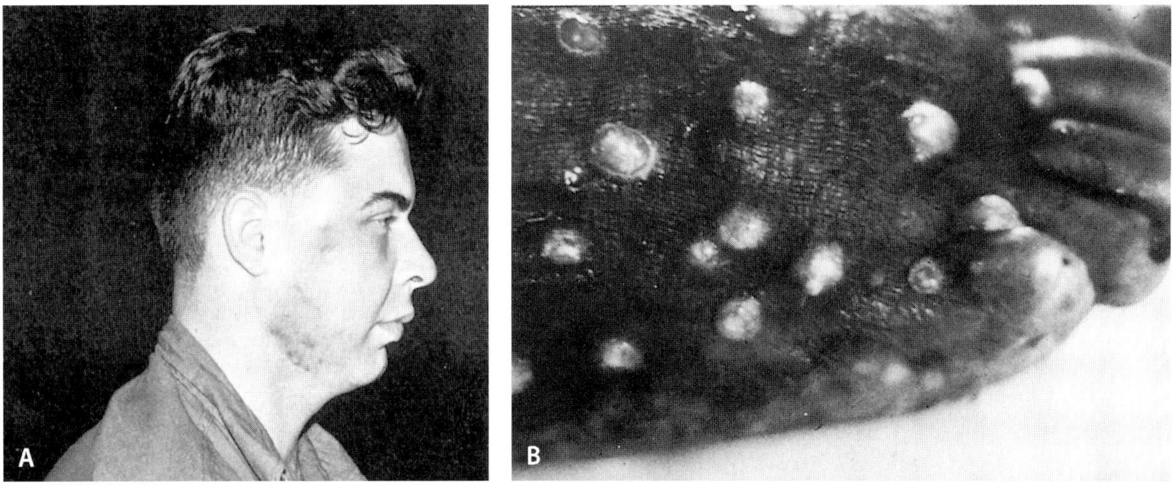

Fig. 6.2 A, B. Multiple sinus tracts are a distinguishing feature of actinomycosis. **A** Actinomycosis affecting the angle of the mandible: the skin is tethered to the bone with some surrounding induration of the subcutaneous tissue and the sinuses are just beginning to appear. AFIP 59-13732-1. **B** Multiple sinus tracts and abscesses in the foot, with the openings raised above the surface (due to *A. madurae*). (**B** from Bittencourt and Londero 1995)

bic bacteria: it has been suggested that these associated bacteria are necessary to initiate an infection. At the edge of the grains, the hyphae are aligned radially and are sometimes coated with Splendore-Hoeppli material, which contains immune complexes, fibrin, and cellular debris. It is important that these actinomyces are differentiated from the aerobic *Nocardia* because treatment differs.

Actinomycosis was first recognized in 1877 in cattle (*A. bovis*), and recognition in humans (*A. israelii*) followed 3 years later; the organism for each is different. There is no racial or sexual predisposition, but actinomycosis is uncommon in children under the age of 10 years.

Actinomycosis is almost always a chronic, fibrosing suppurating infection. There are commonly multiple abscesses of different sizes, with sinus tracts which may interconnect with other abscesses or lead to the skin (Fig. 6.2). The abscesses are limited in size by fibrous tissue. In most patients the sulfur grains (Fig. 6.3) are numerous and easily recognized, but in a few patients a careful search is necessary. Actinomycosis spreads by contiguous expansion and does not respect tissue planes (Fig. 6.4). The fibrosis and infection may produce tumor-like masses, which clinically have been mistaken for malignancy (e.g., within the chest or a frozen pelvis). The destructive process can be severe and disfiguring.

Clinical Characteristics

Actinomycosis is divided by location into three main clinical varieties. Cervicofacial infections account for about 50% of all cases of actinomycosis, abdominal lesions for about 30%, and thoracic lesions for about 15%. Infection in other sites is uncommon.

Cervicofacial Actinomycosis

The organisms, normally present in the mouth, may become invasive after injury to the mucosa, such as a dental extraction or trauma. The overlying skin becomes reddened and inflamed, with hard lumpy swelling either at the site of the infection or at the angle of the jaw. The swollen tissues become thickened, hard, and "woody" and eventually abscesses and sinuses are formed. As some of the sinus tracts heal, new ones form, or the older sinuses may reopen. Trismus is common, even though the site of infection is only slightly painful. The underlying maxilla or mandible may become infected and the infection may extend upwards to involve the meninges or form a brain abscess. The actinomycetes may enter the bloodstream and be carried by macrophages to form metastatic abscesses anywhere in the body. The most important clinical differentiation is from a neoplasm, and the presence of pus and characteristic sinuses is very significant.

Abdominal Actinomycosis

The initial site of infection is usually in the cecum or appendix: only rarely is abdominal actinomycosis associated with cervicofacial actinomycosis. Clinical

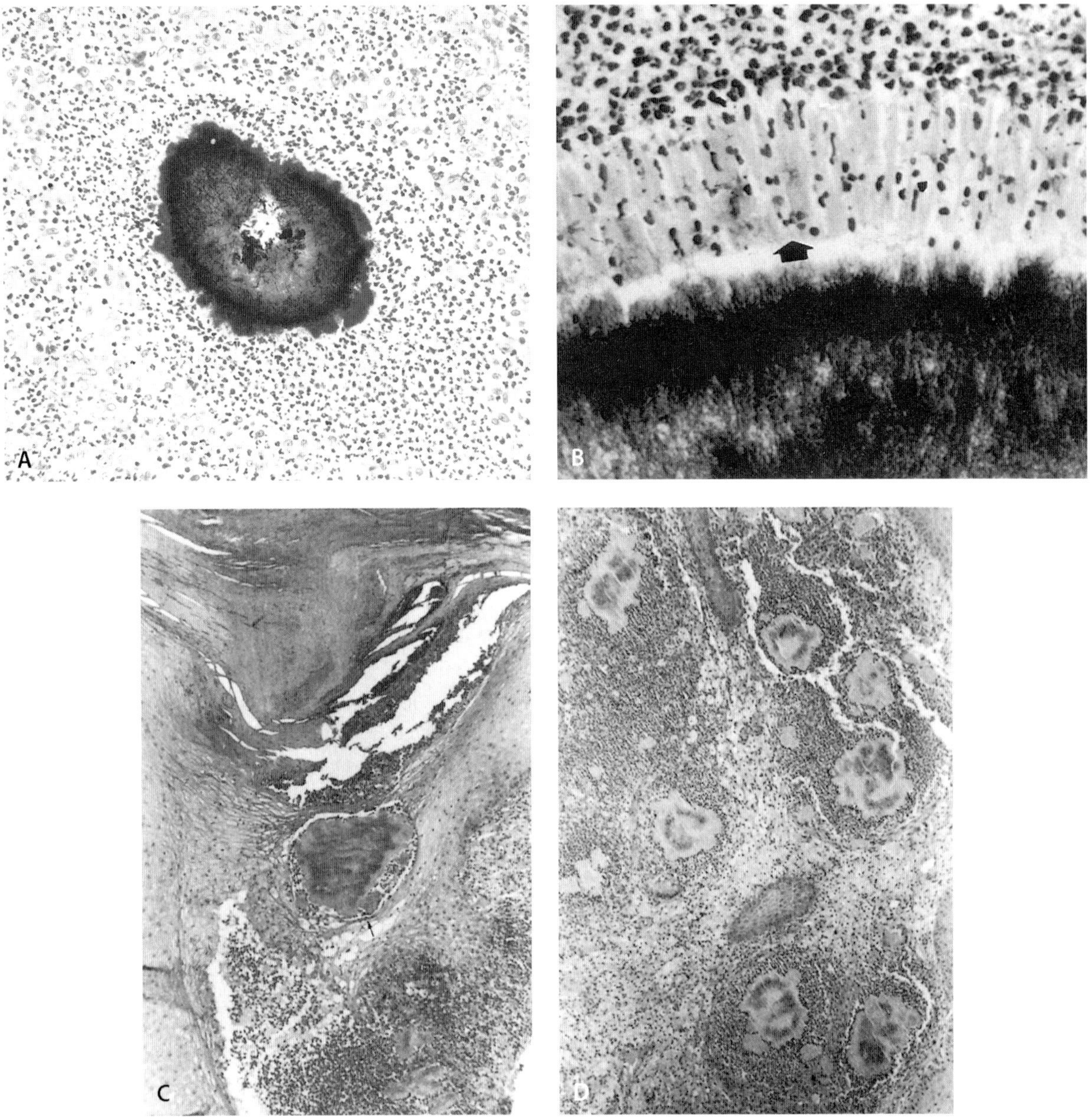

Fig. 6.3 A–D. The histopathology of the actinomycetes. **A** This actinomycotic grain is almost 1.0 mm across and is visible without magnification. Around the perimeter is the Splendore-Hoeppli substance, giving the typical "ray" appearance. There are densely packed filaments centrally and the grain is surrounded by a neutrophil abscess and granulomatous reaction. Brown-Hopps Tissue Gram Stain, ×160. (Courtesy of Dr. Daniel H. Connor) **B** Detail of the Splendore-Hoeppli phenomenon in a grain of *Actinomadura madurae*. **C** A fistulous tract within the epidermis with a large grain of *S. somaliensis* (*arrow*). There is an extensive abscess below it. H & E, ×64. **D** Several other abscesses from the same fungus with multiple filaments around their periphery. H & E, ×64. (**B–D** from Bittencourt and Londero 1995)

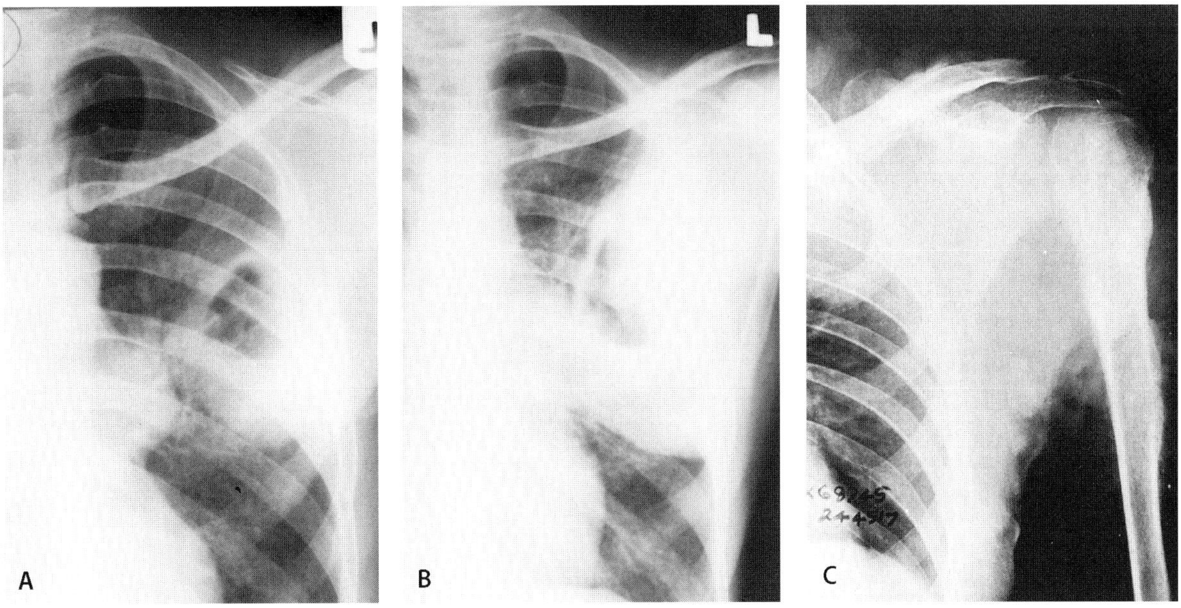

Fig. 6.4 A–C. Actinomycosis is not restrained by tissue planes. **A** A large peripheral lung abscess with an overlying left pleural reaction. There is fluid within the abscess and hilar lymphadenopathy. **B** A few weeks later the abscess had spread through the chest wall, invading the soft tissues and ribs. There is a hypertrophic periosteal reaction along the left clavicle. **C** In a different patient it is impossible to know where the infection started. There is consolidation and fluid in the left apical region, and periosteal new bone around the clavicle, scapula, and humerus. Irregular nodules can be seen in the soft tissues

symptoms suggest appendicitis and there is often a palpable mass before the sinuses appear. This must be differentiated from a mass due to amebiasis, tuberculosis, or a helminthoma: the characteristic grains are not found in any of these other infections. Sinus formation may occur in amebiasis or tuberculosis, but it usually comprises a single tract and occurs late in the infection. There may be direct spread of actinomycosis from the cecal area into the liver or pelvic organs, and even to the urinary tract or pelvic bones: neglected intrauterine devices, left in situ for a long time, have caused uterine, tubo-ovarian actinomycosis. If the infection spreads through the portal system, jaundice may follow. The patient's symptoms may be due to actinomycotic cholecystitis, pyelonephritis, or cystitis. If there are no characteristic lumpy sinus tracts, biopsy may be necessary to establish the correct diagnosis.

Thoracic Actinomycosis

Patients with pulmonary actinomycosis first complain of fever and cough, with yellow sputum: the initial diagnosis may be pneumonia. Abscess cavities in the lungs may suggest a bacterial or tuberculous etiology, but these causes become unlikely if the infection spreads to and through the chest wall and multiple sinuses develop, followed by bone infection and surrounding soft tissue fibrosis. Eventually there is restriction of chest movement. Pulmonary actinomycosis may develop when inhaled bacilli settle in part of a damaged lung, such as a hypoxic fibrotic cavity, bleb, or area of necrosis. It may also reach the lung by spreading through the diaphragm. The mediastinum and pericardium may be involved, causing dysphagia or constrictive pericarditis. Actinomycosis in the chest often seems to progress relentlessly, complicated by anemia and cachexia. Even if successfully treated, there is likely to be significant residual scarring of the lung and chest wall.

Imaging Diagnosis

There are few other infections which spread directly from soft tissues to bone and/or neighboring organs. This, together with the finding of multiple abscesses and sinuses, is an important indicator of actinomycosis at any site.

Cervicofacial Actinomycosis

The soft tissue mass appears before the bony changes, which start with periosteal reaction followed by irregular, moth-eaten bone destruction. As the intraosseous granulomas develop, there will be apparent expansion of periosteal bone around lytic

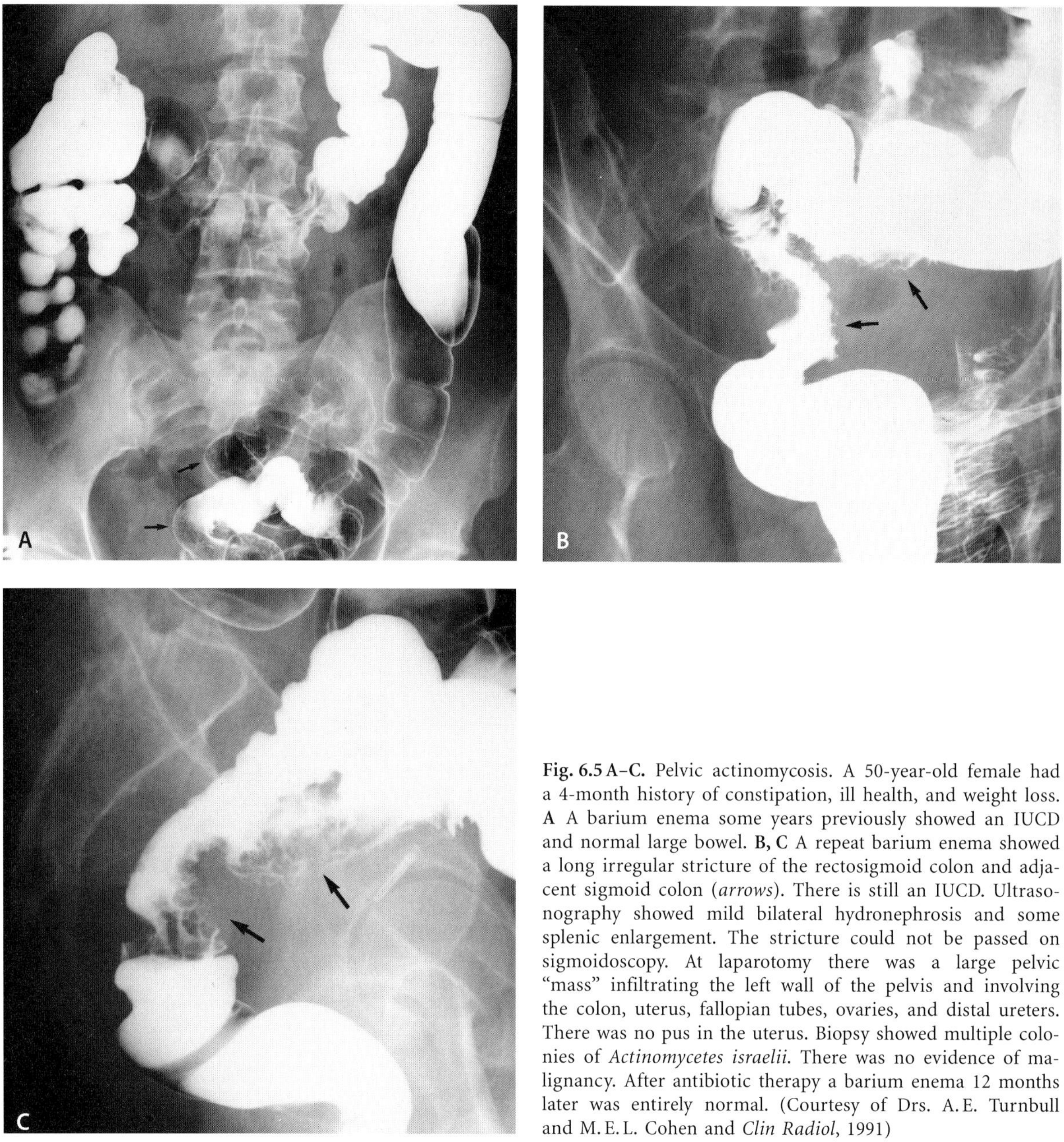

Fig. 6.5 A–C. Pelvic actinomycosis. A 50-year-old female had a 4-month history of constipation, ill health, and weight loss. **A** A barium enema some years previously showed an IUCD and normal large bowel. **B, C** A repeat barium enema showed a long irregular stricture of the rectosigmoid colon and adjacent sigmoid colon (*arrows*). There is still an IUCD. Ultrasonography showed mild bilateral hydronephrosis and some splenic enlargement. The stricture could not be passed on sigmoidoscopy. At laparotomy there was a large pelvic "mass" infiltrating the left wall of the pelvis and involving the colon, uterus, fallopian tubes, ovaries, and distal ureters. There was no pus in the uterus. Biopsy showed multiple colonies of *Actinomycetes israelii.* There was no evidence of malignancy. After antibiotic therapy a barium enema 12 months later was entirely normal. (Courtesy of Drs. A.E. Turnbull and M.E.L. Cohen and *Clin Radiol*, 1991)

lesions. At this stage there will already be sinus tracts between the bone and soft tissues. Early and extensive soft tissue involvement preceding the bone infection, with associated fibrosis and sinus formation, distinguishes actinomycosis from osteomyelitis caused by other pyogenic organisms. Computed tomography (CT) and magnetic resonance imaging (MRI) are important to delineate exactly the location and exent of the infection and to track spread of the infection, particularly upwards through the para-nasal sinuses to the base of the skull, and occasionally even to the meninges and brain. Ultrasonography may be used to show the multiple abscesses within the thick soft tissue tumor and is particularly helpful in the neck. Actinomycosis will result in a thick irregular conglomerate mass, ignoring tissue planes and fixing together all layers as it spreads.

Abdominal Actinomycosis

Actinomycotic granulomas may occur anywhere along the gastrointestinal tract, and be intraluminal, intramural, or outside the bowel. The lumen may be narrowed or distorted by external pressure. Localized stricture formation can be difficult to differentiate from other tropical infections (e.g., amebiasis, schistosomiasis, tuberculosis) or malignancy. Pelvic actinomycosis is common, particularly in women in whom an intrauterine device has been in place for many years (Figs. 6.5, 6.6). *Actinomyces israelii* may be found on cervical smears when there is endometrial or endocervical infection, even when there is no other clinical evidence of systemic disease. Ultrasonography may show tubo-ovarian abscesses, or an apparently unrelated pelvic abscess elsewhere. Almost all other organs in the abdomen and pelvis have been involved (the bowel, bladder, liver, ureters, kidney, gallbladder, and pancreas), as well as the soft tissues. When actinomycosis is suspected, the whole abdomen must be scanned by ultrasonography or CT, including the subphrenic region. Spread through the diaphragm is common in amebiasis, but uncommon in pyogenic infection: only actinomycosis will show multiple sites with abscess formation. Actinomycosis of individual organs may be difficult to diagnose. When the ileum or cecum is infected, there will be distortion due to an abscess or pseudotumor, with internal or external sinuses: the terminal ileum is nearly always involved and partially obstructed. Eventually pelvic actinomycosis will directly involve the pelvic bones, unlike other infections or malignancies.

When the stomach is involved, actinomycosis may present (a) as an infiltrating tumor, (b) as an ulcer or ulcers which may resemble a diverticulum or may penetrate the full thickness of the stomach, or (c) as thickening of the gastric wall without a localized tumor, resembling linitis plastica. The last-mentioned form is least common, but in all three varieties the stomach loses its capacity to expand and becomes locally fixed. Only the multiple sinuses will allow differentiation from carcinoma, lymphoma, tuberculosis, schistosomiasis, and syphilis.

In the duodenum, actinomycosis produces longitudinal ulcers which eventually progress to fistulae and adhesions. It is only the fistulae which will suggest the correct diagnosis and allow exclusion of malignant disease or tuberculosis, but Crohn's disease may cause similar deformities.

Actinomycosis of the colon produces a mass or a stricture, and either may result in obstruction. Perirectal inflammation narrows and distorts the bowel and causes mucosal irregularity and fistulae. This appearance can resemble lymphogranuloma venereum, schistosomiasis, tuberculosis, amebiasis, and Crohn's disease. It is often impossible to make an accurate diagnosis by imaging alone.

Renal actinomycosis may affect one or both kidneys and be mistaken for tuberculosis or malignancy. The calyces are distorted, with enlargement of the kidney or with a localized mass. When there is a sinus tract to the skin, the diagnosis is straightforward, but when there is only renal or perirenal infection the differential diagnosis is difficult, if not impossible.

Actinomycosis of the urinary bladder causes thickening of the bladder wall, and in many cases will be a localized mass, part of which may be intraluminal. At this stage, whatever the method of imaging, the most likely diagnosis will be malignancy. Later there is likely to be involvement of adjacent bone and formation of sinus tracts, simplifying the differential diagnosis (Fig. 6.6 E–F).

Thoracic Actinomycosis

Thoracic actinomycosis often first appears on a chest radiograph as peripheral consolidation, frequently in a lower lobe. There are usually multiple small radiolucent areas, due to the abscesses. These may eventually coalesce into one large lung abscess, with thick walls. Actinomycosis spreads rapidly from the lung into the pleura, causing pleural thickening and eventually an empyema. The infection does not stop there, but spreads into the chest wall, causing osteomyelitis of the ribs, demonstrated radiographically as periosteal reaction and bone destruction (see Fig. 6.4). External sinuses on the chest wall will eventually develop. There is almost always abundant fibrosis, causing loss of lung volume, dense pleural thickening, and restriction of respiratory movement. If healing eventually occures, there may be calcification in the pleura and, less commonly, in the lung.

Both hilar lymphadenopathy and direct extension from the lung into the mediastinum may occur, sometimes with abscess formation. Like blastomycosis, actinomycosis may present as a hilar mass simulating bronchogenic carcinoma. However, outward spread to the chest wall is more characteristic of thoracic actinomycosis.

Skeletal Actinomycosis

Any bone may be involved by direct spread from actinomycosis of the soft tissue (Fig. 6.7): hematogenous spread to bone is unusual. Characteristically there is marked soft tissue thickening beneath which the bone shows marked periostitis and local destruction. When there is intraosseous infection, periosteal expansion occurs. Cartilage is affected less often. Actinomycosis of the vertebrae may cause extensive paravertebral thickening, which may be recognized on scanning before an actual abscess has formed. Multiple vertebrae are commonly involved and show numerous small lytic defects: collapse of the vertebral bodies is common and the intervertebral disc spaces are usually preserved. When healing occurs, bone sclerosis develops and sometimes there is ossification of the intervertebral ligaments.

(Text continues on p. 544)

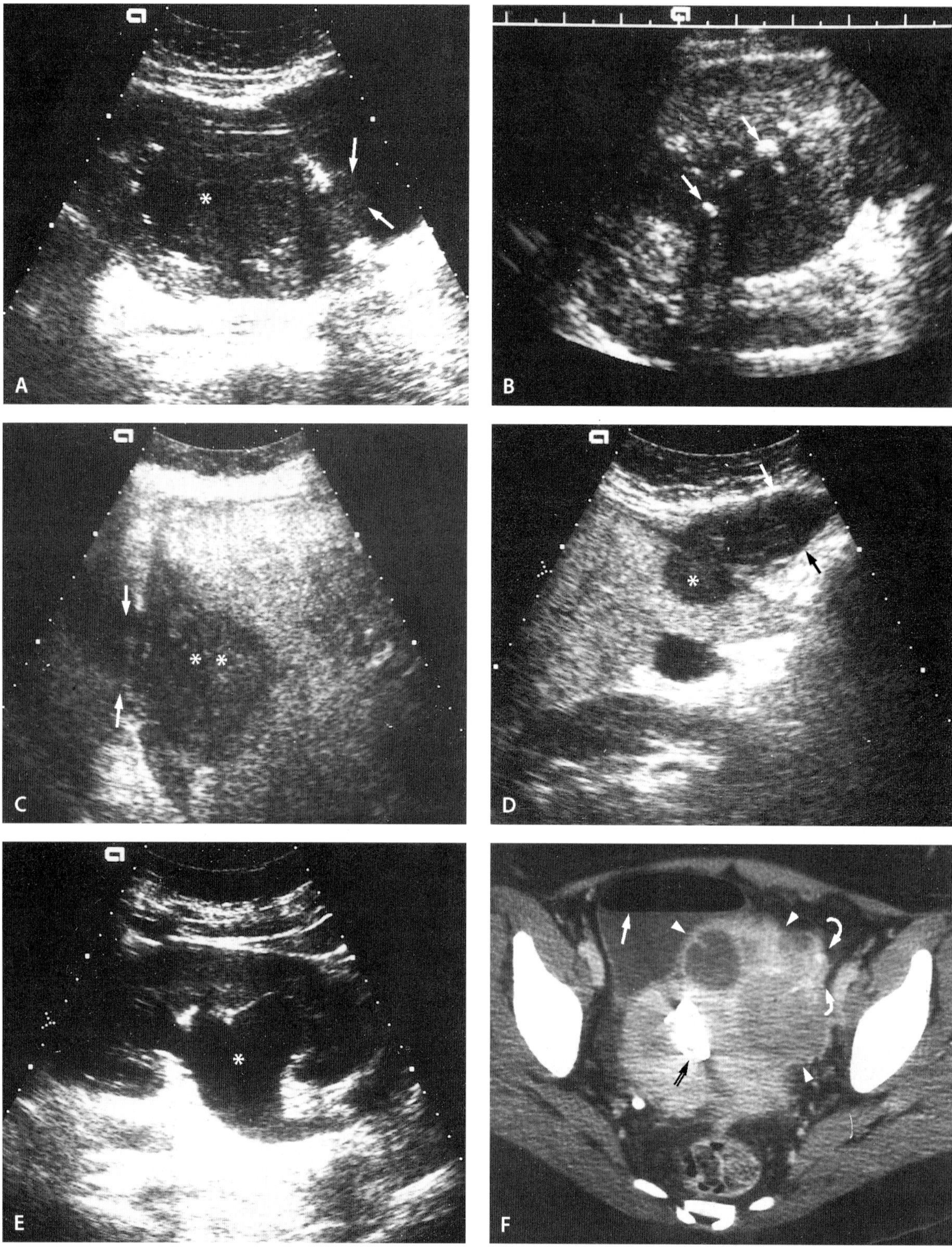

Fig. 6.6 A–H. Pelvic abscesses have many causes but when there is an IUCD, a possibility of actinomycosis should be considered. This 41-year-old woman was febrile and had a left lower quadrant tender mass. **A** Ultrasonography showed that the mass contained fluid and debris (*) and involved the bladder (*arrows*). **B** Transvaginal ultrasonography showed an IUCD (Lippes loop) (*arrows*). **C, D** Scans of the liver showed hypoechoic masses in the right (**) and left (*) lobes with extensions though the liver capsule into the abdominal wall (*arrows*). **E** The left kidney (*) was hydronephrotic due to ureteric involvement. **F** CT scans with contrast showed gas in the bladder (*solid straight arrow*) and the irregular thickened left wall of the bladder, involved with the pelvic mass (*arrowheads*). The IUCD is again shown (*open arrow*). The *curved arrows* show barium in the displaced sigmoid colon. **G, H** see p. 543

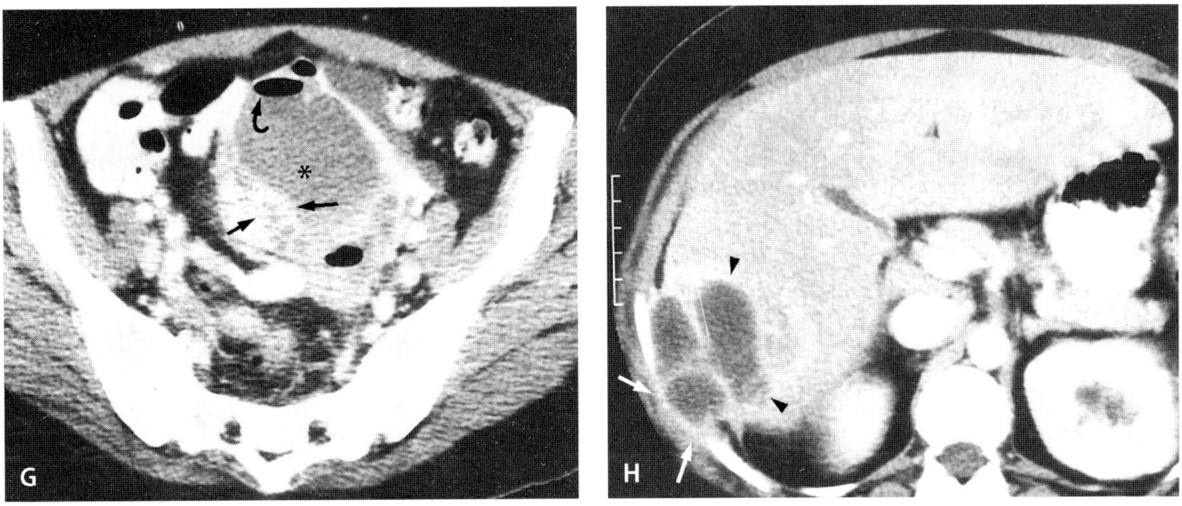

Fig. 6.6 (*continued*). **G** The mass was predominantly fluid (*) and has thick septa (*arrows*). The gas is shown again (*curved arrow*). **H** A liver scan shows a mass in the right lobe (*arrowheads*) with enhancing septa and walls. It extends to the tissues of the abdominal wall (*arrows*). No fistula was demonstrated with other contrast examinations but histopathology confirmed the diagnosis of actinomycosis. (Courtesy of Drs. J.G. Hochsztein, M. Koenigsberg, D.A. Green, and *Radiographics*, 1996)

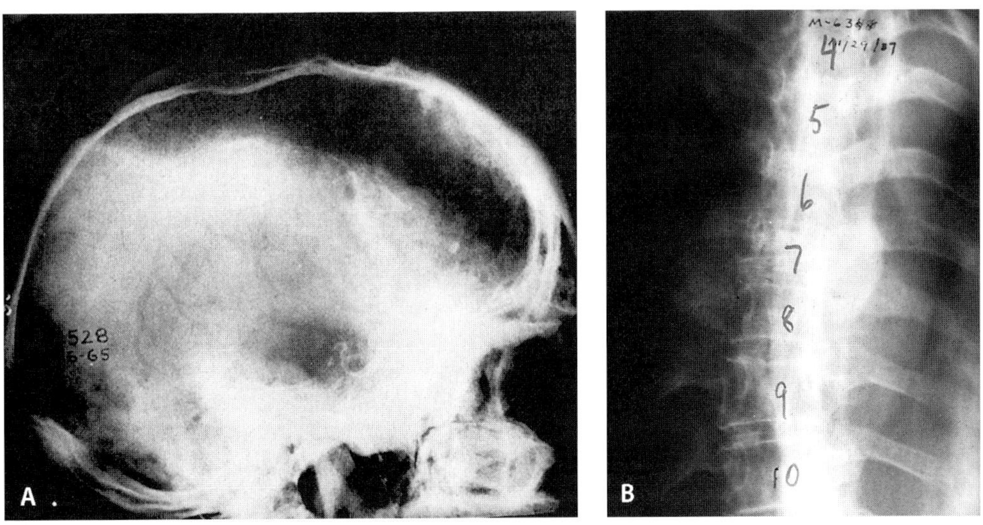

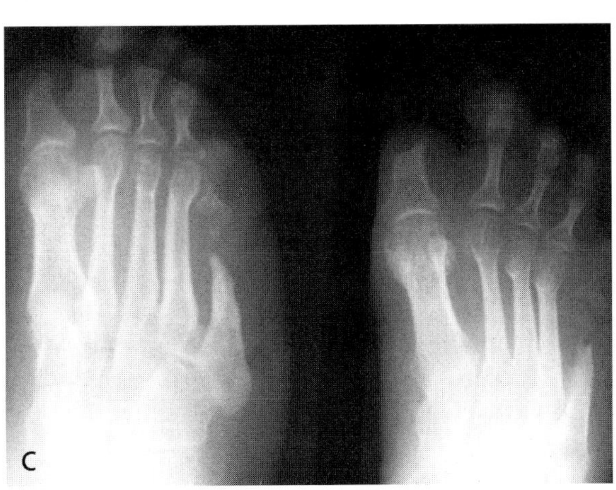

Fig. 6.7 A–C. Actinomycosis in the skeleton. **A** Affecting the frontal bone and cranial vault, extending back to the midparietal region. There is bone destruction with some patchy new bone formation, especially in the frontal bone near the frontal sinus. **B** Infection of the thoracic spine. T7 has partially collapsed and there is a paravertebral abscess on the left side. There is probably more pus running along the spine above and below the affected vertebra. There is a periosteal reaction around the seventh left rib posteriorly. (Courtesy of Dr. Harold G. Jacobson) **C** Oblique and AP projections of the left foot of an African from Zimbabwe. There is partial destruction of the fifth metatarsal digits. There is marked soft tissue swelling and sinus formation. The discharging sinuses with yellow grains made it possible to distinguish this from leprosy

Unless the involvement of the neighboring soft tissues, with fibrosis and sinus formation, is recognized, actinomycosis cannot be differentiated by imaging from most other bone infections.

Aerobic Actinomycetes

The aerobic filamentous bacteria may form grains in tissue only and are divided into four genera. Clinically, however, it is easier to consider two main groups, the *Nocardia* spp. and the *Streptomyces* spp. and to include the very similar *Actinomadura* within this latter group. Laboratory identification can be difficult and is based largely on cell wall differences: taxonomy is complicated because of the similar organisms. The nomenclature adds to the confusion, because the same organism has often been given many names (see *Synonyms* in each section). The clinical history and imaging also have many variations, but it is often possible with careful imaging to suggest which main group is likely to be responsible.

Nocardiosis

Synonyms

Streptothricosis: in the past some authorities have called this actinomycosis. *Nocardia asteroides* has been called *Cladothrix asteroides* and *Actinomyces gypsoides. Nocardia brasiliensis* has been called *Actinomyces mexicana* and *Nocardia transvalensis* (which some believe is a separate species). *Ger*: Nocardiose (Aktinomykose durch *Nocardia asteroides*). *Fr*: Nocardiose. *Sp*: Nocardiosis.

Definition

Nocardiosis is an infection with one of the *Nocardia* spp. within the aerobic schizomycete species. This is usually *N. asteroides*, although *N. brasiliensis* and *N. otitidiscavarium* also infect humans. Even more uncommon is infection with *N. transvalensis*.

Geographic Distribution

The first human infection was described in 1890 and there were few subsequent reports until the last 30 years, when nocardiosis has been recognized more frequently, particularly in patients who are immunocompromised. *N. asteroides* is the most common cause in Japan, but is also found in Africa and tropical America. *N. brasiliensis* is most frequent in South America, and in Mexico may cause 85% or more of all mycetomas. It has also been identified in Africa and Asia.

Epidemiology and Pathology

Nocardiosis occurs in all age groups, particularly in older patients. There are no occupational or racial susceptibilities, but the majority of patients with systemic infection will be male and immunocompromised in some way. Yet, nocardiosis is not common in AIDS patients.

The usual route of infection is through the respiratory tract; less often, infection occurs via ingestion or after tissue damage. In the lungs, patients with chronic pulmonary damage or alveolar proteinosis are most at risk. Suppurating abscesses develop, usually multiple with surrounding fibrous tissue: the pus is odorless and greenish-yellow in color. Histopathologically there are very few epithelioid or giant cells. The infection may be localized, as in the lungs, but may spread to almost any part of the body, most frequently to the brain, peritoneum, muscle, and subcutaneous tissues. In the lungs there is usually chronic pneumonia and multiple abscesses, often involving the pleura and the chest wall. There is no caseation. The partially acid-fast gram-positive filaments are in the pus, sometimes with macrophages, and frequently have invaded adjacent granulation tissue.

The characteristic feature of nocardiosis is multiple abscesses, interlinked by communicating fistulae. There is very little fibrosis and scar tissue: the reaction is mostly inflammatory and suppurative. Less commonly, the fungal colonies (grains) are found in the microabscesses with a surrounding inflammatory edema. This type of infection will probably remain localized and become a nocardial mycetoma. There is no vasculitis and little fibrous tissue proliferation. *Nocardia asteroides* and *N. brasiliensis* are partially acid-fast and can be recognized by this and by the discrete slender branching hyphae (Fig. 6.8). There is an accurate complement fixing test which also can be used for monitoring treatment, but cross-reaction with antigens of some mycobacteria can occur. These are specialized tests and usually require a dedicated laboratory. Culture is easy on Sabouraud's medium. Staining with hematoxylin and eosin (H & E) can be unreliable because individual filaments may not be seen clearly. As with some other fungal and actinomycotic infections, it can be difficult to decide whether the nocardia are causal or a contaminant. Infection by *N. asteroides* may resemble that caused by *Mycobacterium tuberculosis*, particularly when the branching hyphae have broken up, but the tissue reaction and form of the bacteria are distinct and can be recognized histopathologically.

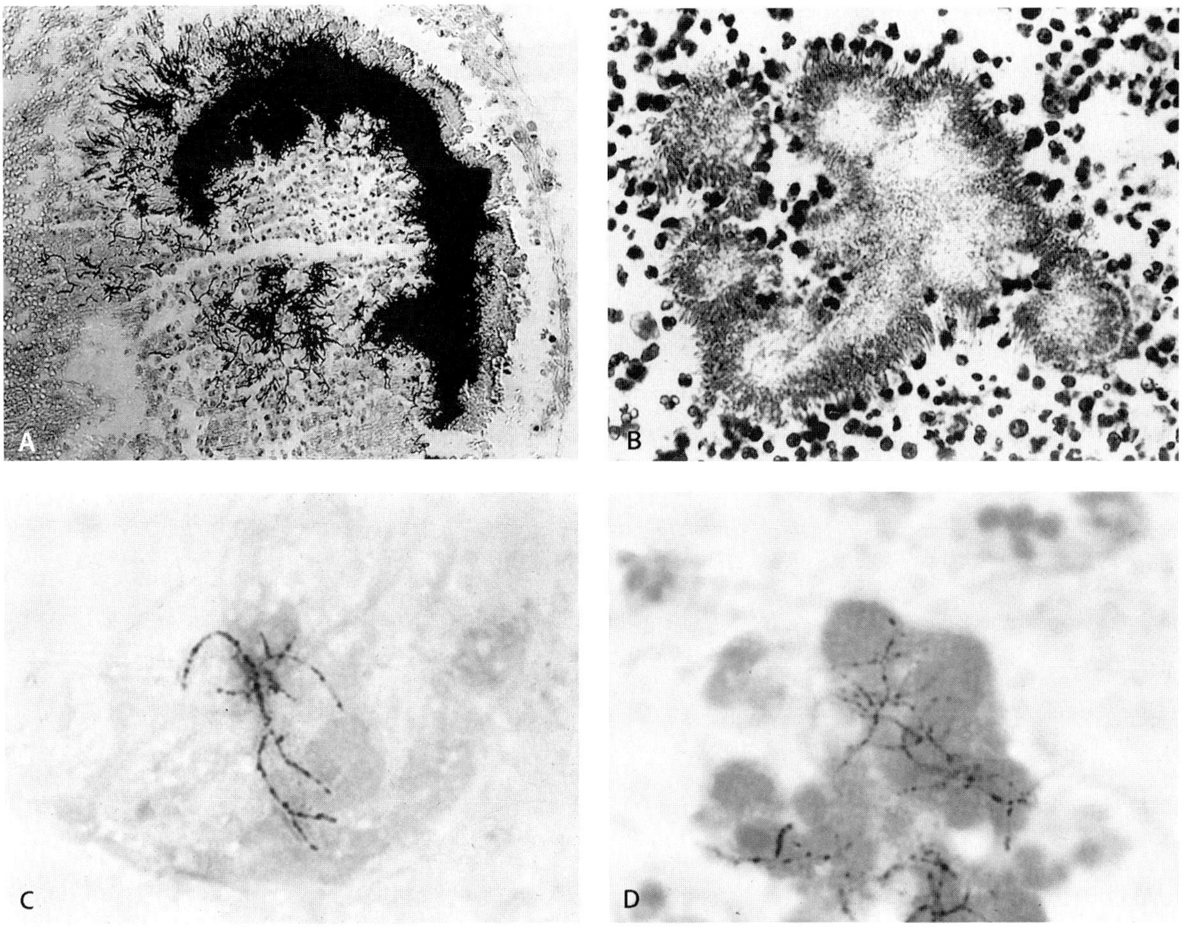

Fig. 6.8. A The very thin filaments of *Nocardia brasiliensis* (Brown-Brenn stain, ×400), and **B** grain showing peripheral eosinophilic clubs (H & E, ×200). **C, D** *Nocardia asteroides* in sputum. (**A, B** from Bittencourt and Londero 1995)

Clinical Characteristics

Some pulmonary infections may have no clinical symptoms and may be self-limiting. In the progressive pattern of infection, the CNS and skin are less commonly infected than the lungs but few parts of the body are immune.

The most striking local clinical features are swelling and sinus formation, with draining pus (Fig. 6.9). When there is systemic infection, these patients present with fever, cough, sputum, chest pain, and symptoms of pneumonia, none of which is specific for nocardiosis. The lungs are the most common site of infection, and when the pleura and chest wall are involved, there will be multiple sinuses but minimal fibrosis. Central nervous system involvement may be asymptomatic or cause headache, a stiff neck, vomiting, convulsions, and, in some patients, mental symptoms or paralysis. This usually indicates a nocardial brain abscess. The eyes (particularly the retina) may be infected. Meningitis is not common and the cerebrospinal fluid does not have any characteristic changes. Spinal involvement, which often causes a paravertebral abscess seen on imaging, may be mistaken for tuberculosis. All the organs, including kidney, liver, spleen, peritoneum, adrenals, and heart, may be involved and there may be multifocal bone involvement. Organ and skeletal involvement can be difficult to recognize clinically, but imaging may provide much more information.

Localized mycetomas are described in detail on pp. 548, 555.

Imaging Diagnosis

Pulmonary Nocardiosis

If not superimposed on damaged lungs, the extent of the infection depends very much on the immune status of the patient. There is usually patchy consolidation in both lungs, with multiple small cavities which coalesce to form larger abscesses.

(Text continues on p. 548)

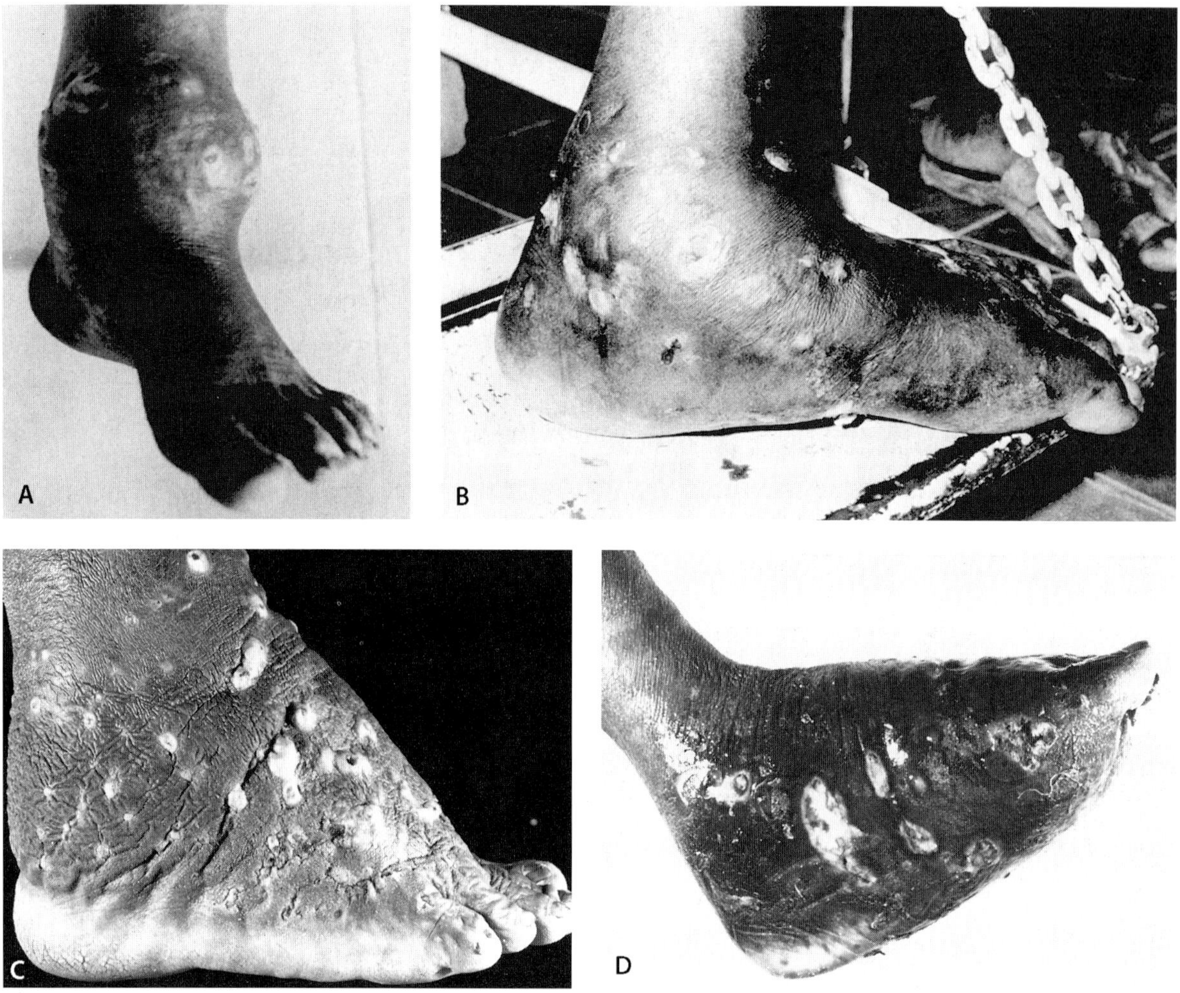

Fig. 6.9 A–D. The clinical appearance of nocardiosis. **A** Localized swelling around the ankle joint with multiple sinuses discharging pus: a patient from West Africa. **B** A similar grossly swollen foot and ankle with multiple sinuses, due to *Nocardia asteroides*: a patient from India. **C** A longstanding, but progressive nocardial infection in the foot of an African from Uganda. This foot was amputated. **D** The very painful chronic infection in the foot of a young woman from Uganda which also had to be amputated. (**C**, **D** courtesy of Dr. Daniel H. Connor)

Fig. 6.10 A–G. A 28-year-old Indian from southern India came to hospital with multiple swellings of the left chest wall. **A** There were multiple sinuses surrounded by heaped-up granulomatous tissue due to nocardiosis. **B** Underlying the soft tissue swelling there was periosteal new bone formation around the clavicles and scapula and some destructive areas in the scapula. There was a pleural effusion under the left upper lobe. **C** Three months later the infection is worse. The left ribs are involved, the clavicles show prolific periosteal new bone formation, there is sclerosis in the scapula as well as areas of destruction, and the pleural thickening and pleural effusion have increased. There is probably infection in the underlying lung. **D** The macroscopic specimen of the lung of a different patient with a similar nocardial infection in the upper lobe. **E** A similar nocardial brasiliensis infection in a patient from South America. In the early stages the outer end of the clavicle shows some periosteal thickening and the scapula is increased in density, with some lytic areas underlying the soft tissue swelling. **F** Later the reaction on the clavicle is more marked and the soft tissue swelling has increased. **G** The right shoulder of a different patient from South America. The whole length of the humerus shows periosteal reaction and multiple lytic areas which have probably spread from the tissue infection around the shoulder and scapula. In this patient the clavicle has remained normal. (**E–G** courtesy of Drs. Harold G. Jacobson and Jorge Ceballas-Labat, Mexico City) ▶

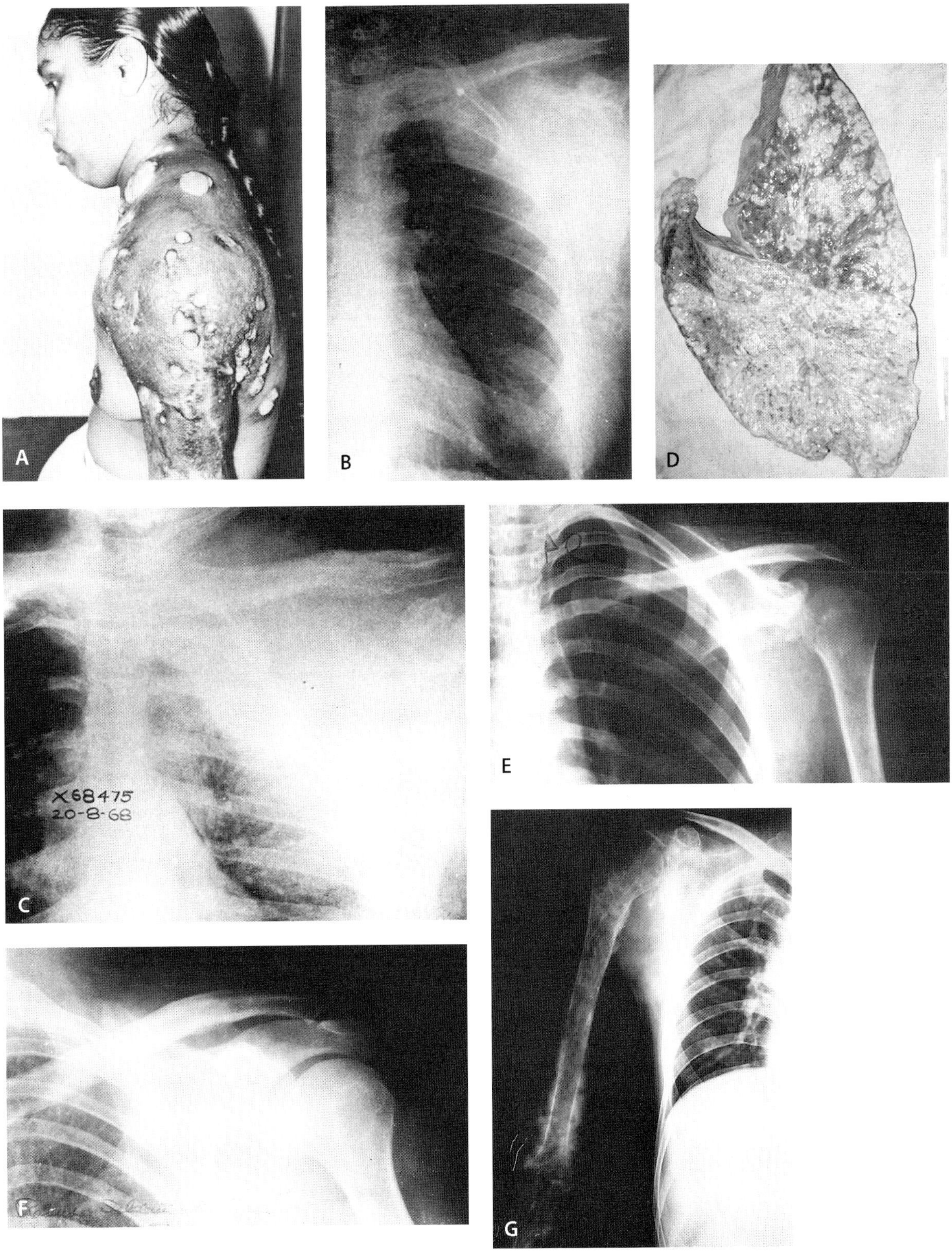
A
B
D
X68475
20-8-68
C
E
F
G

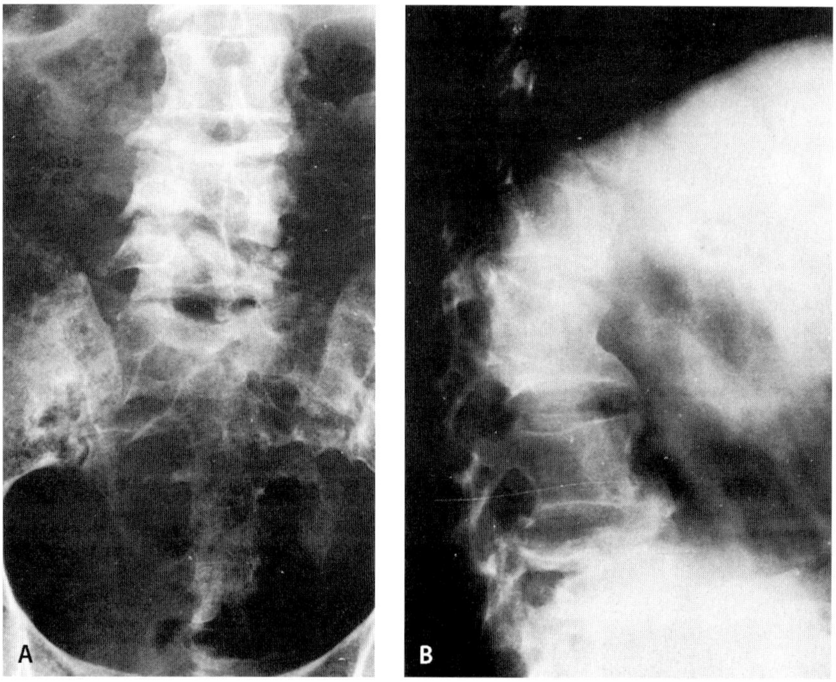

Fig. 6.11 A, B. *Nocardia* affects vertebral bodies the same way as other parts of the skeleton. There are areas of destruction and exuberant new bone formation, but osteoporosis is less common. **A** Anteroposterior and **B** lateral view of the lumbosacral region in a 35-year-old Indian woman who had mistakenly received treatment for tuberculosis. The multiple sinuses which developed allowed a more accurate diagnosis. There is periosteal new bone formation, sclerosis, and partial collapse of several vertebral bodies. There are multiple lytic lesions near the sacroiliac joints. Treatment for nocardiosis provided remarkable clinical improvement and the sinuses dried up after a few months

There may be solitary pulmonary masses, often well defined. These may cavitate: spread to the pleura and into the chest wall is common and results in pleural effusions, empyema, and pleural thickening (Fig. 6.10 A–D). There is less fibrosis than in actinomycosis, but when the ribs are involved, there is an exuberant periosteal reaction and irregular moth-eaten bone destruction. Sinuses develop and subcutaneous nodules may appear, draining the chest wall. Hilar and mediastinal lymphadenopathy and direct spread to the mediastinum occur, but are a little less common than in actinomycosis.

Until there is sinus formation or direct involvement of the chest wall, the differential diagnosis from a pulmonary pyogenic infection or tuberculosis is very difficult. Nocardiosis must be considered whenever there are solitary pulmonary masses, particularly peripheral, or when any lung lesion fails to respond to adequate therapy. Aspiration biopsy may be necessary to establish the diagnosis.

Skeletal Nocardiosis

When the spine is involved a paravertebral abscess may be mistaken for tuberculosis or brucellosis. Nocardiosis infects vertebral bodies, causing bone destruction, compression and loss of vertebral height (Fig. 6.11). There can be sclerosis within the body of the vertebra. The disc space is usually spared, but the pedicles and transverse processes can be infected and become sclerotic. It is difficult to distinguish nocardiosis from tuberculosis and brucellosis, but in the latter the disc space usually narrows early in the infection.

Further examples of skeletal nocardial infections are shown in Figs. 6.10 E–G and 6.12–6.16.

(Text continues on p. 555)

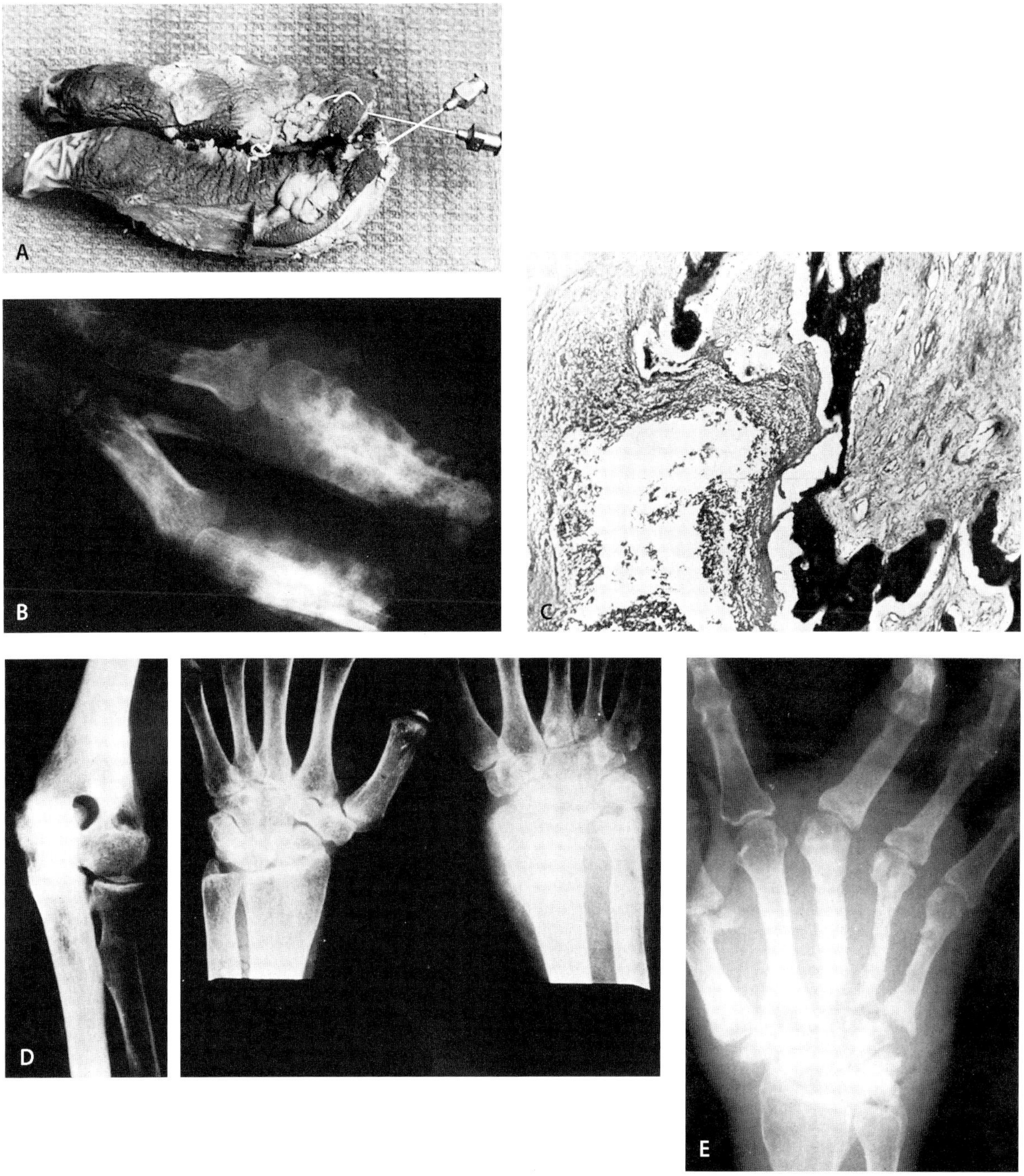

Fig. 6.12 A–E. Nocardial infections of the arm, wrist, and fingers. **A** Specimens of amputated fingers from a patient in India: there are multiple discharging sinuses. **B** The typical exuberant periosteal new bone formation without sequestration: the periosteal new bone and the cortex are perforated by multiple 4- to 7-mm lytic areas. This decompression prevents formation of a sequestrum because the vascular supply to the cortex and the periosteum is maintained (see Fig. 6.18 C–E). **C** Histology of the finger showing lacy (cabbage leaf) periosteal new bone. The fungal abscess perforates through the cortex and periosteum, permitting free drainage from the infected bone. **D** Multiple areas of destruction are typical of nocardial infections, as seen here in the lower end of the humerus and the proximal ulna. The same patient had similar areas of destruction near both wrist joints, with marked soft tissue swelling on the right wrist in particular. This clinically might suggest tuberculosis before the sinuses develop. The periosteal reaction of nocardiosis is proliferative with reactive sclerosis, unlike the osteoporosis of tuberculosis. **E** The end result of incompletely treated nocardiosis. The periosteum has consolidated and the bones have remodeled and become sclerosed, superimposed on the multiple areas of bone and joint destruction

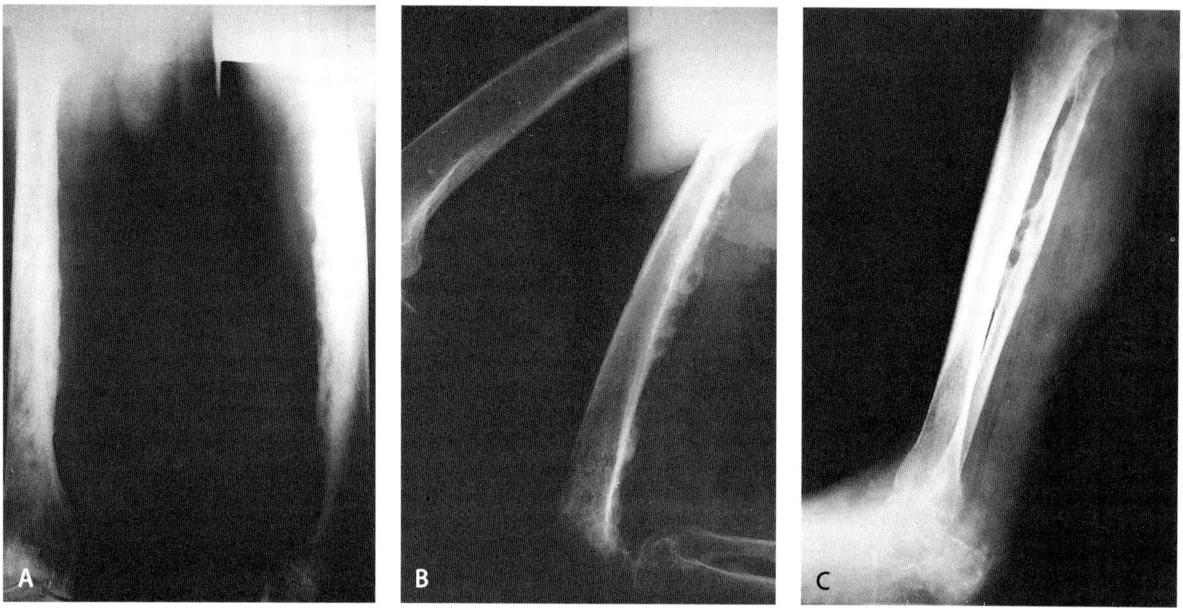

Fig. 6.13 A–C. Nocardial infection of the lower limbs. The femora, fibula, and tibia show the same exuberant periosteal bone reaction with underlying sclerosis. The soft tissue swelling and nodulation can be seen, particularly in the lower leg. (Patients from South America; courtesy of Drs. Harold G. Jacobson and Jorge Ceballas-Labat, Mexico City)

Fig. 6.14 A–F. Nocardiosis of the ankle and feet. **A** A 32-year-old Indian male with swelling of the left foot and multiple nodular sinuses: there was a thick purulent discharge. There were a few sinuses on the right foot also. **B** A radiograph shows multiple areas of destruction in all the bones of the left foot, with intense periosteal new bone, particularly around the metatarsals. There are irregular lytic areas 2–15 mm in diameter. The tarsal joints have been affected. Because the lower leg was infected also, an above-the-knee amputation was planned but the patient absconded with a few month's supply of drugs. **C** On his return most of the sinuses had dried up, the swelling had subsided and the tibia and fibula had improved. He had extensive bilateral pulmonary infection also, but this had regressed. **D–F** This patient was not so fortunate and his foot was amputated, the standard treatment until the difference between the true and the false fungi was recognized. **D** A gross specimen of the foot after amputation. **E** The radiograph shows multiple confluent intercommunicating abscess cavities involving the bones and soft tissues. **F** Cross-sections of the foot show the confluent microabscesses and the multiple smooth wall communicating cavities ▶

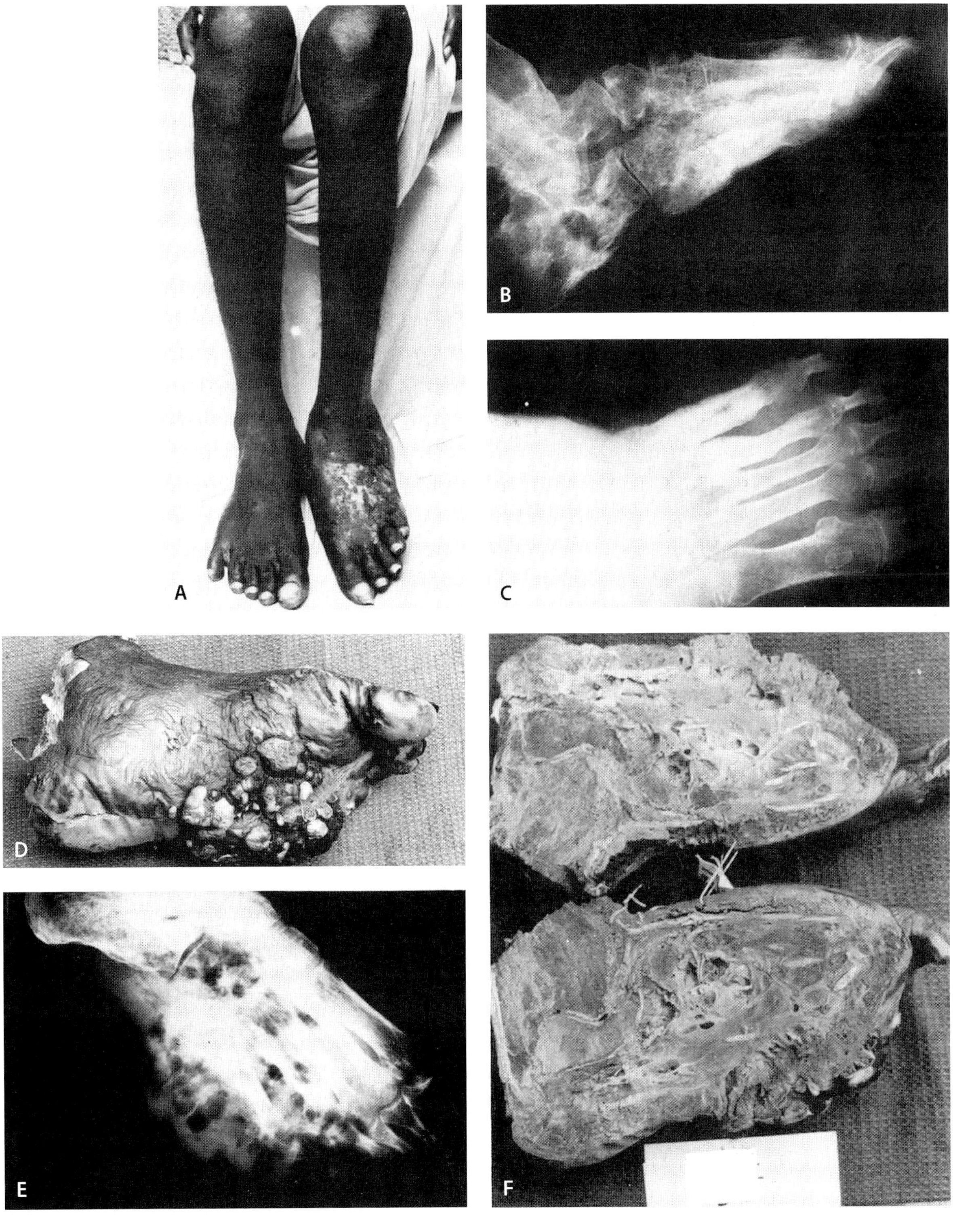
A
B
C
D
E
F

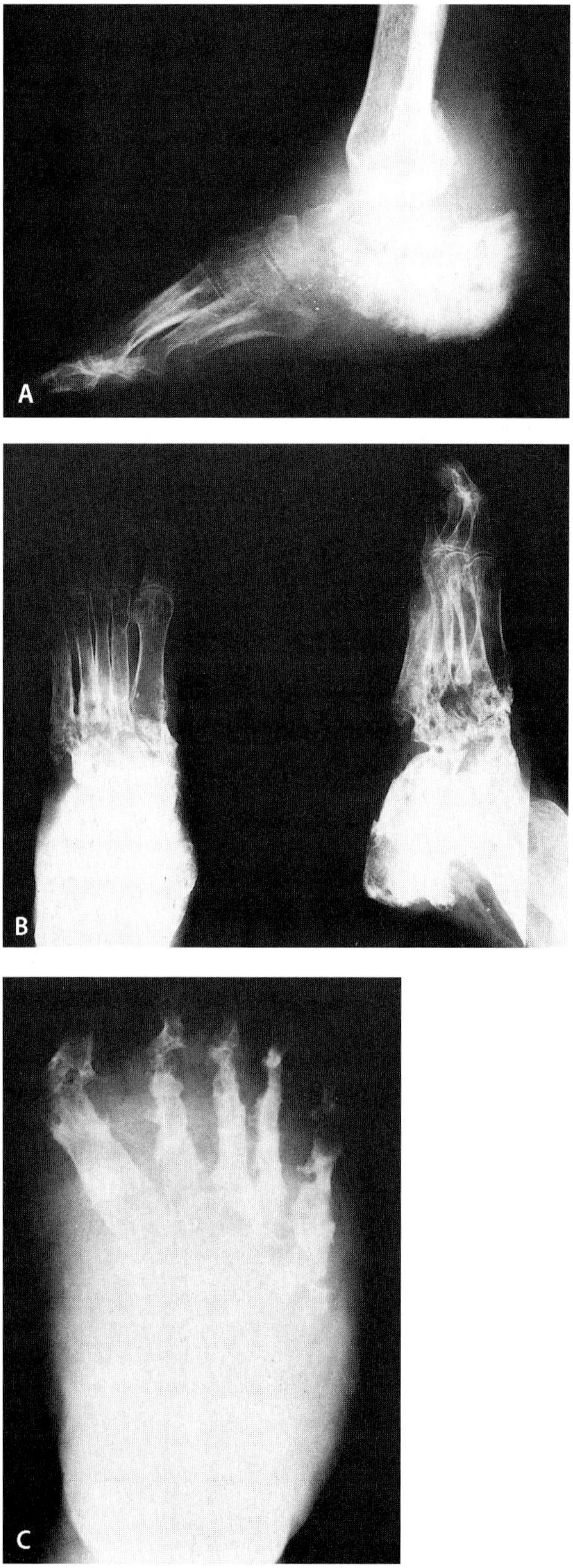

Fig. 6.15 A–C. Three South American patients with severe *Nocardia brasiliensis* infections of the ankle and feet. (Courtesy of Drs. Harold G. Jacobson and Jorge Ceballas-Labat, Mexico City)

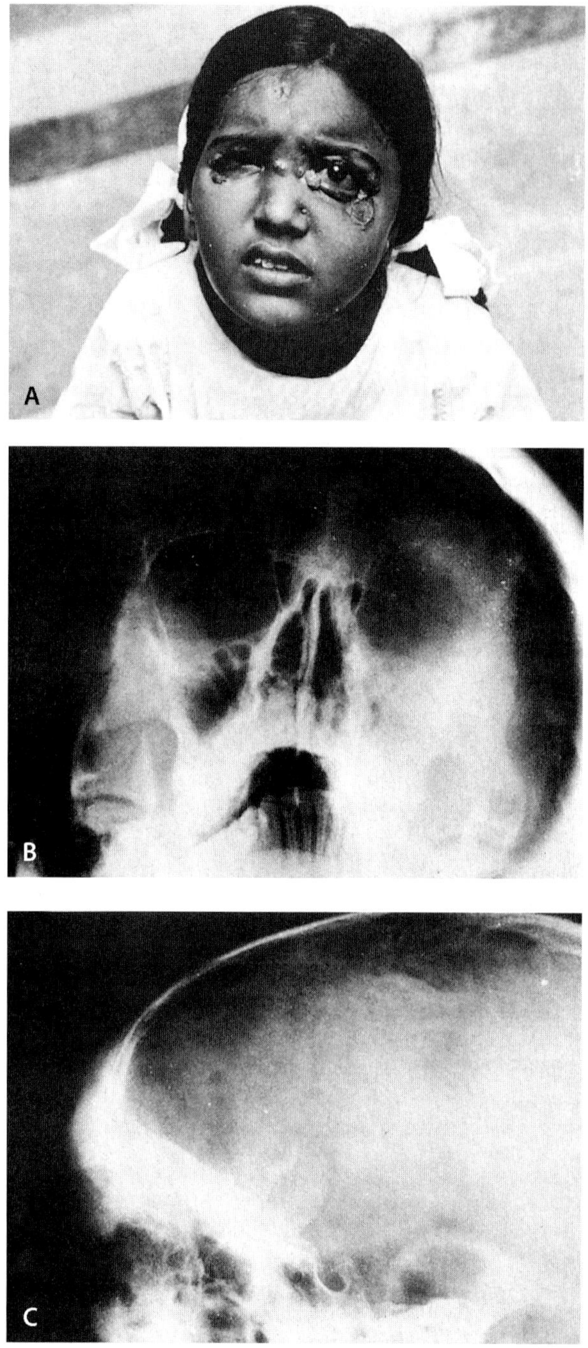

Fig. 6.16 A–I. *Nocardia* often infects the facial bones and paranasal sinuses, and may spread elsewhere in the skull. **A** A young Indian child with a *Nocardia* infection which started in the paranasal sinuses: there is thick granulation tissue discharging pus from multiple sinuses, one of which affects the frontal bone. There is unilateral proptosis, involvement of orbital walls on both sides (**B**), particularly on the left, and thickening of the left maxillary antrum. Part of the bone in the roof of the left orbit has been destroyed and the left orbital fossa has become smaller. As seen in the lateral view (**C**) there is marked sclerosis of the frontal bone. **D–I** see p. 553

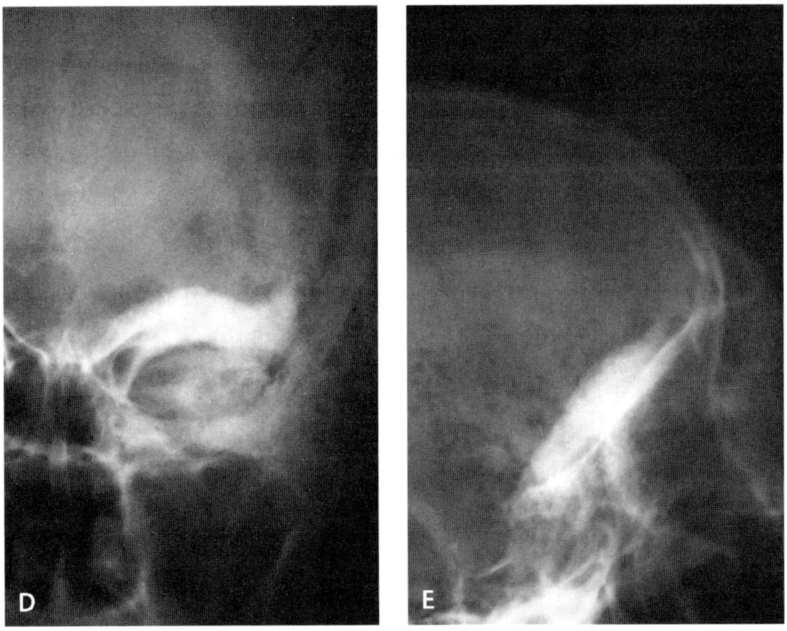

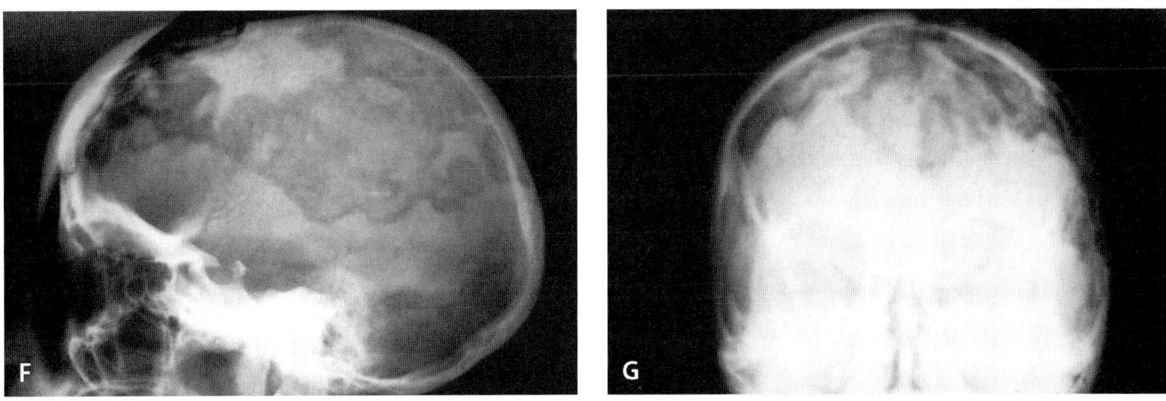

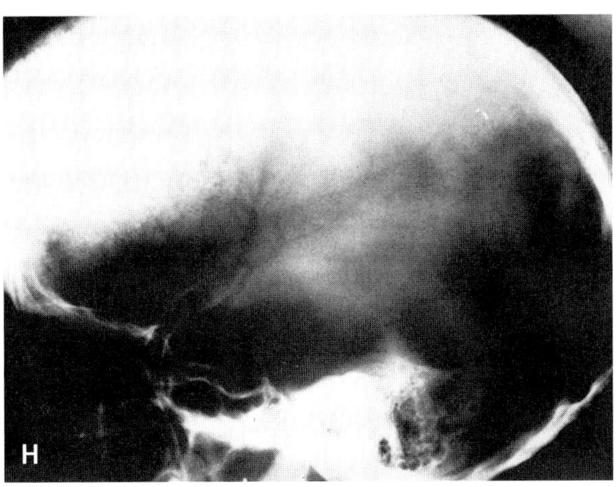

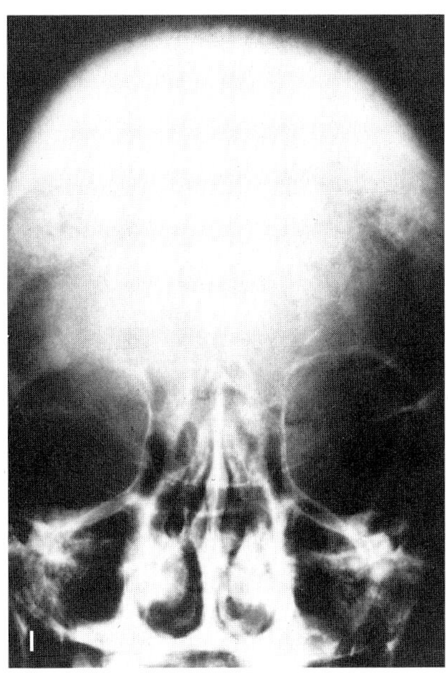

Fig. 6.16 (*continued*). **D, E** Similar supraorbital sclerosis and thickening in a patient from South America. The orbital floor is also beginning to thicken and the orbit is becoming smaller. **F, G** Widespread nocardial infection in the skull of an African patient from Kenya who has Hodgkin's lymphoma. **H, I** Another African patient, from South Africa, with an even more advanced nocardial infection of the skull. (**D, E** courtesy of Dr. Harold G. Jacobson; **H, I** courtesy of the University of Capetown Radiology Library)

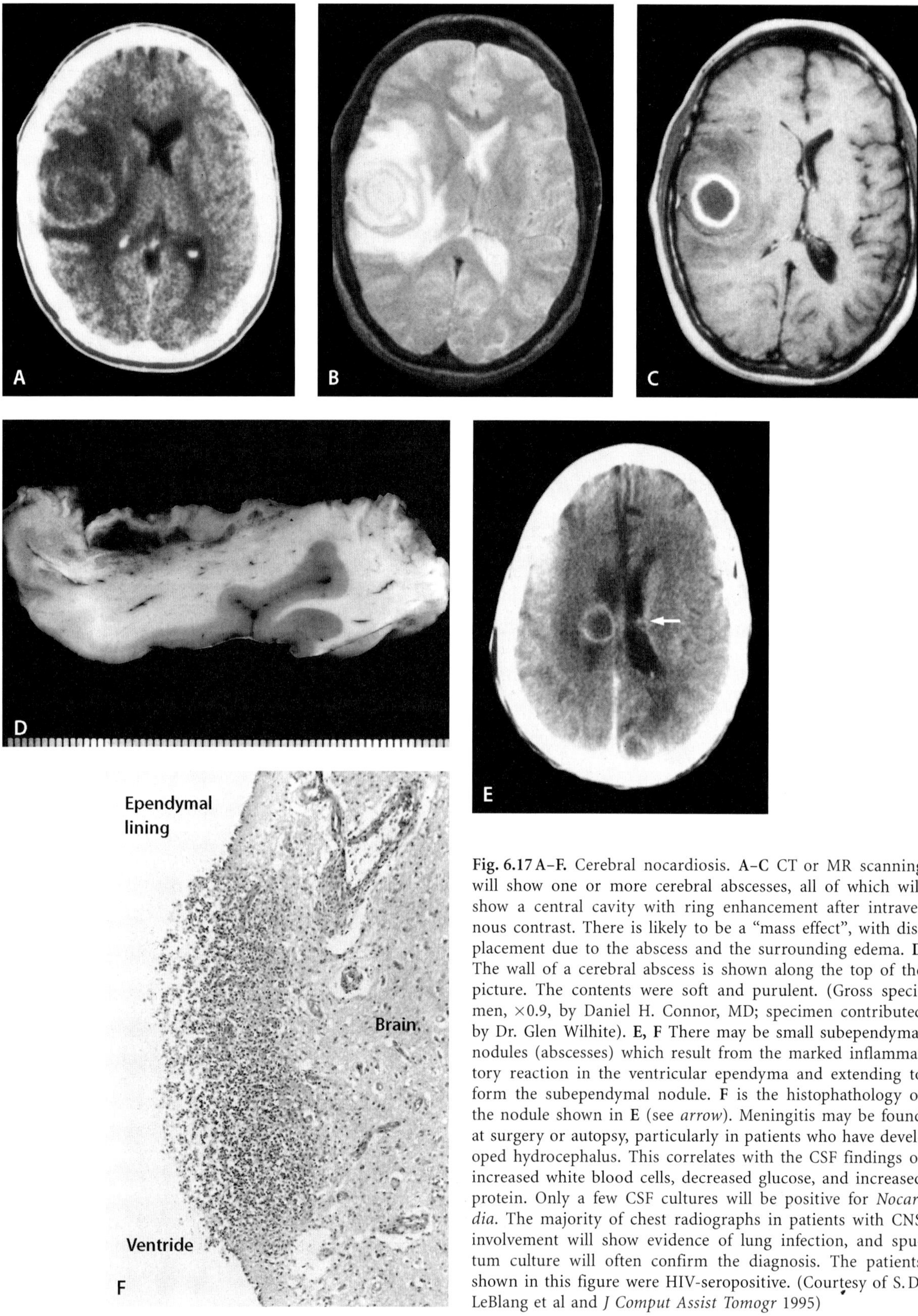

Fig. 6.17 A–F. Cerebral nocardiosis. **A–C** CT or MR scanning will show one or more cerebral abscesses, all of which will show a central cavity with ring enhancement after intravenous contrast. There is likely to be a "mass effect", with displacement due to the abscess and the surrounding edema. **D** The wall of a cerebral abscess is shown along the top of the picture. The contents were soft and purulent. (Gross specimen, ×0.9, by Daniel H. Connor, MD; specimen contributed by Dr. Glen Wilhite). **E, F** There may be small subependymal nodules (abscesses) which result from the marked inflammatory reaction in the ventricular ependyma and extending to form the subependymal nodule. **F** is the histophathology of the nodule shown in **E** (see *arrow*). Meningitis may be found at surgery or autopsy, particularly in patients who have developed hydrocephalus. This correlates with the CSF findings of increased white blood cells, decreased glucose, and increased protein. Only a few CSF cultures will be positive for *Nocardia*. The majority of chest radiographs in patients with CNS involvement will show evidence of lung infection, and sputum culture will often confirm the diagnosis. The patients shown in this figure were HIV-seropositive. (Courtesy of S. D. LeBlang et al and *J Comput Assist Tomogr* 1995)

Table 6.2. Differential diagnosis between *Nocardia*, *Actinomadura pelletieri*, and *Actinomadura madurae*

Nocardia	*Actinomadura pelletieri*	*Actinomadura madurae*
(a) Marked soft tissue involvement (b) Exuberant periosteal reaction (c) Lace-type periosteum with multiple holes 4–6 mm in size (d) Multiple bones involved in proximity (e) Can spread up to leg from the foot (f) Systemic involvement (pulmonary common) (g) Multiple sinuses (h) Mimics tuberculosis but produces more periostitis No sequestra seen	(a) Marked periosteal new bone formation (b) "Holes" 2–4 mm in size (c) Granules are red and very small (d) Aggressiveness and spread not as marked as with *Nocardia* (e) Sesamoids affected (f) Multiple bones involved (g) Joints affected: joints may ankylose	(a) Soft tissue involvement. Bone involvement (b) Moderate periosteal new bone formation: spicules, sun-ray and parallel periosteal reaction (c) Notching of bone, with constriction and moulding (d) "Holes" 5–8 mm in size (e) Large white granules (f) Osteoblastic and osteoclastic activity present (g) Sesamoids affected (h) Splaying and displacement of metacarpal and metatarsal heads

Cerebral Nocardiosis

Cerebral nocardiosis is uncommon, and is always evidence of dissemination except for very rare cases of direct implantation following trauma. Clinically, CNS nocardiosis may be silent, but eventually most patients develop symptoms related to the raised intracranial pressure from the space-occupying inflammatory mass. Brain abscesses may be multiloculated and are often multiple, but of different sizes (Fig. 6.17). Meningeal infections are uncommon. It is not possible to make an accurate etiological diagnosis by imaging alone.

Differential Diagnosis of Nocardial and Other Infections

The basic differences between infections due to *Nocardia, Actinomadura pelletieri*, and *Actinomadura madurae* are shown in Table 6.2. In nocardial infections the clinical finding of multiple sinuses is very significant, together with any bone destruction and periosteal new bone formation. Figure 6.18 C–E (see p. 556) illustrates the difference between pyogenic, fungal, and nocardial osteomyelitis; both the fungi and nocardia easily perforate the periosteum (Fig. 6.18 A, B), whereas in pyogenic osteomyelitis, the periosteum usually remains intact and forms a barrier, being elevated by the pus and lifted off the cortex.

Madura Foot; Mycetoma; Maduromycosis

Progressive swelling of the foot (or occasionally both feet) in those who work without shoes in the fields has been recognized for centuries. It was known that the feet would become lumpy, and there would eventually be draining sinuses with pus containing different colored grains. In the early and mid 19th century the condition was recorded by doctors in small hospitals in India and missionary doctors in East Africa. It was thought to be a manifestation of tuberculosis: the name "Madura foot" followed the first description in 1846 of four cases in Madras, followed in 1859 by another 40 cases from the same area. The bone destruction was soon recognized, and then the "fungus particles." The history and recognition of the multiple organisms which cause the same features is described in "Mycetoma" by E.S. Mahgoub and I.G. Murray (1973).

Synonyms

Mycetoma. Madura foot. Maduromycosis. Carter's foot. Actinomyces foot. Pseudotumors of bone. *Fr.* Madura mycose. *Ger*: Madurafuß. *Sp*: Pie de Madura.

Definition

Madura foot is, strictly, only one form of mycetoma: a true eumycetoma localized to the foot. By common usage for over hundred years, mycetoma and Madura foot became synonymous. Even now, however, Madura foot is not an accurate nomenclature because it describes but one type of mycetoma and, of course, does not only occur in Madras: more over, mycetomas do not only occur in the foot.
Maduromycosis is an indolent infection, most commonly of the foot but occurring also in the upper or lower arm, and rarely in the neck, calvarium, and elsewhere. It is caused by fungi or false fungi of many varieties. The infection slowly spreads through the soft tissues and bone. Multiple sinus

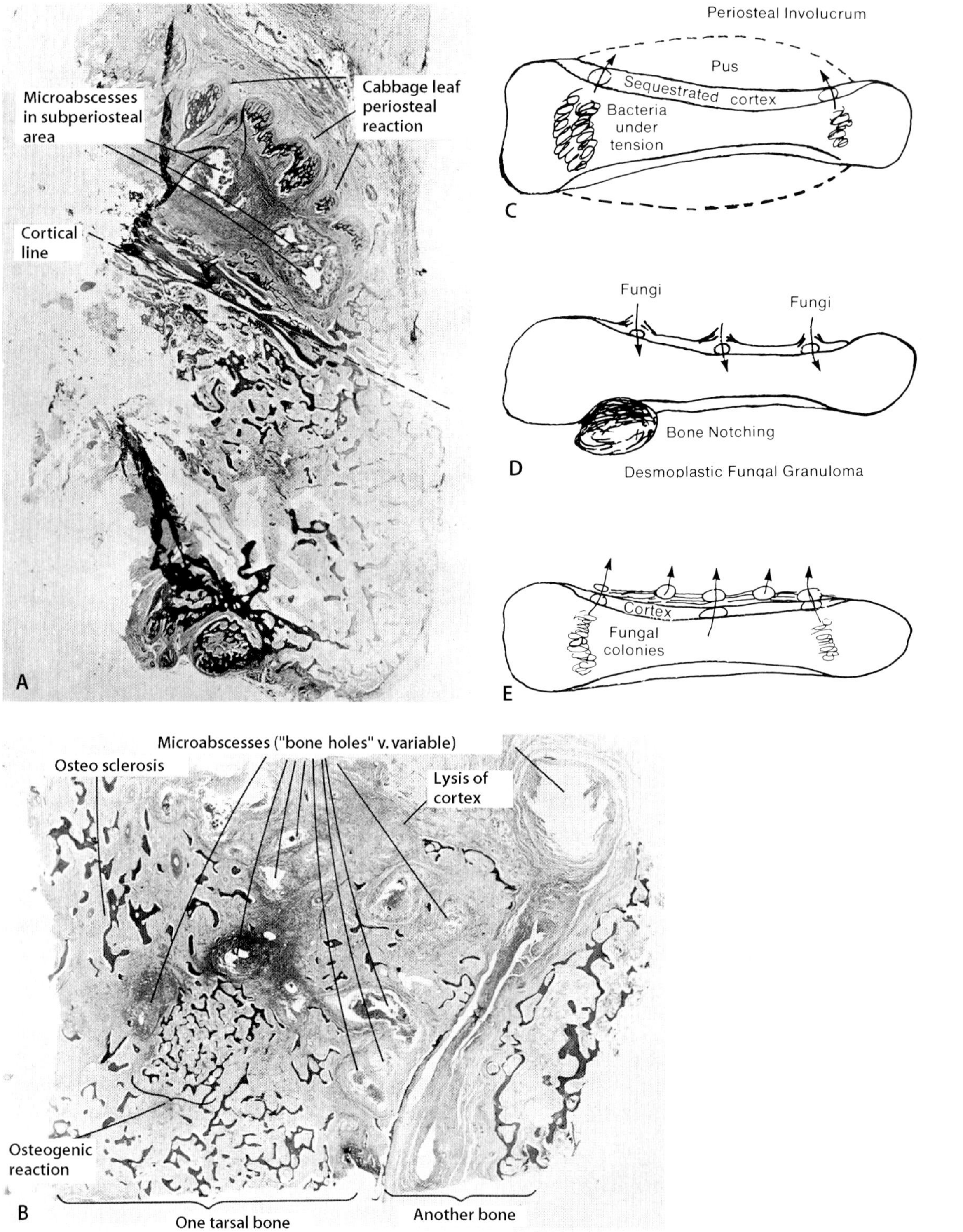

Microabscesses in subperiosteal area
Cabbage leaf periosteal reaction
Cortical line
A
Periosteal Involucrum
Pus
Sequestrated cortex
Bacteria under tension
C
Fungi
Fungi
Bone Notching
D
Desmoplastic Fungal Granuloma
Cortex
Fungal colonies
E
Microabscesses ("bone holes" v. variable)
Osteo sclerosis
Lysis of cortex
Osteogenic reaction
B
One tarsal bone
Another bone

◀ **Fig. 6.18 A, B.** The formation of microabscesses in the subperiosteum in fungal infection. **A** The microabscesses develop when there is a subperiosteal fungal colony which drains externally, giving rise to a periosteal reaction. As the abscesses drain, the periosteum is lifted and punctured, and the sinus forms. **B** When the fungal colonies and the granuloma enter a bone from the adjacent soft tissue, they "lyse" the cortex. As the microabscesses coalesce, they produce a different lucent defect radiographically. (Courtesy of Dr. Sudarisanam, Velore) **C–E** There are major differences between pyogenic, fungal, and nocardial osteomyelitis. **C** Pyogenic osteomyelitis is nearly always a hematogenous infection, so that the infective foci spread from within outwards, through cancellous bone to cortex and up to the soft tissues. Pyogenic infections form pus, but the periosteum is intact and forms a barrier, which is elevated by the pus and stripped off the cortex. This cuts off the vascular supply to the cortex and results in sequestration and devitalization. **D** In fungal osteomyelitis the infection is usually from the outside spreading inwards; the periosteum does not form a barrier and is easily perforated. This permits the visual impression of periosteum with multiple holes in the cortex. Fungal infection is much less purulent and the cortex is not devitalized. Radiologically there will be spicules of periosteal reaction where the bone is invaded, but no sequestrum. This is seen in mycetomas due to eumycetes and the streptomycetes group of schizomycetes. When there is hematogenous spread of the infection, the periosteum is easily perforated and decompression occurs without devitalization of the cortex, in such cases spreading from within outwards. **E** Nocardial osteomyelitis is a more purulent type of infection, but the fungus still easily perforates the cortex and periosteum, effectively allowing periosteal decompression in spite of the diffuse periosteal reaction. The process is the same whether the infection is hematogenous or there is local invasion from the outside into the bone. There is no sequestration in either. A similar pattern is sometimes seen in systemic hematogenous spread from other fungal groups, but for all the periosteum does not form a barrier and is easily punctured and decompressed, so that there is no cortical devitalization. (Drawings in **C–E** courtesy of Dr. A. Chandrahasan Johnson, from the first edition)

tracts drain pus to the skin surface. Madura foot and maduromycosis have become generic names, unrelated to any specific fungus or false fungus.

Geographic Distribution

Localized mycotic infections are fairly common in much of the Indian subcontinent, throughout Africa (particularly south of the Sahara), and in southern Arabia, South America, and Mexico. While occurring most frequently in the geographic zone between 15 °S und 30 °N, mycetomas are quite common in Japan and numerous cases have been reported from the southern United States. Is is difficult to link the infection to any specific climate or rainfall, but the highest incidence of mycetoma is probably in the Sudan, where over 1200 patients with mycetoma were seen during two and a half years and it was thought that 300–400 new cases developed every year. There may be even more on the Indian subcontinent, because many cases are probably not reported. Another country with a high prevalence is Mexico.

Epidemiology and Pathology

Madura foot is common in people who work in the fields and have either poor or no protection for their feet (Fig. 6.19). It has been particularly linked to minor penetrating wounds caused by thorns or splinters (cf. Fig. 6.20 E, F), and such wounds probably account for many of the other limb mycetomas. It is endemic where thorny acacia trees are common. Whether the organisms are in the soil or growing on the acacia thorns is not decided, but thorns have been found deep within mycetomas (including one in the brain of a child). Those who carry baskets of vegetables or wood on their shoulders or head are likely to get mycotic infections in those sites. It is certain that the true incidence of mycetoma is under-recorded, because in many tropical countries patients with mycetomas are seen so frequently that this tpye of infection causes little comment. Because patients do not suffer much pain or disability in the early stages, they are late in reporting to hospital.

The causative organisms of mycetoma form clusters of grains at the center of the lesion, surrounded by a rim of eosinophilic material (Splendore-Hoeppli) which is in turn surrounded by an abscess and granulomatous reaction. Around the grains will be neutrophils and in the older infections, the fungal grains may degenerate and there will be multinucleated giant cells and epithelioid cells. The perimeter is granulation tissue containing lymphocytes, plasma cells, and histocytes. The histopathological changes are similar regardless of the causal organism (Fig. 6.20 D). The fistulae and sinus tracts start in the skin surface, with sinuses opening from nodular bumps on the dorsal and plantar aspects of the foot (or wherever the mycetoma may be situated). The sinuses discharge fungal grains which can be recognized clinically, and clearly seen when pressed between two glass slides.

There is great geographic variation in the etiology of mycetoma. The most frequent organisms are *Madurella mycetomi, Madurella grisea, Pseudallescheria boydii, Leptosphaeria senegalensis, Streptomyces somaliensis, Actinomadura madurae, Actinomadura pelletieri*, and *Nocardia brasiliensis*. Other organisms are very occasionally responsible but it may be impossible to recognize them.

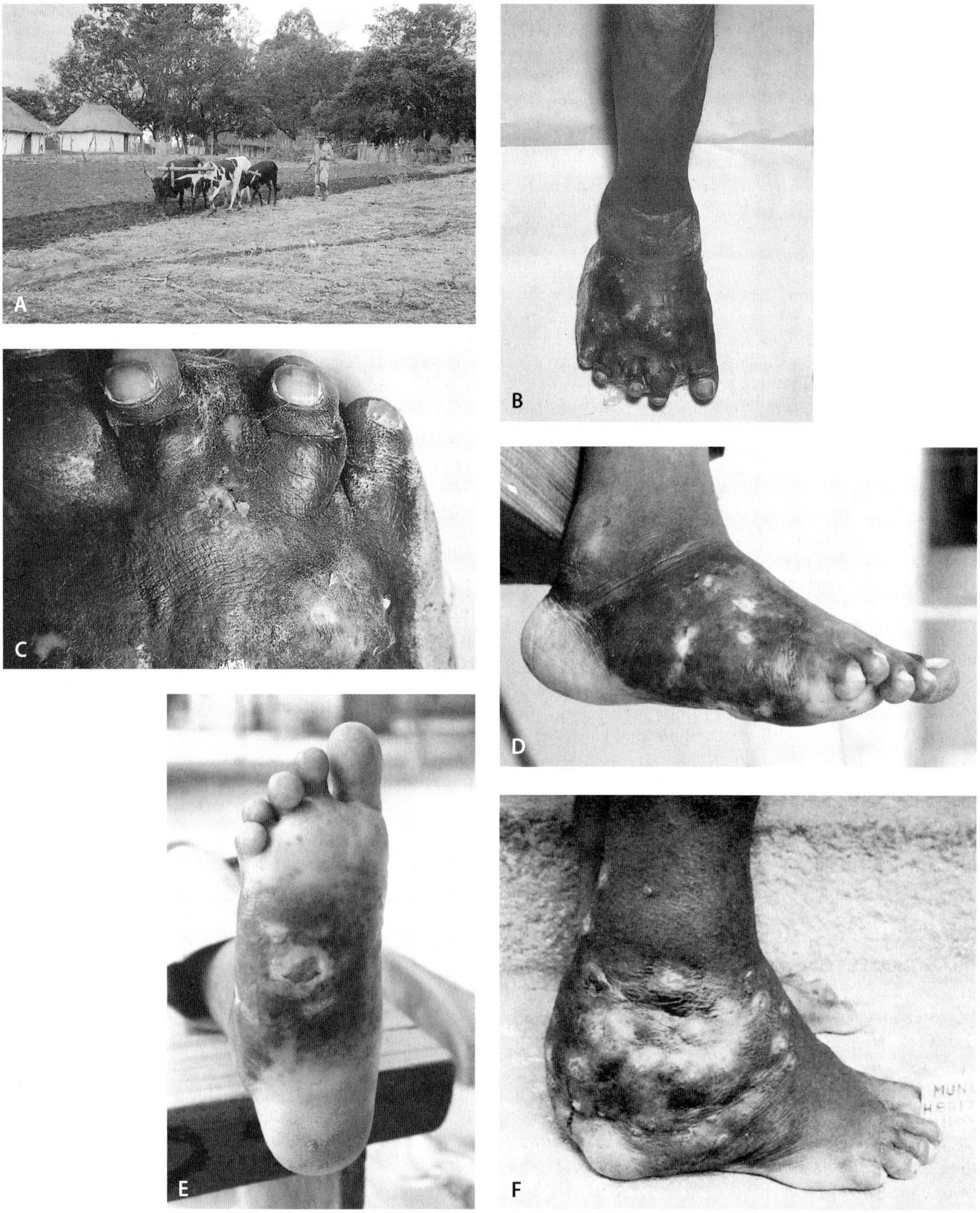

Fig. 6.19. A Agricultural laborers who work without adequate foot protection are the most likely to suffer from a "madura foot", but the clinical presentation is very similar in different countries and with different fungi. **B, C** The swollen foot and ankle of an African from Zimbabwe with multiple discharging sinuses. His main complaint was that it had become a nuisance! **D, E** A similar chronic infection is a 35-year-old African from Tanzania. The large ulcer on the sole of his foot caused very little discomfort. **F** In this Indian patient the ankle is more affected than the foot, but the nodular, grained discharging sinuses are typical of a mycetoma

There is some anatomical variation in the frequency with which the fungi cause infection, for example in the Sudan *M. mycetoma* accounts for the majority of infections of the feet, but *S. somaliensis* is the likely cause of mycetomas around the head and neck. Considering the number of children watching cattle, fetching firewood and playing in soil in which these organisms are frequently found, it is surprising that mycetomas are relatively infrequent in children and females.

Clinical Characteristics

Almost all mycetomas start as a localized nodule or, less commonly, an abscess: all have a long history, often many months or even years. Progress is very slow, but eventually multiple abscesses and sinus tracts develop (Fig. 6.20 A–C). The initial mycetoma usually starts in one foot (or one other localized site) and the whole foot will eventually become swollen. Pain is not significant, and the patient walks on the infected foot, which can carry the full weight of the body. The skin surface will be discolored and as the sinuses start to form, there will also be atrophic scars: the discharge is odorless. There is often secondary bacterial infection, which causes local ulceration and an unpleasant odor.

The sinuses develop in the center of the multiple nodules and are lined by red granulation tissue. The discharge from the sinuses is serosanguinous and purulent with creamy yellowish pus and multiple grains of different colors and sizes. Neither the color nor the size of the grains can be used to recognize the organism, because large, medium, or small grains can come from the same infection. Some grains are soft, others are hard.

The whole infectious process of swelling, nodulation, and sinus formation spreads locally for months and years, usually tracking along some cutaneous fascial planes and causing marked induration. The speed at which the sinuses develop varies greatly: they are seldom apparent in less than 3 months, but by the end of the first 12 months, almost every mycetoma will have discharging sinuses. Once drainage has started, it may continue for a long time, or close spontaneously. The number of sinuses and the amount of swelling provide an indication of the extent but not the duration of the infection.

When bone becomes infected, there is little pain on weight bearing until late in the disease. This lack of pain is probably because the organisms which cause mycetoma penetrate the periosteum and there is no increase in subperiosteal pressure. Tendons, nerves, and muscles are not usually involved so that the movement of the foot (or arm) is often little affected until the infection has spread extensively. There is very little systemic reaction: there is seldom any fever, anemia, weight loss, or other sign of systemic ill health.

Spread along a limb is usually through lymphatics; regional lymph nodes become enlarged, but seldom contain the causative organism. In one series of 949 mycetomas, the typical grains were only found in the regional nodes of 13 patients. Hematogenous spread is very uncommon, so that it is rare to have mycetoma in multiple sites. (This is not true in fungal pulmonary infections.)

If untreated, mycetomas continue to spread for many years, the outcome depending on the organism concerned. The actinomycetes infections often progress more rapidly than infection caused by eumycetes (true fungi).

The clinical differential diagnosis is very dependent on the long history, and the discharging sinuses. The embedded foreign body, if found, provides further evidence. Early lesions have been mistaken to pyogenic granulomas or, in some countries, tuberculosis: some resemble Kaposi sarcoma. If the surface of the skin is unbroken and if bones are not involved, the initial swelling be mistaken for a lipoma. As soon as there are sinuses, and grains are recognized, and particularly when there is bone destruction, the diagnosis of mycetoma is straightforward: defining the causative organism may be more difficult.

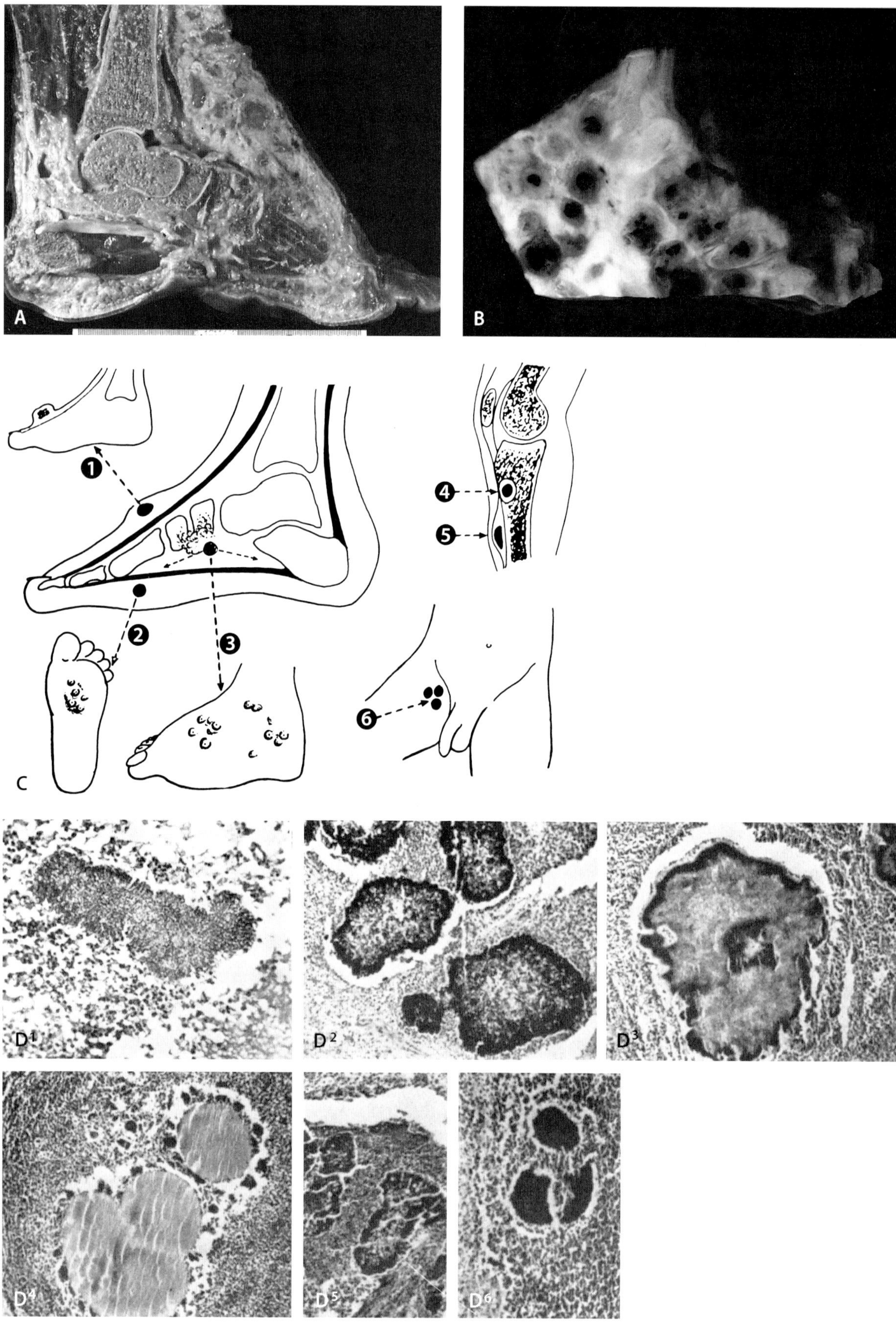
A
B
1
2
3
4
5
6
C
D1
D2
D3
D4
D5
D6

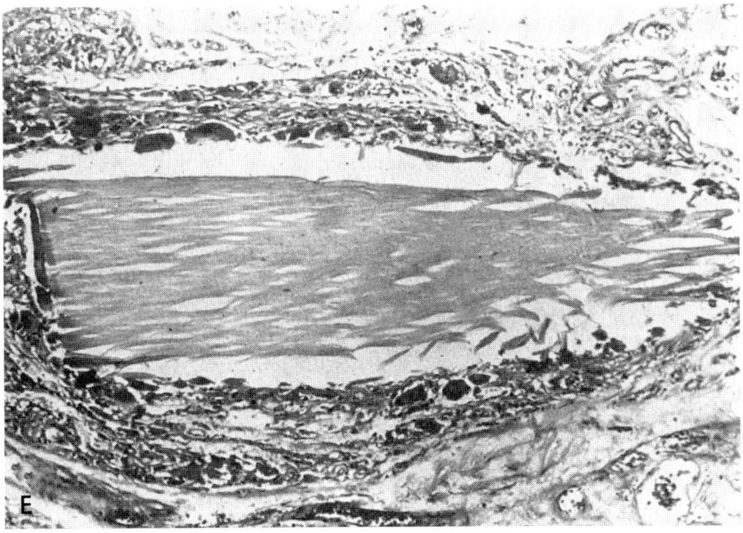

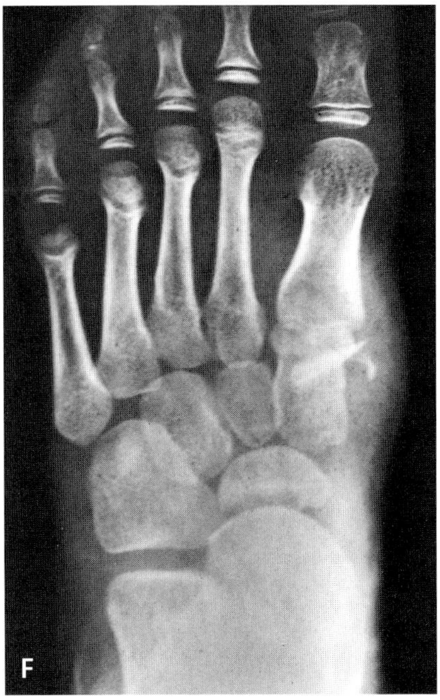

◀ **Fig. 6.20.** **A** The longitudinal section of an amputated foot with severe mycotic infection, causing deep abscesses and marked destruction of all the tissues. (The same patient from Uganda as Fig. 6.9 D.). **B** In this excised specimen from Australia the black grains are surrounded by pyogranulomatous foci. **C** The clinical patterns of mycetoma: *1* A subcutaneous nodule; *2* superficial plantar nodules; *3* nodules deep to the plantar ligament with diffuse bone invasion; *4* primary foci within bone; *5* primary periosteal foci; *6* spread to lymph nodes. **D** The grains of the different fungi are usually easy to recognize on histological section. *1 Actinomadura pelletieri*; *2 Leptosphaeria senegalensis*; *3 Actinomadura madurae*; *4 Streptomyces somaliensis*; *5 Nocardia brasiliensis*; *6 Madurella mycetomi* (sections 1, 4 and 6 courtesy of Prof. R. Camain) **E** Sometimes the cause of the infection can be found, as in the case of this thorn embedded in the soft tissues surrounded by multiple fungal colonies. **F** Occasionally such splinters are visible on radiographs, as on the medial side of the first metatarsal joint of this young African. (**A** courtesy of Dr. Daniel H. Connor; **B** courtesy of Dr. Ian S. Wilkey; **C** from W.W. Davey: *Companion to surgery in Africa*. Edinburgh, E. & S. Livingstone, 1968)

Imaging Diagnosis

The initial well-circumscribed soft tissue nodule can be demonstrated by ultrasonography (or radiographs or MRI) for a long time before any other abnormality develops. An embedded foreign body should be sought. In the foot there will eventually be multifocal osteomyelitis beneath the soft tissue swelling, affecting many of the small bones (Fig. 6.21). A moth-eaten appearance develops, with lucent defects of variable size, ranging in diameter from 3 to 8 mm. Unlike most cases of tuberculosis, there will be abundant periosteal reaction. The periosteum does not form a barrier to the fungi or actinomycetes, which produce multiple lytic defects in the periosteum, allowing the purulent discharge of colonies from within the cancellous bone. Because there is no tension within the periosteum, the blood supply to the bone ist not interrupted and there is no sequestrum (see Fig. 6.18 C–E). Ultrasonography and MRI can show the subcutaneous abscesses beneath the nodules, from which sinuses discharge.

The joint spaces are preserved until late in the disease (Fig. 6.22), but the sesamoid bones can be affected. Eventually the intraosseous microabscesses coalesce and communicate internally, and the articular cartilage becomes involved. In the later stages, due to either fungal arthritis or secondary infection, bony fusion develops across the joint. If the intraosseous or subcutaneous abscesses communicate with sinuses to the skin, air may be found in the smooth, cyst-like cavities from which the contents have been discharged. Arteriography shows that the granulomatous areas are hypervascular. They "blush" because of surrounding granulomatous tissue. The vascularity of these pseudotumors often seems to extend into the bones with a desmoplastic reaction.

As shown in Table 6.3, radiologically there is a difference between the eumycetomas and the actinomycetomas. Another significant difference is that some fungal infections involve only the foot (or other local area), whereas other spread up the leg or limb (Fig. 6.23). This provides an early screening method in the identification of the organisms.

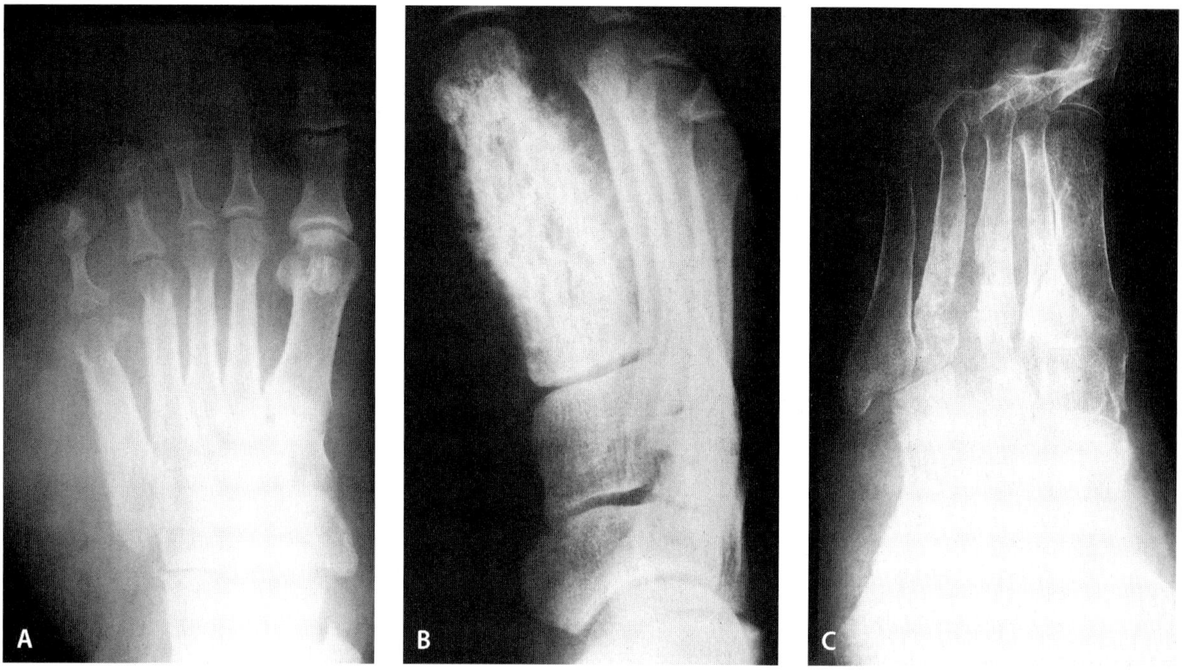

Fig. 6.21 A–C. Madura foot caused by three different types of fungal infection. **A** Marked soft tissue swelling around infection of the fifth metatarsal, spreading to the edge of the fourth metatarsal (*Nocardia*). **B** A spiculated infection of the shaft of the first metatarsal, not involving any other part of the foot (*S. somaliensis*). **C** A destructive infection, but with less periosteal reaction, involving the proximal end of the second metatarsal and spreading up the shafts of the third and fourth metatarsals. The adjoining tarsal bones are also infected (*Madurella*). (Courtesy of University of Capetown Radiology Library)

Table 6.3. True and false fungal infections

	True fungal infections (eumycetomas)	False fungal infections (actinomycetomas)
General course of disease	Less invasive	Highly invasive
Soft tissue changes	(a) Long history (years) (b) Slow spread (c) Significant localized mass	(a) Shorter history (months) (b) Faster spread
Periosteum	Mild to moderate periosteal reaction	Marked to exuberant periosteal reaction
Bone	Marked plastic moulding Fewer and larger "holes" Sesamoid involvement rare Joints rarely involved	Moth-eaten appearance Multiple smaller "holes" Sesamoid involvement common Joints frequently involved Subarticular osteoporosis+

Radionuclide scans are useful because they will demonstrate sites of infection which have not been recognized clinically or radiographically. Unfortunately, as is often the case with radiographs (Fig. 6.24), they do not help in the recognition of the causal fungus.

If treatment is succesful, the extent of healing may be remarkable. The periosteal reaction coalesces, forming a "melting snow" appearance on the cortex of the small bones. Spontaneous remission is not recorded, but in some patients there may be temporary improvement.

Kaposi sarcoma must be considered in the differential diagnosis, especially in those areas where Kaposi sarcoma is common, even in patients who are HIV-negative. In Kaposi sarcoma, one foot may by be swollen, with multiple soft tissue nodules and destruction of the bones of the foot (or insome patients, the hand), and it may be difficult to distinguish between Kaposi sarcoma and mycetoma (cf. Fig. 6.24 A). In most patients with Kaposi sarcoma, further spread of the nodules up the leg, or onto the other leg (or arm), occurs quite rapidly, whereas the progress of mycetoma is slow and extremely chronic. Surgical excision has been advised in some cases of mycetoma to remove the "mass" of infected tissue and, in the end, even amputation may be necessary.

(Text continues on p. 566)

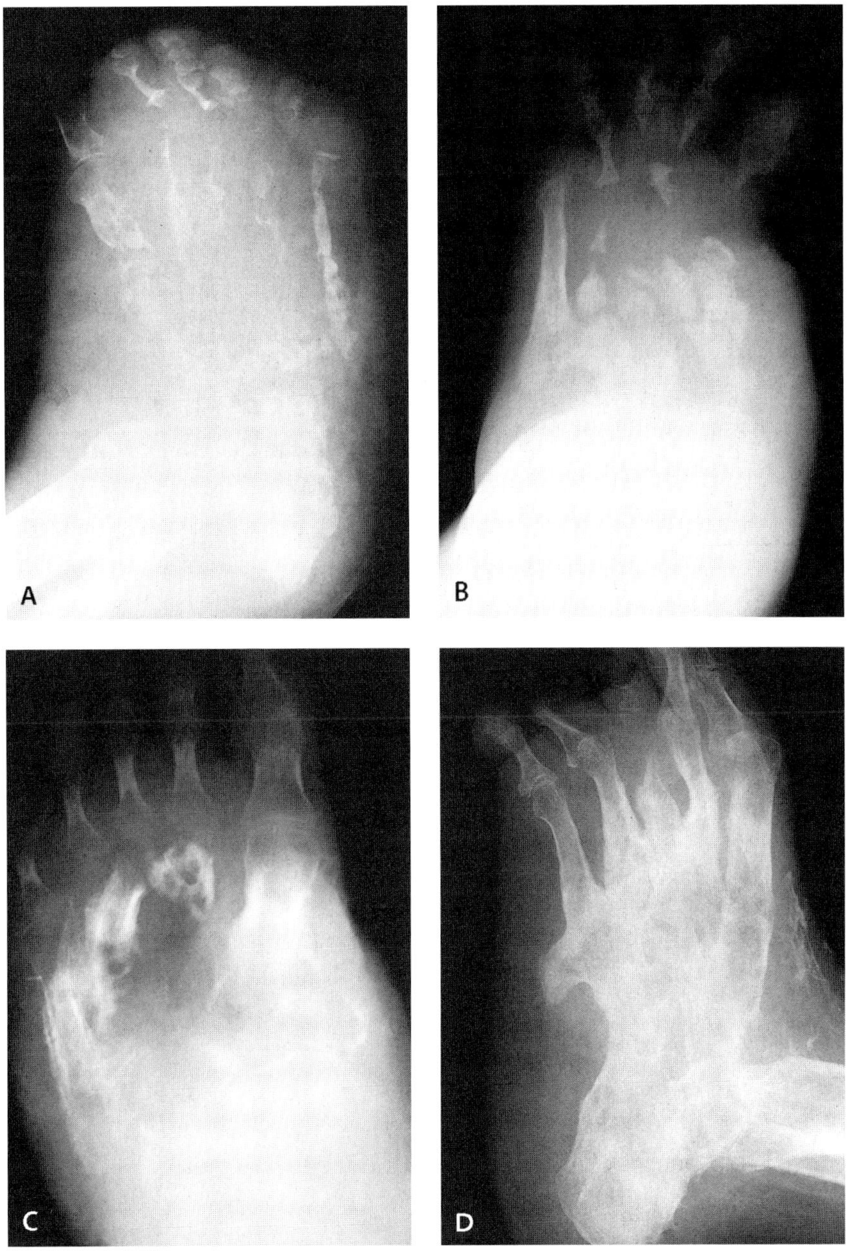

Fig. 6.22 A–D. Advanced madura foot. Tarsal infections can be very destructive of both soft tissues and bone, but many patients complain more of the size of the foot and difficulty in walking, rather than of pain. In **D** the infection may be burned out and there is bony fusion across the joints. This patient was only 34 years old. Patients **A** and **B** came from Zimbabwe and Kenya, patients **C** and **D** from India. (**C**, **D** courtesy of Dr. Harold G. Jacobson)

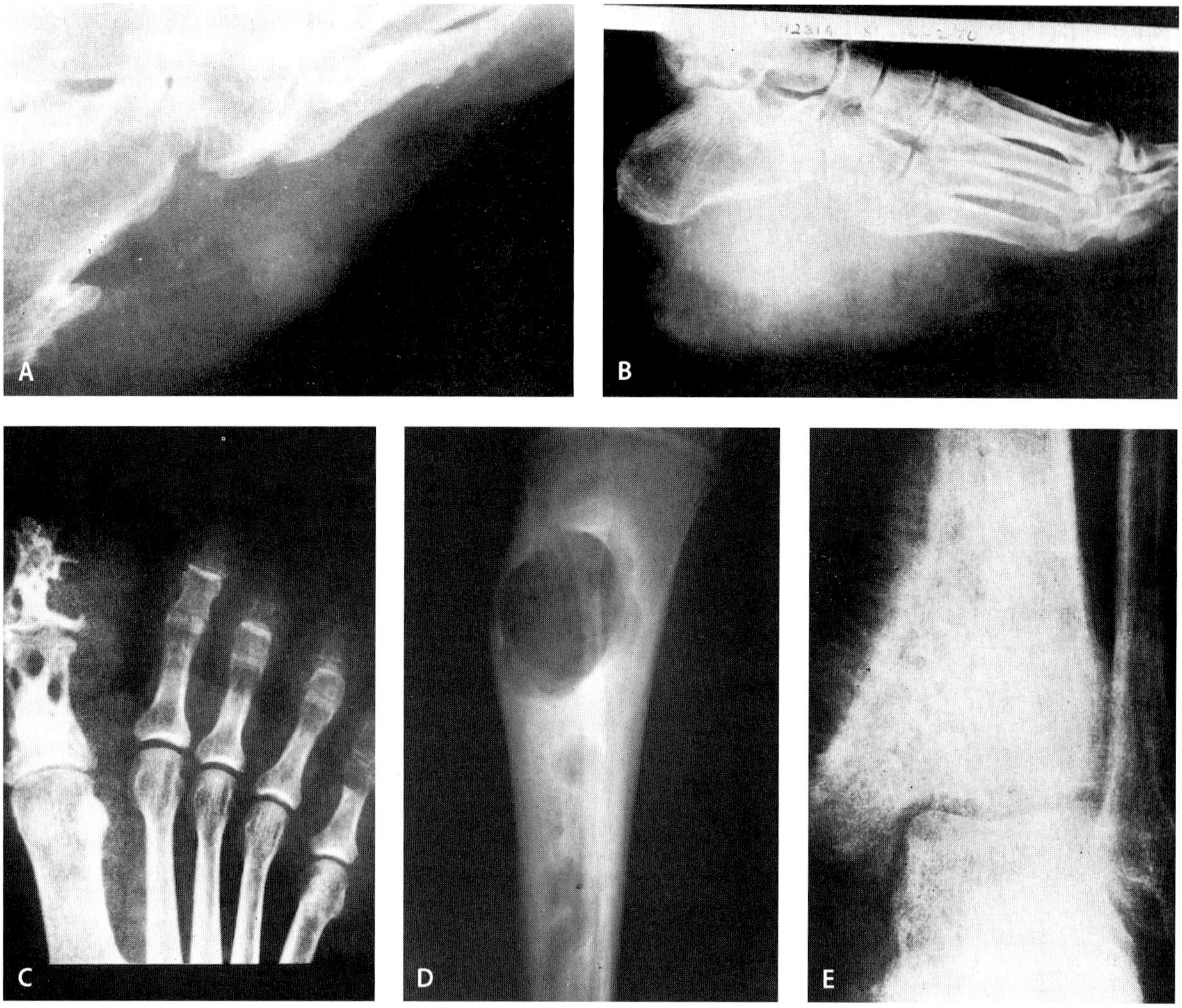

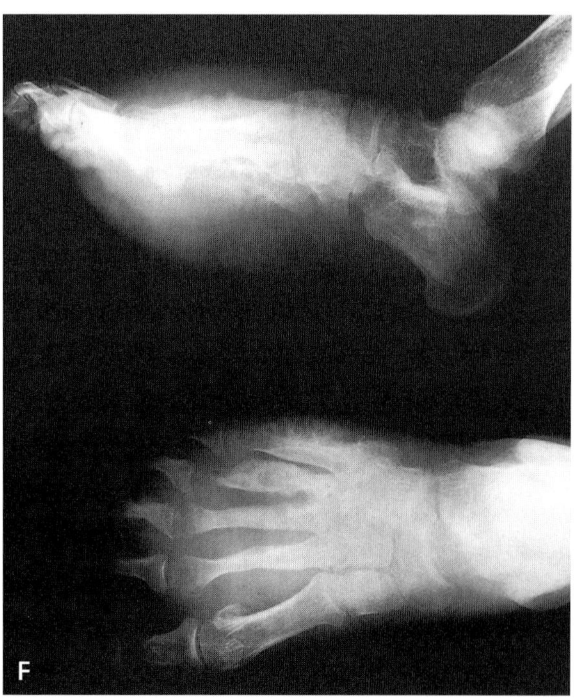

Fig. 6.23 A–F. The pattern of development of madura foot demonstrated by examples of the true fungus *Madurella mycetomi* group. **A** A fungal granuloma on the sole of the foot, superficial to the ligaments. This will stay localized for a long period but can grow to a large size and resemble a tumor. **B** This large fungal mass of *Madurella mycetomi* is deep to the plantar ligament. The bone has not been affected. **C** *Madurella* infection can be localized, involving the soft tissue as well as the bone, which has been molded. There are large circular cavities in the phalanges, surrounded by a dense sclerotic reaction: this usually indicates a secondary infection. There are well-defined periosteal buttresses. **D** An unusual *Madurella* infection in the upper end of the tibia with multiple large defects and only minimal bone reaction. **E** The marked spiculated reaction of *Streptomyces somaliensis* with numerous underlying lucent defects: the lower end of the tibia with some minimal reaction around the fibula. **F** A more extensive *S. somaliensis* reaction affecting soft tissues and bones of the lateral aspect of the foot. (**F** courtesy of Dr. Harold G. Jacobson)

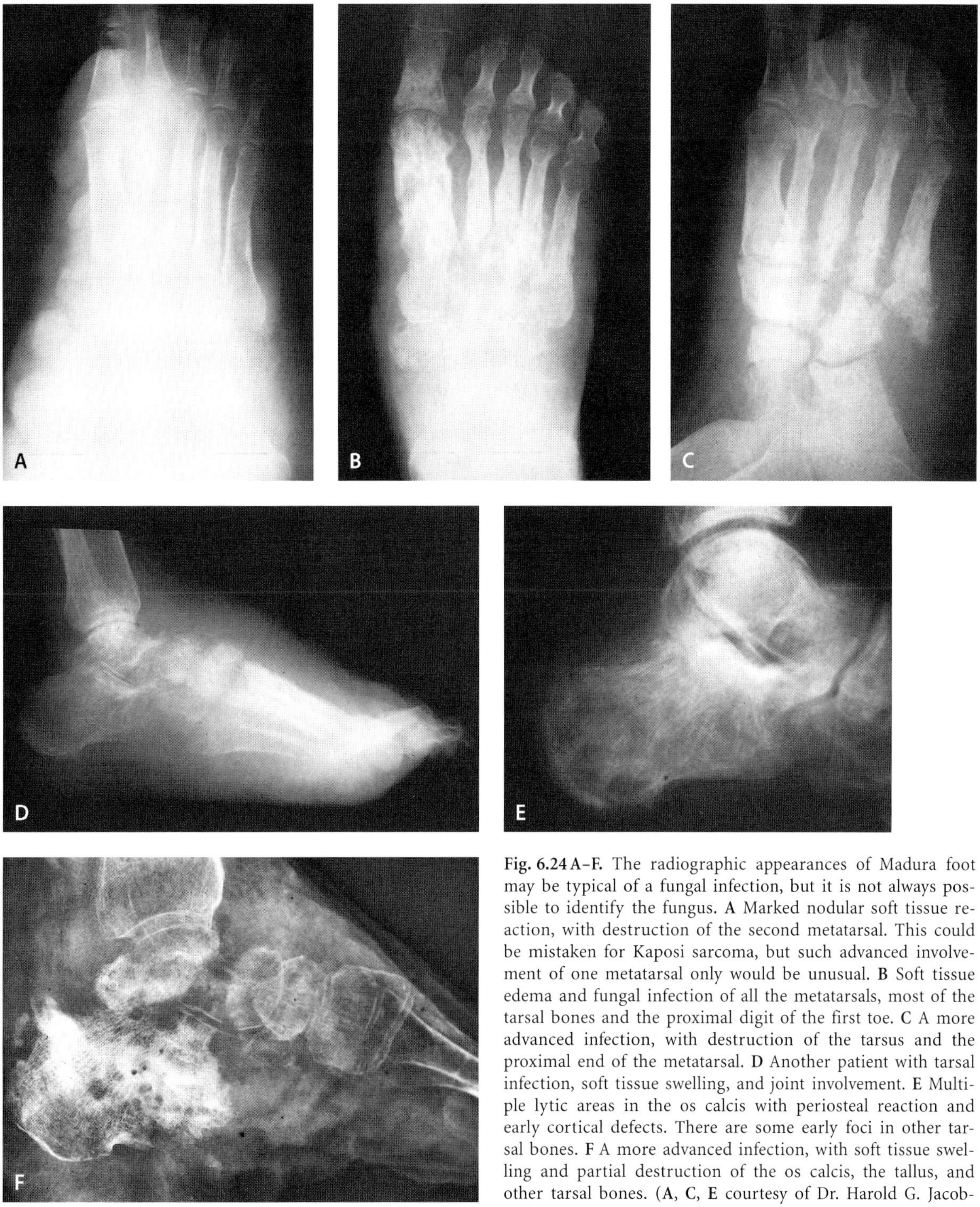

Fig. 6.24 A–F. The radiographic appearances of Madura foot may be typical of a fungal infection, but it is not always possible to identify the fungus. **A** Marked nodular soft tissue reaction, with destruction of the second metatarsal. This could be mistaken for Kaposi sarcoma, but such advanced involvement of one metatarsal only would be unusual. **B** Soft tissue edema and fungal infection of all the metatarsals, most of the tarsal bones and the proximal digit of the first toe. **C** A more advanced infection, with destruction of the tarsus and the proximal end of the metatarsal. **D** Another patient with tarsal infection, soft tissue swelling, and joint involvement. **E** Multiple lytic areas in the os calcis with periosteal reaction and early cortical defects. There are some early foci in other tarsal bones. **F** A more advanced infection, with soft tissue swelling and partial destruction of the os calcis, the tallus, and other tarsal bones. (**A**, **C**, **E** courtesy of Dr. Harold G. Jacobson)

Streptomycosis madurae

Synonyms

Actinomadura madurae. Nocardia indica.

Definition

Streptomycosis madurae is an infection with *Actinomadura madurae*, causing chronic granulomatous suppurative disease, most often localized in one foot and affecting the bones extensively (see previous section).

Geographic Distribution

Actinomadura madurae is very widespread: it is found in India, Africa (especially North Africa), Mexico, and the Mediterranean countries. It is common in South America and has been reported occasionally in other parts of the world.

Epidemiology and Pathology

The mode of entry is through the skin, often of the unshod or poorly protected foot of a farmer or other field worker. The primary lesion is locally invasive and slowly progressive. It forms a hard, localized tumor-like mass which subsequently softens at the center due to necrosis. The necrotic contents are then discharged through a sinus. The infection spreads more deeply, breaching the muscle and fascial planes. As the infection traverses the tissue layers and invades bone, abscesses form aroung the colonies of branching filamentous bacteria, and a granulomatous reaction surrounds the abscess. Sinuses discharge yellow sulfur grains (bacterial colonies) and necrotic tissue. A. madurae grows slowly on artificial media and forms a white or yellow tinted colony.

Clinical Characteristics

The patients are usually in good health: the clinical history starts with tissue damage (from a splinter, bite, or other injury) a few months or even years previously. There is relatively little pain and walking is possible even when the infection is in the foot. The tissues are swollen and covered by multiple nodules, each containing a sinus (see p. 559 for a more detailed description)

Imaging Diagnosis

Imaging shows the soft tissue nodular masses and their extent (Fig. 6.25). When there is a granuloma growing slowly near a bone, there will be a smooth indentation causing progressive notching of the cortex. If this granuloma is situated between closely opposed bones, or joints, such as the metatarsal heads, the bones will be forced apart as the granuloma enlarges. This is a frequent finding. Although the infection may spread widely, remarkably the arch of the foot is usually preserved.
Actinomadura madurae easily invades bone: the periosteum "gives way." Where bone has been invaded, there are spicules of reactive periosteal new bone which can be clearly imaged. Lucent defects develop in the cortex, about 6 mm in diameter and uniform in size in any part of the bone, whether mid-shaft or at the ends (Fig. 6.25 E). There can be large defects in the sesamoid bones. In the later stages the joints become affected (see Table 6.2, p. 555).
Arteriography shows that the granulomas are hyperemic and contain microarteriovenous fistulae. The contrast causes a "blush" and there is early venous return.

Streptomycosis Somaliensis

Infection by *Streptomyces somaliensis* closely resembles the pathological, clinical, and radiological findings due to *A. madurae*. It occurs in the people who live in deserts in the tropics, particularly in East Africa. Colonies grow more rapidly on culture, and are variable in shape and color. The yellow grain is usually very hard, regular, and round or oval.
Skeletal infection causes marked periosteal new bone formation. The holes are slightly smaller than those of infection by *Nocardia* spp. or *A. madurae*. The granules are smaller than those of *A. madurae*, yellow to brown, and hard.

Actinomadura Pelletieri

Synonyms

Nocardia africanus. Micrococcus pelletieri. Madura foot (there are other causes of this condition, see p. 555). *Ger: Nocardia madurae, pelletieri. Fr*: Actinomycete de madurae pelletieri. *Sp. Streptomices pelletieri.*

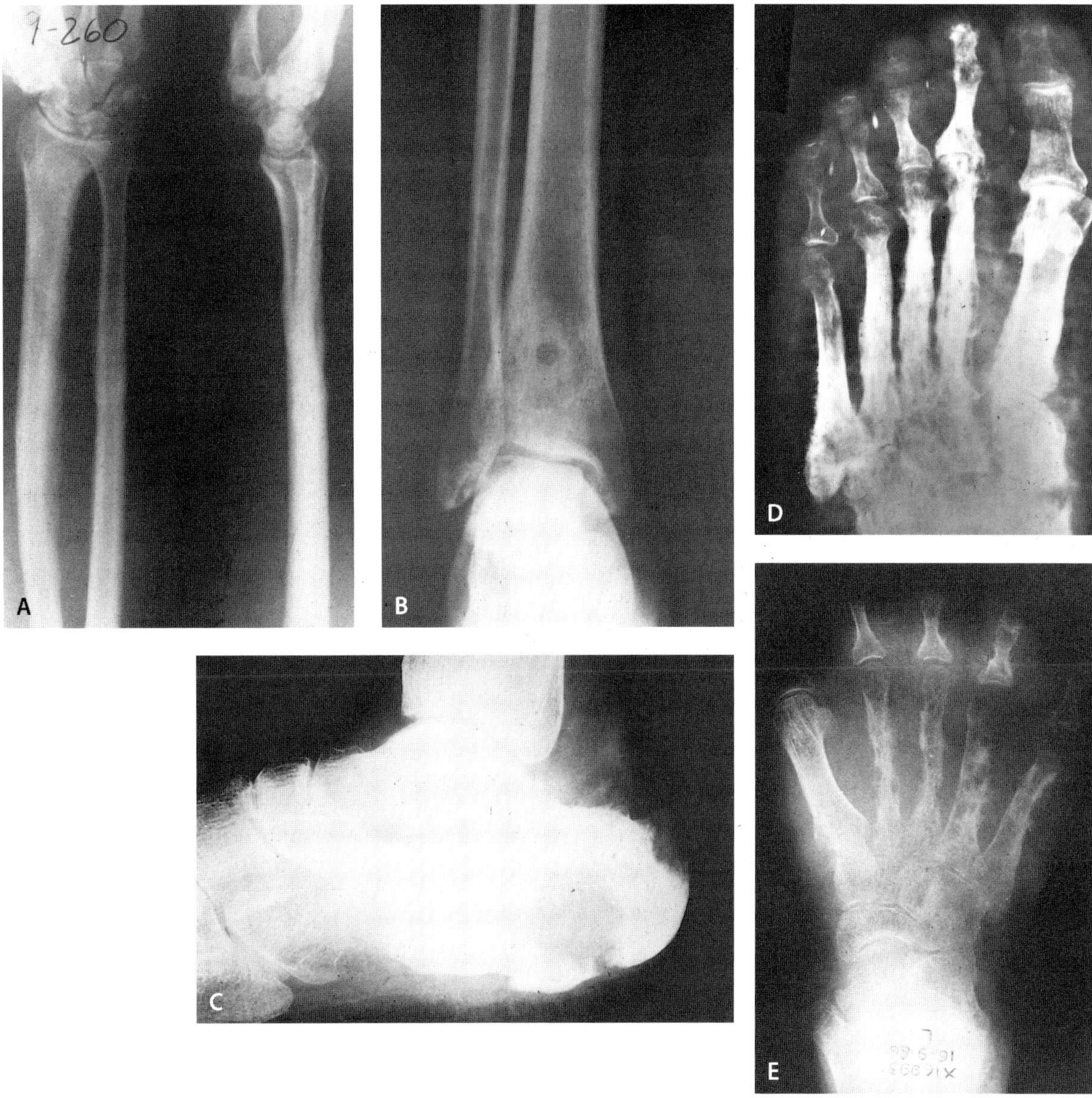

Fig. 6.25 A–E. Infections with *Actinomadura madurae*. **A, B** Early infection in the lower end of the radius (**A**) and the lower end of the tibia (**B**) (different patients). **C** A large abscess in the os calcis causing a lytic lesion and breaking through the cortex inferiorally. There is already loss of trabecular pattern and some increased sclerosis due to multiple microfractures. These can be better demonstrated by standard tomography or CT. **D** An extensive infection of the foot involving all the metatarsals and the adjoining tarsals and spreading through the joints into the second toe. **E** Marked soft tissue swelling and extensive bone involvement. The metatarsal heads are splayed outwards. There are multiple lytic foci (5–6 mm) and the cortex is notched. There are spicules of periosteal new bone and the joints are affected. Most of the tarsal bones, including the os calcis, were also affected in this patient. (**B** courtesy of Dr. Harold G. Jacobson)

Definition

A chronic granulomatous, suppurative mycotic disease usually localized to one foot, caused by *Actinomadura pelletieri*. The deep structures are affected.

Geographic Distribution

This infection is common in India, Africa, Mexico, and countries around the Mediterranean. It is particularly frequent in West Africa and India.

Epidemiology and Pathology

The mode of entry is through the skin. The organism grows slowly in culture. The grains are garnet red and vary from soft to quite firm. Multiple bones and the sesamoids are affected, as are the joints, which may ankylose. *A pelletieri* is more aggressive than *A. madurae*, but less aggressive than *Nocardia* spp. It causes a marked inflammatory reaction.

Clinical Characteristics

The clinical findings are much the same as those of *A. madurae*, but the infection is more likely to extend from the foot up to the leg and is much more locally aggressive. The soft tissue sinus holes are smaller than those in *Nocardia* spp. and *A. madurae* infections.

Imaging Diagnosis

The soft tissue nodules are smaller than those caused by *A. madurae* or *Nocardia* spp. The lucent bone defects are very small, averaging about 2 mm (Fig. 6.26). The periosteal spicules are also smaller but there is intense periosteal new bone, with sclerosis. This results in apparent thickening of the shafts of the metatarsals, which may become double their normal diameter. There is no sequestration, because the multiple lucent areas (the microabscesses) and the sinus tracts effectively decompress the cortex and the periosteum and prevent devitalization of the remaining bone (see Fig. 6.18 D).
Actinomadura pelletieri is the most aggressive of the three streptomyces and frequently extends up the tibia and fibula, whereas *A. madurae* and *S. somaliensis* tend to remain below the level of the ankle. The increased aggressiveness also causes joint involvement, destruction of the articular cartilage, and eventually fusing of the joints by bony ankylosis. Even large joints, such as the ankle, may be fused by *A. pelletieri*.
Table 6.2 (p. 555) assists with the differential diagnosis of bone infection with *Nocardia, A. pelletieri*, and *A. madurae*.

Zygomycosis/Mucormycosis

The best way to start this section is with an extract from Medical Mycology by Drs. Kwon-Chung, and Bennett (Lea and Febiger, Philadelphia, 1992): "The changing terminology for mucormycosis and many of its causative agents has complicated their retrieval from the literature and confused clinicians ... the name mucormycosis has been used extensively and is retained as a medical subhead for indexing ... the older term, phycomycosis is unacceptable because the class of phycomycetes no longer exists. The more recent term zygomycosis ... is usually too imprecise to be helpful (*for an individual patient)*".
It seems probable that not only clinicians are confused?

Synonyms

Mucormycosis, Phycomycosis. Entomophthoromycosis. It is likely that many cases of entomophthoromycosis have been described under headings of infection with mucormycosis (see under definition).

Definition

Zygomycosis is the general term for an infection caused by pathogenic zygomycetes of the orders Murocales and Entomophthorales.
Mucormycosis is a systemic fungal infection caused the genera *Rhizopus, Mucor,* or *Absidia*. Less often it is due to *Cunninghamella* or *Saksenaea*.
Entomophthoromycosis is infection caused by one of the Entomophthorales, usually *Basidiobolus haptosporus* or *Conidiobolus coronatus*, and very rarely *Conidio bolus incongruus*. These infections have epidemiological, clinical, and pathological differences from mucormycosis. It seems very possible that clinical and imaging descriptions have not made a clear differentiation, which may be more important therapeutically than for other reasons.

Geographic Distribution

Zygomycetes are found worldwide: infections have been reported from the Indian subcontinent, Africa, South America, Asia, Europe, and the United States.

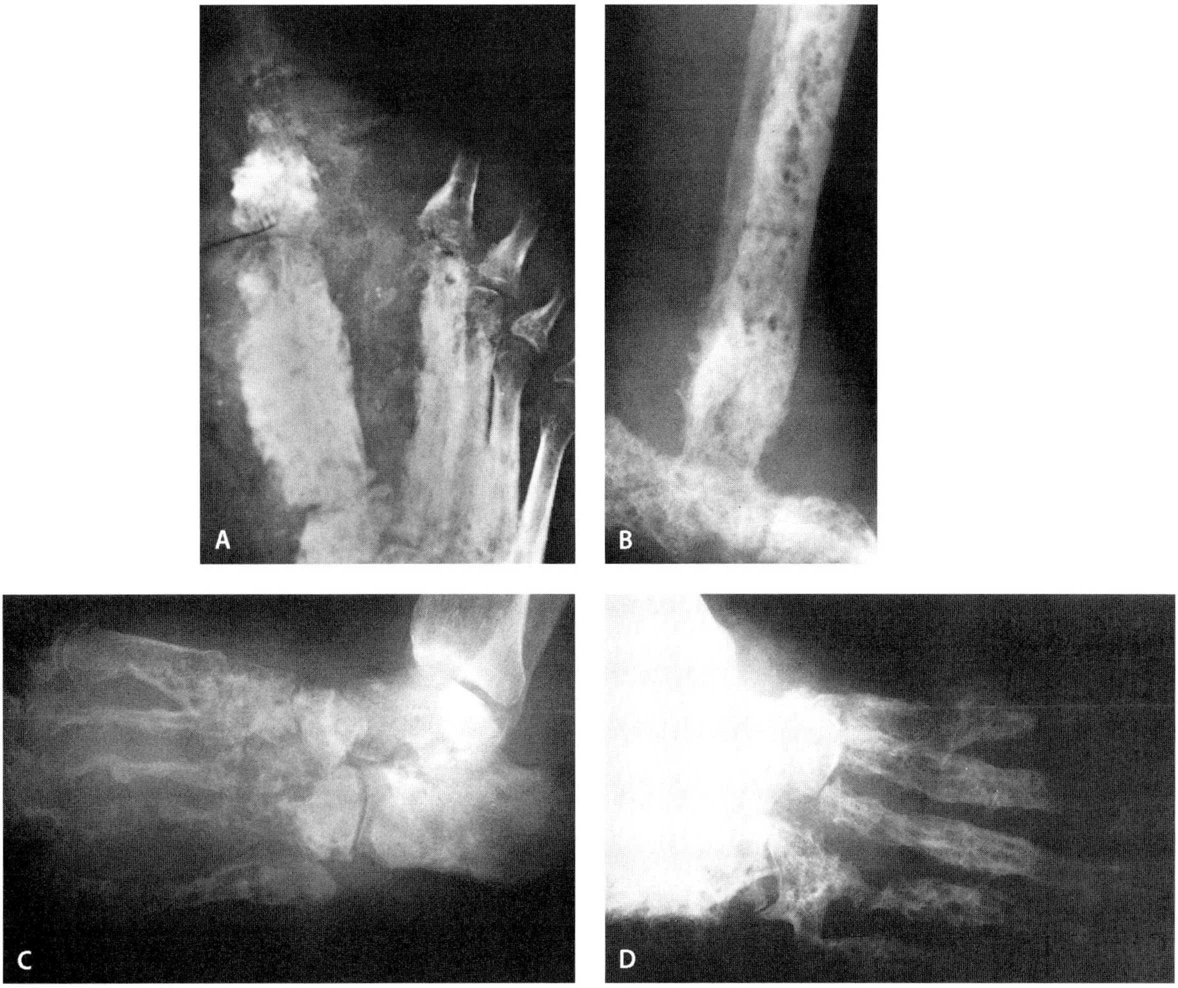

Fig. 6.26 A–D. *Actinomadura pelletieri* is an aggressive fungus: in the foot, multiple small bones are usually affected and show numerous small bony cortical defects and an exuberant periosteal reaction. The average diameter of the holes is 2 mm but they may be obscured as the periosteal and new bone formation develop. The end result shows extensive destruction. **A** Soft tissue swelling, with multiple sinuses visible around infection of the first four metatarsals and adjoining tarsal bones. **B** *A. pelletieri* can extend from the foot into the tibia and fibula, but there is still the same periosteal new bone formation with multiple small 2-mm punched out lesions. As the joint is involved, fusion will occur, as in this case from West Africa. (Courtesy of the late Prof. W. P. Cockshott) **C, D** The end result of *A. pelletieri* infection. Multiple areas of bone destruction with many small holes, joint destruction, and bony fusion. Many patients come to hospital for some other illness rather than their abnormal foot: they have had it so long that they have got used to it, and the need for amputation may be an unwelcome surprise

Epidemiology and Pathology

The zygomycetes are the common molds found on bread, cheese, and fruit. They are also present in decaying vegetation.

Mucormycosis seldom occurs in healthy individuals, although some have been infected while apparently otherwise healthy. It is most common in patients who are immunocompromised for any reason, including diabetes, renal failure, leukemia, the reticulosis, and malnutrition. Mucormycosis is rare in AIDS patients, but both may occur in intravenous drug users. Skin and soft tissue infection has followed local trauma. Intravenous drug abuse is another common factor. Several infections have been linked with contaminated adhesive bandages/tape which have been left in place too long so that the underlying skin has become damaged. Organ transplantation and clinical immunosuppression for any reason increase the risk of infection.

The Entomophthorales are found in the alimentary tract of many amphibians, reptiles, horses, dogs, and chimpanzees but few are clinically infected. A significant difference which affects pathogenicity is that, unlike the members of the Mucorales, the organisms of the Entomophthorales tend not to invade

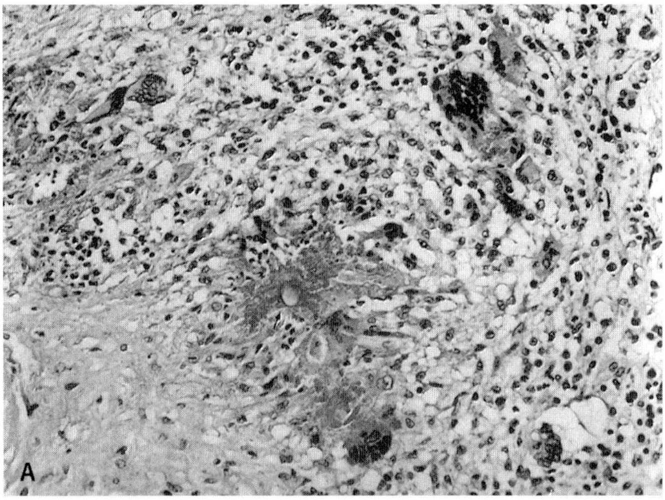

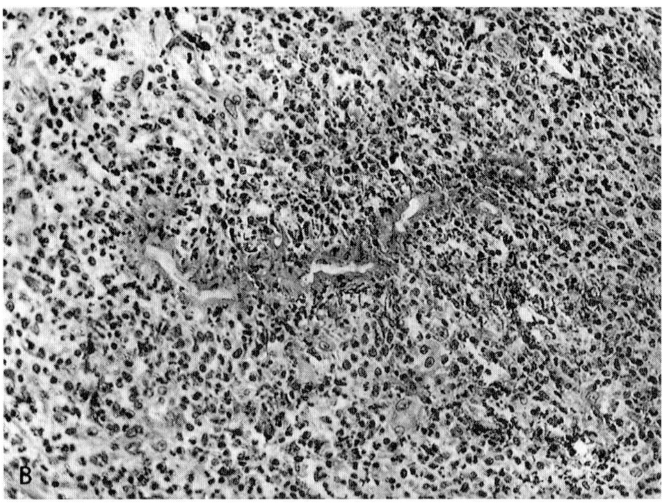

Fig. 6.27 A–D. The histopathology of zygomycosis. **A** The granuloma around a hyphae. There are many epithelioid and giant cells and there are usually plasma cells, macrophages, lymphocytes, and neutrophils. H & E, ×400. **B** Three transverse sections of hyphae and heavy infiltration of eosinophils surrounded by the Splendore-Hoeppli phenomenon. PAS, ×200. **C–D** see p. 571

the wall and lumen of blood vessels (although a few cases of disseminated infection have been recorded). Because vascular invasion is not a feature of the entomophthomycoses, neither septic thrombosis nor infarction and the subsequent necrosis are observed as with mucormycoses. The entomophthomycosis tend to be characterized by indolent local infections, in contrast to the usually quickly disseminating mucormycosis. *Entomophthora coronata* almost always affects only the upper respiratory tract. The hyphae of entomophthoromycoses are septate, while those of mucormycetes are nonseptate; in addition, the hyphae in entomophthomycoses often are enclosed by an eosinophilic sheath (Splendore-Hoeppli phenomenon) not seen in the mucormycoses (Fig. 6.27).

In other respects the infections are similar, with central abscesses surrounded by numerous eosinophils. Biopsy is the best way to establish the diagnosis because serology is unreliable.

Clinical Characteristics

Both types of zygomycetes have similar clinical patterns. Both have a subcutaneous, a mucocutaneous, and a visceral form. Although it is important to differentiate the organisms to provide the correct treatment, it is not possible to do this clinically or by imaging.

The mucocutaneous or subcutaneous forms (Fig. 6.28) present as nodules, or an area of induration involving the limbs or buttocks, increasing steadily and spreading to cause gross disfiguration. The infection begins as a single area of erythematous, thickened and slightly painful cellulitis which quite rapidly develops a central area of black necrosis with a well-defined edge. The appearance may differ if the infection has arisen where there has been previous trauma. The nodules become confluent and in some patients there may be multiple lesions. As the disease advances, it may be mistaken clinically for a malignant tumor. It is usually the

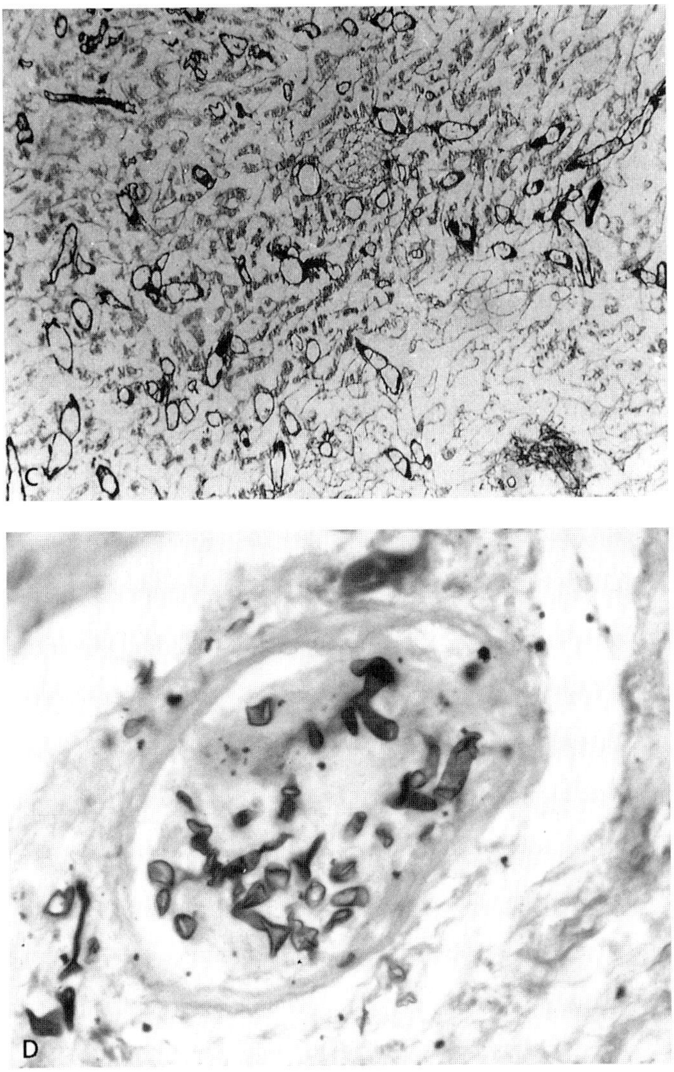

Fig. 6.27 (*continued*). **C** Entomophthoromycosis caused by *Basidiobolus haptosporus*. There are many hyphae, and a few show septations. Gomori methenamine-silver, ×450. **D** A myocardial vessel occluded by a septic thrombosis which contained "twisted ribbon" hyphae characteristic of a zygomycete. Septic thrombosis and septic infarction are common complications of disseminated zygomycosis, and are often fatal, as in the case. Gomori methenamine-silver, ×400. (**A–C** courtesy of Bittencourt and Londero 1995; **D** courtesy of Dr. Daniel H. Connor)

disfiguration (Fig. 6.29 A, B) which brings the patient to the clinic or hospital.

Both subcutaneous and mucocutaneous infections can spread to muscle and underlying bones (Fig. 6.28 D) or to lymph nodes and may even involve adjacent organs. The facial form is good example of this. It has been called rhinocerebral or craniofacial mucormycosis and may originate in the paranasal sinuses. From there it may spread to the orbit, palate, or brain. The initial clinical presentation is acute sinusitis, with fever and sinus headache. There is a purulent nasal discharge in most patients. Progress is rapid over a few days, with increasing edema and areas of black necrosis. The palate may be perforated. The patient may complain of double vision or there may be cranial nerve palsy. Blindness hs been one result: thrombosis of the cavernous sinus or carotid cavernous fistula may occur and the thrombosis may extend to the bifurcation of the carotid artery or cause cerebral embolization or infarction. This is a severe destructive and painful disease, progressing rapidly to death.

Pulmonary infection is usually associated with widespread disseminated disease; however, in some immunosuppressed patients there is direct lung, infection following the inhalation of spores (Fig. 6.29 C). The onset is acute and nonspecific, with cough, fever, shortness of breath, pleural pain, and sputum. The immediate clinical diagnosis will be pneumonia. The infection progresses rapidly, but sputum cultures reveal no bacteria. Fine-needle aspiration biopsy or open lung biopsy may be required to establish the diagnosis. Bronchoscopy may fail to find the organism, particularly when there has been lung infarction.

The visceral form of mucormycosis (Fig. 6.30) starts clinically with loss of weight, abdominal pain, enteritis, and, in some patients, dysuria. In children in

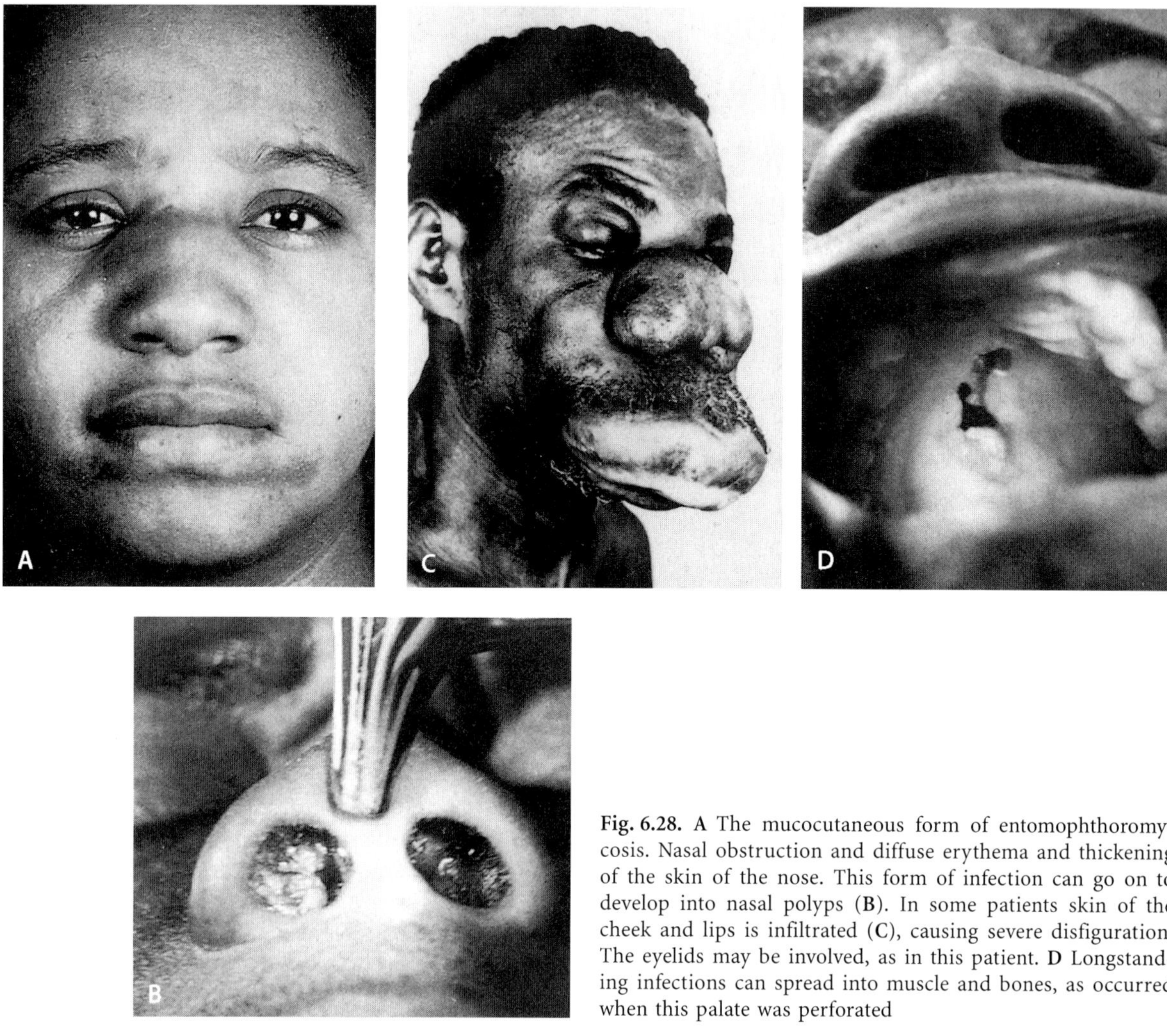

Fig. 6.28. **A** The mucocutaneous form of entomophthoromycosis. Nasal obstruction and diffuse erythema and thickening of the skin of the nose. This form of infection can go on to develop into nasal polyps (**B**). In some patients skin of the cheek and lips is infiltrated (**C**), causing severe disfiguration. The eyelids may be involved, as in this patient. **D** Longstanding infections can spread into muscle and bones, as occurred when this palate was perforated

particular, there may be an abdominal mass and the clinical diagnosis may be lymphoma, schistosomiasis, or tuberculosis. The fungal mass can cause intestinal obstruction or, when the kidneys are involved, hydronephrosis; there may be bladder infection.

In about half the patients with gastrointestinal mucormycosis, the stomach is involved; in about a third, the colon; and less frequently, the esophagus and small intestine. In the stomach there is usually a necrotic ulcer, which may be deeply penetrating. This is the form often seen in malnourished children or in diabetics. The gastric ulcers may perforate, causing pain, which may be the presenting symptom. Localized mucormycotic granulomas can occur anywhere within the bowel and be mistaken for tumors.

Imaging Diagnosis

In the facial form, the full extent of the facial soft tissue swelling can be demonstrated, and radiographs or CT scans of the sinuses are important to show the spread of the infection. Although sinus radiographs provide useful information, CT and MR scans are needed to demonstrate fully the entent of the ethmoid sinus or orbital spread and to show whether there is any intracerebral involvement. Rhinocerebral mucormycosis may be much more extensive than is expected from the clinical examination. All the causal organisms can be very destructive, although *E. coronata* does not usually involve bone.

Imaging can show when the subcutaneous form of zygomycosis involves the underlying bone, because there is usually a reactive periostitis adjacent to the soft tissue granuloma. Ultrasonography, soft tissue radiography, and MRI can demonstrate the superficial or deeper extension of the infection. In the foot or hand, deep infection may displace adjoining

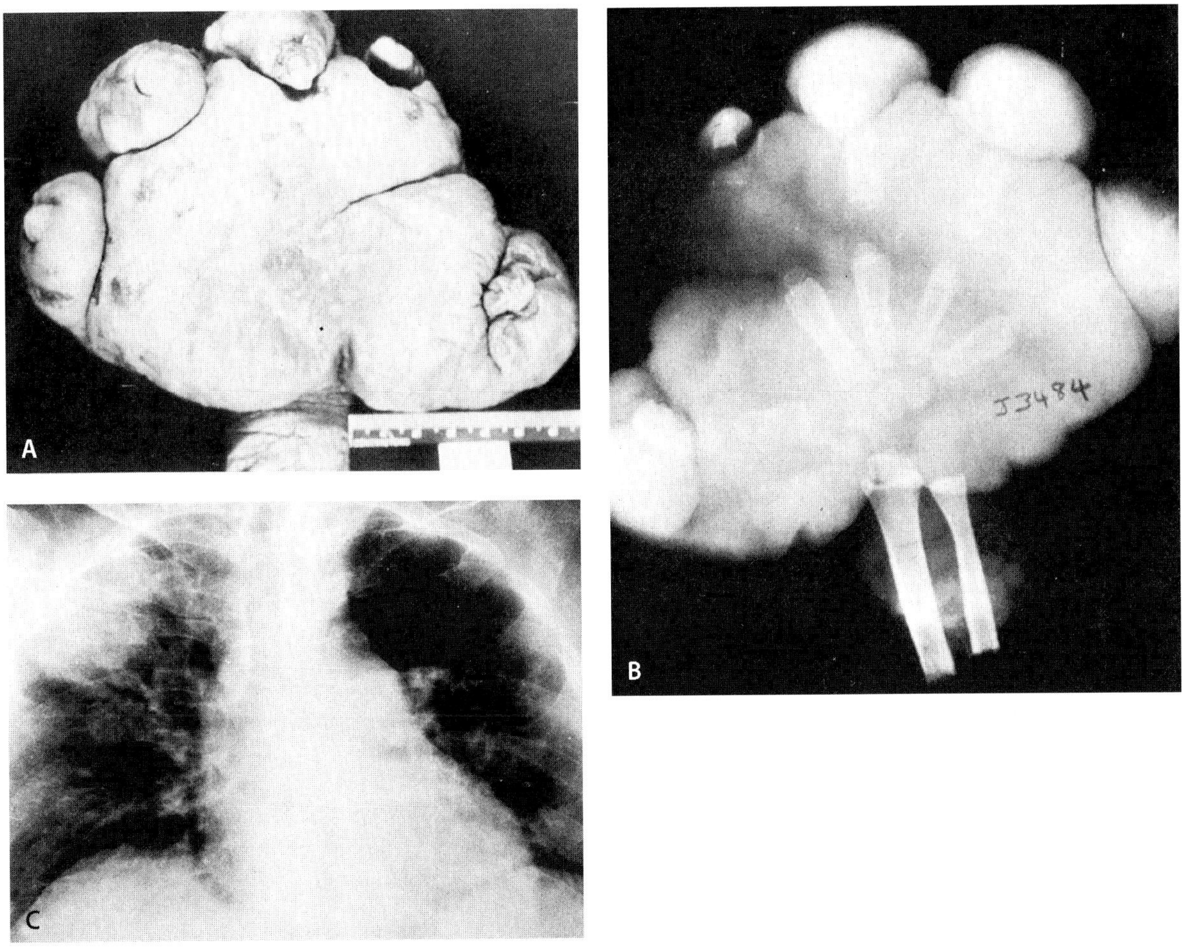

Fig. 6.29 A–C. Mucormycosis can cause gross deformity in any part of the body. **A** The grossly deformed hand of a child and **B** the radiograph of the same hand. The bones are displaced and there is some periosteal reaction, but there is no invasion of any bone. **C** Usually saprophytic fungi can become very virulent and pathogenic in patients who are immunocompromised, such as this 60-year-old Indian man with diabetic ketoacidosis and chronic renal failure, being treated with dialysis. He suddenly became unconscious and delirious: there is consolidation in the right upper lobe

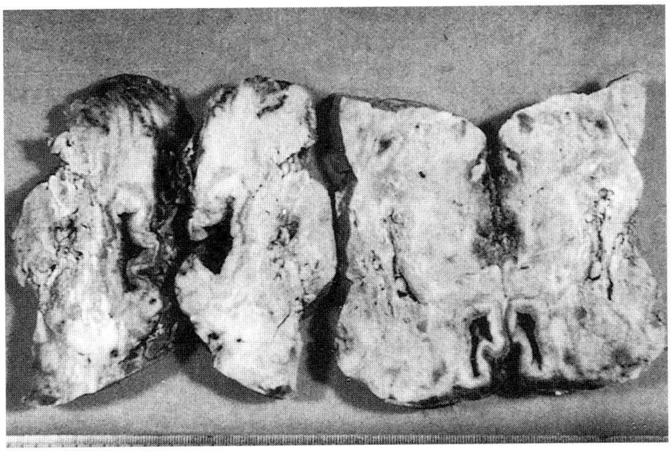

Fig. 6.30. Visceral entomophthoromycosis may present clinically with abdominal symptoms. Although not common, the large bowel may be so involved as to cause obstruction, as shown in this specimen from Brazil. The infection can spread throughout the abdomen, causing hydronephrosis in some patients. (From Bittencourt and Londero 1995, and Dr. Rui Moreira, San Salvador)

bones, shown as separation of the metatarsal or metacarpal heads.

Pulmonary mucormycosis may be very nonspecific. Chest imaging may show patchy or diffuse consolidation, often multifocal (Fig. 6.29C). There may be cavitation, with or without consolidation and there may be small parenchymal nodules, often single. It is not always easy to distinguish consolidation from pulmonary infarction or to be sure whether the abscess is a direct result of the infection or is due to necrosis.

Pleural effusions are relatively uncommon, as is mediastinal involvement. Because mucormycetes invade the large blood vessels, there may be pseudoaneurysms. These may be multiple in the pulmonary artery, best shown by CT or MR scanning and, if necessary, confirmed by pulmonary arteriography. Both the central and the peripheral pulmonary arteries may be involved. When there is peripheral ischemia and infarction, some of the lung tissue may slough and become surrounded by air (pulmonary gangrene). This complication also occurs in aspergillosis, and if the volume of necrotic lung is sufficiently large, the circle of air could be mistaken for a hydatid cyst.

Mucormycotic infection of the bowel can be seen on plain radiographs as dilated bowel, or if there has been perforation, free intraperitoneal or subphrenic gas. Ascites may be recognized with ultrasonography or CT. Partial obstruction from a mucormycetoma can be demonstrated by contrast examination (if the patient is sufficiently well). Any part of the bowel may be involved, and pseudotumors have been reported around the duodenum, mid-ileum, ileocecal valve, and the splenic flexure of the colon. The patients may be too ill for gastrointestinal contrast examination, but ultrasonography or CT scanning may provide useful information. If the lesion can be seen by endoscopy, there is often a black or greenish area of central necrosis.

Cardiac mucormycosis is very uncommon, but has occurred, usually as a complication of disseminated infection.

Mucormycosis is often progressive, with fatal infections in which the diagnosis is only established as the disease progresses into its advanced stages, or not until autopsy. Spontaneous healing has occurred but, even if the underlying immunodeficiency can be rectified, the prognosis in most patients is poor.

Chromoblastomycosis and Phaeohyphomycosis

Previously known as chromomycosis, this is another mycotic infection for which the nomenclature has changed since the first (1981) edition and is still very confusing. To quote "Medical Mycology" again (K.J. Kwon-Chung and J.E. Bennett, 1992), the "nomenclature of many phaeohyphomycotic agents has been complex because of confusion in their classification ... and the different opinions of taxonomists."

This group of infections is described because the fungi have been reported from every continent, with the majority of the patients coming from the rural tropics and subtropics. It is the complications in patients with unusual spread of the fungus which are of importance in imaging. The initial lesions have no specific imaging characteristics.

Synonyms

Chromomycosis. Verrucous dermatitis. Phaeosporotrichosis. (There are numerous other older names.)

Phaeomycotic cyst. This is different clinically and pathologically, and different because it is easily cured by excision. There are no imaging features and it is not discussed further.

Fr: Chromoblastomycose. *Ger*: Chromomykose. Chromoblastomykose. *Sp*: Cromoblastomicosis.

Definition

A chronic infection of the skin and subcutaneous tissue caused by one of the naturally pigmented fungi. Most infections are caused by *Fonsecaea pedrosoi*. The definition is based around the clinical characteristics, which are common to many of these fungal infections, and phaeohyphomycosis is the supporting histopathological definition. Unfortunately, the names chromomycosis and chromoblastomycosis are used differently in different texts, referring to different fungi. There are organisms which can cause both chromoblastomycosis and phaeohyphomycosis, and previously these were included under chromoblastomycosis. Now mycologists are trying to separate the clinical conditions in chromoblastomycosis from those of phaeohyphomycosis.

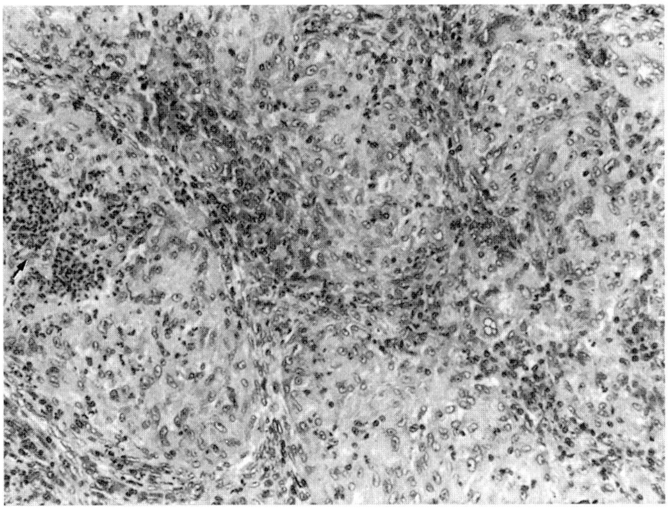

Fig. 6.31. Chromoblastomycosis can resemble squamous cell carcinoma. Histopathologically there is a heavy cellular reaction, with inflammatory cells mixed with epitheloid and giant cells. Microabscesses of neutrophils occur in the center of these granulomas (*arrow*). H & E, ×200. (From Bittencourt and Londero 1995)

Geographic Distribution

Chromoblastomycosis is most common throughout the tropics but may be found anywhere in the world except in the Arctic and Antarctic. There are some areas where the infection is highly endemic, such as the Dominican Republic, Costa Rica, and, in Africa, the Malagasy Republic. In many arid regions, the infection is rare. There is also geographic variation between the causal species.

Epidemiology and Pathology

The organisms are saprophytes found in decaying vegetable matter, on woody plants, and in the soil. The common characteristics of the wide group of fungi which can cause clinical chromoblastomycosis are that they are pigmented (brown, from melanin), muriform, and yeast-like with hyphae which divide by septation (binary fission) and not by budding. They are introduced into tissues by trauma (e.g., with thorns or splinters): transmission from person to person does not occur. The histopathological pattern lies between an infected (suppurative) granuloma and a pseudoepithelioma. There will be many microabscesses in the dermis, a rich infiltrate of eosinophils, many epitheloid cells and giant cells, lymphocytes, and plasma cells. Truly spectacular is the epithelial hyperplasia which frequently resembles squamous cell carcinoma (Fig. 6.31). Fungal elements may be seen in the verrucous lesions, particularly when the skin lesions are flat. Amongst the causal fungi are species of *Fonsecaea, Phialophora verrucosa*, and *Cladosporium (Cladophialophora) carrionii*. All may be seen as groups of thick-walled dark brown "sclerotic cells," either round or angular in shape. *Exophiala dermatitidis* (formerly *Wangiella dermatitidis*) has been included as a further cause of chromoblastomycosis, but does not produce these brown sclerotic "muriform" cells usually found in true chromoblastomycosis.

Clinical Characteristics (Localized Form)

The clinical lesions start with a small papule or ulcer, usually on a lower limb, but sometimes on the hands or elsewhere in the arms. Satellite lesions start if the patient scratches. Progress is very slow, over many months or even years. Eventually they either become smooth or verrucous, tumoral or nodular, with cauliflower-like warty swellings which spread over the years. They may be mistaken for hyperkeratosis or squamous cell carcinoma (Fig. 6.32). When secondary infection occurs there is often a foul discharge. The fungal infection may form large papillomatous growths involving much of the limb. The nodular pattern becomes tumorous, large, rough, and ulcerating. The fungi can be squeezed from the parakeratotic masses. The secondary infection spreads along lymphatics, with satellite lesions: eventually there will be marked fibrosis and so much lymphatic blockage that there can be elephantiasis. There is seldom any regional lymphadenopathy, nor should there be discharging sinuses, although this can occasionally happen after aspiration.

It is emphasized that this a predominantly skin and subcutaneous infection but direct spread to bone has occurred and resulted in chronic osteomyelitis. In phaeohyphomycosis, particularly when due to *Cl. trichoides*, cerebral abscesses may be the commonest complication: there have also been patients with infection of paranasal sinuses. In chromoblastomycosis, cerebral abscesses are rare. (Note: *Cl. trichoides* may have, or soon have, a different name.)

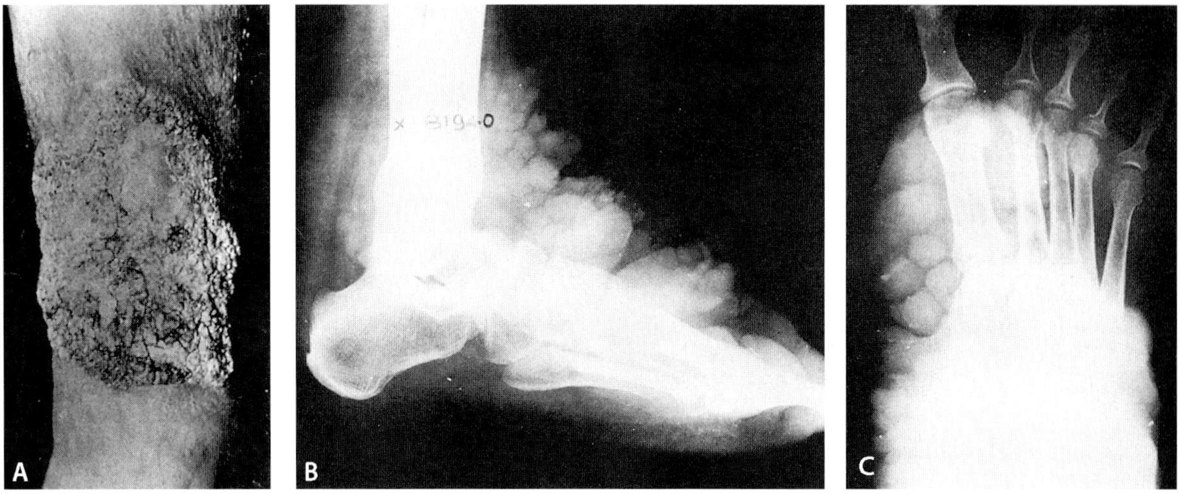

Fig. 6.32. A Chromoblastomycosis on the right leg, mimicking squamous cell carcinoma. **B, C** Radiography shows marked soft tissue swelling of the foot with irregular nodules of different sizes. The infection is confined to the soft tissues and does not involve bone, cause displacement or affect the joints. However, very rarely, this fungus can cause chronic osteomyelitis

Imaging Diagnosis

The cerebral lesions are indistinguishable from any other brain abscess. Plain radiographs of the skull or paranasal sinuses are usually not helpful: CT and MR scanning can demonstrate the brain lesion, which will contrast enhance.

In the peripheral skeleton there are no characteristic changes: the pattern is that of chronic osteomyelitis with one or more central foci.

Summary

For the mycologist, chromoblastomycosis is a fertile source of debate and the allocation and reallocation of fungi into different species. For the radiologicist, it is important to know that this infection can exist, and that it is one of the many causes of cerebral abscess. For the clinician, chromoblastomycosis is a very difficult infection to treat, particularly late in the disease. For the patient, it is a chronic, slowly progressive affliction which seems never to go away and will eventually cause much pain and disability.

Geotrichosis

Definition

Geotrichosis is a rare infection by either of two fungi, *Geotrichum candidum* or *Blastoschizomyces capitatus*. Infection by *G. candidum* is described here.

Synonyms

Oidiomycosis. (*B. capitatus* is also known as *G. capitatum* or *Trichosporon capitatum*). *Fr*: Geotrichose. *Ger*: Geotrichose. *Sp*: Geotrichosis.

Geographic Distribution

Geotrichum candidum occurs worldwide, but is not a common cause of clinical disease.

Epidemiology and Pathology

Geotrichum candidum is an opportunistic fungus most often found in immunodeficient patients. It has been recognized in citrus fruits, milk products, and sewage. It is a filamentous mold which reproduces by segmentation of the hyphae into arthrospores: these may give rise to a yeast-like bud. It is found endogenously in the normal mucosa of the alimentary tract. In those who are immunosuppressed it may become an opportunistic pathogen.

Histopathologically there are multiple microabscesses with a surrounding inflammatory reaction containing the fungi. Recognition of the fungus establishes the diagnosis.

Clinical Characteristics

Most clinical infections are in patients with malignant disease, of either sex and aged 23–79 years. The majority seem to have been acquired following catheterization. Clinically the infection usually appears in the mouth but the lungs or gut can be infected. In the mouth there are white patches, similar to "thrush." When in the lungs, patients present with fever, asthma, or cough, with sputum which is sometimes blood stained and is often very gelatinous. The pulmonary form resembles tuberculosis or chronic *Klebsiella* (Friedländer's) pneumonia.

Gastrointestinal infection causes abdominal pain, diarrhea, blood, and mucus in the stools. The clinical diagnosis is often "colitis." Geotrichosis has caused arthritis following trauma, and resulted in fever and tender swelling of the joints.

Imaging Diagnosis

Only the pulmonary infection has any significant imaging findings. In many patients the chest radiograph will be normal, but some may show peribronchial thickening and a fine nodular mottling at the bases of the lungs. In others there will be air space consolidation, usually in the upper lobes. This may progress to cavitation, usually with thin walls, and the overall pattern resembles tuberculosis. None of these imaging changes is diagnostic.

Adiaspiromycosis

Synonyms

Haplomycosis. Adiasporosis. *Fr: Ger: Sp:* Adiaspiromicosis.

Definition

Adiaspiromycosis is a rare pulmonary infection with *Chrysosporium parvum* var. *crescens* (formerly *Emmonsia crescens*). *C. parvum* var. *parvum* is not known to infect humans. The organisms are dimorphic, forming large spherical cells (200–400 μm) in tissues: mycelial growth occurs in artificial culture medium at 25 °C.

Geographic Distribution

Adiaspiromycosis occurs worldwide.

Epidemiology and Pathology

Chrysosporium parvum var. *crescens* is a dimorphic fungus which grows slowly in culture as a septate, branching mycelium. It causes a very rare fungal infection of the respiratory tract. The fungus frequently infects rodents and small carnivorous animals, and is found in the soil around their habitations. Histopathologically, the organism, *C. parvum* var. *crescens*, forms large spores and provokes a fibrogranulomatous reaction. The granulomas vary in size from 0.5 to 3 mm and may become confluent. In each patient, all are at the same stage of development. Symptoms are probably caused by compression or displacement of the distal airways and alveolar parenchyma.

There is a cutaneous test of unknown reliability, the diagnosis usually being made by identifying the fungus.

Clinical Characteristics

Most patients are asymptomatic; those with disseminated pulmonary disease have general, nonspecific respiratory symptoms, clinically suggesting flu or in more severe infections, pneumonia. Adiaspiromycosis is often a chance finding, even when disseminated nodules are shown on chest imaging. It is not known to have spread beyond the lungs.

Imaging Diagnosis

Chest radiographs may show a single nodule in the lung parenchyma, usually close to a bronchus. Sometimes there are multiple nodules and in some patients there is pneumonic consolidation, seen most commonly in those who have clinical symptoms. When there has been heavy exposure to the fungus, multiple granulomas have resulted. It must be reemphasized that adiaspiromycosis is often an incidental finding and of no clinical significance.

Aspergillosis

The history of aspergillosis is fascinating, the nomenclature is confusing, and the term "aspergillosis" has been said to "describe so many different clinical entities, that, without qualification, the term is almost meaningless" (Kwon-Chung and Bennett, 1992).

Aspergillus candidus was first isolated in 1842 from a bullfinch. *Aspergillus* spp. were then described in various avian species, including a great bustard. Human infection was reported by Virchow in 1856. Since then there have been an increasing number of infections by the various Aspergilli, matched by variations in the names given to them. It was not until 1938 that a pulmonary aspergilloma (fungus ball) was described, and the invasive form was only recognized in the 1950s. Worldwide, the number of invasive infections has increased and continues to grow considerably, helped by the number of patients who are immunodeficient as a result of leukemia, organ transplantation, or corticosteroids; patients with AIDS do not often suffer from aspergillosis.

Synonyms

Ger: Pulmonary aspergillosis = Schimmelpilzerkrankung. *Fr:* Aspergillose (pseudotuberculose aspergillaire). *Sp:* Aspergillosis.

Definition

Aspergillosis describes a disease complex caused by any species of the genus *Aspergillus*, the commonest being *A. fumigatus*. This, and *A. oryzae*, are the pathogenic species most frequently seen in tropical and subtropical regions.

Geographic Distribution

The organism occurs worldwide, with variation only in the prevalence of different species. In Sudan, for example, the most frequently found is *A. flavus*. Elsewhere, *A. niger* causes ear infections and aspergillomas. Sometimes more than one species is found in the same infection (a mixed colony infection). There are many variations on this theme.

Epidemiology and Pathology

There are over 200 species of *Aspergillus*. They are ubiquitous, being found everywhere in the environment. They are most common where there is decaying vegetation, such as compost, hay stacks, and, in some countries, moldy grains. They are found in the soil and in many liquids, and have even been isolated from acids and formalin. They have been identified in roofing material, leather, timber, and food products with high concentrations of salt or sugar (salted meat, jams, and jellies). They frequently cause contamination in laboratory cultures.
The histopathological findings in aspergillosis show that any organ or site can be infected. The fungus may cause:

A) Invasive aspergillosis
Inflammatory granulomas, infarction, edema, and necrotizing lesions of the lungs and other sites, such as the paranasal sinuses
Systemic (and often fatal) disseminated fungemia and infarctions, with tissue invasion

B) Saprophytic aspergillosis
Massive colonies, aspergillomas (fungal balls of entangled mycelial filaments) in preformed cavities (such as those of tuberculosis or any other etiology)

C) Allergic aspergillosis
Allergy to the fungus anywhere in the body, particularly in the bronchi, with toxic effects

The underlying tissue reaction is polymorphic, with macrophages and giant cells containing the separate mycelial filaments. Invasive aspergillosis in any organ is characterized by invasion of vessels, causing septic infarction with necrosis and abscess formation. Within preexisting pulmonary cavities, colonies of *Aspergillus* grow, regardless of the etiology of the cavity, as long as it is dark, moist, aerated, and at least partially sequestered from the body's immune reactions.
There is little systemic reaction to the fungus, other than a moderate eosinophilia, unless there is a specific allergy. Patients with allergic reactions to *Aspergillus* spp. have elevated IgE antibodies but no IgG precipitins, as compared with invasive infections when there are specific antibodies.
The diagnosis of aspergillosis is confirmed by identifying the characteristic branched, septate hyphae and spores in sputum or tissue sections. Culture permits further identification, but the fungus is so ubiquitous that its growth does not necessarily mean that it is responsible for the illness: tissue invasion must be shown. Serological studies help to confirm the diagnosis of intracavitary aspergilloma and allergic bronchopulmonary aspergillosis but these, too, need clinical correlation. The fungi are more often saprophytic than parasitic.

Clinical Characteristics

Aspergillosis presents clinically with a wide spectrum, from peaceful coexistence to severe illness. The clinical symptoms depend on the site, and more particularly on the status of the host's immune system and on whether the patient is granulocytopenic. It is in those who are already severely ill or immunocompromised that there will be dissemination and invasion. Chronic infection and the carrier state occur in atopic individuals, but colonies of the fungus may grow, as in aspergillomas, without any clinical reaction: in some patients, however, an apparently asymptomatic aspergilloma in a cavity provokes high antibody titers to the fungal antigens. In such patients it is probable that the cavity is the result of the fungus infection and did not preexist.
When the lungs are infected, the clinical presentation suggests bronchitis, with increased cough and

sputum. The sputum is often tenacious, leading to poor bronchial drainage and accumulation of pulmonary secretions. This results in secondary atelectasis and bacterial infection, which either causes or complicates bronchiectasis. Even when clinical symptoms are minimal, imaging may show recurrent pneumonia. In other pulmonary infections a predominant symptom is asthma, often associated with fever and cough, and with brown plugs of aspergilli in the sputum. In the early stages of this intrinsic asthma, the airway obstruction is reversible but later there are destructive changes, which may be recognized clinically by the development of the antibodies.

Another common clinical site of infection is a paranasal sinus, often due to *A. flavus* (which is endemic in the Sudan and Middle East). These patients may have no predisposing ill health, and the majority will have normal chest radiographs. The disease progresses slowly and without pain, and frequently presents as unilateral proptosis. Depending on the sinus infected, there may be frontal or facial swelling. The infection can be asymptomatic, but often extends into bone, sometimes into the cranium. The discrepancy between the gross imaging changes and the mild clinical symptoms is important because such spreading infections can be fatal.

Dissemination of the infection by hematogenous spread of the fungus can cause a fulminating disease. Infection may develop anywhere, most commonly in the central nervous system, the gastrointestinal tract, and the myocardium. Dissemination seldom occurs from an aspergilloma, which is usually noninvasive. Almost all disseminated infections originate in the lungs, sometimes following a concomitant infection, such as *Pseudomonas aeruginosa*, which commonly triggers invasive aspergillosis.

Apart from the brain, the urinary tract, particularly the kidneys, is commonly invaded. Bone infection is usually due to spread from a soft tissue focus: for example, when the sinuses are involved there may be periosteal thickening and as the disease progresses, lytic foci develop in the bones. Both clinically and on imaging, malignancy may be suspected because there is little bone sclerosis. The sinuses also have been the primary site of disseminated infections. Among the less common sites are the liver and the thyroid. The cause of death can be severe toxemia, hemorrhage from any site or massive septic pulmonary or other organ infarction.

Imaging Diagnosis

The chest and paranasal sinuses are the most frequent sites of *Aspergillus* spp. infection, from which dissemination originates.

Pulmonary Aspergillosis

In pulmonary aspergillosis the imaging findings depend on the reaction of the patient to the fungus. There are four main categories:

1. Hypersensitive (allergic) aspergillosis
2. Noninvasive aspergillosis
3. Semi-invasive aspergillosis
4. Invasive aspergillosis

1. *Hypersensitive aspergillosis* is, worldwide, probably the most common reaction to the fungus, which in these patients is noninvasive. The host becomes sensitized and, in the lungs, there is a severe inflammatory reaction which leads to bronchitis and bronchiectasis. Many patients are asthmatic, and in many of them there are no clinical symptoms, but there is an abnormal chest radiograph. The imaging diagnosis will be bronchiectasis and the dilated bronchi often appear as linear or Y-shaped "fingers" (cigar or banana densities) because of the thick mucoid material (mucous plugs) within them (Fig. 6.33). This is of relatively high density because of the compacted fungal elements. CT (and bronchography) shows that the bronchiectasis is most marked in the larger bronchi, the more peripheral bronchi being normal. Because of plugging, there will be radiographic evidence of lobar or segmental atelectasis and of obstructive emphysema. The findings are very variable, sometimes changing every day in the same patient. Fibrosis is often the end result.

Aspergillus is one of the less common causes of a hypersensitivity reaction in the lungs (other causes include farmer's lungs, pigeon breeder's disease, byssinosis). In the acute phase there may be pulmonary edema but more commonly there is a fine nodular interstitial pattern throughout both lungs, over which there may be flame or triangular densities, often rapidly appearing. When there are small granulomas surrounding the bronchi (bronchocentric granulomatosis), hyphae of *Aspergillus* spp. can be identified in many of them histologically.

2. *Noninvasive aspergillosis*: the saprophytic form of aspergillosis always occurs in previously damaged lungs, usually in a cavity. Imaging shows a mobile intracavitary, usually indistinct "ball-shaped mass" (Fig. 6.34). On plain radiographs, erect and decubitus frontal projections will usually show movement of the aspergilloma. In some patients either standard tomography or CT will be necessary. Similar round masses may be due to other fungi, a thrombus without infection, a tumor, or Wegener's granulomatosis. A further difficulty is that fungal infection can be superimposed on another underlying cause. Because the cavity may react to the fungus ball, with vascular granulation tissue and in some

(Text continues on p. 582)

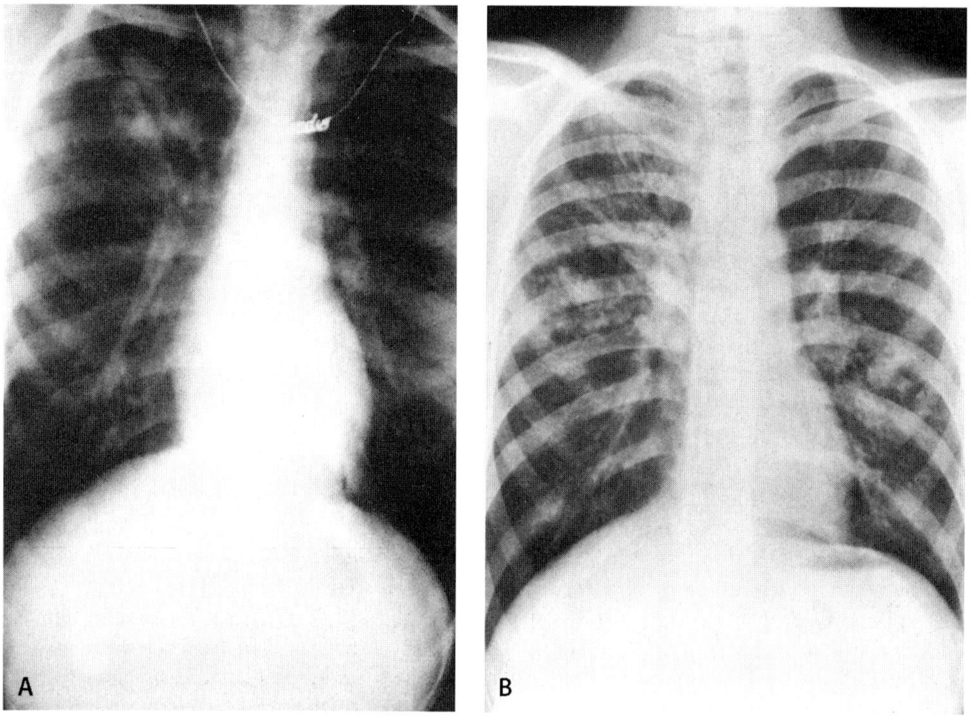

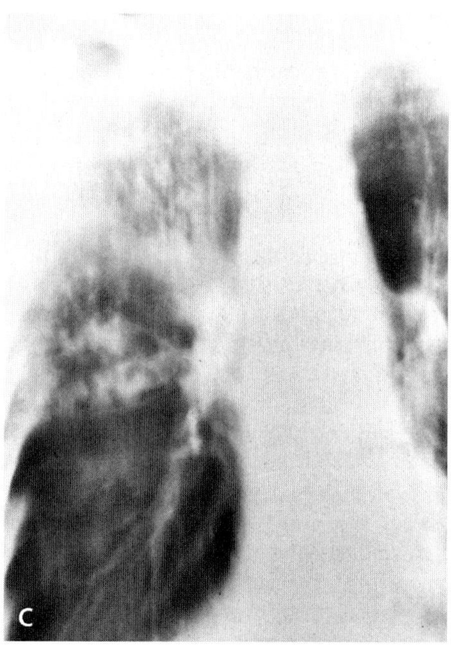

Fig. 6.33 A–C. Hypersensitive pulmonary aspergillosis. **A** The chest radiograph of a teenage. Indian girl with chronic asthma. There are mucoid plugs in the right upper lobe with elongated, cigar-shaped densities. There is some air trapping within them, which must be distinguished from cavitation. These shadows were migratory and transient: chest radiographs taken at other times showed similar branching mucous plugs in other lobes. The lungs are hyperinflated because of asthma. **B** Another patient with chronic asthma, mucous plugs, and the constantly changing linear and round densities. **C** Standard tomography (8 cm) of the same patient. (**B, C** courtesy of Dr. Glenn Lillington)

Fig. 6.34 A–F. Pulmonary aspergillosis is frequently seen as a "fungus ball" within a pulmonary cavity. **A** A thin-walled tuberculous cavity in the right upper lobe of a patient from Tunis: there is a large fungus ball within the cavity, confirmed by the CT scan (**B**). **C, D** Radiographs taken in different positions can be used to show the movement of the fungal ball within the cavity. **C** In the erect position the large fungus ball lies in the bottom of the left apical cavity. **D** When the patient is lying supine with the head downwards, the fungus ball moves to the upper part of the cavity. The apical pleural thickening and fluid, and the contracted left upper lobe are shown on both radiographs. **E** A large fungus ball in the cavity in the right apex of an African patient. There is chronic but active disease elsewhere in the right lung, with another cavity in the right middle lobe. **F** Fungus balls can be bilateral, as in this patient from South Africa. (**A, B** courtesy of Dr. H. Gharbi, Tunis; **E, F** courtesy of the University of Capetown Radiology Library) ▶

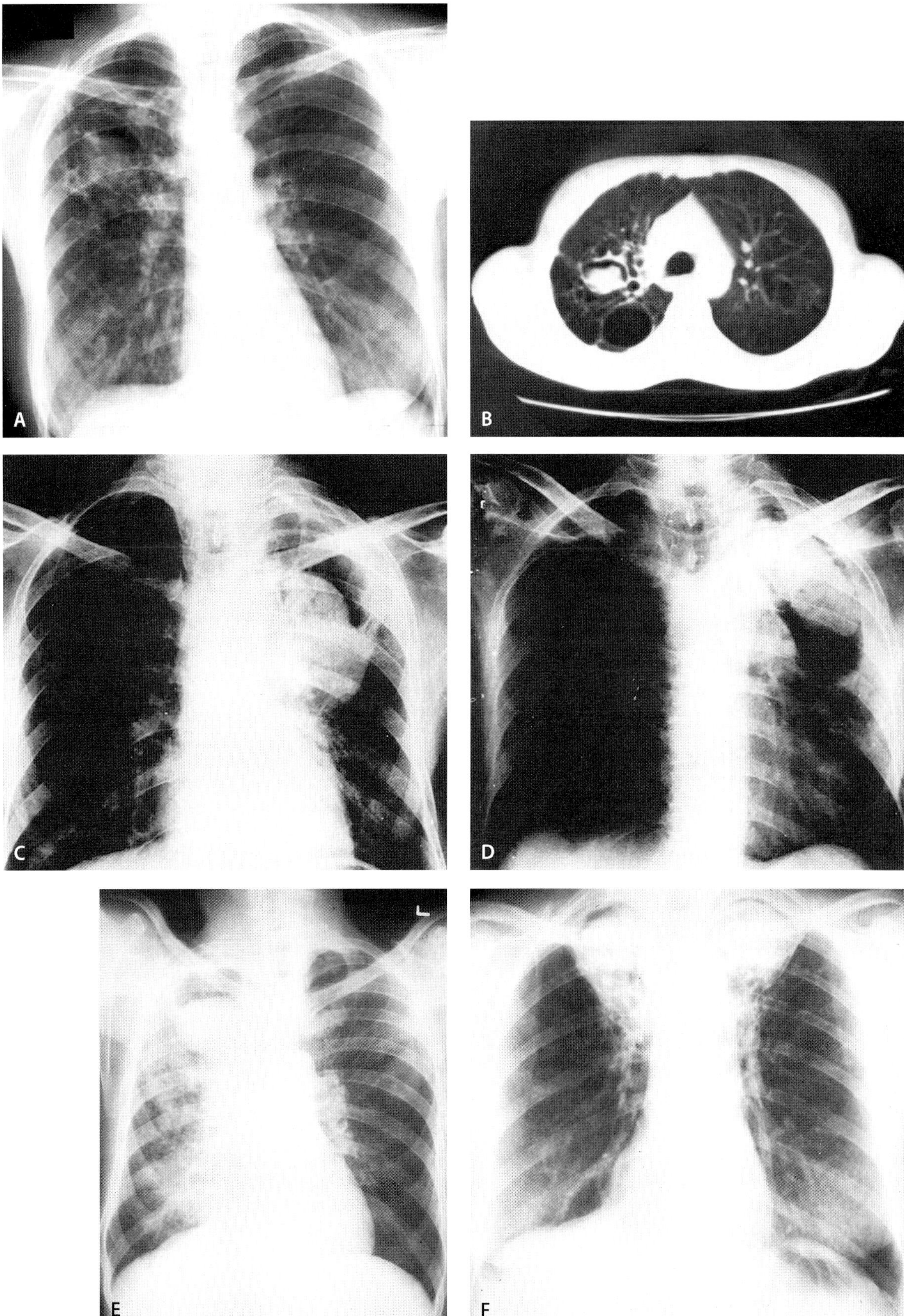
A
B
C
D
E
F

patients a pleural reaction, it is sometimes difficult to be sure that the aspergilloma is still noninvasive. In patients with advanced preexisting tuberculosis or other lung disease, the differentiation between invasive and noninvasive aspergillosis may depend more on the clinical and laboratory tests than on imaging.

3. *Semi-invasive aspergillosis* has only been recognized in the last two decades, and probably occurs only in patients who have a depressed immune system. In this form, it is the *Aspergillus* which creates a chronic cavity and goes on to form an aspergilloma. This is best documented by serial imaging, which usually shows alveolar consolidation which goes on to cavitate as a result of peripheral infarction and necrosis. There is often an extensive pleural reaction. Later a thick-walled, irregular cavity will be seen, which in some patients then becomes thin walled: the lining may be irregular without a fungus ball, or become smoother and eventually contain a typical aspergilloma. Again, it is difficult to decide between the noninvasive and semi-invasive pattern of infection. Clinical and laboratory correlation are important and serial images are equally necessary.

4. *Invasive aspergillosis*: only occurs in immunocompromised patients and results in a wide variety of imaging patterns. The initial diagnosis may be pneumonia, sometimes in more than one lobe, but in many patients there are multiple, ill-defined pulmonary nodules. These are probably the result of pulmonary emboli containing fungi. When there is a large fungal embolus (which is not immediately fatal), consolidation will be found on imaging, which breaks down and cavitates into an abscess. It may be difficult in some patients to decide whether the "mass" is due to necrosis or whether there is now a cavity containing a fungus ball. When the patient is severely ill, the lung may become diffusely involved with multiple irregular (necrotic) spreading nodules: the pleura, pericardium, and even the esophagus and trachea may be involved.

Invasive respiratory tract aspergillosis is a well-recognized complication in severely immunocompromised patients. In the early stages, the chest radiograph may remain normal or show only minimal patchy densities. The airways develop ulcers and inflammatory plaques which do not extend into the lungs. The subsequent pulmonary changes are probably the result of the thick mucus which develops and causes airway obstruction.

In almost all pulmonary infections, the initial problem is to decide whether the *Aspergillus* is a contaminant or a cause. CT scanning of early pulmonary aspergillosis, when there are peripheral nodules, shows a halo of attenuation around these focal areas of bronchopneumonia. This is probably caused by growth of the *Aspergillus* in a ring pattern. The description "target lesions" has been used, and is a consequence of a necrotic center, surrounded by a hyperemic perimeter containing invading hyphae. Part of the blurred ring seen radiographically, and better recognized on CT scanning, may be the result of edema. Nodules and the cavitation within them may be seen on CT scanning but may not be visible on conventional radiographs. Indium-labeled white blood cell scintigraphy may also show infection which cannot be seen on a chest radiograph.

Miliary microabscesses have been reported as a rare form of disseminated aspergillosis: there is no cavitation or infarction. These may be recognizable on high-resolution CT scanning.

CT scanning is the best way to record developing cavitation as the infection progresses. Air within a cavitating mass may indicate shrinkage of the central necrotic tissue and may be an early sign of healing. However, there can be other explanations for this process and the clinical condition of the patient may be a more reliable guide to progress.

In brief, radiographs will clearly show the overall pattern; CT will show the complications more clearly, but the clinical state of the patient and the laboratory results must make the definitive diagnosis.

Extrapulmonary Aspergillosis

The paranasal sinuses are quite a common site for *Aspergillus* infections of patients in the tropics. The underlying histopathology is a sclerosing granuloma which occurs most frequently in the Sudan, India, and the Middle East. There may at first be only a simple aspergilloma in the sinus, but often the infection is invasive and proptosis develops as the fungus spreads from the adjacent sinus. On imaging, there is usually opacification of one or more sinuses. The disease is slow and painless, but CT particularly will show early periosteal reaction causing sclerosis of the antral wall next to the soft tissue granuloma. This closely mimics malignancy, particularly as the "tumor" spreads.

An infection by *A. flavus* (in the Sudan as well as elsewhere) may cause bone destruction which is irregular but quite well defined. Spread may be in any direction, medially or laterally or upwards into the floor of the orbit. CT and MR scanning are very important when there is upward spread, because the frontal bones and meninges may be penetrated and intracranial aspergillosis can be quite extensive (and fatal). Such infections show low attenuation and variable contrast enhancement. MRI will help in the differentiation between paranasal aspergillosis and

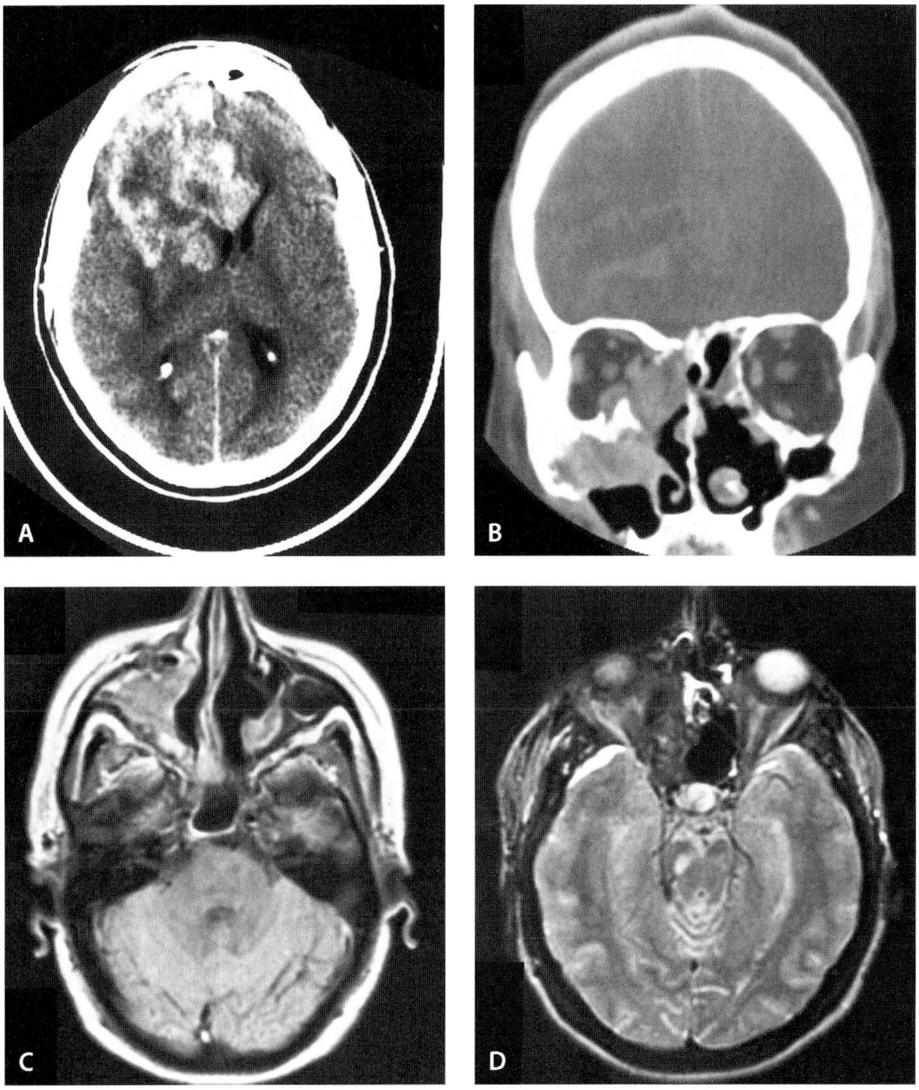

Fig. 6.35 A–D. Frontal aspergillosis complicating a paranasal infection. **A** An axical CT scan after enhancement. There is a mass in the right frontal region obliterating the anterior horn of the right lateral ventricle and compressing the left anterior horn. **B** The same patient. The coronal scan (bone window) shows the soft tissue mass occupying the right maxillary and ethmoidal sinuses: it has destroyed the medial wall and expanded into the orbit, displacing the external ocular muscles. Postoperatively, MRI (T2-weighted) shows a residual mass in the right maxillary antrum (**C**) and in the right ethmoidal sinus and right orbit (**D**). The aspergilloma showed intermediate-low signals in both T2- and T1-weighted sequences. (In **D** there is a rim of fluid over the right temporal region.) The patient was a 39-year-old female from Pakistan with a short clinical history of headache, nausea, vomiting, and deteriorating vision in the right eye. The right antrum had been drained 10 years previously. At the time of **A** and **B** there was right-sided proptosis, right optic atrophy, and left papilledema. Histology showed numerous fungal hyphae of *Aspergillus flavus*. (Courtesy of Dr. A Coulthard et al. and *Clin Radiol*, 1991)

neoplasm. Aspergilloma has a low T2-weighted signal intensity (due to the high iron and manganese content in fungi). Fungi in the nongranulomatous stage have a high T2-weighted signal, as do other inflammatory masses compared with most neoplasms, which show an intermediate signal, with a few giving a high T2-weighted signal. CT and MRI are thus excellent ways to show the extent of bone and soft tissue involvement and should be used whenever spread from the sinuses is suspected (Fig. 6.35). If scanning is not available, linear tomography will also be very helpful. There are almost always large soft tissue polyps and CT (or linear tomography) will demonstrate these. There may be similar polyps within the nose. If the infection spreads downwards, the teeth may be disrupted and appear to "float." In children in some parts of the tropics, Burkitt's lymphoma will have to be excluded as a cause of both proptosis and teeth displacement. In chronic aspergillosis there will be more bone sclerosis, and linear calcification has been reported, most commonly in recurrent infections: neither is likely in Burkitt's lymphoma (see Chap. 41).

Aspergillosis in other sites has no specific imaging characteristics. The granulomas or abscesses may be recognized by scanning, but in almost every patient the clinical and laboratory diagnosis has already been made.

Aspergillosis of the central nervous system may occur from hematogenous spread or, as noted, from direct invasion from the paranasal sinuses. Occasionally aneurysms develop because of fungal infarction. *Aspergillus* granulomas can be recognized on both CT and MR scanning, and are ring enhancing, mimicking tuberculosis, tumors, or other abscesses. Unfortunately, CSF culture following lumbar puncture is usually negative and the diagnosis must be made by tissue biopsy.

Cardiac aspergillosis is very rare and usually indicates immunodepression. Aspergillosis has been cultured from prosthetic valves and spread of the fungus from a valve has caused myocardial abscesses: echocardiography provides helpful information, which will demonstrate these complications in a known case of aspergillosis. As with the CSF, diagnostic blood cultures have a very low positive yield.

Although of little significance for imaging, *Aspergillus* spp (usually *A. niger*) are often present in ear infections: this may be one of the few places in which it can be easily and successfully treated, but occasionally it becomes invasive and spreads into the temporal bone or mastoid. The destruction can be demonstrated by imaging, but as elsewhere, a definitive diagnosis cannot be made, although the clinician's worst fears may be confirmed.

Histoplasmosis Capsulati

Histoplasmosis capsulati is one of the many causes of a "flu-like" illness, with fever, painful muscles, and an irritating cough, which may not really be "just the flu."

Synonyms

Darling's disease. Classic histoplasmosis. Small-form histoplasmosis. Ohio or Mississippi Valley disease. Cave disease. Tingo Maria fever. Reticuloendothelial cytomycosis.

Definition

Histoplasmosis capsulate is a systemic granulomatous disease caused by the dimorphic pathogenic fungus, *Histoplasma capsulatum* var. *capsulatum* (teleomorph: *Ajellomyces capsulatum*). The African form of *Histoplasma, Histoplasma capsulatum* var. *duboisii*, is larger and described separately (see p. 589).

Geographic Distribution

Histoplasma capsulatum is found in tropical and nontropical countries around the world: most cases occur between latitudes 45° north and 30° south. It is most common in the central and eastern United States, in the Mississippi and Ohio Valleys and the Appalachian Mountains, eastern Canada, Mexico, Guatemala, Peru, and Venezuela. While highly endemic in some areas, prevalence can vary widely over short distances.

Epidemiology and Pathology

In the tropics, the fungi are found in both rural and urban areas, in soil around dead or hollow trees, in caves, and anywhere where there are bird or bat excreta. In more temperate climates they are found in the soil of hen houses and farmyards. There are animal reservoirs in dogs, cats, rats, mice, skunks and opossums, bats, and baboons. It is estimated that there are 500 000 new infections annually in the United States alone, but fortunately 90% are asymptomatic and heal without treatment.

The invasive fungi are saprophytic, small (3–4 μm in diameter), and round to oval in shape. After staining with hematoxylin and eosin there may be the false impression of a capsule. Histopathologically, the fungi are located centrally in the granulomas. In patients who are immunodeficient, there will be enormous numbers of organisms concentrated in the cytoplasm of phagocytic cells of the reticuloendothelial system, especially in circulating monocytes and in Kupffer cells, and in phagocytic cells of the spleen, bone marrow, and lymph nodes. In soil, however, the fungus is biphasic, the mycelia producing micro- and macroconidia, which are disturbed when soil is cultivated or excavated. The microconidia are smaller and may be the more infectious. Infection in man is by inhalation, the spores germinate in the alveoli and release yeast forms. Even though dissemination can occur from the lungs, in most patients it is usually well controlled after 2 or 3 weeks. The result is a granuloma containing very few fungi: some may caseate. The residual histoplasmoma is irregular, sometimes with central calcification surrounded by a thick fibrous capsule, within which there are the "ghost" remains of the fungi. The quantity of spores inhaled affects the risk and the severity of the infection, which may also be altered by previous exposure and partial immunity. When many conidia are inhaled, there may be many proliferating yeasts in the alveolae and interstitium of the lungs, resulting in necrosis. In patients who are immunodeficient, the yeast cells divide rapidly and produce large extracellular aggregates. Whatever the site of implantation, regional lymphadenopathy will follow if the infection progresses.

The yeast forms of *H. capsulatum* var. *capsulatum* may be mistaken for *Leishmania* or *Toxoplasma*. Depending on the method of staining, *Torulopsis glabrata* is another source of error. *Penicillium marneffei* can also resemble *H. capsulatum* in vivo.

Laboratory tests include an intradermal sensitivity reaction, which is often positive because of previously unknown infection, and is nonreactive in anergic patients. The skin test is not helpful clinically, but may be useful in epidemiological studies. The skin test can evoke antibody formation (a "false-positive") in individuals who have not been infected earlier. There are complement fixing, precipitin, and fluorescent antibody tests, but serological conversion takes 3–6 weeks, during which time these tests may be negative. In the chronic form of the disease, serological tests remain negative or only become weakly positive in about 50% of all patients.

The diagnosis is made by recognition of the fungus in the sputum or blood, by culture, and in disseminated histoplasmosis, by finding histoplasmal polysaccharide-containing antigen in the urine.

Clinical Characteristics

The clinical spectrum of histoplasmosis capsulati is very broad: fortunately only 5%–10% of all infections result in clinical disease. Pulmonary infections are the most significant, but disseminated infections may be the most serious for the patient. Pulmonary histoplasmosis resembles tuberculosis clinically and on imaging. The clinical syndromes are so varied that constant awareness of histoplasmosis is required to recognize the difference between histoplasmosis and tuberculosis early in the illness: geographical knowledge may be very important when considering the alternatives.

The clinical presentation of the pulmonary infection can be quite asymptomatic or progress through a wide spectrum, including severe acute illness. But pulmonary infection can also appear as a chronic progressive illness. Symptoms vary from mild fever, myalgia, and cough, with increased sputum, to lassitude, pain in the chest, and shortness of breath. These usually start 8–15 days after exposure, and may be accompanied by arthralgia and erythema nodosum. In the majority of patients the disease is self-healing and all that is left clinically after a few weeks is the positive histoplasmin skin test (developing after a few weeks). If there is a known active infection but a persistent negative skin reaction, the prognosis is poor. A rise in titer with complement fixation test is significant, because there can be cross-reactions with North American blastomycosis and some of the other mycoses.

The disseminated form of the infection can be acute or chronic, but is usually progressive. However, there is a silent form of disseminated histoplasmosis recognized where there is splenic calcification in patients who have died for some other reason. Dissemination is most common in children, particularly those who are already ill (e.g., with leukemia or lymphoma) and in the elderly and the immunosuppressed. In such patients it can be acute and fatal. The reticuloendothelial system and bone marrow are affected, resulting in anemia, purpura, and leukopenia. Hepatosplenomegaly and lymphadenopathy develop. Clinically the disseminated infection may closely resemble leishmaniasis or some of the leukemias.

When there is pulmonary progression, this can result in fibrosing mediastinitis, which is often worse than the original pulmonary disease. The mucous membrane of the alimentary tract can be ulcerated and the clinical presentation may be melena. With further systemic spread, cardiac valves, the meninges, brain, and adrenals can be involved. The clinical presentation may then be Addison's disease (*H. capsulatum* may be one of the commonest causes of a cystic mass in the adrenals worldwide). Occasionally oral or laryngeal infections, with laryngeal stricture, can develop. The mortality among patients with the acute dissemination infection is 80% or more unless treated.

However, the disseminated pattern of the disease can also progress slowly in adults, and appear clinically many years (even 30 years) after exposure. Residual nodules are less common in the liver, spleen, and elsewhere than in the lungs. Long-term, slowly progressing pulmonary infection may be more common in those who have been in the tropics or Southeast Asia, but is almost always associated with preexisting chronic obstructive pulmonary disease (emphysema).

The rare subcutaneous form of the disease results in chronic granulomatous ulceration, usually at the site of ulceration.

Imaging Diagnosis

The imaging pattern of histoplasmosis capsulati is so similar to tuberculosis that there is a temptation to refer the reader to Chap. 5. As with tuberculosis, there are acute primary patterns, a chronic reactivation form, a disseminated form and the end results when healed (Fig. 6.36).

Many patients with a positive histoplasmin skin test have multiple calcified nodules in the lung parenchyma, usually in the periphery, and also in the hilar nodes. These are usually incidental findings on a radiograph taken for some other reason. Skin tests sometimes may help to distinguish histoplasmosis from tuberculosis. In a few patients there will be a pulmonary nodule, usually solitary and peripheral (subpleural), well defined, and from a few millimeters to, more commonly, several centimeters across. Some of these nodules slowly enlarge (rather like a tuberculoma): CT scanning is useful to identify calcification, but when seen in older patients this does not always exclude carcinoma. Needle biopsy may be required or even removal of a nodule, particularly when there are several nodules resembling metastases. Even when the needle biopsy shows there is no malignancy, routine follow-up chest imaging to assess any change in the size of any particular nodule may be advisable.

Asymptomatic but enlarged lymph nodes can be calcified, and "eggshell" calcification is a common pattern in histoplasmosis. When the enlarged nodes are not calcified, histoplasmosis cannot be distinguished from any other cause of lymphadenopathy. Pressure from large infected lymph nodes can erode the walls of the bronchi and result in broncholithiasis or, if the nodules are sufficiently large, cause pressure constriction and obstruction: some of the pulmonary radiographic changes may be the result of this. In the more acute primary infection, there will be a "primary complex" with peripheral lung consolidation of varying density and often with associated lymphadenopathy. Parenchymal pneumonic changes may be fleeting, resembling an eosinophilic pneumonia. There is little relationship between the severity of the radiographic changes and the clinical illness. The latter may be mild, even when chest radiographs suggest an extensive process. As the lungs clear, commonly there may be small residual calcified foci. The lymphadenopathy subsides also, but not necessarily in step with the pulmonary improvement.

Acute histoplasmosis is the result of heavy exposure and inhalation, such as may happen when an individual has entered a cave and been the first to disturb accumulated bat droppings. The result can be a severe and often overwhelming illness, causing acute dyspnea, high fever, and fatigue. This is a very dramatic event: in many countries when an important person, such as a king or a priest, has been buried deeply within a cave or in a large, partially closed building, a "curse" is placed on those who may enter and desecrate this sacred resting place. Anyone who ventures to go in search of treasure may develop acute histoplasmosis, which is often fatal in its own right, but especially hazardous for those who believe that they are victims of the supernatural!

In some patients with acute lung infections, the imaging pattern is disseminated miliary nodulation, with lymphadenopathy. These patients are often severely ill, but if they survive and healing occurs, there will be calcified granulomas spread in a "snow storm" pattern throughout both lungs. Such numerous calcified miliary foci are very rarely the result of tuberculosis (but may follow chickenpox pneumonia, especially in adults).

Chronic pulmonary histoplasmosis is almost always superimposed on previous extensive lung disease (e.g., chronic obstructive pulmonary disease and emphysema). Chest radiographs show bullae in the upper lobe, often with contained fluid. The yeast grows in them and eventually spills throughout the bronchial tree, causing pneumonia in different segments of the lungs. This chronic form results in local necrosis, vascular occlusion, and fibrosis. It has been postulated that this is more of an antigen-antibody reaction, rather than the result of the infection. Chronic histoplasmosis is episodic, with symptoms waxing and waning over months, with hemoptysis and shortness of breath often changing but almost always with gradual progression. On imaging, the lung changes can be segmental or lobar, or peripheral opacities. Cavities often become thick-walled but, nevertheless, may continue to enlarge and spread in the adjacent lung. Overall the result is pulmonary fibrosis, very similar to chronic tuberculosis and radiographically indistinguishable (Fig. 6.36 C, D). Other fungal infections, such as aspergillosis, are liable to develop within the damaged lung. At any time this apparently chronic but suppressed histoplasmosis can break down and become more acute.

Fibrosis of the mediastinum is another complication of histoplasmosis which can compress or displace the vena cava, the pulmonary vessels, the trachea and bronchi, and even the esophagus. In endemic areas, histoplasmosis capsulati is probably the commonest cause of mediastinal fibrosis.

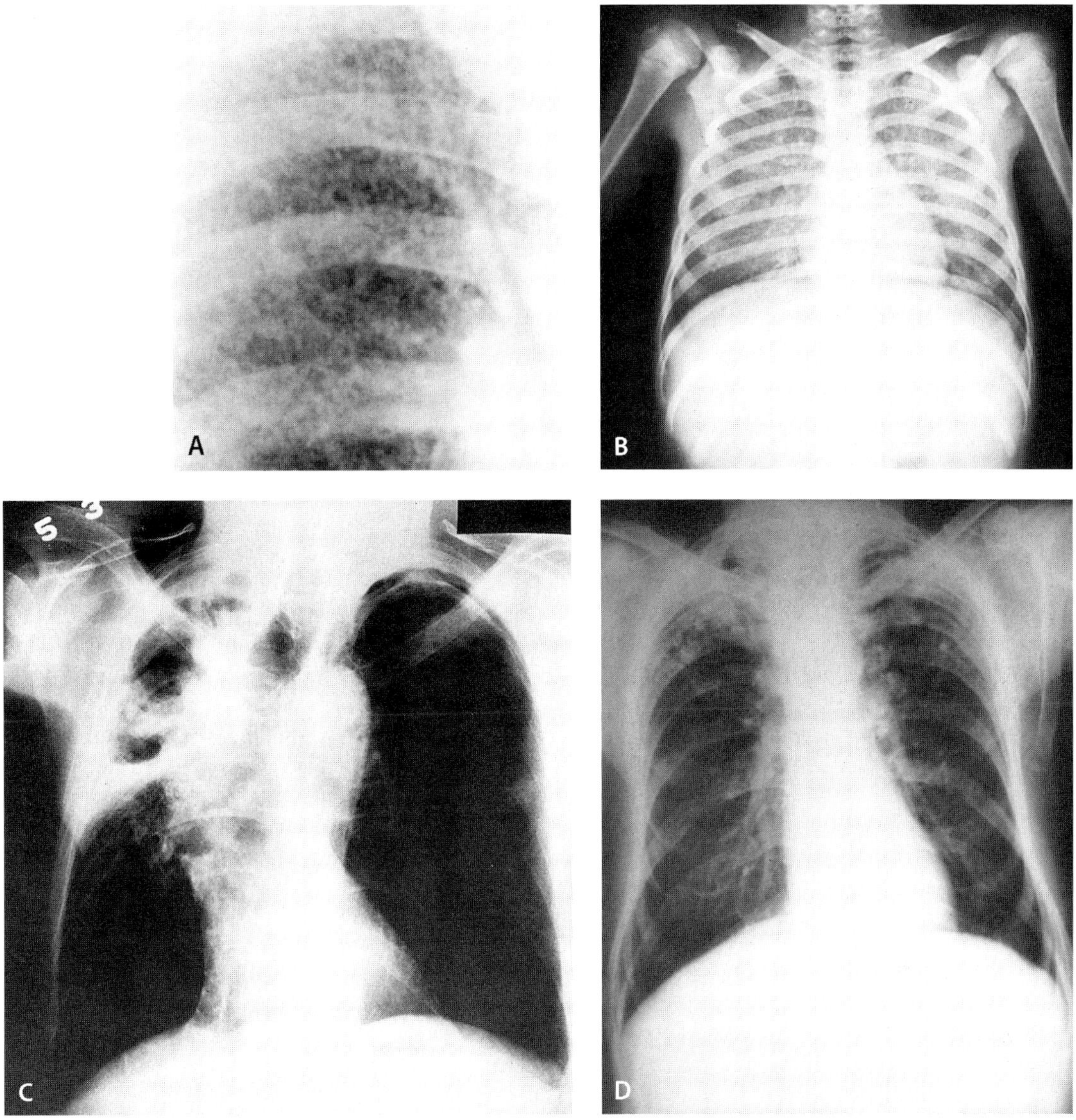

Fig. 6.36 A–G. Histoplasmosis capsulati (due to *H. capsulatum* var. *capsulatum*). **A** The right upper lung of a patient with miliary histoplasmosis: the tiny nodules cannot be accurately distinguished from miliary tuberculosis and many other miliary patterns. **B** Disseminated acute histoplasmosis in a 10-year-old child. **C** Chronic histoplasmosis causing fibrosis, with cavitation in the right upper lobe. There are calcified hilar nodes. Radiologically (and clinically) this is indistinguishable from tuberculosis, but both *Histoplasma capsulatum* var. *capsulatum* and *Aspergillus* were recovered from this lung. **D** Bilateral apical fibrosis from histoplasmosis, again indistinguishable from tuberculosis. **E–G** see p. 588

CT and MR Scanning of Pulmonary Histoplasmosis

A plain chest radiograph provides a great deal of information about histoplasmosis, but however suspicious the findings may be because of local endemicity, the diagnosis can seldom be made firmly. Plain radiographs are usually unable to completely show the complications or the extent of the disease and its resulting fibrosis. CT scanning is the best way to show calcification in the mediastinal mass, particularly the fine stippled pattern which may not be seen on plain radiographs or MRI. CT is also able to demonstrate calcification within lymph nodes or in a peripheral histoplasmoma. It can accurately visualize tracheobronchial narrowing and show the relationship to any adjacent mass. CT can also show when the peripheral lobar and alveolar changes are the result of segmental bronchial blockage. Parenchymal changes, such as pulmonary infarction, which are not clearly seen on a chest radiograph, are better seen with CT, particularly those close to the pleura. In some patients a ventilation-perfusion

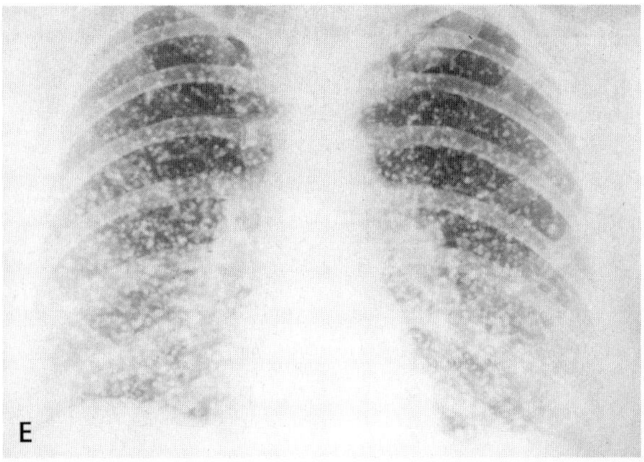
E

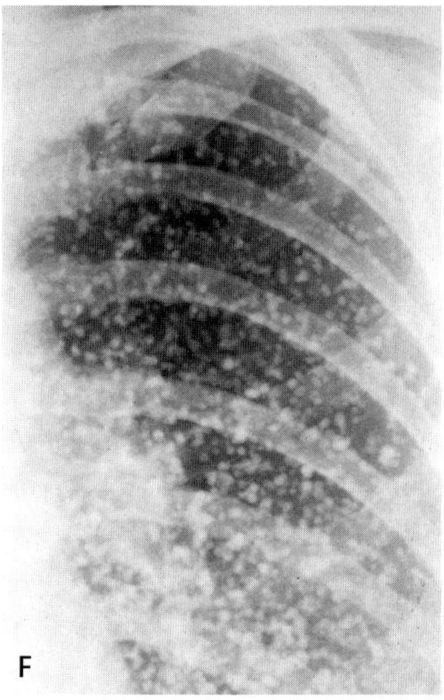
F

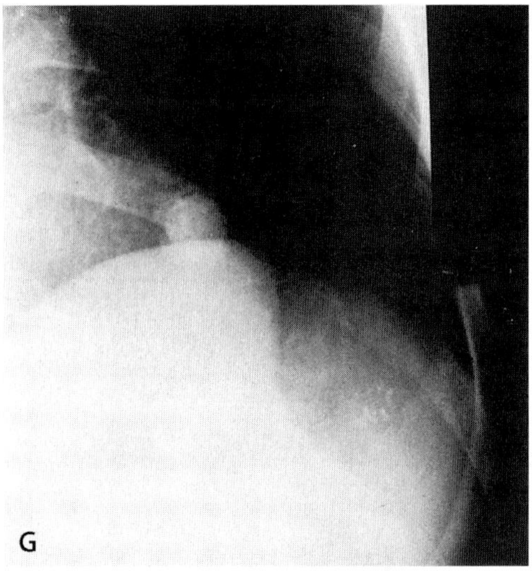
G

Fig. 6.36 (*continued*). **E, F** The characteristic pattern of calcified healed disseminated histoplasmosis. There may be no clinical evidence and the patient may be unaware of having been infected. **G** A histoplasmona in the left lower lobe of an asymptomatic patient. There is central calcification. Histoplasmomas have no diagnositc characteristics and only the histology will establish the diagnosis

radioisotope study showing decreased perfusion to the same area will provide additional evidence of vascular damage. If surgery is contemplated, CT is a useful way to delineate exactly the involved area.

Magnetic resonance imaging is much less accurate than CT at demonstrating calcification, which is an important part of the diagnosis of histoplasmosis, particularly fibrosing mediastinitis. The lymphadenopathy of histoplasmosis has low signal intensity on T2-weighted MR scans. This may indicate benign adenopathy, although histopathological confirmation is required. MRI is particularly useful in assessing vascular compression, which is not clearly seen on CT scanning.

To summarize; the diagnosis of pulmonary histoplasmosis may be considered from plain radiographs, and CT scanning provides additional evidence; MRI is useful to assess vascular complications, but CT should be the first choice if scanning is indicated.

Extrapulmonary Histoplasmosis

In many patients with histoplasmosis, there will be hepatosplenomegaly with coarse miliary or punctate calcification in the liver and the spleen (sometimes found in patients who have no symptoms). CT is the most accurate method of imaging. Other imaging findings include abdominal lymphadenopathy, which on CT may be homogeneous or with more diffuse or central low density. There may be bilateral adrenal enlargement due to diffuse or localized low-density masses. The scanning pattern of hepatosplenomegaly has no specific characteristics in histoplasmosis: calcification is not always found in the abdominal viscera or lymph nodes.

Colonic strictures, mimicking carcinoma, have been reported in histoplasmosis and demonstrated with a barium enema. Other areas of segmental narrowing of the bowel may be difficult to differentiate from amebiasis or tuberculous. In histoplasmosis and tuberculosis there is usually associated regional lymphadenopathy but this seldom occurs in amebiasis: there are really very few distinguishing features

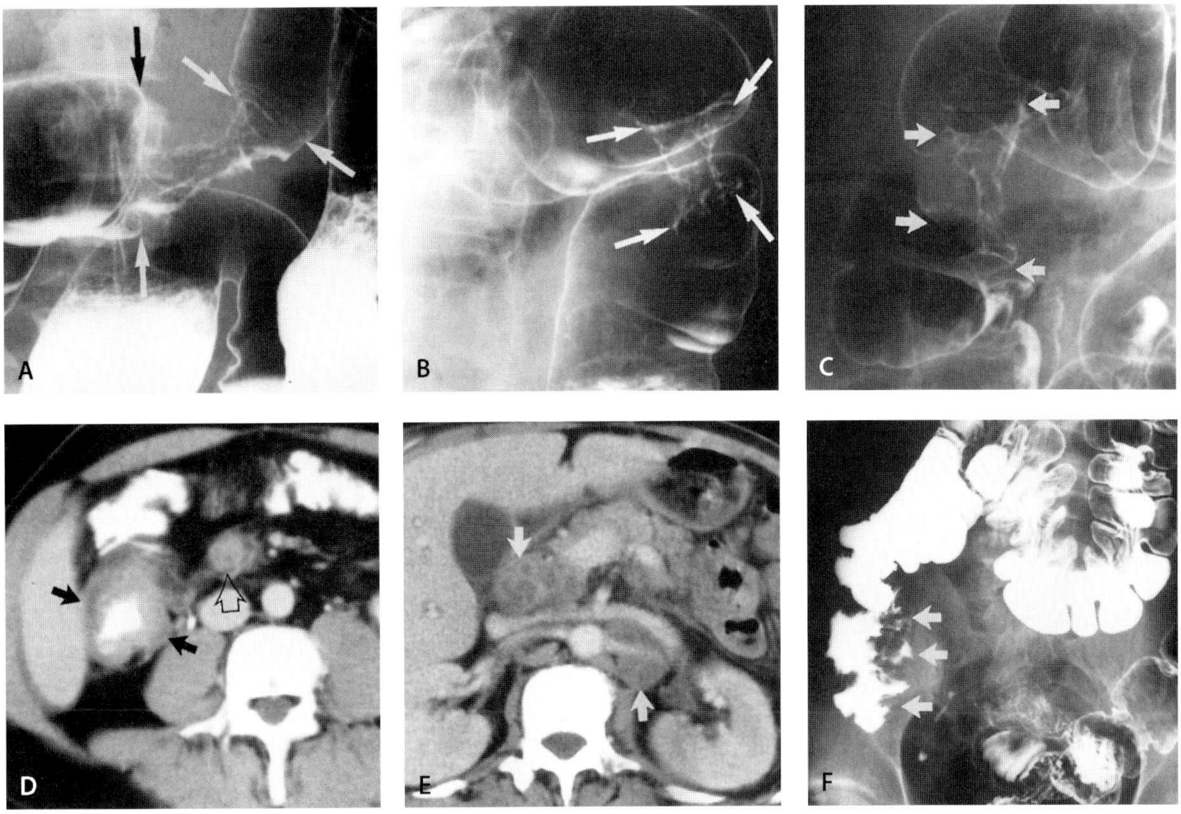

Fig. 6.37 A–F. Disseminated histoplasmosis has many clinical and radiographic presentations, particularly in those who are immunocompromised. **A, B** A double-contrast barium enema showing two apple-core lesions (*arrows*) in the transverse colon of a 39-year-old HIV-positive man. The colon was otherwise normal. **C–E** A similar lesion mimicking a carcinoma of the colon in a different, 50-year-old patient. **C** shows a single narrowed area, and CT scans (**D**) shows the thickening of the bowel wall (*solid arrows*) and enlarged regional lymph nodes (*open arrow*). (**E**) The lymphadenopathy had progressed 8 months later (*arrows*). **F** Histoplasmosis mimicking tuberculosis or amebiasis in the cecum and ascending colon. (Courtesy of Dr. E.G. Balthazar et al. and *AJR*, 1993)

on imaging. Many gastrointestinal lesions due to histoplasmosis may be incidental findings at autopsy: any part of the gastrointestinal tract may be affected, but particularly the terminal ileum and ascending colon. In such lesions there is usually patchy superficial ulceration or raised thickened plaques. Polyps, bowel perforation, and anal fissures have been reported. Many of these can be found during endoscopy but, again, there are no specific imaging characteristics. In most patients gastrointestinal lesions occur as part of known disseminated infection (Fig. 6.37) but rarely they are the first sign that histoplasmosis is beginning to spread.

Skeletal involvement by *Histoplasma capsulatum* var. *capsulatum* is very uncommon and the rare lytic lesions have no specific imaging changes. Involvement of bone marrow is a common feature of disseminated histoplasmosis in immunodeficient patients.

Histoplasmosis Duboisii

Caused by a larger species of *Histoplasma*, histoplasmosis duboisii is clinically, geographically, and histopathologically quite different from the more commonly known and widespread classical histoplasmosis capsulati.

Synonyms

African histoplasmosis. Large histoplasmosis. Large-form histoplasmosis.

Definition

African histoplasmosis is a systemic infection caused by the fungus *Histoplasma capsulatum* var. *duboisii*.

Geographic Distribution

Histoplasma capsulatum var. *duboisii* occurs, with very few exceptions, only on the African continent between the Tropics of Cancer and Capricorn. A few cases of histoplasmosis duboisii have been identified in Madagascar and isolated cases have been recognized in Arabia, parts of Asia, and Japan. It should be emphasized that these cases outside Africa are exceptional. It is suspected that there are clinically silent cases elsewhere, but this is not known for certain because there is no specific skin test. There is no doubt that histoplasmosis duboisii is most common in west and central Africa, particularly Nigeria, Senegal, the Democratic Republic of Congo (formerly Zaire), and Angola.

Epidemiology and Pathology

The *duboisii* variety of *Histoplasma capsulatum* was first described in 1952 (by Vanbreuseghem) named in 1960 (by Ciferri) and fully described as a clinical disease in 1964 (by Cockshott and Lucas). It was obtained from soil mixed with bat guano, as well as the bowel of bats in 1991 (Gugnani et al.). It has been identified in two species of baboons from Guinea and Senegal. The yeast cells of *Histoplasma capsulatum* var. *duboisii* average about 10 µm in diameter, about twice the size of *H. capsulatum* var. *capsulatum*. They are thick walled and round or oval. They reproduce by a single bud which can equal the size of the parent cell, giving an hourglass appearance. Thus, in tissue, the two varieties vary in size.
H. capsulatum var. *duboisii* may remain viable for many years within tissues without clinical evidence of disease. Infection is spread by inhalation and affects all age groups, but particularly persons in their second decade. There is no significant racial or gender predominance. Histopathologically, the fungus is both extra- and intracellular, but tends to accumulate within large macrophages, which may contain up to 30 fungal cells, all apparently continuing to grow and bud. The fungus may also lie free within the tissues. The reaction is granulomatous, with very large giant cells full of fungi and surrounded by inflammation and fibrosis (Fig. 6.38). Caseation occurs, but unlike in histoplasmosis capsulati, calcification is not a feature. In some patients, particularly the immunodeficient with disseminated disease, the yeasts are found in large numbers within the tissue but without any significant inflammation: the extent of the reaction in each patient depends very much on their immune status. Different histological lesions can be seen at the same time in one patient, but the reason for this is unclear.

Diagnosis depends on the recognition of the fungus from a biopsy specimen or from pus or exudates. Culture may be required and there is also an immunofluorescent test.

Clinical Characteristics

There are two main clinical presentations: localized and disseminated.
Localized form: The lesions are isolated skin, bone, or lymph node infections.
They are chronic and may not become clinically apparent until after long incubation. On the skin there are small painless papules which may form plaques or nodules (Fig. 6.39), ulcerate, or become cold abscesses with a tendency to break down. The skin lesions can be single or multiple and some have a surrounding pigment halo. They may heal spontaneously, develop exuberant granulation tissue, or invade underlying bone. Lymph nodes may suppurate and bone infections occur in one-third of all patients, developing into chronic osteomyelitis with draining sinuses. Infection of the lungs, mucous membranes, or intestinal tract is uncommon except in the rapidly progressive disseminated form of histoplasmosis duboisii.
Disseminated form: There is fever, anemia, and weight loss, as well as abdominal pain and jaundice in some patients. Multiple cutaneous lesions are usually present all over the body, together with subcutaneous abscesses. Lumps may develop over the head with underlying lytic lesions of the skull, radiographically resembling multiple myeloma or tuberculosis. Multiple lymph nodes enlarge and the liver and spleen may be infected and enlarged. Infections of the urinary bladder and large bowel have been reported and have a poor prognosis. As the infection worsens, pulmonary lesions will develop. Unless treated, the patient will die.
Skin lesions are the most common clinical presentation, but bones and joints are frequently infected, the joints being involved by spread from bone lesions. The femora, ribs, skull, upper arms, and vertebrae are the bones most commonly affected.
African histoplasmosis often arises in patients already suffering from tuberculosis, schistosomiasis, malnutrition, leishmaniasis, or AIDS.

Imaging Diagnosis

Histoplasma capsulatum var. *duboisii* infections usually arise in the metaphyses of the long bones, the small bones of the hand, and the flat bones. The earliest lesion is a small lytic area, as occurs in multiple myeloma, skeletal metastases, or, in some pa-

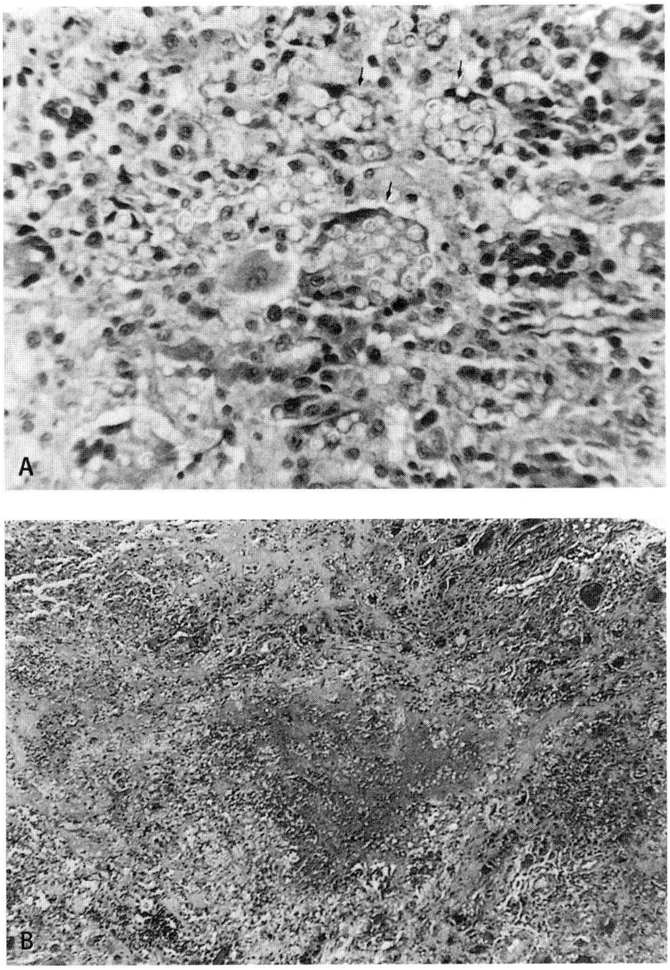

Fig. 6.38 A, B. *Histoplasma capsulatum* var. *duboisii*. **A** The histopathology shows granulomas with many huge giant cells, up to 200 µm in diameter, packed with large yeast cells. H&E,×200. **B** Caseous necrosis surrounded by fibrosis with only a few giant cells. H & E, ×80. (**A**, **B** from Bittencourt and Londero 1995; **B** was provided by Prof. Kaschula, Capetown)

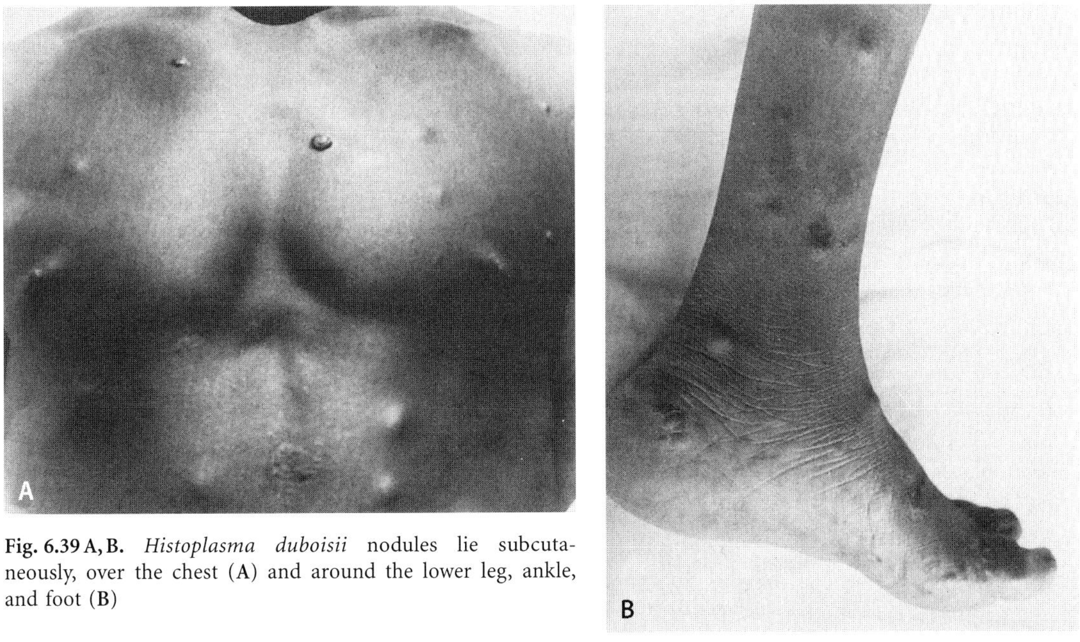

Fig. 6.39 A, B. *Histoplasma duboisii* nodules lie subcutaneously, over the chest (**A**) and around the lower leg, ankle, and foot (**B**)

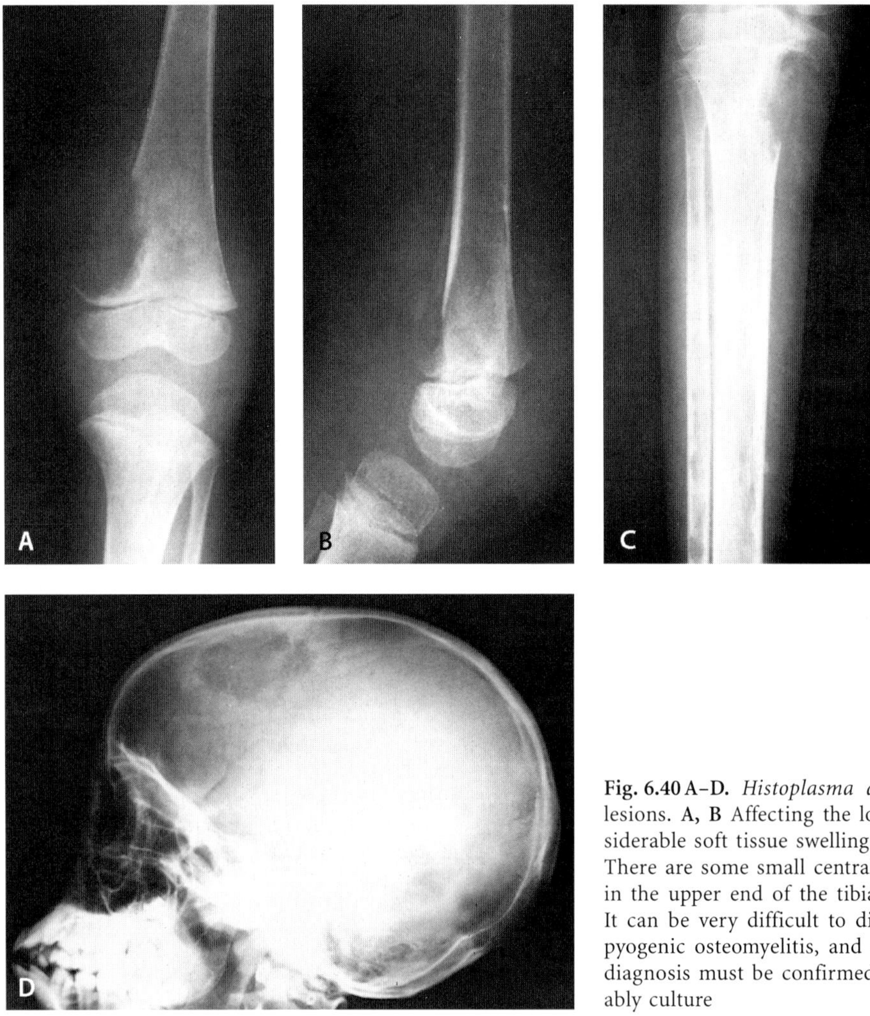

Fig. 6.40 A–D. *Histoplasma duboisii* causes destructive bone lesions. **A, B** Affecting the lower end of the femur, with considerable soft tissue swelling and elevation of the periosteum. There are some small central lytic foci. **C** Similar destruction in the upper end of the tibia and **D** several foci in the skull. It can be very difficult to distinguish between this fungal or pyogenic osteomyelitis, and in some patients, neoplasm. The diagnosis must be confirmed clinically, by biopsy and preferably culture

tients, tuberculosis. These lesions are often quite diffuse, and in small bones there may be a lattice-like area. The center of these bone infections becomes necrotic and can drain into the soft tissues, forming a subcutaneous abscess which may persist deeply or connect with the skin. Although there is some periosteal reaction, this is often made worse by secondary pyogenic infection acquired through a draining sinus.

Infection of bone can be widespread and dramatic, involving the whole length of long bones. Paraplegia from vertebral involvement has been reported, with the discs usually remaining intact (as occurs in other infections, e.g., actinomycosis and coccidioidomycosis). Paraspinal abscesses may develop and drain through sinuses.

In the disseminated pattern, the pulmonary lesions are difficult to distinguish from tuberculosis or from histoplasmosis capsulati. In one patient diffuse miliary nodules were observed radiographically, and at autopsy granulomatous nodules were found throughout both lungs and within enlarged and necrotizing lymph nodes. This pattern has been seen in other patients, and has responded to treatment. Direct spread to other systems is uncommon.

The imaging diagnosis of histoplasmosis duboisii is in many ways easier than that of other fungal or pyogenic bone infections, though distinction from neoplasm may be difficult (Fig. 6.40). The extent of the bone destruction and the multiple bones involved as the disease progresses result in a characteristic pattern (Fig. 6.41).

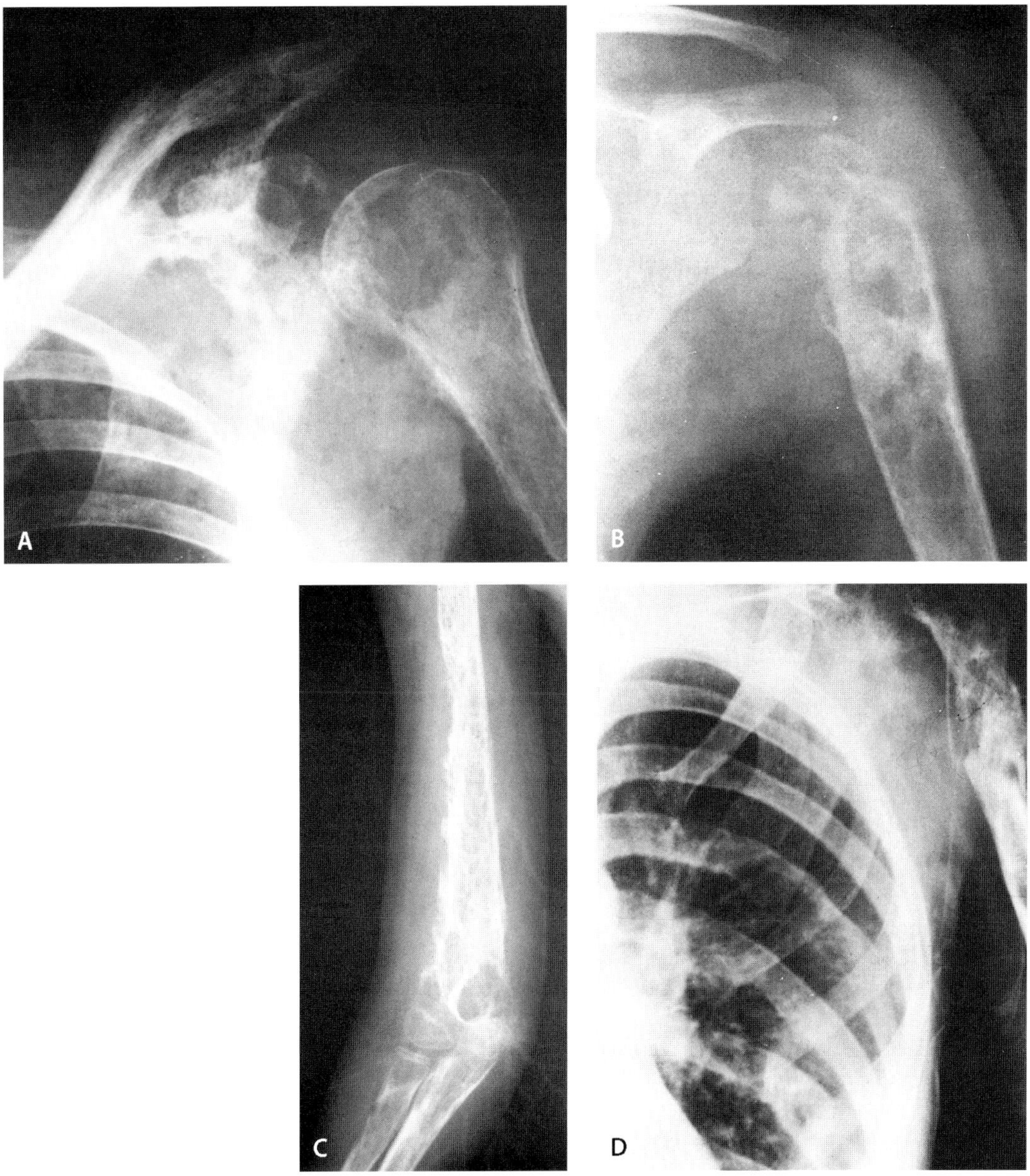

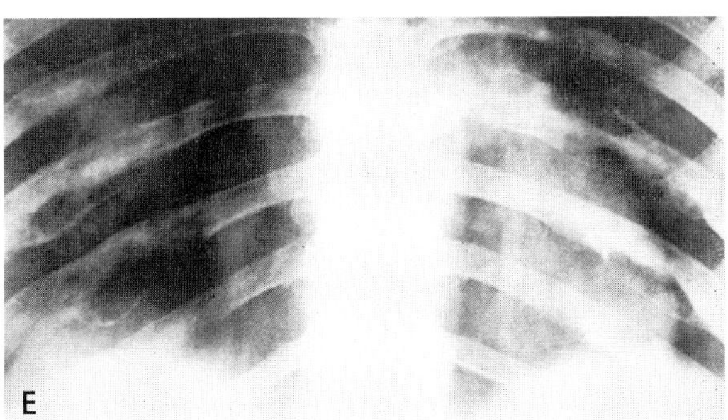

Fig. 6.41 A–E. Histoplasmosis duboisii should always be considered (where geographically likely) when there are multiple irregular areas of bone destruction, often with suprisingly little periosteal reaction. **A** A large lytic lesion in the upper end of the humerus with minimal periosteal elevation. There are multiple areas of bone destruction in the scapula, some showing reactive sclerosis. **B** Multiple quite large destructive foci in the upper end of the humerus, with disruption of the humeral head. There is soft tissue swelling. **C** Another patient with multiple lytic areas in the lower half of the humerus, destruction of the elbow joint, and further foci in the upper end of the radius and ulna. The humerus shows more periosteal reaction than is usual. **D** The shoulder joint of this patient has been completely destroyed and there are multiple lytic foci in the humerus and the remains of the scapula. There are also many foci in the ribs. **E** A different patient with multiple lytic areas in many of the ribs on both sides. All the patients in Fig. 6.40 and 6.41 came from West Africa. (Courtesy of the late Prof. W. P. Cockshott)

Coccidioidomycosis

Coccidioidomycosis is an infection which causes a varying response from the authors of textbooks on tropical diseases, as it does in patients. The causative fungus, *Coccidioides immitis*, occurs naturally only in some part of the Western Hemisphere. Some tropical texts ignore the disease completely, but in others it is described at length. As with many other diseases in this book, it can occur in both tropical and subtropical regions, particularly in those which are relatively arid.

Synonyms

Valley fever. Desert rheumatism. The bumps. California disease. Posada's disease. Wernicke's disease. Coccidioidal granuloma. San Joaquin fever. *Fr:* Coccidioidomycose. *Ger:* Kokzidioidomykosa. Talfieber. Wüstenfieber. *Sp:* Coccioidomicosis.

Definition

Coccidioidomycosis is a mycotic infection caused by *Coccidioides immitis* (the species name, "immitis" means "not mild").

Geographic Distribution

The infection is hyperendemic in the southwestern United States (in some regions of the San Joaquin Valley up to 97% of children may have positive skin reactions). It is also endemic in Mexico, Guatemala, Honduras, Colombia, Venezuela, Bolivia, Paraguay, Argentina, and Brazil, particularly where there are semiarid or desert regions. Sporadic infections have been identified in Europe, Japan, Asia, Canada, and Australia amongst individuals who have been exposed in the endemic areas or to products from those areas.

Epidemiology and Pathology

The first patient was described in 1891, a soldier with a skin infection in Northern Argentina. He survived for over 11 years, during which time he was studied by Posadas and Wernicke: hence the synonyms. The infection has been studied extensively since then, and there are at least five textbooks titled "Coccidioidomycosis." There are innumerable reports and reviews in general and specialized medical journals: here is yet another!

Coccidioides immitis is found as a saprophytic mold in soils in endemic areas. The molds produce infective arthroconidia or arthrospora. Infections are usually the result of inhalation of fungus from dust. Rarely, traumatic introduction of the fungus into the skin has resulted in disease. Many mammals have been infected, some wild, but also those housed in zoos in the endemic areas. Wild rodents and rattle and gopher snakes have been infected in nature.

In endemic areas, dust is laden with highly infective chlamydospores which are round, nonbudding, thickwalled spherules containing numerous endospores: these develop into branching, septate filamentous hyphae which form anthrospores, found in both nature and culture. The chains of thick-walled barrel-shaped arthrospores (arthroconidia) which grow on cultures alternate with empty cells, which is an important though nonspecific diagnostic characteristic.

Coccidioides immitis is a dimorphic fungus. When inhaled, the arthrospores enlarge and become rounded to produce spherules. The spherules produce as many as 800 endospores; these, when released into tissues, can mature into new spherules and the lifecycle starts again. When infected tissue or body fluid is cultured, the hyphae form develops from the spherule-endospore form. The tissue reaction is both suppurative and granulomatous, with caseation and granulomas formed of giant cells and macrophages. As healing occurs, there is fibrosis and calcification. The extent of the necrosis and the pace of healing depend on the size of the infected dose and the immune status of the patient. Thus, it is in the immunosuppressed that severe pulmonary or disseminated infections are likely to occur. Nevertheless, clinically silent infections, recognized only by positive skin reactions, are very common in endemic areas.

Patients with competent cell-mediated immunity convert their coccidioidin skin test within 2–21 days after clinical symptoms begin. Conversion is a useful way to make a diagnosis, but it must be confirmed histopathologically, by culture, or serologically. Positive skin tests may revert to negative (anergy) if the patient's immunity fails, which usually indicates that the infection is disseminated. Unfortunately, the cutaneous test is not completely reliable because cross-reactions with other fungal infections can occur or the test may be negative despite frank disease.

There are serological preciptin, complement fixation and immunodiffusion tests which can help with the diagnosis and assessment of progress and treatment. When infections are asymptomatic, less than 10% of the patients will have positive complement fixation titers. When there is meningitis, antibodies will be found in the spinal fluid, with reduced sugar, elevated proteins, and cells. When there is pulmonary infection, sputum culture is frequently positive. Urine samples may yield the organism in some patients with disseminated disease.

Clinical Characteristics

Coccidioidomycosis can cause a wide variety of signs or symptoms or have no clinical affect. In most individuals the only result of exposure to *C. immitis* is conversion of the skin test without any symptoms. In some patients there may be a tiny calcified granuloma or fibrotic scar or cavity, visible on a routine chest radiograph and representing a pulmonary residuum.

In patients in whom there are clinical smyptoms, the common diagnosis is "flu," with a mild fever, pleuritic chest pain, generalized aches and pains, night sweats and chills, and a cough. Some patients may have a fine diffuse transient erythematous rash covering the body and limbs, and may develop erythema nodosum or erythema multiforme. These are "the bumps," itchy, tender nodules of varying size. There is often arthralgia, without effusion (desert rheumatism). In such patients the skin test often causes a violent reaction. Most patients improve clinically and return to health after 3 or 4 weeks. If symptoms persist for 6–8 weeks, there is said to be persistent coccidioidomycosis.

A few patients develop the rare primary cutaneous lesions, which resemble a chancre at the site of inoculation. This is followed by regional lymphadenopathy. However, most cutaneous lesions (nodules, ulcers, and pustules) are the result of dissemination of infection from a primary pulmonary site. Such dissemination may result in single or multiple cutaneous lesions, some of which may spread extensively over the skin. Pulmonary cavities may persist without general dissemination, but with recurrent complaints of cough and hemoptysis, and may lead to a pneumothorax.

The most serious pattern of infection is extrapulmonary dissemination, which is more common in some communities than in others. It is ten times more common in blacks, Filipinos, other Asians, Eskimos, and American Indians. It is much less common in Caucasian females than in Caucasian males, but if the patient is pregnant, then the later the infection starts, the more likely is dissemination and the prognosis worsens accordingly.

Any immunodeficient patient is liable to develop disseminated coccidioidomycosis: not only those with AIDS, but immunosuppressed transplant patients, and those receiving corticosteroid or chemotherapy. It has been suggested that the size of the initial dose of spores is significant, with a heavy load increasing the risk of subsequent dissemination. This has not been verified in humans.

Disseminated coccidioidomycosis usually involves the bones (Fig. 6.42 A), joints, skin (Fig. 6.42 B), me-

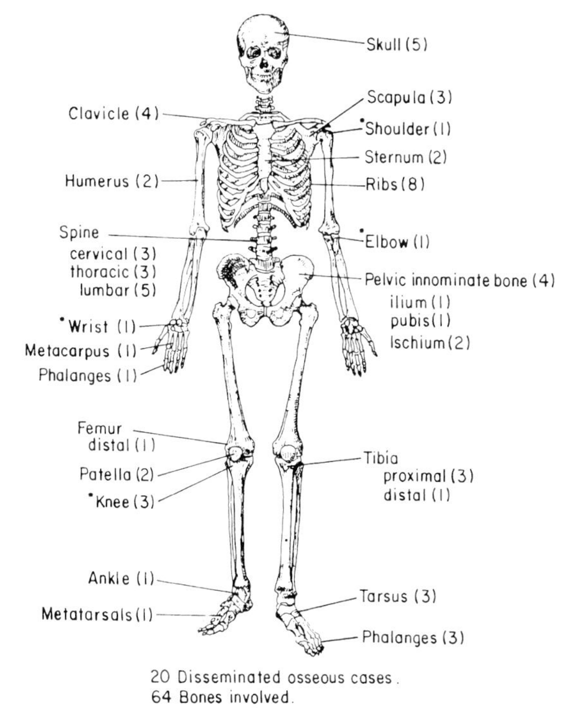

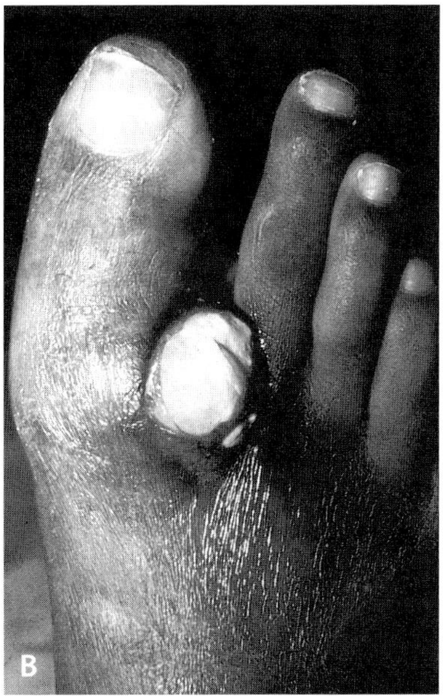

Fig. 6.42. A The distribution of skeletal lesion in 20 patients with disseminated coccidioidomycosis. **B** A cutaneous lesion in disseminated coccidiodomycosis: there are usually well circumscribed and contain many fungi. (A courtesy of Dr. J. P. McGahan, Sacramento)

ninges, and the urinary tract. It can involve any organ in the body although the gastrointestinal tract and endocardium are seldom infected. Chronic meningitis develops in about 30% of those with disseminated infection, but the onset may be difficult to recognize: the early symptoms are ill health, personality change, and headache. The brain is seldom involved, but without treatment the meningitis is invariably fatal.

Imaging Diagnosis

The small calcified granulomas or scars seen in the lung in asymptomatic coccidioidomycosis have already been noted: another finding on a plain chest radiographs is localized pleural thickening.

When the patients has symptoms, the chest radiograph often shows consolidation, commonly in the upper lobes, or fleeting nodular or bronchopneumonic densities in the middle and lower lobes: these may coalesce to lobar consolidation or break down into small but multiple cavities (Fig. 6.43). Pneumonia may persist, or become fibrotic and, with healing, can develop calcification. If the disease is progressive, the small cavities are joined by tissue breakdown into one large cavity: this may persist or heal with fibrosis. However, some of the linear densities, particularly in basal regions, may be peribronchial or lymphatic thickening and not fibrosis.

At all stages, hilar lymphadenopathy is common (Fig. 6.43 A); the mediastinal nodes are enlarged less frequently. There can be lymphadenopathy even when there is no visible parenchymal lesion (Fig. 6.43 C) and this may persist for months: the etiology of such lymphadenopathy cannot be recognized by imaging alone.

Pleural involvement, with pleural effusion and thickening, is quite common and a pneumothorax and empyema can also occur.

A solitary nodule, a coccidioidoma (Fig. 6.43 F), is often clear in outline and very similar to a tuberculoma. Such nodules can be 0.5–2 inches (1–5 cm) in diameter, and are usually single but occasionally multiple. CT or standard tomography sometimes shows central calcification. Aspiration biopsy is necessary to establish the diagnosis. It has been suggested that the location of these nodules in different parts of the lung is a way to distinguish them from tuberculomas. Unfortunately, both coccidioidomas and tuberculomas may occur in any part of the lung, and both may remain unchanged for months and may either grow slowly or cavitate. Calcification can occur in both infections. In tuberculosis, changes in the patient's immunity can result in breakdown of the nodules with local or distant spread: this is rare in coccidioidomycosis. A coccidioidoma does not represent the threat of bronchogenic spread which occurs with a tuberculoma.

All patterns of the disease can be unilateral or bilateral. As already noted, there may be linear densities, particularly in basal regions, which may be peribronchial or lymphatic thickening. Miliary lesions in the lung (Fig. 6.43 B) usually denote hematogenous spread and are usually accompanied by extrapulmonary dissemination. A reticulonodular pattern, resembling but larger than that in miliary tuberculosis, can be seen in AIDS patients with coccidioidomycosis: if there is cavitation, the prognosis is poor.

In the chronic, benign pattern of pulmonary infection, the most characteristic finding is a thin-walled cyst, with or without bronchial communication. These "grape skin" cavities (Fig. 6.43 D) have no apparent surrounding parenchymal reaction, but the wall of the cavity is often several millimeters thick. Serial films may show progression from thick- to thin-walled cysts, and rapid inflation and deflation. These cysts may be secondarily infected, contain a fungus ball, heal with fibrosis, be filled with blood by internal hemorrhage, or rupture and produce a pneumothorax. Although strongly suggestive of coccidioidomycosis, similar thin-walled cavities occur in tuberculosis, melioidosis, and dirofilariasis. In some patients, the cavities are thick walled and even less specific, but a very thick-walled cavity with a central lucency (a "doughnut cavity") may favor the diagnosis of coccidioidomycosis.

Healing is by fibrosis, often with residual bronchiectasis and in some patients, parenchymal and nodal calcifications. The imaging pattern of pulmonary coccidioidomycosis closely mimics that of tuberculosis (Fig. 6.43) and histoplasmosis: the distinction can often only be made by histopathology. All three infections can be complicated by other fungi (e.g., the formation of fungus balls in the cavities), and also by pyogenic secondary infection.

Extrapulmonary coccidioidomycosis can be fatal. It may occur when the patient is apparently recovering from the initial infection. Bone lesions occur in about 20% of patients with disseminated disease; the most common sites are the vertebrae, skull, pelvis, hands, feet and the ends of the long bones (Fig. 6.44 A–C, 6.45, 6.46). As occurs in many other fungal infections, such as blastomycosis, sporotrichosis, and madura mycosis, the foci of osteomyelitis are often juxta-articular. Joint infection usually follows spread from a nearby bone lesion and is most common in the wrist, elbow, and ankle. In infants, the mid shaft of bones may be affected. The bone foci are usually sharply marginated and punched out; they are lytic at first, but later become sclerotic. Coccidioidomycosis in bones and joints is quite destructive and resembles tuberculosis or even malignancy.

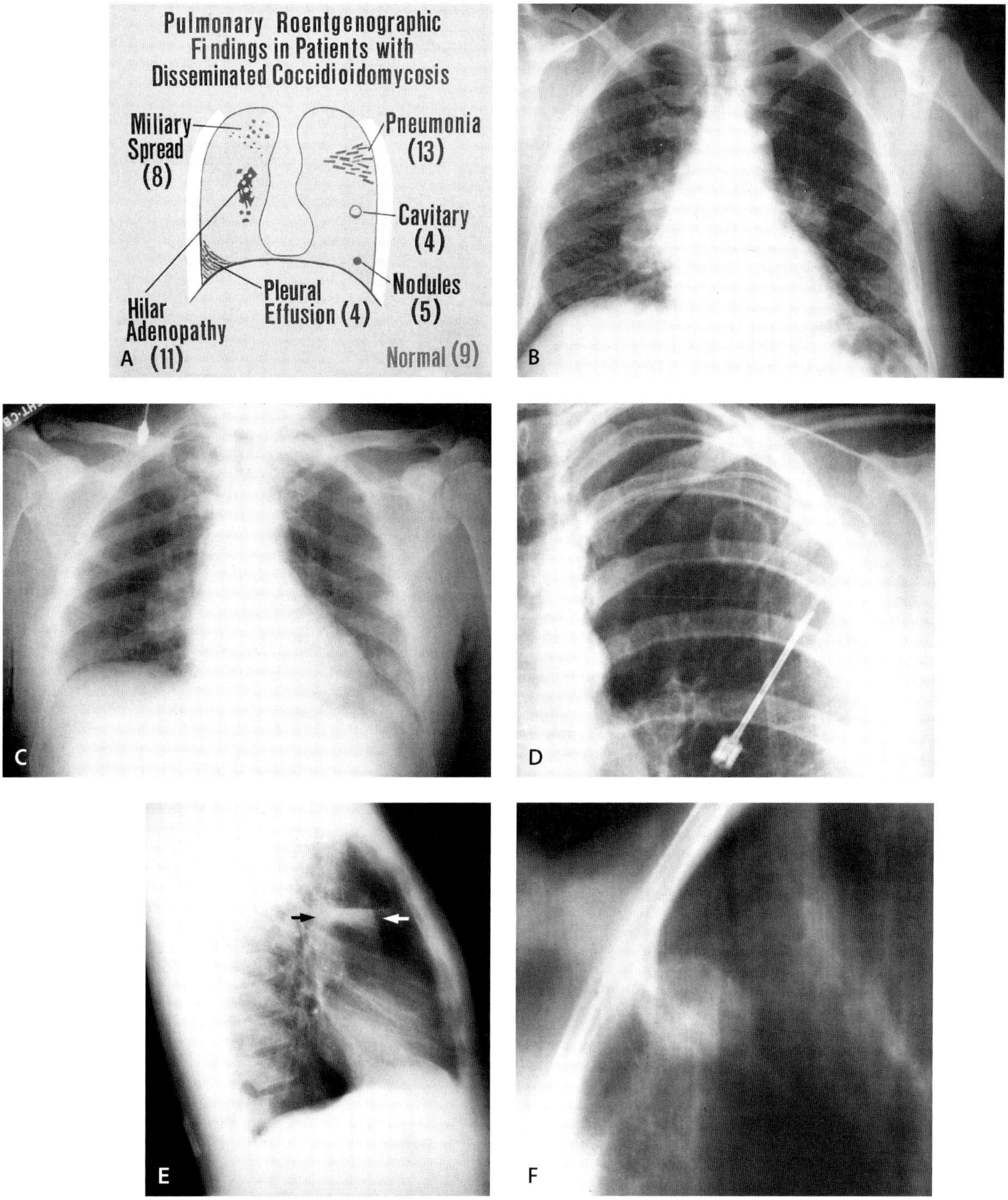

Fig. 6.43. Coccidioidomycosis mimics tuberculosis in the variety and multiplicity of images which may be seen, a few of which are illustrated in this and the next four figures. **A** The pulmonary lesions in 54 patients. **B** Miliary spread throughout both lungs with marked hilar and mediastinal lymphadenopathy. **C** Lymphadenopathy without obvious pulmonary foci. **D** The ring, "grape skin" cavity which is so typical of this infection. **E** A large fluid-containing cavity in an upper lobe, seen in a lateral projection (*arrows* show fluid-level). **F** A peripheral coccidiodaoma with a small pleural effusion. (**A** courtesy of Dr. J.P. McGahan, Sacramento; **D** courtesy of Dr. J.P. McGahan et al. and *AJR*, 1981)

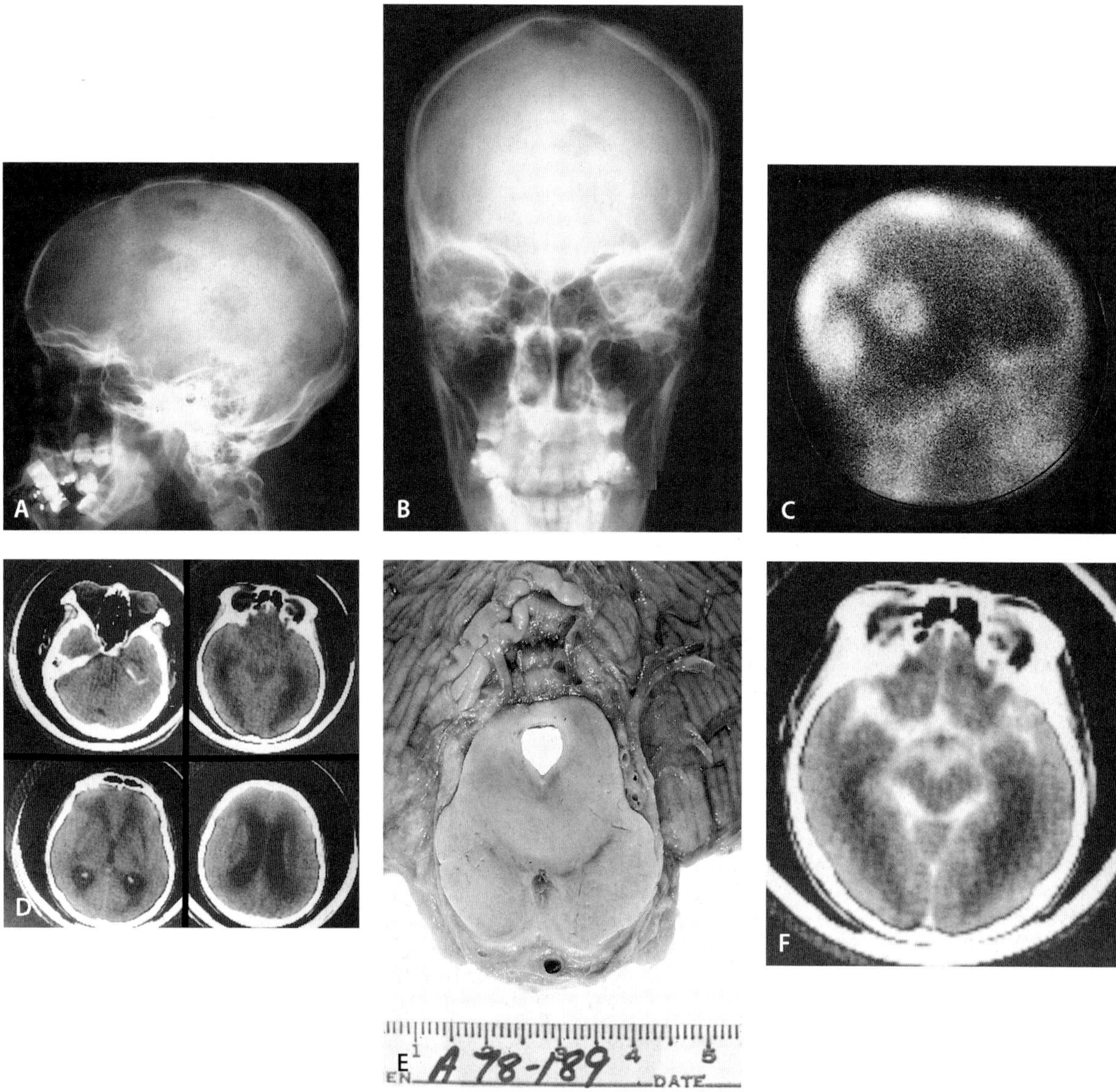

Fig. 6.44 A–F. Cranial and cerebral coccidioidomycosis. **A, B** Multiple well-circumscribed lytic defects in the skull. **C** Increased uptake of 99 mTc-methylene diphosphonate in bony lesions in the skull: some of these may not be suspected clinically or on radiographs. **D** CT scan showing hydrocephalus associated with coccidioidal meningitis. **E** Basal meningeal thickening seen at autopsy. **F** Post contrast enhancement in the basal meninges in coccidioidomycosis. (**A–D, F** courtesy of Dr. J.P. McGahan et al. and *AJR*, 1981)

A paravertebral abscess may develop from a spinal lesion and there may be complete obstruction on myelography: involvement of the intervertebral disc is infrequent. Scintigraphy is useful when dissemination is first suspected, because many bone lesions will be clinically silent for some time. CT is helpful in the spine in demonstrating the exact extent of the vertebral involvement and any abscess. MRI is useful to show an abscess and any involvement of the spinal cord.

Cerebral coccidioidomycosis causes granulomatous thickening of the leptomeninges (Fig. 6.44 E). Arteritis is an uncommon complication. CT demonstrates diffuse leptomeningitis in most patients with cerebral coccidioidomycosis. This is characterized by obliteration of the CSF spaces, particularly at the base around the mid brain: when actively infected, there will be contrast enhancement of the meninges, particularly around the brain stem (Fig. 6.44 F). Hydrocephalus complicates the infection in about 50% of the patients (Fig. 6.44 D) even when the meningitis has been treated. Granulomas within the brain are uncommon, but seem to have a predilection for the cerebellum. They may be demonstrated by CT

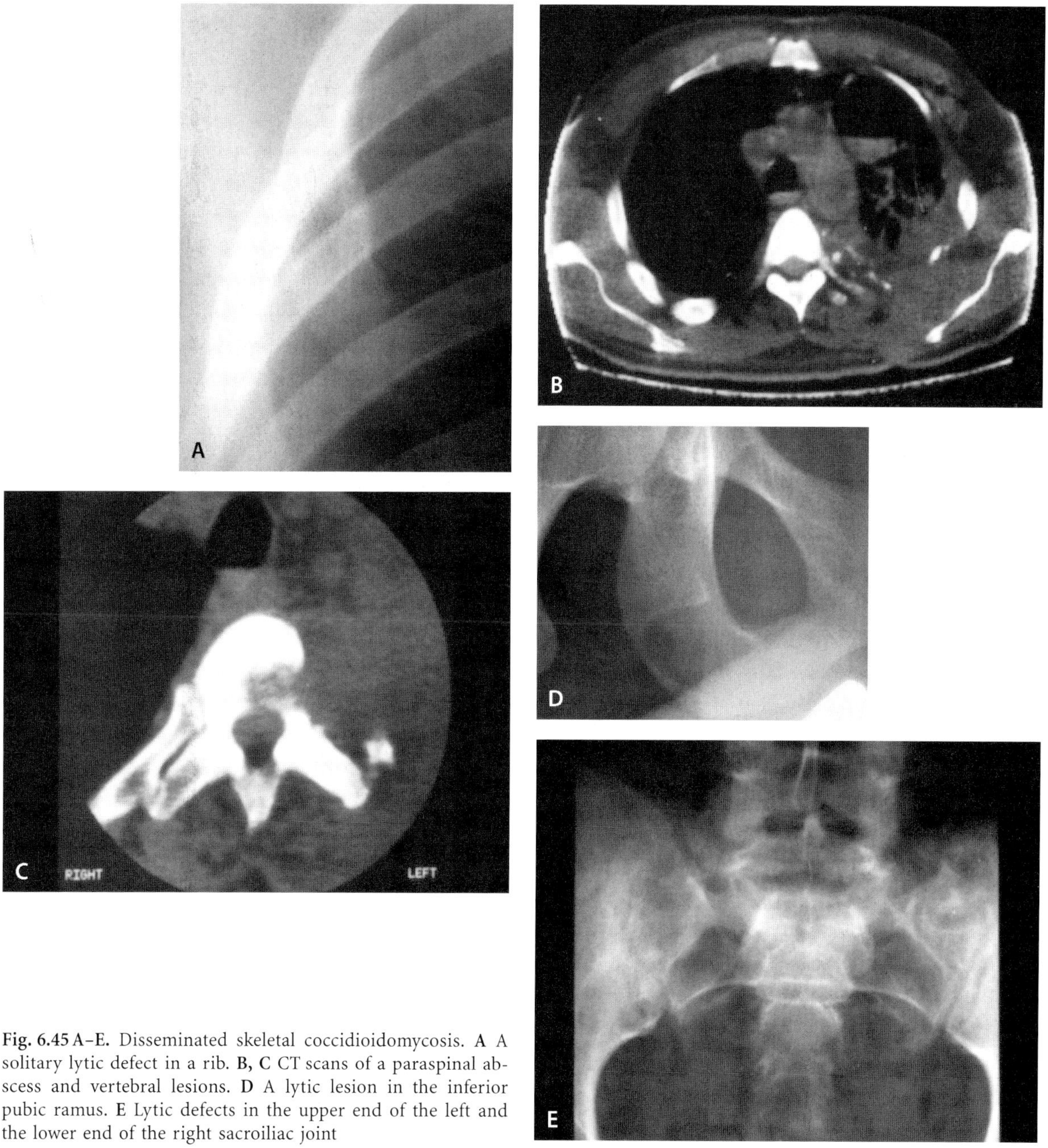

Fig. 6.45 A–E. Disseminated skeletal coccidioidomycosis. A A solitary lytic defect in a rib. B, C CT scans of a paraspinal abscess and vertebral lesions. D A lytic lesion in the inferior pubic ramus. E Lytic defects in the upper end of the left and the lower end of the right sacroiliac joint

or MRI as discrete, peripheral, enhancing masses. Encephalomalacia may follow treatment, particularly after amphotericin-B-methyl ester. The most important reasons for cerebral scanning are to establish the pattern of meningeal infection, and to monitor the hydrocephalus and its response to treatment. Only occasionally will an intracerebral granuloma be of clinical importance.

Abdominal coccidioidomycosis is quite common but difficult to recognize unless the patient is known to have the infection. Lymphadenopathy (Fig. 6.47) occurs often and is recognized by radionuclide scanning, ultrasonography, CT, or MRI. About half the patients with disseminated disease will have liver involvement, which may not be clinically apparent. Radionuclide scanning of the liver shows diffuse patchy uptake and all methods of scanning can show focal lesions. Similarly, the spleen is often involved, with small, 1- to 3-mm, focal granulomas. Renal infections are usually in the parenchyma, with calyceal swelling and distortion of the collecting system: this closely resembles tuberculosis and can be demonstrated by ultrasonography, CT, MRI, or radionuclide scanning. Abdominal abscesses occur, but the imaging findings are very nonspecific.

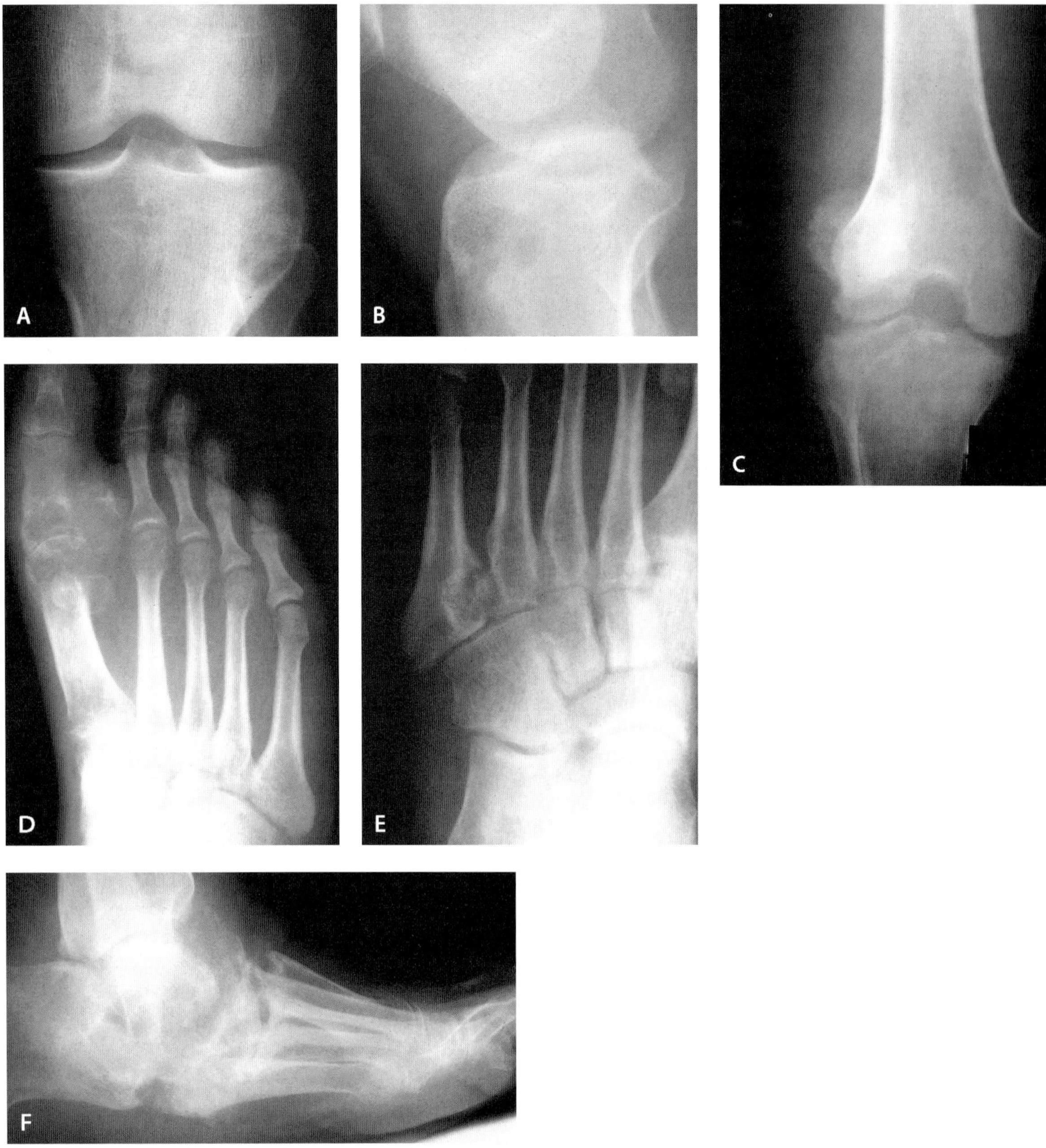

Fig. 6.46 A–F. Skeletal coccidioidomycosis in the lower limb. **A, B** A lytic lesion in the lateral tibial condyle. **C** Ill-defined lesions in the lower end of the femur medially, and in the patella. **D** A granuloma causing destruction on both sides of the first metatarsophalangeal joint, with an associated soft tissue mass. There are early lesions in the distal phalanx and the proximal end of the first metatarsal. **E** A more "punched-out" lytic lesion in the proximal end of the fifth metatarsal. **F** Almost complete destruction of the mid-tarsal bones and the proximal ends of the first four metatarsals, with soft tissue swelling. (**D** courtesy of Dr. J.P. McGahan et al. and *AJR*, 1981)

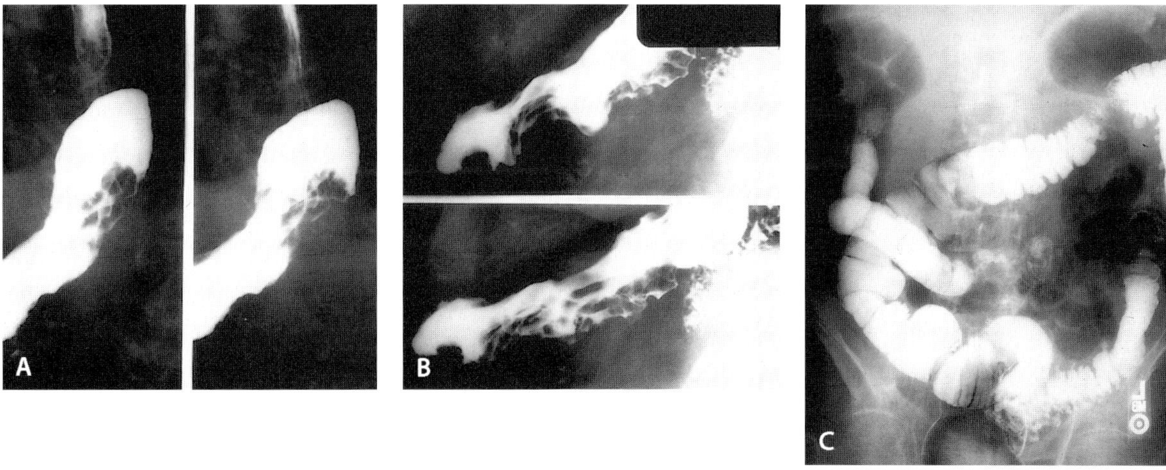

Fig. 6.47 A–C. Abdominal coccidioidomycosis. Although the liver, spleen, and kidneys can be affected in disseminated coccidioidomycosis, lymphadenopathy is also a frequent finding. **A, B** Distortion of the stomach and duodenum by enlarged lymph nodes, with localized adhesions and direct spread. **C** A different patient with lymphadenopathy and adhesions causing partial intestinal obstruction in the mid and lower abdomen

Sporotrichosis

Although this is primarily a cutaneous fungus, it is important for radiologists because disseminated forms occur, involving not only the lungs but also the genitourinary tract, bones, joints, muscles and meninges. It is quite a common infection in parts of the world.

Synonyms

Schenck's disease. Beurmann-Gougerot's disease. *Ger*: de Beurmann Krankheit. *Fr*: Maladie de Beurmann-Gougerot. *Sp*: Esporotricosis.

Definition

Sporotrichosis is infection with the dimorphic fungus *Sporothrix schenckii*. There is a less common variety, *S. schenckii* var. *luriei*.

Geographic Distribution

Sporothrix schenckii is found worldwide, particularly in the soil. *S. schenckii* var. *luriei* was first described in 1969 and has been isolated in South Africa and Europe. There is a varying incidence of human infection. Sporotrichosis is quite common in Mexico and parts of Central and South America (El Salvador, Brazil, Uruguay, Venezuela, Colombia), particularly where there is high humidity and moderate temperature. It is found in Japan and elsewhere in Asia, and in Australia and southern Africa. It is uncommon in dry or cold regions.

Epidemiology and Pathology

Sporotrichosis usually results from traumatic inoculation, either while working with soil, or from thorns or splinters. Epidemics have occurred: for example, 3000 cases in the Witswatersrand, South Africa, where the timber used as pit props in the mines was heavily contaminated with *S. schenckii*. Gardeners, florists and others working with plants are at risk. In Uruguay, 80% of patients have been infected by the claws of armadillos: other animals and even human fingernails are another source of infection. Infection has occurred after handling a burrowing fish, presumably from contact with the soil and contamination of wounds. There is no gender or race predilection, but sporotrichosis is more frequent in children and young adults, probably as a result of increased exposure to soil and vegetation. Alcoholics are at particular risk for the pulmonary and disseminated forms. It is not contagious, but familial cases occur from exposure to a common source.

The systemic form probably results from inhalation. Histopathologically, as with other mycoses, there is a diffuse inflammatory pyogranulomatous reaction, with progression to fibrosis. The fungus may not be found easily in the involved tissue, and culture may be necessary to identify it. In the lung there may be hyperplasia of the mucosa, described as pseudocarcinomatous. In the disseminated disease there may be both yeast forms and hyphae. The histopatholo-

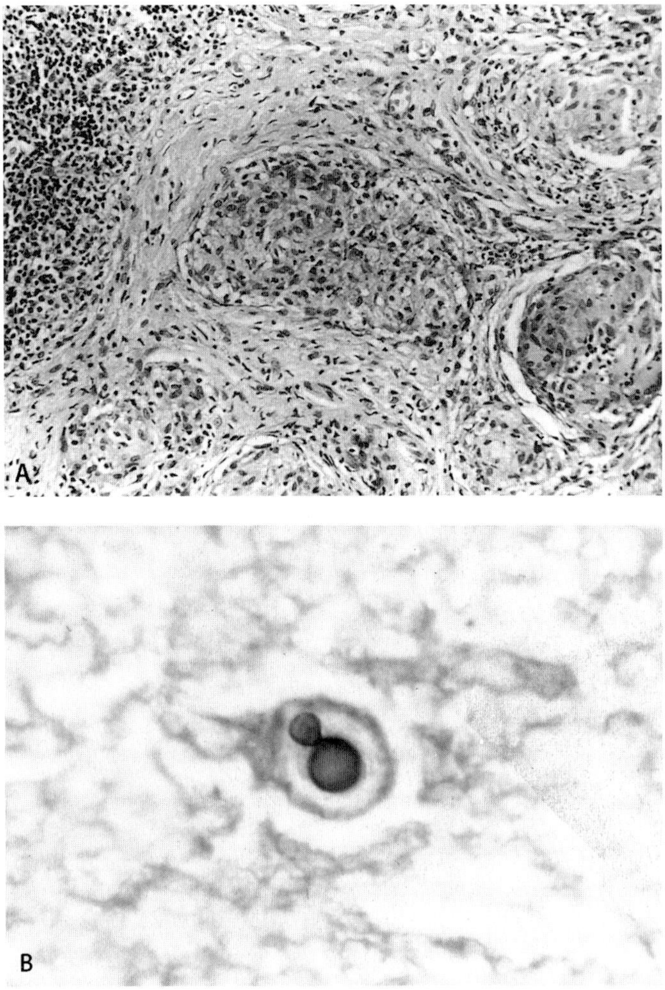

Fig. 6.48 A, B. The histopathology of sporotrichosis. **A** Several well-circumscribed granulomas with diffuse infiltration of neutrophils around them and, on the *left*, a heavy mononuclear infiltration. H & E, ×160. **B** Although it is often difficult to demonstrate *Sporothrix schenckii*, the appearance is characteristic. There is a "narrow neck," budding, and a surrounding layer of Splendore-Hoeppli material. Gomori methenamine-silver, ×1300. (**A** from Bittencourt and Londero 1995; **B** courtesy of Dr. Daniel H. Connor)

gical findings (Fig. 6.48) vary with different strains of the fungus and the patient's immune status.

Progressive lesions in the lung develop as nodules, cavities, or diffuse infiltration. Both the lung tissue and regional lymph nodes may undergo caseating necrosis. Spontaneous remission may occur as a result of a strong immunological response.

The laboratory diagnosis depends on recognition of the fungus, either in scrapings form the edge of the lesions or by culture of exudates or biopsy specimens. Agglutination, immunoassay, and immunofluorescent tests are valuable, particularly in disseminated infections. There is a sporotrichin skin test which is very reliable, but because asymptomatic infections occur, a positive reaction does not always indicate active infection.

Clinical Characteristics

The cutaneous form of infection (Fig. 6.49) is the commonest, developing as a subcutaneous nontender nodule 1 week to 6 months after inoculation. The skin becomes blackened (and the lesion may be mistaken for anthrax) and then ulcerates, resembling a gumma. In some localities, 75% of the infections are on the upper limbs. In most patients the regional lymph nodes enlarge and multiple nodules form along the lymphatics: these nodules may become indurated and may eventually ulcerate, but other lymphatics become acutely inflamed. The skin lesion may persist for many years, and some do not develop lymphatic spread, remaining without change, localized where they started. This is the most common pattern in children, where the infec-

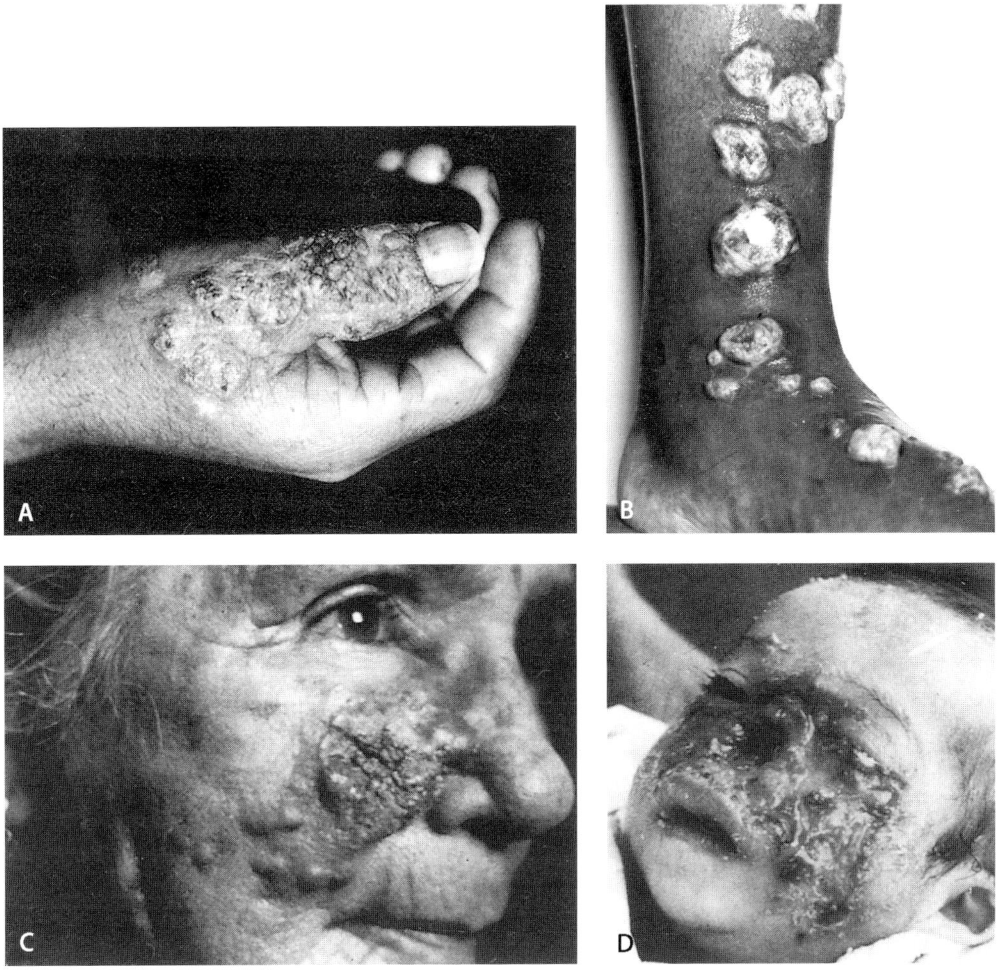

Fig. 6.49 A–D. Sporotrichosis can be localized or show lymphocutaneous spread. **A** A verrucous infection on the thumb, resembling chromoblastomycosis. **B** A more characteristic pattern of lymphocutaneous spread in the skin and subcutaneous tissues of the leg. **C** A verrucous lesion on the face, with small satellite nodules. **D** A large ulcerative mucocutaneous lesion in a 6-month-old child: this was misdiagnosed as leishmaniasis. (**A**, **C**, **D** from Bittencourt and Londero 1995; **B** courtesy of Dr. Daniel H. Connor)

tion may be found on the face and the early lesion can resemble verrucous warts. There is an uncommon mucocutaneous infection, involving the nose, mouth pharynx, and even the vocal cords.

In other patients, the cutaneous infections may spread directly to underlying bones or joints and there may be an effusion into a joint. Tenosynovitis often affects the elbows of knees. However, systemic spread may also occur without any apparent initial cutaneous or pulmonary lesions. This usually occurs in immunodepressed patients, who have not only multiple hard subcutaneous nodules but infection in the bones, viscera, heart, and even meninges. The clinical symptoms depend on the site of the infection.

When the lungs are involved (which is in less than 20% of cases), the clinical complaints are of general malaise, chronic cough with sputum, and hemoptysis, accompanied by fever, dyspnea, and chest pain, Eventually there may be chest wall involvement, with infection of the ribs and draining sinuses, but this occurs less commonly than in actinomycosis or nocardiosis. Apart from the draining sinuses, pulmonary sporotrichosis is indistinguishable from other granulomatous infections, such as tuberculosis, sarcoidosis, and histoplasmosis capsulati. Some patients with pulmonary infection may be asymptomatic.

Imaging Diagnosis

There are no specific or diagnostic imaging findings in sporotrichosis.

The primary lung infection is progressive and usually bilateral and destructive, with either cavita-

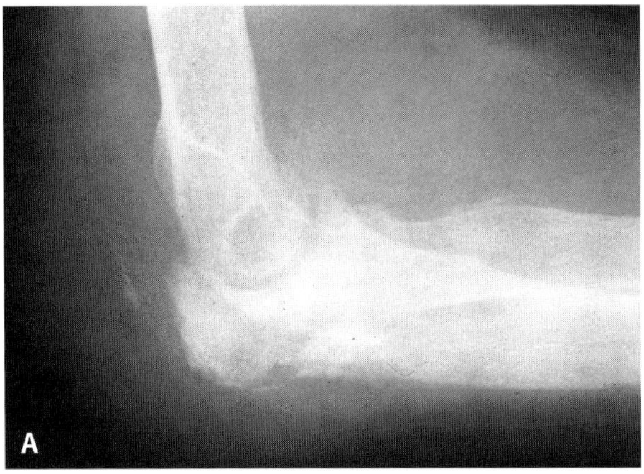

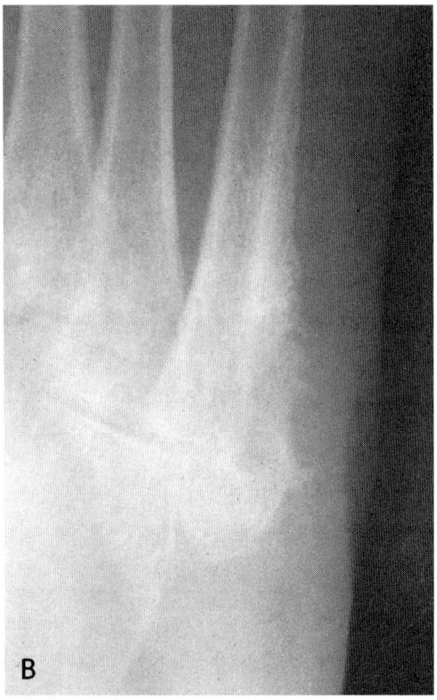

Fig. 6.50 A, B. Disseminated sporotrichosis. **A** A destructive lesion starting in the ulna and spreading to affect the upper end of the radius and the elbow joint. There is marked tissue swelling. **B** A more localized, spiculated lesion at the proximal end of the fifth metatarsal. (**A, B** courtesy of Dr. Harold G. Jacobson)

tion or consolidation. The lesions are often apical and mistaken for tuberculosis. The infection can be localized and nodular, or segmental, or there may be miliary spread which becomes confluent in patches. If the infection persits, thin-walled cavities appear and there will be fibrosis. If untreated, this becomes a massive density with central necrosis and cavitation. Pleural effusion and pleural thickening may occur, but are not very common: the infection may spread into the chest wall and cause osteomyelitis of the ribs, with sinus tracts and fistulae.

Mediastinal lymphadenopathy is common, and may be the presenting feature. The hilar lymph nodes enlarge rapidly and may compress a bronchus. This is most often mistaken for primary tuberculosis or sarcoidosis, or lymphadenopathy from one of the other mycotic infections. The diagnosis cannot be made by imaging, but needs appropriate skin and laboratory tests.

Computed tomography and MRI will demonstrate mediastinal lymphadenopathy and the pulmonary lesions, but there are no specific findings.

Skeletal involvement is common (Fig. 6.50), usually underlying the cutaneous and subcutaneous lesions: occasionally there is no obvious primary site. Bone infection causes an intense periosteal reaction and destructive osteomyelitis, with lytic lesions in the metaphyses. Neighboring joints develop infections by direct spread, with effusions and destruction of the articular surfaces and periarticular tissue. There can be serious skeletal involvement even without symptoms, and scintigraphy is useful to detect these cases, particularly in the spine in patients with severe infections.

Systemic spread is usually a complication of pulmonary infection. Although almost any organ or site may be involved, there are no specific imaging findings allowing the diagnosis of sporotrichosis.

Blastomycosis

Previously known as North American blastomycosis, because this is where it was first described and most cases occur, blastomycosis has now been reported throughout Africa, in the Middle East, and in some parts of Europe.

Synonyms

Gilchrist's disease: Chicago disease. *Fr.* Blastomycose. *Ger:* Blastomykose. *Sp*: Blastomicos Norté Americana.

Definition

Blastomycosis is an infection caused by the fungus *Blastomyces dermatitidis.*

Geographic Distribution

Blastomycosis is most commonly found in North America, from Canada through Mexico and parts of Central America. It is endemic in the Mississippi River Basin, around the Great Lakes and in the southeastern United States. It is now also recognized in many other parts of the world, particularly in Africa a (large number of cases are reported from Zimbabwe).

Epidemiology and Pathology

Only recently has *B. dermatitidis* been isolated from the soil of river banks. Man is infected by inhalation of mycelia or rarely through the skin. This fungus is an occupational hazard for microbiologists and pathologists. Dogs, cats, and cows are infected, but no man to man or animal to man transmission is known except from dog bites and possibly in one case in which a man with a urinary tract infection was probably the source of pelvic blastomycosis in his wife. Inhalation of the infectious conidia of the mycelial form results in alveolitis with exudation of fluid and inflammatory cells, which can be localized or diffuse. Initially, there is an inflammatory predominantly suppurative pyogranulomatous reaction, in which fungal cells are extracellular. Subsequently there may be an abscess and foci of necrosis. In the more chronic pattern the appearance varies with the age of the lesion and the immune status of the patient. In the lungs there may be compact granulomas or confluent, suppurative granulomas with central necrosis. Healing occurs with fibrosis and sometimes cavitation: calcification and caseation are uncommon. Blastomycosis eventually causes a chronic granulomatous inflammation, with hyalinization: fibrosing mediastinitis is a complication, but less often than in histoplasmosis capsulati.

Cutaneous blastomycosis causes a pseudoepitheliomatous hyperplasia with intraepidermal and dermal microabscesses, containing fungal colonies surrounded by epithelioid giant cells. There may be similar hyperplastic lesions in the larynx. When dissemination occurs, the skin, the mucosa of the respiratory tract, the genitourinary tract, bones, and the CNS may all be affected. Unlike in paracoccidioidomycosis, the gastrointestinal system is seldom involved. In patients with a poor immune status, the fungal cells may proliferate heavily and there is minimal inflammatory response.

Clinical Characteristics

The patient usually presents with cough, fever, night sweats, and general weakness and may be thought to have tuberculosis. The sputum may be blood stained and purulent, again suggesting tuberculosis.

The cutaneous form of infection presents as papules which progress to crusty ulceration, with raised edges: they may assume a warty verrucous appearance and steadily enlarge (Fig. 6.51). Skin lesions are often multiple and most commonly appear on the face and limbs. They are usually painless and may be mistaken for squamous cell carcinoma. Sometimes they have a serpiginous advancing border which causes a mutilating deformity. Atrophic scars develop where there have been old lesions. The underlying bones are affected and sinuses form: there is regional lymphadenopathy. Other lesions can occur in the mucous membranes of the nose, mouth, larynx, and vagina.

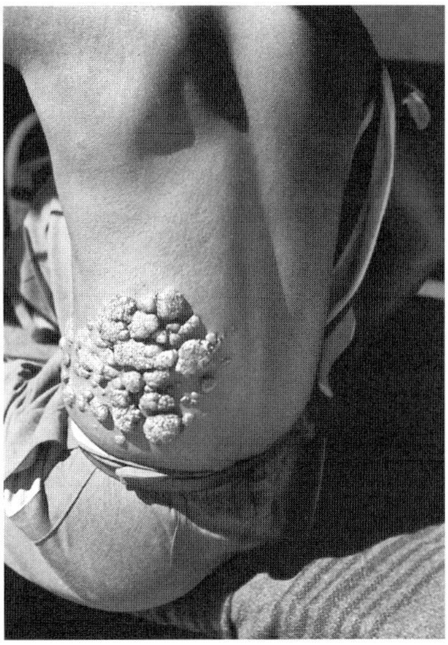

Fig. 6.51. Cutaneous blastomycosis with a spreading verrucous, ulcerative lesion which had progressed slowly over a number of years. An African man from Zimbabwe

Skeletal lesions can occur in up to 25% of all infected patients. The infection can involve any organ, but usually this happens in patients who already have skin or pulmonary blastomycosis.

Systemic infection begins in the lungs and may remain pulmonary or disseminate to cause meningitis, spinal abscess, epididymo-orchitis, prostatitis, osteomyelitis, or arthritis, or to infect any other organ system. Apart from the prostate, *B. dermatitidis* does not often affect the urinary tract and, even more rarely, the gastrointestinal tract. Dissemination may not develop for years after the initial inoculation. Because there are no reliable laboratory or skin tests, it is difficult to know how many asymptomatic cases there are, or whether reactivation occurs. Overwhelming primary blastomycosis may occur, even in immunocompetent individuals. Diffuse lung infection can lead to adult respiratory distress syndrome (ARDS). If untreated, over 90% of patients will die of the infection.

Imaging Diagnosis

The changes on imaging are very nonspecific and extremely variable.
In pulmonary blastomycosis, the chest images strongly resemble tuberculosis: there may be a primary complex with a small focus of infection in the lung and hilar lymphadenopathy. This may heal. In some patients there is nonsegmental pneumonia, most frequently in the upper lobes. The air space disease is patchy and confluent, with indistinct outlines: lobar pneumonia is less common. A distinguishing feature from pyogenic pneumonia is the very slow rate of change.
Solitary focal masses are quite common; such masses are usually well defined and distinct and may be up to 10 cm in diameter (Fig. 6.52 A–C). Unlike in some of the other fungal infections, these large solitary nodules are often found around the hila or close to the mediastinum, and may mimic bronchogenic carcinoma.
In other patients there is bilateral and diffuse interstitial thickening, which usually indicates further progression of the infection. Cavitation is perhaps a little less common than in tuberculosis, but may occur in almost any part of the lung (Fig. 6.52 D): there may be single or multiple cavities with thick or thin walls. In the disseminated pattern of the infection there may be miliary pulmonary nodules.
The pleura can be infected, resulting in either thickening or effusion, or both. All patterns of the infection can result in fibrosis.
Lymphangitis and lymphadenopathy (Fig. 6.52 D) are unusual in blastomycosis, occurring in less than 10% in most series. Even less common is spread of the pleural infection into the chest wall.
Musculoskeletal imaging shows that many patients with cutaneous pseudoepithelioma have underlying skeletal involvement. In disseminated infections, multiple bones and joints are affected and scintigraphy is a useful preliminary imaging procedure. There may be skin sinuses, but these are uncommon. The flat and short bones and the ends of the long bones show irregular bone destruction and some have reactive new bone formation.
Soft tissue abscesses may occur and can be accurately delineated by ultrasonography. They are subcutaneous, and occur anywhere throughout the body, not only in the limbs and trunk but also internally. Abscesses have been recorded in the liver, adrenals, pericardium, and myocardium, and within the orbit.
Joints are usually affected by direct spread from a nearby focus because the foci of osteomyelitis are often juxta-articular (as with other fungus infections): cartilage is destroyed. Joint effusions increase the joint space at the start of the infection, but later there is loss of articular and periarticular tissues and subluxation may result. In the end there may be bony fusion.
Spinal involvement resembles tuberculosis, with infection of the vertebral bodies and quite early of the intervertebral disc space. Paravertebral abscesses can develop.
Computed tomography and MR scanning clearly demonstrate the spectrum of blastomycosis. Ulcerating masses within the larynx have been demonstrated, and simulate malignancy. Miliary pulmonary nodules, small granulomas, and patches of pneumonia may be demonstrated a little more clearly by CT than with routine chest radiography. Previously unsuspected calcification in pulmonary foci or in lymph nodes may be seen by CT scanning. MRI is useful in vertebral infections to show the extent of any abscess and to exclude cord involvement.
Unfortunately, all imaging changes are very nonspecific and seldom strengthen a suspected diagnosis of blastomycosis. A history of visiting or living in the endemic regions is a reason to include blastomycosis in the differential diagnosis.

Paracoccidioidomycosis

With Luiz Fellipe Dequeiros Mattoso

Formerly known as South American blastomycosis and still most frequently found in Latin America, the generally accepted terminology is now paracoccidioidomycosis.

Synonyms

South American blastomycosis. Brazilian blastomycosis. Lutz-Splendore-Almeida's disease. Paracoccidioidal granuloma. Para. *Ger*: Parakokzidioidomykose. *Fr*: Paracoccidioidomycose. *Sp.* Paracoccidioidmicosis. Blastomicosis Sudamericana.

Definition

Paracoccidioidomycosis is infection with the thermal dimorphic fungus *Paracoccidioides brasiliensis* (formerly *Blastomyces brasiliensis*).

Geographic Distribution

Paracoccidioidomycosis occurs in Brazil and other countries of South and Central America and is the most common systemic mycosis in that region. Where it is endemic, perhaps over 10% of the population has been infected. Only three cases have been

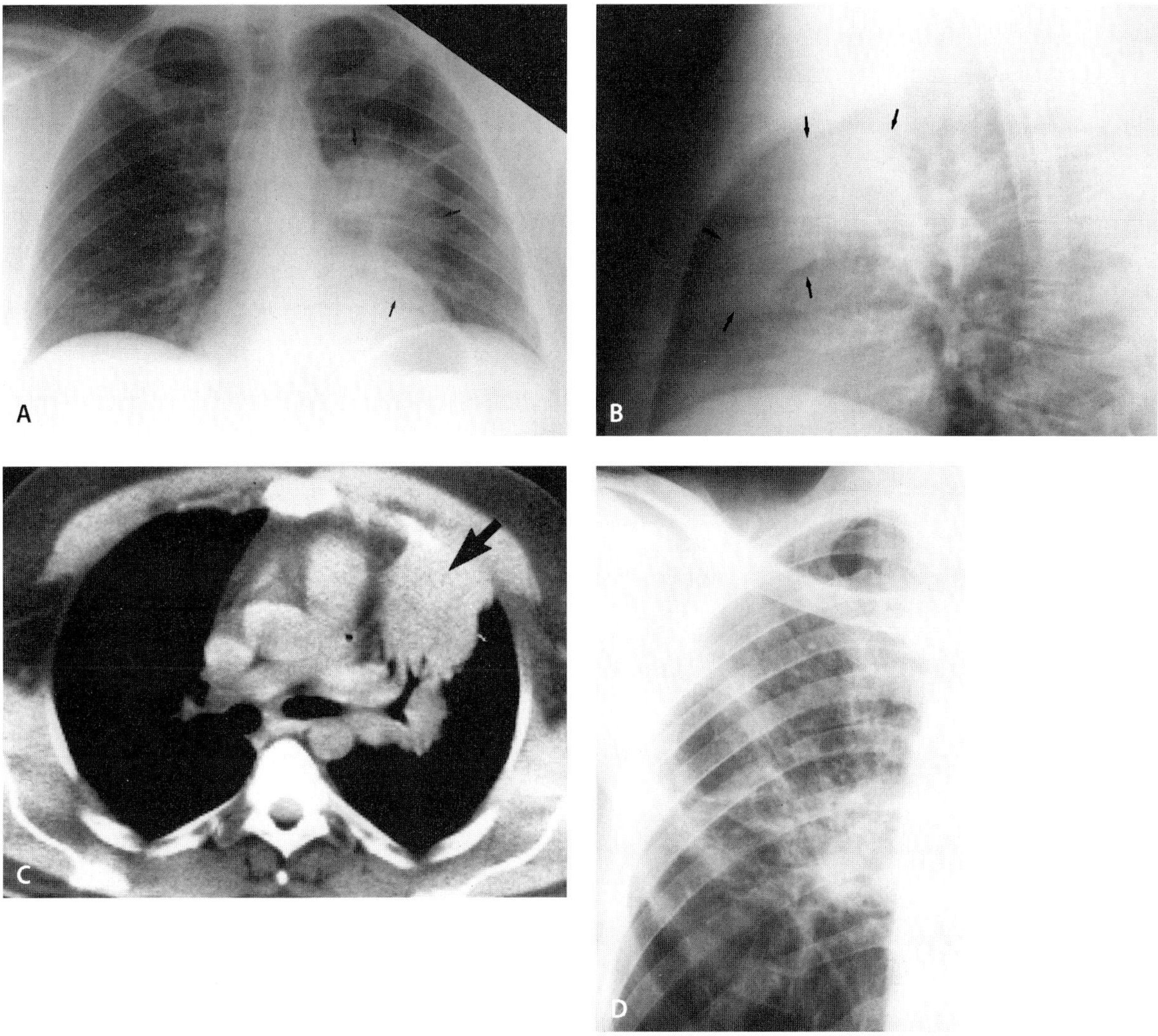

Fig. 6.52 A–D. Pulmonary blastomycosis. **A, B** A large mass in the left upper lobe (*arrows*). **C** The same mass on a CT scan (*arrows*). This was removed surgically and was found to be a granulomatous mass within which was evidence of blastomycosis: the patient was a 39-year-old man with a 9-month history of cough. **D** A progressive infection in the right upper lobe, with cavitation and pleural reaction: there is hilar lymphadenopathy. (**A–C** courtesy of Dr. L. R. Brown et al. and *Mayo Clin Proc* 1991; **D** courtesy of Dr. Harold G. Jacobson)

reported from the Caribbean, and the infection is rare or nonexistent in French Guiana, Guyana, Belize, Nicaragua, and Surinam. Isolated cases have been reported from the United States, Japan, Europe, and Africa, but each of these patients has lived previously where the infection is endemic.

Epidemiology and Pathology

The ecology and natural habitat of *P. brasiliensis* are unknown: it is probably a saprophyte in rural surroundings, particularly wet tropical and subtropical regions, and those with dryer, temperate winters. It is difficult to prove this, because the fungus has seldom been isolated from the soil, although the mycelial phase has been grown in the laboratory on various vegetation, dust, and even coffee leaves. The fungus has been found in the testes of a guinea pig following soil inoculation and also from soil with an acid pH in coffee plantations. It has been identified in dog food, but this was probably contaminated. It has been isolated from the gastrointestinal tract of bats and armadillos, but the significance of this is unknown. It may be unique compared with other mycoses in that natural infections occur only in mankind.

Human to human transmission is unknown. Indeed, it is not agreed amongst experts exactly how the infection does occur. A high incidence of lesions in

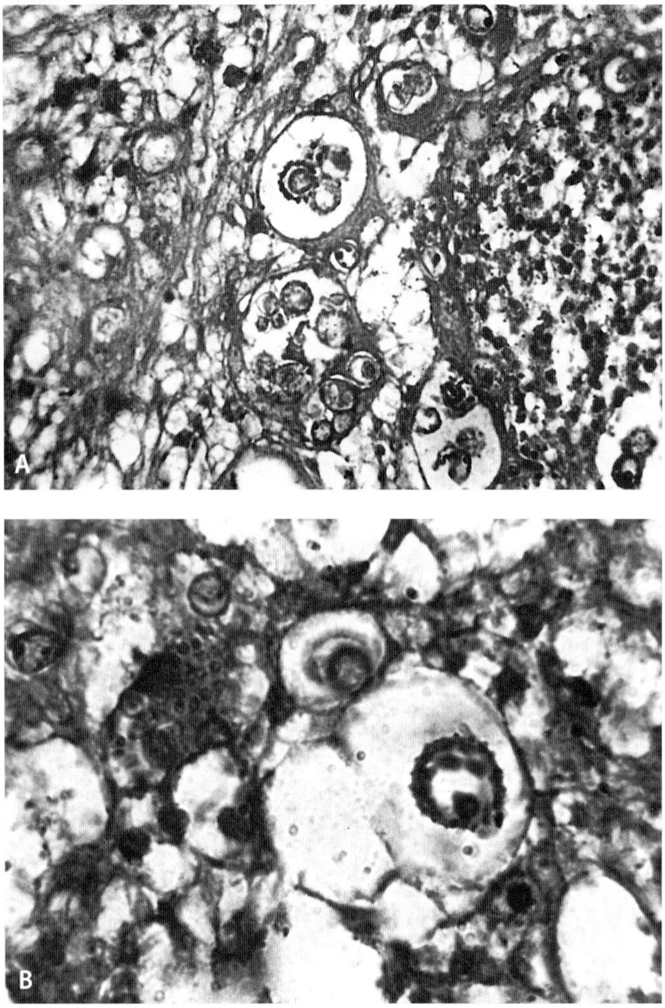

Fig. 6.53 A, B. The histopathology of paracoccidiodiomycosis. **A** Rounded fungi with peripheral budding, giving a "ship's wheel" appearance which is typical of *P. brasiliensis* with a surrounding inflammatory infiltrate. H & E, ×100. **B** Binary and peripheral budding, again with the "ship's wheel" outline. The multiple buds which give the nodular "ship's wheel" appearance are very characteristic. Grocott-Gomori methenamine-silver stain, ×400. (Courtesy of Dr. I.L. Aymor, Rio de Janeiro)

the mouth suggests mucosal infection as the source, but it seems more likely that it is inhaled, because lesions are limited to the lungs in about one-third of patients with the progressive form of the infection. To add further confusion, chest radiographs may be normal even though *P. brasiliensis* has been isolated from the sputum or bronchial washings of the same patient. It is established that a patient's immunity is to some extent genetic and that the male predominance may be related to an inhibitory effect of estrogen on the in-vivo yeast phase, but whatever the mechanism, the majority of patients with a positive skin reaction have not developed clinical infection.

Paracoccidioidomycosis is common in children of both sexes but the asymptomatic form shows up more frequently over the age of 30 years. In older patients, it is more common in men.

The histopathology (Fig. 6.53) explains the pattern of the infection. When localized, the reaction is mainly granulomatous and the yeasts are inside giant cells. When disseminated, the granulomatous reaction is much less significant, and there is more edema and suppuration, with some localized areas of necrosis and occasional microabscesses. It is unusual to find hyphae. There are more yeast phase cells including extracellular organisms.

In acute paracoccidioidomycosis there are widespread necrotic foci, mainly in lymph nodes, spleen, intestines, bones, and paranasal sinuses. The fungus seems to have a predilection for the lymphoid tissue of the mucosa and the regional lymph nodes. In the small intestine the lesions begin in Peyer's patches, but eventually involve the full thickness of the bowel wall. Lymphadenopathy can be marked and enlarged lymph nodes may coalesce.

When the disease is disseminated, it is the cervical and mediastinal lymph nodes which are most frequently involved, often becoming caseous. Nodules in any organ can also become necrotic. In patients with disseminated infections, the adrenals are infected in about half those who come to autopsy, but overt adrenal insufficiency is uncommon.

In the more chronic infections, the skin, lungs, lymph nodes, stomach, small intestine, adrenals, CNS, spleen, and liver are common sites.

In the lungs there may be various tissue reactions, including acute alveolitis, early granulomas, mature granulomas and pulmonary fibrosis. This fibrosis involves also the lymph nodes and bronchi, as well as the major branches of the pulmonary vessels.

In the chronic form of paracoccidioidomycosis, cerebral (CNS) infection may be asymptomatic or, alternatively, the only site with clinical significance. The meninges are involved at the base of the brain and if there is a granulomatous cerebral lesion, it is usually well circumscribed. In the chronic pattern of infection, the thickening of the instestinal mucosa may be such that obstruction may occur in the jejunum, ileum, or colon. Wherever chronic foci occur, as healing progresses they go on to extensive fibrosis.

The diagnosis is made by identifying the fungus in sputum, pus, or other fluids, or in tissue sections. Immunodiffusion tests are useful for diagnosis and screening; immunoelectrophoresis is more sensitive but less practical. Skin tests are unreliable.

Clinical Characteristics

The clinical presentation varies between children and adults.

Juvenile infections are often subacute but progressive and equally common in girls and boys. Many children have abdominal symptoms: pain, diarrhea, palpable masses, and even symptoms of an acute abdomen. There may be hepatosplenomegaly, fever, and weight loss. Lymphadenopathy may be generalized, and the majority of children will have enlarged lymph nodes in the neck or submandibular area, often with draining sinuses. Chest radiographs will show mediastinal and hilar lymphadenopathy; sputum culture may be positive even when there is no clinical evidence of chest infection. Because of fungemia, there may be acute and relapsing episodes and multiple skin lesions (Fig. 6.54 A, B). The acute form in younger patients can be rapidly fatal.

Paracoccidioidomycosis in adults tends to run an indolent course, sometimes causing illness many years after departure from the endemic area. Oral mucous membrane infection is common, affecting the gums, tongue, lips, or palate (Fig. 6.54 D–F). The mucosal granulomas on the soft palate have a "mulberry" pattern, the tongue becomes nodular and there may be painful ulcers in the mouth, making eating difficult. Pharyngeal infection may cause hoarseness and the nasal cartilage may be infected. Coexisting skin lesions occur but less commonly than those in the mouth. When the skin is infected, it is usually on the face, but in severe infections lesions may appear anywhere on the body: the majority will be papular with small central ulcers, but these may enlarge into an elevated plaque, ulcer (Fig. 6.54 C) or dry warty area.

Lymphadenitis does not seem to be related to the site of mucocutaneous lesions. Clinical examination may show enlarged cervical and submandibular lymph nodes, but imaging often reveals similar lymphadenopathy in the mediastinum, axilla, and femoral regions.

Pulmonary infection is quite common at autopsy but seldom presents clinically: if apparent, the complaints then are of cough, sputum, and hemoptysis, clinically suggesting tuberculosis.

In the disseminated disease, almost any organ can be involved, including the adrenal glands, small and large bowel, liver, and meninges. Infection occurs in bones and joints, either separately or under skin lesions. The first clinical evidence of infection may be at any of these sites and a lung focus may be found subsequently. Involvement of the CNS by granulomas, arteritis, or thrombosis will result in clinical symptoms related to the site.

Imaging Diagnosis

When the lungs are involved, there can be two patterns: a benign self limiting form and another in which there is slow progression (Fig. 6.55).

"Benign" Pulmonary Form. In many patients the chest radiograph is normal. In others there may be bilateral air space consolidation, often more than is expected clinically, but with no specific distribution. Thin-walled cavities may develop. There is often quite marked hilar adenopathy. As healing takes place there is local fibrosis and an increased interstitial pattern. Calcification either in the lungs or lymph nodes is unusual.

High-resolution CT is the most accurate way to image early paracoccidioidomycosis: scans show peribronchial and septal thickening and later will confirm the cavitation, alveolar consolidation, scarring, and associated emphysema (Fig. 6.56). Micronodules may be seen and hilar adenopathy is clearly demonstrated.

(Text continues on p. 612)

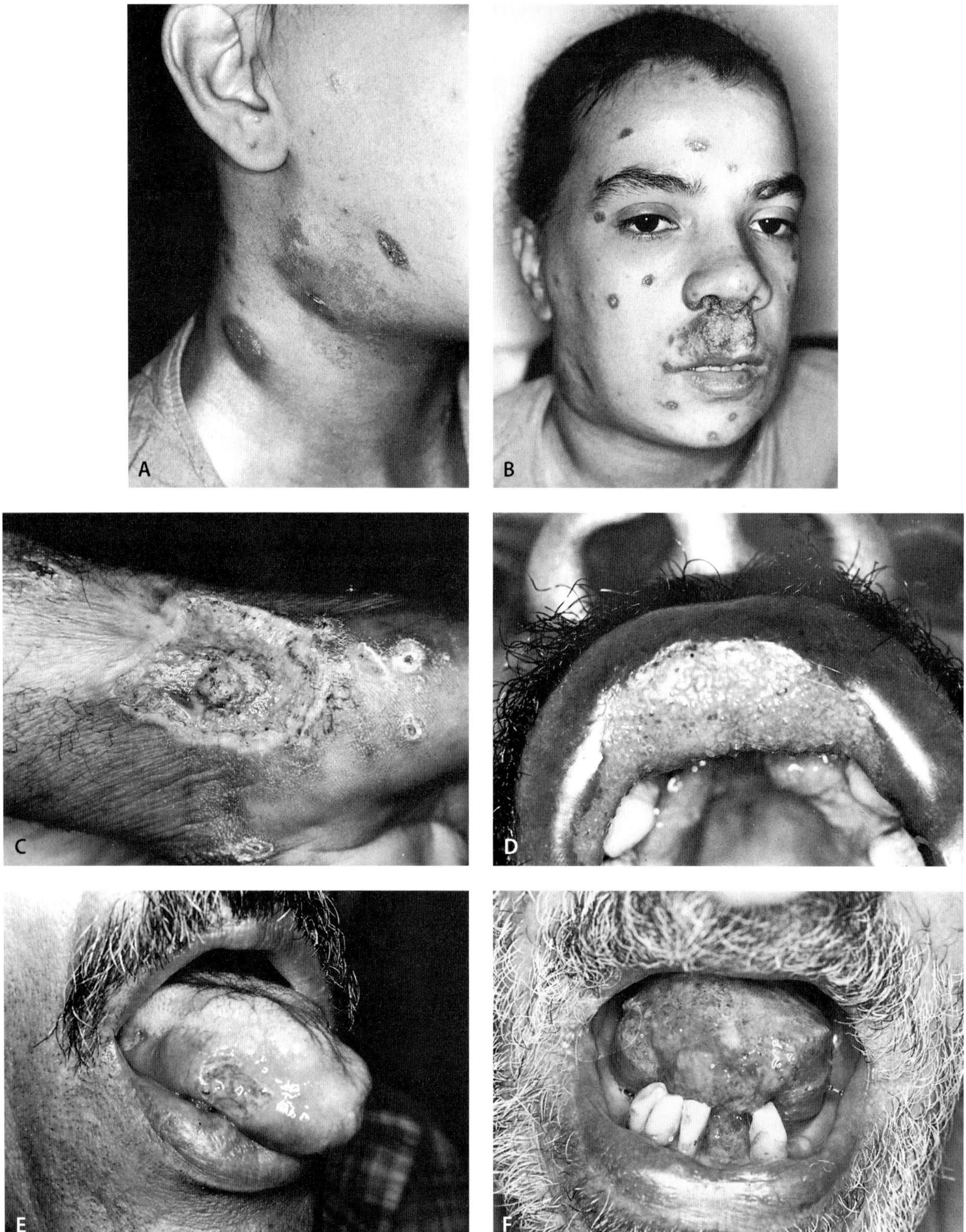

Fig. 6.54 A–F. The clinical appearance of paracoccidioidomycosis. **A** Subacute disseminated infection with multiple small ulcerating nodules on the face and neck, and associated cervical lymphadenopathy. **B** Multiple small ulcerating lesions around the face and a mucocutaneous, more extensive lesion on the upper lip. **C** An ulcerating granulomatous lesion near the elbow with multiple small nodules around it. **D** A mucocutaneous lesion across the upper lip. **E** A large solitary ulcerating lesion on the side of the tongue. **F** Multiple small ulcerating lesions under the tongue. (Courtesy of Drs. A.C. Francesconi do Valle and R.R. Guimaras, Rio de Janeiro)

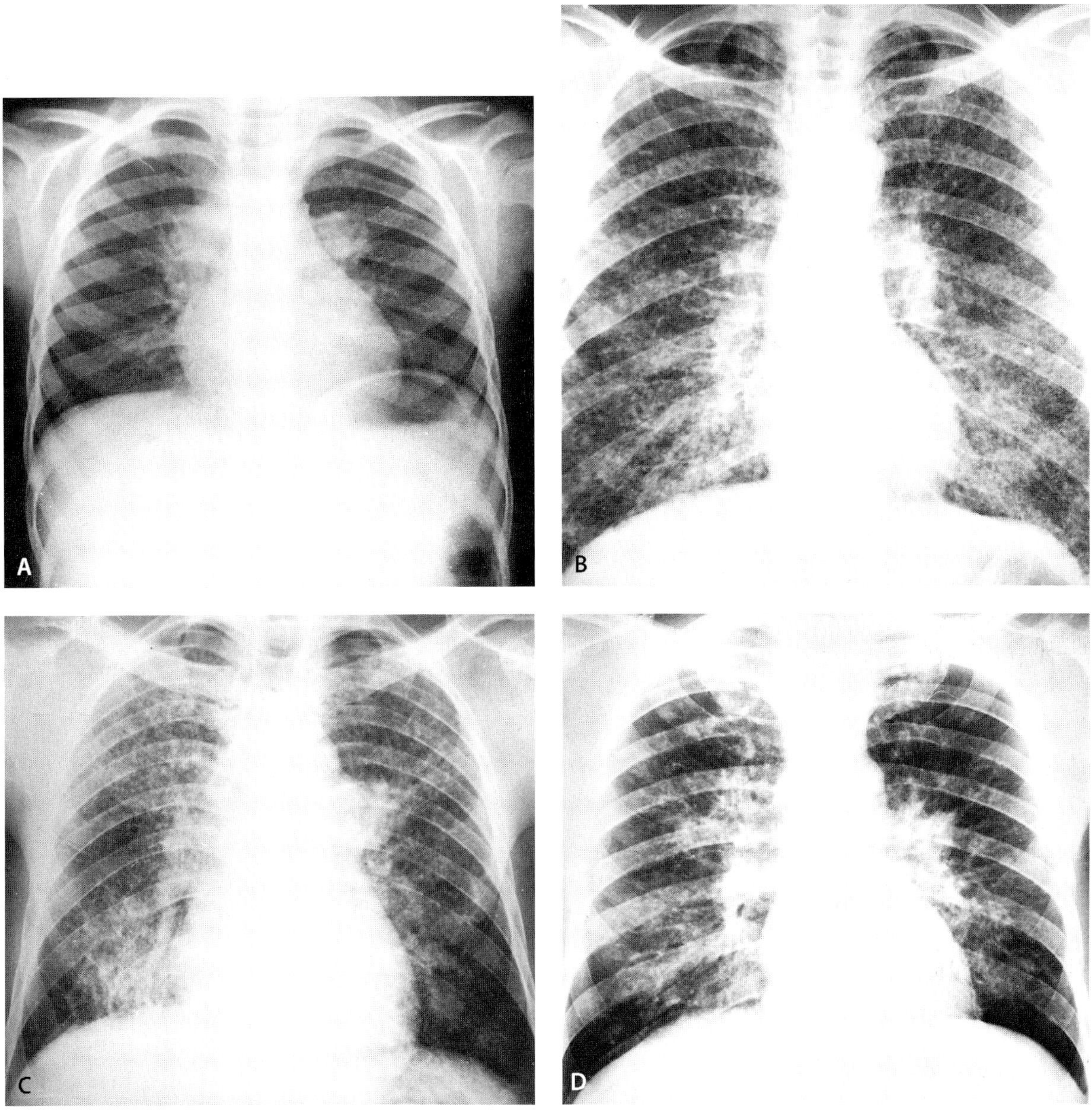

Fig. 6.55 A–F. Pulmonary paracoccidioidomycosis. **A** Bilateral hilar and mediastinal lymphadenopathy in a young boy. This is a primary infection, which is unlikely to be seen in adults. **B** Hematogenous "miliary" nodules throughout both lungs. **C** Multiple small nodules with hilar and mediastinal lymphadenopathy, with some linear streaking due to peribronchial and septal thickening. There is some patchy consolidation in the right lower lobe. **D** Interstitial thickening particularly in the perihilar regions: there is bilateral lymphadenopathy. **E, F** see p. 612

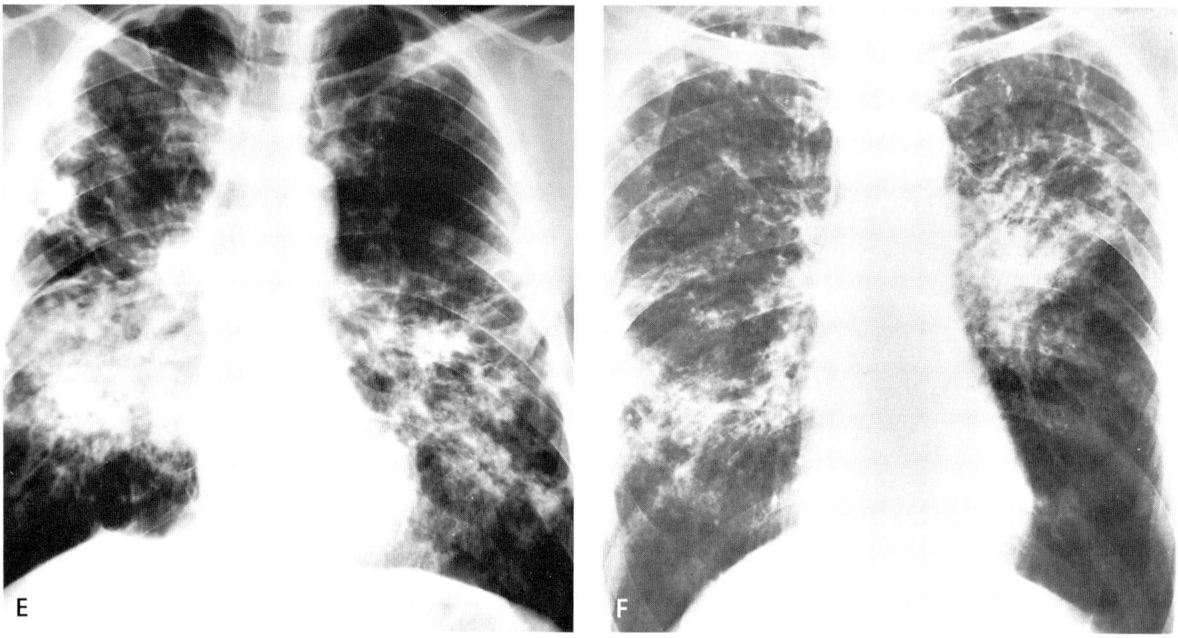

Fig. 6.55 (*continued*). E Diffuse interstitial and alveolar consolidation, with fibrosis and some peripheral large nodules. These are mainly in the mid lung field, the lower zones being spared: this is very characteristic of the chronic form of the infection. F Bilateral interstitial fibrosis, with multiple dense nodules and some upper lobe contraction. The lower lobes, particularly the left, have become emphysematous. All these chest radiographs could be misdiagnosed as tuberculosis. (Courtesy of Drs. A.C. Francesconi do Valle and R.R. Guimaras, Rio de Janeiro)

Progressive Pulmonary Form. Chest imaging shows slowly progressive, bilateral patchy alveolar consolidation, with nodulation in some patients. Solitary pulmonary nodules are uncommon. The lower lobes may be slightly more affected than other parts of the lungs, but there is no characteristic distribution. In some patients the lung lesions are the result of aspiration pneumonia from the buccal ulceration. It has been suggested, but not proven, that this is one of the reasons for the slightly predominant basal location. There is lymphadenopathy, but it is not so marked as in the benign form. Pulmonary fibrosis may progress significantly to cause cor pulmonale. Pleural effusions are uncommon.

In general, the radiographic appearance of the chest resembles tuberculosis or other fungal infections (Fig. 6.55).

Gastrointestinal Form. In some patients there is a palpable abdominal mass, but plain radiographs of the abdomen are normal: ultrasonography shows lymphadenopathy. In other patients, abdominal radiographs show distended loops of bowel with fluid levels, suggesting partial obstruction. In disseminated infections, ultrasonography shows ascites and marked mesenteric lymphadenopathy. Lymph node calcification has been noted, but the pattern is nonspecific.

Contrast studies of the small intestine in the early stages of infection show mucosal nodulation, sometimes with central ulceration. There may be segmental small bowel spasm and there is often hypersecretion. As the infection progresses, lengths of bowel become thickened and rigid, with irregular spiky and edematous mucosa. Several centimeters of bowel may show distorted mucosa, eventually becoming narrow and rigid, with decreased peristalsis, but with almost normal intervening segments of bowel (Fig. 6.57 A–D). Later in the infection, strictures develop and are usually localized, the result of scarring. Ileocolic and ileocecocolic intussusceptions may occur. An inflammatory mass may develop in the ileocecal region, causing the cecum to contract or, in some cases, distend. The cecal outline may become conical. In the colon there is a similar pattern, with localized or diffuse narrowing, particularly in the ascending colon (Fig. 6.57 E). Any part of the colon may be involved; in some patients almost the whole large bowel is affected, but in others there are intervening normal segments. Stenosed areas can be single or multiple, and may be found at any level, including the rectum (Fig. 6.57 F). There may be pseudodiverticuli and fistulae.

Regardless of the extent of the abdominal infection, standard chest radiographs may initially be normal, but high-resolution CT may show changes previously unsuspected on routine chest radiographs.

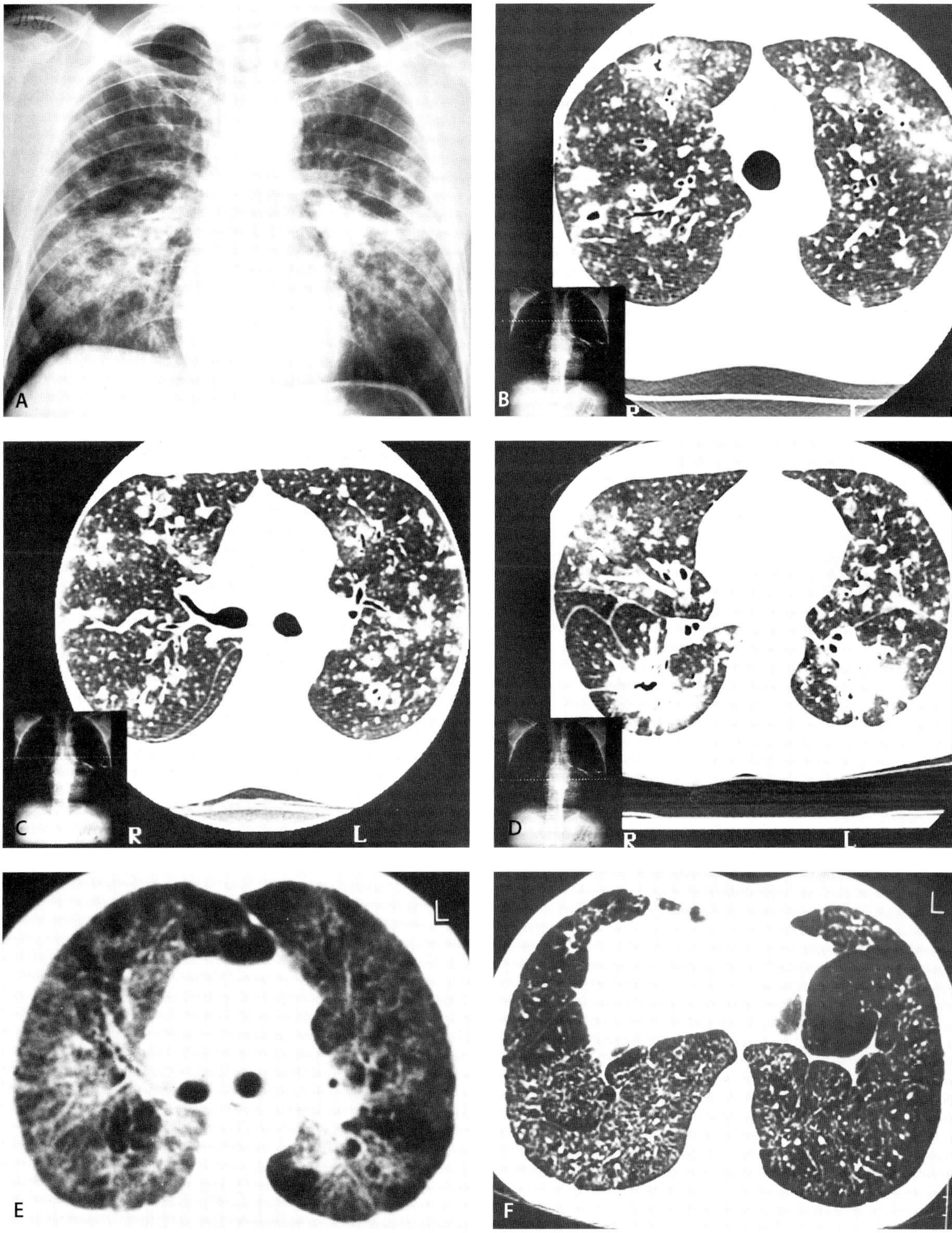

Fig. 6.56 A–F. CT scanning of the chest will often show the changes of paracoccidioidomycosis more clearly. **A** The chest radiograph and **B–D** the CT scans of the same patient showing the multiple interstitial, nodular and linear densities. Many of the nodules are rough in outline: thick-walled cavities can be seen. In other areas the infection has coalesced, forming large masses. **E, F** CT scans of a different patient showing particularly the peribronchial thickening and interstitial fibrosis, with the well-marked emphysematous areas at the lung bases

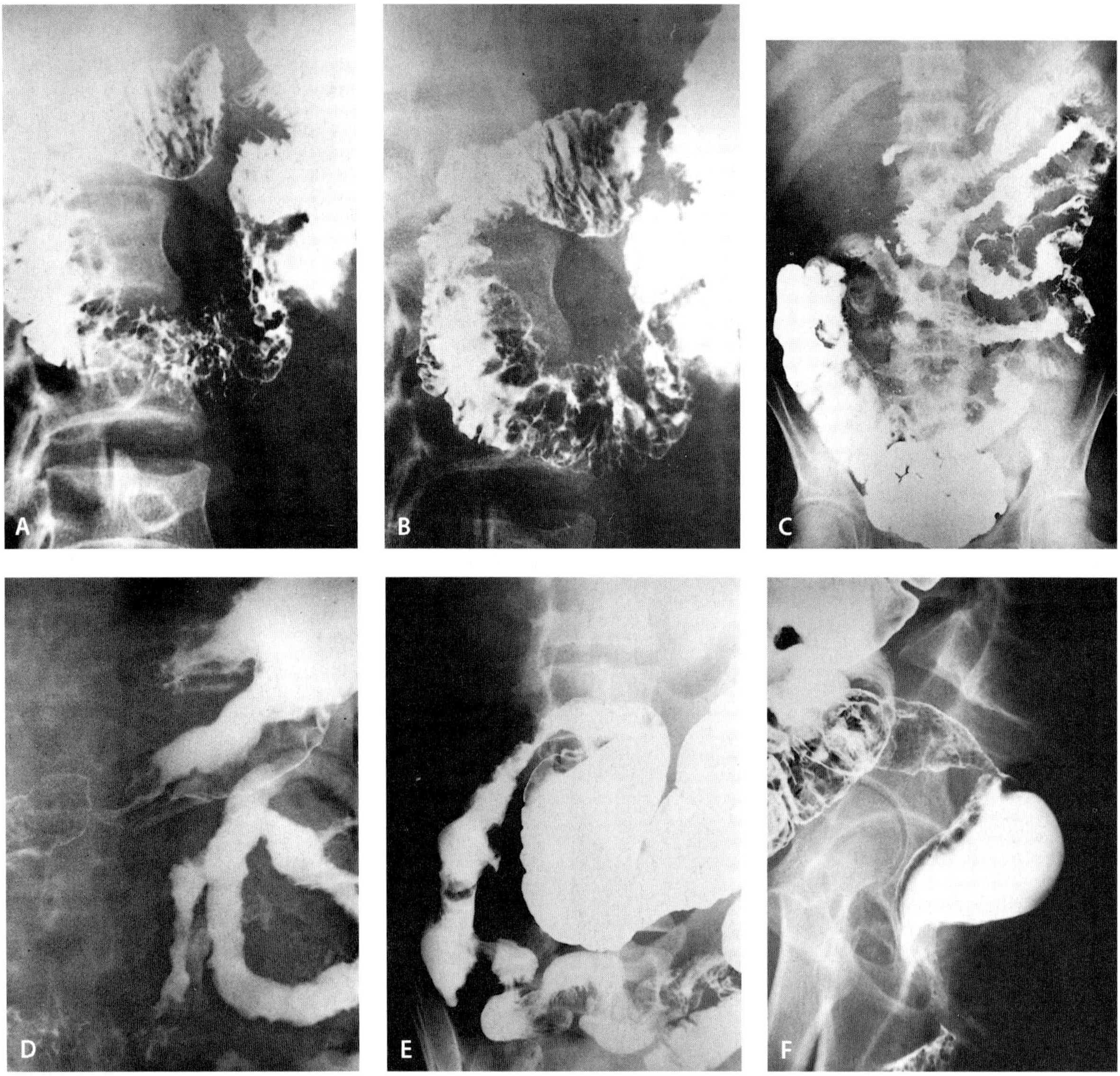

Fig. 6.57 A–F. Paracoccidioidomycosis of the alimentary tract. **A, B** Barium contrast studies showing nodular thickening of the duodenum and proximal jejunum. The normal mucosal pattern has been lost. **C** More extensive jejunal and ileal involvement, with diffuse thickening and loss of the normal mucosal pattern. There are some sections with marked narrowing and thickening of the mucosa, and some small pseudodiverticuli have developed. **D** Loops of jejunum and upper ileum in which the normal pattern has disappeared: some segments are dilated and others narrowed. The lower ileum is still normal. **E** Diffuse narrowing of the entire cecum and the ascending colon, as far as the hepatic flexure. The mucosal pattern has been replaced with nodulation. The terminal ileum and transverse colon appear normal. **F** Severe localized stenosis of the upper rectum, with nodular mucosa above and below it. All these patients are adult males

Involvement of Other Sites. Paracoccidioidomycosis does not usually infect the urinary tract primarily, but distortion or displacement of the ureters and occasionally the kidneys can be caused by retroperitoneal infection. Ultrasonography is the most useful survey examination, but excretory urography will show the ureteric status more accurately and is another way to exclude hydronephrosis. Bladder infection is only likely to occur after contamination, e. g., following catheterization.

Hepatic, splenic, and adrenal granulomas may be recognized by MRI, CT, or ultrasonography. Similarly, cerebral granulomas or meningeal infection are well shown on MRI or CT scanning (Fig. 6.58).

Skeletal involvement by paracoccidioidomycosis is rare, even in the widely disseminated systemic infections. Lytic lesions may develop in the most vascular part of any bone (Fig. 6.59).

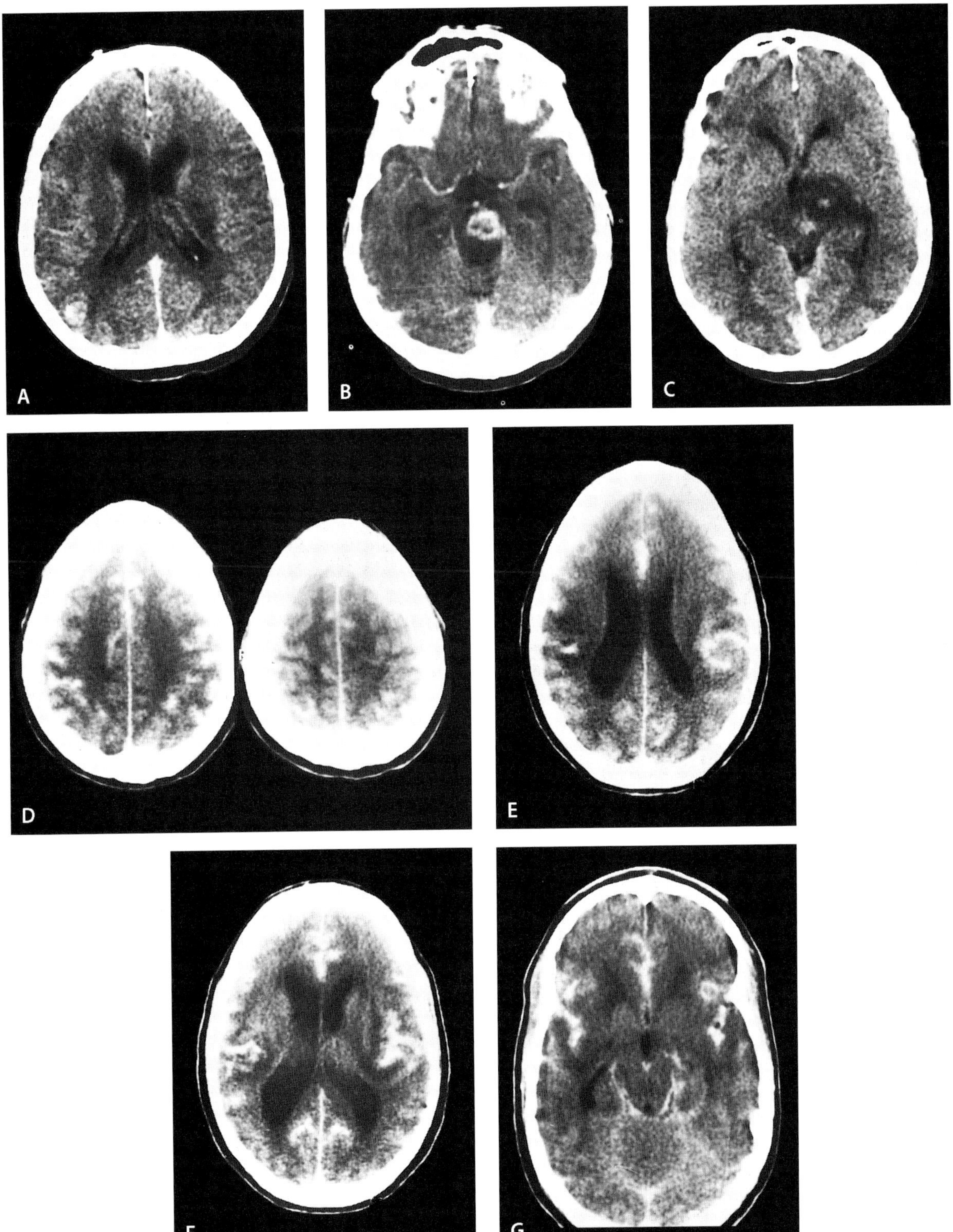

Fig. 6.58 A–G. Cerebral paracoccidioidomycosis. CT scanning will often show enhancing nodules, some with a peripheral rim of enhancement such as **A** in the parietal cortex, or **B** in the brain stem. **C** A thalamic lesion which is small and surrounded by marked edema. The lesions in **A–C** are all cerebral granulomas. **D–G** are scans of a different patient and show enhancement of the meninges and cortical gyri, particularly in the basal cysterns. A small nodule with peripheral enhancement is present in the left frontal lobe (**G**) and there is also ventricular enlargement. These changes are due to meningoencephalitis. (Courtesy of Drs. A.C. Francesconi do Valle and R.R. Guimaras, Rio de Janeiro)

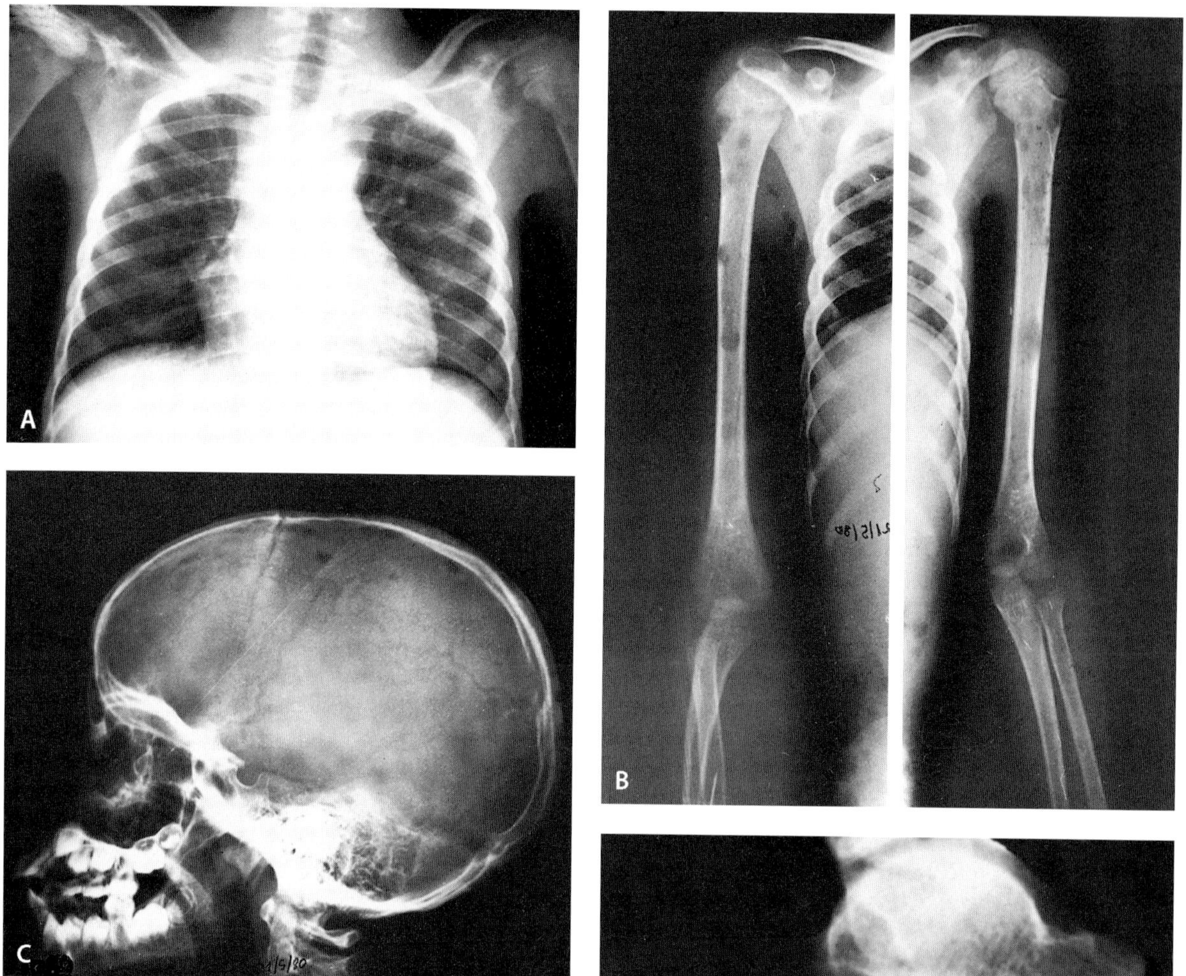

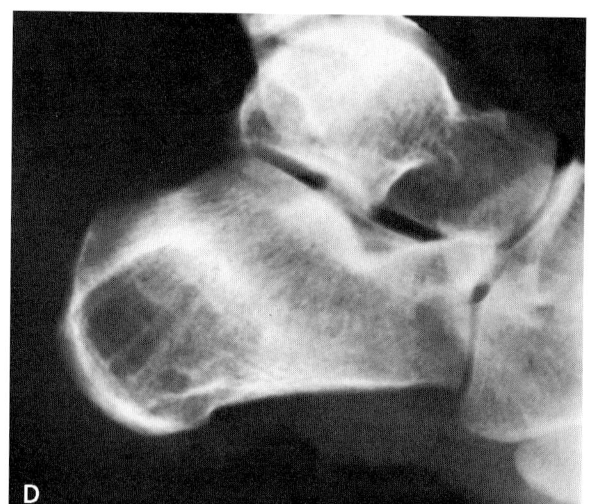

Fig. 6.59 A–D. Skeletal paracoccidioidomycosis. **A** The chest radiograph of an 11-year-old boy with mediastinal enlargement and multiple osteolytic foci in the scapula, upper humerus, and ribs. **B** The same patient: there are multiple sharply demarcated cortical osteolytic lesions in the humeri and scapulae. The shoulder joints, particularly the left, are also infected and there is a lytic focus in the right acromium. There is no evidence of sclerosis around any of these lytic lesions. **C** The skull of the same patient also shows multiple small osteolytic lesions. **D** A different patient, an adult male, with a large osteolytic lesion in the os calcis. It is possible that this is the result of a wound in the heel, allowing direct inoculation. (Courtesy of Dr. I.L. Aymore, Rio de Janeiro)

In the mandible and maxilla there may be rarefaction and loss of clarity of the alveolar margin: if the infection is extensive, teeth may be lost. There are no characteristic imaging findings, and it is very unlikely that bone infection will occur in the absence of systemic disease.

Differential Diagnosis

In an endemic area it is not difficult to establish the diagnosis; however, elsewhere it is not easy to distinguish paracoccidioidomycosis from other mycotic infections or from amebiasis, tuberculosis and, in the abdominal form, Crohn's disease (regional ileitis). The finding of disseminated skin lesions, including perianal or penile nodules, or involvement of bones or joints makes the diagnosis more likely.
Nevertheless, microscopy and identification of the fungus is essential.
The most important factors in making the diagnosis of paracoccidioidomycosis are epidemiology and a high index of suspicion.

Lobomycosis

Lobomycosis is discussed because it is a variety of paracoccidioidomycosis. It was first discovered in 1931 by Jorge Lobo in the Amazon region.

Synonyms

Keloid blastomycosis (queloidiform blastomycosis). Cheloidal (keloidal) blastomycosis. Jorge Lobo's disease. Amazonian blastomycosis. Blastomycoid granuloma. Pseudo leprosy. *Fr*: Lobomycose. *Ger*: Lôbo Krankheit. *Sp*: Lobomicosis.

Definition

Lobomycosis is an infection with the fungus *Loboa loboi* (*Paracoccidioides loboi*, probably a variation of *Paracoccidioides brasiliensis*).

Geographic Distribution

Lobomycosis is found in the Amazon valley (with an very high prevalence in Ciaibi Indians), Surinam, and other parts of South and Central America. It has been recognized in France.

Epidemiology and Pathology

Lobomycosis is most common in thickly vegetated tropical climates. More than 300 cases have been confirmed in humans. There is no racial preference, but depending on the pattern of work, men in some areas and women in other areas are more affected. The infection occurs in humans and dolphins, but the fungus has not yet been cultured. The mode of entry is presumed to be through skin abrasions, particularly in agriculture workers. Most patients are therefore rural inhabitants or living in jungles. The clinical course is so slowly progressive that patients seldom remember when or how it started. Transmission from human to human has not occurred, though transmission from human to dolphin has been observed (the incubation period was 3 months).
The infection causes subepidermal nodules which histopathologically are granulomas with multiple hyaline fibers, histiocytes, and giant cells (Fig. 6.60). There is very little inflammatory reaction or suppuration.
The diagnosis is made by clinical observation of the characteristic skin lesions, or by finding the fungus on tissue sections (Fig. 6.60 C, p. 618). So far, skins tests and serology are not available. This is important, because as there is no specific treatment, the best hope of cure is early excision.

Clinical Characteristics

There are no systemic symptoms. Patients present with freely mobile subepidermal nodules which may coalesce to form large masses, covered by thinly stretched overlying epidermis. They closely resemble hard shiny keloids and cause little discomfort (see Fig. 6.1 A, p. 534; Fig. 6.60 A, p. 618). They can be hyperesthetic or anesthetic. Mucosa and internal organs are not involved. Eventually, some of the nodules may fungate or ulcerate and sometimes spread to lymphatics. They seldom heal spontaneously: squamous cell carcinoma has developed in chronic lesions. Remote elevated crusted plaques are probably caused by auto-inoculation.

Imaging Diagnosis

There are no imaging findings of significance. Lobomycosis is included because it is often discussed in reference to blastomycosis and radiologists must be aware that there is such an infection and, if asked, that there is no reason for imaging because spread beyond the obvious lesion is not known to occur.

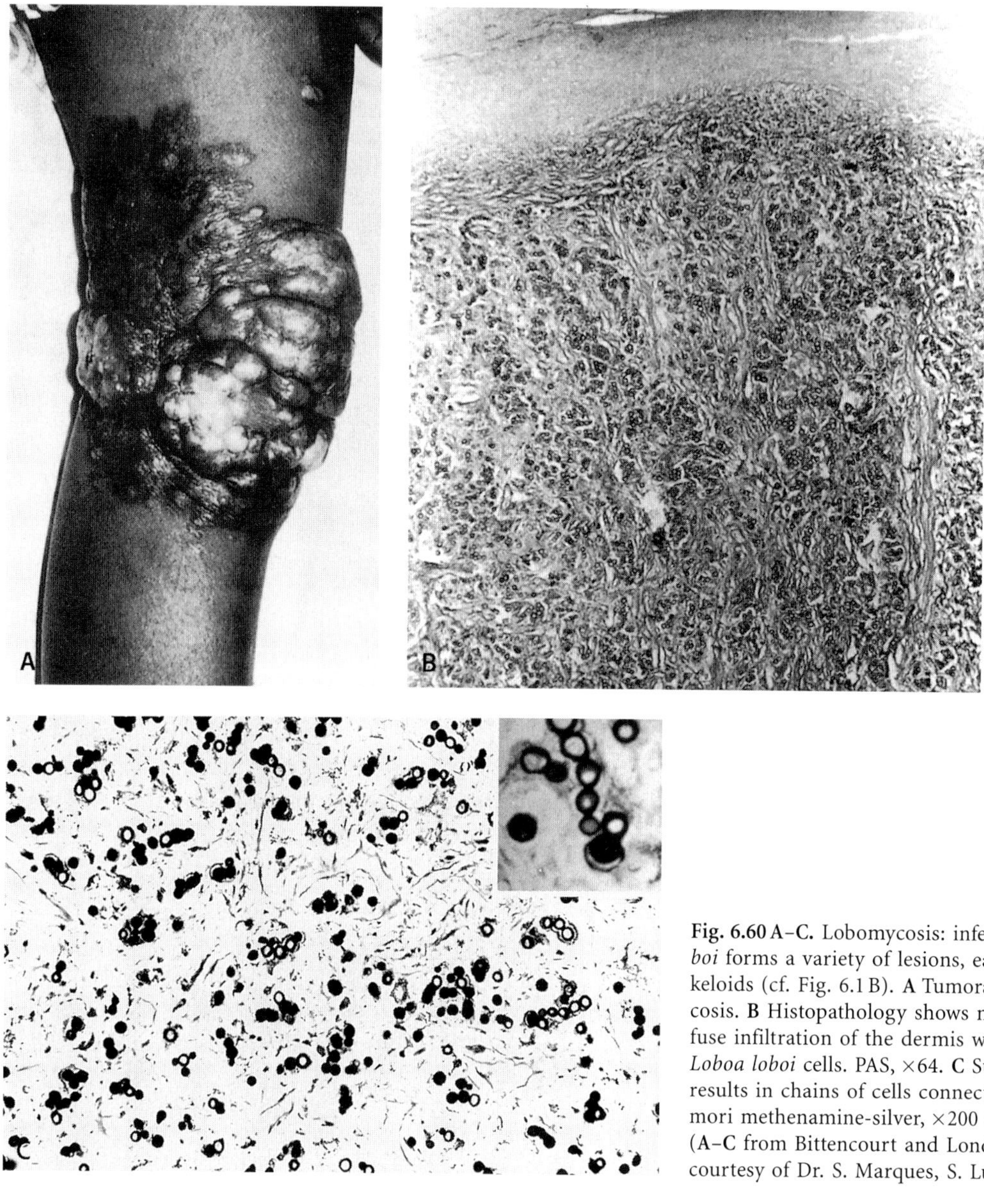

Fig. 6.60 A–C. Lobomycosis: infection with *Loboa loboi* forms a variety of lesions, easily mistaken for keloids (cf. Fig. 6.1 B). **A** Tumoral form of lobomycosis. **B** Histopathology shows no fibrosis but diffuse infiltration of the dermis with many *Loboa loboi* cells. PAS, ×64. **C** Successive budding results in chains of cells connected together. Gomori methenamine-silver, ×200 (*inset*, ×500). (A–C from Bittencourt and Londero 1995; A also courtesy of Dr. S. Marques, S. Luis)

Cryptococcosis

Synonyms

Torulosis. Busse-Buschke's disease. European blastomycosis. Torulosis histolytica. *Ger*: Cryptococcosis neoformans (Erreger der europäischen Blastomykose). *Fr*: Cryptocoque neoforme. *Sp*: Criptococosis neoformans.

Definition

A subacute or chronic fungus infection caused by *Cryptococcosis neoformans.*

Cryptococcosis neoformans occurs in two variants, distinguished by serology: *C. neoformans* var. *neoformans* (serotypes A, B, and AD) and *C. neoformans* var. *gattii* (serotypes B and C).

Geographic Distribution

C. neoformans var. *neoformans* is a common pathogen which occurs worldwide: *C. neoformans* var. *gattii* only occurs in tropical and subtropical countries: the serotype C infections are limited to southern California.

C. neoformans var *neoformans* is an opportunistic, saprophytic yeast which is widely distributed, particularly in old pigeon droppings, but also in the

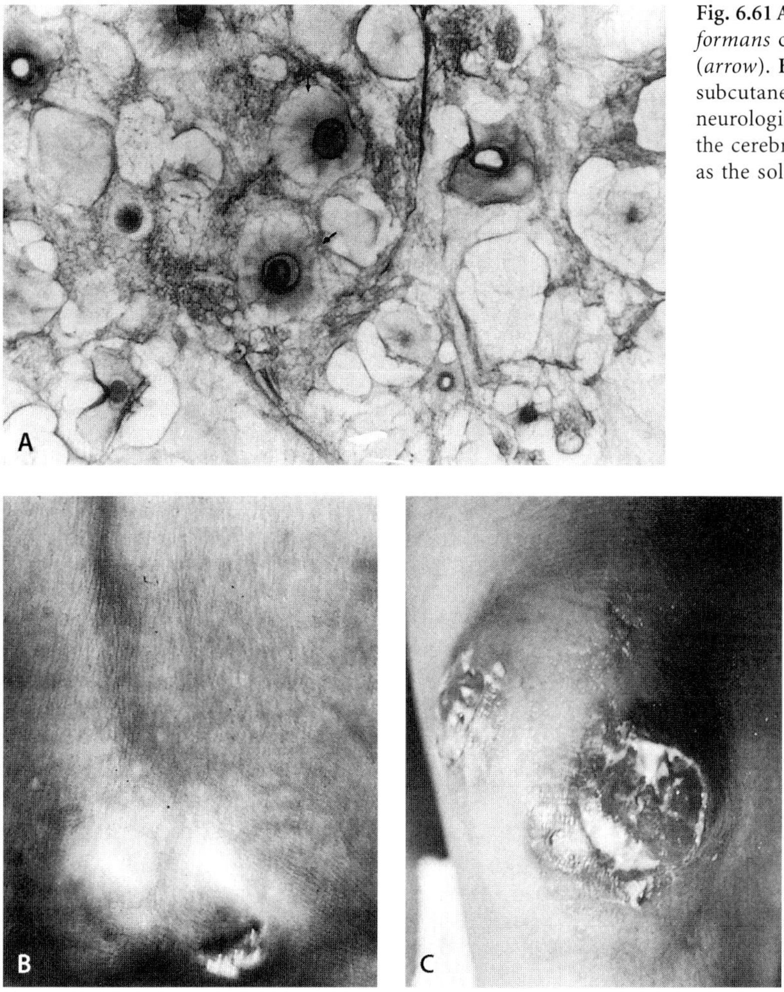

Fig. 6.61 A–C. Cryptococcosis. **A** *Cryptococcus neoformans* cells with a thick capsule and spiculation (*arrow*). **B** A nodule skin lesion and an ulcerating subcutaneous "tumor.". Although the patient had no neurological symptoms, the fungus was found in the cerebrospinal fluid. **C** Subcutaneous tumefaction as the sole manifestation of cryptococcosis

droppings or in soil contaminated by droppings from some other birds. It has been cultured from abandoned houses, woods, and soil. *C. neoformans* var. *gattii* has been cultured from under the bark and around flowering eucalyptus trees and also in bat droppings. *C. neoformans* can survive passage through the alimentary tract of birds which are not actually infected themselves. The fungus has also been found on fruit and in milk, e.g., milk from cattle with cryptococcal mastitis.

Infection occurs by inhalation, not by contact: very rarely, fungus may be accidentally inoculated into the skin. Infections by *C. neoformans* var *neoformans* occur throughout the year, particularly in cities and towns: infections by *C. neoformans* var. *gatti* are more seasonal and more common in rural communities. *C. neoformans* var. *gatti* is a little more common in children and young adults whereas *C. neoformans* var *neoformans* is more frequent in older (30 to 60-year-old) urban dwellers.

Cryptococcosis has been found in many domestic and wild animals. As will be discussed later, *C. neoformans* var neoformans is associated with immunosuppression (it is the fourth leading infectious cause of death in patients with AIDS in the United States) and chronic debilitating diseases, while *C. neoformans* var *gatti* is found in immunocompetent patients.

The histopathological findings depend on the immune status of the patient. In those who are immunocompetent, pulmonary infections are granulomatous. Yeasts are both extra- and intracellular, and surrounded by a granulomatous reaction including giant cells, epithelioid cells, macrophages, and plasma cells. The extent of necrosis is variable. In more chronic infections, fibrosis develops and residual pulmonary granulomas occur. There is seldem any calcification: these granulomas (cryptococcomas) are usually an incidental finding at autopsy or mistaken for neoplasms on chest radiographs.

In those with deficient immunity, there is minimal if any inflammatory reaction: for example, enormous numbers of yeasts accumulate in the meninges. They have thick mucinous capsules and fill and expand the subarachnoid space. There is no suppuration and no evidence of any granulomatous reaction: it is difficult to detect any host reaction at all. The large number of fungal cells with mucoid capsules are shiny and slimy macroscopically (Fig. 6.61 A). In patients who are severely immunodeficient, the large extracellular aggregates distort the normal architecture of any organ. These masses may be so large that they resemble a tumor, with an irregular outline. In other patients there may be multiple small "miliary" nodules. In patients with progressive pulmonary disease, there will be hilar and mediastinal lymphadenopathy. When necrosis occurs, the larger nodules may show central cavitation, but this does not occur in the miliary pattern. The numerous yeasts in the lung may give the appearance of lobar pneumonia. The diagnosis can be confirmed by finding the organisms in sputum, lung biopsy specimens, and cultures. However, *C. neoformans* var *gattii* may be found in the sputum or bronchial washing of normal patients and it does not always mean there is active infection.

Meningeal infection is very common and causes thickening of the subarachnoid meninges, especially at the base of the brain and over the cerebellum. There may be a mucoid exudate: the fungi will be seen in the cerebrospinal fluid or may be cultured from it. In those who are severely immunodeficient, the fungal masses in the leptomeninges may be large enough to displace the brain, while in other patients there may be meningeal adhesions. The diagnosis can be confirmed by finding cryptococcal polysaccharide antigen in the cerebrospinal fluid, using latex agglutination. This is a very sensitive test, reliable in over 90% of patients with cerebral infections.

Clinical Characteristics

There are three ways in which cryptococcosis presents clinically. Meningitis (or meningo-encephalitis) ist the most common, pulmonary infection is almost as frequent but may be undetected, and there may be hematogenous dissemination to various sites, including bone, prostate and the eyes.

As already noted, the patient's susceptibility is increased by the preexistence (or coexistence) of Hodgkin's disease or other reticulosis, leukemia, sarcoidosis when treated with steroids, diabetes, immunosuppressive drugs, or AIDS. Rarely, apparently healthy patients with no detectable immunodeficiency develop cryptococcal meningitis, but why this should happen to these individuals and not to thousands of others who are exposed to the organism is an unsolved problem.

Primary pulmonary infections are often undetected and subclinical infections are common: many pigeon handlers have positive serological evidence for cryptococcosis and are quite unaware of having had any infection. There may be a vague history of illness during childhood, clinically thought at the time to be an upper respiratory virus or bronchitis. Small cryptococcomas may be found on chest imaging or autopsy without having been clinically suspected. Such cryptococcomas are either small nodules close to the pleura or solitary circumscribed lesions in the lung parenchyma (Fig. 6.62, p. 622). Those with clinical symptoms complain of cough, sputum, pain in the chest, loss of weight, and fever. There may be hemoptysis and night sweats, a clinical spectrum varying from influenza to tuberculosis. When the patient is immunocompromised there may be reactivation of a previously unknown focus or a new infection. Even immunocompromised patients may be asymptomatic or have nonspecific chest symptoms, such as cough and shortness of breath. These may persist a long time and often slowly worsen. However, in the majority of immunocompromised patients there is an acute, rapidly progressing pulmonary infection, with pleural effusions and disseminated disease. Many of the symptoms are caused by the large fungal masses and when these rupture into a bronchus, the sputum will be copious and gelatinous.

Many immunocompromised patients go on to have meningeal symptoms, complaining of headache, vomiting, and a stiff neck: this may be followed by raised intracranial pressure, coma, and death. The cerebrospinal fluid will contain monocytes and the initial diagnosis may be tuberculous meningitis (Fig. 6.63, p. 623). In other patients, the onset of CNS cryptococcosis is insidious and it is only later that focal neurological signs appear. Clinically a solid intracranial cryptococcoma mimics a cerebral tumor.

Cutaneous cryptococcosis may present as ulcers, granulomas, nodules, or spreading cellulitis (Fig. 6.61 B, C). Both cutaneous and meningeal cryptococcosis are features of immunodeficiency and dissemination: approximately half of the patients with skin infection will progress to meningitis, even if they have previously been without clinical signs.

Cryptococcal bone infection is usually painful: the skull and the vetebrae are common sites, but there may be infection anywhere in the skeleton. Most bone and cutaneous lesions are multiple. Lesions in the liver, spleen, and kidneys are also part of disseminated disease in patients who are severely immunocompromised. In patients with AIDS, other clinical presentations have been of arthritis, peritonitis, and myocarditis. Without treatment, disseminated or meningeal cryptococcosis is eventually fatal.

Imaging Diagnosis

The chest images reflect the different patterns of the infection.

Peripheral pleural fungal collections may be found in patients who are asymptomatic: these appear as multiple subpleural masses, often bilateral. Granulomas may also occur in the lung parenchyma, particularly in the lower lobes: they are best imaged by CT scanning. On plain radiographs they are from 0.5 to 4 cm in diameter and appear solid, almost always without cavitation or calcification. However, on lung biopsy (which is the most likely way to establish the diagnosis) there will probably be some central necrosis. CT or standard tomography may show air bronchograms in some of these masses. These well-circumscribed granulomatous nodules have been called "toruloma" in some publications.

In patients who presented clinically with chronic flu-like symptoms or more severe illness, chest radiographs may show unilateral or bilateral consolidation, which can be segmental or lobar. There may be a discrepancy in the appearance between frontal and lateral projections (Fig. 6.62 D, E). Because this "consolidation" is fungal rather than inflammatory, air bronchograms may be seen on standard tomography or, better, by CT scanning. Patients with cryptococcal pneumonia may have hilar or mediastinal lymphadenopathy.

In patients who are immunocompromised, and in a few patients in whom the apparent balance between the infection and host is unexpectedly disturbed, dissemination of the infection may occur. There is usually clinical evidence that the patient's illness has worsened. The chest radiographs will then show miliary or diffuse reticulonodular patterns: interstitial thickening may be found on high-resolution CT scanning before it is recognized on chest radiographs.

Cryptococcosis then becomes a more severe and acute disease, and few patients remain relatively asymptomatic. In the majority there is rapid progression both clinically and radiographically. Disseminated lung disease, pleural effusions, and lymphadenopathy are common and in a few patients cavitation may be recognized in some of the pulmonary or subpleural nodules. Lymphadenopathy without any visible pulmonary lesions may occur, but is uncommon.

The extent of the pneumonic consolidation depends on the severity of the infection and the patient's immune response. In some, the consolidation is extensive and diffuse, but in others, with a poor response, the disease is more rapidly progressive and consolidation is less significant. Adult respiratory distress syndrome may develop.

Cryptococcal meningitis is the most frequent complication of disseminated infection in those who are immunocompromised. Many patients have only CNS symptoms and their chests are clinically and radiographically normal. In these patients, CT scanning may show a pulmonary focus and at autopsy there is almost always a pulmonary lesion even when the clinical presentation has been meningeal.

Magnetic resonance imaging and CT scanning may show focal meningitis, dilated perivascular spaces, and multiple cryptococcomas. In the basal ganglia and midbrain there is usually symmetrical perivascular infection with multiple miliary nodules. There can be cryptococcomas in the brain, apparently without meningeal involvement; more commonly, both parenchymal and meningeal infections coexist.

Perivascular invasion is best seen on MRI: on T1-weighted sequences it will appear symmetrical, bilateral, and hypointense or isointense, and on T2-weighted sequences as hyperintense areas. The appearance in the basal ganglia, thalamus, and substantia nigra has been described as "soap bubbles." Gadolinium-enhanced T1-weighted sequences will identify miliary nodules more clearly. Cryptococcomas are hypointense on T1-weighted scans and hyperintense on T2-weighted scans, which often show surrounding edema. Following intravenous gadolinium contrast, there may be ring enhancement (T1-weighted scans).

Plain skull radiographs are of no significant value in the diagnosis of cryptococcosis, but may show well-circumscribed osteolytic lesions, with very little periosteal reaction. The same osteolytic pattern is found whenever any bone is involved. The gelatinous material from these bone lesions may spread into the subcutaneous tissues and resemble a tuberculous abscess. It can be imaged by ultrasound or MRI. Skeletal infections can be detected by radioisotope scanning. Fortunately, such skeletal lesions seldom, if ever, occur unless there is disseminated cryptococcosis, because there are no specific diagnostic findings on imaging.

Candidiasis

Hippocrates recognized oral thrush in the fourth century B.C. and described a disseminated form in two patients. By the eighteenth and nineteenth centuries there were many descriptions and further confirmation that this could become a systemic disease, even involving the brain. By 1877 it was known that the fungus was dimorphic, appearing as either yeast or mycelia: 20 years later it was realized that the different forms depended on environmental conditions. From then on the number of different species recognized and named grew considerably:

(Text continues on p. 624)

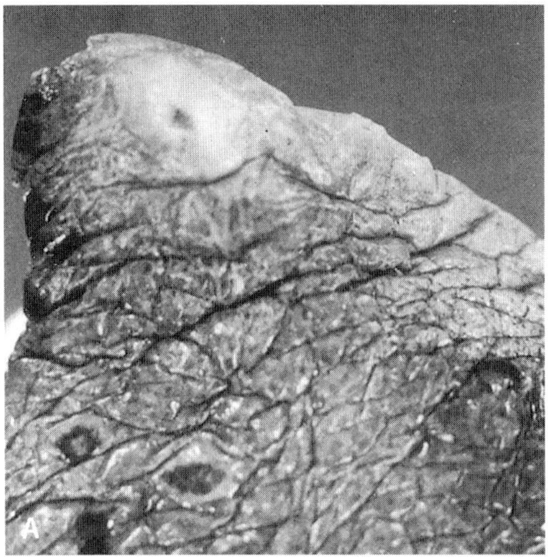

Fig. 6.62 A–G. Pulmonary cryptococcosis. **A** Multiple pulmonary subpleural nodules seen at autopsy. **B** A cut section of the lung showing that there are confluent nodules in the lung parenchyma. **C** A solitary pulmonary lesion, well circumscribed but not encapsulated. A granuloma due to *Cryptococcus neoformans*, a primary infection, most of which are undetected. **D, E** PA and lateral radiographs of the chest of a 22-year-old male complaining of fever: his neck was stiff and he was slightly disorientated. There is a large solitary mass in the basal segment of the left lower lobe, close to the pleura. The outline is irregular, especially anteriorly (better seen on the lateral view). The differential diagnosis includes tuberculosis or other lung granulomas or pneumonia. F, G see p. 623

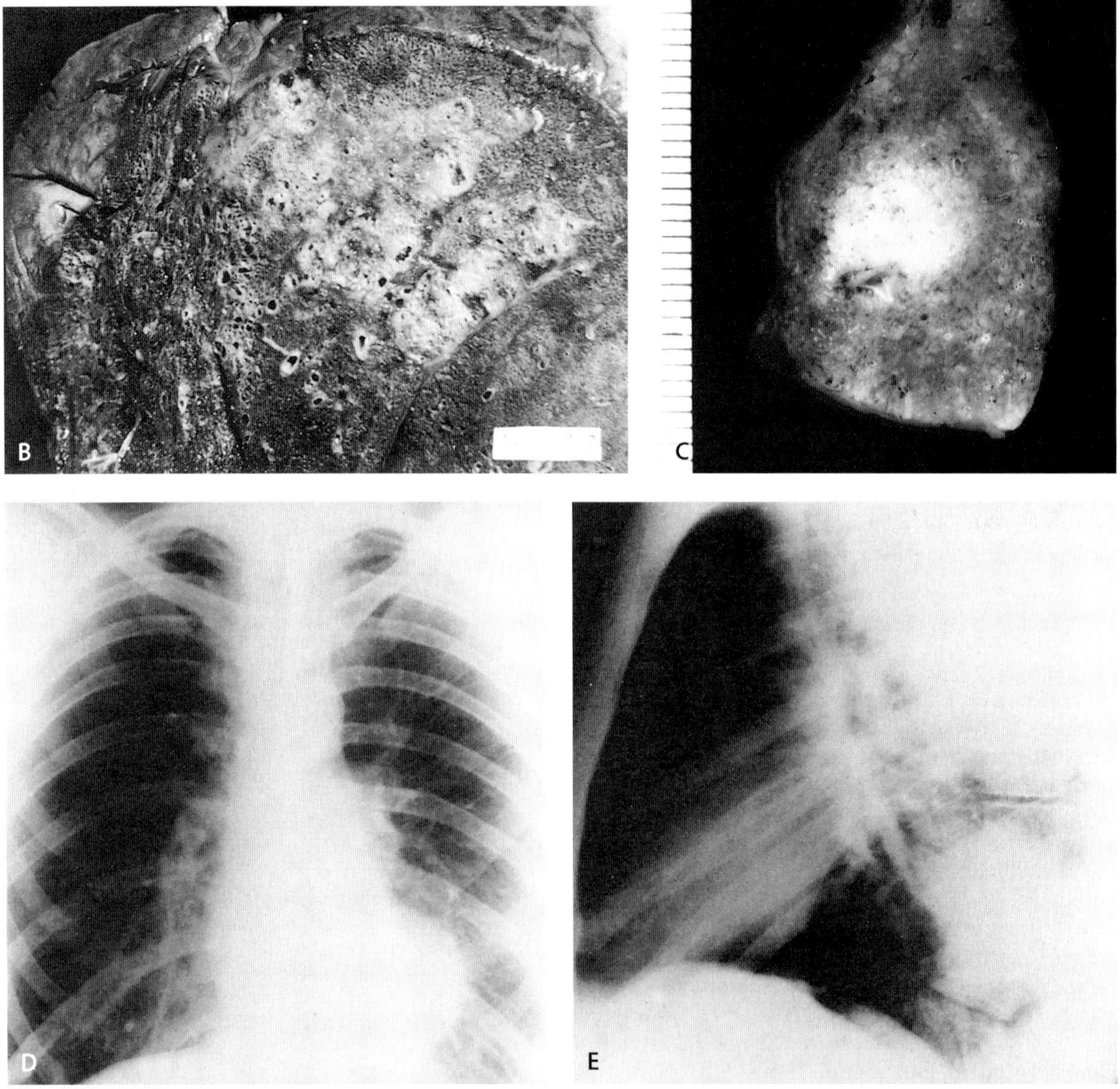

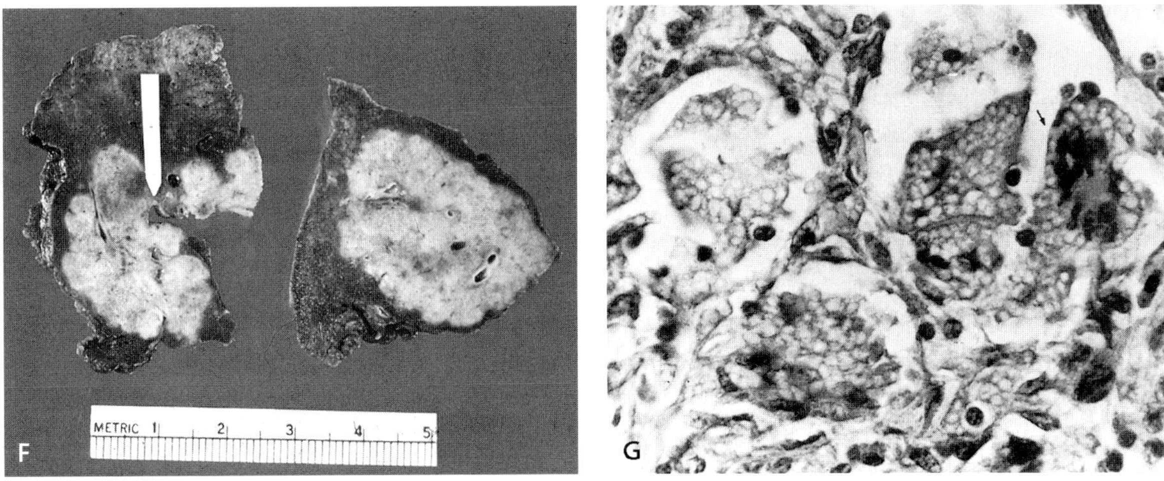

Fig. 6.62 (*continued*). **F** A surgical specimen shows the lobulated, irregular contour of a large cryptococcal granuloma. AFIP 1239772. **G** Multiple fungal cells with macrophages and giant cells. Mucicarmine, ×200. (**A, B, G** from Bittencourt and Londero 1995; **C** specimen contributed by Drs. D. Rulon, Ohio and Daniel H. Connor)

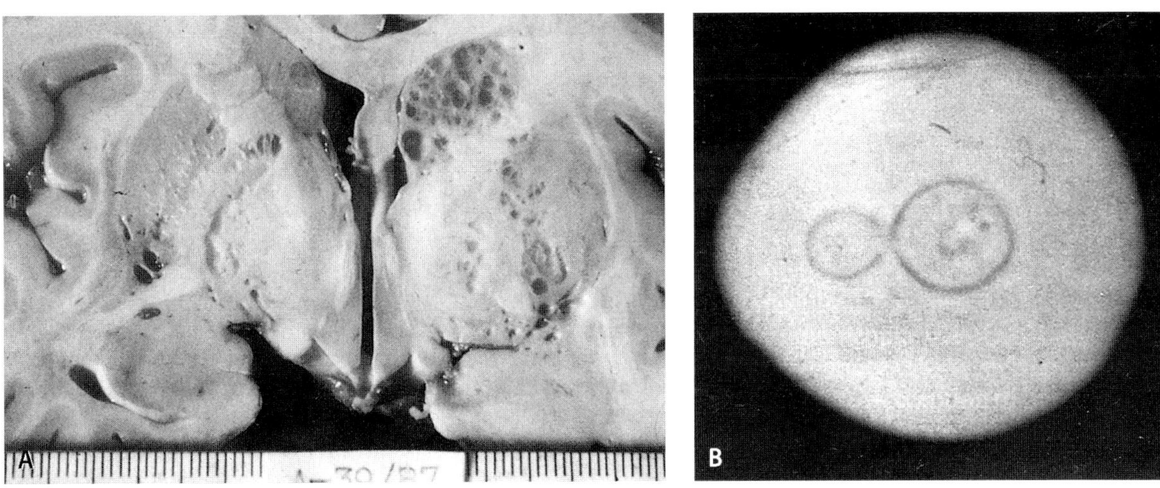

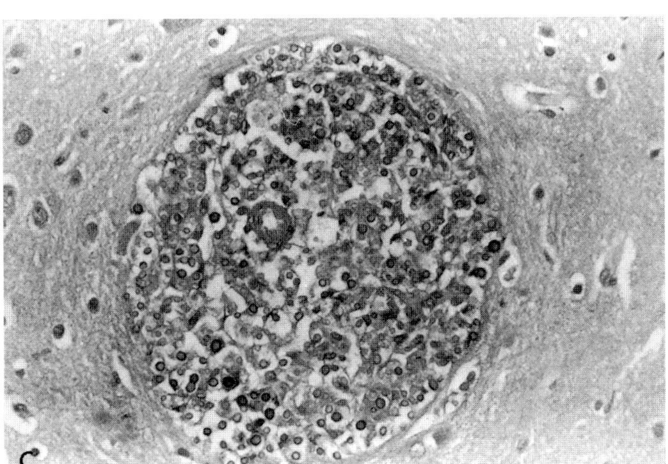

Fig. 6.63 A–C. Cerebral cryptococcosis. **A** A section of the brain showing multiple cystic lesions. **B** Cryptococcus neoformans cell in cerebrospinal fluid. India ink,×1200. **C** A small cryptococcal lesion in the brain: there is no inflammatory reaction, the lesion consists of small capsule-deficient cryptococcus cells. Mayer's mucicarmine, ×256. **A–C** from Bittencourt and Londero 1995)

moniliasis was the name used by many experts but in 1954 *Candida* became the agreed generic name. In the first edition on this textbook there was a separate small section on *Torulopsis glabrata*, but the species has now been reclassified as *C. glabrata*: the group name *monilia* has also been discarded. One may perhaps wonder what any of these fungi will be called if there is ever a third edition of this book!

Synonyms

Moniliasis. Thrush. Bronchomycosis. Tea taster's cough. Mycotic vulvovaginitis. *Ger*: Candidiasis. *Fr*: Candidiose. *Sp*: Candidiasis.

Definition

Candidiasis is an infection by one of the group of fungi of the genus *Candida*. Most of the *Candida* spp. are commensal and part of the normal flora in the mouth, pharynx, colon, vagina, and skin. Its presence therefore does not imply a pathological state unless there is evidence of tissue invasion or there has been an overwhelming increase in the number of fungi.

Geographic Distribution

The yeast and hyphae which cause candidiasis are everywhere, associated with warm-blooded animals. They have been extensively studied in the mouth, rectum, vagina, and skin of healthy people. There is no significant geographic variation.

Epidemiology and Pathology

There are more than 80 species of *Candida*, but only a few are pathogenic in humans. The commonest cause of candidiasis is *Candida albicans*, a normal commensal in the mouth and upper respiratory and intestinal tracts. Another common fungus is *C. tropicalis*. The various species probably have a predilection for different clinical sites: for example, *C. albicans* and *C. parapsilosis* are the most common causes of endocarditis, while *C. tropicalis* frequently causes disseminated infections in immunosuppressed patients and many of those with hematological malignancies. *C. krusei* infects neutropenic patients and gives children diarrhea. It is invasive in patients with septicemia. Many other species have been occasionally isolated and have been cultured from a very wide range of environmental sources. *Candida* spp., particularly *C. albicans*, have been isolated from animals. If found in food or drinks (fruit juices are often contaminated) this is a reflection of the packaging and processing rather than the fruit juice. While the risk posed to healthy individuals is slight, for those who are immunosuppressed the risk is considerable and the infection can be fatal.

Candida are larger than bacteria and are gram-positive; all species can reproduce by budding, forming blastospores. Elongation of these yeast cells, with branching, can produce hyphae, the species varying in the way that these are produced. *C. albicans* can produce cylindrical germ tubes, which are rudimentary hyphae, from blastospores. *Candida* grows on a wide variety of common culture media, but most often is grown on Sabouraud's agar. There is a skin test which indicates prior sensitization by *C. albicans*, but many healthy adults react positively so that the test has little clinical use. The *Candida* spp. are opportunistic: they can produce toxic effects and potentially tissue-digesting enzymes such as protease and phospholipase. Gram stains and the periodic acid-Schiff stain show the fungi in tissue sections. Sometimes the tissue reaction is suppurative and without a contrast stain the fungi may be overlooked; in other cases the reaction is granulomatous and suggests tuberculosis, so it is important for pathologists to utilize special stains for fungi whenever there is any possibility of a mycosis.

Candidiasis may be cutaneous, mucocutaneous, or systemic. The papular dermatitis produced by *C. albicans* has no imaging characteristics. There is a marked inflammatory response causing an edematous, shiny erythema. This may be acute or chronic and is often extensive and progressive. This infection does not spread to deeper underlying tissues, but there may be vascular invasion and dissemination.

Mucocutaneous candidiasis is most commonly seen as oral thrush or vaginal, penile, or rectal infections. Again, there are no specific imaging findings. The systemic candidal infections do cause changes which are important for the imaging department.

Clinical Characteristics

Candidiasis is seldom a disease of healthy people, though candida vulvovaginitis may occur in healthy women and oral thrush may be found in apparently normal newborn infants. Cutaneous candidiasis appears on damaged skin but also in moist, hot surfaces such as the creases and folds in the axilla or inguinal regions, or under heavy breasts. Infections are common in the extremes of age, premature infants, and the elderly.

The status of the immune system is the most significant factor in the natural history of the disease. Those most at risk are immunocompromised, because of AIDS, diabetes, leukemia, or chronic ill health or malnourishment. Other patients will have been on prolonged antibiotic, steroid, or cytotoxic therapy: some have had a prior bacterial infection. Drug addicts are heavily at risk of intravenous self-inoculation. Sickle cell disease has been associated with candidiasis. There are no occupations with particular risk, apart from tea tasting.

Candida spp. are invasive, which accounts for hematogenous spread. Pulmonary candidiasis causes pneumonia, usually bilateral and particularly at the lung bases. There are no characteristic clinical signs or symptoms.

Gastrointestinal candidiasis may be completely asymptomatic or cause retrosternal pain. Esophagoscopy may show white mucosal plaques along the whole length of the esophagus, particularly the distal third. In between the plaques, the esophageal mucosa is edematous and red. As the infection progresses, the esophagus may ulcerate, the ulcers being lined with a shaggy, gray base: bleeding is common. In severe infections swallowing is affected and perforation may occur. There are quite often complicating concomitant infections, particularly in AIDS patients.

In the stomach, candidiasis causes superficial gastric erosion and the symptome are those of gastritis. Ulceration may develop in the small intestine and colon. The lesions may be extensive, and invade blood vessels, spreading to the liver, spleen, and gallbladder (perhaps spreading directly also). Candidal peritonitis more commonly follows contaminated dialysis, causing abdominal pain, tenderness, and a low-grade fever. Candidal peritonitis can also follow abdominal surgery. Pancreatic abscesses have been reported.

Candidiasis of the urinary bladder usually follows catheterization, but hematogenous spread can occur, with the kidneys, ureters, and bladder being infected. *Candida* infection may occur whenever the bladder does not empty properly, particularly in a neurogenic bladder, and following pelvic irradiation. Clinically, these infections are often asymptomatic but may precipitate complete urinary obstruction. When there is pyuria, it is probably due to a secondary infection or underlying bladder disease rather than to candidiasis. In the kidney, *Candida* pyelitis also follows obstruction or surgical interference, including ureteric catheterization. Renal papillary necrosis following such infection is another cause of renal pelvic and ureteric obstruction. Urine cultures can be used as evidence of *Candida* dissemination, but must be interpreted carefully because they may be falsely positive or negative.

Candidiasis is a common cause of septicemia, particularly in long-stay hospital patients with numerous catheters and heavy antibiotic therapy. Scattered candidal skin lesions may develop when there is fungemia, even when it is difficult to isolate *Candida* spp. from the blood. When disseminated, the site of clinical infection depends on many factors, but particularly on tissue damage from previous surgery, radiotherapy, the passage of calculi, or catheterization. When the liver and spleen are infected, the patient will have a low-grade fever, upper quadrant abdominal pain, hepatomegaly, splenomegaly, and, sometimes, jaundice. Liver function tests may become abnormal. Biopsy or autopsy will show multiple small abscesses throughout the liver and/or spleen: their centers may be necrotic, with hyphae, pseudohyphae, and yeasts growing in them.

Candidal septicemia often causes acute and subacute endocarditis, particularly if there is a valvular abnormality or previous surgery. Intravenous or pulmonary artery catheters are a common source of infection. *Candida* spp. can usually be grown from blood which is taken from these patients. Retinal infections can result from candidemia.

Badly damaged joints, e.g., from rheumatoid arthritis or following joint replacement, may become infected by *Candida* spp., usually by hematogenous spread, but occasionally directly at the time of surgery. Bone infection may be by direct or hematogenous spread; the lumbar vertebrae seem to be the most commonly affected.

Candidal meningitis afflicts neonates, particularly those of low birth weight. Adults may develop candidal cerebral abscesses, but most cerebral candidal infections follow surgery or trauma to the head.

The clinical findings in candidiasis have been summarized by Rippon (Table 6.4, p. 626).

Imaging Diagnosis

Only the pulmonary and disseminated infections, such as those of the alimentary tract, are of importance to imaging. Except in the esophagus, it is difficult if not impossible to make a firm imaging diagnosis of candidiasis by any imaging technique.

Pulmonary Candidiasis

Patients who are only moderately immunosuppressed may have candidal bronchitis, with bronchial wall thickening and hyperemia of the mucosa, indistinguishable from bronchial or viral bronchitis. The secretions may cause transient atelectasis.

More commonly, there is pneumonia – either scattered bronchopneumonia with ill-defined nodular

Table 6.4. Clinical findings in candidiasis, as summarized by Rippon

I. Infectious form
  A. Mucocutaneous involvement
    1. Oral: glossitis, stomatitis, cheilitis, perlèche (fissures at angle of mouth)
    2. Vaginitis: balanitis
    3. Bronchial and pulmonary lesions
    4. Alimentary: esophagitis, enteric and perianal infections
    5. Chronic mucocutaneous candidiasis
  B. Cutaneous involvement
    1. Intertriginous and generalizd candidiasis
    2. Paronychia, onychomycosis
    3. "Diaper" disease (napkin candidiasis)
    4. Candidal granuloma
  C. Systemic involvement
    1. Urinary tract infections
    2. Endocarditis
    3. Meningitis
    4. Septicemia
    5. Iatrogenic candidemia
II. Allergic form
  A. Candidids
  B. Eczema
  C. Asthma
  D. Gastritis

shadows throughout both lungs, or, much less commonly, lobar penumonia, which suggests that the candidiasis complicates bacterial pneumonia. There may be fleeting changes in the radiographic appearances of the chest when the plugs of thickened mucus are coughed up, resembling bronchial casts. Miliary dissemination also occurs, causing soft and faint miliary nodulation throughout the lungs.
Pleural effusions and lymphadenopathy are uncommon: fibrosis and calcification are rarely seen.
In some patients with septicemia, the chest remains normal.

Candidiasis of the Alimentary Tract

The earliest sign of esophageal candidiasis is abnormal motility, with decreased peristalsis, aperistalsis, and some areas of spasm. The esophagus may widen and if the deeper muscularis layers are involved, remain distended. Because the mucosa is ulcerated, with contrast the esophagus appears rough and shaggy (like a carpet) (Fig. 6.64). The ulcers caused by the pseudohyphae trap the barium and retain it for a long period, unlike the normal rapid mucosal clearing. The fungal granulomas in the mucosa produce multiple small "negative" defects, which might be mistaken for small esophageal varices, but the ulcers of candidiasis are most numerous in the upper part of the esophagus and de-

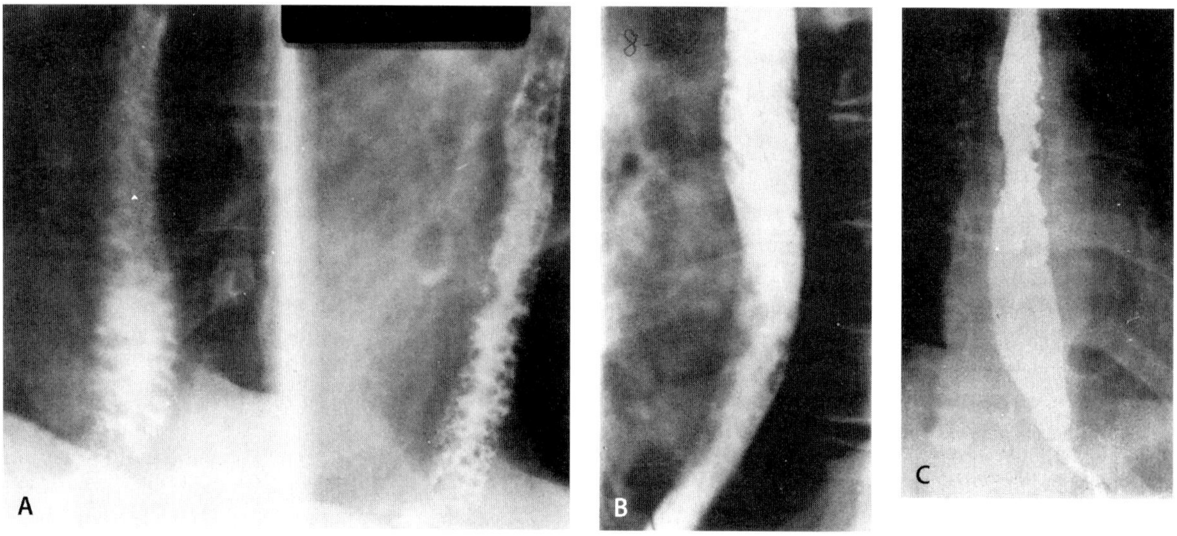

Fig. 6.64 A–C. Candidiasis of the esophagus. **A** The barium-filled esophagus of a patient with chronic leukemia on steroid therapy. There are multiple nodules along the esophagus caused by granulomas and a matrix of hyphae and yeast forms. These may retain the barium for 30–60 min. The esophagus is edematous and normal peristalsis is lost. Both the mucosa and the peristalsis will return to normal within a few days of appropriate therapy. AFIP 229498-250. **B** A similar but less severe infection in a 79-year-old man who also had leukemia. AFIP 239498-249. **C** A man from India with marked esophagitis. The radiological appearance mimics varices, but when due to candidiasis the nodules are most prominent at the top of the esophagus whereas varices occur in the lower half. (C courtesy of Dr. A. Gajaraj, Madras)

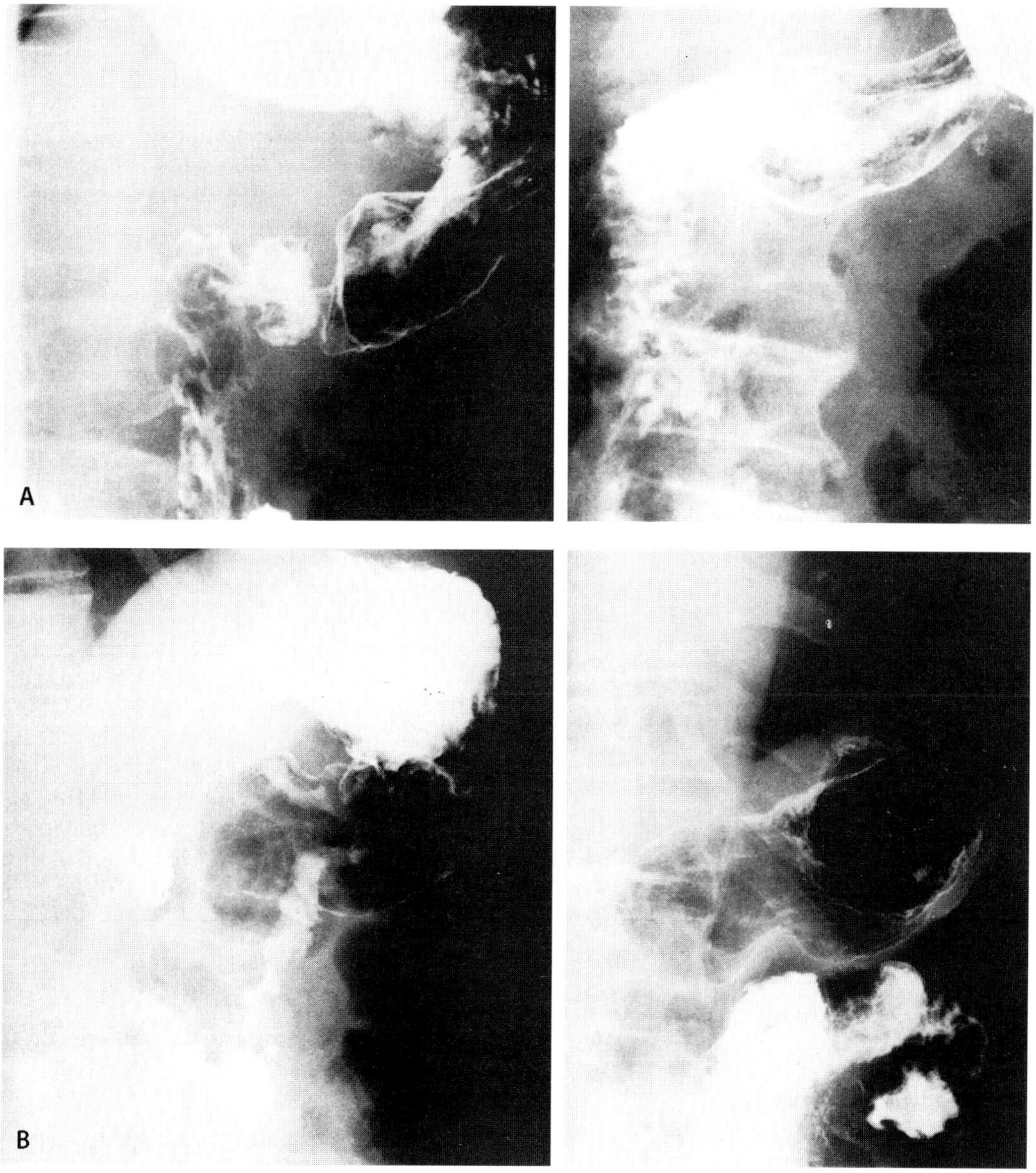

Fig. 6.65 A, B. Candidiasis of the stomach. **A** Barium contrast study showed decreased peristalsis in the stomach, with rigidity and narrowing of the body and pylorus. The mucosal folds are lost: the barium coats the fungal membranes in the stomach and the appearance suggests that there are food particles and even gastric ulcers. This patient was a severe diabetic who had not taken anything by mouth for weeks. Endoscopy showed a membrane in the stomach and multiple small ulcers. **B** The patient after 2 weeks of treatment: the peristalsis has returned and the gastric mucosa is normal. It may take some weeks before recovery is complete

crease towards the cardia, which is the converse of esophageal varices (Fig. 6.64 C).

The mucosal reaction can produce small polyps, diverticula, and even larger polyps resembling carcinoma. When patients have achalasia, e.g. from Chagas' disease or scleroderma, the obstruction at the cardia increases the likelihood of esophageal candidiasis, and the appearance may resemble retained food. Some of the fungus can be dislodged, and fungus balls in the esophagus have been described.

Candidiasis of the stomach is not common: it causes decreased peristalsis (Fig. 6.65). The larger mucosal folds are partially preserved but the minor folds are effaced and there is prolonged retention of barium in the shaggy carpet-like membrane which covers the mucosal lining. Discrete polypoid nodules may develop, and ulcerate centrally. The appearance can be mistaken for Kaposi sarcoma or lymphoma. If the patient is successfully treated, the stomach may return to an almost normal state.

There are no specific images in the small intestine: in the large bowel the appearances resemble those of an irritable colon or even early ulcerative colitis.

Candidiasis of the Biliary Tract and Liver

Candidiasis of the biliary tract is unusual. Fungus balls may be shown by cholangiography or ultrasonography. It is difficult to distinguish the images from any other cholangitis.
In the liver, *Candida* causes microabscesses from hematogenous spread. These can be demonstrated by ultrasonography or CT, and some will enhance with intravenous contrast. Four patterns of hepatosplenic candidiasis have been described on ultrasonography. The early abscesses are surrounded by a hypoechoic ring which surrounds an inner hyperechoic ring: the outer zone is fibrous tissue, the inner is inflammatory cells. There is a central hyperechoic necrotic area, caused by the fungi. Larger abscesses have a more typical target appearance (bull's eye), but when most patients are scanned, these stages will be past and the finding on ultrasonography will be of multiple hypoechoic foci. Later again, as healing occurs there is further fibrosis and calcification. The foci become more echogenic and there may be acoustic shadowing in some cases.
The CT findings are similar: the microabscesses show as multiple low attenuated foci scattered throughout the liver and spleen. As they heal, calcification may be detected. MRI shows the same pattern, but the calcification may not be recognized.

Candidiasis of the Genitourinary Tract

The most common of all fungal infections of the urinary tract is *Candida*: On scanning (ultrasonography CT, or MRI), the same pattern of microabscesses seen in the liver will be found in the kidneys. In acute candidiasis, the findings resemble any acute pyelonephritis. The fungi may produce filling defects on the mucosa of the renal collecting system (Fig. 6.66 A), mimicking small radiolucent calculi, blood clots, or even epithelial tumors. In immunodeficient patients, particularly diabetics, the fungal mass can be large enough to cause obstruction (Fig. 6.66 B, C). CT or ultrasonography will show these changes clearly and demonstrate that the renal outline is deformed. In neonatal renal candidiasis, ultrasonography is not a reliable way to indicate the need for treatment or assess its success and need for continuation. There is no correlation between the sonographic findings and apparent deterioration during treatment. If there have been renal abscesses which heal, calcification may follow, as in the liver or spleen. A few patients have had candidal interstitial cystitis, causing trabeculation and thickening of the urinary bladder and dilatation of the collecting system.
None of these imaging changes are really diagnostic in the urinary tract: urinary tests may be misleading and percutaneous aspiration biopsy may be necessary.

Intracerebral Candidiasis

Intracerebral candidiasis is almost always the result of dissemination. CT and MRI will show multiple microabscesses, with enhancing ring or nodular lesions. These are indistinguishable from any other infection, and do not have any specific distribution.

Rhinosporidiosis

Rhinosporidium seeberi is included with the fungi although it has not been successfully cultured in artificial culture medium and the taxonomic position is uncertain.
This organism was originally thought to occur in the nostrils (hence its name) but has now been found in the ears, eyes, mouth, and larynx, as well as the urethra. Dissemination has occurred, with multiple skin and subcutaneous infections, as well as in the liver, spleen, lung, and kidneys. Bone infections in the hands and feet serve to emphasize that rhinosporidiosis is not restricted to the nostrils.

Definition

Rhinosporidiosis is infection with *Rhinosporidium seeberi* (*Coccidium seeberi*).

Geographic Distribution

The infection is found worldwide but is particularly common in Sri Lanka and in some areas of India. It is common in Madras (in southern India), rare in Central India. The next highest prevalence is in South America, where there are endemic foci, and in Africa; it has been reported from the United States. It is much less common in Europe and more temperate climates.

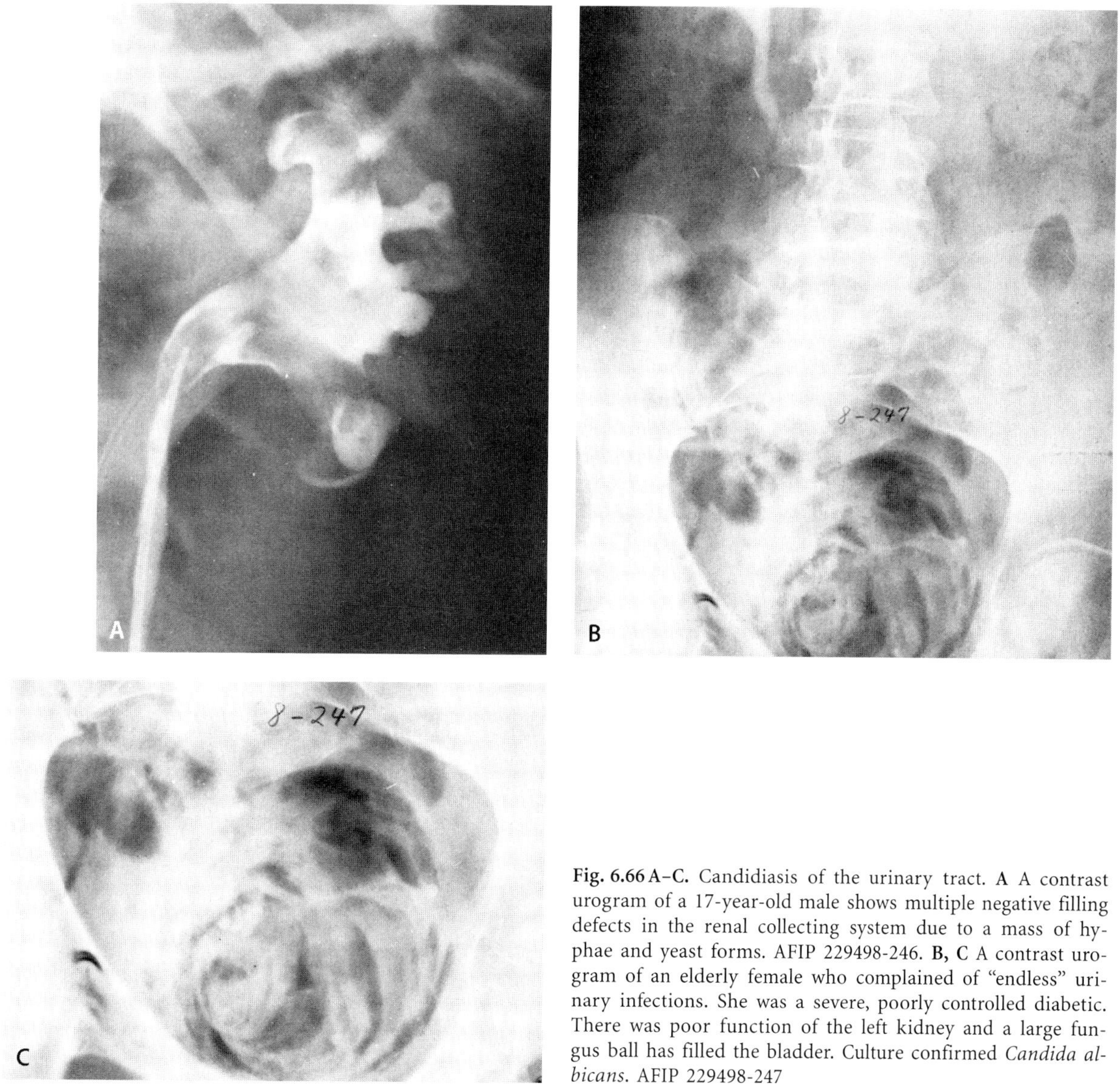

Fig. 6.66 A–C. Candidiasis of the urinary tract. **A** A contrast urogram of a 17-year-old male shows multiple negative filling defects in the renal collecting system due to a mass of hyphae and yeast forms. AFIP 229498-246. **B, C** A contrast urogram of an elderly female who complained of "endless" urinary infections. She was a severe, poorly controlled diabetic. There was poor function of the left kidney and a large fungus ball has filled the bladder. Culture confirmed *Candida albicans*. AFIP 229498-247

Epidemiology and Pathology

The organism has not been cultured, except in association with living cells, nor has it been identified other than in humans and some animals, particularly dogs and horses. Its natural habitat and the routes of infection and transmission are still unknown, although trauma is thought by some to be essential before the infection can start. Human eye infection has been linked to bathing in stagnant water or working in paddy fields. Nasal infection seem to be more common where there are storms or in those who work in sandy river beds. Not surprisingly, it is therefore more common in males from 20 to 40 years old.

Transmission from human to human is unknown. Although infections have been recognized in the female genital tract and rectum, sexual transmission has not been documented. Mucocutaneous lesions usually occur in the nose or eye. Thus, although the epidemiology is well documented, the source and ways of transmission remain a mystery.

The tissue reaction is a chronic inflammation with occasional foreign body giant cells. Hyperplastic growth of overlying epithelium gives rise to friable polyps and the spherical fungi (sporangia) may be clinically visible as white spots (Figs. 6.67, 6.68 A). The thick-walled sporangium contains hundreds of endospores developing at different rates. The underlying fibromyxomatous connective tissue may be hyperemic. Regional lymph nodes are not usually affected.

The diagnosis is made by recognition of the fungus, either from the surface of the polyp or by histo-

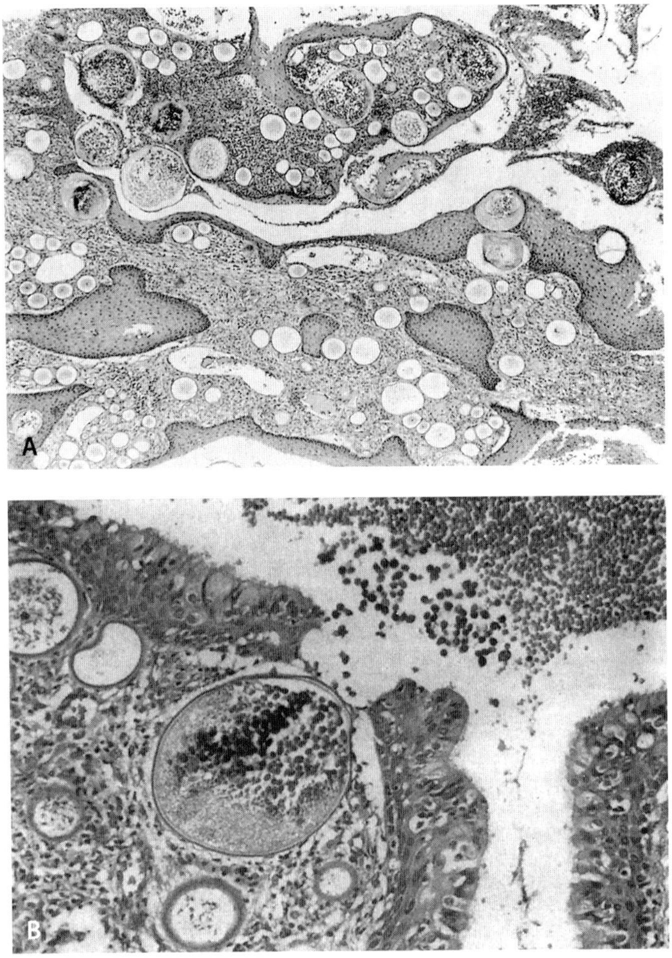

Fig. 6.67 A, B. Rhinosporidiosis commonly presents with nasal polyps. A The cut section of a nasal polyp in which there is squamous metaplasia of the epithelium. There are numerous spherical strictures within the chorium and outside the mucosa. H & E, ×40. Eventually a granulomatous reaction occurs and B mature spherules discharge the endospores through the lining epithelium. H & E, ×160. (A, B from Bittencourt and Londero 1995)

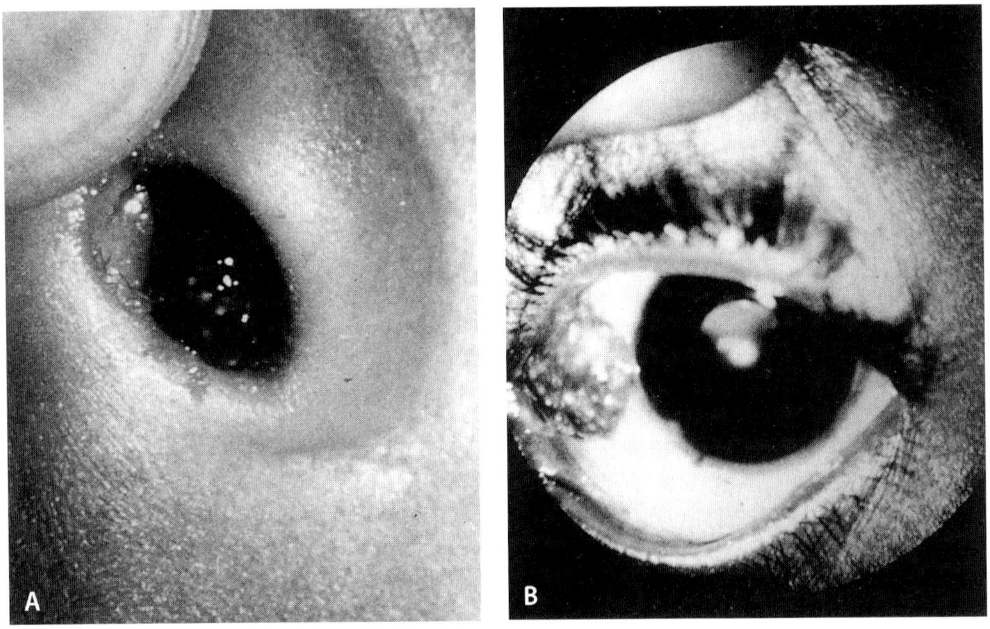

Fig. 6.68. A A nasal polyp with tiny white spots in an 11-year-old child. B A conjunctival lesion. In India about 90% of patients have nasal polyps whereas in Brazil more than half have conjunctival lesions, and this is the pattern in Africa. (A courtesy of Dr. I. Campbell; B courtesy of Prof. R. Marback; both from Bittencourt and Londero 1995)

pathology. The sporangia of *R. seeberi* are much larger than and thus easily differentiated from the spherules of *Coccidioides immitis*. Serology and animal inoculation are not helpful.

Clinical Characteristics

Rhinosporidiosis in children is equally common in males and females, but in adolescents and adults it is much more common in males: this probably reflects an occupational association. Wherever the infection occurs, it appears clinically as soft, friable, vascular polyps, from pink to red to violet in color. On the skin, early lesions are flat. The polyps are lobulated and bleed easily. Under the epithelium there are tiny white spots, which are the sporangia. On the skin the papillomatous lesions may become warty. The infection may persist for 30 years or more, yet dissemination is uncommon. New lesions are usually clost to the original sites, and auto-inoculation is suspected. The polyps may become significantly pedunculated and when in the nose they may block the ostia into the sinuses: on the conjunctiva they can be large enough to evert the lid.

Two-thirds of the reported infections are in the nose, and present clinically as nasal obstruction or bleeding. They are not painful, but may cause irritation. As they grow, there is a profuse mucoid nasal discharge. Pedunculated polyps may extend backwards into the pharynx and spread onto the palate. However, the most common site is anteriorly in the nose, particularly along the septum.

As noted, the palpebral conjunctiva is the next most common site (Fig. 6.68 B). The patient may complain of a foreign body in the eye or of a blood-stained discharge. This is worsened if the lacrimal ducts are occluded.

Similar lesions in the larynx cause hoarseness: on the tongue and palate a common presentation is a sessile granuloma.

In the urethra, rhinosporidiosis is much more common in men than in women. A similar friable, pink discrete painless polyp protrudes from the urethral meatus. Multiple lesions in the urethra have presented further posteriorly. Hematuria, intermittent bleeding, and discharge are the reasons that the patients come for treatment. Similar polypoid or flat lesions occur in the vagina, vulva, or rectum, but, as noted already, sexual transmission has not been recorded.

Spread to the liver, spleen, lungs, and kidneys is excessively rare. There is likely to be ascites and in some patients, peripheral edema. Osseous lesions have been identified in only two patients: one with a granuloma in the scapula and another with osteolytic foci in the hands and feet.

If there are systemic clinical symptoms in a patient with rhinosporidiosis, it should suggest an accompanying pyogenic infection. Only in the very rare, widely disseminated infection is there likely to be fever, wasting, and perhaps, death.

Imaging Diagnosis

The soft tissue masses do not require imaging. Blockage of the paranasal sinuses or in the nasopharynx can be demonstrated and in very long-standing infections there may be deformity of the facial bones. In a few patients, the polypoid masses in the trachea or bronchi have caused mild obstruction with air trapping.

There are no specific imaging findings: rhinosporidiosis is another cause of an opaque antrum or other sinus, of a mass in the airways, and occasionally of pulmonary atelectasis. The bone changes are nonspecific: the urethral polyps are more likely to be of concern to patients than to require imaging.

Acknowledgements. We are grateful to Dr. Demosthenes Pappagianis, MD, PhD, Professor of Medical Microbiology and Director of the Coccidioidomycosis Serology Laboratory, School of Medicine, University of California, Davis, Calif., USA, who was kind enough to advise us on the many details of mycology in this chapter.

Bibliography

General Mycology

Baker RD, et al: *Human Infection with fungi, actinomycoses and algae.* Springer, Berlin Heidelberg New York, 1971

Bearse P: Mycotic infections of the stomach. *Am J Dig Dis* 5:674–676, 1938

Bennett JE, et al: Fungal diseases. In: Warren KS, Marmoud AAF (eds) *Tropical and geographical medicine, part 6.* McGraw-Hill, New York, 1984, pp 889–980

Binford CH, Dooley JR: Diseases caused by fungi and deep mycoses. In: Binford CH, Connor DH (eds) *Pathology of tropical and extraordinary diseases.* Armed Forces Institute of Pathology, Washington DC, 1976, pp 551–609

Bittencourt AL, Londero AT: *Tropical mycotic disease.* In: Doerr W, Seifert G (eds) *Tropical pathology.* Springer, Berlin Heidelberg New York, 1995, pp 707–798

Chandler FW, Kaplan W, Ajello L: *A colour atlas and textbook of the histopathology of mycotic disease.* Wolfe, London, 1980

Chandler FW, Watts JC. *Pathologic diagnosis of fungal infections.* ASCP Press, Chicago, 1987, pp 279–286

Crotty JM: Systemic mycotic infections in Northern Territory Aborigines. *Med J Aust* 1:184–186, 1965

Goldberg HI, Reeder MM: Infections and infestations of the gastrointestinal tract. In: Margulis AR, Burhenne HJ (eds) *Alimentary tract roentgenology.* C.V. Mosby, St. Louis, 1973, pp 1588–1590

Halde C: Mycotic diseases. In: Goldsmith R, Heyneman D (eds) *Tropical medicine and parasitology.* Appleton and Lange, Norwalk, 1989, pp 198–223

Jain SK, et al: A clinico-radiological study of secondary mycoses in pulmonary tuberculosis. *Ind J med Sci* 45:81–84, 1991

Kwon-Chung KJ, Bennett JE: *Medical mycology*, Lea and Feliger, Philadelphia, 1992

Litzky LA: The pathology of fungal disease in the lung. *Semin Radiol* XXXI:4–13, 1996

MacKenzie DWR, et al: The mycoses. In: Strickland GT (ed) *Hunter's tropical medicine, 7th edn.* Saunders, Philadelphia, 1991, part IV, pp 501–545

McAdams HP, et al: Thoracic mycoses from endemic fungi: radiologic-pathologic correlation. *Radiographics* 15:255–270, 1995

McAdams HP, et al: Thoracic mycoses from opportunistic fungi. Radiologic-pathologic correlation. *Radiographics* 15:271–286, 1995

Mycoses. Scientific publication No. 304. Pan American Health Organization, Washington DC, 1975

Odds FC, et al: Nomenclature of fungal disease: a report and recommendation from the sub-committee of the International Society of Human and Animal Mycology (ISHAM). *J Med Vet Mycol* 30:1–10, 1992

Pena CE: Deep mycotic infections in Colombia. A clinicopathologic study of 162 cases. *Am J Clin Pathol* 47:505–520, 1967

Rippon JW: Medical mycology. The pathogenic fungi and the pathogenic actinomycetes. Saunders, Philadelphia, 1974

Rippon JW: Pathology and epidemiology of opportunistic mycotic infections. A review. *Am J Med Technol* 43:226–228, 1977

Ross MD, Gelfand M: Deep fungal infections in Rhodesia. A 10 year study. *Cent Afr J Med* 24 & 25:208–212, 1978

Symmers W: Deep-seated fungal infections. *Am J Clin Pathol* 46:514–517, 1966

Uflacker R, et al: Parasitic and mycotic causes of biliary obstruction. *Gastrointest Radiol* 7:173–179, 1982

Wentworth BB: *Diagnostic procedures for mycotic and parasitic infections, 7th edn.* Am Pub Health Assoc, 1995

Actinomycosis

Armitage G, Smith E: Abdominal actinomycosis, case report and review of antibiotic treatment. *Br J Surg* 42:77–80, 1954

Baron R, Arduino LJ: Primary actinomycosis. *J Urol* 62:410–416, 1949

Bates M, Cruickshank G: Thoracic actinomycosis. *Thorax* 12:99–124, 1957

Blain AW: Primary actinomycosis of the stomach. *JAMA* 127:168–172, 1933

Brewrer NS, et al: Primary anorectal actinomycosis. JAMA 228:1397–1400, 1974

Brogden J: Actinomycosis of Gl tract – 14 cases. *J Lab Clin Med* 8:180–188, 1922

Chan Y, Cheng CSK, Ng P: Mesenteric actinomycosis. *Abdom Imaging* 18:286–287, 1993

Chandler FW, Connor DH: Actinomycosis. In: Connor DH, et al (eds) *Pathology of infections diseases.* Stamford. Appleton and Lange. Ch. 40. pp 391–396. 1997

Cruickshank JG, et al: Nocardiosis and actinomycosis in the Mashonaland province of Rhodesia. *Cent Afr J Med* 21:152–158, 1975

Desai G, Nath S: Concomitant infection of the large bowel by actinomycosis and *Ent. histolytica. Cent Afr J Med* 31:196–197, 1985

Fife TD, Finegold SM, Grennan T: Pericardial actinomycosis: case report and review. *Rev Infect Dis* 13:120–126, 1991

Frank P, et al: Pulmonary actinomycosis: *Br J Radiol* 47:373–378, 1974

Fry GA, et al: Primary actinomycosis of the rectum with multiple perianal and perineal fistulae. *Mayo Clin Proc* 40:296–299, 1965

Fuller C, Wood H: Actinomycotic granuloma of the stomach. *JAMA* 139:1163–1168, 1945

Goldwag S, Abbitt PL, Watts B: Case report – percutaneous drainage of periappendiceal actinomycosis. *Clin Radiol* 44:422–424, 1991

Ha HK, Lee HJ, Kim H, et al: Abdominal actinomycosis: CT findings in 10 patients. *AJR* 161:791–794, 1993

Hadjipetros K, et al: Primary actinomycosis of the stomach. *Germ J Surg* 159:234–239, 1920

Halvorsen RA, Korobkin M, Foster WL, et al: The variable CT appearance of hepatic abscesses. *AJR* 141:941–946, 1984

Harris LA, DeCosse JJ, Dannenberg A: Abdominal actinomycosis evaluation by computed tomography. *Am J Gastroenterol* 84:198–200, 1989

Hochsztein JG, Koenigsberg M, Green DA: U.S. case of the day (actinomycotic pelvic abscess) Secondary to I.U.D. *Radiographics* 16:713–716, 1996

Keebler C, Chatwant A, Schwartz R: Actinomycosis infection associated with intrauterine contraceptive devices. *Am J Obstet Gynecol* 145:596–599, 1983

Kuo TY, et al: Lesions of the lungs, chest wall, and ribs. *JAMA* 230:1051–1052, 1974

Maloney JJ, Cho SR: Pelvic actinomycosis. *Radiology* 148:388, 1983

Mazuji MK, et al: Gastric actinomycosis. *Arch Surg* 94:292–293, 1967

McNeil MM, Brown JM: The medically important aerobic actin mycetes; epidemiology and microbiology. *Clin Microbiol Rev* 7:357–417, 1994

Morson BC: Primary actinomycosis of the rectum. *Proc R Soc Med* 54:723–724, 1961

Niethammer JG, Gould HR, Nelson HS Jr: Anorectal actinomycosis: CT evaluation. *J Comput Assist Tomogr* 14:838–845, 1990

Olsen MC, Demos TC, Tamayo JP: Actinomycosis of the retroperitoneum and an extremity: CT features. *Abdom Imaging* 18:295–297, 1993

Olsson T: Angiography in actinomycosis of the abdomen. Report of 2 cases. *Am J Roentgenol Radium Ther Nucl Med* 122:278–280, 1974

Perlow JH, Wigton Y, Yordan EL, Graham J, Wood N, Wilbanks GD. Disseminated pelvic actinomycosis presenting as metastatic carcinoma: association with the Progestasert intrauterine device. Rev Infect Dis 13:1115–1119, 1991

Pesqueira V, Engelking B: Actinomycosis of the bladder and urachus. *J Urol* 62:163–167, 1949

Rabinowitz L: Ulceration of the duodenum from actinomycotic infection. *N Engl J Med* 209:236–239, 1933

Roesler PJ Jr., Wills JS: Hepatic actinomycosis: CT features. *J Comput Assist Tomogr* 10:335–337, 1986

Shah JK: Actinomycosis: a 1-year review. *East Afr Med J* 48:496–501, 1972

Shearburn E: Actinomycosis of the stomach and duodenum. *Surgery* 14:38–46, 1943

Tseng CK, et al: A case report of abdominal actinomycosis. *Jurume Med J* 12:168–172, 1965

Turnbull AE, Cohen MEL: Case report: pelvic actinomycosis with the development and resolution of a recto-sigmoid stricture. *Clin Radiol* 43:420–422, 1991

Tytgat H, et al: A propos de l'actinomycose du colon droit. *Acta Chir Belg* 64:425–432, 1965

Urdaneta W, et al: Intramural gastric actinomycosis. *Surgery* 62:431–435, 1967

Webb WR, Sagel SS: Actinomycosis involving the chest wall: CT findings. *AJR* 139:1007–1009, 1982

Wheeler H: Actinomycosis ulceration of the duodenum and jejunum. *Br J Surg* 15:430–437, 1927

Nocardiosis

Baghdadlian H, et al: *Nocardia transvalensis* pneumonia in a child. *Pediatr Infect Dis J* 8:470–471, 1989

Bross JE, Gordon G: Nocardial meningitis: case reports and review. *Rev Infect Dis* 13:160–165, 1991

Carlsen ET, et al: Nocardiosis and alveolar proteinosis. *Ann Intern Med* 60:275–281, 1964

Chandler FW. Nocardiosis. In: Connor DH, et al (eds) The pathology of infectious diseases. Appleton and Lange, Stamford, 1997, pp 701–708

Kramer MR, Uttamchandaui RB: The radiographic appearance of pulmonary nocardiosis associated with AIDS. *Chest* 98:382–385, 1990

Krick JA et al: Nocardia infection in heart transplant patients. *Ann Intern Med* 82:18–26, 1975

LeBlang SD, et al: CNS Nocardia in AIDS patients: CT and MRI with pathologic correlation. *J Comput Assist Tomogr* 19:15–22, 1995

Murray JF, et al: The changing spectrum of nocardiosis. A review and presentation of nine cases. *Am Rev Respir Dis* 83:315–330, 1961

Nocard E: Note sur la maladie de boeufs de la guadeloupe: connue said le non de farcie. *Ann Inst Pasteur* 2:293–294, 1888

Padron S, et al: Lymphocutaneous *Nocardia brasiliensis* infection mimicking sporotrichosis. *South Med J* 66:609–612, 1973

Seabury JH, et al: Mycetoma mandibularis due to *Nocardia pelletieri*. *Am J Med* 55:846–850, 1973

Smego RAJ, Gallis HJ. The clinical spectrum of *Nocardia brasiliensis* infection in the United States. *Rev Infect Dis* 6:168–180, 1984

Torre NP, Kim BK. Septic arthritis due to *Nocardia caviae*. *Ann Rheum Dis* 50:968–969, 1991

Twun-Danso K, et al: Nocardial pulmonary infection in a noncompromised patient. *Omani Med J* 13:26–30, 1996

Mycetoma (Madura Foot)

Abbott P: Mycetoma in the Sudan. *Trans R Soc Trop Med Hyg* 50:11–24, 1956

Arredondo HG, Ceballos TH. Unusual location of mycetomas. *Radiology* 78:72–76, 1962

Bendl BJ, et al: Mycetoma in Saudi Arabia. *J Trop Med Hyg* 90:51–59, 1987

Bezer H: Bone lesions of mycotic infections of the foot – Madura foot. *Presse Med (Suppl)* 15:142–144, 1961

Chandler FW, Ajello L: Mycetoma. In: Connor DH, et al (eds) Pathology of infectious diseases. Appleton and Lange, Stamford 1997, pp 1035–1044

Cockshott WP: Mycetoma. In: Middlemiss JH (ed) Tropical radiology. Intercontinental Medical Books, New York, 1961, pp 38–51

Cockshott WP: In: Schintz HR (ed) *Roentgen diagnosis (Am 2nd edn), vol 3*. Grune & Stratton, New York, 1961, p 623

Davey WW: Mycetoma. In: *Companion to surgery in Africa*. E & S Livingstone, London, 1968, pp 54–66

Davies AGM: The bone changes of Madura foot: observations on Uganda Africans. *Radiology* 70:841–847, 1958

Destombes P: Histopathologie des mycetomes. *Ann Soc Belge Med Trop* 82:261–276, 1972

Fahal AH, et al: Abdominal wall mycetoma: an unusual presentation. Trans R Soc Trop Med 88:78–80, 1994

Grantham-Hill C: Some clinical observations on mycetoma. *Trans R Soc Trop Med Hyg* 25:39–48, 1931

Green W, Adams H: Mycetoma in the U.S. *Am J Clin Pathol* 42:75–91, 1964

Klokke AH, et al: The causal agents of mycetoma in South India. *Trans R Soc Trop Med Hyg* 62:509–576, 1968

Latapi F. Micetoma. Análisis de IOO casos estudiados en la Ciudad de México. Mem III. Cong. ibero-latinoam de dermatol, 1959

Lynch JB: Mycetoma in the Sudan. *Ann R Coll Surg Engl* 35:319–340, 1964

Mahgoub ES, Murray IG: *Mycetoma*. Heinemann, London

Mariat F, Destombes P, Segretain G: The mycetomas: clinical features, pathology, etiology and epidemiology. *Contrib Microbiol Immunol* 4:1–39, 1977

Pagenstecher GA: Madurae foot. *JAMA* 78:1363–1365, 1922

Peyron JP, et al: Interet de la radiologie dans le diagnostic des mycetomes. *Med Trop* 39:27–29, 1979

Reeder MM: Tropical diseases of the foot. *Semin Roentgenol* 15:378–390, 1970

Reeder MM: Tropical diseases of the soft tissue. *Semin Roentgenol* 8:47–71, 1973

Seabury JH, et al: Mycetoma mandibularis due to *Nocardia pelletieri*. *Am J Med* 55:846–850, 1973

Segretain G, Mariat F: Mycetoma. In: Warren KS, Marmoud AAF (eds) *Tropical and geographical medicine*. McGraw-Hill, New York, 1984, pp 934–941

Sharif HS et al: Mycetoma: comparison of MR imaging with CT. *Radiology* 178:865–870, 1991

Ur-Rahaman N et al: Cranial and epidural mycetoma caused by *Streptomyces somaliensis*. *Neuroradiology* 29:95–97, 1987

Zygomycosis

Backer W, et al: Mucormycosis of the digestive tract. *Arch Pathol* 63:176–182, 1957

Balsulrahmanyan M: Case of pulmonary mucormycosis. *Indian J Pathol Bact* 6:60, 1983

Bartrum RJ, Warnick M, Herman PG: Roentgenographic findings in pulmonary mucormycosis. *Am J Roentgenol* 117:810–815, 1973

Bigby TD, et al: The clinical spectrum of pulmonary mucormycosis. *Chest* 89:435–439, 1986

Chandler FW, Watts JC: Zygomycosis (mucormycosis) In: Connor DH, et al (eds) *Pathology of infectious diseases*. Appleton and Lange, Stamford, 1997, pp 1113–1119

Cockshott WP, et al: Upper respiratory infection due to *Entomophthora coronata*. *Radiology* 90:1016–1019, 1968

Funada H, et al: The air crescent sign of invasive pulmonary mucormycosis in acute leukemia. *Cancer* 53:2721–2723, 1984

Lake F, McAleer, Tribe A: Pulmonary mucormycosis without underlying systemic disease. *Med J Aust* 149:323–326, 1988

Loevner LA, Andrews JC, Francis IR: Multiple mycotic pulmonary artery aneurysms: a complication of invasive mucormycosis. *AJR* 158:761–762, 1992

McDevitt GR Jr, Brantley JM, Cawthon MA: Rhinocerebral mucormycosis: a case report with magnetic resonance imaging findings. *Clin Imaging* 13:317–320, 1989

Murphy RA, Miller WT Jr.: Pulmonary mucormycosis. *Semin Roentgenol* XXXI:83–87, 1996

Ramon Y, et al: Extensive maxillary sequestration resulting from rhinocerebral mucormycosis. *J Oral Surg* 35:989–991, 1977

Restrepo A, et al: Subcutaneous phycomycosis: report of the first case observed in Colombia, South America. *Am J Trop Med Hyg* 16:34–39, 1967

Sugar A: Mucormycosis. *Clin Infect Dis* 145:126–129, 1992

Tedder M, et al: Pulmonary mucormycosis: results of medical and surgical therapy. *Ann Thorac Surg* 57:1044–1050, 1994

Terk MR, et al: MR imaging in rhinocerebral and intracranial mucormycosis with CT and pathologic correlation. MRI 10:81–87, 1992

Zagoria RJ, Choplin RH, Karstaedt N: Pulmonary gangrene as a complication of mucormycosis. *AJR* 144:1195–1196, 1985

Chromoblastomycosis

Coulanges P: La chromomycose a Madagascar. *Ann Int Pasteur Madagascar* 48:69–95, 1979

McGinnis MR, Chandler FW: *Chromoblastomycosis*. In: Connor DH, et al (eds) *Pathology of infectious diseases*. Appleton and Lange, Stamford, 1997, pp 971–976

McGinnis MR: Chromoblastomycosis and phaeohypho mycosis: new concepts, diagnosis and mycology. *J Am Acad Dermatol* 8:1–16, 1983

Tsai T, et al: Systemic chromoblastomycosis. *Am J Clin Pathol* 46:103–113, 1966

Geotrichosis

Chang WWL, Buerger L: Disseminated geotrichosis. *Arch Intern Med* 113:356–360, 1964

Fishbach RS, White ML, Finegold SM: Bronchopulmonary geotrichosis. *Am Rev Respir Dis* 108:1388–1392, 1973

Ghamande AR, Landis FB, Snider GL: Bronchial geotrichosis with fungemia complicating bronchial carcinoma. *Chest* 59:98–101, 1971

Hardy DB, Nassar NN, Rinaldi MG: Traumatic joint infection due to *Geotrichum candidum*. *Clin Infect Dis* 20:468–469, 1995

Heinic GS, MacPhail LA, Greenspan JS: Oral *Geotrichum candidum* infection associated with HIV infection. A case report. *Oral Surg Oral Med Oral Pathol* 73:726–728, 1992

McGinnis MR, Chandler FW: Geotrichosis. In: Connor DH, et al (eds) *Pathology of infectious diseases*. Appleton and Lange, Stamford, 1997, 1003–1005

Sheehy TW, Honeycutt BK, Spency JT: *Geotrichum* septicemia. *JAMA* 235:1035–1037, 1976

Adiaspiromycosis

Bambirra EA, Nogueira AMMF: Human pulmonary granulomas caused by *Chrysosporium parvum* var. *crescens (Emmonsonia crescens)*. *Am J Trop Med Hyg* 32:1184–1185, 1983

Binford CH, Connor DH: Adiaspiromycosis. In: *Pathology of tropical and extraordinary diseases*. Armed Forces Institute of Pathology, Washington, D.C., 1976, pp 594–596

Knoblich R: Pulmonary granulomatosis caused by vegetable particles. So-called lentil pulse pneumonia. *Am Rev Respir Dis* 99:380–389, 1969

Kodousek R, et al: Pulmonary adiaspiromycosis in man caused by *Emmonsia crescens*. Report of a unique case. *Am J Clin Pathol* 56:394–399, 1971

Watts JC, et al: Human pulmonary adiaspiromycosis. *Arch Pathol* 99:11–15, 1975

Watts JC, Chandler FW: Adiaspiromycosis. In: Connor DH, et al (eds) *Pathology of infectious diseases*. Appleton and Lange, Stamford, 1997, pp 929–932

Aspergillosis

Albelda GM, et al: Bronchopulmonary fistula complicating invasive pulmonary aspergillosis. *Am Rev Respir dis* 126:163–167, 1982

Altman AF: Thoracic wall invasion secondary to pulmonary aspergillosis. *Am J Roentgenol* 129:140–148, 1977

Butz RO, Zoetina JR, Leininger BJ: Ten years experience with mycetoma in patients with pulmonary tuberculosis. *Chest* 87:356–358, 1985

Carette MF, Isnard F, Mayaud C, Valade S, Akoun AG, Helenon C, Bigot JM: Radiologic aspects of acute invasive pulmonary aspergillosis in 18 immunosuppressed patients (in French). *J Radiol* 67:381–389, 1986

Cartoni C, et al: *Aspergillus* osteomyelitis of the rib. Sonographic diagnosis. *J Comp US* 20:217–220, 1992

Coulthard A, Ghokar A, Sengupta RP: Case report. Frontal aspergilloma – a complication of paranasal aspergillosis. *Clin Radiol* 44:425–427, 1991

Dahniya MH, et al: Appearances of paranasal fungal sinusitis on computed tomography. Pictorial review. *Br J Radiol* 71:340–344, 1998

DeShazo RD, Chapin K, Swain RE: Current concepts: fungal sinusitis. *N Engl J Med* 337:254–259, 1997

Diedrich S, et al: Chest radiographic findings of *aspergillus* infection in the early postoperative period in lung transplant patients. Proc 18 Int Congr Radiol, S 119

Freundlich IM, Israel HL: Pulmonary aspergillosis. *Clin Radiol* 24:248–253, 1973

Glimp RA, Bayer AS: Fungal pneumonias: allergic bronchopulmonary aspergillosis. *Chest* 80:85–94, 1981

Hofken W: Aspergilloma of the lung. *Forstchr Geb Roentgenstr Nuklearmed* 84:397–401, 1956

Kanyerezi BR, Rwabugahya RH: Pulmonary aspergillosis. *East Afr Med J* 47:179–184, 1970

Kaufman DM, et al: Central nervous system aspergillosis in two young adults. *Neurology* 26:484–488, 1976

Kemper CA, et al: Ulcerative and plague like tracheobronchitis due to infection in patients with AIDS. *Clin Infect Dis* 17:344–352, 1993

Klein DL, Gamsu G: Thoracic manifestations of aspergillosis. *Am J Roentgenol* 134:543–552, 1980

Kuhlman JE, et al: Invasive pulmonary aspergillosis in acute leukemia. The contribution of CT to early diagnosis and aggressive management. *Chest* 92:95–99, 1987

McAdams HP et al: Thoracic mycoses from opportunistic fungi: radiologic-pathologic correlation. *Radiographics* 15:271–286, 1995

Miller WT: Aspergillosis: a disease with many faces. *Semin Roentgenol* XXXI:52–66, 1996

Miller WT Jr, et al: Pulmonary aspergillosis in patients with AIDS. Clinical and radiographic correlations. *Chest* 105:37–44, 1994

Montone KT, Litzky LA: Rapid method for detection of *Aspergillus*-55 ribosomal RNA using a genus-specific oligonucleotide probe. *Am J Clin Pathol* 103:48–51, 1995

Neeld DA, et al: Computerized tomography in the evaluation of allergic bronchopulmonary aspergillosis. *Am Rev Respir Dis* 142:1200–1205, 1990

Novey HS, Wells ID: Allergic bronchopulmonary aspergillosis. *West J Med* 130:1–5, 1979

Patel PJ, et al: CT findings in paranasal aspergillosis. *Clin Radiol* 45:319–321, 1992

Potente G: Computed tomography in invasive aspergillosis. *Acta Radiol* 30:587–590, 1989

Roberts CM, Atron KM, Strickland B: Intrathoracic aspergilloma. Role of CT in diagnosis and treatment. Radiology 165:123–128, 1987

Rudwan MA, Sheikh HA: Aspergilloma of the paranasal sinuses: a common cause of unilateral proptosis in the Sudan. *Clin Radiol* 27:497–502, 1976

Schwartz S, Thiel E: Palate destruction by *Aspergillus*. Images in clinical medicine. *N Engl J Med* 337:241, 1997

Thompson BH, et al: Varied radiologic appearances of pulmonary aspergillosis. *Radiographics* 15:1273–1284, 1995

Van Ede AE, et al: Pneumopericardium complicating invasive pulmonary aspergillosis. *Infection* 22:102–105, 1994

Watts JC, Chandler FW: Aspergillosis. In: Connor DH, et al (eds) Pathology of infectious diseases. Appleton and Lange, Stamford, 1997, pp 933–942

Zinreich SJ, et al: Fungal sinusitis. Diagnosis with CT and MR imaging. *Radiology* 196:439–444, 1988

Histoplasmosis Capsulatum

Balthazar EJ, Megibow AJ, Barry M, Opulencia JF: Histoplasmosis of the colon in patients with AIDS: imaging findings in four cases. *AJR* 161:585–587, 1993

Bank S, et al: Histoplasmosis of the small bowel with "giant " intestinal villi and secondary protein loosing enteropathy. *Am J Med* 39:492, 1965

Brown AE, et al: Histoplasmosis: report of case. *Proc Staff Meet Mayo Clin* 15:812, 1940

Chandler FW, Watts JC: Histoplasmosis capsulati. In: Connor DH, et al (eds) *Pathology of infectious diseases.* Appleton and Lange, Stamford, 1997, pp 1007–1016

Conces DJ, Tarver RO, Vix VA: Broncholithiasis: CT features in 15 patients. *Am J Radiol* 157:249–253, 1991

Conces DJ, et al: Disseminated histoplasmosis in AIDS: findings on chest radiographs. *Am J Roentgenol* 160:15–19, 1993

Conces DJ Jr: Histoplasmosis. Semin Roentgenol XXXI:14–27, 1996

Connel JV, Muhm JR: Radiographic manifestations of pulmonary histoplasmosis: a 10 year review. *Radiology* 121:281–285, 1976

Coss KC, et al: Esophageal fistula complicating mediastinal histoplasmosis. *Am J Med* 83:343–346, 1987

Dabke V, et al: Histoplasmosis simulating carcinoma. A case report with review of Indian literature. *Indian J Cancer* 11:116–119, 1974

Dietz MW: Ileocecal histoplasmosis. *Radiology* 91:285, 1968

Felson B: Less familiar roentgen patterns of pulmonary granulomas. *Am J Roentgenol* 81:211, 1959

Gelfand M: The curse of the pharaohs. Editorial. *Cent Afr J Med* 21:199, 1975

Ginder DR: Patterns of pulmonary histoplasmosis. *J Maine Med Assoc* 65:35–39, 1974

Goodwin RA, et al: Disseminated histoplasmosis: clinical and pathological correlations. *Medicine* 59:1–33, 1980

Gross BH, Schneider HJ, Proto AV: Eggshell calcification of lymph nodes: an update. *Am J Roentgenol* 135:1265–1268, 1980

Henderson RG, et al: *Histoplasma capsulatum* as cause of chronic ulcerative enteritis. *JAMA* 118:885, 1942

Jenkins DW, Fisk DE, Byrd RB: Mediastinal histoplasmosis with esophageal abscess: two case reports. *Gastroenterology* 70:109–111, 1976

Landay MJ, Rollins NK: Mediastinal histoplasmosis granuloma: evaluation with CT. *Radiology* 172:657–659, 1989

Lee KR, et al: The radiology corner. Gastrointestinal histoplasmosis, roentgenographic, clinical and pathological correlation. *Am J Gastroentrol* 63:255–265, 1975

McAdams HP, et al: Thoracic mycoses from endemic fungi: radiologic pathologic correlations. Radiographics 15:255–270, 1995

Mugerwa JW: *Histoplasma* infections in Uganda. *East Afr Med J* 54:227–231, 1977

Negroni P: Histoplasmosis: diagnosis and treatment (rev. ed.) Charles C Thomas, Springfield, Jll., 1965, p. 28

Palayew MJ, et al: Benign progressive multinodular pulmonary histoplasmosis. A radiological and clinical entity. *Radiology* 111:311–314, 1974

Park HM, Jay SJ, Holden RW: Pulmonary scintigraphy in fibrosing mediastinitis due to histoplasmosis. *J Nucl Med* 22:349–351, 1981

Perez CA, et al: Some clinical and radiographic features of gastrointestinal histoplasmosis. *Radiology* 86:482, 1966

Radin DR: Disseminated histoplasmosis: abdominal CT findings in 16 patients. *AJR* 157:955–958, 1991

Rholl KS, Levitt RG, Glazer HS: Magnetic resonance imaging in fibrosing mediastinitis. *Am J Roentgenol* 145:255–259, 1985

Rosenthal J, et al: Rheumatologic manifestations of histoplasmosis in the recent Indianapolis outbreak. *Arthritis Rheum* 26:1065–1070, 1983

Rubin SA, Winer-Muram MT: Thoracic histoplasmosis. *J Thorac Imaging* 7:39–50, 1992

Shull HJ: Human histoplasmosis: disease with protean manifestations often with digestive system involvement. *Gastroenterology* 25:582, 1953

Sutaria MK, Polk JW, Reddy P: Localized pulmonary histoplasmosis (coin lesion). A report of 58 cases. *Chest* 61:361–364, 1972

Weinstein JB, Aronberg DJ, Sagel SS: CT of fibrosing mediastinitis: findings and their utility. *Am J Roentgenol* 141:247–251, 1983

Weiss ED, Haskell BF: Anorectal manifestations of histoplasmosis. *Am J Surg* 84:541, 1952

Wieder S, et al: Pulmonary artery occlusion due to histoplasmosis. *Am J Radiol* 138:243–251, 1980

Histoplasmosis Duboisii

Adekunle OO, Sudhakaran P, Timeyin ED: African histoplasmosis of the jejunum: report of a case. *J Trop Med Hyg* 81:88–90, 1978

Ajello L: Histoplasmosis – a dual entity: histoplasmosis capsulati and histoplasmosis duboisii. *Igiene Moderna 79:3–10, 1983*

Arendt V, Coveman-Pelsenor V, Gottleib R: African histoplasmosis in a Belgian AIDS patient. *Mycoses* 34:59–61, 1991

Brown KGE, et al: Disseminated histoplasmosis duboisii in Malawi: partial response to sulfonamide-trimethoprim combination. *East Afr Med J* 51:584–590, 1974

Butler TM, Gleisser CA, Bernal JC: Case of a disseminated African histoplasmosis in a baboon. *J Med Rheumatol* 17:153–161, 1988

Chandler FW, Ajello L: Histoplasmosis duboisii. In: Connor DH, et al (eds) Pathology of infectious diseases. Appleton and Lange, Stamford, 1997, pp 1017–1022

Clark BM, Greenwood BM: Pulmonary lesions in African histoplasmosis. *J Trop Med Hyg* 71:36–40, 1968

Cockshott WP: Dactylitis and growth disorders. *Br J Radiol* 36:19–25, 1963

Cockshott WP, Lucas AO: African histoplasmosis. *Q J Med* 33:223–245, 1964

Cole ECE, et al: Bowel infections with *Histoplasma duboisii. J Trop Med Hyg* 68:92–96, 1965

Coulanges P: Existence of histoplasmosis with *Histoplasma duboisii* outside continental Africa (on the first Malagash case). *Bull Soc Pathol Exot Filiales* 75:400–403, 1982

Coulanges P: L'histoplasmose a grandes formes (*M. duboisii*) a Madagascar. Apropos de trois cas. *Arch Inst Pasteur Madagascar* 56:169–174, 1989

DeVroey C: Epidemiology of African histoplasmosis. *Ann Soc Belge Med Trop* 52:407–419, 1972

Gentilini M, et al: African pulmonary histoplasmosis due to *M. duboisii. Ann Med Interne (Paris)* 128:451–455, 1977

George AJ, Ravisse P, Drocihet E: Identification specifique d'*Histoplasma duboisii* par immunofluorescence sur coupe histologiques. *Bull Soc Fr Mycol Med* 9:121–123, 1980

Gugnani HC, et al: A natural focus of *Histoplasma capsulatum* var. *duboisii* is a bat cave. *Mycopathologia* 127:151–157, 1994

Lanceley JL, Lunn NF, Wilson AMM: Histoplasmosis in an African child. *J Pediatr* 59:756–764, 1961

Lodell DM, Copiello MA, Riccio FJ: African histoplasmosis in Connecticut. *Conn Med* 46:187, 1982

Lucas AO: Cutaneous manifestations of African histoplasmosis. *Br J Dermatol* 82:435–447, 1970

Lunn HF: A case of histoplasmosis of bone in East Africa. *J Trop Med Hyg* 63:175–180, 1960

Oddo D, Etchart M, Thompson L: Histoplasmosis duboisii (African histoplasmosis). An African case reported from Chile with ultrastructural study. *Pathol Res Pract* 186:514–517, 1990

Olurin O, Lucas AO, Oyediran ABO: Orbital histoplasmosis due to *Histoplasma duboisii. Am J Opthalmol* 68:14–18, 1969

Risson RP, Evans EQV: Enlarged cervical lymph node due to African histoplasmosis. *J Laryngol Otol* 102:954–956, 1988

Walter J, Spooner ETC: Natural infection of the African baboon (*Papio papio*) with the large cell form of histoplasmosis. *J Pathol Bacteriol* 8:436–439, 1960

Williams AO, Lawson EA, Lucas AO: African histoplasmosis due to *Histoplasma duboisii. Arch Pathol* 92:306–318, 1971

Coccidioidomycosis

Batra P: Pulmonary coccidioidomycosis. *J Thorac Imaging* 7:29–38, 1992

Batra P, Batra RS: Thoracic coccidioidomycosis. *Semin Roentgenol* XXX:28–44, 1996

Beller TA, Mitchell DM, Sobonya RE: Large airway obstruction secondary to endobronchial coccidioidomycosis. *Am Rev Respir Dis* 120:939–942, 1979

Birsner JW: The roentgen aspects of five hundred cases of pulmonary coccidioidomycosis. *Am J Roentgenol Radium Ther Nucl Med* 72:556–573, 1954

Craig JR, et al: Disseminated coccidioidomycosis: diagnosis by needle biopsy of liver. *West J Med* 122:171–174, 1975

Dalinka MK, et al: Roentgenographic features of osseous coccidioidomycosis and differential diagnosis. *J Bone Joint Surg [Am]* 53:1157–1164, 1971

Eller JL, Siebert PE: Sclerotic vertebral bodies; an unusual manifestation of disseminated coccidioidomycosis. *Radiology* 93:1099–1100, 1969

Goldstein E, et al: Ventricular fluid and the management of coccidioidal meningitis. *Ann Intern Med* 77:243–246, 1972

Larsen RA, et al: Acute respiratory failure caused by primary pulmonary coccidioidomycosis. Two case reports and a review of the literature. *Am Rev Respir Dis* 131:797–799, 1985

Loeb M, et al: Coccidioidomycosis of the thyroid. *Ann Intern Med* 91:409–411, 1979

Lopez AM, Williams PL, Ampel NM: Acute pulmonary coccidioidomycosis mimicking bacterial pneumonia and septic shock. A report of 2 cases. *Am J Med* 95:236–239, 1993

McAdams HP, et al: Thoracic mycoses from endemic fungi. Radiologic-pathologic correlation. *Radiographics* 15:255–270, 1995

McGahan JP, Graves DS, Palmer PES: Coccidiodial spondylitis. Usual and unusual radiographic manifestations. *Radiology* 136:5–9, 1980

Nykamp PW: Vertebra plana: two cases due to disseminated coccidioidomycosis. *Ariz Med* 28:165–167, 1971

Pappagianis D: Epidemiology of coccidioidomycosis. *Curr Top Med Mycol* 2:199–238, 1988

Pappagianis D, Chandler FW: Coccidioidomycosis. In: Connor DH, et al (eds) Pathology of infectious diseases. Appleton and Lange, Stamford, 1997, pp 977–988

Pappagianis D, Zimmer BL: Serology of coccidioidomycosis. *Clin Microbiol Rev* 3:247–268, 1990

Pickney L, Parker BR: Primary coccidioidomycosis in children presenting with massive effusion. *Am J Roentgenol* 130:247–249, 1978

Sargent EN, Balchum E, Freed AL: Multiple pulmonary calcifications due to coccidioidomycosis. *Am J Roentgenol Rad Ther Nucl Med* 109:500–504, 1970

Stadalnik RC, et al: Diagnostic value of gallium bone scans in evaluation of extrapulmonary coccidioidal lesions. *Am Rev Respir Dis* 121:673–678, 1980

Stevens DA: Coccidioidomycosis. *N Engl J Med* 332:1077–1082, 1995

Wesselius LJ, Brooks RJ, Gall EP: Vertebral coccidioidomycosis presenting as Pott's disease. *JAMA* 238:1397–1398, 1977

Winn RE, Johnson R, Galgiani JN: Cavitary coccidioidomycosis with fungus ball formation. *Chest* 105:412–416, 1994

Sporotrichosis

Brook CJ, Ravikrishnan KP, Weg JG: Pulmonary and articular sporotrichosis. *Am Rev Respir Dis* 116:141–143, 1977

Chandler FW, Watts JC: Sporotrichosis. In: Connor DH et al (eds) *Pathology of infectious diseases.* Appleton and Lange, Stamford, 1997, pp 1089–1098

Comstock C, Wolson AH: Roentgenology of sporotrichosis. *Am J Roentgenol Radium Ther Nucl Med* 125:651–655, 1975

Cox PA, et al: Sporotrichosis of the thumb. A case report. *Med Ann DC* 42:182–184, 1973

England WM, Hochholzer L: Primary pulmonary sporotrichosis: report of 8 cases with clinico-pathologic review. *Am J Surg Pathol* 9:193–204, 1985

England WM, Hochholzer L: Sporothrix infection of the lung without cutaneous disease. Primary pulmonary sporotrichosis. *Arch Pathol Lab Med* 111:298–299, 1987

Evers RH, et al: Pulmonary sporotrichosis. *Chest* 66:91–92, 1974

Landero AT, Ramos CD: Sporotrichosis in Rio Grande do Sui (Brazil). 3 decades of observation (in Portuguese). *An Bras Dermatol* 64:307–310, 1989

Lurie HI: Five unusual cases of sporotrichosis from South Africa, showing lesions of muscles, bones and viscera. *Br J Surg* 50:585–591, 1963

Marrocco GR, et al: Granulomatous sinovitis and osteitis caused by *Sporothrix schenckii. Am J Clin Pathol* 64:345–350, 1975

Scott EN, et al: Serological studies in the diagnosis and management of meningitis due to *Sporothrix schenckii. N Engl J Med* 317:935–940, 1987

Blastomycosis

Brown LR, et al: Roentgenologic features of pulmonary blastomycosis. *Mayo Clin Proc* 66:29–38, 1991

Chandler FW: Blastomycosis. In: Connor DH, et al (eds) Pathology of infectious diseases. Appleton and Lange, Stamford, 1997, pp 943–952

Cush R, et al: Clinical and roentgenographic manifestations of acute and chronic blastomycosis. *Chest* 69:345–349, 1976

Davidson L, Gelfand M: North American blastomycosis in Rhodesia. *Cent Afr J Med* 18:129–137, 1972

Frean J, Blumberg L, Woolf M: Disseminated blastomycosis masquerading as tuberculosis. *J Infect* 26:203–206, 1993

Halvorsen RA, et al: Pulmonary blastomycosis. Radiologic manifestations. *Radiology* 150:1–5, 1984

Jacobs SJ: Medical grand rounds from Touro infirmary. Blastomycosis. *J LA State Med Soc* 126:373–377, 1974

Koen AF, Blumberg LH: North American blastomycosis in South Africa simulating tuberculosis. *Clin Radiol* 54:260–269, 1999

Kuzo RS, Goodman LR: Blastomycosis. *Semin Roentgenol* XXXI:45–51, 1996

Matta M, et al: North American blastomycosis. Report of a case encountered in Lebanon and probably originating in Gambia. *Dermatologica* 146:346–349, 1973

McAdams HP: Thoracic mycoses from endemic fungi: radiologic-pathologic correlation. *Radiographics* 15:255–270, 1995

Meyer KC, McManus EJ, Maki DG: Overwhelming pulmonary blastomycosis associated with adult respiratory distress syndrome. *N Engl J Med* 329:1231–1236, 1993

Neuzil KM, et al: Extrapulmonary thoracic disease caused by *Blastomycosis dermatitidis Chest* 106:1885–1887, 1994

Rabinowitz JG, et al: Pulmonary manifestations of blastomycosis: radiological support of a new concept. *Radiology* 120:25, 1976

Riegler HF, et al: Blastomycosis osteomyelitis. *Clin Orthop* 100:225–231, 1974

Sarosi GA, et al: Clinical features of acute pulmonary blastomycosis. *N Engl J Med* 290:540–543, 1974

Sheflin JR, Campbell JA, Thompson GP: Pulmonary blastomycosis: findings on chest radiographs in 63 patients. *Am J Roentgenol* 154:1177–1180, 1990

Wiener-Muram HT, Beales DH, Cole FH Jr: Blastomycosis of the lung: CT features. *Radiology* 182:829–832, 1992

Paracoccidioidomycosis (South American Blastomycosis)

Avritchir Y, Peroni AA: Radiological manifestations of small intestinal South American blastomycosis. *Radiology* 127:607–609, 1978

Guerrini RM, et al: High resolution CT of pulmonary paracoccidioidomycosis. Proc 18th In Congr Radiol, Singapore, S 120

Hughes WT, Franco S, Oh MHK: Systemic blastomycosis in childhood. Case report and reviews. *Clin Pediatr* 8:597–601, 1969

Londero AT, Chandler FW: Paracoccidioidomycosis. In: Connor DH, et al (eds) Pathology of infectious diseases. Appleton and Lange, Stamford, 1997, Ch 114

Londero AT, Fischmann O: Perianal and rectal lesions in South American blastomycosis. *Mycopathol Appl* 32:231–236, 1967

Londero AT, et al: Progressive pulmonary paracoccidioidomycosis. A study of 34 cases observed in Rio Grande Do Sul (Brazil). *Mycopathologia* 63:53–56, 1978

Magalhaes A: Paracoccidioidomycosis (South American blastomycosis). Radiological Aspects. *Rev Hosp Clin Fac Med Sao Paulo* 35:147–155, 1980

Meyer TN: Duodenal obstruction due to South American blastomycosis. *R Ass Med Bra* 28:73–74, 1982

Moraes CR de: Calcifações intra-abdominais na Blastomicose Sul-Americana. *Rev Inst Med Trop Sao Paulo* 13:428–432, 1971

PAHO: The Pan-American symposium on Paracoccidioidomycosis. Washington: Pan American Organisation Scient. *Publ* 254, 1972

Paracoccidioidomycosis. Scientific publication no 254. Pan American Health Organization, Washington, DC, 1972

Penna FJ: Blastomycosis of the colon resembling clinically ulcerative colitis. *Gut* 20:896–899, 1979

Pereira AH: Paracoccidioidomicose gastro-entérica. Estudo radiologico. Thesis: Faculty of Medicine, University of Rio de Janeiro, 1983

Restrepo A, et al: Paracoccidioidomycosis (South American blastomycosis). A study of 39 cases observed in Medellin, Colombia. *Am J Trop Med* 19:68–76, 1970

Lobomycosis

Azulay RV, et al: Keloidal blastomycosis (Lobo's disease) with lymphatic involvement (case report) *Int J Dermatol* 15:90–92, 1976

Binford CH, Dolley JR: Lobo's disease. In: Binford CH, Connor DH (eds) *Pathology of tropical and extraordinary disease.* Armed Forces Institute of Pathology, Washington, DC, 1976, pp 583–584

Dias LB, Sampaio MM, Silva D: Jorge Lobo's disease. Observations on its epidemiology and some unusual morphological forms of the fungus. *Rev Inst Med Trop Sao Paulo* 12:8–15, 1970

Lucaz CS, Barruzzi RG, Rosa MCB: Jorge Lobo's Disease (in Portuguese). USP, Sao Paulo, 1986

Lobo J: Queloidiform blastomycosis. Jorge Lobo's disease. *Proc 7th Int Congr Trop, Med and Malaria* 3:93–94, 1964

Nikolaidis G, Rosen T: Lobomycosis. In: Connor DH, et al (eds) *Pathology of infectious diseases.* Stamford, Appleton and Lange, 1997, pp 1023–1028

Symmers WC: A possible case of Lobo's disease acquired in Europe from a bottle-nosed dolphin (*Tursiops truncator*). *Bull Soc Pathol Exot Filiales* 76:777–784, 1983

Cryptococcosis

Andreula CF, Burdi N, Carella A: CNS cryptococcosis in AIDS: spectrum of MR findings. *J Comput Assist Tomogr* 17:438–441, 1993

Bateson EM, Yaksich IP: The radiological features of cerebral torulosis (*Cryptococcus neoformans*). *Australas Radiol* 20:216–224, 1976

Briggs DR, et al: Nasal cryptococcosis. *Arch Otolaryngol* 100:390–392, 1974

Chandler FW, Watts JC: Cryptococcosis. In: Connor DH, et al (eds) *Pathology of infectious diseases.* Stamford, Appleton and Lange, 1997, pp 989–998

Chechani V, Kamholz SL: Pulmonary manifestations of disseminated cryptococcosis in patients with AIDS. *Chest* 98:1060–1066, 1990

Conces DJ Jr, Vix VA, Tarver RD: Pleural cryptococcosis. *J Thorac Imaging* 5:84–86, 1990

Cox LB, Tolhurst JC: Human torulosis (cryptococcosis). A clinical, pathological and microbiological study with a report of 13 cases. Melbourne University Press, Melbourne, 1946

Fujito NK, et al: Cryptococcal intracerebral mass lesions. The role of CT and nonsurgical management. *Ann Intern Med* 94:382–388, 1981

Gordonsson J, et al: Pulmonary cryptococcosis. *Radiology* 112:557–561, 1974

Henson DJ, Hill AR: Case report. Cryptococcal pneumonia. A fulminant presentation. *Am J Med Sci* 288:221–222, 1984

Khoury MB, et al: Thoracic cryptococcosis: immunologic competence and radiographic appearance. *AJR* 141:893–896, 1984

McAdams HP, et al: Thoracic mycoses from opportunistic fungi: radiologic-pathologic correlation. *Radiographics* 15:271–286, 1995

Miller WT Jr, Edelman JM, Miller WT: Cryptococcal pulmonary infection in patients with AIDS. Radiographic appearance. *Radiology* 175:725–728, 1990

Patz EF, Goodman PC: Pulmonary cryptococcosis. *J Thorac Imaging* 7:51–55, 1992

Ramsay GC, et al: Cavitary fungus disease of the lungs. *Radiology* 109:29–32, 1975

Sider L, Westcott MA: Pulmonary manifestations of cryptococcosis in patients with AIDS: CT features. *J Thorac Imaging* 9:78–84, 1994

Tien RD, et al: Intracranial *Cryptococcus* in immunocompromised patients. CT & MR findings in 29 cases. *AJNR* 12:283–289, 1991

Wilhelm JP, et al: Brain scanning and cisternography in cryptococcosis. *Radiology* 109:121–124, 1975

Woodring JM, et al: Pulmonary cryptococcosis. *Semin Roentgenol* XXXI:67–75, 1996

Yoon DY et al: Extensive cervical lymphadenopathy in a healthy child; an unusual manifestiation of cryptococcosis. *Br J Radiol* 54:133–137, 1999

Zlupko GM, Fochler FJ, Goldschmidt ZH: Pulmonary cryptococcosis presenting with multiple pulmonary nodules. *Chest* 77:575, 1980

Candidiasis (Monilisiasis)

Berman LH, et al: Assessment of sonography in the diagnosis and management of neonatal renal candidiasis. *Clin Radiol* 40:577–581, 1989

Bodey GP (ed) Candidiasis: pathogenesis, diagnosis and treatment, 2nd edn Raven, New York, 1993

Brabander JO, et al: Intestinal moniliasis in adults. *Can Med Assoc J* 77:478, 1957

Buff SJ, et al: *Candida albicans* pneumonia: radiographic appearance. *Am J Roentgenol* 138:645–646, 1982

Chisholm EB, Hutch JA: Fungus ball (*Candida albicans*) formation in bladder. *J Urol* 86:559, 1961

Cohen HL, et al: Renal candidiasis of the infant: ultrasound evaluation. *Urol Radiol* 8:17–21, 1986

Craig JM, Farber S: The development of disseminated visceral mycosis during therapy for acute leukemia. *Am J Pathol* 29:601, 1953

Gefter WB, et al: Candidiasis in the obstructed esophagus. *Radiology* 138:25–28, 1981

Goldberg HI, Doods WJ: Cobblestone esophagus due to monilial infection. *Am J Roentgenol* 104:608–612, 1968

Gottlieb S, et al: Echocardiographic diagnosis of the aortic valve vegetation in *Candida* endocarditis. *Circulation* 50:826–830, 1974

Kassner EG, et al: Pulmonary candidiasis in infants. Clinical, radiological and pathological features. *Am J Roentgenol* 137:707–716, 1981

Kaufman SA, et al: Monilial esophagitis in a patient with hemoglobic SC disease: demonstration of esophageal motor abnormality by cineradiofluorography. *Ann Intern Med* 57:650, 1962

Levine MS et al: Opportunistic esophagitis in AIDS: radiographic diagnosis. *Radiology* 165:815–820, 1987

Lipman J, Saadia R: Fungal infections in critically ill patients. Editorial. *Br Med J* 315:266–267, 1997

Lipton SA, et al: Candidal infection in the central nervous system. *Am J Med* 76:107–108, 1984

Luna MA: Candidiasis. In: Connor DH, et al (eds) *Pathology of infectious diseases.* Stamford, Appleton and Lange, 1997, pp 953–964

McAdams HP, et al: Thoracic mycoses from opportunistic fungi: Radiologic-pathologic correlation. *Radiographics* 15:271–286, 1995

Mindell HJ, Pollack HM: Fungal disease of the ureter. *Radiology* 146:46, 1983

Murray JG, Buckley HR: Serological study of *Candida* species. In: Winner HI, Hurley R (eds) Symposium on *Candida* infections. E & S Livingstone, London, 1966

Pastakia B, et al: Hepatosplenic candidiasis: wheels within wheels. *Radiology* 166:417–421, 1988

Pugh TF, Fitch SJ: Invasive gastric candidiasis. *Pediatr Radiol* 16:67–68, 1986

Rippon JW: *Medical mycology: the pathogenic fungi and the pathogenic actinomycetes.* Saunders, Philadelphia, 1974

Roberts L, et al: Adult esophageal candidiasis: a radiographic spectrum. *Radiographics* 7:289–307, 1987

Rogers KB: *Candida* infections in paediatrics. In: Winner HI, Hurley R (eds) Symposium on *Candida* infections. E & S Livingstone, London, 1966

Samuels BI, Bodey GP, Libshitz H: Imaging in candidiasis. *Semin Roentgenol* XXXI:76–82, 1996

Sanders E, et al: Monilial esophagitis in a patient with hemoglobin SC disease: demonstration of esophageal motor abnormality by cineradiogluorography. *Ann Intern Med* 57:650, 1962

Semelka RC, et al: Detection of acute and treated lesions of hepatosplenic candidiasis: comparison of dynamic, contrast enhanced CT and MR imaging. *J Magn Reson Imaging* 2:341–345, 1992

Shirkhoda A: CT findings in hepatosplenic and renal candidiasis. *J Comput Assist Tomogr* 11:795–798, 1987

Silverman EM, et al: The diagnosis of systemic candidiasis in smears of venous blood. *Am J Clin Pathol* 60:473–475, 1973

Smith JM: Mycoses of the alimentary tract. *Gut* 10:1035, 1969

Stephan JC: Radiology seminar CXXXXIII: esophageal moniliasis. *J Miss State Med Assoc* 15:406–407, 1974

Winner HI: General features of Candida infections: In: Winner HI, Hurley R (eds) Symposium on *Candida* infections. E & E Livingstone, London, 1966

Rhinosporidiosis

Acharya PV, Gupta RL, Darbasi BS: Cutaneous rhinosporidiosis. *Indian J Dermatol Venereal* 39:22–25, 1973

Binford CH, Connor DH: *Pathology of tropical and extraordinary diseases.* Armed Forces Institute of Pathology, Washington, CD, 1976, pp 597–599

Chitravel V, et al: Cell mediated immune response in human cases of rhinosporidiosis. *Sabourandia* 19:135–142, 1981

Mills AE, et al: Rhinosporidiosis in Rhodesia. *Cent Afr J Med* 24:187–189, 1978

Ousor R, Wamukota WM: Rhinosporidiosis in Uganda: a review of 51 cases. *East Afr Med J* 55:582–586, 1978

Satyanarayana C: Rhinosporidiosis with a record of 255 cases. *Acta Otolaryngeal (Stockh)* 51:348–366, 1960

Watts JC, Chandler FW: Rhinosporidiosis. In: Connor DH, et al (eds) *Pathology of infectious diseases.* Stamford, Appleton and Lange, 1997, pp 1085–1088

Wright IG et al: Rhinosporidiosis in Rhodesia: a report of three cases. *Cent Afr J Med* 24:55–56, 1979

7 Taeniasis, Cysticercosis, Sparganosis, Other Tapeworm Infections

Taeniasis and Cysticercosis

The literature on tapeworms and the larval stage of *Taenia solium*, the cysticercus, is considerable and venerable. Aristophanes mentions the parasite in one of his plays, written about 400 B.C.; cerebral cysticercosis was discussed by Ramier in 1558. The first radiological report identifying the calcified larval cysts of *Taenia solium* appeared in the 1890s, but it was another 50 years before an adult *Taenia saginata* was recognized in a small bowel series.

There are many myths about tapeworms, which is not surprising since they are the longest worms to parasitize man, extending in some patients to a length of 30 feet. Some African tribes believe that it is necessary to have a tapeworm to ensure virility. We have been unable to trace any reports to confirm this; on the contrary, the worms may cause ill health and debility. The remedies and cures that have been devised and offered for elimination of the worm are almost as mythical, yet tapeworms are far from being an endangered species; they live in millions of people all over the world. At some stage in their life cycles, either alive or dead, both *T. solium* and *T. saginata* may have clinical significance, and their radiological recognition becomes important to the patients and their physicians.

By far the most important of these tapeworm infections is cysticercosis, caused by the larval stage of *T. solium*, the pork tapeworm. The larval stage begins after the ingestion of eggs passed in feces by the adult worm. These larvae, or cysticerci, develop in various body tissues with an affinity for muscles and the central nervous system (neurocysticercosis), where the most significant clinical manifestations appear, with no age predilection. *T. solium* infection is endemic in parts of Asia, India, Africa, Europe, and Latin America. Until recent years, there were only sporadic cases in the United States. However, due to increased immigration from Central America and travel to endemic areas, cysticercosis is on the rise in the United States, especially in California, Arizona, New Mexico, Texas, and Colorado. An understanding of the epidemiology, pathophysiology, and current laboratory and imaging methods, including computed tomography (CT) and magnetic resonance imaging (MRI) is needed to accurately diagnose neurocysticercosis. Imaging manifestations of the different types and stages of neurocysticercosis are reviewed in a separate section below, providing important information for the management of this infection.

Synonyms

Tapeworm: Taeniasis saginata. Taeniasis solium. Beefworm. Porkworm. *Sp:* Taenia saginata/solium. *Fr:* Taenia inerme/arme. *Ger:* Taenia saginata/solium.

Cysticercosis: Sp: Cisticercosis. *Fr:* Cysticercose. *Ger:* Blasenwurmkrankheit.

Definition

Taeniasis is infection of man by the beef tapeworm, *Taenia saginata*, or the pork tapeworm, *Taenia solium*. Other species of tapeworms which infect humans are described at the end of this chapter.

Cysticercosis is infection by the larval stage of the pork tapeworm, *T. solium*. (There is no acceptable report of infection of man by the larval stage of *T. saginata*.)

Geographic Distribution

The beef tapeworm, *Taenia saginata*, is found in Latin America, Africa, Russia, Asia, and throughout the Moslem world. It is said to be "universal" in Ethiopia. It is estimated that about 40 million persons are infected worldwide.

The pork tapeworm, *Taenia solium*, is a parasite of humans and pigs. It is less common, infecting about 3 million people, and is likely to be rare in Islamic (Moslem) and Jewish communities. It is most common where raw or insufficiently cooked pork is eaten. Infected pigs are common in Central and South America (especially Mexico, Venezuela, and Chile), in Portugal and Eastern Europe, Russia, Manchuria, China, India, Pakistan, Madagascar, and parts of Africa, especially West Africa. It is sometimes thought that the parasite is called "*T. solium*" because there is usually only one adult worm in a patient, but in fact it is given this name because the rostellum (the hook-bearing part of the scolex) resembles the conventional image of the sun. Although in many patients the adult worm is solitary, as many as 11 worms have been found in one person. In southern Africa, up to 50% of those infected have two worms. Mixed infections with both species of *Taenia* can occur.

Cysticerci are commonly found in cattle or pigs, but they occur also in cats, rats, monkeys, dogs, giraffes, buffalos, lamas, and some antelopes.

Although of common origin, taeniasis and cysticercosis are clinically and radiologically two quite separate diseases and will be discussed individually.

Taeniasis

Epidemiology and Pathology

Man acquires adult tapeworms (taeniasis) by eating undercooked or raw infected meat ("measly pork" or beef). The cysticercus in the ingested meat is released by the digestive juices and evaginates, and the larva attaches itself to the mucosa of the small bowel and develops into an adult tapeworm in 5–12 weeks (Fig. 7.1). The tapeworm inhabits the jejunum of man and obtains its nourishment from the food of the host. The head (scolex) of the worm is attached to the bowel by hooklets and suckers; there may be several hundred segments (or proglottids) liberating eggs as they mature (Figs. 7.2, 7.3). The pork tapeworm (*T. solium*) averages 6–20 feet in length and the beef tapeworm (*T. saginata*) 15–30 feet.

The life cycle of both worms is similar except for the intermediate host. Each gravid segment of *T. solium* inhabiting the bowel of man contains 30 000–40 000 eggs. When the proglottids are released, they travel down the gut and, with the help of independent movement, pass through the anus. On the ground they disintegrate, releasing their eggs, which may survive for several weeks, during which time they must be ingested by the intermediate hosts, pigs (*T. solium*) or cattle (*T. saginata*), to complete their life cycle. The eggs hatch in the intestines of their host with the help of digestive juices, liberating their active embryos (oncospheres), which penetrate the wall of the gut with the aid of hooks, and probably also by means of lytic secretions. The oncospheres travel in the blood (and probably the lymphatics) to the muscles and elsewhere through-

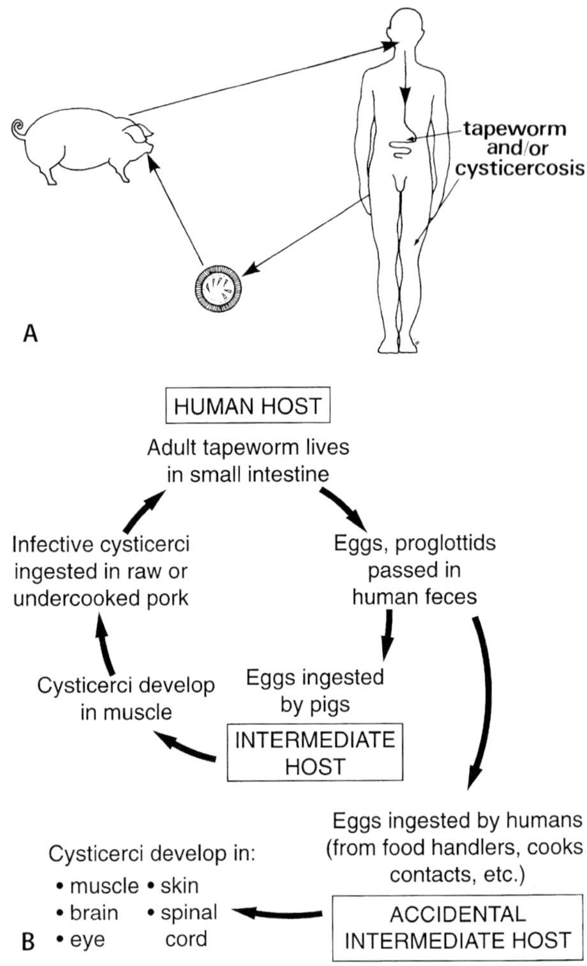

Fig. 7.1 A, B. Life cycle of *Taenia solium*

out the body. In the tissues, the hooks are shed and the oncospheres develop into larvae (cysticerci), completing the life cycle. Man is an accidental intermediate host and, like the pig, may develop larval taeniasis.

The life cycle of *T. saginata* is the same as for *T. solium* except that cattle are the intermediate hosts, and the eggs released are even more numerous (594 million per annum – an astronomical thought for a radiologist!); moreover, the worms can live nearly 30 years.

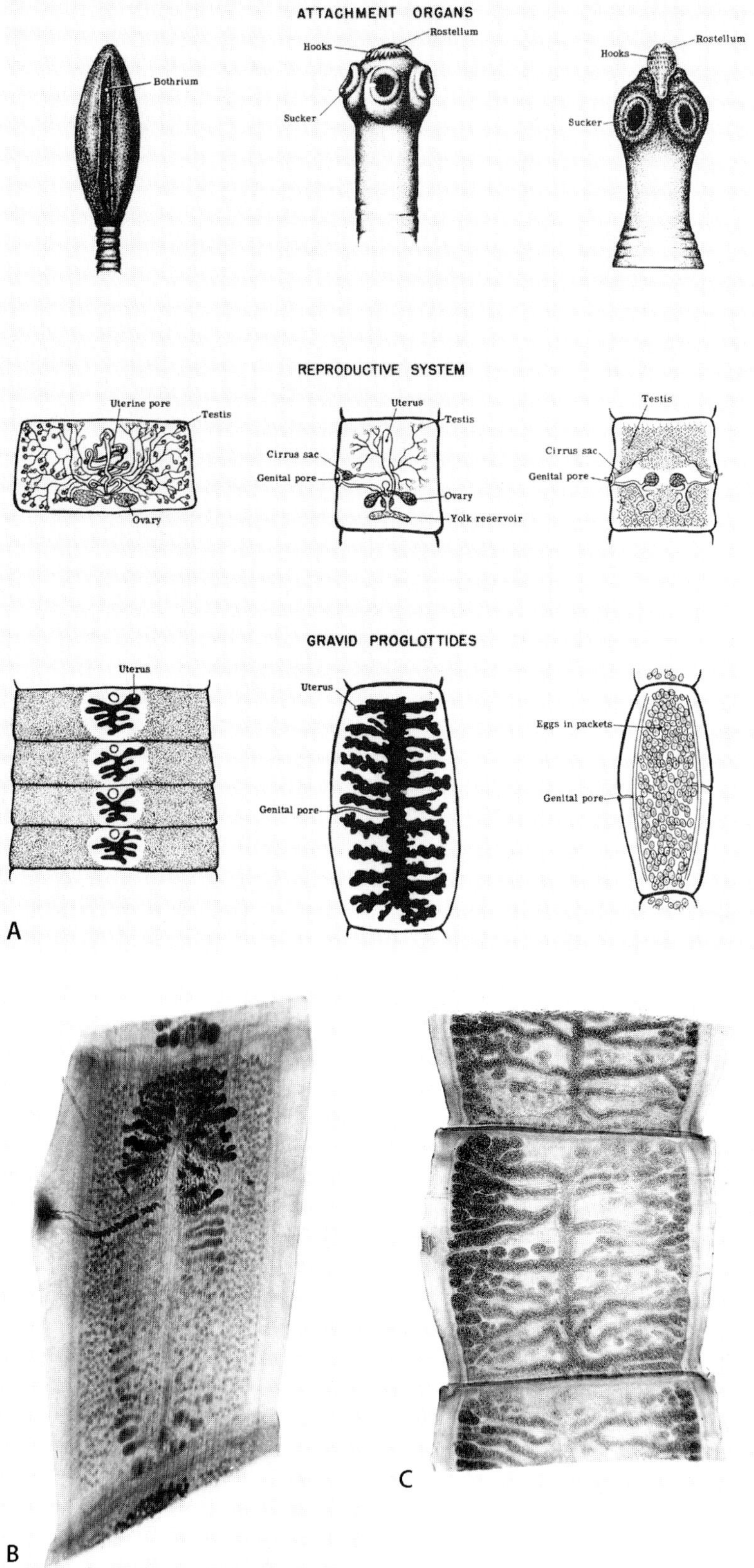

Fig. 7.2. A Morphology of adult tapeworms. (Courtesy of U.S. Naval Medical Corps) **B** Gravid proglottid segment of *T. saginata* showing branching uterus and genital pore (*left center*). ×7.5. AFIP 56-3320. **C** Similar proglottids of *T. solium*. ×7.5. AFIP 56-7108

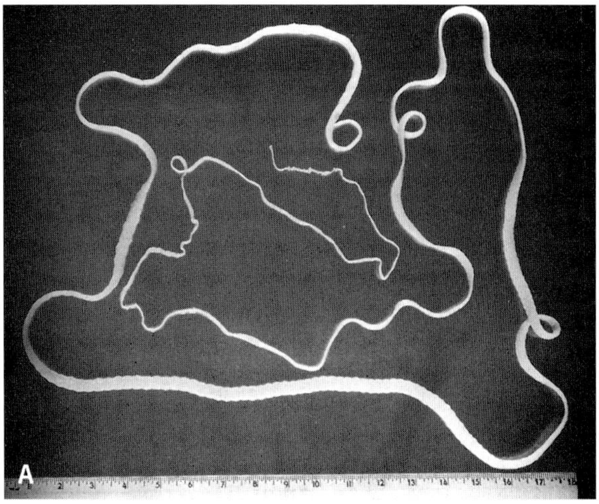

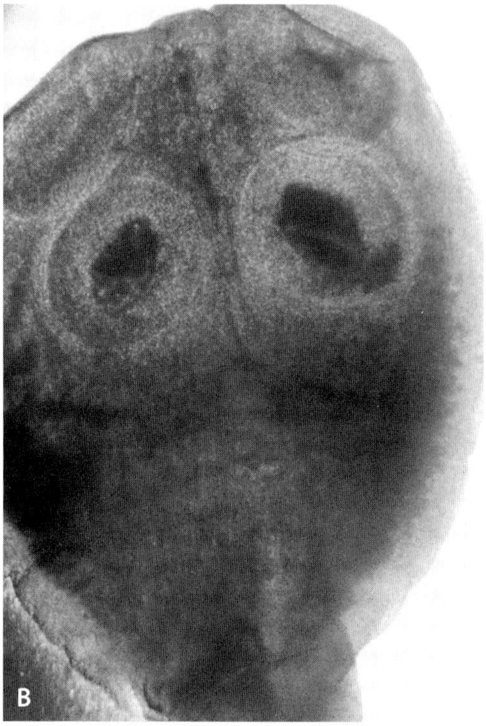

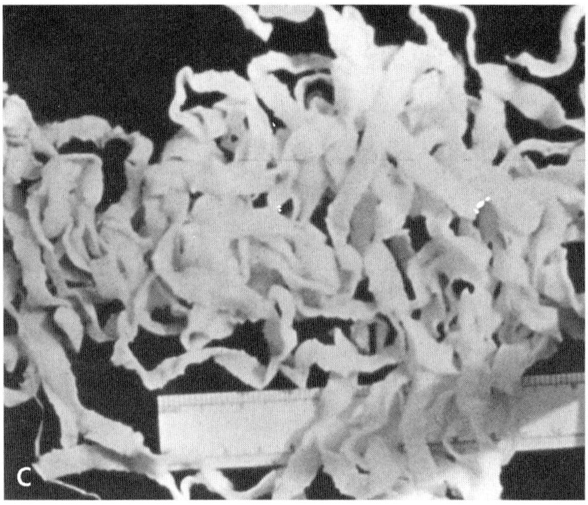

Fig. 7.3. A Adult *T. saginata* worm. Note the tiny head (scolex) and neck of the worm (*center*), with the worm gradually widening into hundreds of proglottid segments. **B** Magnified view of the scolex of *T. saginata* showing the suckers to good advantage. AFIP 68-1462-6. **C** Adult *T. solium* worm showing the numerous proglottids. (Courtesy of Dr. Herman Zaiman)

Laboratory Diagnosis

The laboratory diagnosis is made by identifying ova or proglottids in stool. Enzyme-linked immunosorbent assay (ELISA) techniques for antigen or antibody can reveal *T. solium* in the stools of tapeworm carriers even in the absence of proglottids. DNA probes can be useful in differentiating *T. saginata* and *T. solium*.

Clinical Characteristics

Most patients infected with the adult worm have few clinical symptoms: the worms are a chance finding on defecation. Abdominal discomfort, anorexia, malaise, weight loss, indigestion, diarrhea, and even constipation can occur. Patients may have up to 10% eosinophilia. Obstruction has been reported in some patients with multiple worms. Pruritus ani occurs in up to 25% of patients.

Fig. 7.5. A Taeniasis saginata. Small bowel series reveals a solitary beef tapeworm of great length outlined by barium as a continuous radiolucent structure running through multiple loops of jejunum and ileum. Unlike *Ascaris*, a tapeworm has no alimentary canal and thus does not ingest barium. **B** Adult *T. saginata* recovered intact following its passage after a vermifuge was administered. Note the extraordinary length of this worm, which may at times reach 20–30 feet. The patient was a U.S. soldier seen at Tripler Army Medical Center in Honolulu, Hawaii with a history of extensive travel ▶

Radiological Diagnosis

Despite the ubiquitous presence of *T. saginata* throughout the world, it is seldom demonstrated radiologically on small bowel barium studies. Characteristically it appears in the lower jejunum or ileum as an unusually long and gradually widening radiolucent line within the barium column (Figs. 7.4, 7.5). It widens from 1–2 mm in diameter at its neck to 12 mm at its distal end. It may be folded on itself because of its great length, but it still appears as a continuous structure.

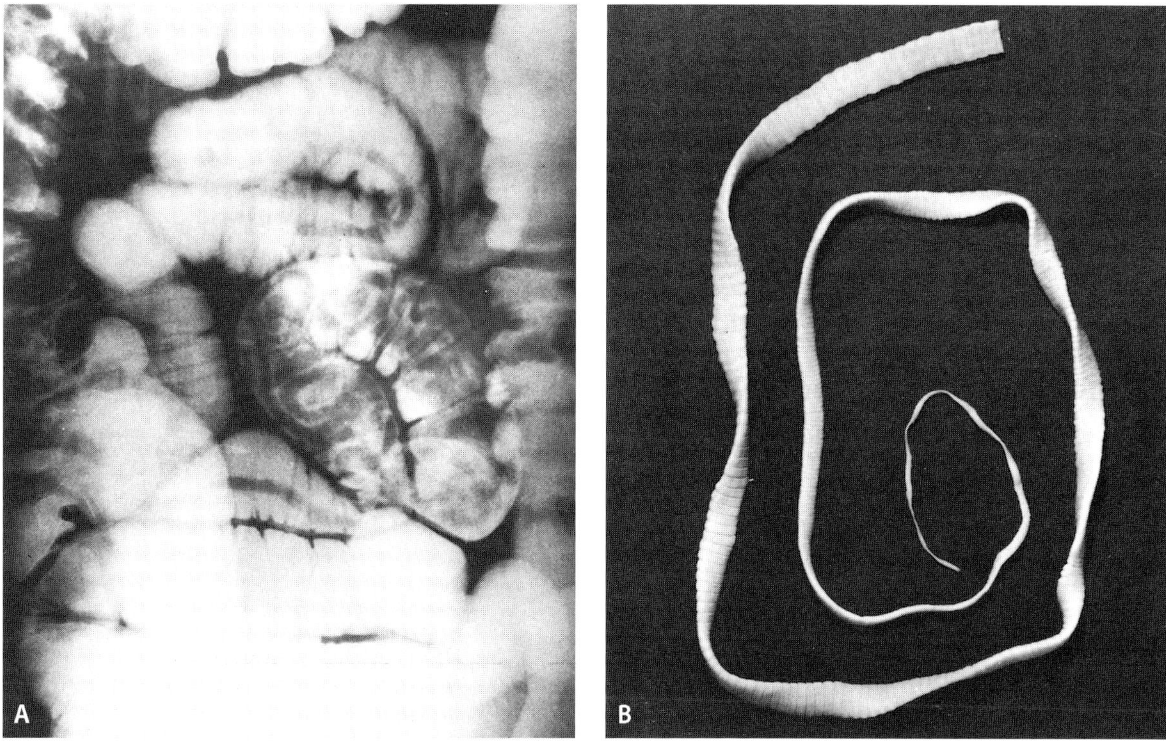

Fig. 7.4. A Adult *T. saginata* in the ileum of a 25-year-old Lebanese admitted to hospital with acute abdominal pain, which was intermittent and severe. Reflux of barium into the terminal ileum during a barium enema examination revealed a markedly elongated ribbon-like radiolucent shadow representing the adult tapeworm, which was coiled upon itself through part of its course. The patient was given a vermifuge and 210 cm of worm, including the scolex, was passed. (Courtesy of Dr. Lawrence E. Fetterman, Mobile) **B** Adult *T. saginata* showing the slender head and neck (*center*) and numerous proglottid segments

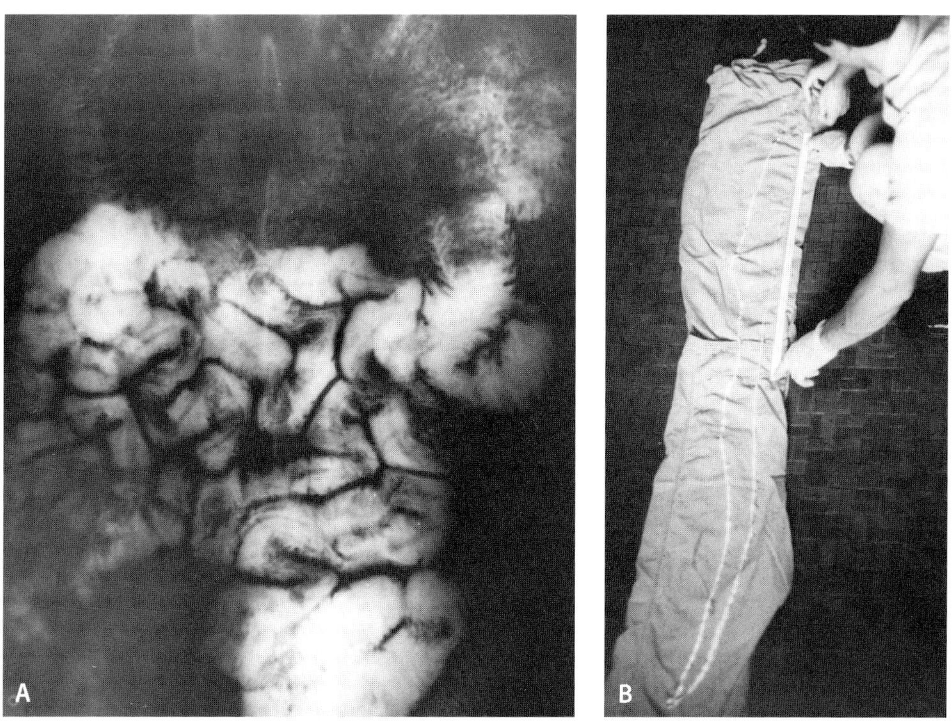

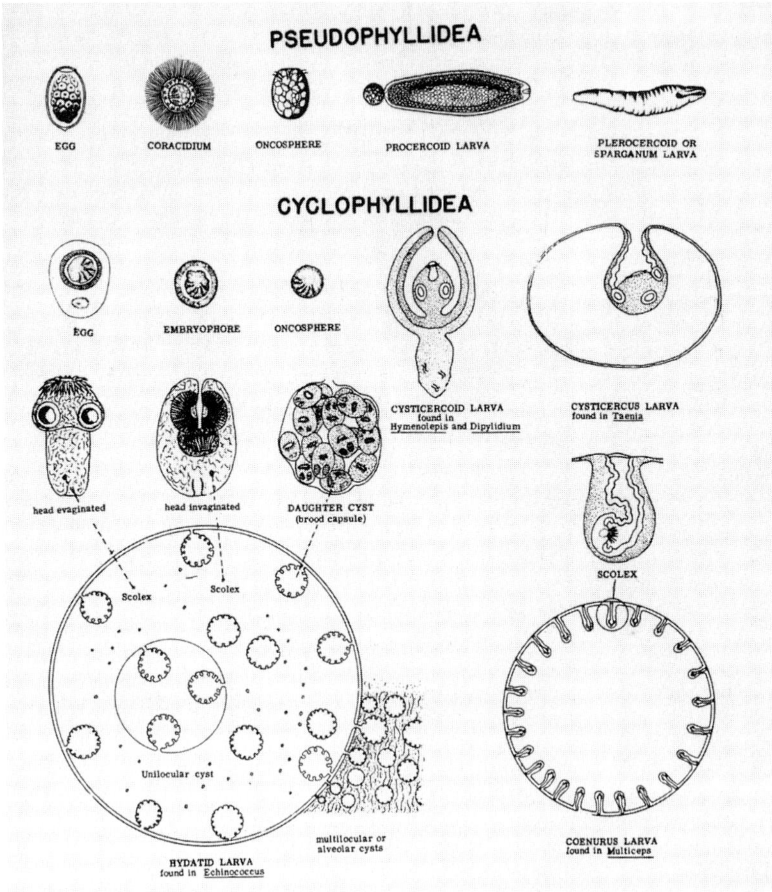

Fig. 7.6. Immature stages of human tapeworms: *Sparganum (top); Hymenolepis* and *Taenia* cysticerci (*middle*); *Echinococcus* larva (*bottom left*); *Coenurus* larva (*bottom right*). (From Medical Parasitology, U.S. Navy)

Unlike the roundworm *Ascaris*, tapeworms have no alimentary canal; each proglottid absorbs nutrients instead through its tegument. *Ascaris* may have a characteristic thread-like strand of barium within its alimentary tract and is much shorter.

Taenia solium has not been identified radiographically; presumably its appearance would resemble that of *T. saginata*, but it would be shorter.

Differential Diagnosis

Recognition of the adult *T. saginata* in the small bowel is not difficult, once seen: it is usually many feet in length and cannot be mistaken for the much shorter *Ascaris* or anything else. It must be emphasized, however, that it is uncommon for the worm, even when lengthy, to be demonstrated, and a normal upper gastrointestinal study and small bowel series do not exclude the possibility of a tapeworm.

Cysticercosis (Outside the Central Nervous System)

Epidemiology and Pathology

Man acquires cysticercosis by ingesting food, water, or feces containing eggs of *T. solium* (Figs. 7.6, 7.7). Autoinfection can occur from contaminated hands or, less commonly, by regurgitating proglottids of an adult tapeworm from the gut into the stomach during a bout of nausea; this may occur spontaneously or in association with antihelminthic therapy. Oncospheres (larvae) released from their shells in the gut penetrate the mucosa and spread throughout the body, developing into cysticerci, most commonly in the voluntary muscles and brain, but also in the orbits, heart muscle, liver, and lung. Oncospheres may invade the eye and be seen clearly moving in the anterior or posterior chamber. Infections vary from a single cysticercus to many hundreds (Fig. 7.8), and may be limited to one organ or be generalized.

The resting cysticercus grows to a stable size of 1–2 cm within 3–4 months. Intact cysticerci provoke mild inflammation and fibrosis that "walls them off." As long as the parasite remains alive, equilib-

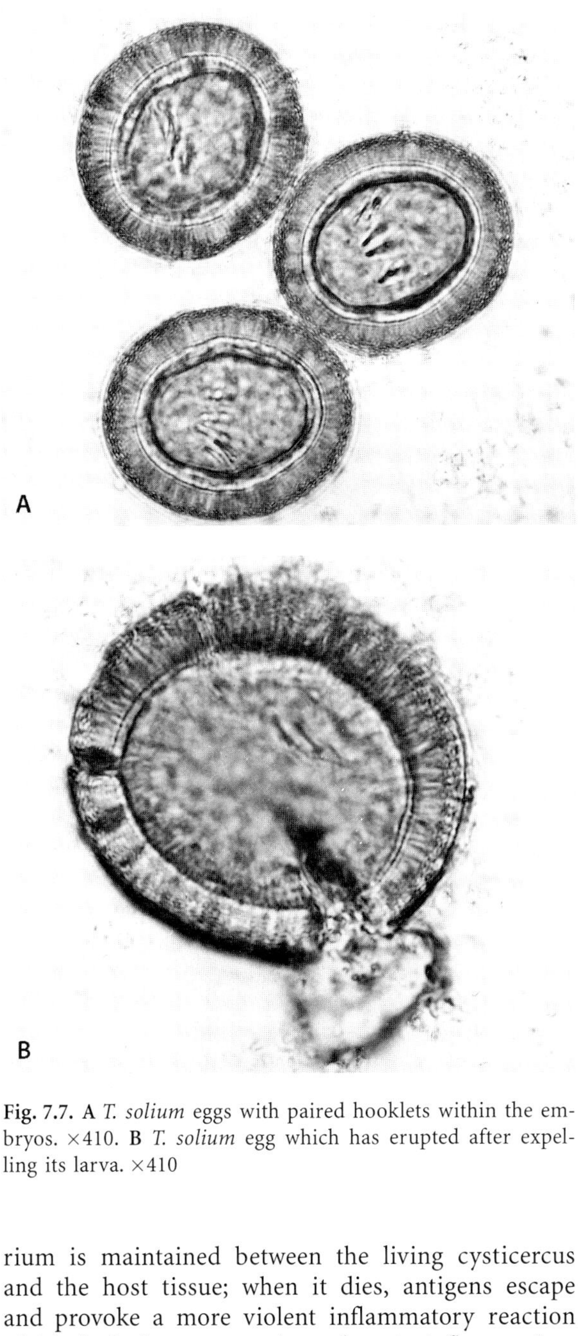

Fig. 7.7. **A** *T. solium* eggs with paired hooklets within the embryos. ×410. **B** *T. solium* egg which has erupted after expelling its larva. ×410

rium is maintained between the living cysticercus and the host tissue; when it dies, antigens escape and provoke a more violent inflammatory reaction which includes suppuration, chronic inflammation, and eventually a foreign body granulomatous reaction to the tegument, hooklets, and calcareous corpuscles. Finally, after a few months, the lesion resolves as a calcified scar. Such calcification may not affect the cyst capsule or its contents, and the shape may be maintained unless pressure causes collapse, flattening the calcified cyst into a spindle shape. The life of the cyst may vary within wide limits, and both dead calcified cysts and living parasites may coexist in the same individual and even in the same organ. The parasites usually die in 3–6 years, although they may live longer. In body tissues, it takes several months to 3 years to develop calcification, but within the brain calcification is less common and takes even longer to develop.

Laboratory Diagnosis

A positive pathological diagnosis is made when the cysticercus is excised and identified microscopically. However, the radiological appearance is usually so characteristic that it provides a reliable way of establishing the diagnosis. In cerebral cysticercosis, the cerebrospinal fluid (CSF) may show a significant eosinophilia with lymphocytosis and raised protein albumin; these changes are nonspecific. ELISA can reveal antigens in the CSF and in serum, but false negatives can occur in HIV-positive individuals. Enzyme-linked immunoelectrotransfer blot (EITB) exhibits higher specificity and sensitivity than ELISA.

Clinical Characteristics

It may be difficult to establish the date of infection, but it is rare for individuals to have clinical signs in less than 2 years after visiting an endemic area. While the cysticercus is growing, there are mild and transient manifestations such as headache, irregular fever, myalgia, and a transient eosinophilia. In most patients, however, these symptoms are completely absent. The larvae in muscle give rise to few symptoms: palpable cystic soft tissue swellings can develop around them (Fig. 7.9). Some collapse and disappear within a few days and others may develop over a dozen or more years. The impression may be that these palpable swellings migrate, but the ability to feel them depends on distention of the cyst capsule with fluid after the parasite dies. Cysts occur almost anywhere over the body, but are rarely palpable in the hands or feet even when demonstrable radiologically.

Heart block has been reported as a result of a cysticercus impeding cardiac conduction (Fig. 7.10 A). Cysticerci may remain alive and unencapsulated in either chamber of the eye and may cause interruption of vision, retinitis, uveitis, and palpebral conjunctivitis. The clinical and imaging signs of neurocysticercosis (Fig. 7.10 B) will be discussed later.

(Text continues on p. 650)

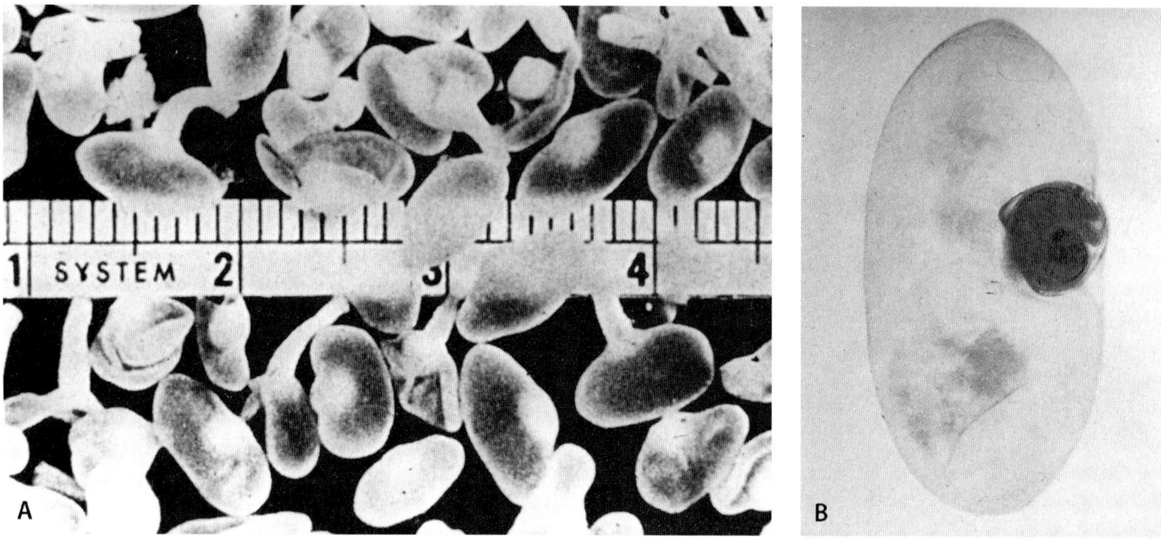

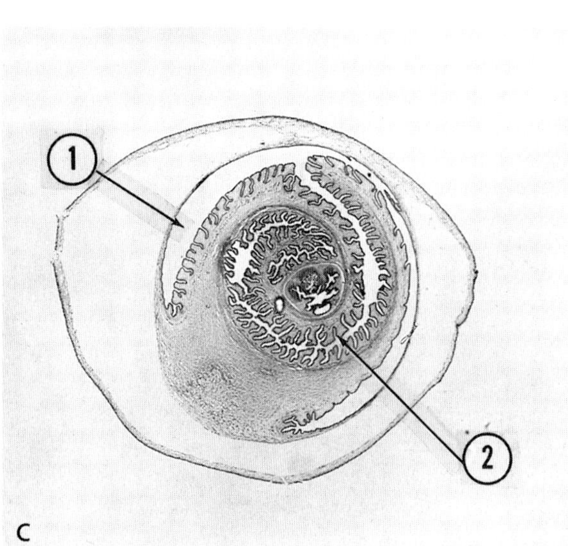

Fig. 7.8. **A** Multiple cysticerci of *T. solium* digested free from cattle muscle. (Courtesy of Dr. Herman Zaiman) **B** Encysted cysticercus with its scolex. Note the characteristic oval shape. ×4. **C** Section through cysticercus of *T. saginata*. The cysticercus is a bladder (*1*) containing a scolex (*2*) formed by invagination of the proliferating wall. ×10. AFIP 68-5273

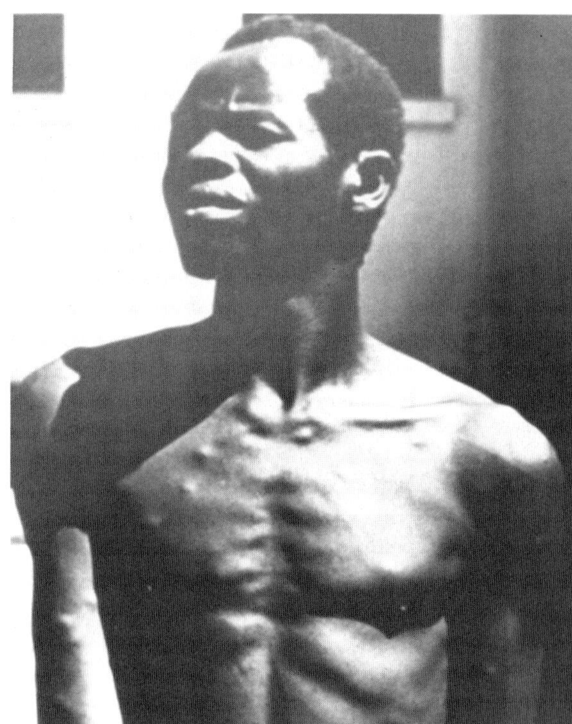

▶

Fig. 7.9. Cysticercosis in an adult African man showing numerous subcutaneous swellings caused by the larval stage of *T. solium*. (Courtesy of Dr. Herman Zaiman)

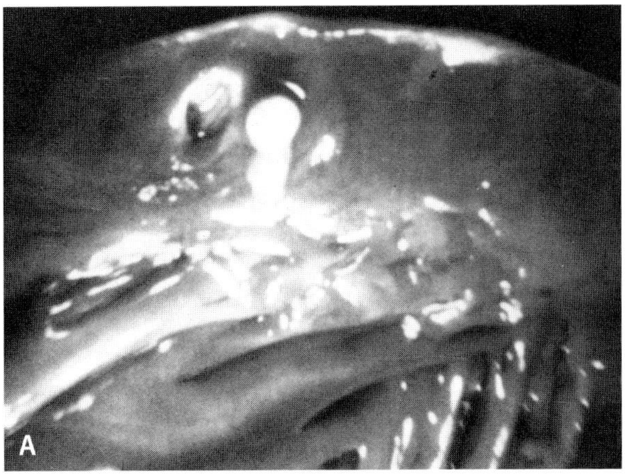

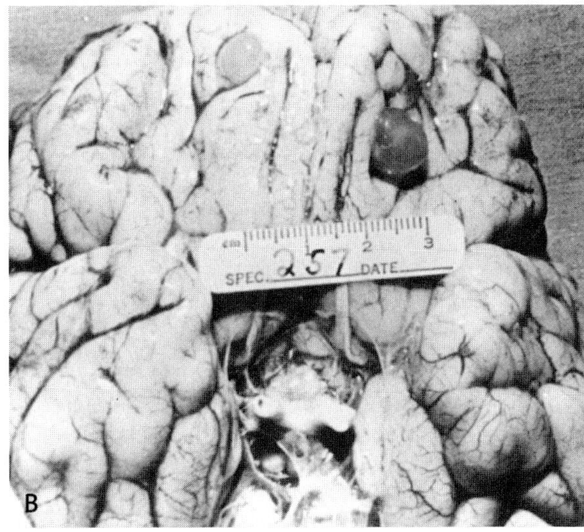

Fig. 7.10. **A** Multiple cysticerci in the myocardium of the left ventricle. **B** Cerebral cysticercosis of the base of the brain. (**A, B** courtesy of Dr. Herman Zaiman)

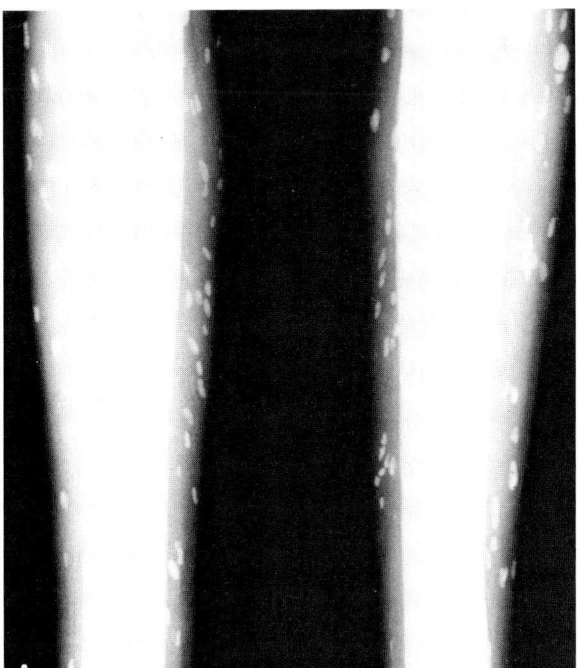

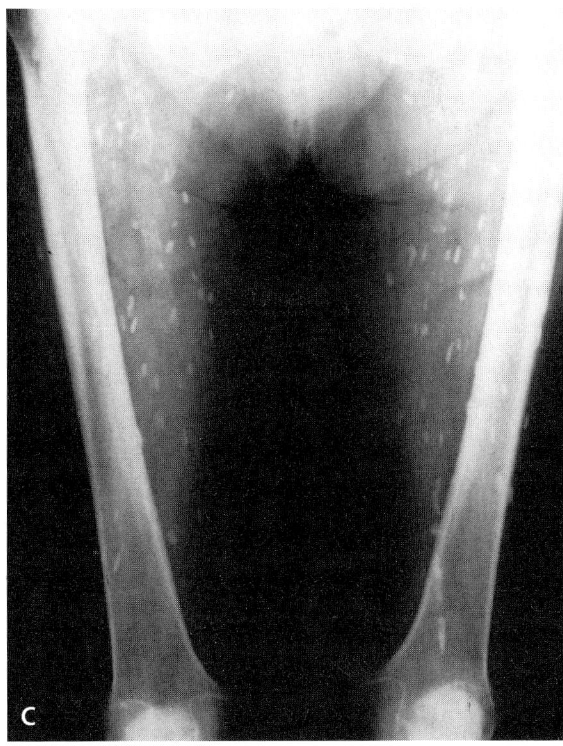

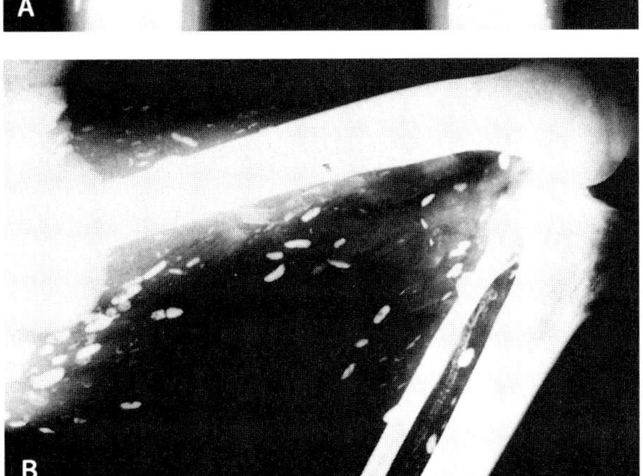

Fig. 7.11 A–C. Cysticercosis in three patients showing typical rice grain calcifications in the soft tissues and muscles of the lower extremities. Note that the oval and linear cysticerci are aligned with their long axes in the plane of the muscle bundles of the legs. Note also the variation in size and shape of the cysticerci, although the majority are approximately 10 mm in length by 4 mm in width

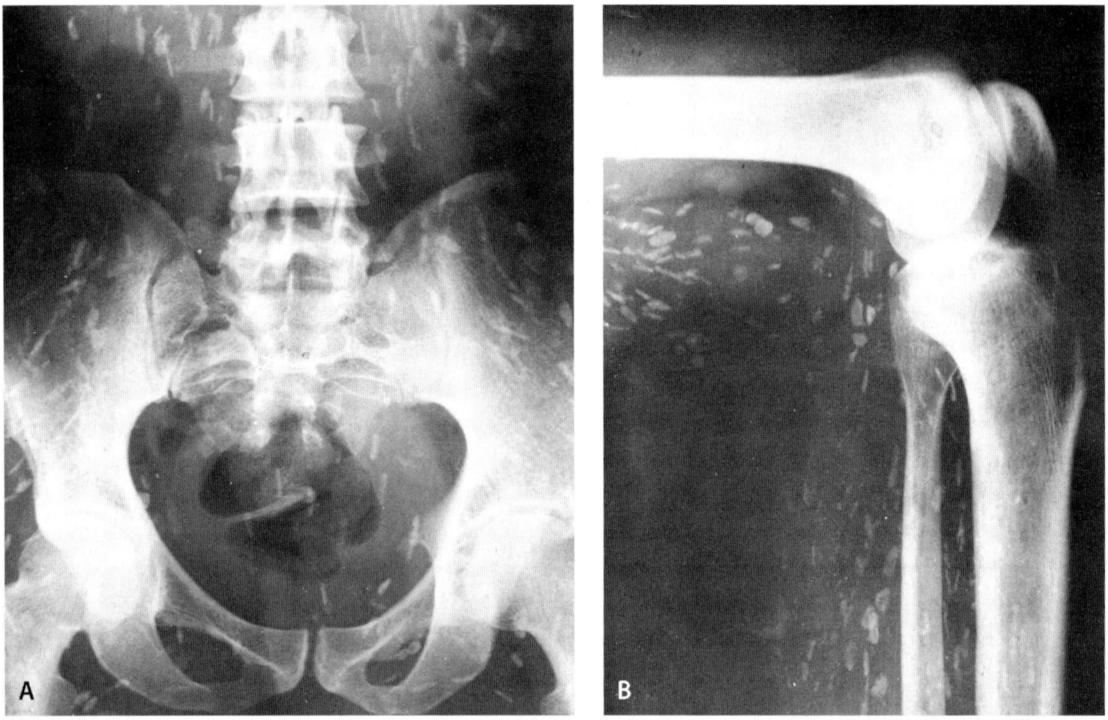

Fig. 7.12 A, B. Cysticercosis of the muscles of the back, abdomen, buttocks, and lower extremity of another patient. Note the alignment of the calcified cysticerci in the axes of the muscle fibers and their variation in shape from elongate and linear to more plump oval or elliptical configurations. Many of the calcifications have a small lucent center and, when viewed from the side, may resemble ring calcifications

Imaging Diagnosis

The calcified cysticercus produces single (rarely) or multiple (often several hundred) calcifications in the soft tissues, which are linear or oval in shape and usually measure 4–10 mm or more in length and 2–5 mm in width. Cysts as large as 23 mm have been reported. The calcified cysts will have their long axes in the plane of the surrounding muscle bundle (Figs. 7.11–7.14).

In some series, calcified larvae have been demonstrated in up to 97% of patients examined 5 or more years after infection; such a high rate of detection is not to be expected routinely. Some patients with cerebral cysticercosis will have no evidence of calcified cysts in the muscles and are unaware of their infection.

Partially calcified cysts and even noncalcified cysts have been demonstrated by soft tissue radiography. The technique is useful when there is a localized (clinical) swelling, but as a method of "search" it is unreliable and unjustified.

Cysticerci may be seen in the lungs, where they are about 3–6 mm in diameter. The outer shell is calcified, with a somewhat lighter and softer center. In the lungs, the cysts remain more nearly round compared with the oval or elongate calcified cysts in muscle.

In the liver, the cysticercus is larger and has been described as the size of a cherry (1 cm in diameter). If a cyst is seen in the liver and there are other calcified cysts in the muscles or lungs, the diagnosis is reasonably reliable; but if cysts are seen in either the lung or liver solely (a rarity), they cannot be differentiated from other causes of small calcified nodules.

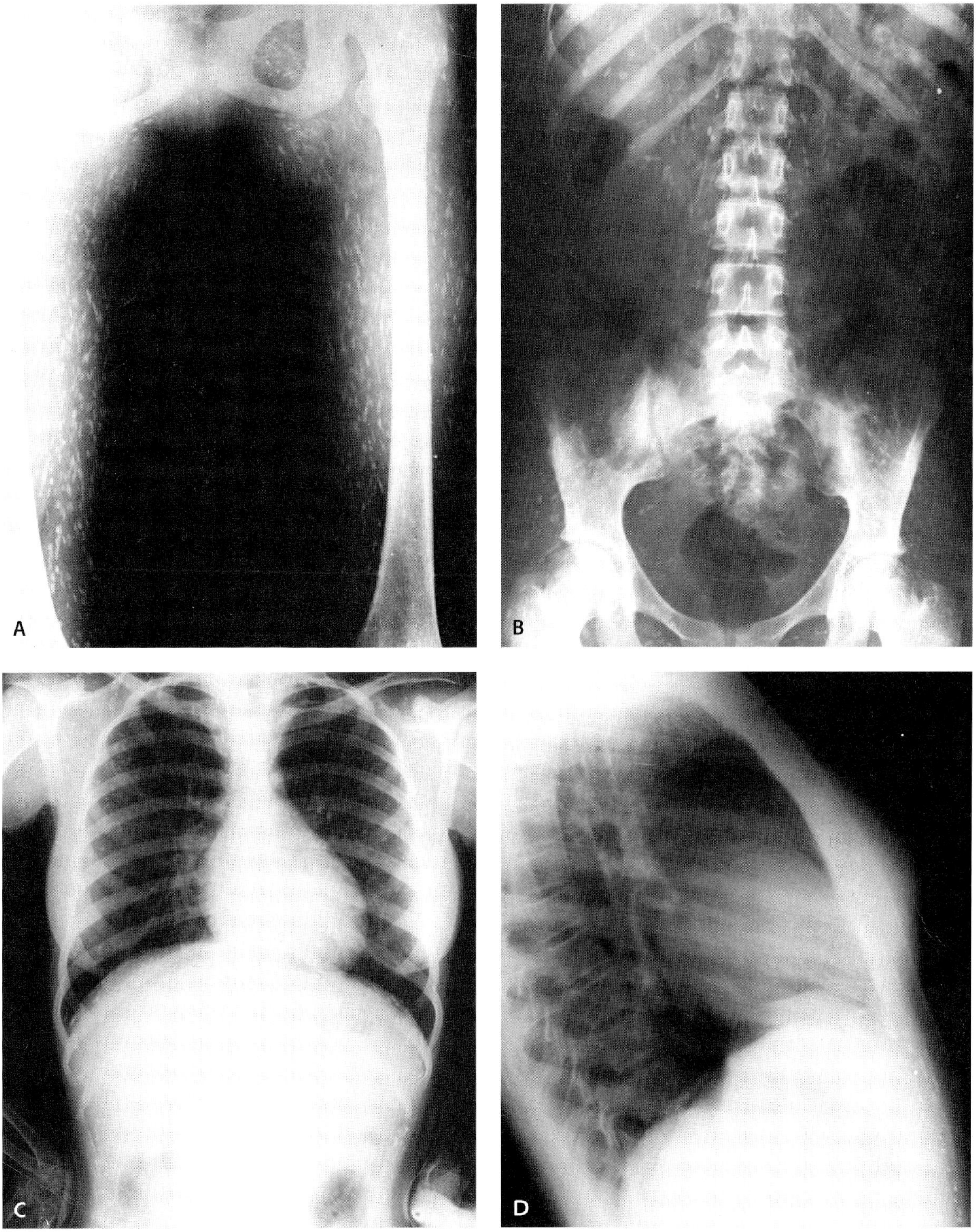

Fig. 7.13 A–D. Extensive cysticercosis of the soft tissues, muscles, diaphragm, and lungs in a 13-year-old Colombian woman. Note in B–D that the rice grain calcifications overlying the abdomen are actually in soft tissues and muscles of the buttocks, flanks, anterior abdominal wall, and back. In C and D calcified larvae can be seen in the diaphragm as well as in the muscles of the chest and abdominal wall, axillae, and neck. (Courtesy of Dr. William Thomas, McLean)

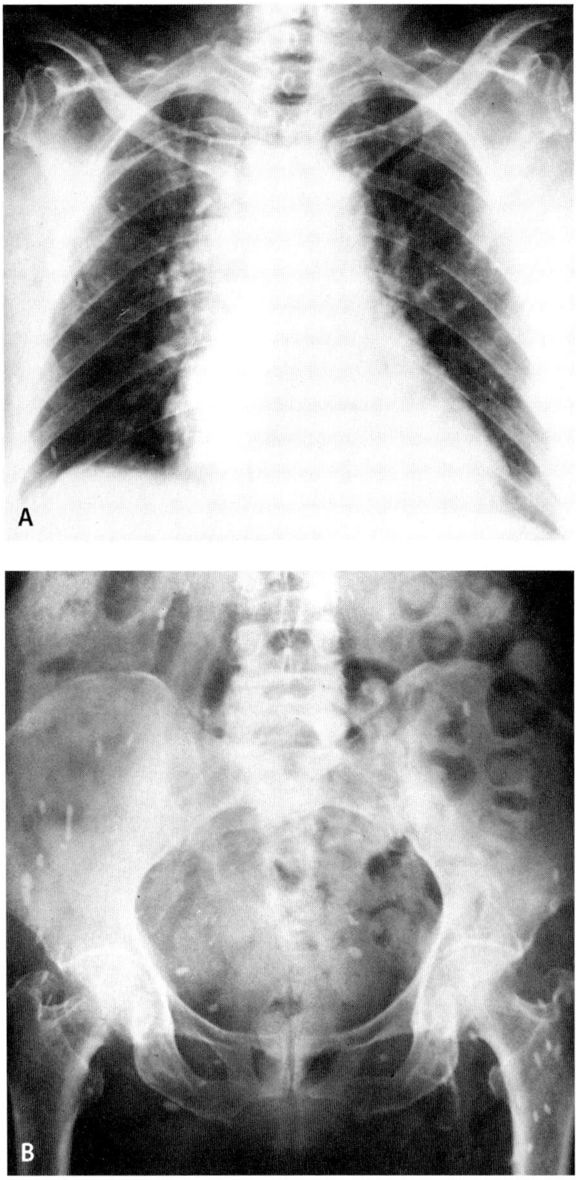

Fig. 7.14 A, B. Cysticercosis involving the muscles of the neck, axillae, and chest wall (**A**) and the back, buttocks, abdominal wall, and thighs (**B**) of another patient

Neurocysticercosis

With Enrique Palacios

Pathology

The pathological findings of cysticercosis within the brain differ slightly from those elsewhere in the body. The cysticercus develops to form a small, firmly encapsulated cyst. Several pathological forms are found: the cyst may develop in the brain parenchyma or it may be mobile, lying in the ventricles or in the aqueduct. Alternatively, there may be a racemose cyst, a large delicate, thin-walled, translucent, ramifying body (usually sterile) lying in the ventricular system, cisterna magna, or cerebellopontine angle. It may even extend through the foramen magnum into the upper cervical region. In other patients, neither of these forms may exist; instead there may be a basal arachnoiditis without any obvious cysticercus in immediate relationship.

In the brain, the cysticercus becomes surrounded by neuroglia; degeneration leads to a walled-off and discolored ring of glial tissue. Inflammation does not develop until the cysticercus dies and degenerating cysticerci stimulate infiltration of neutrophils, eosinophils, and macrophages. A granulomatous reaction eventually ensues, characterized by foamy macrophages with occasional epitheloid cells and foreign body giant cells. The lesions subsequently become fibrotic and may calcify.

Five types of neurocysticercosis are recognized according to their location: (1) parenchymal, (2) arachnoidal, (3) ventricular, (4) spinal, and (5) mixed.

Parenchymal cysticercal larvae undergo degeneration, and various stages can be identified: (a) *vesicular stage*, viable cysticerci with immune tolerance by the host; (b) *colloidal stage*, nonviable cysticerci with the host's immune system reacting against the degeneration of the parasite; (c) *granular nodular stage*, nonviable cysticerci with immune response and deposition of mineral salt; and (d) *calcified stage*, the sequelae of nonviable nodular granulomas. The lesions may also be found simultaneously in different stages in the same individual. Another pattern of parenchymal cysticercosis is the *miliary* or *encephalitic* type, where numerous small lesions produce severe acute or chronic inflammatory reaction with diffuse brain edema and symmetrical compression of the ventricles.

Arachnoiditis, vasculitis with infarcts, cranial nerve involvement, and impairment of CSF circulation with obstructive communicating hydrocephalus result with involvement of the basal cisterns. Obstruction of the ventricular system may occur from intraventricular lesions and reactive ependymitis.

Involvement of the spinal canal is rare and may give rise to myelopathies when the spinal cord is affected and radiculopathies when the subarachnoid space and leptomeninges are involved by space-occupying lesions or arachnoiditis.

Laboratory Diagnosis

Because of the wide range of nonspecific clinical findings in neurocysticercosis, the diagnosis can be confirmed only with imaging and CSF studies. Both of these methods have dramatically improved diagnostic accuracy because they provide evidence of the location and stage of the cysticerci and the degree of host inflammatory reaction.

False-positive results in immune tests are sometimes seen in individuals from endemic areas because of contact with the parasite without development of the disease. False-negative results in serum can occur because of local production of antibodies without a parallel increase in peripheral blood, and also in HIV-positive patients. In CSF, there is objective evidence of a host reaction against cysticerci within the subarachnoid space, with the degree of inflammation manifested by elevated cells and/or proteins, and a positive immunological reaction to cysticercal antigens in ELISA or complement fixation tests, both of which may have 80% sensitivity and 96% specificity values. These tests are reliable and specific in meningeal cysticercosis and somewhat less useful in cases of parenchymal and ventricular neurocysticercosis, particularly in noninflammatory cerebrospinal fluid.

Clinical Characteristics

Most of the clinical manifestations of cysticercosis occur when the central nervous system (CNS) is affected. The presence of cysticercus in the CNS can incite a mild or extensive host response, almost always triggered by death of the cyst and resultant inflammatory reaction. Extraparenchymal lesions (ventricular, subarachnoid, spinal, and mixed) have a poorer prognosis than parenchymal lesions. Symptoms depend on the size, number, and location of lesions and include headaches, jacksonian epileptic seizures, focal neurological deficit, loss of vision, mental disturbances, and neuropsychiatric problems produced by brain parenchymal mass effect, reactive edema, and glial scarring. Meningitis, hydrocephalus, ischemic cerebrovascular disease, cerebellar ataxia, spinal cord compression, and transient paralytic episodes can occur at times.

In parenchymal-type cysticercosis, some affected individuals may remain asymptomatic. On the other hand, infection of the brain can be so overwhelming that death occurs from fulminating disease within a week of onset of symptoms and closely resembles an acute encephalitis.

The cysts can present as cerebral tumors (Fig. 7.10 B), with clinical signs varying according to their location. Apart from intermittent raised intracranial pressure from cysts within the ventricular system, those affecting the meninges over the base of the brain can also raise the intracranial pressure by obstruction to the flow of CSF.

Imaging Diagnosis

The possibility of neurocysticercosis should be remembered in every patient with recent onset of epilepsy or other unexpected cerebral symptomatology. Residence in, or travel to, an endemic area 3 or more years previously should alert physicians to this possibility. About 10% of patients known to have cysticercosis will show one or more cerebral calcifications on routine radiographs of the skull (Figs. 7.15, 7.16). Over 75%, and in some series nearly 100%, will have calcifications in muscles or elsewhere in the soft tissues; however, failure to demonstrate calcified soft tissue cysticerci does not exclude cerebral cysticercosis because it is possible to have parasites in only one organ. Intracranial cysticerci calcify later and much less often than those in the muscles and soft tissues. In the brain, they occasionally show calcium deposition in their investing capsules; there may be an area of radiolucency inside and, in the very center, a tiny calcified scolex may sometimes be seen on careful inspection (Fig. 7.15). Rarely, cysts may produce areas of bony erosion in the cranial vault. These are smooth and well defined and may be demonstrated as increased translucency of the skull rather than "cystic" defects. Prior to the advent of CT and MRI, pneumoencephalography was the most reliable examination for neurocysticercosis (Fig. 7.17). The cysts may be located anywhere within the brain and will mimic cerebral tumors. Free-floating cysts may block the ventricular system, causing a symmetrical internal hydrocephalus and dilatation of the aqueduct of Sylvius without deviation. There may be only partial obstruction, which may vary with the position of the patient. Complete obliteration of the aqueduct is rare. In some patients the outline of the cysticercus within the ventricles or aqueduct may be seen. The ventricles may show irregular margins and cysticerci may be seen attached to the ventricular walls. Demonstration of the clear cysts has been described (Filipov's sign) as spherical or ovoid translucent areas, with very clear centers and darker edges and with sharply defined outlines.

Cysticerci may be seen anywhere around the periphery of the brain, including the basal cisterns. In a small proportion of patients, there will be basal leptomeningitis, demonstrated as severe hydrocephalus, and there may be signs of cortical atrophy. In some patients, positive contrast ventriculography may be helpful, particularly in posterior fossa cysticercosis. The demonstration of the rounded defects is more reliable utilizing positive contrast media (see Fig. 7.43 B).

Cerebral arteriography has little part to play in the diagnosis of cerebral cysticercosis where CT and MRI are available. It may help in demonstrating the mass effect but is far less accurate in providing the diagnosis than CT and MRI.

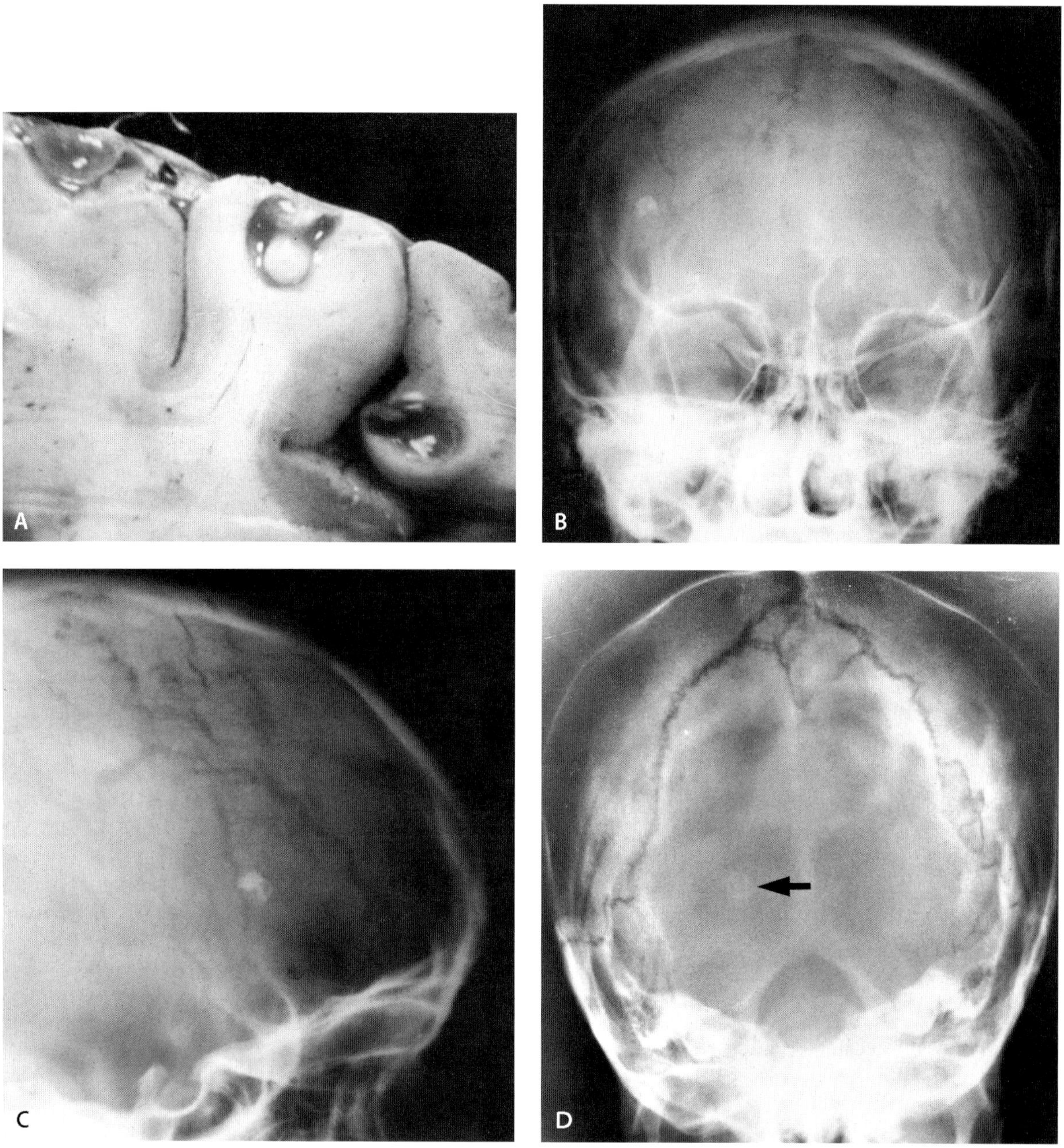

▲ **Fig. 7.15.** A Cysticercus of *T. solium* in the brain. (Courtesy of Dr. Herman Zaiman, Valley City, North Dakota) **B** Posteroanterior view and **C** right lateral view of the skull reveal a solitary calcified cysticercus in the right frontal lobe of a patient from Colombia. Note the typical 2-mm calcification representing the scolex within a central radiolucency surrounded by a partially calcified sphere 1 cm in diameter, which is the body of the encysted larva. **D** Anteroposterior Townes' view of the skull reveals a solitary calcified cysticercus in the left cerebral hemisphere of a 3-year-old Colombian girl with mongolism and a history suggestive of convulsions. Note again the target-like appearance of the calcification with a central density (scolex) surrounded by a lucent area and finally a ring of calcification around the outside of the cysticercus cyst (*arrow*). (B–D courtesy of Dr. William Thomas, McLean)

Fig. 7.17. Huge cysticercus cyst in the left cerebral hemisphere protruding into the left lateral ventricle on **A** frontal and **B** lateral views from a 1960s pneumoencephalogram. There is moderate hydrocephalus and a slight shift of the ventricular system towards the right in this U.S. airman, who had visited Mexico previously. **C** Tomographic cuts from the same pneumoencephalogram clearly outline the large mass impinging on the left lateral ventricle. Occasionally cysticerci attain such great size, although much more commonly they are considerably smaller, often measuring about 1 cm. (Courtesy of Dr. Dennis Chalus, Denver) ▶

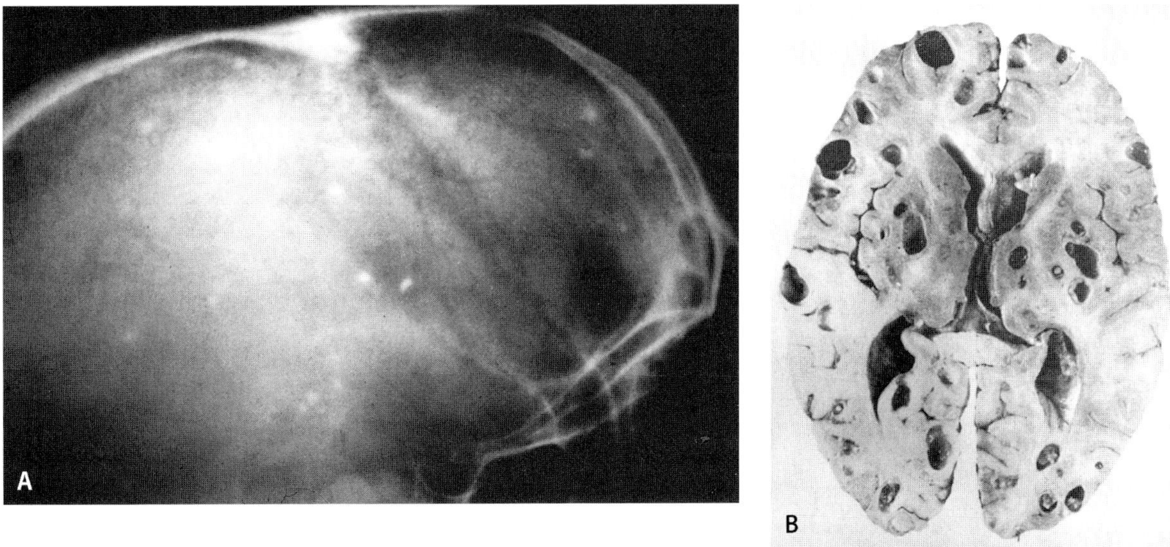

Fig. 7.16. **A** Cerebral cysticercosis in an 11-year-old Colombian girl with a history of grand mal seizures. There are numerous 2- to 4-mm calcifications scattered throughout the brain compatible with, but not diagnostic of, cysticercosis since several other diseases such as tuberculosis may give similar calcifications. **B** Autopsy specimen of the brain of another patient with fatal cerebral cysticercosis showing multiple cysticerci of varying size and shape in the cortex and ventricular walls of the brain. In the brain, cysticerci are thin-walled cysts, each of which is filled with clear fluid and contains a scolex

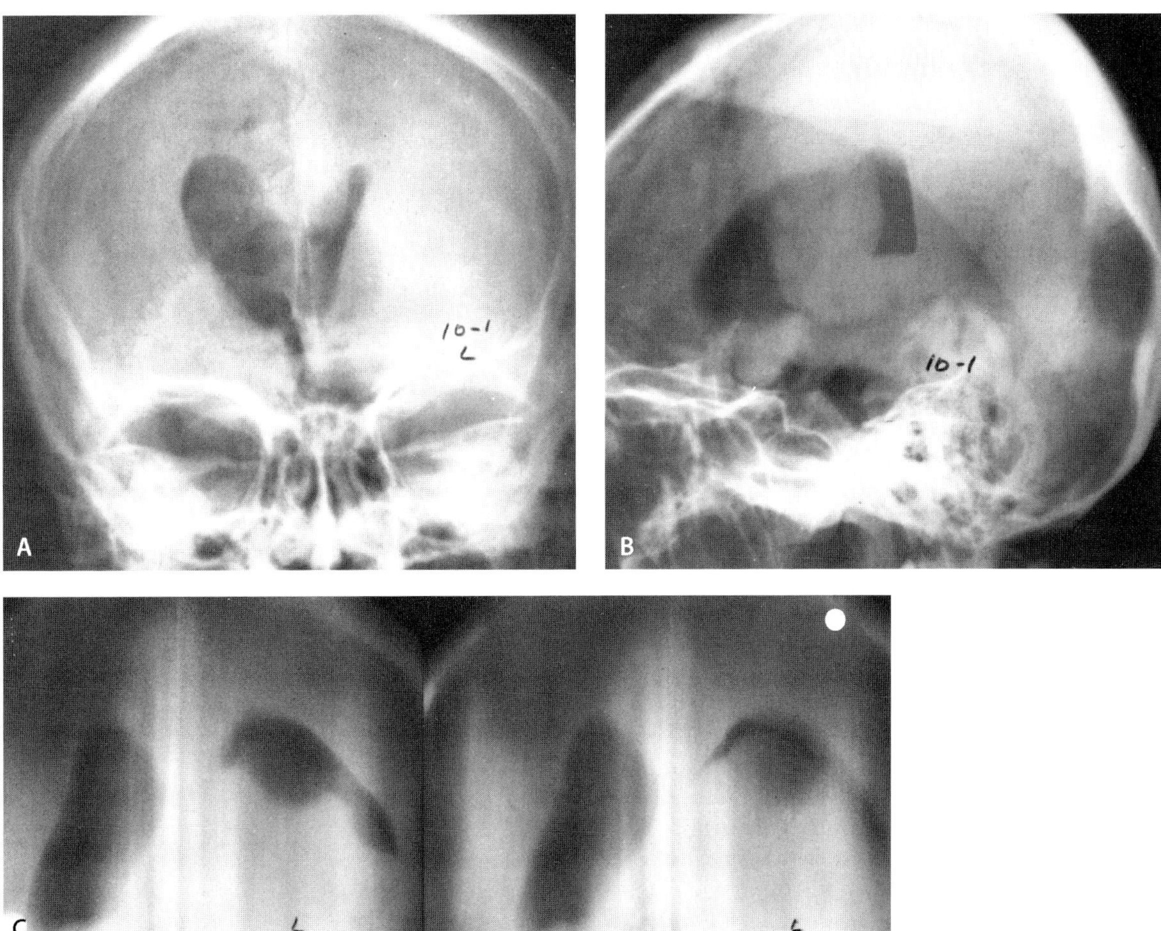

Computed tomography and MRI performed before or after administration of intravenous contrast media are the imaging methods of choice in neurocysticercosis, giving reliable information about the location and activity of the cysts. CT will not only demonstrate both calcified and uncalcified cysts, but also free-floating cysts and hydrocephalus in many patients. The findings are characteristic, and the multiplicity of lesions will strongly suggest cysticercosis. However, solitary cysts may occur. MRI with different pulse sequences and with multiplanar capability, aided by intravenous contrast enhancement, is of great value in the diagnosis of neurocysticerosis, particularly in patients with lesions at the base of the brain, temporal lobes, and brain stem, as well as associated vascular insults. However, CT imaging is still a valuable diagnostic tool, especially in detecting small calcified lesions which can be overlooked with MRI.

Classification in Neuroimaging

In the CNS, the cysticercus, by way of the bloodstream, initially invades the subarachnoid space and then the cortical brain, especially at the junction of gray and white matter. On MRI or CT, the lesion may be demonstrated as an ill-defined nodule with minimal enhancement following injection of intravenous contrast medium, indicating the initial inflammatory reaction (Fig. 7.18). Following this, the cysticercus evolves into the *vesicular stage*, which is the viable stage of the parasite and appears as a low-density cyst on CT with minimal peripheral or no contrast enhancement (Fig. 7.19). On MRI, it appears as a hypointense lesion on the T1-weighted image and hyperintense on T2-weighted image with similar intensity to CSF; this lesion may or may not enhance with contrast media and may be associated with surrounding edema (Figs. 7.20–7.25). Commonly, on MRI a central or mural nodule is identified representing the scolex, which is isointense on T1- and T2-weighted images and measures approximately 1–2 mm in diameter (Figs. 7.21–7.25, 7.28).
The cysticercal larva continues to undergo degeneration into the *colloidal stage*, where the cyst enlarges, the vesicular fluid turns dense, and the capsule becomes thickened and lobulated (Figs. 7.26, 7.27). There may be a host inflammatory reaction with formation of perilesional edema and peripheral contrast enhancement. Occasionally, in this stage the lesion can simulate an abscess or a glioma. In the *nodular-granular stage* (Fig. 7.28), there is retraction of the larva with secondary mineralization. On MRI, the lesion may be isointense on T1-weighted images with nodular or ring-like enhancement with perilesional edema. On T2-weighted images the lesion is hypointense with central hyperintensity. In this stage, MRI is more sensitive than CT, and the lesion may simulate a granuloma, a tuberculoma, or a fungal lesion.
In the *calcified stage*, the lesions are small and hyperdense on CT (Fig. 7.29). This is the sequela of nonviable granulomas commonly seen in asymptomatic individuals. On MRI, small calcified lesions may be overlooked. The *miliary type* of parenchymal cysticercosis is seen in childhood and adolescence, and may give rise to clinical encephalitis. This encephalitic form is demonstrated as numerous and diffuse lesions, associated with marked edema. On CT and MRI, these lesions appear small (about 3–5 mm in size), nodular, cystic, and associated with variable degrees of edema, with nodular or ring contrast enhancement (Figs. 7.30–7.32).
The *racemose type* of cysticercosis is a conglomerate of vesicles appearing as multiloculated cystic masses in the subarachnoid basal and sylvian cisterns attaining large size, lacking scolices, and producing significant compromise of the adjacent structures (Figs. 7.33–7.35).
Occasionally, when there is meningeal involvement, an intense inflammatory leptomeningeal reaction and fibrotic thickening producing arachnoiditis occur. In this *arachnoidal type*, the cysticercus cysts are isodense or isointense to CSF on CT and MRI respectively, and may be difficult to detect if they are small. The diagnosis may be inferred by focal deformity of the subarachnoid cisterns. Contrast enhancement of the meninges and obstructive communicating hydrocephalus may be seen on CT and MRI (Figs. 7.36, 7.37). Vasculitis may lead to brain infarcts, most commonly in the distribution of the middle cerebral artery. Digital angiography may be the method of choice to confirm the diagnosis.
In the *intraventricular type*, the cysticercus cyst may be found anywhere in the ventricles, commonly in the midline leading to obstructive hydrocephalus, either acute or chronic (Figs. 7.38–7.43). The wall of the cyst may enhance, secondary to ependymal reaction (Fig. 7.40), and the scolex can be identified at times (Fig. 7.41). The intraventricular lesions may be isodense or isointense with CSF and there may be focal deformity of the affected ventricle (Fig. 7.42). Occasionally, when there is clinical suspicion of ventricular cysticercosis and with no obvious CT and MRI findings of its presence, other studies such as CT ventriculography may be useful to confirm the diagnosis (Fig. 7.43).

(Text continues on p. 669)

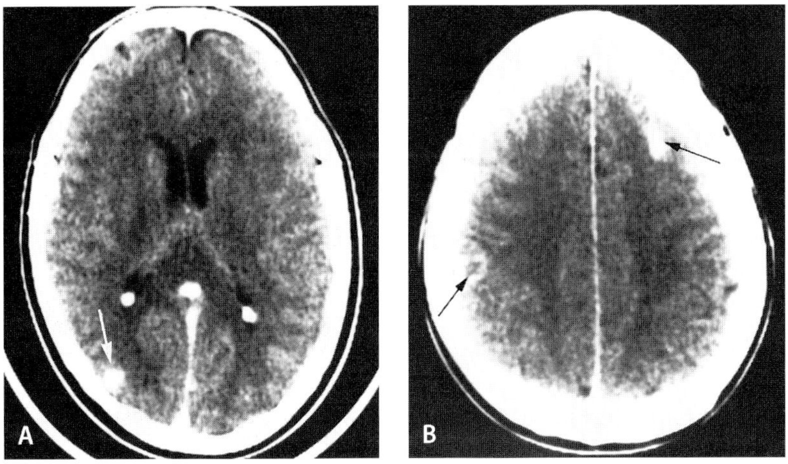

Fig. 7.18 A, B (*left, middle*). Early cortical intraparenchymal cysticercal lesions, prior to vesicular stage. CT axial, postcontrast. **A** Enhancing lesion in the right occipitoparietal area (*arrow*) **B** Enhancing lesions (*arrows*) in another patient. (Courtesy of Dr. Enrique Palacios, Berwyn)

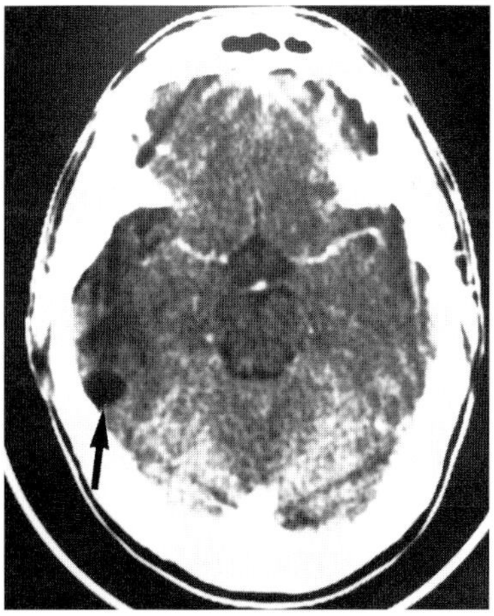

Fig. 7.19 (*right*). Cysticercosis, vesicular stage. CT axial, postcontrast. Cystic lesion in the right temporal area (*arrow*). (Courtesy of Dr. Enrique Palacios, Berwyn)

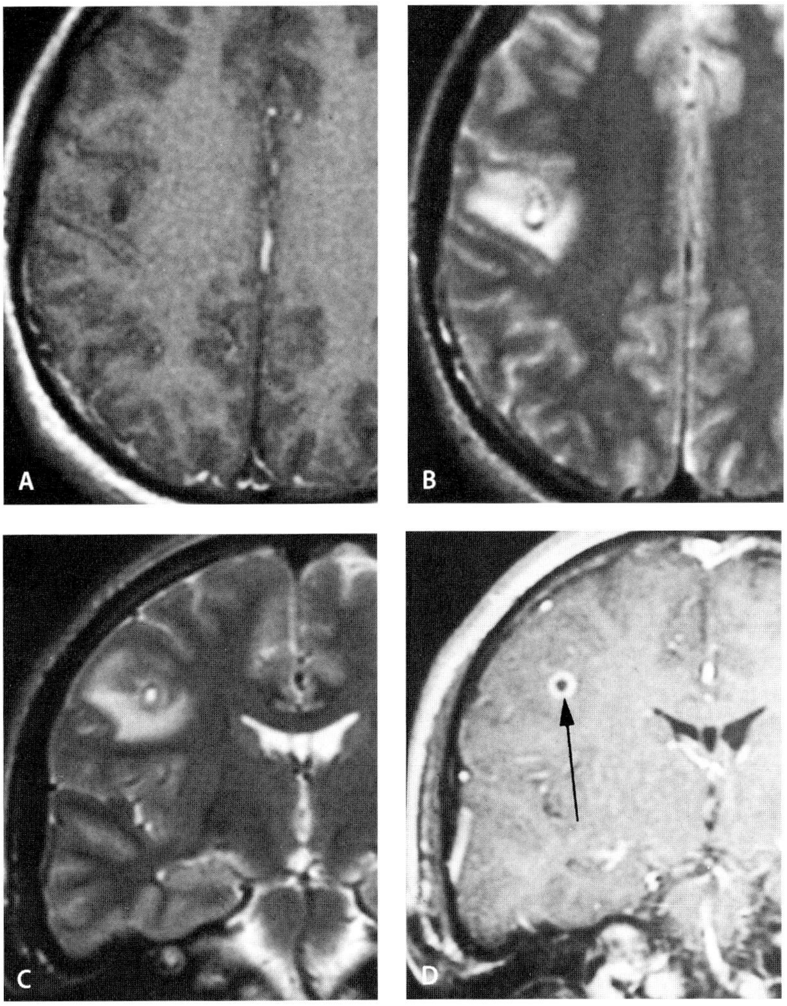

Fig. 7.20 A–D. Cysticercosis, vesicular stage, right parietal area. MRI. **A** Axial T1-weighted image showing a hypointense lesion. **B, C** On axial and coronal T2-weighted images, the lesion is hyperintense and associated with surrounding edema. **D** Coronal T1-weighted image, postcontrast, showing peripheral enhancement of the lesion (*arrow*). (Courtesy of Dr. Enrique Palacios, Berwyn)

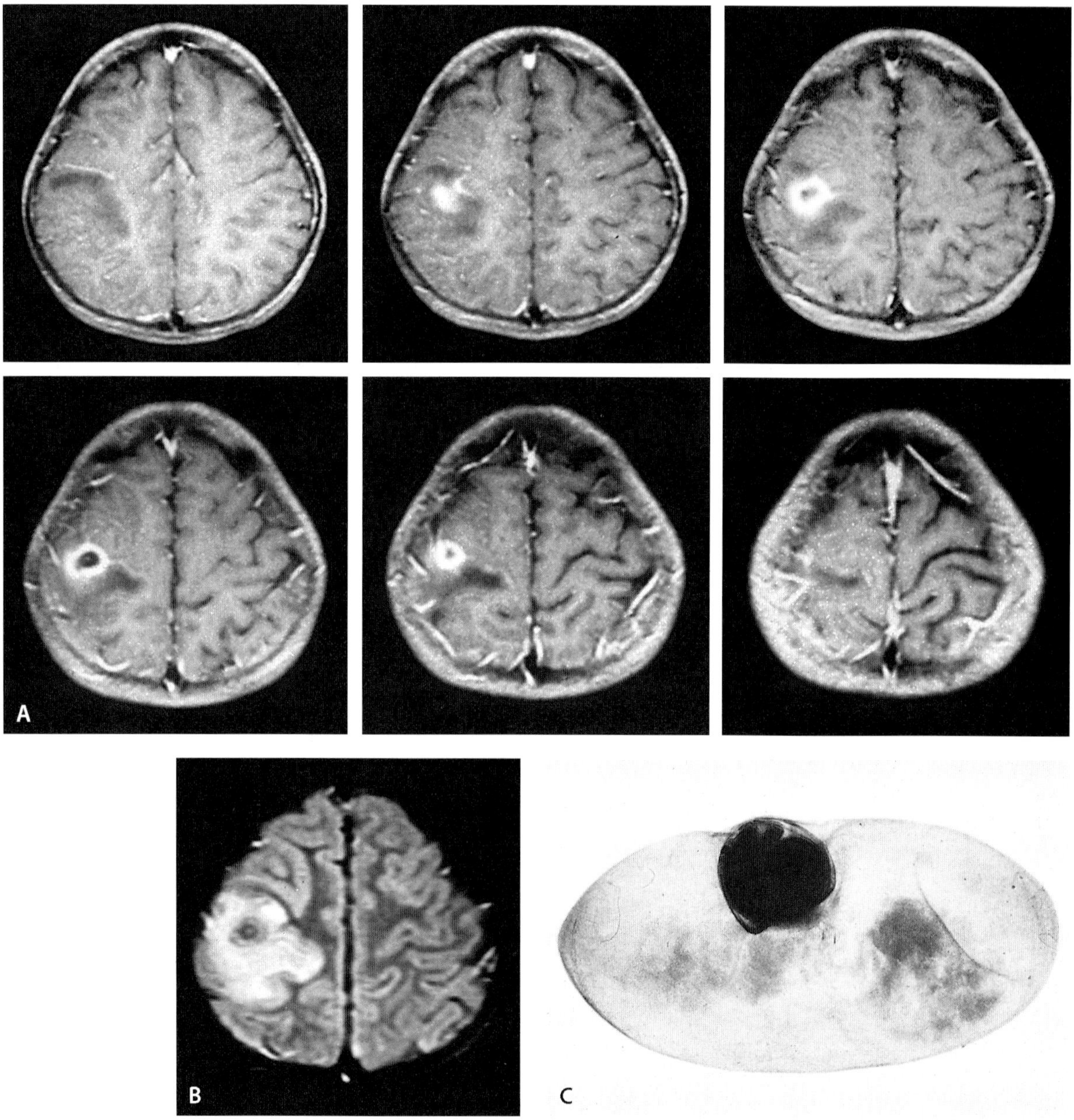

Fig. 7.21 A–C. Neurocysticercosis, vesicular stage, in a Mexican adult. **A** T1-weighted MRI sequence before and after gadolinium enhancement. There is a low signal intensity zone of edema surrounding a single cysticercus, which shows ring enhancement after gadolinium injection. **B** T2-weighted MR image shows intense high-signal edema around the cysticercus. The tiny 2-mm scolex of the cysticercus is visible within the cyst. **C** Cysticercus of *T. solium* with scolex (*top*). (**A**, **B** courtesy of Dr. George Leopold, San Diego)

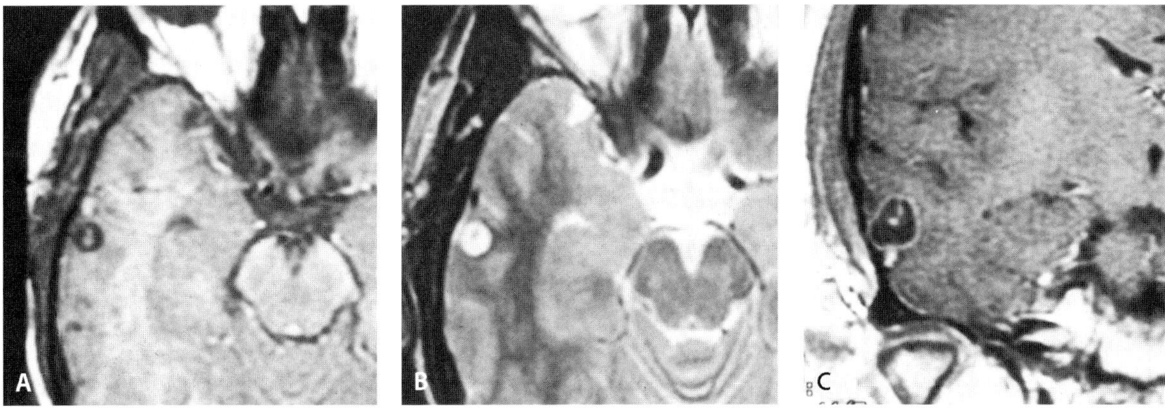

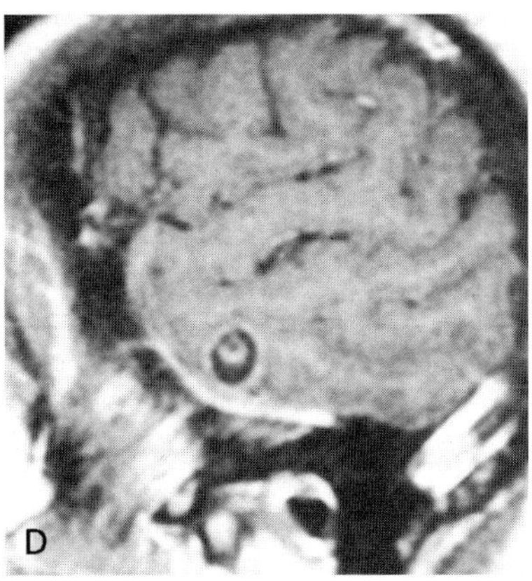

Fig. 7.22 A–D. Single cysticercus, vesicular stage, right temporal cortex. MRI. **A** Axial T1-weighted, **B** axial T2-weighted, **C** coronal T1-weighted, postcontrast, and **D** sagittal, postcontrast images. Note scolex within the cyst. (Courtesy of Dr. Enrique Palacios, Berwyn)

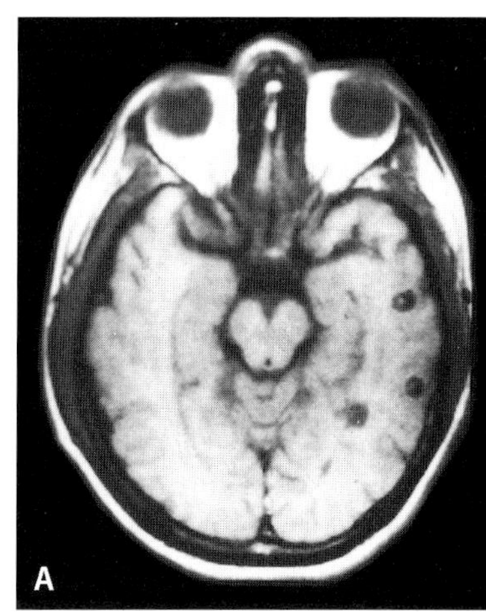

Fig. 7.23 A–D. Cysticercosis, vesicular stage. MRI axial images showing multiple bilateral lesions, including one in the superior fourth ventricle. **A**, **B** T1-weighted images show scolices within the lesions. **C**, **D** T2-weighted images reveal cystic lesions. (Courtesy of Dr. Enrique Palacios, Berwyn)

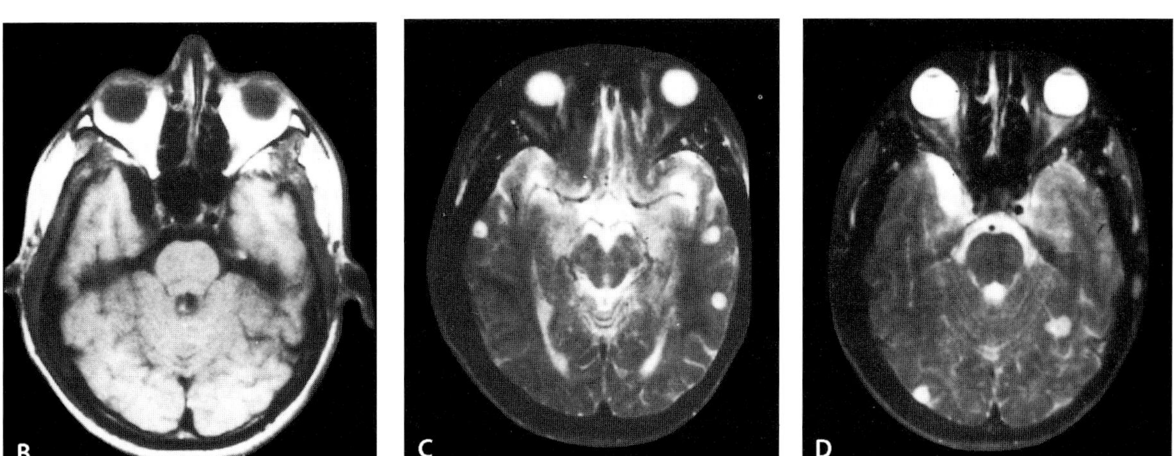

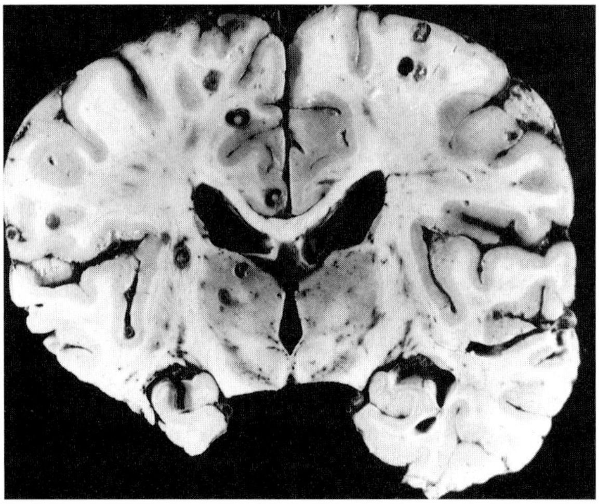

Fig. 7.24. Parenchymal cysticercosis, multiple lesions. Pathological specimen in coronal plane. The cysticerci in the vesicular stage are scattered in both gray and white matter, including the right thalamus. (Courtesy of Dr. Enrique Palacios, Berwyn)

Fig. 7.25 A–D. Neurocysticercosis with numerous cystic parenchymal lesions, vesicular stage, throughout the brain of a middle-aged Norwegian sailor who had traveled throughout the world. He was admitted to Queen's Medical Center in Honolulu, Hawaii for evaluation of multiple neurological symptoms. T1-weighted coronal (**A**) and axial (**B**) MR images reveal multiple small cysts approximately 1 cm in size scattered throughout the cerebral hemispheres and basal ganglia. Some cysticerci are in paraventricular locations and others contain a well-defined 2-mm scolex within the cyst contents (*arrow* in **B**). **C** Coronal image obtained after gadolinium injection shows ring enhancement of many cysticerci. The cerebellum and midbrain are involved as well as the cerebral hemispheres. Note the paraventricular cysticercal nodules. **D** T2-weighted axial view shows numerous cysticercal cysts containing high signal intensity fluid, as well as intense high-signal edema surrounding many cysts in the brain parenchyma. (Courtesy of Drs. Stephen Holmes and Michael Meagher, Honolulu)

▼

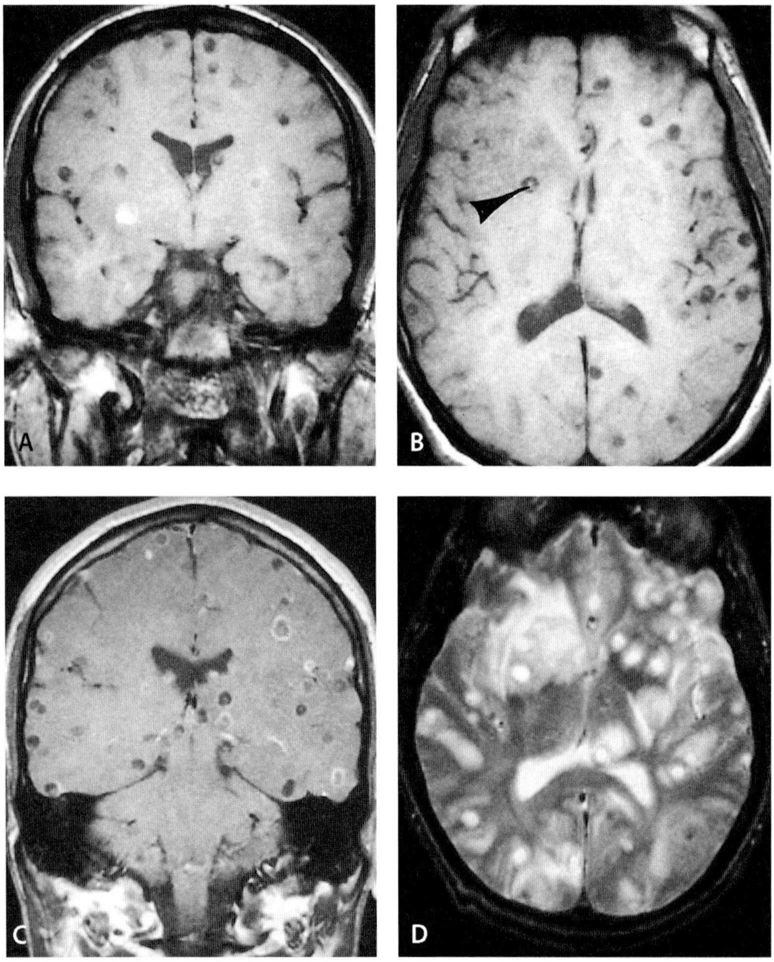

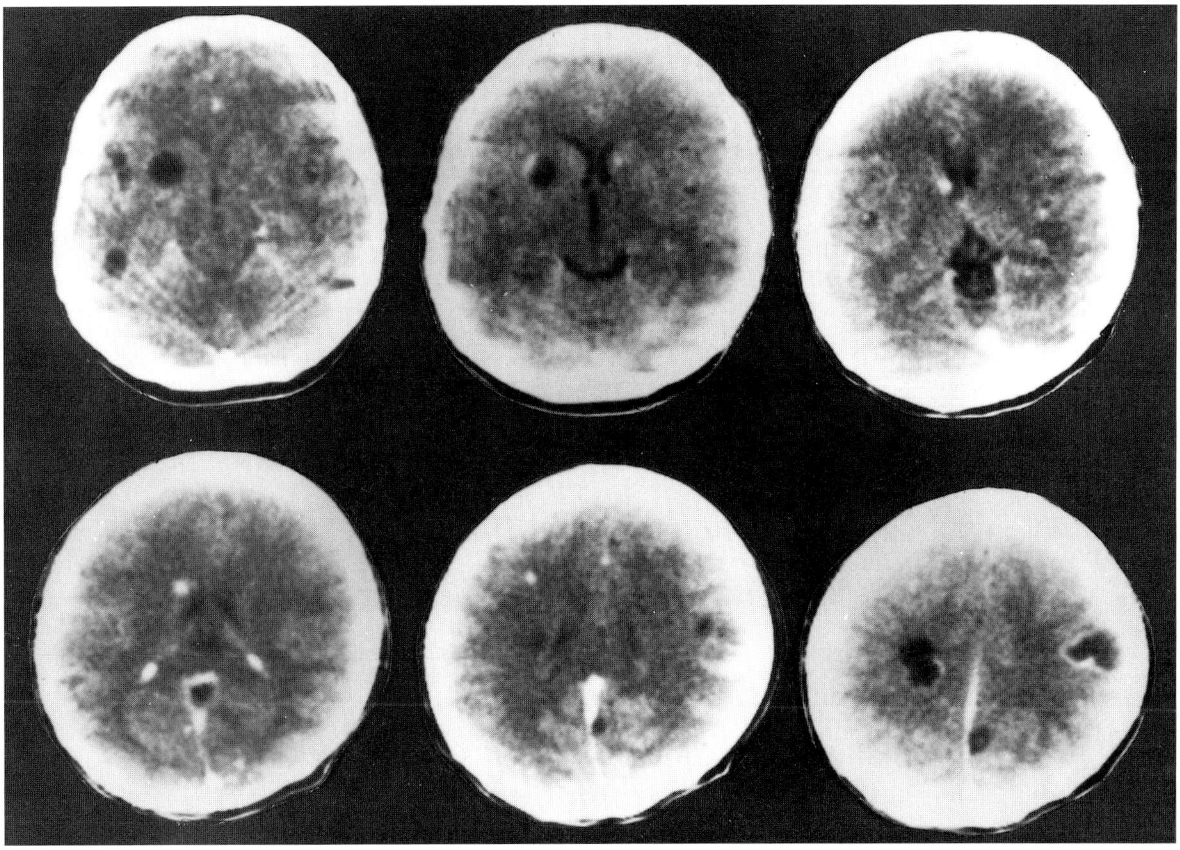

▲
Fig. 7.26. Bilateral cystic parenchymal lesions, vesicular and colloidal stages, with minimal enhancement. CT axial plane, multiple sections, postcontrast. Note also other calcified cysticerci. (Courtesy of Dr. Enrique Palacios, Berwyn)

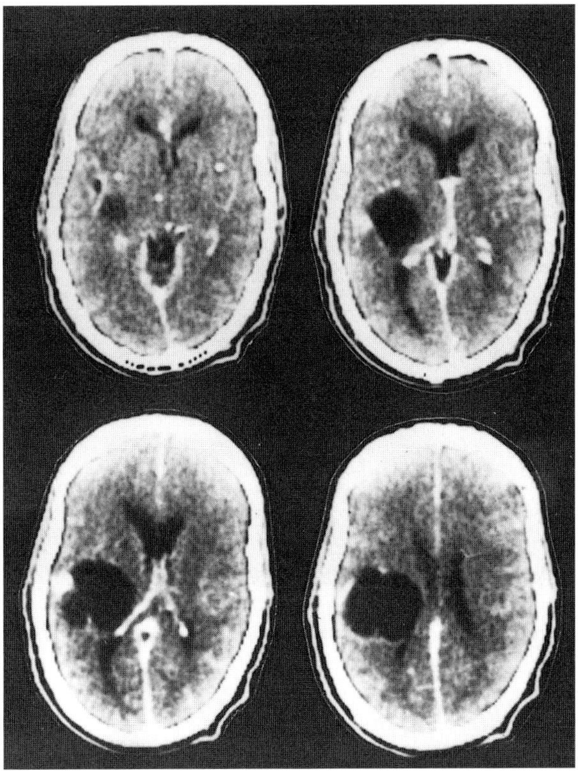

◀
Fig. 7.27. Cysticercal lesion, colloidal stage. CT axial, multiple sections, postcontrast. Large lobulated cyst in the right temporal area extending into the posterior basal ganglia with peripheral enhancement. (Courtesy of Dr. Enrique Palacios, Berwyn)

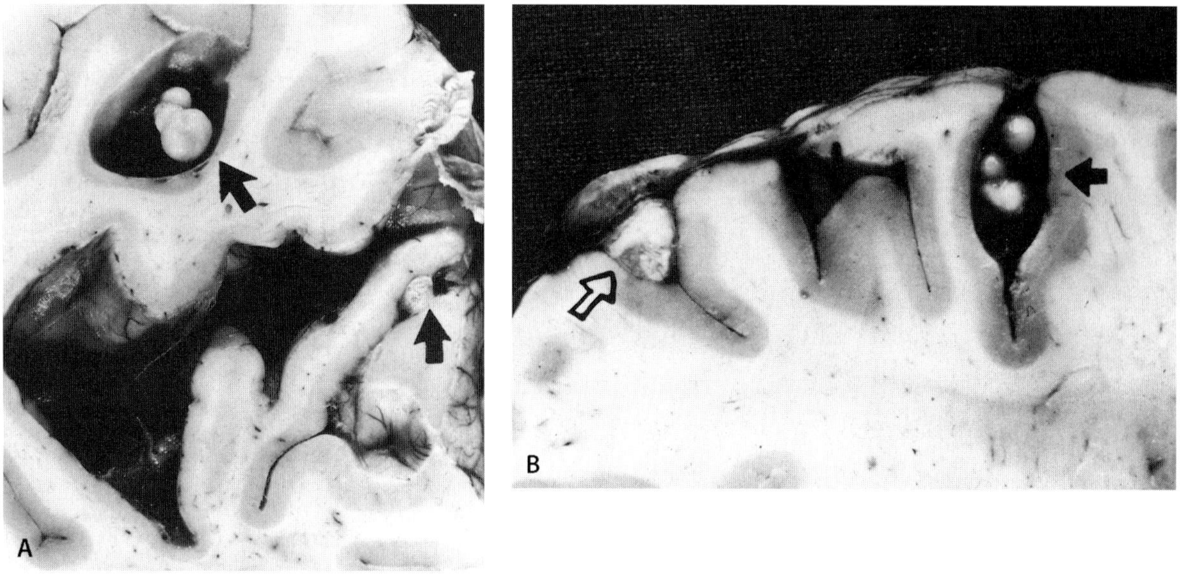

Fig. 7.28 A, B. Cysticerci, vesicular and nodular-granular stages, pathological specimens. **A** One vesicular cyst showing its larva lies burrowed between convolutions of the brain (*upper arrow*). A second cysticercus is undergoing hyalinization and mineralization corresponding to the nodular-granular stage (*lower arrow*). **B** A live cysticercus in the vesicular stage lies burrowed between two convolutions, showing its larva (*solid arrow*). There is also a cysticercus undergoing mineralization corresponding to the nodular-granular stage (*open arrow*). (Courtesy of Dr. Alfonso Escobar)

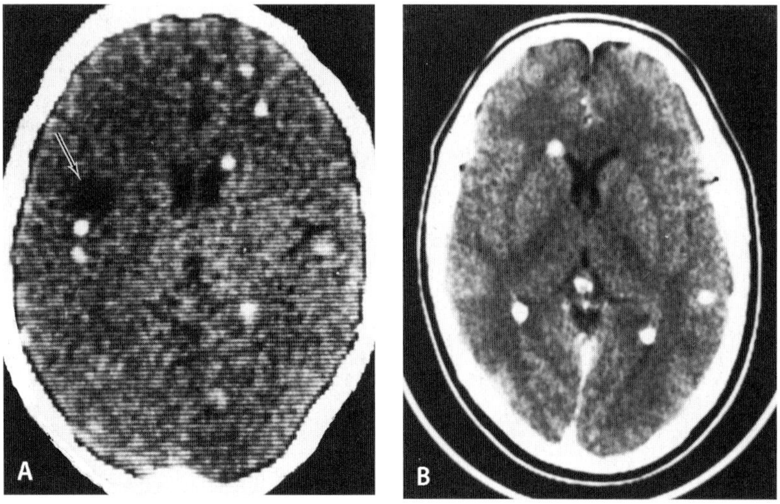

Fig. 7.29 A, B. Cysticercosis with multiple scattered lesions in the calcified stage. **A** CT axial. An associated lesion in the vesicular stage is also present on the right (*arrow*). **B** CT axial, postcontrast, in a different patient. Calcified lesions are present in the right frontal and left temporo-occipital areas. (Courtesy of Dr. Enrique Palacios, Berwyn)

Fig. 7.30 A, B. Diffuse miliary or encephalitic type cysticercosis. CT axial, multiple sections. **A** Precontrast enhancement. There is extensive symmetrical edema. **B** Postcontrast study reveals numerous bilateral enhancing lesions. (Courtesy of Dr. Enrique Palacios, Berwyn) ▶

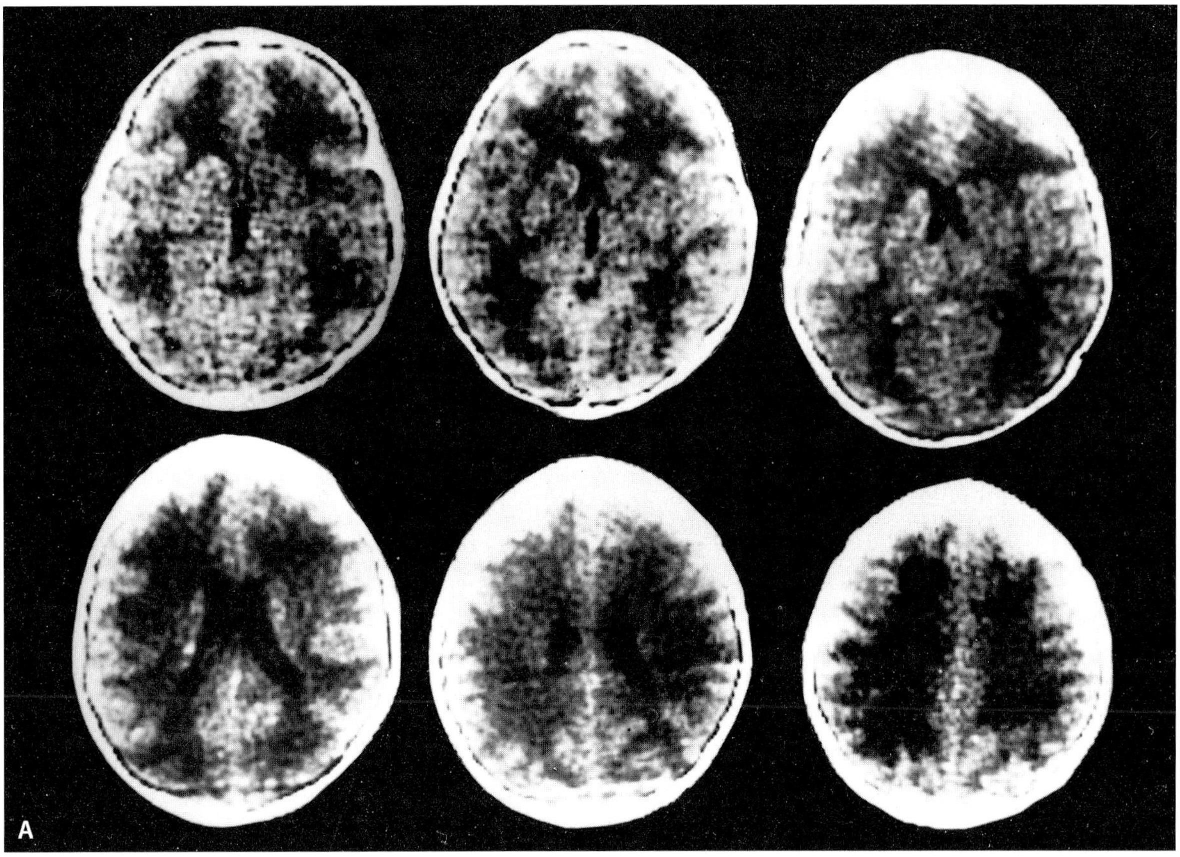
A

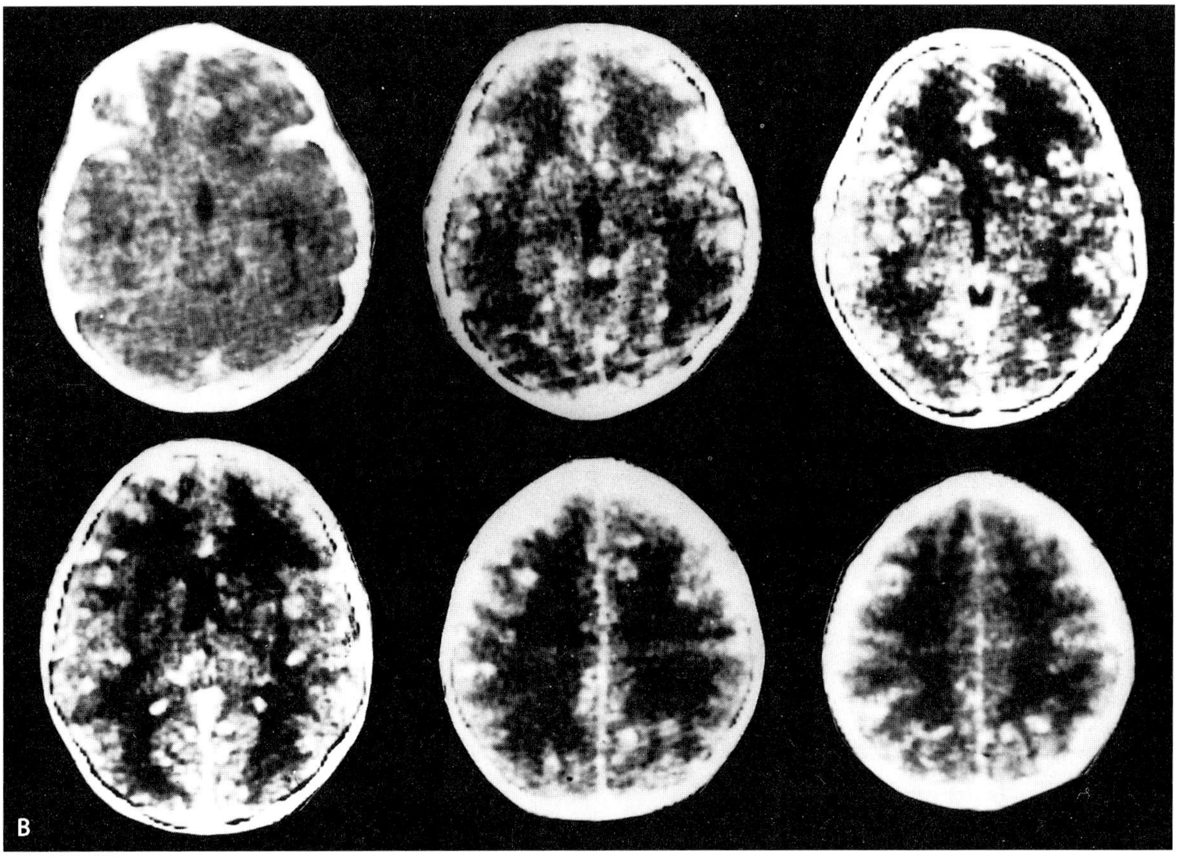
B

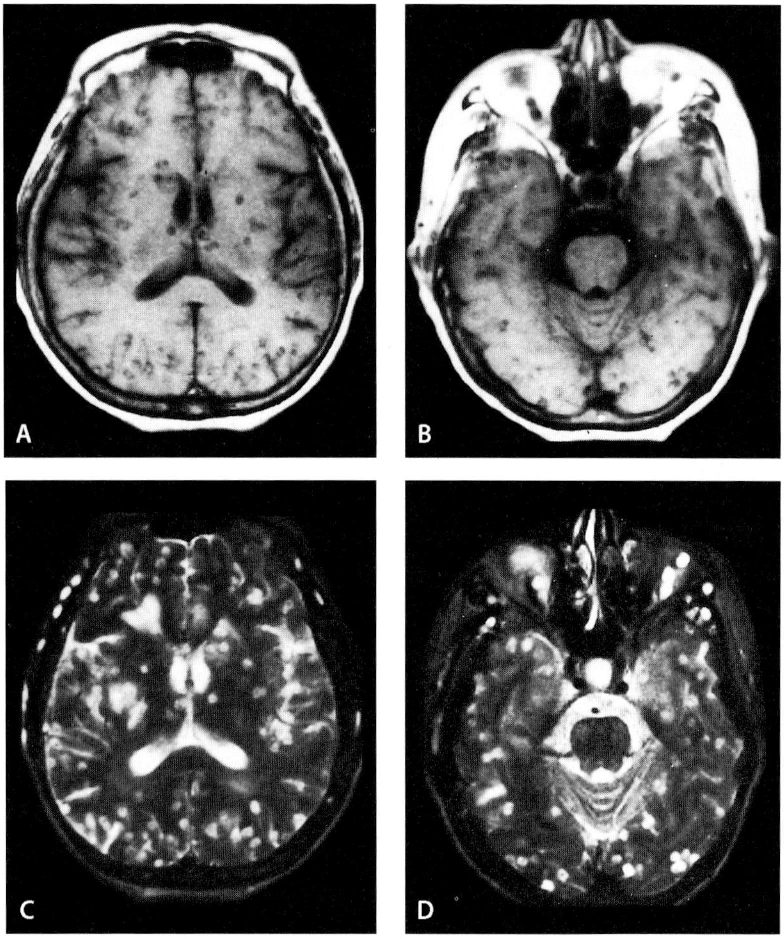

Fig. 7.31 A–D. Parenchymal cysticercosis, diffuse miliary type. MRI axial. Numerous cysticerci are noted bilaterally after a diffuse edema subsided. Lesions are also present in the orbits and subcutaneous soft tissues. **A, B** T1-weighted images; **C, D** T2-weighted images. (Courtesy of Dr. Enrique Palacios, Berwyn)

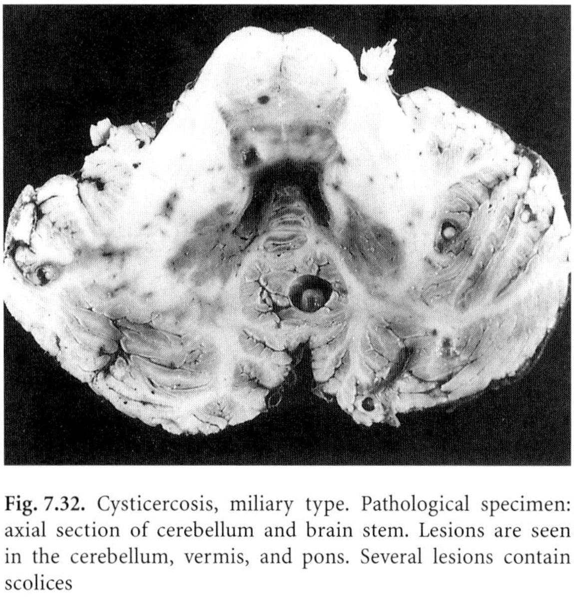

Fig. 7.32. Cysticercosis, miliary type. Pathological specimen: axial section of cerebellum and brain stem. Lesions are seen in the cerebellum, vermis, and pons. Several lesions contain scolices

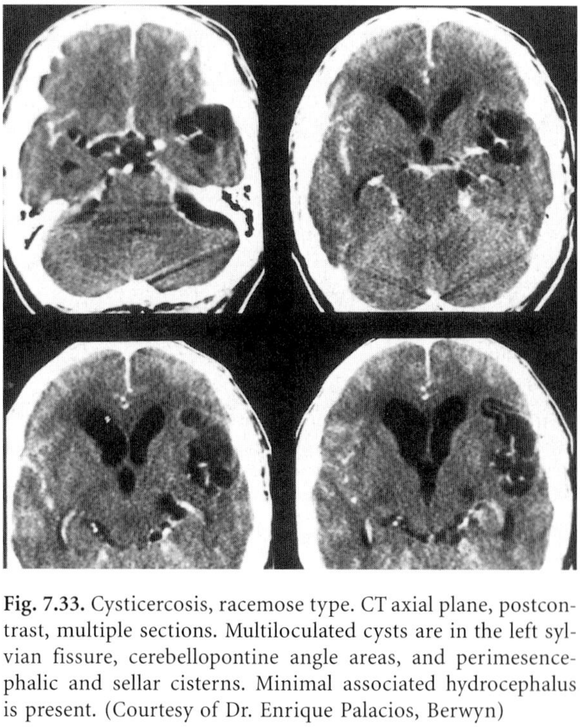

Fig. 7.33. Cysticercosis, racemose type. CT axial plane, postcontrast, multiple sections. Multiloculated cysts are in the left sylvian fissure, cerebellopontine angle areas, and perimesencephalic and sellar cisterns. Minimal associated hydrocephalus is present. (Courtesy of Dr. Enrique Palacios, Berwyn)

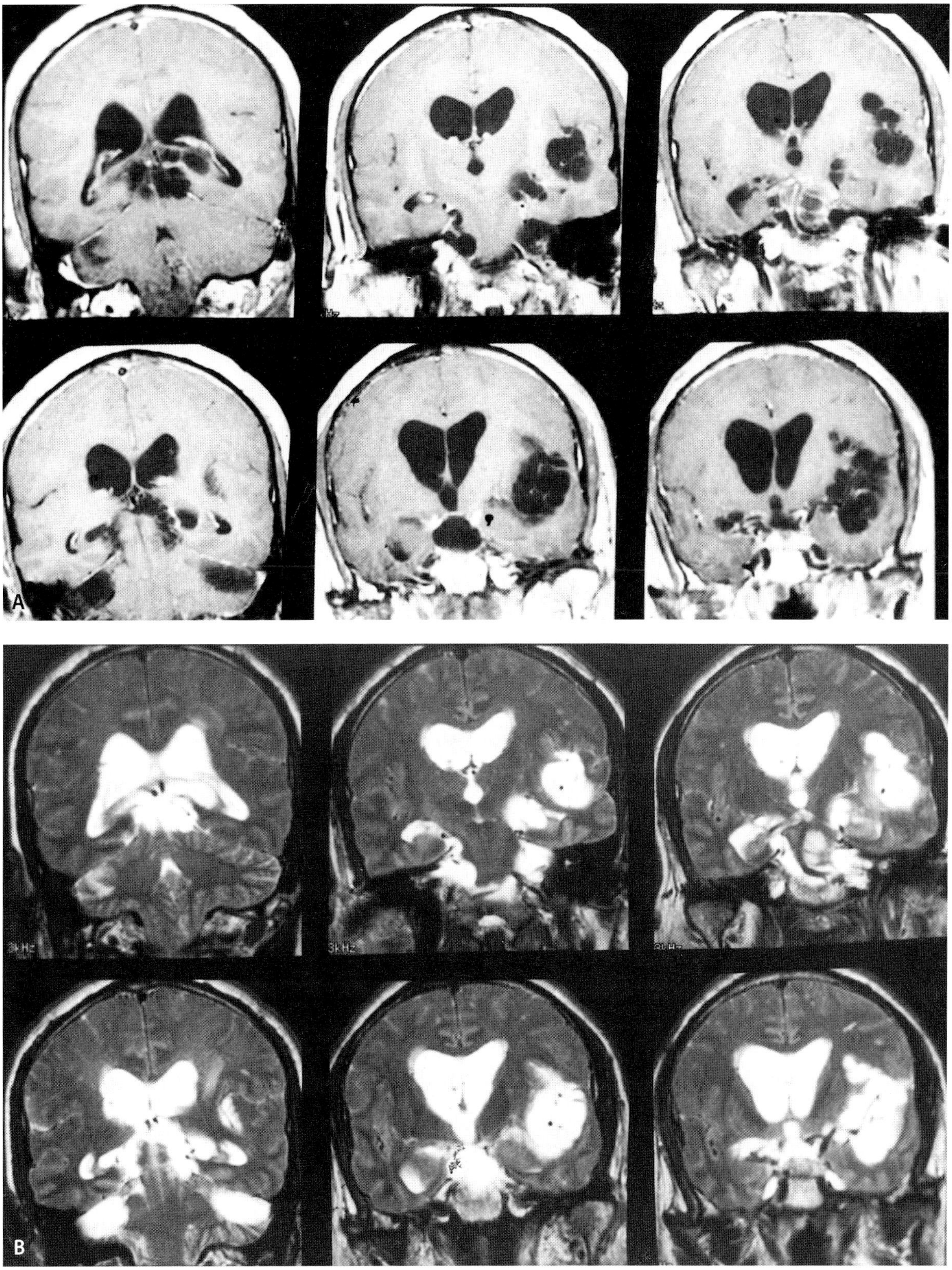

Fig. 7.34 A, B. Cysticercosis, racemose type. Same patient as in Fig. 7.33. MRI coronal, multiple sections. **A** T1-weighted, post-contrast images. **B** T2-weighted images. (Courtesy of Dr. Enrique Palacios, Berwyn)

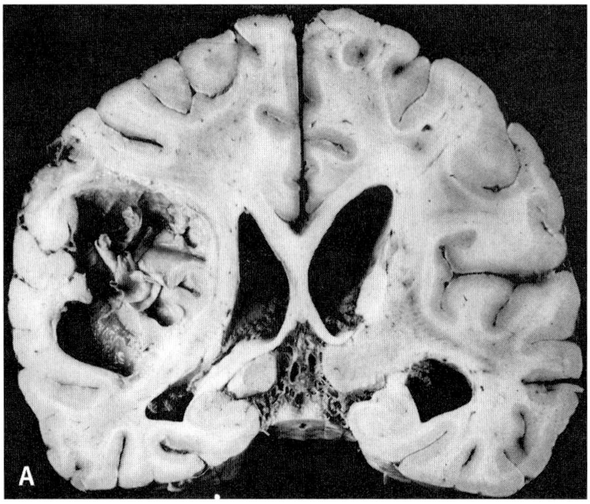

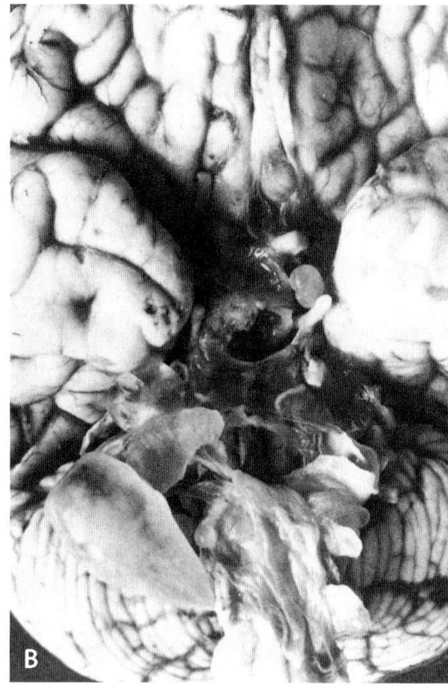

Fig. 7.35 A, B. Racemose type cysticercosis. **A** Specimen of brain in coronal plane reveals a large lobulated cystic mass in the right sylvian fissure. There is marked expansion of the fissure with compression of the adjacent structures. **B** Specimen of base of brain reveals numerous cystic lesions in the posterior fossa, cerebellopontine angle, and sellar areas. (Courtesy of Dr. Alfonso Escobar)

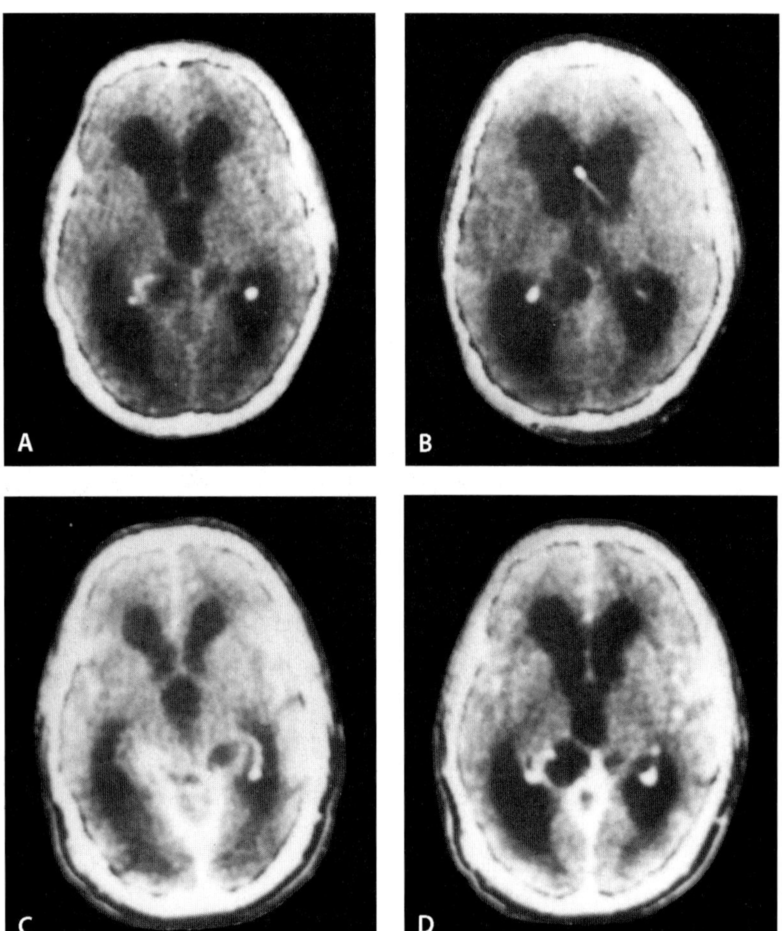

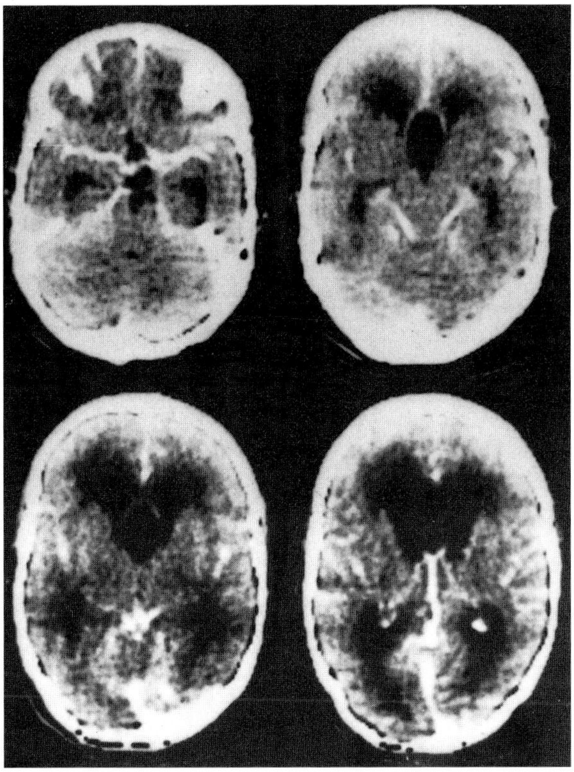

Fig. 7.37. Arachnoidal and intraventricular cysticercosis. CT axial, multiple sections, postcontrast. A cysticercus cyst in the anterior third ventricle has produced obstructive hydrocephalus. Note also contrast enhancement of the tentorium and perimesencephalic cisterns secondary to meningeal involvement. (Courtesy of Dr. Enrique Palacios, Berwyn)

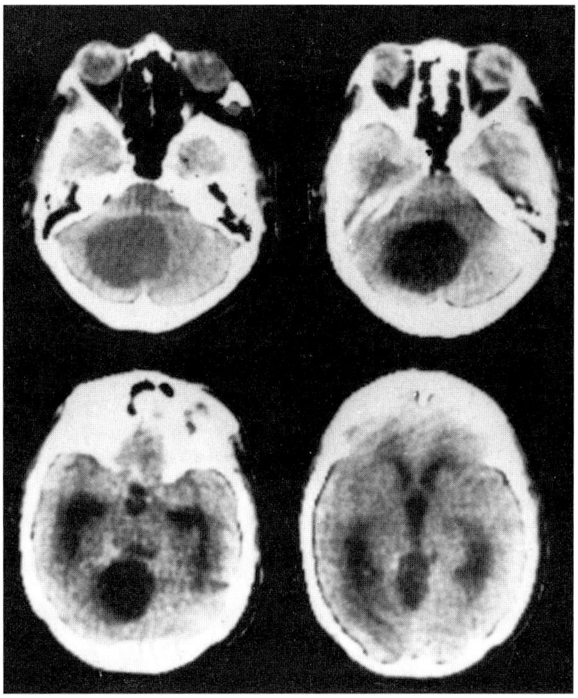

Fig. 7.38. Intraventricular cysticercosis. A large cysticercus occupies the fourth ventricle causing obstructive hydrocephalus. CT axial, multiple sections. (Courtesy of Dr. Enrique Palacios, Berwyn)

◀ **Fig. 7.36 A–D.** Arachnoidal type cysticercosis. CT axial. **A, B** Precontrast. **C, D** Postcontrast. Perimesencephalic lesions are identified with marked enhancing meningeal reaction producing obstructive communicating hydrocephalus. (Courtesy of Dr. Enrique Palacios, Berwyn)

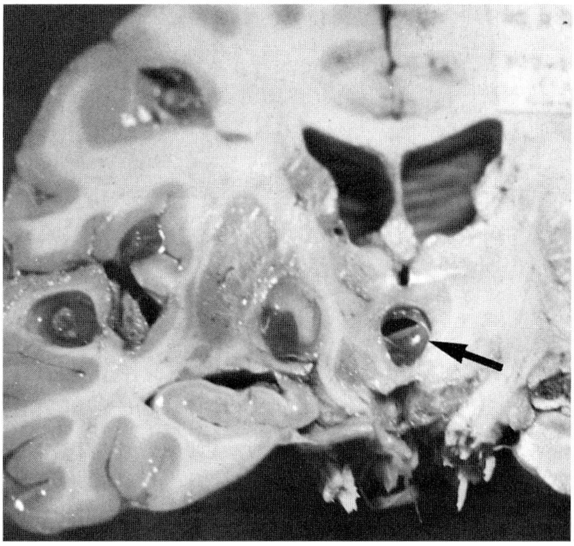

Fig. 7.39. Intraventricular and parenchymal cysticercosis. Pathological specimen, coronal section. Lesions are seen in the right temporal area, basal ganglia, and third ventricle (*arrow*). (Courtesy of Dr. Enrique Palacios, Berwyn)

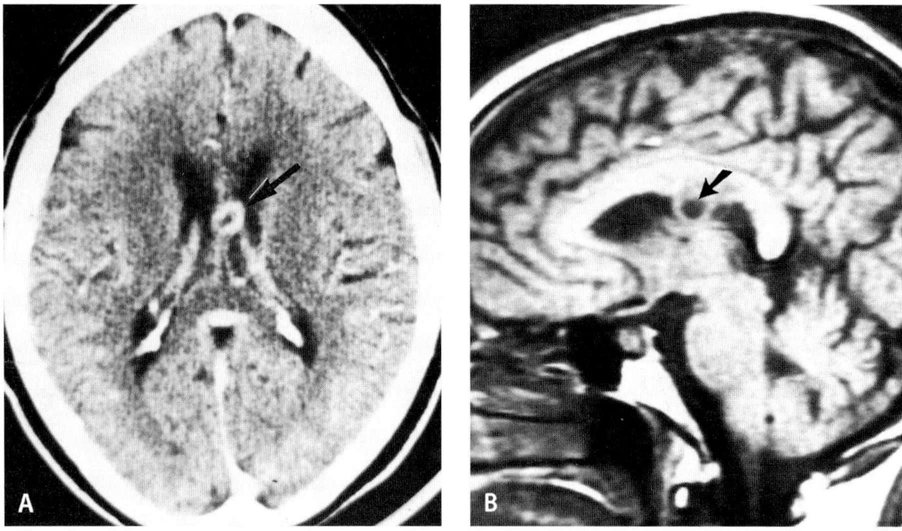

▲

Fig. 7.40 A, B. Small cysticercus cyst in the roof of the third ventricle. **A** Axial CT, postcontrast study, showing ring enhancement of the lesion (*arrow*). **B** Sagittal MRI, T1-weighted image, confirms the location of the cyst (*arrow*). (Courtesy of Dr. Enrique Palacios, Berwyn)

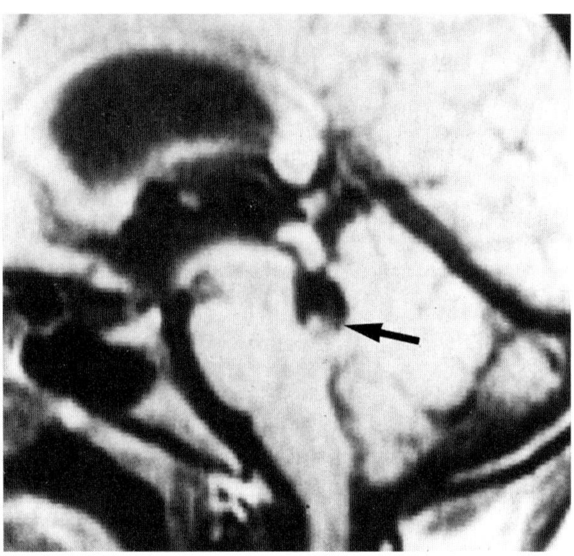

◀

Fig. 7.41. Intraventricular cysticercosis. Small cyst in the fourth ventricle producing hydrocephalus. MRI sagittal plane, T1-weighted image. Note scolex in the inferior portion of the cyst (*arrow*). (Courtesy of Dr. Francisco Garcia)

Fig. 7.42 A, B. Large cysticercus cyst in the trigone of the right lateral ventricle identified on MRI. **A** Sagittal T1-weighted and **B** axial T1-weighted images, postcontrast. There is significant compression of the quadrigeminal plate and posterior third ventricle. (Courtesy of Dr. Enrique Palacios, Berwyn)

▼

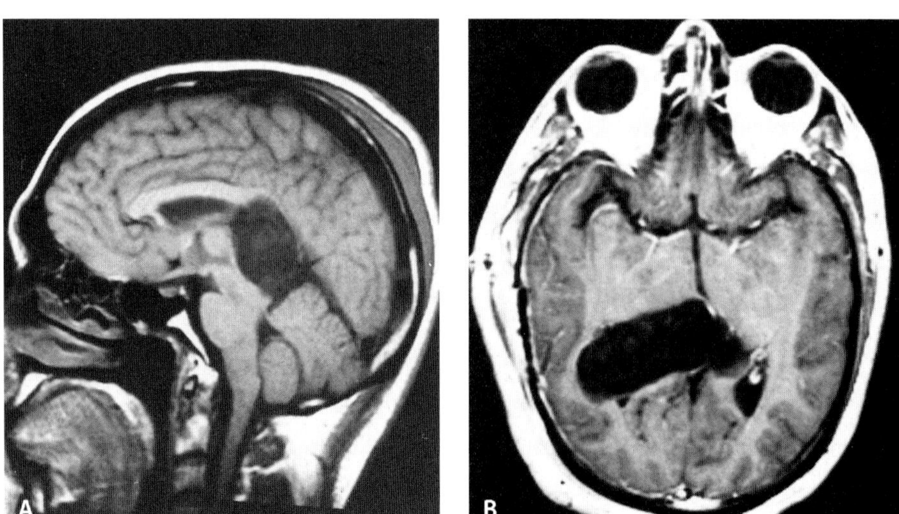

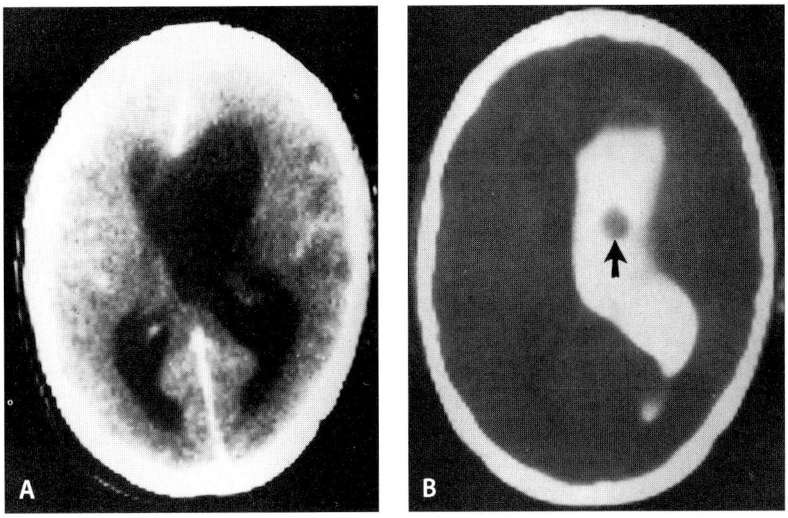

Fig. 7.43 A, B. Intraventricular cysticercus cyst within the left lateral ventricle with ipsilateral dilatation from obstruction of the foramen of Monro. A Axial CT. B CT ventriculogram: following opacification of the left lateral ventricle, a cysticercus cyst is evident (*arrow*). (Courtesy of Dr. Enrique Palacios, Berwyn)

Intraspinal neurocysticercosis is very rare (less than 1% of patients with neurocysticercosis) and may occur in combination with cerebral infection or separately. Conventional radiographs of the spine do not show any abnormality. Myelography may demonstrate intradural, extramedullary filling defects of different sizes, but more or less spherical in shape. In other patients, there will only be marked irregularity, deformity, or fragmentation of the column of contrast material, secondary to arachnoiditis. Complete obstruction may occur, probably associated with the nonspecific arachnoiditis, similar to basal arachnoiditis in the skull. It is helpful that, in most patients, complement fixing tests on CSF will be positive.

Magnetic resonance imaging is the diagnostic method of choice in patients suspected of having intraspinal cysticercosis. The cysticerci are more commonly found in the subarachnoid space and appear as cystic or lobulated masses, isointense or hyperintense to spinal fluid (Figs. 7.44–7.46). Occasionally, because of its isointensity, the lesion may be difficult to locate, particularly when there is associated inflammatory reaction and arachnoiditis. In these cases, when clinically indicated, myelography and CT postmyelography may complement the MRI study. An intramedullary cysticercus appears as a cystic mass on T1-weighted images, with peripheral enhancement with contrast medium. Mural enhancement and a nodule corresponding to the scolex may also be seen (Fig. 7.47).

Although there are no specific findings in spinal cysticercosis, this possibility should be considered where there are smooth, spherical intradural defects found on myelography, or lobulated or cystic masses on CT or MRI, particularly where the disease is endemic or in those who have been exposed to the possibility of infection.

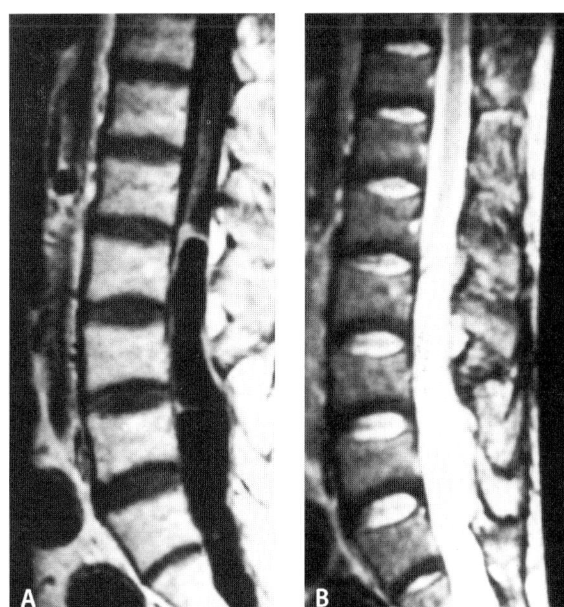

Fig. 7.44 A, B. Intraspinal cysticercosis, lumbar area. Multiple large cystic lesions within the subarachnoid space, isointense to spinal fluid. MRI sagittal plane. A T1-weighted and B T2-weighted images. (Courtesy of Dr. Alavaro C. Magalhaes)

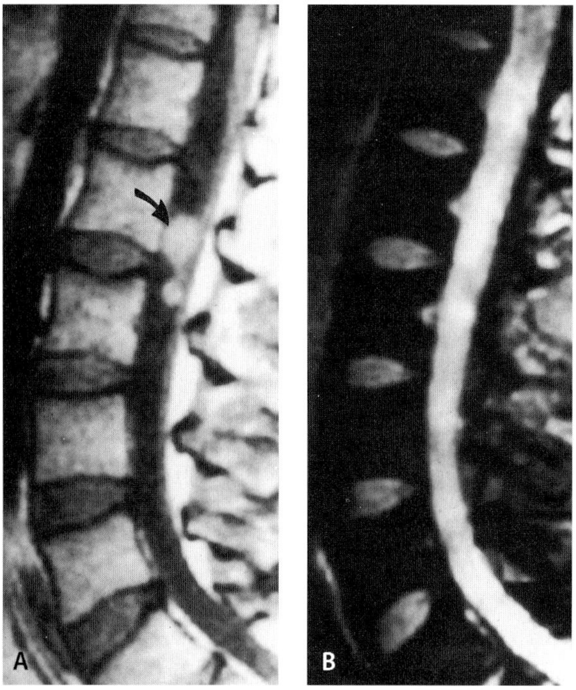

Fig. 7.45 A, B. Intraspinal cysticercosis, lumbar area. MRI sagittal plane. **A** T1-weighted image identifies a lobulated mass (*arrow*) in the subarachnoid space, isointense to the conus medullaris. **B** On a T2-weighted gradient-echo image, the mass is slightly hyperintense to spinal fluid. The lesion was demonstrated to move in position on subsequent examinations. (Courtesy of Drs. David Garza Cruz, Olivia Jimenez Flores, and Hugo Arredondo Estrada)

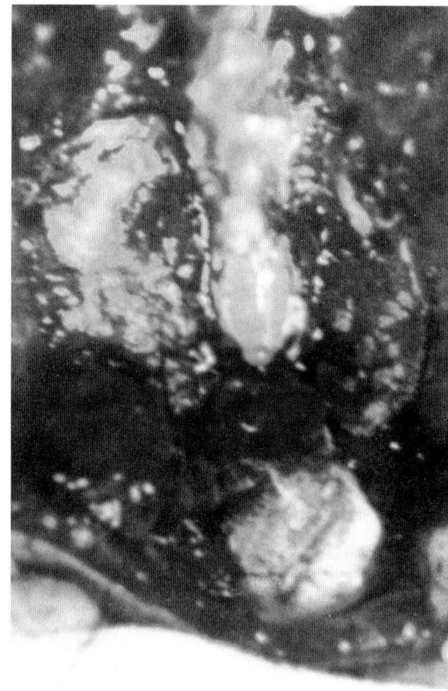

Fig. 7.46. Intraspinal cysticercosis in a Mexican patient. Photograph taken at the time of surgical removal shows a large cysticercus cyst (*center*) bulging from the spinal canal at the operative site. (Courtesy of Dr. Jorge Ceballos-Labat, Mexico City)

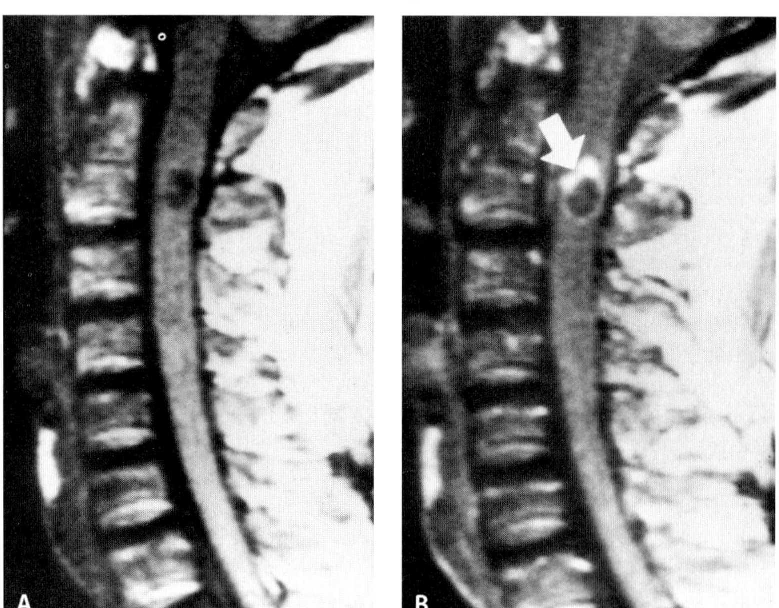

Fig. 7.47 A, B. Intraspinal cysticercosis, proximal cervical area. MRI sagittal plane. **A** T1-weighted image reveals an intramedullary cystic lesion with a scolex within the cyst. **B** T2-weighted postcontrast image shows marked mural enhancement (*arrow*). (Courtesy of Drs. K.H. Chang, S.Y. Cho, J.R. Hesselink et al. and *Neuroimaging Clin North Am*, 1991)

Challenges in Treatment

Neurocysticercosis remains a very challenging clinical and socioeconomic problem in endemic areas. Medical treatment using cysticidal drugs, e.g., praziquantel (a pyrazinoisoquinolone compound) and albendazole (a benzimidazole compound), and surgical intervention continue to evolve. Neuroimaging undoubtedly plays an important role in the understanding of the pathophysiology and in the management of this disorder. However, much work remains to be done, particularly in the areas of sanitation and education in the epidemiology of cysticercosis.

Differential Diagnosis

When calcified cysticerci are clearly seen in muscle planes, their oval or ellipsoid shape is unlikely to be mistaken for other calcifications (e.g., granulomas or other parasites such as *Sparganum, Armillifer,* or *Loa loa*). When seen "end on," the cysticerci cannot be identified as such. Difficulty occurs in the brain when there is no calcification and the cysts cause a cerebral "mass effect"; in such patients, CT and/or MRI with contrast enhancement will usually suggest the correct etiology.

Sparganosis

Until a few years ago, sparganosis was of no real interest to radiologists. In the first edition of this book it was discussed in six lines because there were no significant images. However, CT and MRI have altered that by making the worm and its surrounding chronic and granulomatous inflammation visible within the brain. Sparganosis must now be added to the differential diagnosis for patients with severe headaches, seizures, hemiparesis, or other CNS symptoms and signs.

The first human infection by a sparganum was detected by Manson in 1882, a discovery acknowledged by the name given to the responsible tapeworm, *Spirometra mansoni* (and also to a second species, *S. mansonoides*, not recognized until 1935). Although the CNS infections are the most dramatic, there are many other presentations which, if not of prime radiological importance, are more than a minor irritation for the unfortunate patients. Prevention is relatively easy, treatment is not; the foibles and tastes of humanity so often ignore caution that this tapeworm must be added to the list of those which, if they live in the patient long enough, can cause death, at least in those unfortunate individuals infected with the rare *S. proliferum* species.

Synonyms

Cestodiasis (a general term). Spirometrosis. Sparganum infection. Larval diphyllobothriasis (an older term).

Definition

Sparganosis or spirometrosis is infection by a sparganum, the second stage (plerocercoid) larva of a pseudophyllidean tapeworm of the genus *Spirometra* of the family *Diphyllobothriidae*. There are at least three species of *Spirometra* (and about 13 of the genus *Diphyllobothrium*) which infect humans. The more common nonproliferative form of sparganosis is caused by *Spirometra mansoni* or *S. mansonoides*. The proliferative, systemic form of sparganosis is caused by *S. proliferum* and is very rare. The exact definition of an infection in a patient should specify the causative species.

Geographic Distribution

Human sparganosis is found worldwide, but most frequently in China, Korea, Japan, Taiwan, and elsewhere in Southeast Asia. Infections have been reported in the Southeastern United States, and elsewhere in the Americas, and from East Africa. The adult tapeworms are found in domestic cats and in wild carnivores in tropical and subtropical regions of America, Asia, Australia, and Africa. Frogs, snakes, birds, and small mammals can also be infected.

Spirometra mansoni is the usual cause of infection in China, Japan, and Southeast Asia, whereas *S. mansonoides* is the more likely cause in the Americas. The rare *S. proliferum* is found in Japan and Southeast Asia, with at least three cases reported in the Americas.

Epidemiology and Pathology

The life cycle of the *Spirometra* involves several hosts. The definitive hosts are dogs, cats, and wild carnivores and the *Spirometra* live in their intestines. Eggs are shed in the feces and hatch in stagnant fresh water: the motile, ciliated coracidia which are released are eaten by the first intermediate host, a cyclops in which they develop into procercoid larvae. When these tiny crustaceans are eaten by fish, snakes, amphibians, or mammals, including humans (the second intermediate hosts), the larvae penetrate the intestinal wall, becoming plerocercoids, and spread throughout the body, especially to muscles and subcutaneous tissues. Here the plerocercoid or sparganum develops and encysts, awaiting completion of its life cycle when a dog, cat, or other carnivore consumes the infected flesh. The sparganum then develops into an adult tapeworm within the small intestine of its final host. Adult worms are variously estimated to survive from 10 to 30 years. Human sparganosis is acquired in three different ways:

1. By drinking contaminated water in which there is an infected cyclops, the most common method of transmission in the United States.
2. By eating infected raw or undercooked flesh containing spargana.
3. By use of a poultice of raw infected flesh applied to skin, conjunctiva, or mucosa. This is a common treatment in parts of Asia where the poultice may be applied to an open wound, allowing the worm in the infected flesh to crawl directly into human tissues, thus making the patient an unwitting intermediate host. Raw pork, frogs, and snakes used in this way, or eaten, are the most likely reservoirs for spargana.

There are two forms of sparganosis, the proliferative and the nonproliferative. In the much more common nonproliferative form, when the worm is alive there is little tissue reaction as the sparganum migrates through the host. There may be eosinophilia or leukocytosis. A live sparganum may be seen as a white glistening and slowly undulating flat, ribbon-like worm, from 2 mm to 10 cm or more in length (Fig. 7.48). Each sparganum varies in width, having some broad areas and other narrow, string-like areas (Fig. 7.49 A). The worm, which moves slowly and less often encysts in the abnormal human host, can leave a track of focal necrosis surrounded by chronic inflammation and numerous eosinophils. If the sparganum dies, a granuloma or an abscess surrounds the carcass. There is a fibrous tissue and chronic inflammatory reaction also, including focal areas of eosinophilia and often Charcot-Leyden crystals.

In the CNS, the granulomatous reaction is similar, with adjacent gliosis, which may be dense, and associated acute and chronic inflammation. The dead sparganum is usually found centrally within the lesion. Worms have also been found in the subarachnoid space.

The proliferative form of sparganosis produces similar granulomas, but these are much more widespread; there may be thousands of granulomatous cysts within the infected tissues, including the CNS. These granulomatous cysts match the size of the sparganum they contain. Some descriptions of *S. proliferum* refer to continuous branching and budding, unorganized and without symmetry. Some

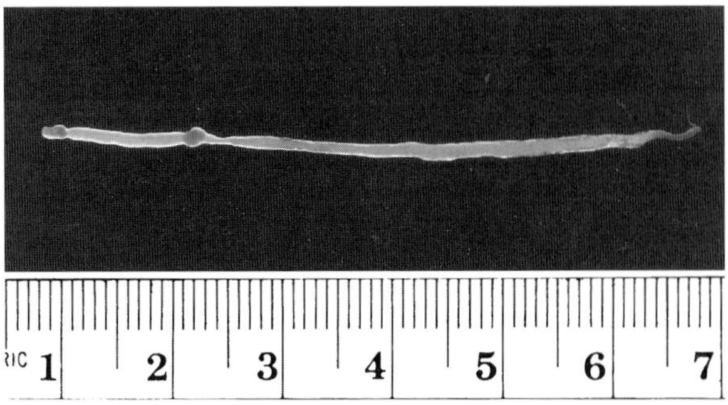

Fig. 7.48. Sparganum, the larval phase of the tapeworm *Spirometra*, can survive in damp surroundings for several days, which is why contaminated poultices used in wound dressings may lead to human sparganosis. This plerocercoid larva, or sparganum, was removed from the skin of the abdomen of a white tree frog (*Litoria caerulea*), a native of Australia. It was kept in tap water and tied itself in two knots. (Courtesy of Prof. J.H. Theis, Davis)

authorities believe that *S. proliferum* is an aberrant type of the nonproliferative sparganum, but recent studies have shown it to be a unique species of sparganum. The adult worm has not been identified.

Laboratory Diagnosis

An accurate diagnosis can be made in two ways: either by identifying the sparganum (Fig. 7.49 B) or by the antisparganum IgG antibody enzyme-linked assay that is over 96% sensitive and specific. However, MRI and CT cerebral scanning have a significant role in establishing the diagnosis. Both can show unilateral or bilateral lesions that vary in size and shape, and often change in position on subsequent scans.

Clinical Characteristics

The more common nonproliferative form of sparganosis is clinically the same whether caused by *S. mansonoides* or *S. mansoni*. There is usually a single discrete, tender, slowly growing subcutaneous nodule, which may migrate over a considerable distance. These nodules can persist for a long time, but patients usually request that they be excised. Spargana in the subconjunctiva cause considerable pain and irritation, edema, and excess tears. If they are in the periorbital tissues, there will be swelling and occasional proptosis which may result in blindness. Most spargana, however, are in the subcutaneous tissues or muscles of the chest and abdominal walls or limbs. Others may be in the scrotum and epididymis. Following ingestion, any of the ab-

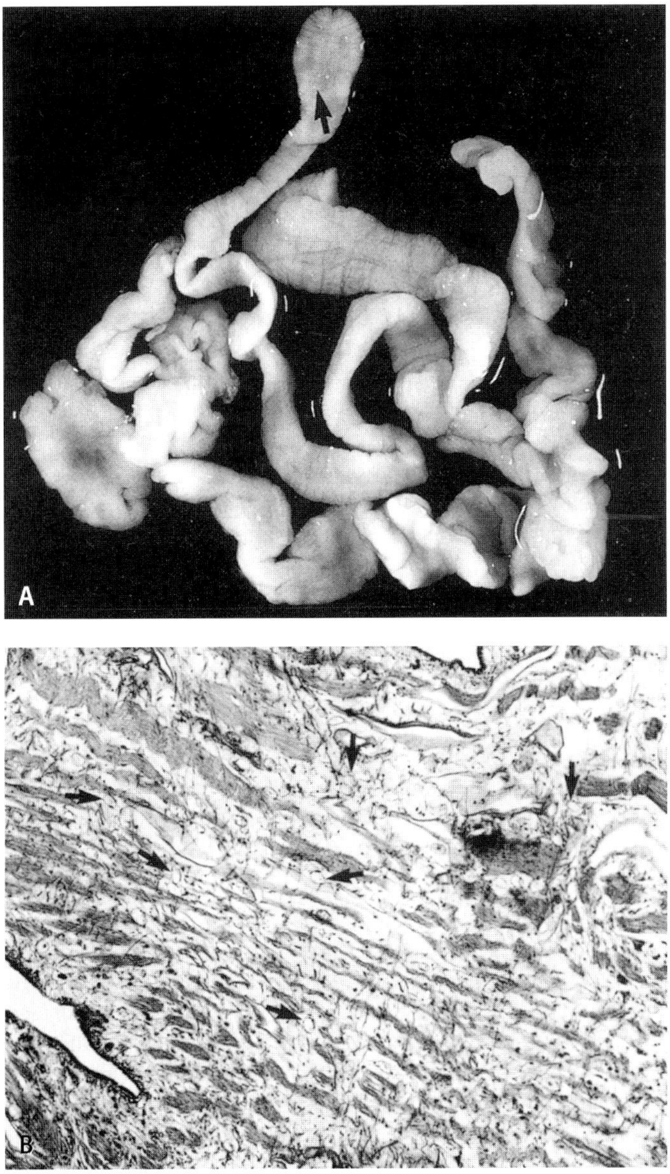

Fig. 7.49. **A** The sparganum from a subcutaneous nodule. The *arrow* indicates the flattened anterior end. The ribbon-like body varies in thickness and shows pseudosegmentation. ×2. **B** High magnification (×50) of a sparganum showing loose stroma with fluid-filled spaces, calcareous corpuscles (*arrows*), mesenchymal fibers, and longitudinal bundles of smooth muscle. (Courtesy of Marty and Andersen 1995)

dominal viscera and the pleura may be affected. Peritonitis has occurred when the intestine has been perforated.

Sparganosis has caused eosinophilic cystitis with a localized mass in the bladder wall. The histopathology was similar to infections elsewhere, with a sinuous necrosis following the track of the worm. The tunnels were plugged with an amorphous necrotic eosinophilic mass; Charcot-Leyden crystals were present. On cystoscopy the bladder was hyperemic and the mass was movable. At surgery there were adhesions and necrosis between the vesicoureteric pouch and colon. Contrast urography showed the mass in the wall of the bladder, which was confirmed on CT as being 3 cm in size. The serum IgG titers and the peripheral blood eosinophilia returned to normal after surgical removal of the mass. The route by which the sparganum reaches the CNS is unknown, but may be through the skull foramina or in the connective tissue surrounding vessels and nerves. The clinical presentation depends on the site and size of the lesion. A seizure, often without localizing neurological signs, is the most common presentation, but there may be gradual onset of hemiparesis, progressing over several years. Similarly, severe headaches may persist for years or there may be sensory changes and, in some patients, memory loss, mental deterioration, dizziness, difficulty with speech and swallowing, hemianopsia, and other CNS symptoms.

Proliferative sparganosis is rare, with probably less than 20 confirmed cases. The majority have occurred in Japan and Southeast Asia. The sparganum of *S. proliferum* is very invasive and spreads throughout the body by continuous branching and budding; even small pieces of tapeworm left behind after attempted excision may spread and infect distant sites. *S. proliferum* is most common in the CNS, but is also found in skeletal muscle and elsewhere. Because there are sometimes thousands of spargana, the clinical presentation is often of slowly growing multiple nodules, most of which are painful; there may also be a single branching lobulated mass that is highly invasive. Later in the infection, the skin and fascia over the worm become thickened, resembling elephantiasis and containing thick slimy lymph. Massive infiltration can cause disintegration and failure of the infected organs. Because the larvae can live for 10 or 20 years and the worm may continue to infiltrate tissues, death is virtually inevitable. Attempts at surgical removal of the *S. proliferum* are unsuccessful because of the ability of the spargana to proliferate so widely. Some unexpected clinical presentations have included pulmonary embolism and intestinal obstruction. While surgical removal of the sparganum (provided it is complete) can cure the nonproliferative form, there is as yet no way to treat proliferative sparganosis.

Sparganosis can be avoided by not eating raw fish, frogs, or snakes, by drinking only clean water, by deworming pet cats and dogs, and, of course, by choosing a poultice which does not include raw flesh.

Imaging Diagnosis

Except in the CNS, imaging shows no specific findings. Calcification has occurred in some of the spargana granulomas, and can be mistaken for cysticercosis. It is probable that the larger larvae could be recognized within a subcutaneous nodule by ultrasonography, but no reports of this have been found. An uncommon clinical presentation is eosinophilic urinary cystitis, with a localized mass (the granuloma around the worm) that can be recognized on ultrasonography, urography, or CT/MR scanning. Worm granulomas have also occurred in the testes and epididymis, presenting a difficult differential diagnosis unless movement and change in position on rescanning are recognized. Indeed, wherever the "mass" is recognized clinically or by imaging, its mobility helps to establish the diagnosis (although sparganosis is not the only parasitic infection in which the area of interest moves around). The clinical finding of raised peripheral eosinophilia and serum titers will confirm the diagnosis in these patients.

In the CNS, CT will show low-density areas in the cerebral white matter. The majority are unilateral, but the lesions can be bilateral and there may be localized cortical atrophy in the same areas. The lesions can be scattered in any part of the brain. At the same time there can be one or more small punctate or nodular calcifications, associated with the low-density area. Contrast enhancement shows nodular, linear, irregular or amorphous lesions: a ring appearance may be present (Fig. 7.50 A). These lesions are avascular on contrast angiography. Follow-up CT scans can show that these nodules are moving to different parts of the brain. Over a period of years there can be slight progression or degeneration of the existing lesions. It is likely that the CT findings reflect a longstanding inflammation, with active granulomas and areas of degeneration, probably mirroring the status of the worm.

Magnetic resonance imaging is, however, the most reliable diagnostic modality and is more sensitive than CT in imaging cerebral sparganosis. MRI better demonstrates the difference between the normal and abnormal tissue and can show lesions not identified by CT scanning. In more than half the patients, MRI will show localized cortical atrophy, particularly along the gyri: this may not be so well seen on CT. Another characteristic finding on both CT and MRI is associated ventricular dilatation. This also can be unilateral and is not due to a mass effect.

T1-weighted MRI scans show mildly hypointense areas of cerebral white matter, which on proton and T2-weighted images are hyperintense in the periphery of the lesion with a relatively hypointense central focus (Figs. 7.50 B, 7.51 A). With gadolinium enhancement, the cortical or subcortical lesions are reliably demonstrated as round, nodular, irregular, or conglomerate masses, some being ring-shaped or beaded, two patterns that are better seen by MRI than by CT (Figs. 7.51 B, 7.52). Nevertheless, the multifocal lesions do show on CT as areas of low attenuation, and in many patients there will be small punctate calcifications, which are perhaps due to cortical petechial hemorrhage, that are better seen by CT than by MRI. Many of these will be in the same area as the lesions shown by contrast enhancement, but some will be remote and not related. Although the actual calcification may not be recognized by MRI, T1-weighted and proton density images may show focal hypointense lesions, becoming more hyperintense on T2-weighted images.

The combination of the CT or MRI findings, the ELISA results, and the history of eating raw flesh or using a contaminated poultice will strongly suggest the correct diagnosis of sparganosis. Should the diagnosis be in doubt, the change in the location of the lesions on subsequent scans (CT or MRI) should

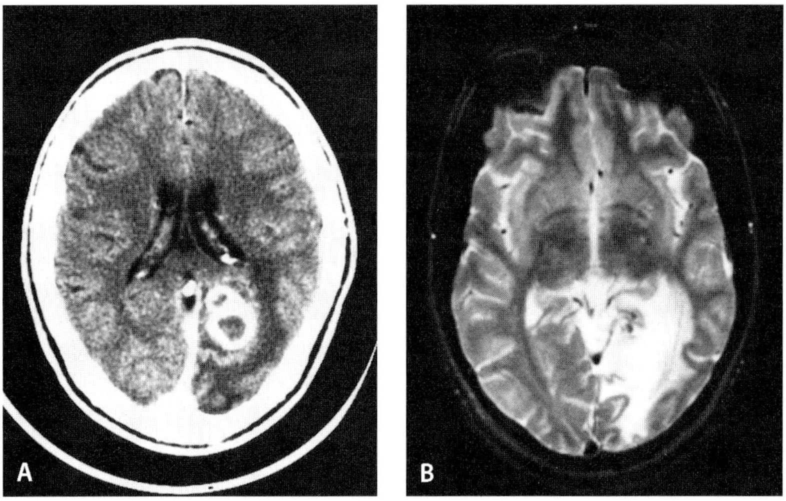

Fig. 7.50. A Contrast-enhanced CT of the brain of a 21-year-old man from India who presented with generalized tonic-clonic seizures and right homonymous hemianopsia. There is a 5-cm cystic lesion in the left occipital lobe showing ring enhancement. B MRI of the same patient shows considerable bright edema surrounding the cystic lesion. The mass was surgically excised and within the cavity were found a small amount of tan exudate and a live undulating white 10 by 1 mm sparganum. Postoperatively, the patient's seizures and visual deficit resolved. [Photographs provided by Dr. M. Holodniy. From Connor DH, Chandler FW, et al (eds): *Pathology of infectious diseases*. Stamford, Conn., Appleton & Lange, 1997]

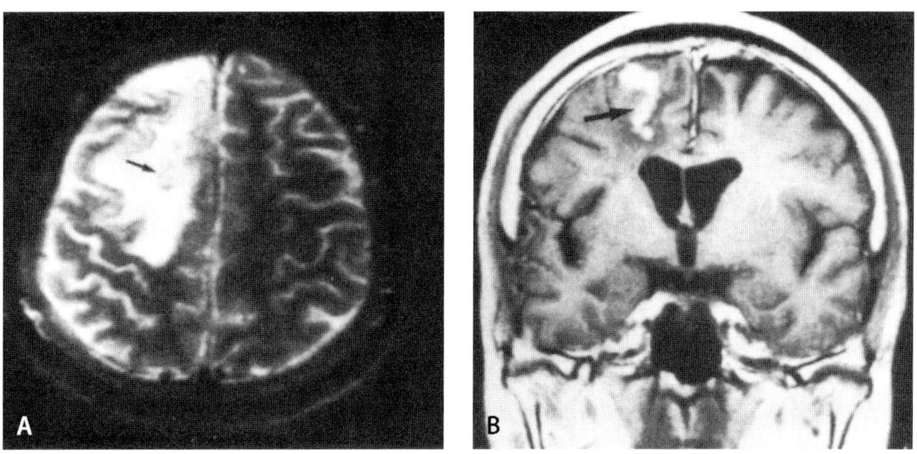

Fig. 7.51. A T2-weighted MRI showing a wide area of subcortical hyperintensity in the right frontal region, with some cortical shrinkage. The *arrow* indicates a hypointense region within the hyperintense area due to a granuloma. B Gadolinium-enhanced MRI showing the tortuous linear, beaded granuloma (*arrow*) extending down to the periventricular region. There is a surrounding hypointense area of edema or, perhaps, encephalomalacia: there was a similar region in the left frontal cortex. Three live worms were found at surgery. (Courtesy of Dr. W.K. Moon et al and *Radiology*, 1993)

be sufficient to indicate movement of the worm and establish the probable diagnosis. It is the mobility of the lesions which distinguishes these granulomas from those of other etiology; also, other granulomas do not show the same pattern of enhancement and associated ventricular dilatation.

Differential Diagnosis

Sparganosis must be differentiated from all other infectious granulomas, particularly tuberculosis and paragonimiasis. Calcified foci might be mistaken for cysticercosis. However, the location of the low-density areas of extensive degeneration along the white matter bundles, with adjacent ventricular dilatation, the presence of single or multiple nodular lesions, beaded or irregular in outline, and the mobility of

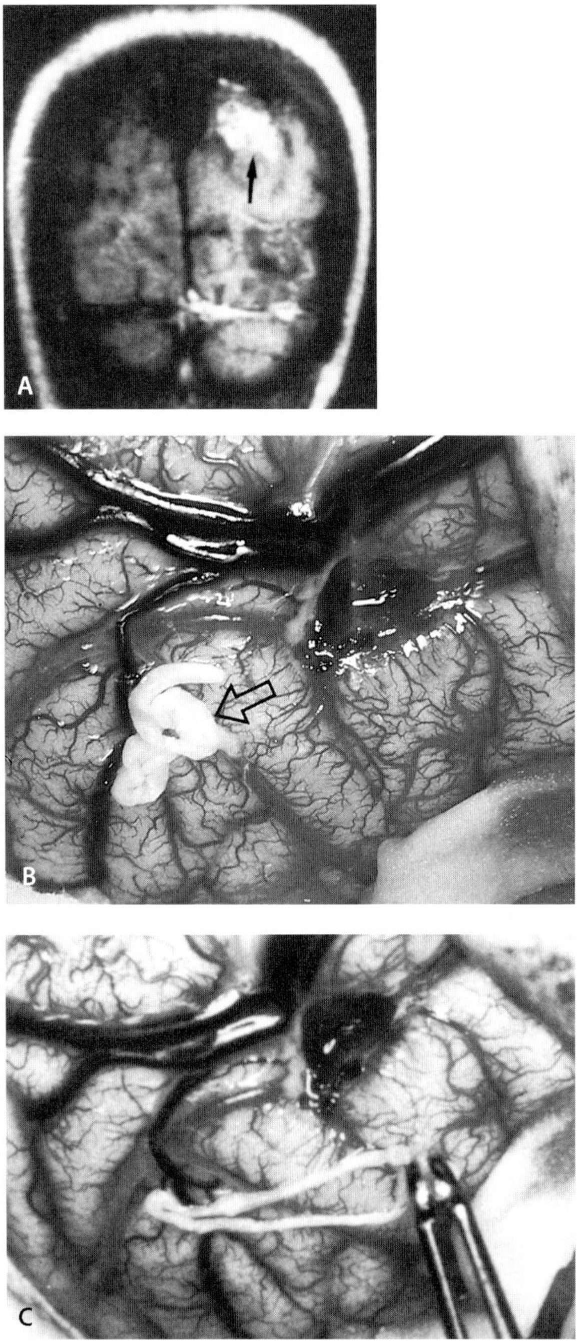

Fig. 7.52. **A** Gadolinium-enhanced MRI shows an irregular enhancing lesion with a ring shape and beaded contours (*arrow*) in the left parietal cortex of a 19-year-old man who had a headache for 7 months. **B, C** At surgery, a live worm (*open arrow* in **B**) moved slowly from the brain: it was 10 cm long. (**A, C** courtesy of Dr. W.K. Moon et al and *Radiology*, 1993; **B** from C.L. Carroll, in D.H. Connor, ed. *The pathology of infectious diseases*. Stamford, Conn., Appleton & Lange, 1997; **B, C** photographed by Dr. K.H. Chang)

the lesions suggest sparganosis rather than tuberculosis or other granulomatous diseases. Metastatic malignant nodules are usually well defined and round and are very unlikely to cause adjacent ventricular dilatation. However, some cases of sparganosis show a mass effect and must be distinguished from a neoplasm: this is somewhat more common within a few months of the start of the infection. The long history and the memory of eating raw flesh, particularly fish, frogs, or snakes, are also significant in making the diagnosis. They provide a warning, once again, that raw flesh is better not eaten, and it is certainly undesirable as a component of a poultice.

Other Tapeworm Infections

Many other species of tapeworm may infect man. The majority have no imaging significance, but radiologists should be aware of the following infections, as they may cause clinical symptoms and important imaging findings in patients who are referred for radiological investigation.

Coenurosis: *Taenia multiceps* (Bladderworm)

Human coenurosis represents infection by a coenurus, the larval stage of any one of four species of tapeworm: *Taenia multiceps, T. serialis, T. brauni,* and *T. glomerata*. The coenurus, or larval stage of these four species, has multiple protoscolices, which microscopically distinguishes it easily from the cysticercus of *T. solium*, which has only a single scolex. These adults of *Taenia* spp. live in the intestines of dogs and other canines and pass eggs which are then ingested by grazing animals, usually sheep, goats, and rabbits. Oncospheres escape from the eggs and form coenuri in various tissues. Localization in the CNS of sheep causes the "staggers."

Most human infections resulting in cerebral coenuri have occurred in West, East, and South Africa, France, England, Brazil, and the United States. Coenuri cysts in the brain may cause ventricular obstruction, giving rise to raised intracranial pressure. Patients with coenurosis present with headache and papilledema. The cysts have been responsible for jacksonian epilepsy, hemiplegia, monoplegia, and cerebellar ataxia. When the spinal cord is affected, there may be spastic paraplegia. Ventriculography, CT, or MRI may show dilatation of the ventricles, but there are no specific diagnostic findings. On CT scans viable cysts appear as lucent lesions surrounded by a contrast-enhanced peripheral rim. Multiple echo MRI sequences reveal that the intensity of the cyst contents is similar to that of CSF.

Diphyllobothrium latum (Fish or Broad Tapeworm)

The genus *Diphyllobothrium* includes more than 50 species of tapeworm. *Diphyllobothrium latum* was the first to be recognized and is most common in Northern Europe; however, the same name is used to describe the cause of clinical diphyllobothriasis in North America, regardless of which of the 13 species found in humans is responsible. This is not an uncommon infection, with perhaps over 9 million cases occurring worldwide. The experts debate whether *Diphyllobothrium* belong to the same genus as *Spirometra*.

The infection is also known as fish tapeworm disease or broad tapeworm disease. Although most common in the Northern Hemisphere, particularly in Europe and the more northern American and Canadian states and provinces, the tapeworm has a worldwide distribution and in the tropics has been found in East and West Africa (Botswana, Angola, Uganda, Madagascar), Indonesia and New Guinea, and parts of South America. The intermediate hosts are freshwater crustaceans and freshwater fish. Infection of fish and subsequently fish-eating mammals (bears, dogs, and other carnivores) and humans may occur wherever sanitation is poor and human waste is dumped into rivers and lakes. The transport of unfrozen fish from infected waters has caused infection in humans who are far from the endemic areas. When a human (the normal definitive host) or other mammal eats raw infected fish, the encysted sparganum or larva within the fish musculature is released and develops into an adult tapeworm within the intestine. Adult worms can live for up to 29 years.

Fortunately, the fish tapeworm's only significance for radiologists is that it should be recognized as yet another cause of eosinophilia and anemia and that heavy infection with the long (3–10 m) adult worms may cause mechanical intestinal obstruction.

Hymenolepis nana, Hymenolepis diminuta, and *Inermicapsifer madagascariensis*

These tapeworms are widespread in the tropics and all may affect man (*Hymenolepis nana* has no other host except mice); in many tropical countries they are more common than either *T. solium* or *T. saginata*. There are no clinical symptoms or radiological signs unless the worm load is very heavy, in which case anorexia, diarrhea, abdominal pain, and headache may occur. Rarely, seizures have been reported. At least one-third of patients will have eosinophilia. Intestinal obstruction from blockage or volvulus has occurred, because there may be thousands of these tiny worms within the human intestine.

Acknowledgement. The authors are indebted to Drs. Perla Salgado Lujambio and Rafael Rojas Jasso for their contributions to the Neurocysticercosis section of this chapter.

Bibliography

Taeniasis and Cysticercosis

Almeida-Pinto J, Veiga-Pires JA, Stocker A, et al: Cysticercosis of the brain. The value of computed tomography. *Acta Radiol* 29:625–628, 1988

Antonov IP, et al: X-ray diagnosis of cysticercosis of the brain [abstracted in English]. *Vestn Roentgenol Radiol* 6:72–78, 1974

Arseni C, Samitca DC: Cysticercosis of the brain. *Br Med J* II:494–496, 1957

Barkovich AJ, Citrin CM, Klara P: Magnetic resonance imaging of cysticercosis. *West J Med* 145:687–690, 1986

Benston, et al: Computer tomography in intracranial cysticercosis. *JCAT* 1:464–471, 1977

Bhargava S: Radiology – including computed tomography – of parasitic diseases of the central nervous system. [Review]. *Neurosurg Review* 6:129–137, 1983

Bickerstaff ER, et al: Cysticercosis of the posterior fossa. *Brain* 79:622–634, 1956

Brailsford JF: *Cysticercus cellulosae*: its radiographic detection in the musculature and central nervous system. *Br J Radiol* 14:79–93, 1941

Brinkmann U: Megacities. *Time Magazine*, Jan 11, 1993, p 36

Brooks AM, Essex WB, West RH: Cysticercosis of superior oblique muscle. *Aust J Ophthalmol* 11:119–122, 1983

Byrd E, Locke GE, Biggers S, Percy AK: The computed tomographic appearances of cerebral cysticercosis in adults and children. *Radiology* 144:819–823, 1982

Carbajal JR, Palacios E, Azar-Kia B, et al: Radiology of cysticercosis of the central nervous system, including computed tomography. *Radiology* 125:127–131, 1977

Carmault JE, et al: Spinal cysticercosis. *West J Med* 123:311–313, 1975

Carpio A, Placencia M, Santillan F, Escobar A: A proposal for classification of neurocysticercosis. *Canad J Neurol Sci* 21:43–47, 1994

Castillo M, Quencer RM, Post MJD: MR of intramedullary spinal cysticercosis. *AJNR* 9:393–395, 1988

Chang KH, Kim WS, Cho SY, et al: Comparative evaluation of brain CT and ELISA in the diagnosis of neurocysticercosis. *AJNR* 9:125–130, 1988

Chang KH, Lee JH, Han MH, Han MC: The role of contrast-enhanced MR imaging in the diagnosis of neurocysticercosis. *AJNR* 12:509–512, 1991

Chang KH, Cho SY, Hesselink JR, Han MH, Han MC: Parasitic diseases of the central nervous system. *Neuroimaging Clin North Am* 1:159–178, 1991

Cockshott P, Middlemiss H: *Clinical radiology in the tropics.* Churchill Livingstone, Edinburgh, 1979

Colli BO, Martelli N, Assirati Junior JA, et al: Cysticercosis of the central nervous system. I. Surgical treatment of cerebral cysticercosis: a 23 years experience in the Hospital das Clinicas of Ribeirao Preto Medical School. [Review]. *Arquivos de Neuro-Psiquiatria* 52:166–186, 1994

Colli BO, Assirati Junior JA, Machado HR, et al: Cysticercosis of the central nervous system. II. Spinal cysticercosis. [Review]. *Arquivos de Neuro-Psiquiatria* 52:187–199, 1994

Cook GC (ed): *Manson's tropical diseases, 20th edn.* Saunders, London, 1996

Corona T, Pascoe D, Gonzalez-Barranco D, et al: Anticysticercus antibodies in serum and cerebrospinal fluid in patients with cerebral cysticercosis. *J Neurol Neurosurg Psychiatry* 49:1044–1049, 1986

Creasy JL, Alarcon JJ: Magnetic resonance imaging of neurocysticercosis. *Top Magn Reson Imaging* 6:59–68, 1994

Cruz I, Cruz ME, Teran W, et al: Human subcutaneous *Taenia solium* cysticercosis in an Andean population with neurocysticercosis. *Am J Trop Med Hyg* 51:405–407, 1994

Danziger J, Bloch S: Tapeworm cyst infestations of the brain. *Clin Radiol* 26:141–148, 1977

Davis LE, Kornfeld: Neurocysticercosis: neurologic, pathogenic, diagnostic and therapeutic aspects. *Eur Neurol* 31:229–240, 1991

Del Brutto OH, Zenteno MA, Salgado P, Sotelo J: MR imaging in cysticercotic encephalitis. *AJNR* 10:18–20, 1989

Del Brutto OH: Cysticercosis and cerebrovascular disease: a review. [Review]. *J Neurol Neurosurg Psychiatry* 55:252–254, 1992

Del Brutto OH: Single parenchymal brain cysticercus in the acute encephalitic phase: definition of a distinct form of neurocysticercosis with a benign prognosis. *J Neurol Neurosurg Psychiatry* 58:247–249, 1995

DeVilliers PD: Cerebral cysticercosis. *S Afr Med J* 27:1097–1098, 1953

DiLoreto DA, Kennedy RA, Neigel JM, Rootman J: Infestation of extraocular muscle by *Cysticercus cellulosae. Br J Ophthalmol* 74:751–752, 1990

Dixon HBF, Hargreaves WH: Cysticercosis (*Taenia solium*); a further 10 years' clinical study, covering 284 cases. *Q J Med* 13:107–121, 1944

Dorfsman J: Radiological aspects of spinal cysticercosis. *Acta Radiol* 5:1003–1006, 1966

Edington GM, Gilles HM: *Pathology in the tropics, 2nd edn.* Williams & Wilkins, Baltimore, 1976, pp 194–201

Escobar A, Nieto D: Cysticercosis. In: Minckler J (ed) *Pathology of the nervous system, vol. 3.* McGraw-Hill, New York, 1972, pp 2507–2515

Escobar A: The pathology of neurocysticercosis of the central nervous system. In: Palacios E, Rodriguez-Carbajal J, Taveras JM (eds) Cysticercosis of the central nervous system. Charles C. Thomas, Springfield, Ill., 1983, pp 27–54

Estanol B, Corona T, Abad P: A prognostic classification of cerebral cysticercosis: therapeutic implications. *J Neurol Neurosurg Psychiatry* 49:1131–1134, 1986

Fetterman LE: Radiographic demonstration of *T. saginata*: an unexpected cause of abdominal pain. *N Engl J Med* 272:364–365, 1965

Flisser A, Willms K, Laclette JP, et al (eds) *Cysticercosis. Present state of knowledge and perspectives.* Academic Press, New York, 1982

Freyer B: Roentgenologic diagnosis of cerebral cysticercosis. *Fortschr Geb Roentgenstr Nuklearmed* 94:394, 1961

Garretto U: Radiological picture of noncalcified cysticercus in muscles. *Radiol Med* 35:1938

Ginier BL, Poirier VC: MR imaging of intraventricular cysticercosis. *AJNR* 13:1247–1248, 1992

Gold BM, Meyers MA: Radiologic manifestations of *Taenia saginata* infestation. *AJR* 128:493–498, 1977

Gonzales Morantes, Rangel Guerra R, Campa Nunez HK, Vogel H: Cysticercosis cerebralis in the computed tomogram. [In German; English summary]. *CT Sonographie* 3:87–92, 1983

Guilberto M, Ferreira MVC: Computed tomography in neurocysticercosis. *J Neurol Neurosurg Psychiatry* 46:936–942, 1983

Hahn A: A case of cysticercus of the lungs. *Radiol Glasnik* 3:86–89, 1939

Hamilton JB: *Taenia saginata. Radiology* 47:64–65, 1946

Handler LC, Mervis B: Cerebral cysticercosis with reference to the natural history of parenchymal lesions. *AJNR* 4:709–712, 1983

Isidro-Llorens A, Dachs F, Vidal J, Sarrias M: Spinal cysticercosis. Case report and review. *Paraplegia* 31:128–130, 1993

Jampol LM, Caldwell JBH, Albert DM: Cysticercus cellulosae in the eyelid. *Arch Ophthalmol* 89:319–320, 1973

Jena A, Sanchetee PC, Gupta RK, et al: Cysticercosis of the brain shown by magnetic resonance imaging. *Clin Radiol* 39:542–546, 1988

Jena A, Sanchetee PC, Tripathi R, et al: MR observations on the effects of praziquantel in neurocysticercosis. *Magn Reson Imaging* 10:77–80, 1992

Keats TE: Cysticercosis: a demonstration of its roentgen manifestations. *Mo Med* 58:457–459, 1961

Kramer LD, Locke GE, Byrd SE, Daryabagi J: Cerebral cysticercosis: documentation of natural history with CT. *Radiology* 171:459–462, 1989

Lenczner M, Wollin DG: Multiple infarcts and necrosis in bone. *Can Med Assoc J* 78:344–345, 1958

Lotz JW, Hewlett R, Alheit B, Bowen R: Neurocysticercosis: correlative pathomorphology and MR imaging. *Neuroradiology* 30:35–41, 1988

MacArthur WP: Cysticercosis as seen in British army with special reference to the production of epilepsy. *Trans R Soc Trop Med Hyg* 27:343, 1934

Machado LR, Nobrega JP, Barros NG, et al: Computed tomography in neurocysticercosis: a 10-year long evolution analysis of 100 patients with an appraisal of a new classification. *Arquivos de Neuro-Psiquiatria* 48:414–418, 1990

Malde HM, Shroff MM, Gadkari SS, et al: Ocular and orbital cysticercosis. *Australas Radiol* 37:279–280, 1993

Malik SRK, Gupta AK, Choudry S: Ocular cysticercosis. *Am J Ophthalmol* 66:1168–1171, 1968

Martinez HR, Rangel-Guerra R, Elizondo G, et al: MR imaging in neurocysticercosis: a study of 56 cases. *AJNR* 10:1011–1019, 1989

Martinez HR, Rangel-Guerra R, Arredondo-Estrada JH, et al: Medical and surgical treatment in neurocysticercosis. A magnetic resonance study of 161 cases. *J Neurol Sci* 130:25–34, 1995

Marty AM, Andersen EM: *Taeniidae* and cysticercosis. In: Doerr W, Seifert G (eds) Tropical pathology, 2nd edn. Springer, Berlin Heidelberg New York, 1995, pp 848–857

McCormick GF: Cysticercosis – review of 230 patients. *Bull Clin Neurosciences* 50:76–101, 1985

Medina MT, Rosas E, Rubio-Donnadieu F, Sotelo J: Neurocysticercosis as the main cause of late-onset epilepsy in Mexico. *Arch Intern Med* 150:325–327, 1990

Mervis B, Lotz JW: Computed tomography (CT) in parenchymal cerebral cysticercosis. *Clin Radiol* 31:521–528, 1980

Minguetti G, Ferreira MC: Computed tomography in neurocysticercosis. *J Neurol Neurosurg Psychiatry* 46:936–942, 1983

Monteiro L, Coelho T, Stocker A: Neurocysticercosis – a review of 231 cases. *Infection* 20:61–65, 1992

Mukherjee A, Roy T, Mukherjee S, et al: Neurocysticercosis. *J Assoc Physicians of India* 41:287–289, 1993

Neal JH: An endoscopic approach to cysticercosis cysts of the posterior third ventricle. *Neurosurgery* 36:1040–1043, 1995

Obrador S: Clinical aspects of cerebral cysticercosis. *Arch Neurol Psychiatry* 59:457–468, 1948

O'Neill DP, Connor DH: Cysticercosis. In: Connor DH, Chandler FW (eds) *Pathology of infectious diseases, vol 2.* Appleton & Lange, Stamford, Conn., 1997, pp 1365–1371

Palacios E, Lujambio PS, Jasso RR: Computed tomography and magnetic resonance imaging of neurocysticercosis. *Semin Roentgenol* 32:325–334, 1997

Palacios E, Rodriguez-Carbajal J, Taveras JM: Neuroradiology of cysticercosis of the central nervous system. Charles C. Thomas, Springfield, Ill., 1983, pp 101–143

Palmer PES, et al: Tropical diseases. In: Pettersson H (ed) *Radiology of abdominal and tropical diseases.* The NICER Institute, Oslo, 1995, pp 288–291

Percy AK, Byrd SE, Locke GE: Cerebral cysticercosis. *Pediatrics* 66:967–971, 1980

Reddy DG, Ramamurthy B: Ventriculographic changes in cysticercosis of the brain. *Br J Surg* 41:11–12, 1953

Reeder MM: Tropical diseases of the soft tissues. *Semin Roentgenol* 8:47–71, 1973

Reeder MM, Palmer PES: Infections and infestations of the gastrointestinal tract. In: Freeny PC, Stevenson GW (eds) *Margulis and Burhenne's alimentary tract roentgenology, 5th edn.* Mosby, St. Louis, 1994, pp 1475–1542

Revuelta R, Juambelz P, Balderrama J, Teixeira F: Contralateral trigeminal neuralgia: a new clinical manifestation of neurocysticercosis: case report. *Neurosurgery* 37:138–139, 1995

Rhee RS, Kumasaki DY, Rodriguez-Carbajal J, et al: Radiology of cysticercosis of the central nervous system including computed tomography. *Radiology* 125:127–131, 1977

Rhee RS, Kumasaki DY, Sarwar M, et al: MR imaging of intraventricular cysticercosis. *JCAT* 11:598–601, 1987

Rodacki MA, Detoni XA, Teixeira WR, et al: CT features of cellulosae and racemous neurocysticercosis. *JCAT* 13:1013–1016, 1989

Rodriguez-Carbajal J, Flisser A, Rubio-Donnadieu F, et al: Human cysticercosis in Mexico. [Spanish]. *Gaceta Medica de Mexico* 124:191–208, 1988

Rodriguez-Carbajal J, Salgado P, Gutierrez R, Escobar A, Aruffo D, Palacios E: The acute encephalitic stage of neurocysticercosis; computed tomography manifestations. *AJNR* 4:51–55, 1983

Rosas N, Sotelo J, Nieto D: ELISA in the diagnosis of neurocysticercosis. *Arch Neurol* 43:353–356, 1986

Ruiz MB, Haughton VM: A new plain film finding in cysticercosis. *Neuroradiology* 33:79–80, 1991

Samuel E: Roentgenology of parasitic calcification. *Am J Roentgenol Radium Ther Nucl Med* 63:512–522, 1950

Santin G, Vargas SJ: Roentgen study of cysticercosis of central nervous system. *Radiology* 86:520–528, 1966

Savoirado M, Cimino C, Passerini A, La Mantia L: Mobile myelographic filling defects: spinal cysticercosis. *Neuroradiology* 28:166–169, 1986

Sen DK: Cysticercus cellulosae in the eyelid, orbit and lacrimal gland. *Acta Ophthalmol (Copenh)* 58:144–147, 1980

Sharma BS, Banerjee AK, Kak VK: Intramedullary spinal cysticercosis. Case report and review of literature. *Clin Neurol and Neurosurg* 89:111–116, 1987

Sotelo J, Escobedo F, Rodriguez-Carbajal J, et al: Therapy of parenchymal brain cysticercosis with praziquantel. *N Engl J Med* 310:1001–1007, 1984

Sotelo J, Guerrero V, Rubio-Donnadieu F: Neurocysticercosis: a new classification based on active and inactive forms. A study of 753 cases. *Arch Intern Med* 145:442–445, 1985

Suh DC, Chang KH, Han MH, et al: Unusual MR manifestations of neurocysticercosis. *Neuroradiology* 31:396–402, 1989

Suss RA, Maravilla KR, Thompson J: MR imaging of intracranial cysticercosis: comparison with CT and anatomorphologic features. *AJNR* 7:235–242, 1986

Teitelbaum GP, Otto RJ, Lin M, Watanabe AT, Stull MA, Manz HJ, Bradley WG Jr: MR imaging of neurocysticercosis. *AJNR* 10:709–718, 1989

Thornton H, et al: Taeniasis and cysticercosis with special reference to Rhodesia. *Cent Afr J Med* 15:45–52, 1969

Van As AD, Joubert J: Neurocysticercosis in 578 black epileptic patients. *S Afr Med J* 80:327–328, 1991

Vanijanonta S, Bunnag D, Riganti M: The treatment of neurocysticercosis with praziquantel. *Southeast Asian J Trop Med & Public Health* 22 Suppl:275–278, 1991

Vasantha S, Ravikumar BV, Roopashree SD, et al: Neuroanatomy of *Cysticercus cellulosae* (Cestoda) as revealed by acetylcholinesterase and nonspecific esterase histochemistry. *Parasitol Res* 78:581–586, 1992

Vatopoulos G, Cotsilimbas D: On ten cases of cerebral cysticercosis. *Evangelismos Hosp Rev* 22:645–659, 1960

Venkataraman S, Roy AK, Dhamija RM, Sanchetee PC: Cysticercal meningoencephalitis: Clinical presentation and autopsy findings. *J Assoc Physicians of India* 38:763–765, 1990

Vijayan GP, et al: Neurological and related manifestations of cysticercosis. *Trop Geogr Med* 29:271–278, 1977

Waki K, Oi H, Takahashi S, et al: Successful treatment of *Diphyllobothrium latum* and *Taenia saginata* infection by intraduodenal 'Gastrografin' injection. *Lancet* 2(8516):1124–1126, 1986

Yang SY, Wang ML, Xue QC: Cerebral cysticercosis. *Surg Neurol* 34:286–293, 1990

Zavala JT: Etiology of cysticercosis. In: Palacios E, Rodriguez-Carbajal J, Taveras JM (eds) Cysticercosis of the central nervous system. Charles C. Thomas, Springfield, Ill., 1983, pp 18–26

Zee CS, Segall HD, Ahmadi J, et al: CT myelography in spinal cysticercosis. *J Comput Assist Tomogr* 10:195–198, 1986

Zee CS, Segall HD, Boswell W, et al: MR imaging of neurocysticercosis. *J Comput Assist Tomogr* 12:927–934, 1988

Zee CS, Segall HD, Destian S, et al: MRI of intraventricular cysticercosis: surgical implications. *J Comput Assist Tomogr* 17:932–939, 1993

Zee CS, Segall HD, Miller C, et al: Unusual neuroradiological features of intracranial cysticercosis. *Radiology* 137:397–407, 1980

Zimmerman RA, Bilaniuk LT, Sze G: Intracranial infection. In: Brant-Zawadski M, Norman D (eds) Magnetic resonance imaging of central nervous system. Raven, New York, 1987, pp 235–257

Zur G: Cysticercosis of the lung and liver. *Fortschr Geb Roentgenstr Nuklearmed* 75:186–193, 1951

Sparganosis

Anders K, et al: Intracranial sparganosis: uncommon infection – case report. *J Neurosurg* 60:1282–1286, 1984

Campbell EW, Beals C: Striking eosinophilia in sparganosis. *Postgrad Med J* 62:138–140, 1977

Carroll CL, Connor DH: Sparganosis. In: Connor DH, et al (eds) *Pathology of infectious diseases.* Appleton & Lange, Stamford, Conn., 1997, pp 1559–1565

Chang KH, et al: Cerebral sparganosis: CT characteristics. *Radiology* 165:505–510, 1987

Chang KH, et al: Parasitic diseases of the central nervous system. *Neuroimaging Clin North Am* 1:159–178, 1991

Chang KH, et al: Cerebral sparganosis: CT features in 34 cases. *Neuroradiology* 34:1–8, 1992

Fan K-J, Pezeshkour GH: Cerebral sparganosis. *Neurology* 36:1249–1251, 1986

Holodniy M, et al: Cerebral sparganosis: case report and review. *Rev Infect Dis* 13:155–159, 1991

Landero A, et al: Cerebral sparganosis caused by *Spirometra mansonoides*: case report. *J Neurosurg* 75:472–474, 1991

Liao SW, et al: Proliferating sparganosis of the lumbar spine. Case report. *J Formos Med Assoc* 81:603–611, 1983

Marty AM, Anderson EM: Helminthology. In Doerr W, Siefert G (eds) *Tropical pathology.* Springer, Heidelberg Berlin New York, 1995, pp 841–847

Moon WK, et al: Cerebral sparganosis: MR imaging versus CT features. *Radiology* 188:751–757, 1993

Mueller JF: The life history of *Diphyllobothrium mansonoides* (Mueller, 1935), and some consideration with regard to sparganosis in the United States. *Am J Trop Med Hyg* 18:41–66, 1938

Mueller JF, Strano AJ: *Sparganum proliferum*, a sparganum infected with a virus? *J Parasitol* 60:15–19, 1974

Norman SH, Kreutner A Jr: Sparganosis: clinical and pathologic observations in ten cases. *South Med J* 73:297–300, 1980

Oh SJ, Chi JG, Lee SE: Eosinophilic cystitis caused by vesical sparganosis: a case report. J Urol 149:581–583, 1993

Sze G, Zimmerman RD: Magnetic resonance imaging of infections and inflammatory disease. *Radiol Clin North Am* 26:839–859, 1988

Zhang HL, et al: Ocular sparganosis-caused blindness. *Chin Med J* 96:73–75, 1983

Coenurosis

Pau A, Turtas S, Brambilla M, et al: Computed tomography and magnetic resonance imaging of cerebral coenurosis. *Surg Neurol* 27:548–552, 1987

Pau A, Perria C, Turtas S, et al: Long-term follow-up of the surgical treatment of intracranial coenurosis. *Brit J Neurosurg* 4:39–43, 1990

8 The Acquired Immunodeficiency Syndrome (AIDS) in the Tropics

With Elizabeth H. Moore and Erik H.L. Gaensler
Advised by Benjamin Imalingat, Paul Reeve, and M.W. Wachira

Almost any discussion of AIDS, verbal or written, generates controversy and strong opinions. The disease has been blamed on the colonial powers, "God's punishment for promiscuity, sexual deviation or intravenous drug usage," "a genetically altered virus pioneered in a military laboratory", abnormal human contact with monkeys or apes in Central Africa, the vaccination programs against smallpox, polio and other infections, or some unknown factor in the border trade between Tanzania and Uganda. Some believe that it is being spread by walking in the footsteps of a sick person. Alternatively, AIDS "does not exist," is "an invention of the western media," is the result of witchcraft, or "is not infectious." Symptoms may be ascribed to diabetes or dysentery rather than to AIDS. The acceptance of the diagnosis can be fatalistic, "*Acha inuiwe dawa sina*" ("I have no medicine, so let it kill me"), or practical "we have no money" (Chairman of national AIDS committee). Innovative theories regarding AIDS prevention have been suggested: "Women with AIDS should be shot" (a member of parliament), or less final, "anyone with AIDS should be isolated" or banned from school, games, work, and public places or not allowed into the country.

Official response has often been energetic and occasionally unconventional. At one time it was noted that a Malawian trucker, crossing the border from Mozambique to Zimbabwe, could expect officials to examine his passport, his vehicle's papers, and his genitals. The scientific press is not always more helpful, as is exemplified by a statement in 1986 from the Pasteur Institute in France that "many insects in central Africa are infected with the AIDS virus," to which the Center for Disease Control in the USA replied in 1987, if "mosquitoes are indeed transmitting AIDS, they are being very selective about whom they bite." Only a few percent of AIDS cases are devoid of any identifiable risk factor for transmission.

Researching the literature to establish the incidence of AIDS is equally interesting, particulary looking back over the past 15 years. This illustrates not just the rapid spread of the virus, but the slow process by which people and their governments have come to terms with this epidemic. Many governments denied that there were patients in their countries. Reports, estimates, and authoritative statements abound, and are corrected, amended, and contradicted with great rapidity. The literature is confused and confusing. There is, for example, a report on AIDS in Africa by a medical group from China: however, there are few reports from anyone concerning AIDS in China, and certainly none from an African medical group.

Amidst the plethora of literature on the subject, why a review of AIDS in the tropics? Few doctors anywhere can be unaware of AIDS, yet not all may be aware of how much AIDS varies in its presentations and complications. Most publications on the subject of AIDS have centered around patients in the Western world, often homosexuals or intravenous drug abusers living in urban settings. The vast majority of AIDS patients worldwide do not fit this profile. Over the past 10 years, increasingly numerous reports detailing the presentation of AIDS in the developing countries have appeared, making it clear that the natural history of AIDS differs depending on the microbiological and nutritional environment, as well as the societal behavior and local customs of the population affected.

In this chapter, the complications of AIDS will be reviewed for various tropical populations. When possible, the reasons for the patterns of illness encountered will be analyzed. In addition, many, if not most of these opportunistic diseases have altogether different clinical and radiological manifestations when they affect an HIV-infected host instead of a normal host. This chapter will emphasize these differences, reviewing the radiographic manifestations of the common opportunistic infections and malignancies as they appear in the AIDS patient. All of this information is needed to produce a geographically and radiologically appropriate differential diagnosis.

In the past, data collection on the frequencies of various complications of AIDS in the tropics has been hampered by the relative lack of diagnostic equipment, laboratories, and sophisticated imaging technology. Even though computed tomography (CT) scanning and magnetic resonance imaging (MRI) are increasingly available in the tropics, few

Table 8.1. Worldwide estimates of current infection (1999)

AIDS	34.6 million
Liver and lung flukes	70 million
Malaria	3–500 million (of whom 1 million die every year in Africa)
Schistosomiasis	250 million
Whipworm	360 million
Hookworm	1.25 billion
Amebiasis	600 million
Ascariasis	1.38 billion
Tuberculosis	20+ million

From Who reports.

studies are performed on known AIDS patients. A diagnosis of HIV infection frequently ends diagnostic studies and even therapeutic intervention, since scarce resources are assigned instead to patients with potentially curable conditions. The problem of defining complications of AIDS in the tropics has been partially resolved by thorough and carefully performed autopsy studies (for example, those of Lucas and colleagues in the Ivory Coast).

Comparative Statistics: the Relative Scope of the Problem

If numbers alone are the trigger for media attention and medical expenditure, then AIDS is unfairly privileged. The estimated incidence figures for many of the diseases described in this book exceed by many times those of AIDS (Table 8.1). Most of these other diseases can be effectively treated or cured if the resources are available, and their incidence is relatively stable; by contrast AIDS is not curable at present and there has been an exponential increase in the numbers affected.

Synonyms

Human immunodeficiency virus infection (HIV). AIDS. Acquired immunodeficiency syndrome. Retroviral disease in man. SIDA. Slim disease. Ukimwi. The wasting syndrome. Lentivirinae infection.

Definition

An infection with one or more of the retroviruses, Retroviridae, subgroup Lentivirinae, causing progressive immunodeficiency in humans and directly damaging many tissues, e.g., the central nervous and the reticuloendothelial systems. These are the direct (primary) cytopathic effects; the secondary effects are changes in immune status, opportunistic infections, and malignancies. Various retroviral infections exist in animals (e.g., feline leukemia, equine infectious anemia, caprine arthritis, and encephalitis) but the causative retroviruses are genetically and phenotypically different from the human T-lymphotropic virus, type III (HTLV-III), more generally known as the human immunodeficiency virus, HIV-I, or the AIDS virus.
The clinical definition of AIDS is on p. 687.

Geographic Distribution

Infections by HIV occur worldwide; different subtypes of the virus involve different geographic areas. Currently the highest incidence of AIDS occurs in sub-Saharan Africa, Southeast Asia, and the Caribbean. Even within these broad regions there are major differences; for example, a high rate is found in Haiti, Bermuda, and the Bahamas but a low rate is reported from Cuba. The largest population affected is in Africa, where in some countries 30% of the high-risk population (age 15–50) are infected. Groups such as the military, the elite, diplomats, and businessmen may have even higher rates; 85% of prostitutes in Nairobi are HIV positive. The World Bank and WHO in Africa estimate that 25% of the sub-Saharan workforce will die in the next 20 years, that the average life span, which had been increasing to 58–63 years, will fall to 47 years and that 3 million children will die. Worldwide perhaps 14 million children will be orphaned or without one parent, and 30% of all neonates will be HIV positive unless education is effective and treatment or prevention becomes available. The social outcome in some countries is already devastating.

Patterns of Spread

The World Health Organization has defined three patterns of spread for the AIDS epidemic. A type 1 pattern, exemplified by the United States and Western Europe, is characterized by disease spread primarily by homosexual behavior and intravenous drug abuse. A type 2 pattern, exemplified by Africa, describes primarily heterosexual spread. It has been estimated that 80% of HIV infections in East Africa are heterosexually transmitted. Homosexuality and drug abuse are rare. A type 2 pattern is also currently seen in the Caribbean and parts of Latin America, although homosexuality and drug abuse are also contributing factors in these areas. A type 3 pattern of spread occurs in areas with recent introduction of HIV by spread from countries with type 1 or type 2 patterns via blood products or sexual contact, often prostitution. The regions thus affected include Eastern Europe, North Africa, the Middle East, and Asia.

Whether AIDS is spread by homosexuals, heterosexuals, bisexuals, intravenous drug users, or transfusion of blood products, it makes little difference to the clinical course of the disease, with some notable exceptions. More important are the individual's general health and hygiene and the bacterial, viral, and parasitic cohabitants of the world in which the patient lives and has lived.

Africa

The first cases of AIDS in black Africans were identified in the 1980's, occurring in young heterosexuals with chronic wasting, opportunistic infections, and/or Kaposi's sarcoma. However, it seems probable that AIDS in Africa has a much longer history: see p. 685. Currently, AIDS is the most common cause of death in many African cities. The highest rates of infection worldwide are in sub-Saharan Africa, particularly Malawi, Zambia, Tanzania, Uganda, Rwanda, Burundi, and Zimbabwe. In sub-Saharan Africa, the trans-Africa highway provides an interesting lesson in social geography. The truck drivers from the coast in Tanzania and Kenya and the prostitutes along the highway form an almost unbroken chain of infection deep into the heart of Africa, from which the epidemic spreads into the countries which are supplied by the trucks. (There is an exactly similar pattern of spread by lorry drivers in India.) In Atzori's revealing Tanzanian survey, the level of HIV seroprevalence was directly correlated with the distance between the subject's home village and the nearest main road.

In Africa, the common occurrence of ulcerative venereal diseases, such as chancroid, and the lack of male circumcision increase heterosexual transmission (see below). Condom use is not favored ("no one eats a sweet with the wrapper still on"); men's dislike of condoms was the major reason for not using them reported by women in a study from Tanzania. In Malawi, with the highest rate of HIV infection in the world, traditional beliefs hold that women require frequent sexual intercourse, the semen acting as a vitamin to restore blood lost during menses (a proposed benefit which would be negated by condom use). Unfortunately, while initiating an educational compaign against AIDS in the new century, the President of one african country forbade mention of condoms.

Contaminated blood products, medical injections with unclean needles, and maternal-fetal spread are also important routes of transmission. Transfusion has contributed an estimated 10%–15% to AIDS transmission in Africa, particularly affecting children with malaria, women with pregnancy-related anemia, trauma victims, and patients with sickle cell disease. Improving standards in blood banking may reverse this trend. Between 5% and 15% of AIDS is perinatally transmitted.

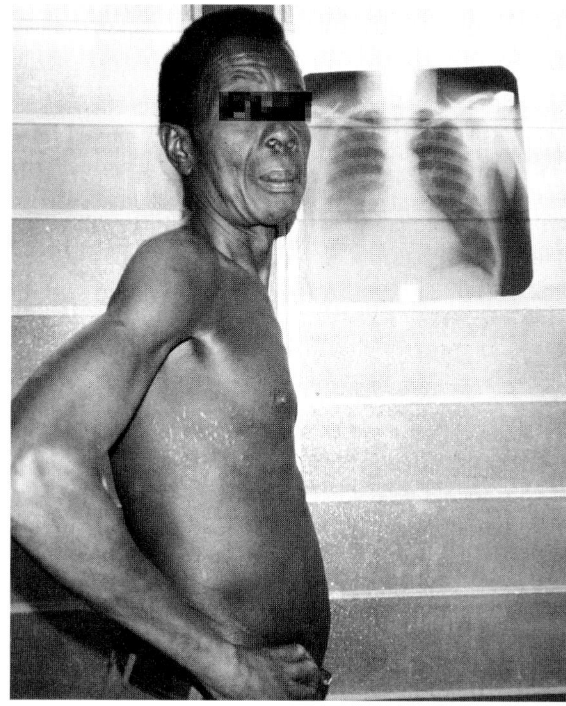

Fig. 8.1. Traditional medical treatment of tuberculous pleurisy by scarification over the right lower chest. The chest film in the background shows a right-sided pleural effusion at the exact site the traditional healer has applied his or her treatment. Such procedures place the individual at risk for transmission of blood borne diseases, including AIDS

Certain cultural practices may also promote the heterosexual spread of AIDS in Africa. There is a tradition of multiple wives or sexual partners. Networks of concurrent sexual partners, a common situation in sub-Saharan Africa, facilitate transmission. Prostitution is considered more acceptable than in some other parts of the world. Scarification (Fig. 8.1), tattooing, the rites of passage into manhood or womanhood [circumcision, female circumcision (genital mutilation) infibulation], blood letting and blood brotherhood, use of ritual and medicinal enemas given through a dirty reed or horn, and even close head or body shaving, all entail risk of transmission of HIV if, as is almost inevitable, only one instrument is shared by a group.

Heterosexual spread is enhanced by multiple births in rapid succession, with cervicitis, recurrent infection, and scarring. In some societies the surviving spouse after the death of her husband must free the spirit of the deceased by having sex with the nearest relative.

Intensive educational programs have been launched in almost all countries of Africa, with varying success. Knowledge is spreading ("sex is no fun if you are dead" – a high school pupil), but sometimes "knowledge is excellent: behavior is abysmal". However, there is some recent evidence that education may be changing behavior. The first report of decreasing seroprevalence of HIV-1 in Uganda young adults, 13–24 years old, was published in 1995 by Mulder and colleagues. A Ugandan behavioral study published in 1997 by Asiimwe-Okiror and colleagues comparing behavioral patterns in 1989 and 1995 showed increasing condom use, a 2-year delay in the age of first sexual intercourse, and, over the same period, a 40% decline in HIV seroprevalence in women attending antenatal clinics. Similarly, a study of Tanzanian urban factory workers registered a marked decrease in those reporting sex with multiple partners as well as those reporting casual sex partners between 1991 and 1994.

Common opportunistic infections and malignancies seen in African AIDS include tuberculosis, bacteremia, cerebral toxoplasmosis, pyogenic pneumonias, cytomegalovirus, Kaposi's sarcoma, and nonspecific enteritis (see pp. 690, 716).

Asia

HIV and AIDS rates in Asia vary substantially between countries. Japan demonstrates a very low rate, with the majority of AIDS cases occurring in hemophiliacs infected by blood products produced elsewhere. Homosexuality is rare, as is intravenous drug abuse, and condoms are widely used for contraception. However, some Japanese men participate as customers in the sex trade countries of Asia, such as Thailand, where a high percentage of prostitutes are infected, providing a possible avenue of infection. Korea demonstrates low levels of seropositivity in all groups. Officially reported statistics of AIDS in the People's Republic of China describe extremely low rates, but the reliability of these reports is unknown. The level of knowledge about sexually transmitted diseases appears to be low: in a 1994 survey involving rural Chinese villagers, only 18% had heard of AIDS, and only 25% and 28% respectively had heard of sexually transmitted diseases or condoms.

Hong Kong appears to have a type 1 or Western distribution of infections, with the majority in homosexuals and bisexuals. *Pneumocystis carinii* and tuberculosis are common opportunistic infections. Singapore appears to have a relatively low level of HIV infection. In Vietnam, the infected population primarily comprises male intravenous drug abusers and female sex workers. Thailand has experienced three major HIV epidemics, in intravenous drug users, sex workers, and male sexually transmitted disease (STD) patients. Efforts to limit the epidemic have been ineffective. Two-thirds of the intravenous drug abusers in Myanmar (formerly Burma) are thought to carry the virus. The three most common opportunistic infections encountered in the AIDS population in Southeast Asia are extrapulmonary tuberculosis, cryptococcosis, and *Penicillium marneffei*, a fungal pathogen endemic to the region.

The first cases detected in India by surveillance were in 1986. The Ministry of Health, plagued by budget cuts, is as yet poorly equipped to handle a large number of AIDS patients. An AIDS epidemic is predicted for India primarily because of the large number of prostitutes, many of whom are infected (47% in a sampling from 1997). Although only 4.4% of respondents to a 1997 Delhi survey had participated in sex outside or before marriage, most positive respondents were males who frequently sought sex with commercial sex workers. Almost half had never used a condom during extramarital or premarital encounters.

The male to female infection ratio in India is 5:1, with female cases being primarily seen in prostitutes. The typical route of infection among males is heterosexual contact with female sex workers, while in women who are not prostitutes, the most common source of infection is their husband. Large numbers of blood donors are HIV positive, particularly professional blood donors.

In the study by Chacko et al. of 61 AIDS patients in Vellore, India, the most common presenting symptoms included weight loss, fever, and chronic diarrhea. Common secondary infections included tuberculosis, both pulmonary and/or extrapulmonary, oropharyngeal candidiasis, and cryptococcal meningitis. Kaposi's sarcoma was not seen in any patient. The mean duration from AIDS diagnosis to death was 4.5 months. In another study, tuberculosis and candidiasis were the most common secondary infections. Secondary infections by virulent bacteria are also common, as are cryptococcosis, cryptosporidiosis, and cytomegalovirus. Although *Pneumocystis carinii* pneumonia was not observed in one Indian study, in another 9% of patients expired with *P. carinii* as a terminal infection, with a mean CD4 count of 6 cells/mm^3. In a small study of interstitial pneumonia in Bombay, three of five patients were bronchoalveolar lavage or transbronchial biopsy positive for *P. carinii*. Among Indian AIDS patients examined at autopsy for gastrointestinal disease, 71% of those with diarrhea yielded an organism, as compared with 29% of those without diarrhea. The most frequent pathogens were cytomegalovirus, parasites, fungi, and *Mycobacterium tuberculosis*.

Screening of a high-risk population at a sexually transmitted disease clinic in Bombay also revealed a high incidence of HIV-2 infection, usually occurring as a co-infection with HIV-1. However, in another study by Saran and Gupta of all seropositives tested for both viruses, 31% were HIV-2 positive only. Thus, India joins the group of HIV-2 epidemic countries, which has included Western Europe, West Africa, Brazil, and the United States.

Cuba and the Caribbean

A large screening study within Cuba has revealed that the overall prevalence of infection in that country is extremely low, with higher rates in visiting foreigners and in homosexuals. Those infected are isolated to contain the epidemic.

Other Caribbean countries differ greatly from Cuba. In these countries transmission appears to be primarily homosexual, bisexual, and heterosexual, with a minor contribution of intravenous drug abuse. Bisexuality is generally believed to be common in the Caribbean because homosexuality is not well tolerated; therefore many homosexuals are married with families. Subsequent spread to the general heterosexual population has occurred, and pediatric AIDS has resulted. Further spread of HIV in the community has been promoted by cultural patterns of multiple sexual partners and a propensity for unprotected sex.

Quinn's study of 4000 women attending a prenatal clinic in Port au Prince, Haiti, demonstrated a 9.2% HIV infection rate. High rates of infection have also been seen in the English-speaking Caribbean countries such as the Bahamas and Bermuda.

Co-infection with HTLV-1 may occur, and this appears to speed progression to AIDS and shorten survival.

Histoplasmosis capsulati is endemic in much of the Caribbean, and AIDS patients are at risk for disseminated disease: there are also high rates of tuberculosis.

Central and South America

In Latin America, HIV infection is most common in Brazil and Mexico. Initial infections appeared in homosexual and bisexual males with subsequent spread to the heterosexual community via bisexuals. Intravenous drug abusers contribute to spread in a limited fashion, particularly in Argentina and Brazil. Unlike Africa and Asia, prostitution does not appear to be a major factor. Mexico is an endemic area for coccidioidomycosis, and Central America is an endemic area for histoplasmosis capsulati. Protozoal infections such as toxoplasmosis, cryptosporidiosis, and isosporiasis are common in South America. Fungal and mycobacterial innfections are more common in Brazil than *P. carinii* or viral infections.

Australia

The patterns of HIV infection is type 1, with initial cases seen in homosexual and bisexual males in urban centers. Subsequent transmission to the heterosexual population has occurred. Education of the public and the prostitute population and increased condom use have diminished the spread of a variety of sexually transmitted diseases including gonorrhea. Unfortunately, participation as sex tourists in Asian countries by Australian males has produced persistent seeding of penicillinase-producing strains of gonorrhea from Southeast Asia, with obvious implications for the importation of HIV. Opportunistic infections appear to be similar to those encountered in the United States, with a high prevalence of *P. carinii* infection and a preponderance of atypical mycobacterial infection as compared with *M. tuberculosis*.

Epidemiology

Human retroviral infection was first documented in 1980, with the discovery of what is now termed HTLV-1. This virus is recognized as the cause of certain T-cell leukemias and lymphomas, as well as tropical spastic paraparesis, characterized by advancing spasticity and weakness with sensory disturbances. Another retrovirus, HTLV-II, appears closely associated with intravenous drug use, but its role in human disease remains unclear. It is most common in West Africa, but has been seen in Europe, North America, and recently in India. It is closely related to the simian immunodeficiency virus (SIV) and also causes a similar immunodeficiency syndrome. There are five subtypes. Recent studies have suggested that the clinical course of HIV-2 may be more indolent than that of HIV-1 (Markovitz) and that the complications may differ from those of HIV-1, with increased rates of cytomegalovirus, HIV encephalitis, and cholangitis (Lucas et al). Furthermore, a study of prostitutes in Dakaar, Senegal, indicates that HIV-2 is less easily transmitted sexually than HIV-1 (Kanki et al). Perinatal transmission appears to be rare (Markovitz). Some patients are co-infected with HIV-1 and HIV-2, or with HIV-1 and HTLV-1.

HTLV-III, redesignated HIV-1, the cause of AIDS, has spread worldwide in epidemic proportions. There are two major groups, M (containing ten subtypes, subtype B being the most common worldwide) and O (containing various heterogeneous viruses). There is some evidence that when an individual is co-infected with multiple subtypes, in vivo genetic recombination may occur, creating hybrid genomes, resulting in further antigenic diversity (and thus a potential threat to vaccine development).

No one can be sure when the AIDS mutation occurred. The HIV has now been identified in blood samples from Zaire as far back as 1959. Because an early poliomyelitis vaccine is known to have been contaminated with at least one monkey virus, SV 40, some have speculated that that HIV represents a mutation of SIV, introduced into the human population by a contaminated poliomyelitis vaccine used in Africa in the 1950s. Genetic analysis suggests that mutation occurred in the late 1940s or 1950s. Regardless of its origins, there is no clinical evidence that AIDS developed as a significant clinical disease before the mid 1970s. Blood samples from central and southern Africa from 1970 to 1974 are negative for HIV. The autopsy services at major medical centers in Africa were active, taking part in extensive and careful 5-year cancer surveys. There was no evidence of an AIDS-like syndrome or "slim disease." Significant numbers of AIDS cases did not develop until the mid 1970s. It can only be concluded that since the first edition of this book, a new disease has come to the fore, replacing a disease (smallpox) which has been eradicated.

Pathology

HIV may be found in serum and plasma, lymphocytes, semen, cervical and vaginal secretions, saliva, cerebrospinal fluid, tears, urine, amniotic fluid, breast milk, and body tissues. After entry into the body, HIV preferentially infects and kills a specific group of T-helper lymphocytes known as CD4 cells. A viral surface glycoprotein binds the virus to the CD4 receptor, allowing viral RNA to enter the cell. The viral genetic information becomes incorporated into the host cell nucleus, resulting in production of more copies of the virus and destruction of the host T-helper cell. A decrease in the number of these cells impacts their role in the activation of B lymphocytes, monocytes, and natural killer cells. When counts fall too low, opportunistic infections will provide clinical evidence of immunosuppression. For this reason, CD4 lymphocyte counts are used to monitor the degree of immunosuppression as HIV infection progresses. AIDS is diagnosed when the CD4 count falls below 200 cells/mm^3, or when an AIDS-defining opportunistic infection or malignancy develops. As immunosuppression worsens, the CD4 count can be used to predict the types of opportunistic infections and malignancies for which the patient is at risk, allowing the timely institution of prophylactic measures if available.

Some individuals may not be susceptible to AIDS. For instance, an inactive allele of chemokine receptor 5, a cell entry co-factor for HIV, confers resistance when homozygous, and slows progression when heterozygous. This mutation is present in 1% of Caucasians in the homozygous form but is rare in other racial groups tested. However, because other heavily exposed individuals lacking this mutation remain HIV negative, other forms of resistance are presumed to exist. There is a so far unexplained small group of very high risk prostitutes in Nairobi who have remained HIV negative for years.

The laboratory results can be correlated with the clinical stages of AIDS. Immediately after infection, there is an asymptomatic carrier stage. This is antibody negative but the virus itself can be detected. After about 2–4 weeks, some patients may experience an acute self-limiting illness characterized by fever, malaise, a rash, arthralgia, and often generalized lymphadenopathy. These nonspecific viral symptoms fade into a healthy antibody-positive carrier state, which may last for as long as 10 years while the immune system does silent but ferocious battle with the virus. Eventually, a significant loss of the CD4 T-helper lymphocytes becomes clinically recognizable when there is development of the opportunistic infections, neoplasms, and/or neurological symptoms characteristic of AIDS. In Europe and the United States, between 2% and 8% of serum-positive homosexuals develop clinical illness each year. After 12–13 years about 65% will be AIDS patients.

There is some evidence that chronic immune activation due to antigenic stress by parasitic infestation or other chronic infections common in the tropics may increase the risk of seroconversion after exposure to HIV and increase the rate of disease progression to AIDS and death. In a laboratory experiment designed by Weissman and colleagues to examine the relationship between immunostimulation and susceptibility to AIDS infection, immunostimulated lymphoid cells required 100 times less HIV to produce infection than nonimmunostimulated cells. It has been demonstrated in Uganda that progression from HIV infection to clinical AIDS is more rapid than for similar patient cohorts in developed countries.

If the individual is otherwise healthy, the rate of progression from HIV infection to AIDS is surprisingly uniform in different parts of the world. When AIDS does develop, however, progress towards death is often more rapid in the tropics than in Europe or the United States. This may be due to a delay in seeking health care, or none may be available; in addition there may be increased exposure to other infections such as dysentery or tuberculosis in the tropics, and ill health may be complicated by malnutrition.

The clinical history is different for those who, following the initial viral stage, become symptomatic and have a persistently low helper/suppressor (CD4/

CD8) ratio. These patients often have persistent lymphadenopathy or one or more other symptoms and signs without the complete AIDS syndrome. This is ARC, or AIDS-related complex. Their progress is more rapid, and 20%–50% of patients deteriorate to AIDS within a year.

The standard criteria for AIDS diagnosis are a positive laboratory test for HIV antibodies, specific histological or microbiological confirmation of an HIV-defining disease, and documentation of CD4 cell counts of less than 200 cells/µl. In some cases, diagnostic imaging (such as a CT scan) may be used for the nonpathological confirmation of the complications of the disease.

Routine serological testing with an enzyme-linked immunosorbent assay (ELISA) should be confirmed when positive with a Western blot. Alternative laboratory testing protocols, such as substituting two ELISA tests for an ELISA and a Western blot, will generate what may be an unacceptable level of both false-negative and false-positive results. For example, an Indian study by Chattopadhya and colleagues compared two serial ELISA tests with a Western blot test: samples positive by a first serological screening test and negative by a second serological screening test, results considered negative by the World Health Organization (WHO) protocol, were found to be HIV positive by Western blot in 8.7% of cases. But if two samples were positive on ELISA screening, 3.2% were HIV negative by Western blot.

The HIV-2 retrovirus cross-reacts with SIV serological testing, but is not always detected by HIV-1 serological tests, so in some geographic areas, two types of screening test are required. Testing for viral load is predictive of prognosis and useful for monitoring antiviral therapy.

Progression to AIDS may also be monitored by following CD4 cell counts, as well as total lymphocyte counts (TLC). Post and colleagues have determined that a TLC of <1250/µl predicts disease progression as accurately as a CD4 count of <200/µl and may be used to initiate prophylaxis.

The Clinical Patterns

HIV infection causes essentially the same immunosuppression in all of its hosts, but the clinical presentation and complications of AIDS in the tropics differ because of preexisting conditions in the host and the host's environment, many of which also contribute to immunosuppression. These include poor hygiene, poor living conditions, preexisting infections (especially parasites), chronic debilitating, diseases, nutritional deficiencies, reduced accessibility to diagnosis and treatment and, possibly but unlikely, unknown factors such as genetic predisposition. This variable background also affects the patterns of spread and the progression from infection to AIDS, as well as the time from the development of AIDS to death.

When AIDS does develop, almost any system may be involved. There may be myocarditis, pericarditis, and endocarditis, and opportunistic infections presenting as oral thrush, esophagitis, gastritis, and colitis. Lymphadenopathy, particularly abdominal, may be nonspecific or tuberculous or from atypical mycobacteriosis. There may be cystitis, pyelonephritis, renal abscesses, nephropathy, and renal insufficiency. HIV-neuropathy causes various neurological syptoms, such as microcephaly, delayed development, ataxia, seizures, dementia and coma.

In much of the tropics, tuberculosis and the gastrointestinal manifestations of AIDS predominate. *M. tuberculosis* is the most common significant pathogen and gastrointestinal disease the most common clinical presentation. Common Western pathogens, such as *P. carinii* and atypical mycobacteria are rare in many regions, but both groups, tropical and temperate, share other complications such as Kaposi's sarcoma, although not always in the same way.

Children with AIDS have their own diagnostic problems. Many of the clinical signs and symptoms resemble common childhood complaints (see p. 688).

Clinical Definitions of AIDS

Clinical criteria to define AIDS have been developed by the World Health Organization for use in sub-Saharan Africa and elsewhere to allow the diagnosis of AIDS without laboratory testing. Clinical definitions vary considerably in different locations depending on the local prevalence of opportunistic diseases and the sophistication of diagnostic procedures available. The sensitivity of the clinical definition developed for sub-Saharan Africa has ranged from about 33% to 65%, with a specificity of 78%–90%.

Relying on clinical criteria alone has certain drawbacks. For example, in Africa, the present system includes persistent cough as one of the minor criteria, and severe weight loss and persistent fever as major criteria, making it difficult to distinguish patients with tuberculosis from those with AIDS. Even in patients known to be HIV positive, the presence of pulmonary tuberculosis and the accompanying symptoms need not indicate progression to AIDS. As another example, a common manifestation of AIDS in Africa is "slim disease," manifested by weight loss, chronic diarrhea, and chronic fever. This was incorporated into one definition of the HIV-related wasting syndrome, but only if not associated with other conditions such as cryptosporidiosis or tuberculosis which might cause similar findings. However, in many cases, these other diseases are related to HIV and it is often difficult in Africa to exclude such concurrent diseases. It has been suggested that in Africa, the HIV-related wasting syndrome might better be defined as requiring greater than 10% weight loss, chronic diarrhea for at least 30 days, and chronic fever for at least 30 days, whether or not there are concomitant diseases which might be responsible for these findings.

A population study in Tanzania by Todd and colleagues showed that the proportion of adult deaths attributable to HIV was 35% overall and 53% in the 20–29 age group. However, the applicable WHO clinical case definition of AIDS was satisfied for only 18% of deaths occurring in HIV-positive patients because many signs and symptoms associated with HIV deaths were nonspecific.

A clinical definition of AIDS has been developed for South America, applicable to developing countries with adequate serological facilities but without other sophisticated diagnostic procedures. Clinical criteria in South America differ from those used in Africa: diarrhea and weight loss are less common in South American patients, so cachexia was substituted. The South American definition also has the advantage of including symptoms of central nervous system dysfunction. Using a complex scoring system of symptomatolology and documented diseases, this system achieves relatively high specificity and sensitivity.

Clinical definitions of AIDS should ideally be equated with a laboratory standard such as a CD4 count of less than 200 cell per mm^3. However, it is unlikely that even tailored clinical definitions can be accurate in locations where there are high endemic rates of diseases which are also HIV associated, such as tuberculosis and Kaposi's sarcoma.

Infants, Children, and AIDS

Thirty percent or more of children born to HIV-seropositive mothers will themselves become seropositive, and their AIDS incubation period will be shorter, with clinical signs and symptoms appearing relatively quickly. However, HIV-1 serological tests in infants must be interpreted with caution because maternal antibodies may persist for as long as 15 months. Thus, if there are no clinical indications of disease, a positive serological test in an infant under 15 months may not indicate infection and may revert to negative. If the child is antibody positive after age 15 months, he or she is probably infected. When available, viral culture, *in vitro* production of antibodies, or polymerase chain reaction testing can resolve this dilemma.

Children with AIDS have their own special diagnostic problems. Many of the clinical signs and symptoms of the disease are similar to other common childhood complaints, such as measles (often a severe disease in the tropics), malaria, failure to thrive, chronic cough and fevers, recurrent diarrhea, and respiratory disease. The difficulties are exemplified by pneumonia, which in the developing world is the cause of death of 30% of children under the age of 5 years, even without AIDS. Distinguishing between bacterial pneumonia and tuberculosis and determining which patient might harbor HIV is a major diagnostic challenge, especially where laboratory and imaging facilities are limited or nonexistent. In some regions, Burkitt's lymphoma and acute Kaposi's sarcoma of childhood are endemic and their presence is not AIDS defining.

In the study by Vetter et al. of children hospitalized in Abidjan, Ivory Coast, the most common reasons for hospital admission in HIV-positive children were respiratory infection and malnutrition. Mortality was 2.4 times higher in HIV-positive children compared with HIV-negative hospitalized children. Most pneumonias in pediatric AIDS are caused by common bacterial pathogens, but if there are severe respiratory signs with any interstitial pneumonia, and a poor response to antibiotics, *P. carinii* pneumonia should be considered, even though it is rare in some countries. On the other hand, lymphocytic interstitial pneumonitis, a persistent interstitial micronodular pulmonary parenchymal pattern, may have minimal respiratory signs.

In an autopsy study of children with AIDS, also from Abidjan, respiratory infections, *P. carinii* pneumonia, and measles were common as compared with HIV-negative deaths, while pyogenic meningitis was common in both groups. Surprisingly, in HIV-positive children, tuberculosis, lymphocytic interstitial pneumonitis, and HIV encephalitis were rarely found at autopsy. In a study from Zambia, high HIV rates were found in children with tuberculosis (69%), malnutrition (41%), pneumonia (28%), and diarrhea (24%). HIV may be responsible for various neurological symptoms in children, including microcephaly, delayed development, ataxia, seizures, and coma.

Malaria and Transfusion-Related AIDS

Malaria, particularly infection with *Plasmodium falciparum*, is an immense public health problem in Africa and many other tropical countries, made worse by the increase in drug-resistant strains. Fortunately, concomitant HIV infection does not seem to increase the chances of clinically significant malarial episodes, or change the rate of progression from HIV to AIDS. Indeed, there has even been some evidence that malaria or the chloroquine used to treat malaria may have some effect against HIV. An elegant longitudinal study from Mama Yemo Hospital in Kinshasa, Zaire, showed no difference in malarial rates in a group of children who had been exposed to HIV in utero, some of whom were HIV positive, some of whom had advanced AIDS, and some of whom were HIV negative or had reverted to the HIV-negative state after birth. These findings are confirmed by numerous other studies.

However, the severe anemia caused by malaria may necessitate transfusion, which presents a substantial risk for AIDS and other blood-borne diseases. For example, 87% of transfusion in Kinshasa are performed for malaria and 6% of the blood donors are HIV positive. Chikwem et al's study of donated blood in Nigeria revealed that among 364 healthy donors, 14.9% showed hepatitis B, 5.8% HIV-1, 4.1% *Plasmodium falciparum*, and 3.6% *Treponema pallidum*. Worldwide, HIV-positive blood is transfused either because the blood is not properly tested or because blood must be given in an emergency whether or not it has been tested, and testing may be a lengthy process. Needles may be reused without effective sterilization. The risk of transfusion-related AIDS is found over much of the malarial world, compounded in some regions (such as West Africa), by the high prevalence of hemoglobinopathies which also require transfusion.

Falciparum malaria is the most common cause of anemia of pregnancy in sub-Saharan Africa. Malarial parasitemia is highest in the 13th–16th weeks of pregnancy and, for unknown reasons, the rise is most significant in the primigravida patients. It is not, however, the only cause of anemia: parasites, malnutrition, high fertility rates, and chronic ill health all contribute. In Zaire, examination of 2950 untreated pregnancies revealed that 72% of patients had a moderate anemia (hemoglobin level 7–11) and 3.7% of patients had severe anemia (hemoglobin under 7). A 50% mortality is observed when the hematocrit is less than 13% and there is concomitant heart failure. Because the anemia of pregnancy is often treated by transfusion with inadequately screened blood, it is an important cause of AIDS in the maternal and fetal populations.

Leprosy and AIDS

Although far less common than *Mycobacterium tuberculosis, Mycobacterium leprae* is still a significant public health problem in sub-Saharan Africa, India, and other developing countries in Asia, the Middle East, the Caribbean, and Haiti (see Chap. 34). There has been concern that, due to immunosuppression, HIV may increase susceptibility to leprosy. Data are mixed on this subject. A study in Zambia demonstrated a markedly increased incidence of HIV infection in new leprosy patients as compared with controls, whereas a larger study of leprosy patients in the Ivory Coast, Senegal, and Yemen noted equal HIV-positivity rates. In a primate model of leprosy, inoculation led to increased leprosy infection rates in those animals which were SIV positive. It has been postulated (but not proven) that HIV infection may accelerate the development of clinical leprosy: however, active chronic infection with leprosy may accelerate the course of HIV disease due to the preexisting immune response. In Haiti, although HIV-positive rates in leprosy patients were the same as in the general population, the HIV-positive leprosy patients progressed to symptomatic AIDS more rapidly than would be expected. It also appears that leprosy relapses are more common in HIV-infected individuals.

Maternal/Fetal AIDS

Maternal-fetal HIV transmission may occur at three stages during the perinatal period: pregnancy, delivery, and nursing. Overall, the rate of perinatal transmission varies from 20% to 60%. Rates of HIV-1 and HIV-2 transmission are similar. Intrauterine transmission probably occurs in 20%–30% of HIV-positive mothers, but this rate can be modified if the mother receives antiviral therapy (e.g. zidovudine). Rates of transmission to the fetus are probably higher if the mother becomes infected during her pregnancy and becomes viremic at that time rather than being infected before she becomes pregnant. Transmission during delivery occurs; the risks are unknown but thought to be high. For comparison, 90% of hepatitis B transmissions are known to occur during delivery, and therefore delivery is likely to be a significant risk period for HIV transmission as well. The transmission of AIDS postpartum also occurs, since the virus is found in breast milk. A 15% increase in perinatal HIV transmission has been documented in infants breast fed exclusively, as compared with formula-fed infants. The risk of transmission increases with the number of months of breast feeding. However, without breast feeding, many babies in the tropics will likely be malnourished or develop diarrhea due to poor hygiene. While HIV-positive mothers in Europe and America are advised not to breast feed their babies, if babies in the tropics are not breast fed, the increase in infant mortality may exceed mortality from AIDS.

In July 1998 the United Nations changed their policy and recommended that women who were HIV-positive should not breast feed their infants. The UN acknowledged that this is a very controversial policy and would be against well-established social customs in many countries. But in 1997 UNAIDS estimated that 30% (200,000) of the 600,000 children in the world who became HIV infected, acquired their infection from breast feeding. Recent studies have shown that as many as 70% of the women at prenatal clinics may be HIV positive, and 30% or more of women in six African countries were infected. The major problem with the new policy is that 90% of women in developing countries do not know whether or not they are infected and worldwide at least 30% of pregnant women receive no antenatal care.

Women who have symptomatic HIV infections or AIDS have a significantly increased rate of miscarriage, low-birth-weight infants, intrauterine fetal death, and preterm delivery; however, asymptomatic HIV-positive infections have not been associated with increased complications of pregnancy, according to the work of Kumar and colleagues. Placental size may be larger in HIV-infected mothers, a nonspecific sign seen in numerous infections.

Although it had been previously believed that a single pregnancy does not adversely affect the course of HIV disease in the mother, a recent controlled study by Kumar and colleagues from India refutes this. HIV-infected pregnant and nonpregnant women were matched for CD4 counts, age, and parity. The mean survival time was about 19 months for the pregnant women and about 23 months for the nonpregnant women. Many of the infants were delivered preterm, with high infant mortality.

Multiple pregnancies in the HIV-infected mother are thought to speed progression towards clinical AIDS. A possible mechanism for this is the activation of latently infected helper cells by the circulating paternal antigens from the fetus, viral production being stimulated by each successive pregnancy.

HIV Transmission and Other Sexually Transmitted Diseases

Key to the understanding of different patterns of spread worldwide are differences in the relative efficiency of heterosexual transmission of AIDS. In the United States, heterosexual contact is relatively inefficient in spreading HIV, with a possibility of conversion estimated at approximately 0.2% with a single sexual contact. In comparison, an infected prostitute in Nairobi may have an HIV transmission rate of 8% with a single sexual contact, rising to 28% if the male was uncircumcised and a genital ulcer was acquired at the same time.

The rate of heterosexual AIDS transmission is significantly increased if the couple (or one partner) already has an ulcerative sexually transmitted disease. This may affect HIV transmission in one of three ways. First, genital ulcers may increase the infectivity of the donor because of blood or serum from the ulcerated area. Second, open sores may increase the susceptibility of the recipient, both due to nonintact skin or mucosa and also because there may be an increased number of CD4 cells at the ulcer site, making cross-infection easier. Finally, various diseases may be cofactors in any HIV initial infection or progression from increased activation of T4 lymphocytes leading to increased production of HIV-infected cells and viral copies.

The sexually transmitted diseases associated with increased HIV infection include syphilis, chancroid, lymphogranuloma venereum, and herpes simplex. These are all common in most areas in which heterosexual tansmission occurs. *Chlamydia trachomatis* is a possible cofactor. Gonorrhea and genital warts, as well as various other nonulcerative sexually transmitted diseases, probably do not increase susceptibility to or transmission of HIV. The incidence of non-AIDS sexually transmitted diseases observed in antenatal clinics in Malawi has been measured by Maher and Hoffman at 42%, with a 32% HIV positive rate.

Men who have not been circumcised are at increased risk of HIV infection (odds ratio 4.8), with countries in which circumcision is rare closely matching the countries of the "AIDS belt" in Africa. The effect may be due to an increased incidence of ulcerative STDs such as chancroid in uncircumcised males, as well as other factors related to hygiene or a more favorable environment for viral survival and transmission. The relative risk is so striking that some believe circumcision should be considered as an intervention strategy for AIDS control.

Complications of AIDS in the Tropics

Many diseases present in the tropics can hasten the development of AIDS, change its clinical course, or attack a host weakened by AIDS. Many of these diseases will have different manifestations than when encountered in the normal host. As already described (p. 687), the clinical presentation and complications of AIDS differ mainly because of preexisting conditions in the host and the host's environment. Some complications of AIDS in the tropics are never seen in Western patients. For example, the protozoan responsible for leishmaniasis has emerged as an AIDS-related pathogen in South America, India, Central Asia, and around the Mediterranean, including North Africa, and penicilliosis is seen exclusively in Southeast Asia.

There is no evidence that amebiasis, malaria, purulent meningitis, schistosomiasis, tetanus, cholera, malignancies (other than Kaposi sarcoma and lymphoma), and nondisseminated strongyloidiasis are increased in HIV-positive individuals or individuals with AIDS.

As the CD4 count falls, reflecting increasing immunosuppression, the patient will become susceptible to increasingly opportunistic organisms. For instance, thrush may appear when CD4 counts have only fallen to 300–400 cells/mm^3. As long as CD4 lymphocyte counts remain above 200 cells/mm^3, common bacterial pneumonias and *Mycobacterium tuberculosis* predominate. With increasing immunosuppression (CD4 counts less than 200 cells/mm^3), unusual bacterial pathogens and *Pneumocystis carinii* appear. With further declines, disseminated fungal infections and Kaposi's sarcoma are seen. At CD4 counts of below 50 cells/mm^3, lymphoma, cytomegalovirus, and atypical mycobacteria become more likely. Patients in the tropics are likely to die from infections associated with AIDS such as tuberculosis, intestinal parasites, or bacterial pathogens even before a profound level of immunosuppression is reached. This explains why some of the complications of AIDS which are common in more temperate climates are rarely encountered in the tropics. The mean CD4 count of AIDS patients at death in the large autopsy series by Lucas and colleagues from West Africa was 141 cells/mm^3.

With worsening immunosuppression, some less opportunistic organisms may present with unusual clinical or radiological features, reflecting the diminished ability of the immune system to control the infection. For example, with CD4 counts below 200/mm^3, the body can no longer mount a granulomatous response: tuberculosis is then less likely to form localized granulomas or cavities and more likely to produce patchy airspace disease or undergo hematogenous dissemination. Similarly, pulmonary cryptococcosis presents as a diffuse pneumonia rather than as well-circumscribed lung nodules.

Categorization of the many pathogens which affect AIDS patients in the tropics is difficult because the majority involve more than one body part or organ system. In the following summary of imaging findings, organisms have been loosely grouped by the region involved. Whenever possible, illustrative radiographs have been obtained from AIDS patients living in or who have recently emigrated from the tropics.

Organisms Causing Pulmonary Infections

Tuberculosis

The mycobacterial infection most commonly associated with AIDS in the tropics is tuberculosis. In the autopsy series of Lucas and colleagues from the Ivory Coast, the most common cause of death in HIV-positive patients was tuberculosis, disseminated in the vast majority of cases. In 32% it was the cause of death, while in an additional 6%, active tuberculosis was present but not the primary cause of death. Fifty-four percent of HIV-positive patients with AIDS-defining pathology had tuberculosis. The disease was disseminated in almost all of these patients and tuberculous meningitis and tuberculous enteritis were common extrapulmonary manifestations.

Even prior to the onset of the AIDS epidemic, tuberculosis was an extremely common cause of morbidity and mortality in the tropics, with a prevalence of infection much greater than 50% (see Chap. 5). In the tropics, it is probable that many people are already infected with *M. tuberculosis* before becoming HIV positive, but those with HIV have a greatly increased risk of developing or reactivating tuberculosis as compared with seronegative patients. For example, the study by Leroy and colleagues of women in Kigali, Rwanda, demonstrated an 18.2-fold increase in the incidence of active tuberculosis in HIV-positive patients after 4 years of follow-up as compared with HIV-negative controls. As has been confirmed by recent DNA fingerprinting studies, the majority of HIV-associated active tuberculous infections, even those occurring after adequate treatment, are the result of reactivation, although primary infection or reinfection also occurs. HIV-infected tuberculosis patients have a higher incidence of fever, tuberculin skin test anergy, and positive blood cultures than normal hosts.

The interaction between tuberculosis and HIV may have consequences for both epidemics. Cases of tuberculosis have increased twice as fast in countries with high HIV seropositivity as compared to countries with low seropositivity. In very broad terms, about a third of tuberculosis cases can be attributed to HIV. Poor cell-mediated immunity in HIV leads to greater susceptibility to tuberculous infection, and these individuals then transmit the disease to others, further increasing the epidemic. The risk of reactivation of tuberculosis in an AIDS patient over the course of 1 year approximates the risk of reactivation in an HIV-negative patient over a lifetime. The rapid progression to clinical tuberculosis in AIDS patients contributes to the development of resistant strains of tuberculosis. There is increasing evidence that tuberculosis speeds the clinical course of pre-existing HIV infection, and recent studies have suggested that treatment for tuberculosis will actually increase CD4+ cell counts in some AIDS patients.

The prevalence of HIV in patients with tuberculosis in sub-Saharan African countries ranges from 20% to 67%: in Mexico it is about 25%, in Central America and South America about 20%–30%. In Central Africa about 40% of HIV-positive autopsies show disseminated tuberculosis. Of those patients dying with "slim disease," 44% had disseminated tuberculosis at autopsy. Among patients with extrapulmonary tuberculosis, the majority will be HIV positive. Extrapulmonary tuberculosis has been found in 70% of patients with tuberculosis who have CD4 counts of less than 100 cells/mm^3.

As previously noted, the high incidence of tuberculosis can confuse AIDS statistics. Where only clinical criteria are used for the diagnosis of AIDS, there may be overdiagnosis of AIDS in patients who only have tuberculosis. The same clinical findings may be seen in both, such as weight loss exceeding 10% of body weight, with fever and cough for a month or more. Many patients with untreated tuberculosis, particularly those who are undernourished or in chronic ill health from parasites, will meet the clinical criteria for AIDS without actually having the disease. On the other hand, AIDS patients infected with tuberculosis often have no sputum, negative sputum smears, or negative chest radiographs, making the diagnosis of tuberculosis more difficult.

Extrapulmonary tuberculosis may produce extensive lymphadenopathy in patients with AIDS, often with low-density or hypoechoic necrotic centers seen on CT or ultrasound scanning. It may be impossible to differentiate between tuberculosis and lymphoma, and both may exist together. Tuberculous lymphadenitis in HIV patients (as well as HIV-related lymphadenitis) tends to be bilateral and symmetrical, involving many nodal groups, while tuberculous lymphadenitis in the normal host is usually asymmetrical, focal, and often cervical. Other extrapulmonary manifestations, such as pleural, pericardial, abdominal, meningeal and miliary spread, are very common in AIDS patients. Unfortunately, they are also common in undernourished and chronically unwell individuals without AIDS.

In one study, HIV-2 infection appeared to be associated with a lower tuberculosis mortality than HIV-1 infection or dual infection. However, in Abidjan, patients infected with HIV-2 and tuberculosis showed wasting, diarrhea, candidiasis, and lymphadenopathy, similar to patients with HIV-1. Among those patients presenting with newly diagnosed tuberculosis, 30% were HIV-1 positive, 4% HIV-2 positive, and 9% positive for both strains. It is worthy of note that 25%–30% of these patients with active tuberculosis were PPD (purified protein derivative) negative.

Tuberculosis, provided it is not drug resistant, can be successfully treated even when the patient has AIDS, although a slow response may be expected in advanced HIV infections and the death rate will be much higher in HIV-positive or AIDS patients. Nevertheless, chemoprophylaxis with isoniazid in Zambia resulted in a ninefold decrease in AIDS-related tuberculosis. Although there was no change in the mortality statistics within this group, it can be expected that there would have been a decrease in new cases amongst contacts.

Tuberculosis remains an enormous public health problem, and not only in the developing world. There are similar epidemics in eastern Europe and increasing numbers of cases throughout the developed world due to immigration, AIDS, and the emergence of resistant strains. It is estimated (1998) that about three million people die of tuberculosis every year, and these figures are probably underestimates.

Imaging Findings

Chest radiographs are not routinely taken in many third world countries for the diagnosis of tuberculosis except in severely ill patients or if a pneumothorax or pleural effusion is suspected. Thus, the diagnosis of tuberculosis relies mainly on examination of the sputum, but sputum is often scant or absent in the AIDS patient. Conversely, AIDS patients may have acid-fast bacilli (AFB) on sputum smears but a normal chest radiograph. Even if sputum is produced, negative AFB smears do not rule out tuberculosis as the cause of an abnormal chest radiograph. In an African study of AIDS patients, bronchoscopy of AFB smear-negative pneumonias which were unresponsive to penicillin yielded a diagnosis of tuberculosis in 39% of cases.

The appearance of tuberculosis on a chest radiograph is dependent on the immune status of the patient. Early in AIDS infection, tuberculosis presents in the typical pattern of the immuno-competent patient, with upper lobe densities and cavities (Fig. 8.2). Later in the infection, the immune system is no longer able to mount a granulomatous reaction, and "typical" upper lobe densities and cavitation are less common; diffuse, patchy transbronchial spread without definite granuloma formation is more common (Figs. 8.3, 8.4). There may be mediastinal or hilar lymphadenopathy, sometimes massive (Figs. 8.5–8.7). The appearance may resemble "primary" tuberculosis, but the vast majority of these cases, particularly in third world populations, represent progressive or reactivation tuberculosis.

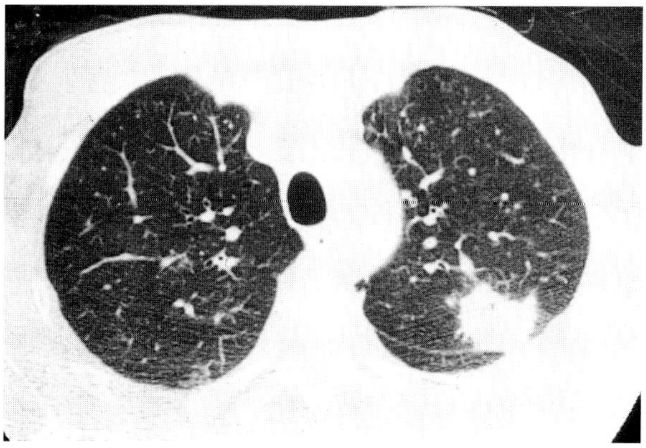

Fig. 8.2. In the earlier stages of AIDS, before the onset of profound immunosuppression, the appearance of pulmonary tuberculosis may be similar to that in the non-AIDS patient, with upper lobe nodules or cavities

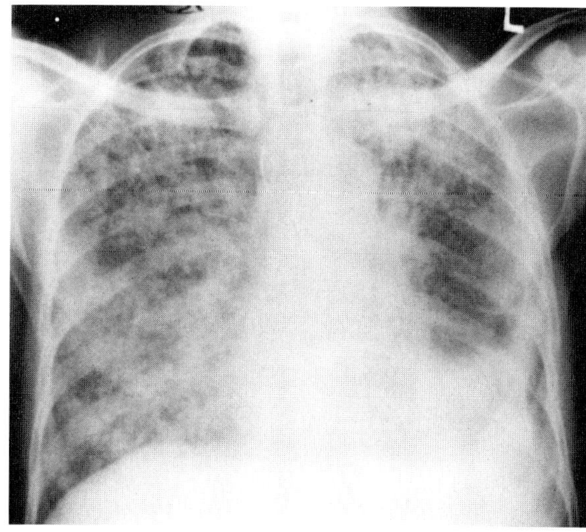

Fig. 8.3. Extensive transbronchial spread of tuberculosis from upper lobe foci

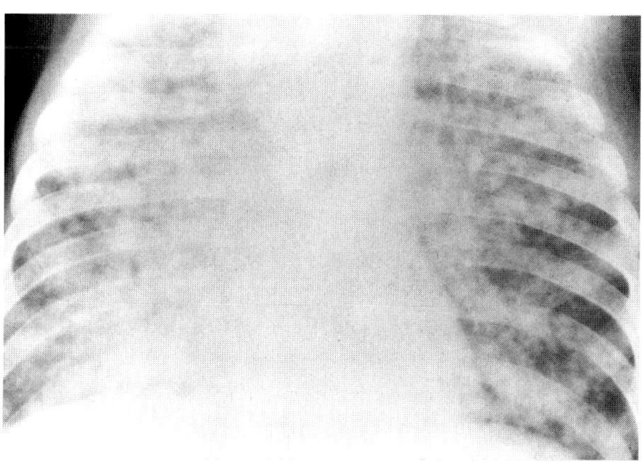

Fig. 8.4. Rapidly progressive bilateral nodular disease in a child with extensive transbronchial spread of tuberculosis

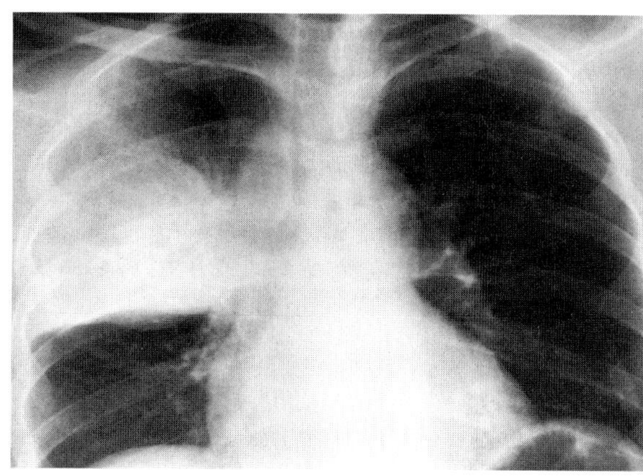

Fig. 8.5. In the AIDS patient, tuberculosis may resemble "primary" tuberculosis, as in this patient with upper lobe consolidation and massive right paratracheal lymphadenopathy

Lobar consolidation in atypical locations may be seen and progression may be unusually rapid (Fig. 8.8). Miliary disease, which ordinarily may result either from primary nonimmune or progressive primary disease, is more common in patients with AIDS than in HIV-negative patients (Fig. 8.9).

Long's comparison of radiographic findings of tuberculosis in Haitians with and without HIV or AIDS shows that a typical reactivation pattern was seen in 80% of HIV-negative patients, 51% of HIV-positive non-AIDS patients, and 20% of AIDS patients. Similarly, a typical "primary" pattern was seen in 80% of AIDS patients, 30% of HIV-positive non-AIDS patients, and 11% of HIV-negative patients.

A study of chest radiographic findings in Zambia and Zaire by Tshibwabwa-Tumba and colleagues confirms that HIV-infected tuberculosis patients, as compared to with those who are HIV-negative, have a higher incidence of lymphadenopathy (26% vs 13%), pleural effusions (16% vs 7%), miliary disease (10% vs 5%), interstitial pattern (12% vs 7%), and consolidation (10% vs 3%), but a lower incidence of atelectasis (12% vs 24%) and a much lower incidence of cavitation (33% vs 78%).

AIDS-related tuberculosis is an important cause of empyema. Two-thirds of the empyemas treated in surgical units at a Zambian Hospital were from AIDS-related tuberculosis. Pericardial effusions are also common.

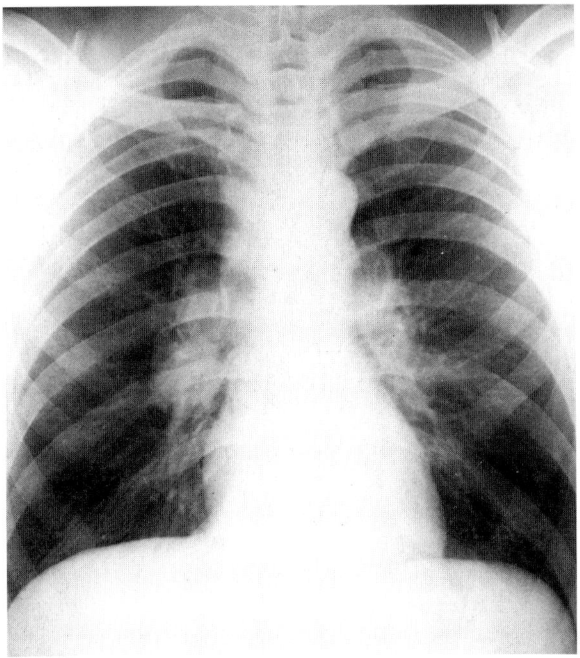

Fig. 8.6. Enlarged hilar and mediastinal lymph nodes may be the only manifestations of tuberculosis in AIDS

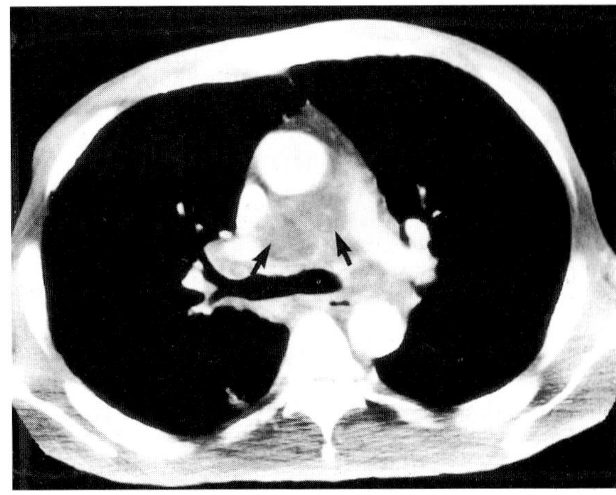

Fig. 8.7. Extensive mediastinal lymphadenopathy with some necrosis (*arrows*)

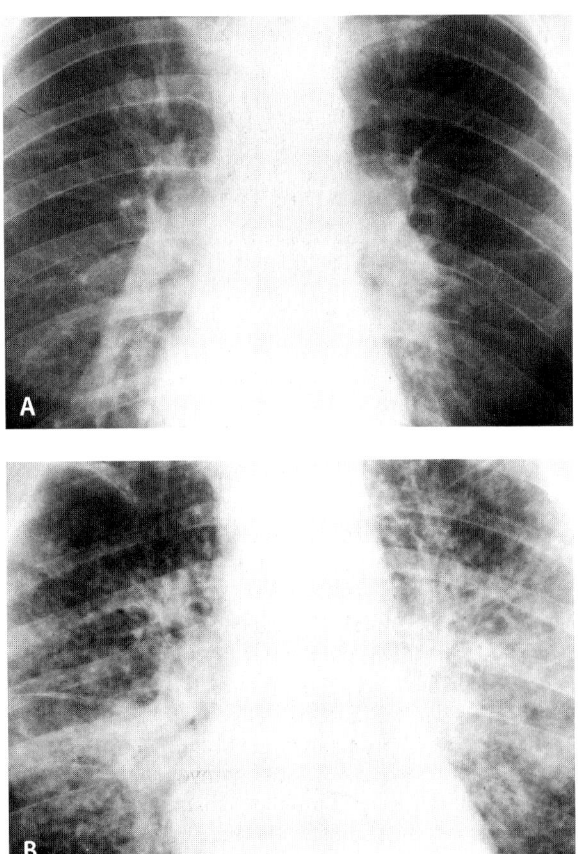

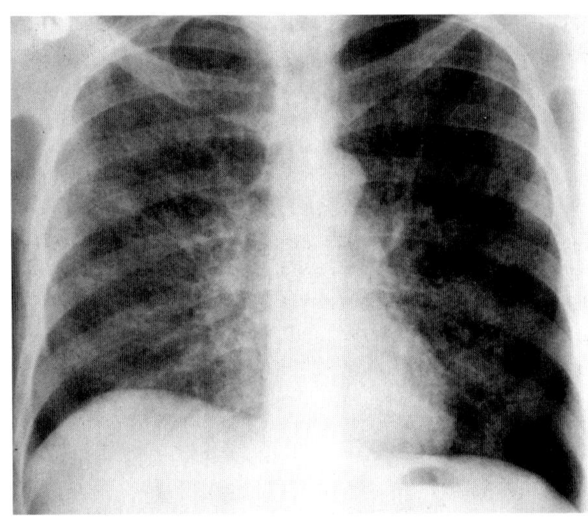

Fig. 8.9. Miliary tuberculosis is characterized by innumerable very small nodules. This condition is seen in AIDS more often than in the normal HIV-negative host, and can result either from "primary" or postprimary progressive tuberculosis

◄

Fig. 8.8 A, B. Hilar and mediastinal lymphadenopathy (A) progressing to diffuse parenchymal nodularity (B) over a 5-day period in this profoundly immunosuppressed patient

Atypical Mycobacteria

Ten strains of atypical mycobacteria cause clinical disease, but *M. avium-intracellulare*, also known as MAC (*Mycobacterium avium* complex) is a particularly common opportunistic organism in AIDS. The atypical mycobacteria are present in the environment worldwide. High rates of infection have been found in Australian AIDS patients, which is not surprising because a high prevalence has been noted there before the AIDS epidemic. In Brazil, atypical mycobacterial isolates from bone marrow aspirates are more than twice as common as *Mycobacterium tuberculosis* in AIDS patients with persistent fever, anemia, and leukopenia. In the United States, the atypical mycobacteria are one of the most common manifestations of AIDS, but clinical atypical mycobacterial infections are relatively rare in African AIDS patients. For example, in the autopsy study of Lucas and colleagues in the Ivory Coast, atypical mycobacterial infections were only seen in 3% of HIV-positive patients, and were not primarily responsible for any death. As von Reyn et al.'s culture of environmental and water supply samples from the United States, Finland, Zaire, and Kenya showed, African samples were less likely to be contaminated with atypical mycobacteria than those from the United States or Finland. Although one study found atypical mycobacteria in 13% of African AIDS patients, these infections did not appear to be clinically relevant. Similarly, atypical infections are not often encountered in most South America countries, other than Brazil.

In the developed world, most patients do not develop clinically relevant atypical mycobacterial infection until CD4+ counts fall below 100 cells/mm^3, below the mean value at death in the tropics. However, this would not seem to completely explain the marked disparity in the numbers of cases encountered, so it has been theorized that prior infection with tuberculosis, very common in the African HIV population and elsewhere in the tropics, may produce some class resistance to the development of clinically significant atypical infections. This is contrary to the commonly accepted belief held before AIDS that there is no cross-resistance between *M. tuberculosis* and the atypical mycobacteria.

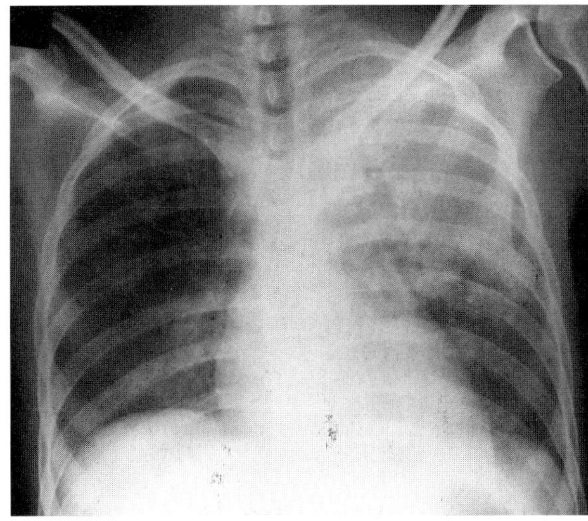

Fig. 8.10. Atypical mycobacterial infection (*Mycobacterium avium* complex) has produced extensive airspace disease in this patient with advanced AIDS

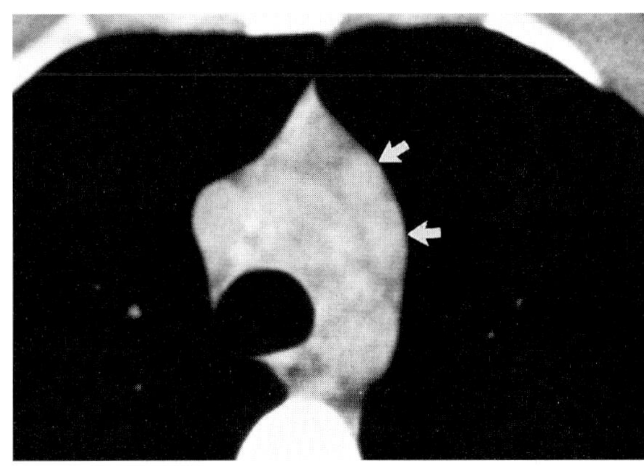

Fig. 8.11. Enlarged lymph nodes (*arrows*) caused by atypical mycobacterial disease are usually (though not necessarily) of soft tissue density

Imaging Findings

Atypical mycobacterial infection in the AIDS patient is often a disseminated infection, with correspondingly variable radiographic presentations. Chest disease may be manifested by nodules, localized airspace disease, bronchiectasis, and diffuse patchy interstitial and/or airspace disease (Fig. 8.10). The chest radiograph may also be normal in AIDS patients with documented pulmonary *M. avium* complex infection. Enlarged lymph nodes, effusions, and cavities are less common than with tuberculosis (Fig. 8.11). Extrathoracic involvement is very common (Figs. 8.12, 8.13).

It must be remembered that inspite of the differences in the chest images of HIV+ve and HIV–ve patients, it is not possible to use the imaging findings to make the diagnosis of AIDS. Many HIV-ve patients in the tropics show similar patterns of both M. tuberculosis and atypical (MOTT) infections because they are immunocompromised for other reasons (see Chap. 5, pp. 398–422).

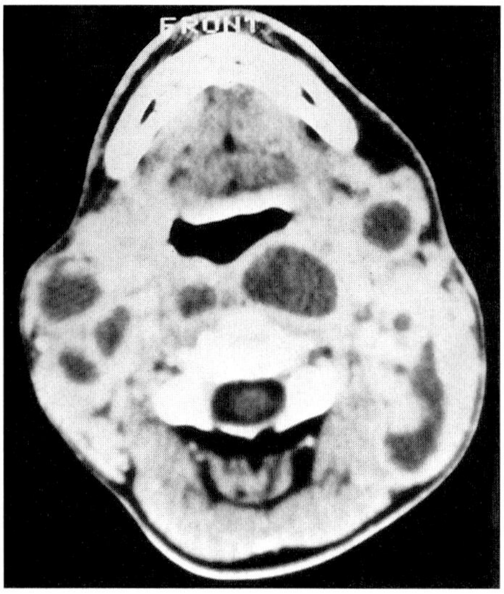

Fig. 8.12. Extensive cervical lymphadenopathy due to *Mycobacterium avium* complex showing the unusual finding of extensive necrosis

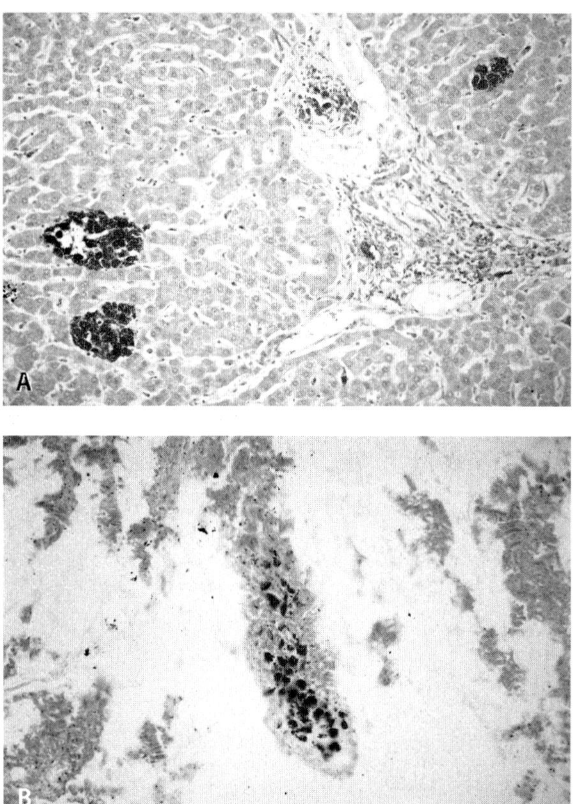

Fig. 8.13 A, B. Infection with *Mycobacterium avium* complex can result in widely disseminated lesions, as in this case: **A** In the liver and **B** in the small intestine. (Courtesy of Dr. Daniel H. Connor)

Pyogenic Infections

Frequently overlooked in discussions of AIDS-related infections are the common organisms which cause pneumonias and other infections in all patients, but for which AIDS patients are at far greater risk. In the autopsy study of Lucas and colleagues in the Ivory Coast, pyogenic pneumonias were present in 30% and were the primary cause of death in 8% of HIV-positive patients. The causative organism were equally divided between gram-positive cocci and gram-negtive rods. In a study by Gilks and colleagues of sex workers in Nairobi, 79 episodes of invasive pneumococcal disease were seen in 587 HIV-positive women, as opposed to one episode in 132 seronegative women (relative risk 17.8). Occult bacteremia was also seen in this study, a finding not usually encountered in normal adult hosts with pneumococcal pneumonia. HIV-infected patients in Kenya who later developed pneumococcal bacteremia had a significantly lower antibody level towards pneumococcal antigen (pneumolysin) compared with seronegative controls. Prevention of AIDS-associated pneumococcal disease by means of vaccination has not been attempted in the developing world.

In a study of Zimbabwean children with bacterial infections, HIV-positive children were more likely to exhibit bacteremia, particularly enterobacteremia, and more likely to die if bacteremic. Pathogens encountered were staphyloccocci (coagulase negative, followed by *S. aureus*) and *Streptococcus pneumoniae*. Nontyphoidal *Salmonella, E. coli*, and *Klebsiella* were the most frequent gram-negative isolates. Two cases of *Rhodococcus equi* pneumonia were seen, a zoonosis causing pneumonia in foals known to infect AIDS patients.

Bacteremia was present in 16% of HIV+ patients, and was responsible for 11% of deaths in the autopsy series of Lucas and colleagues (Ivory Coast). It was the second most common cause of death after tuberculosis. Etiology of the sepsis, in descending order, included pyelonephritis, pneumonia, enteritis, hepatobiliary disease, and gynecological infections.

Pyogenic pulmonary, blood, gastrointestinal, renal, sinus, CNS, skin, muscle, soft tissue, bone and joint infections, as well as endocarditis, are seen with a greater frequency in AIDS patients than in normal hosts.

Imaging Findings

In the AIDS patient, common organisms may have unusual clinical and radiographic presentations. *Streptococcus pneumoniae* is very common in the AIDS patient (Fig. 8.14). and is more likely to be as-

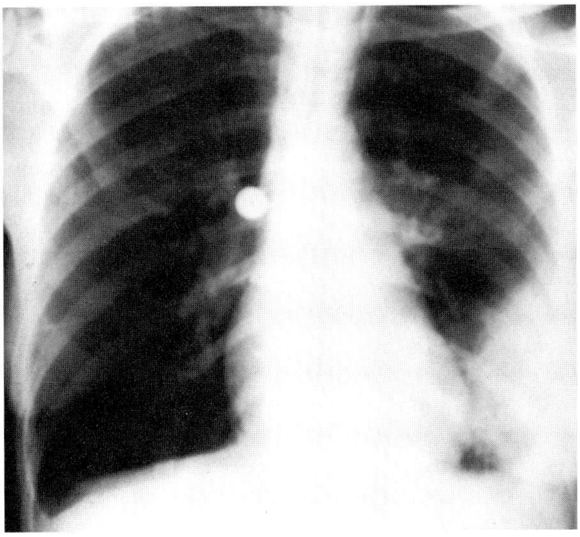

Fig. 8.14. AIDS patients are particularly susceptible to *Streptococcus pneumoniae* infection, with a higher incidence of cavitation, spread to other sites, and emypema formation as compared to the normal HIV-negative host

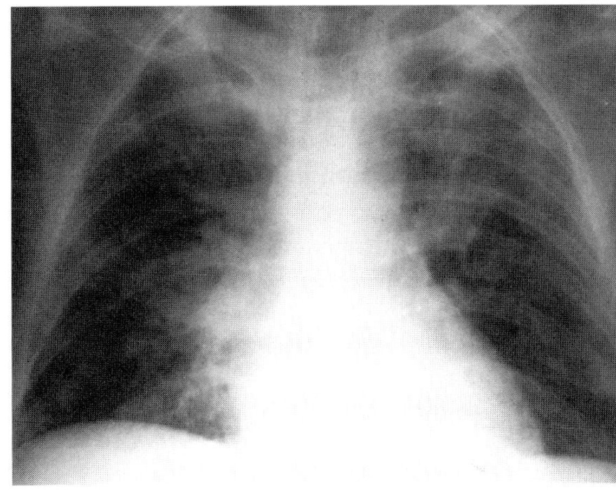

Fig. 8.15. Common pathogens such as *Pseudomonas aeruginosa* may affect AIDS patients as well as normal HIV-negative hosts, and may then have a more severe course. (Courtesy of Dr. Jeffrey Klein)

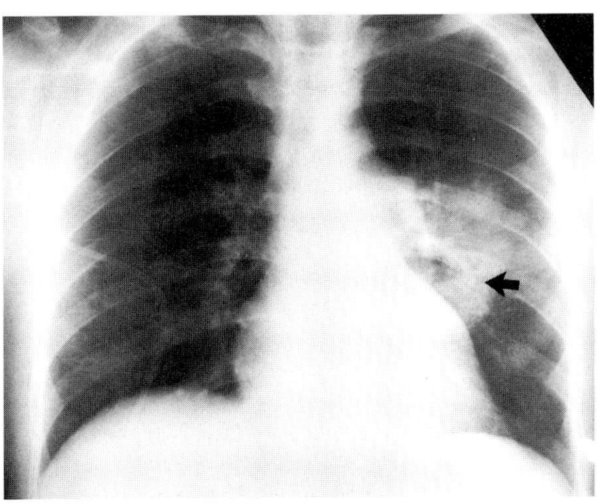

Fig. 8.16. *Rhodococcus equi*, usually encountered in equine foals, can produce mass-like areas of consolidation which may cavitate (*arrow*) in the AIDS patient. (Courtesy of Dr. Charles White)

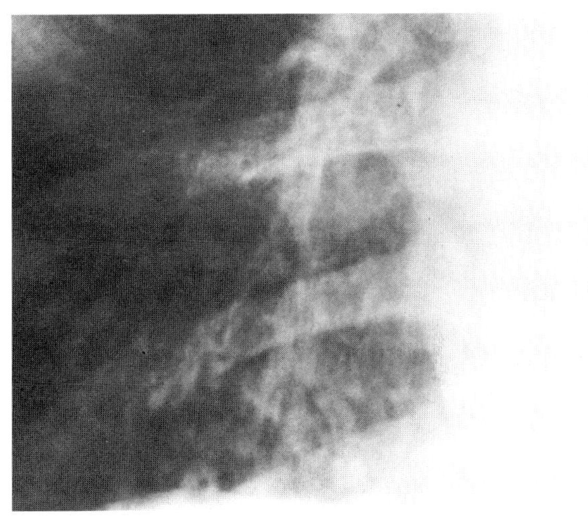

Fig. 8.17. Pyogenic airways disease may produce bronchial wall thickening and bronchiectasis, favoring the lower lobes

sociated with aggressive spread and multilobar involvement, cavitation, empyema formation, and sepsis than in the normal host.

Pseudomonas bronchopneumonia in the AIDS patient may present with a reticular or reticulonodular pattern, as well as alveolar consolidation (Fig. 8.15). *Staphylococcus aureus, Haemophilus influenzae,* and *Streptococcus monocytogenes* are other common pathogens. Nontyphoid strains of *Salmonella* pneumonia may cavitate, form abscesses, or be associated with bacteremia.

Rhodococcus equi pneumonia is characterized by dense pulmonary consolidation with or without cavitation, as well as mediastinal lymphadenopathy and pulmonary nodules (Fig. 8.16).

Pyogenic infection of the airways is increasingly recognized as a complication of AIDS, causing bronchial wall thickening, impacted bronchioles, and/or bronchiectasis, and primarily involving the lower lobes (Fig. 8.17).

Bacillary Angiomatosis

Bacillary angiomatosis is a cause of angiomatous skin nodules in AIDS patients, but the infection is not confined to the skin and almost any organ can be involved, particularly at mucocutaneous junctions. The infection is caused by bacillae of the genus *Bartonella*, particularly *B. henselae*, and *B. quintana*, an organism commonly found in cats (24% of cats in Zimbabwe) and also found in fleas and ticks. Clinically the infection presents with fevers, anemia, and angiomatous skin lesions which have an erythematous scale collar. The number of skin lesions seems to reflect the degree of immunosuppression. The individual skin lesions vary considerably but some resemble Kaposi's sarcoma, except that these nodules are painful, while those of Kaposi's sarcoma seldom are.

Bacillary angiomatosis responds rapidly to a variety of antibiotics, but resolution may take many weeks and there may be recurrence when therapy is discontinued. Cases of bacillary angiomatosis have been reported wherever there is AIDS, from the Americas, Africa, Europe, and Asia; however, because the disease is so easily confused with Kaposi's sarcoma, the real incidence is difficult to quantify accurately.

Imaging Findings

Multiorgan involvement is common, with lung nodules, mediastinal lymphadenopathy, pleural effusions, and ascites (Figs. 8.18–8.21). The liver and spleen may be infected and severe hemorrhage can occur. The associated, often pronounced lymphadenopathy and soft tissue masses show dramatic contrast enhancement because the lesions contain well-formed, functional vascular structures (Fig. 8.22). This does not always help in the differential diagnosis from Kaposi's sarcoma, as these nodules will also blush on angiography and show enhancement on CT (see Chap. 42). Intracerebral and ophthalmic infections also occur and in some patients the endobronchial, tracheal, and esophageal lesions may become life threatening. There may be lytic lesions of bone. Because bacillary angiomatosis can be satisfactorily treated, it is important to distinguish this infection from Kaposi's sarcoma: this is best done by histopathology or isolation of the organisms from the lesions or from blood.

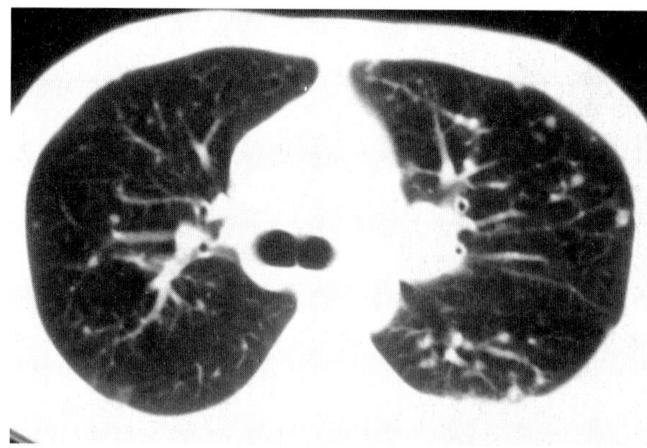

Fig. 8.19. The CT image of smaller pulmonary nodules, due to bacillary angiomatosis, in another patient. (Courtesy of Dr. Jeffrey Klein and *Radiology*, 1995)

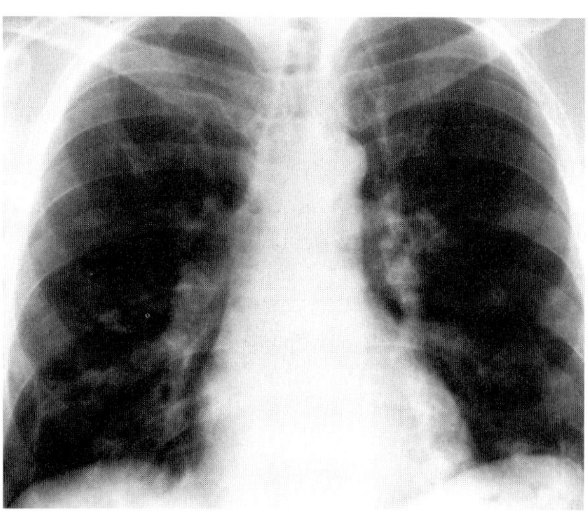

Fig. 8.18. *Bartonella henselae*, the cause of bacillary angiomatosis, may present as numerous small to moderate sized pulmonary nodules. (Courtesy of Dr. Jeffrey Klein and *Radiology*, 1995)

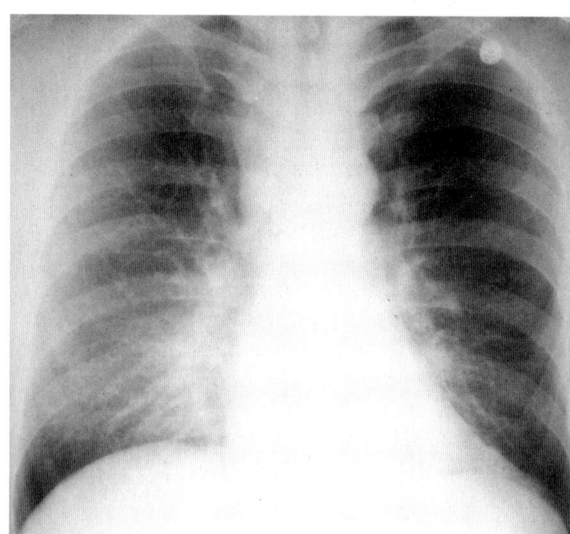

Fig. 8.20. Mediastinal and right hilar lymphadenopathy associated with bacillary angiomatosis

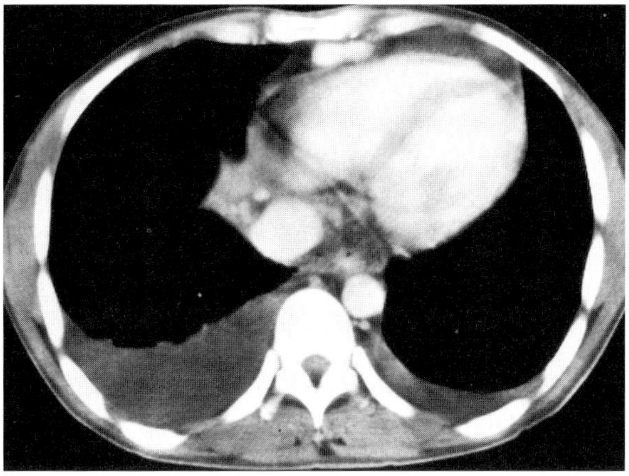

Fig. 8.21. Pleural effusions occur frequently in bacillary angiomatosis. Note also the enhancing cardiac lymph node in the retrosternal area

◄

Fig. 8.22 A, B. Marked enhancement after contrast injection, equal to the density seen in vascular structures, is characteristic of bacillary angiomatosis. CT images precontrast (**A**) and postcontrast (**B**) showing lymph nodes in the neck (*arrows*)

▼

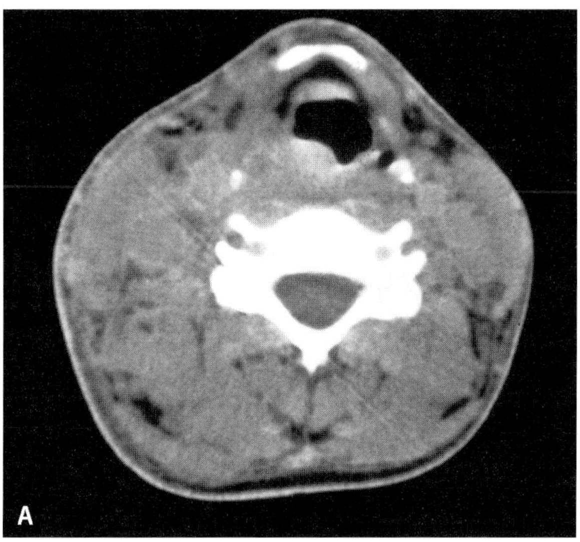

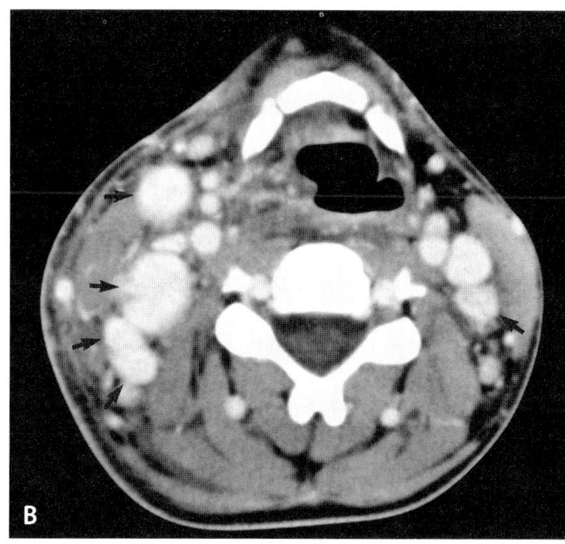

Nocardiosis

A very uncommon manifestation of AIDS in the developed countries, nocardiosis appears to be more common in the tropical world. In an autopsy study from Abidjan, Ivory Coast of HIV-positive patients, there was a 4% incidence of nocardiosis, which was thought to be the cause of death in 2%. The majority of infections were disseminated. Pulmonary disease is most common, followed by cerebral abscesses. Involvement of other organs is rare, but adrenal abscesses have been reported. It is possible that some patients with "smear-negative sputum" for tuberculosis actually have nocardiosis.

Imaging Findings

The manifestations of nocardiosis are protean. The disease may present as multiple nodules which may cavitate, as well as lobar or even diffuse airspace disease, or as a combination thereof. There may be mediastinal lymphadenopathy, pleural effusions, or pleural thickening (Fig. 8.23). Cerebral involvement is most commonly recognized by ring-enhancing abscesses, frequently associated with subependymal nodules and hydrocephalus. (See also Chap. 6 and AIDS and the central nervous system p. 722).

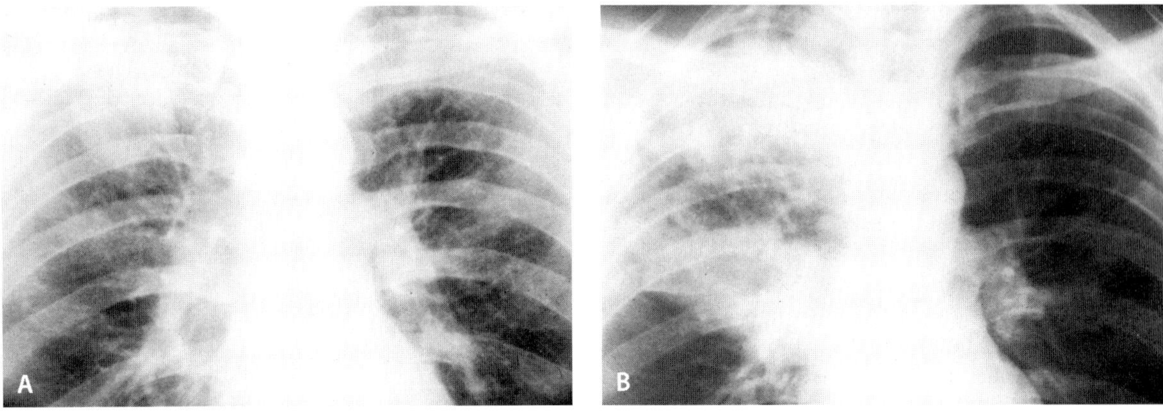

Fig. 8.23 A, B. In pulmonary nocardiosis there may be progressive involvement, with abscesses and lymphadenopathy. Lobar consolidation and pleural effusions are also common

Viral Pathogens

Cytomegalovirus

A member of the herpes virus group, cytomegalovirus is present in many HIV-1 patients in both the developed and nondeveloped worlds. Immunosuppression leads to reactivation of this common latent infection. However, it has been thought to be an uncommon cause of clinically significant AIDS-related disease in the tropics, perhaps since it is generally seen with CD4+ counts below $50/mm^3$. This does not seem to be the case in patients with HIV-2, in whom severe cytomegalovirus infections appear to be more common. Recent autopsy studies of African infants have shown that cytomegalovirus is a common isolate from lung and liver at the time of death, although the significance of this finding is unclear. Along with *P. carinii*, cytomegalovirus is a common isolate at autopsy in pediatric patients in Chiang Mai, Thailand.

Cytomegalovirus infection has an immunomodulating effect, further encouraging the development of superinfections by other organisms in these patients. Thus, it is often part of a multiorganism infection.

The most common manifestation of cytomegalovirus is retinitis, which if untreated may lead to blindness. Less common manifestations include esophagitis, gastritis, colitis, and pneumonia.

Varicella and herpex simplex are other viral pathogens affecting the lungs and other organs in AIDS.

Imaging Findings

Pulmonary involvement by cytomegalovirus is characterized most commonly by a diffuse reticular or reticulonodular pattern, or ground glass density, and may progress to frank airspace disease. It may also produce localized masses, usually 1–3 cm in size. Other findings such as pleural effusion or lymphadenopathy are rare. Pulmonary involvement is usually accompanied by clinically significant disease at other sites, such as retinitis, esophagitis, colitis, or cholangitis.

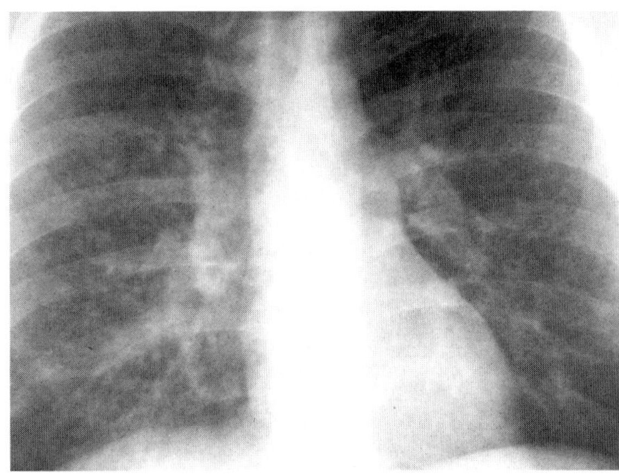

Fig. 8.24. Varicella pneumonia in the AIDS patient produces a diffuse small nodular pattern. Pulmonary involvement is uncommon in the normal host, but common in anyone who is immunosuppressed

AIDS patients share the same propensity to disseminated varicella infection as other immunocompromised hosts. The appearance in the lungs is similar – a diffuse small nodular pattern (Fig. 8.24).

Herpes simplex pneumonia presents with diffuse airspace disease.

Pneumocystis carinii

Although *P. carinii* pneumonia is the most common complication of AIDS in the United States and in Western Europe, occurring in 65%–85% of homosexual AIDS patients, it is far less common in Africa and other parts of the world. It may be underestimated because of the lack of availability of diagnostic bronchoscopy, but this does not fully explain the difference. Even within Africa, there is substantial variation. For example, in Burundi the rate of pneumocystosis was found to be 3% and in the Democratic Republic of Congo, 12%–21%. In an autopsy study from the Ivory Coast, pneumocystosis was only found in 9% of HIV-positive autopsies. Numerous other studies from sub-Saharan Africa show that even where there are adequate diagnostic facilities, i.e., bronchoalveolar lavage, transbronchial biopsy, or autopsy, pneumocystosis rates will range between 3% and 22% (the highest value being from Zimbabwe). However, the autopsy study by Jeena et al. of African infants suggests that it is more common than previously thought, occurring in 78% of samples of lungs tested.
Similarly, a recent African study of bronchoscopy isolates in AIDS-related pneumonias unresponsive to penicillin and AFB smear-negative revealed a 33% incidence of pneumocystosis. In this study, the median CD4 count for these cases was $134/mm^3$, while for tuberculosis it was $206/mm^3$. Pneumocystosis is uncommon in Haitian AIDS but has been noted to be relatively common among the urban homosexual population in southern Brazil, in Mexico, and in Hong Kong. In a pediatric autopsy study in Thailand, *P. carinii* was a common isolate.

As has been speculated to explain the situation for atypical mycobacteria, it has been proposed that African AIDS patients die of other, less opportunistic infections prior to onset of the profound immunosuppression required to develop pneumocystosis. It is also possible that *P. carinii* is a much less prevalent organism. Because of these statistics, prophylactic therapy against pneumocystosis may be of little value in many tropical regions.

Imaging Findings

The earliest manifestations of *P. carinii* infection may be extremely subtle, and the radiographs may seem to be normal, though on CT scanning, ground glass opacities may be visible. The earliest finding visible on chest radiography is usually the development of poor definition of the borders of the vascular markings. Subsequently, a diffuse interstitial pattern appears, followed by a "ground glass" appearance, with hazy consolidation of the pulmonary parenchyma (Figs. 8.25, 8.26).
As the disease progresses, consolidation becomes denser with the development of air bronchograms (Fig. 8.27). The infection is usually diffuse, but often has a lower lobe predominance. Radiographic findings reported in African AIDS have included lobar, multilobar, and diffuse airspace disease. A lobar distribution is rare, and is more likely to be caused by *Streptococcus pneumoniae* or *M. tuberculosis*. Parenchymal nodules are a variant appearance which is not uncommon (Fig. 8.28). These may cavitate and form pneumatoceles, which may enlarge and rupture if peripheral, leading to pneumothorax

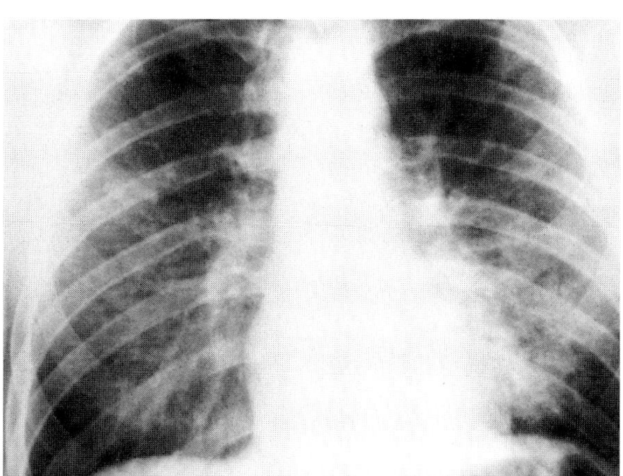

Fig. 8.25. Early *P. carinii* pneumonia is characterized by an interstitial pattern which results in ill-defined borders of the lung vascular markings (*right base*), progressing to ground glass opacities (*left base*)

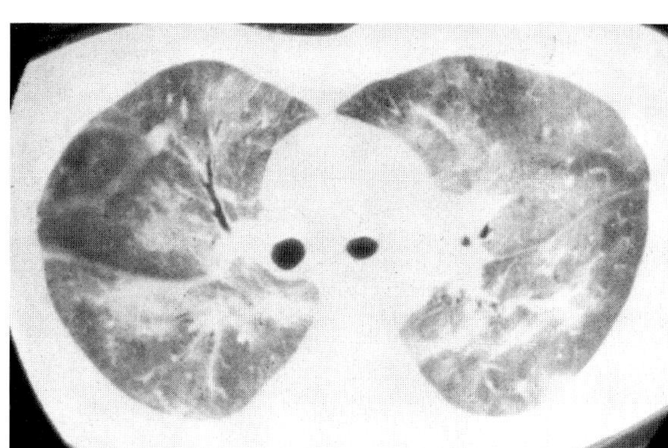

Fig. 8.26. CT scanning in patients with *P. carinii* pneumonia clearly demonstrates a diffuse ground glass pattern

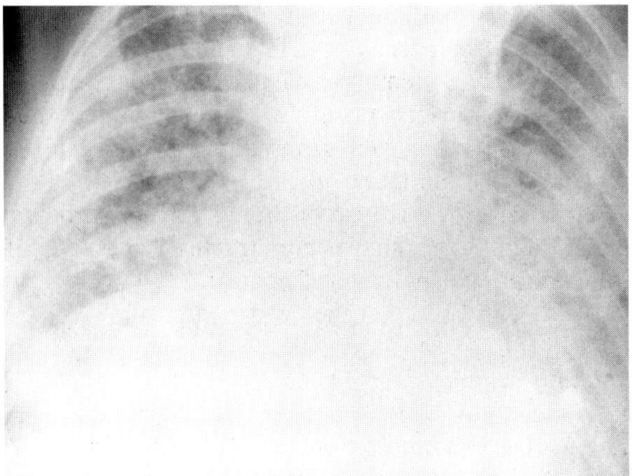

Fig. 8.27. Severe *P. carinii* pneumonia may also cause diffuse airspace disease

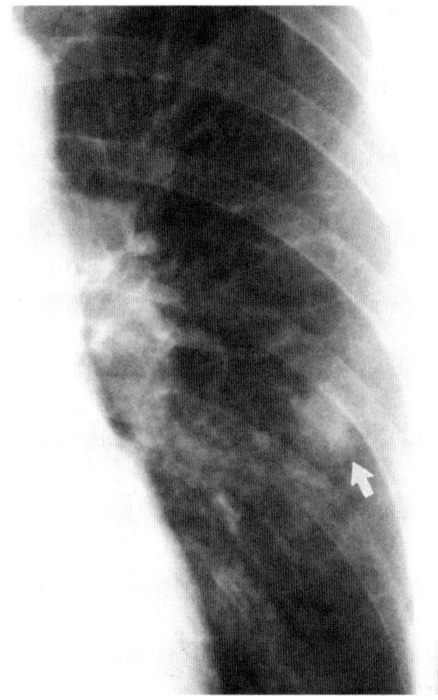

Fig. 8.28. A discrete nodular pattern is unusual in *P. carinii* pneumonia. The cause of this pulmonary nodule (*arrow*) was confirmed by needle biopsy

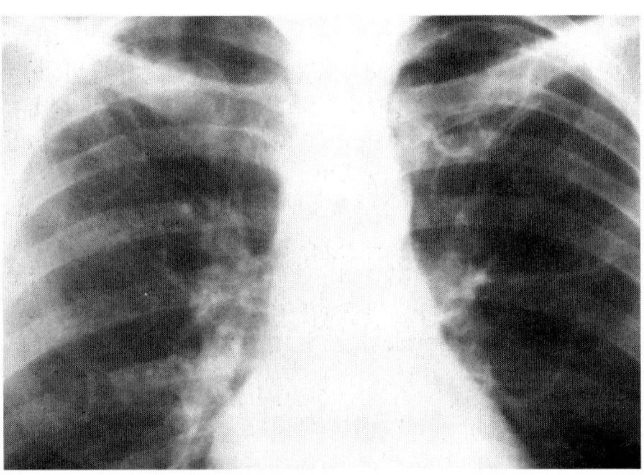

Fig. 8.29. *Pneumocystis carinii* nodules may excavate, creating pneumatoceles, which may trap air and become very large

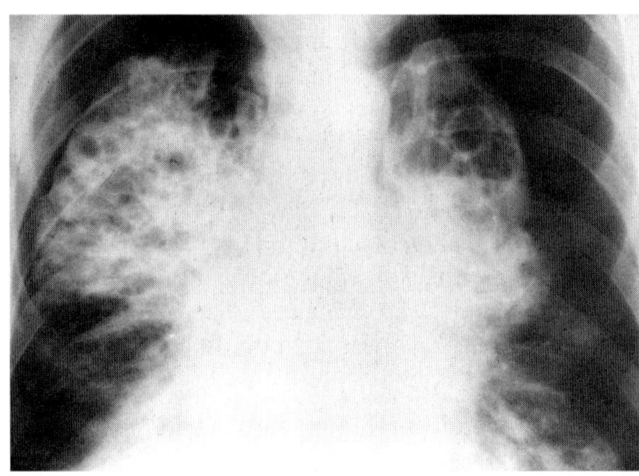

Fig. 8.30. When *P. carinii* results in numerous peripheral cystic lesions, bilateral pneumothorax may result. The cystic lesions in this patient are best visualized in the periphery of the collapsed left upper lobe. Persistent air leaks may occur after chest tube placement and are a frequent management problem

(Figs. 8.29–8.31). Associated adenopathy and pleural effusions are rare. Extrapulmonary involvement may occasionally include spleen, bone marrow, abdominal lymph nodes, peritoneum, or liver (Fig. 8.32). Extrapulmonary involvement may produce calcification in rim-like or punctate fashion.

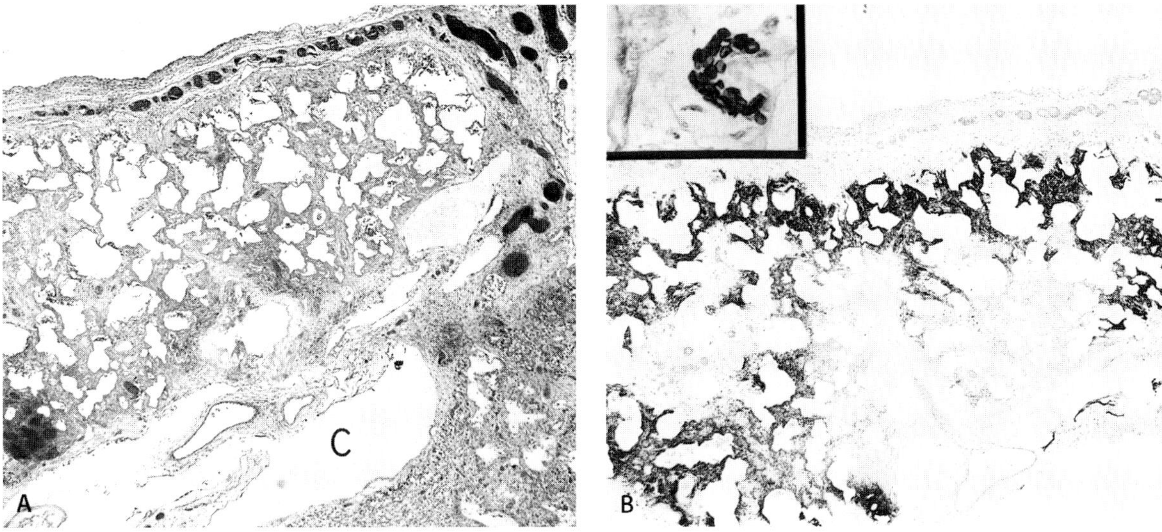

Fig. 8.31 A, B. The cysts of *P. carinii* pneumonia. **A** A section of the lung showing a cyst (*C*) and subpleural necrosis. The air spaces are dilated. H & E, ×80. **B** The same area of necrosis showing dystrophic calcification and, in the *inset*, P. carinii embedded within the calcified area. von Kossa's stain, ×80; *inset*: Gomori methenamine-silver stain, ×2000. (From M.A. Greco and D. Zagzag, in D.H. Connor, ed. *The pathology of infectious diseases.* Stamford, Appleton and Lange, 1997, pp 169–181)

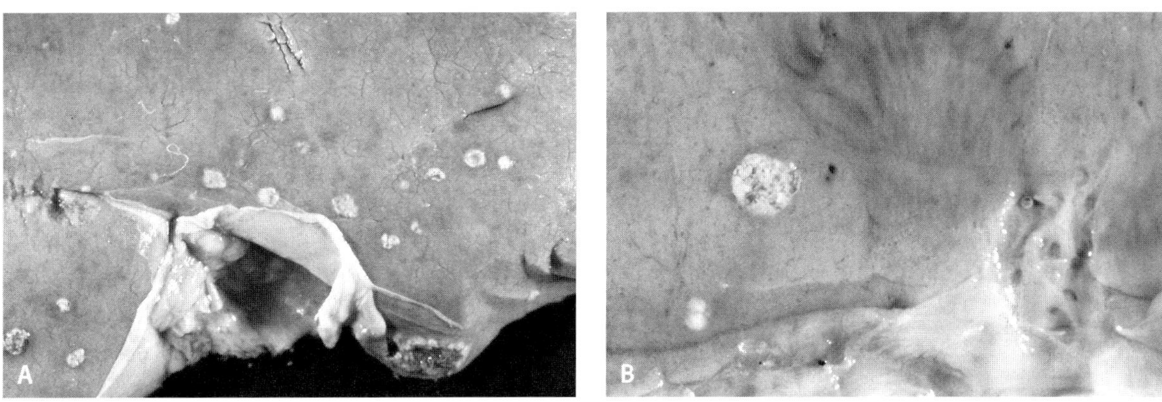

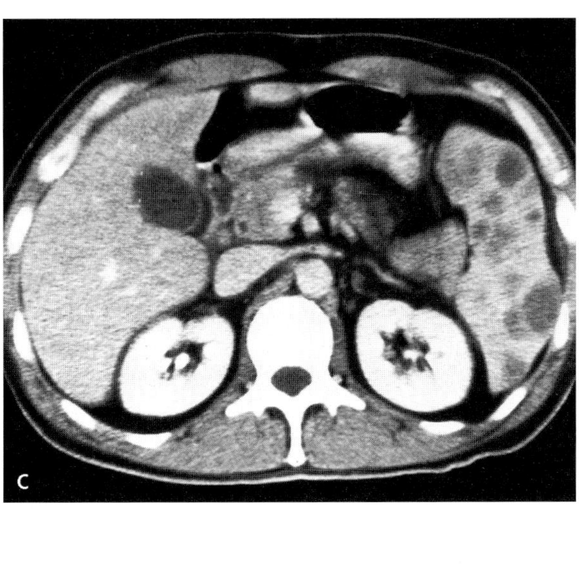

Fig. 8.32 A–C. When *P. carinii* is disseminated, any organ can be affected. **A, B** Macroscopically there are gray or white nodules, as in this kidney. **C** CT scanning shows low-density lesions, particularly in the spleen in this patient

Fungal Disease and AIDS

Cryptococcosis

Cryptococcus neoformans is an important central nervous system (CNS) pathogen in AIDS. Bird droppings are an extraordinarily rich source of this ubiquitous fungus. Entry into the body if from a pulmonary source; all patients with pulmonary cryptococcosis must be investigated for CNS involvement by examination of the cerebrospinal fluid (CSF). Clinically, meningitis is the commonest presentation, but pseudocysts or cryptococcomas may cause symptoms. A study from Rwanda showed that there was primary pulmonary cryptococcosis in 13% of AIDS patients with pulmonary disease of unknown etiology: it was best diagnosed by bronchoalveolar lavage because the associated symptoms of cough, weight loss, fever, dyspnea, chest pain, and headache were nonspecific. Treatment of the pulmonary disease appears to prevent the further dissemination of cryptococcal disease.

Imaging Findings

Pulmonary cryptococcosis in the AIDS patient does not form the typical well-circumscribed nodules seen in the normal host who is capable of a healthy granulomatous response; rather, it is usually characterized by diffuse disease (Fig. 8.33). The most common manifestations documented in Rwanda (Batungwanayo) include a diffuse interstitial infiltrate (76%), an alveolar pattern (19%), mediastinal and/or hilar lymphadenopathy (11%), nodules (5%), and pleural effusions (5%). A miliary pattern of small nodules may also be seen.

Computed tomography scans in CNS cryptococcosis are frequently normal but there may be low-density lesions, occasionally showing contrast enhancement,

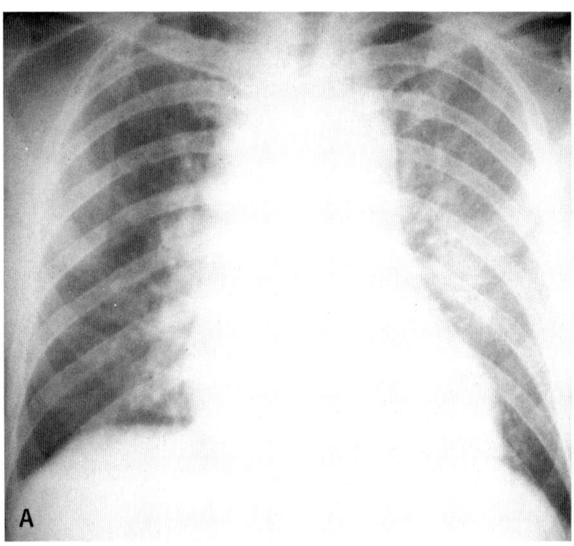

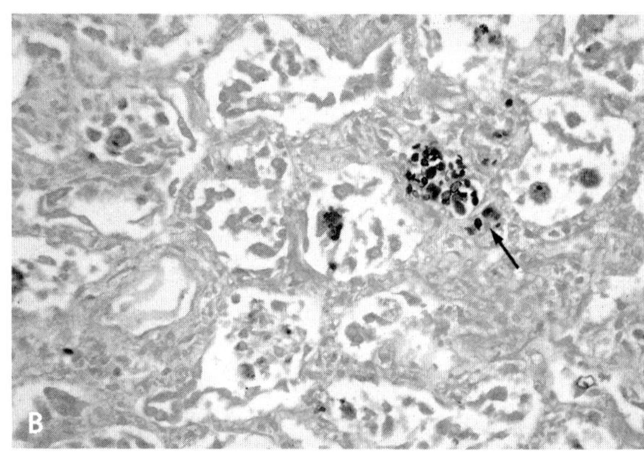

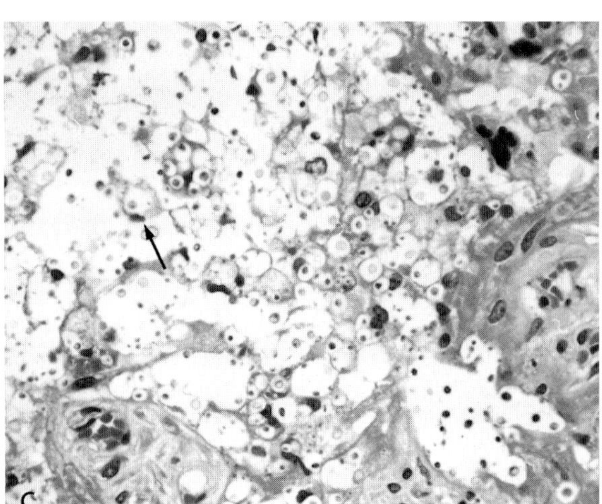

Fig. 8.33 A–C. In the immunocompromised host, *Cryptococcus* involving the lung will present as a diffuse interstitial or airspace pattern, best seen here in the left lung (**A**). Enlarged lymph nodes may also be seen, as in this patient. **B** Pulmonary cryptococcus in an AIDS patient. There is very little inflammatory reaction. The patient also had *P. carinii* infection. Gomori methenamine-silver stain, ×72. **C** Placental enlargement occurs in HIV-positive pregnant women, but added to this may be infections: the intervillous spaces in this placenta contain cryptococci. H & E, ×40. (**B** courtesy of Dr. Daniel H. Connor; **C** from C.R. Abranowsky, in D.H. Connor, ed. *The pathology of infections diseases.* Stamford, Appleton and Lange 1997, p. 170)

particularly in the basal ganglia. There may occasionally be larger masses, which may enhance (see pp. 618–623, 725).

Histoplasmosis

Histoplasma capsulatum (var. *capsulatum*) occurs in many african and south-east asian countries, as well as parts of the United States, Central and South America (see p. 584). Disseminated histoplasmosis is an indicator disease for AIDS. All patients living in or migrating to endemic areas are at risk. Patients tend to be in a relatively advanced stage of the disease, with CD4 counts characteristically under 100 cells/mm^3.

Histoplasmosis had not been considered a significant pathogen in Africa, but cases of disseminated "African" histoplasmosis due to *Histoplasma capsulatum* (var. *dubosii*) in HIV-infected African patients have recently been reported. It was found in 3% of patients who died from AIDS in the Ivory Coast.

Imaging Findings

Focal areas of airspace disease, nodules and effusions may be seen. Enlarged lymph nodes are seen less often than in the normal host. Disseminated histoplasmosis presents in AIDS as a small nodular pattern on chest radiography similar to any disseminated fungal disease (Fig. 8.34) (see p. 586). Histoplasmosis duboisii often affects the skeleton (see pp. 589–593).

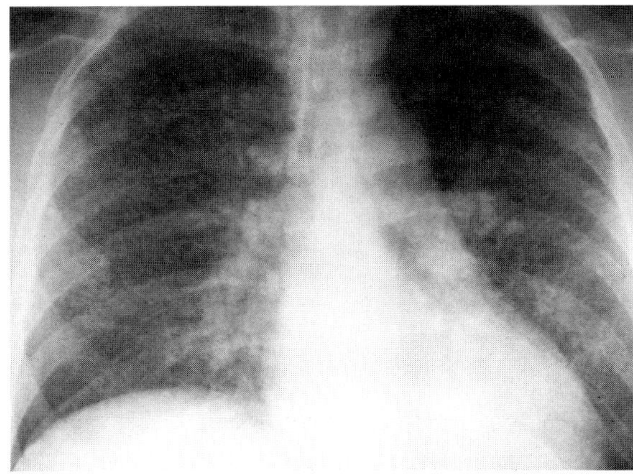

Fig. 8.34. Disseminated histoplasmosis produces a small nodular pattern in the lung, as do most hematogenously disseminated fungal infections. Associated bowel involvement is common in AIDS patients

Penicilliosis

Penicillium marneffei is a fungal infection involving AIDS patients living in or traveling to Southeast Asia. The reservoir for the fungus is the bamboo rat, a root rat living in tunnels in the high plateaus of Southeast Asia, and other rodents. In endemic areas, infection in more frequent in the rainy season than the dry season. It has been known as "Chinese histoplasmosis."

Penicilliosis is the third most common opportunistic infection in HIV disease in parts of Southeast Asia (after extrapulmonary tuberculosis and cryptococcal meningitis). It can clinically resemble tuberculosis, molluscum contagiosum, cryptococcosis, or histoplasmosis. Clinical features include fever, weight loss, hepatosplenomegaly, anemia, skin lesions with central umbilication, lymphadenopathy, pulmonary symptoms, and rarely, gastrointestinal symptoms such as colitis. In AIDS patients, the symptoms are more acute in onset and more intense. The organism can be isolated from skin, blood, bone marrow, and other organs. In the study of Bhoopat and colleagues from Thailand, it affected 20% of AIDS patients undergoing autopsy. Treatment with parenteral amphotericin B or itraconazole has been successful.

Imaging Findings

Chest radiographs may show a diffuse reticulonodular, a localized alveolar, a diffuse alveolar, or a localized interstitial pattern. Parenchymal masses, which may cavitate, and enlarged lymph nodes may be seen, though calcification is unusual. There may be pleural or pericardial involvement. Abscesses may also involve the skin, liver, subcutaneous tissues, and lymph nodes. Lytic bone lesions and joint infections may occur.

Aspergillosis

Although a less common pathogen in AIDS than in the neutropenic chemotherapy patient, *Aspergillus* occasionally involves AIDS patients. It was present in 3% of AIDS deaths in the Ivory Coast.

Imaging Findings

The most common radiologic manifestations are thick-walled cavitary lesions and, less commonly, nodules, consolidation, and pleural effusion (see pp. 577–584).

Coccidioidomycosis

Endemic to the southwestern United States, Mexico, and portions of Central America, coccidioidomycosis is a substantial risk for AIDS patients residing in or traveling to endemic areas. While usually localized to the lung in the normal host, in AIDS patients dissemination is common.

Imaging Findings

Radiographic manifestations include cavitary masses, localized areas of consolidation, and pleural effusion or empyema. Hematogenous dissemination results in a small nodular pattern, often heralded by pronounced lymphadenopathy (Fig. 8.35). There may be lytic lesions of bone (see pp. 594–601).

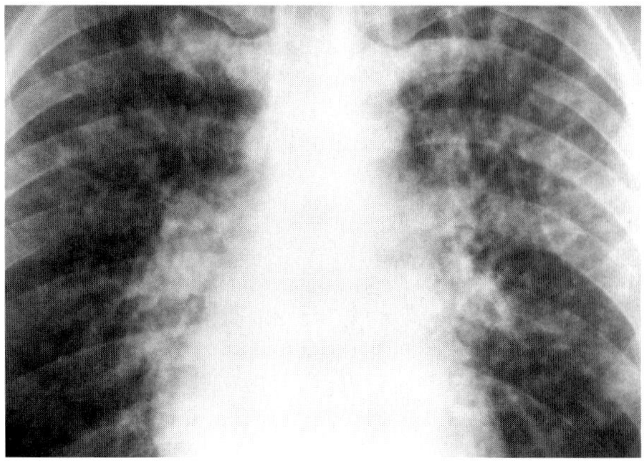

Fig. 8.35. Disseminated coccidioidomycosis produces a pattern of small parenchymal nodules, usually preceded by the development of hilar and/or mediastinal lymphadenopathy

Candidiasis

Though usually confined to the gastrointestinal tract, *Candida* pneumonias and disseminated candidiasis may occur in AIDS.

Imaging Findings

Candida pneumonia produces a nonspecific pattern of airspace disease, often accompanied by pleural effusion. Disseminated candidiasis resembles any hematogenously disseminated fungal infection, producing a small nodular pattern (Fig. 8.36) (see pp. 621–629).

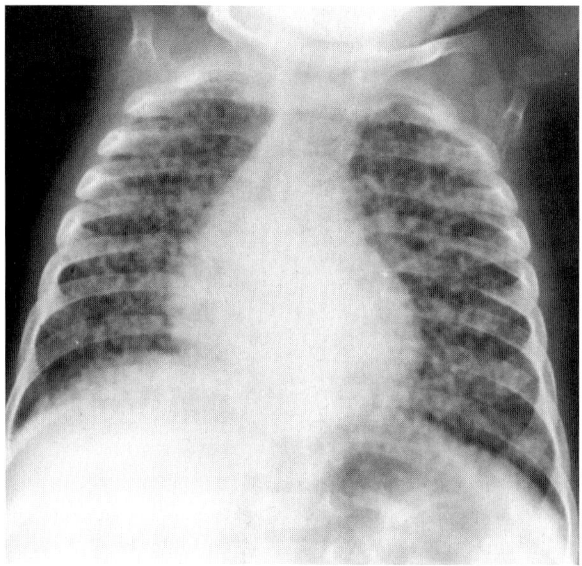

Fig. 8.36. This 9-month-old infant presented with cough and failure to thrive. The chest radiograph demonstrates a diffuse small nodular appearance due to disseminated candidiasis

Nonspecific Interstitial Pneumonitis

In a large percentage of patients with AIDS and pulmonary symptoms (38% in a study from Rwanda), no cause can be identified even after numerous investigations including open lung biopsy.

Imaging Findings

These patients will demonstrate an interstitial pattern on chest radiograph and nonspecific interstitial pneumonitis on lung biopsy. It has been speculated that this may represent the direct effect of HIV on lung tissue.

Lymphocytic Interstitial Pneumonitis

An AIDS-related polyclonal lymphoproliferative disorder known as lymphocytic interstitial pneumonitis is particularly common in the pediatric age group (25% of children with AIDS), but it seldom progresses to lymphoma in the AIDS patient The lungs are predominately affected (hence the name lymphocytic interstitial pneumonitis), but it is now known to be a systemic process, with lymphoid infiltrates in many organs. Patients may also seem to have chronic mumps because the salivary glands are often involved.

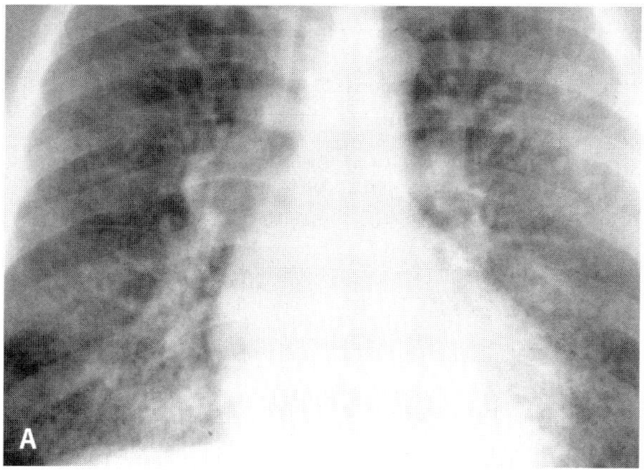
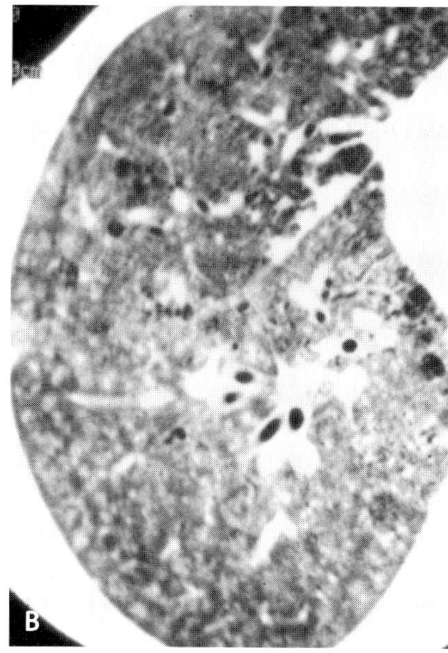

Fig. 8.37. Lymphocytic interstitial pneumonitis, a polyclonal lymphoproliferative process, produces a pattern of many small nodules, seen here on **A** chest radiograph and **B** CT image

Imaging Findings

On chest radiographs, lymphocytic interstitial pneumonitis appears as an interstitial or reticulonodular pattern, as small nodules (2–4 mm), or as subsegmental consolidation (Fig. 8.37). In some cases, the reticulonodular pattern in the lungs clears as the CD4 counts fall to very low levels, this being considered a poor prognostic sign.

Cardiac Disease in AIDS

Cardiac lesions associated with AIDS include pericardial effusions (often tuberculous, but also viral or fungal), metastases, and cardiomyopathy. In a series from Rwanda of patients with pericardial effusion, 81% were HIV positive; 91% of those with documented tuberculous pericarditis were HIV positive. An AIDS autopsy study from Puerto Rico showed an unexpectedly high rate of cardiac involvement, at 32%. *Histoplasma capsulatum, Toxoplasma gondii, Mycobacterium tuberculosis,* cytomegalovirus, *Cryptococcus neoformans* and atypical mycobacteria were all isolated. Nonspecific myocarditis was also identified.
There may be multiple Kaposi's sarcoma nodules affecting the heart and pericardium. The AIDS virus itself may produce a dilated congestive cardiomyopathy in roughly 17% of patients,which may be rapidly progressive: children are often affected.

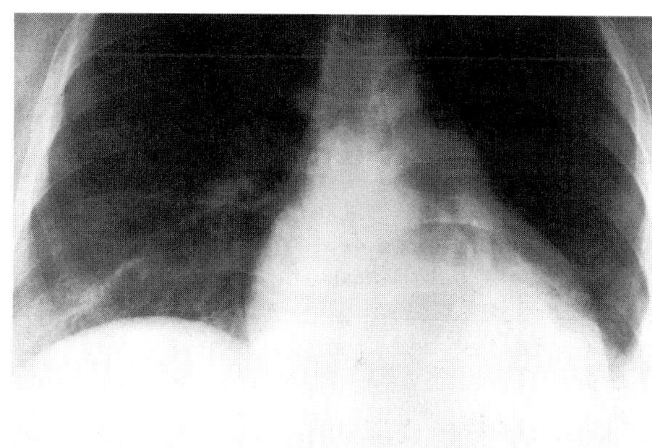

Fig. 8.38. Marked cardiac enlargement occurring over the course of only a few months in a patient with AIDS cardiomyopathy

Imaging Findings

In HIV-related myocarditis, a dilated cardiomyopathy causes increasing cardiac size and, eventually, congestive heart failure (Fig. 8.38). An enlarged cardiac silhouette may also indicate pericardial effusion (Fig. 8.39). In such cases, the classic bag-shaped heart may be seen, with straightening of the left heart border to the level of the transverse portion of the aorta, the superior extent of the pericardium. Ultrasonography will confirm the diagnosis, because it is very difficult to distinguish cardiomyopathy from pericardial fluid radiographically (see p. 301).

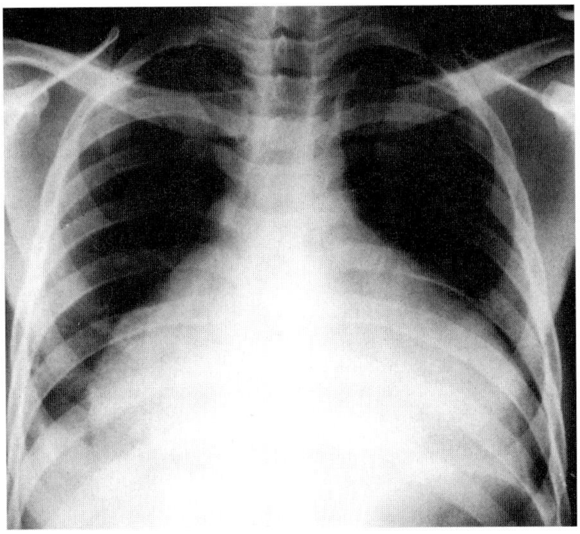

Fig. 8.39. Severe cardiomegaly, with a silhouette which strongly suggests a large pericardial effusion: in this AIDS patient it was due to tuberculous pericarditis. Without ultrasonography or other scanning this may be difficult to distinguish from some of the tropical cardiomyopathies

Differential Diagnosis of Thoracic Disease

The radiographic pattern of disease may indicate the likely diagnosis, especially when correlated with the level of immunosuppression and local frequencies of infections or malignancies. In general, common causes of nodules in the lung in AIDS include pneumocystosis, tuberculosis, cytomegalovirus infection, cryptococcosis, aspergillosis, nocardiosis, Kaposi's sarcoma, and non-Hodgkin's lymphoma. Pleural effusions are most commonly caused by bacterial pneumonias, tuberculosis, and Kaposi's sarcoma. Cavitary lung lesions are common in invasive aspergillosis, *Pseudomonas* infection, nocardiosis, and rhodococcosis. Tuberculosis is more likely to cavitate in earlier stages of AIDS. Less common causes of cavities include cryptococcosis, coccidioidomycosis, and histoplasmosis. Kaposi's sarcoma and non-Hodgkin's lymphoma may occasionally cavitate. Thoracic lymphadenopathy suggests tuberculosis, atypical mycobacteria, cryptococcosis, Kaposi's sarcoma, lymphoma, or bacillary angiomatosis. When bronchoscopy is not available, transthoracic needle biopsy of pulmonary masses or pneumonias has been proposed as an efficient means of diagnosis.

AIDS-Related Neoplasms

AIDS-related neoplasms may involve the thorax, the abdomen, and other sites.

AIDS-Related Lymphomas

AIDS-related lymphomas are non-Hodgkin's lymphomas: intermediate or high-grade B-cell lymphomas, including diffuse large cleaved and noncleaved cell, large cell immunoblastic and small noncleaved cell Burkitt's or non-Burkitt's lymphomas (Fig. 8.40). Over 60% are high-grade lymphomas, especially of the small non-cleaved Burkitt's, non-Burkitt's, or immunoblastic types. These are commonly extranodal; 76% are entirely extranodal, while 98% have some involvement of an extranodal site such as the central nervous system, the bone marrow, the gastrointestinal tract, or mucocutaneous junctions. Twenty percent are primary lymphomas of the brain. Many authors believe that AIDS-related lymphomas are related to the Epstein-Barr virus.

Lymphoma associated with AIDS usually presents clinically at an advanced stage. It is important that these lymphomas be distinguished from lymphadenopathy due to tuberculosis or other causes. It is also important to separate true lymphoma from the progressive generalized lymphadenopathy which is commonly seen in AIDS. In Lucas et al.'s recent study of HIV-associated lymphoma in Africa, 2.8% of HIV+ve hospital deaths had non-Hodgkin's lymphoma (1.6% visceral and 1.2% primary cerebral lymphoma).

About 50% of AIDS patients with lymphoma have had previous (or have concomitant) opportunistic infections. Symptoms of fever and weight loss are frequent. Early diagnosis is of little importance, since the treatment of HIV-related lymphomas is unsatisfactory. The CNS lymphomas have the worst prognosis and are not as radiosensitive as non-HIV-related brain lymphomas: high-grade extracranial lymphomas may show a response to a combination of chemotherapy and radiotherapy. Better results may be seen with large noncleaved cell lymphomas. Compared with lymphomas in the non-HIV patient, complete response is unusual. The mean survival time of patients with AIDS-related lymphomas undergoing chemotherapy is 5.5 months, far less than in other hosts.

Classic pediatric Burkitt's lymphoma is not an AIDS-associated tumor in Africa. Pediatric non-Hodgkin's lymphoma is rare, probably because the children do not survive long enough to develop this malignancy.

Although the incidence of Hodgkin's disease is also increased in the HIV-positive patient group in many settings, this trend has not been observed in an African study by Sitas and colleagues, in which the only cancers to show increased frequency were Kaposi's sarcoma and non-Hodgkin's lymphoma, the latter somewhat less than reported in developed countries.

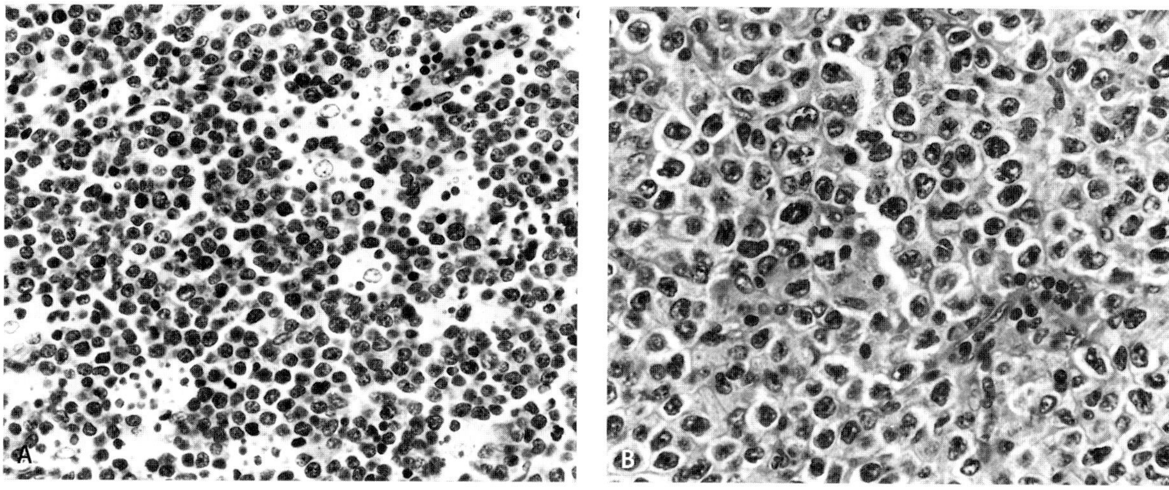

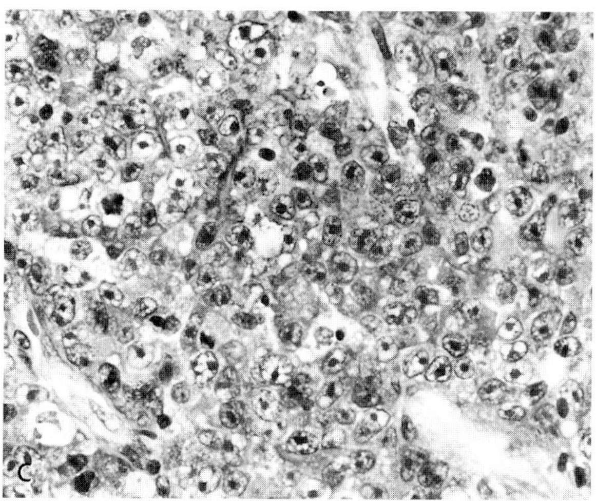

Fig. 8.40 A–C. The histopathology of the three most common types of HIV-associated malignant lymphoma (all at ×400). **A** The "starry sky" appearance of small non-cleaved malignant lymphoma. There is a high mitotic rate in the lymphoid cells. **B** Diffuse large cell malignant lymphoma. **C** The plasmacytoid type of large cell immunoblastic lymphoma. There is a single prominent nucleoli in the lymphoid cells, and the cytoplasm is eccentric. (From R.J. Siegel, in D.H. Connor, ed. *The pathology of infectious diseases.* Stamford,, Appleton and Lange, 1997, pp 161–168)

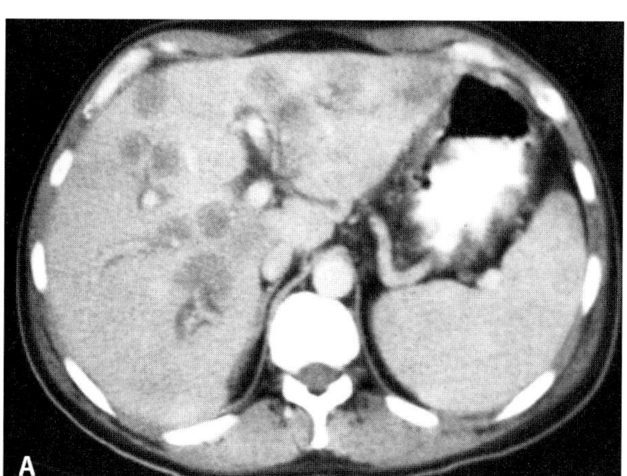

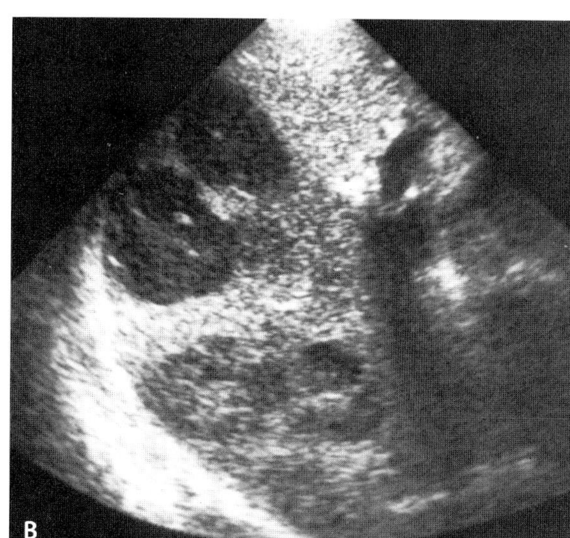

Fig. 8.41. A A CT scan of the liver showing multiple low-density lesions due to non-Hodgkin's lymphoma. **B** On ultrasonography these are hypoechoic

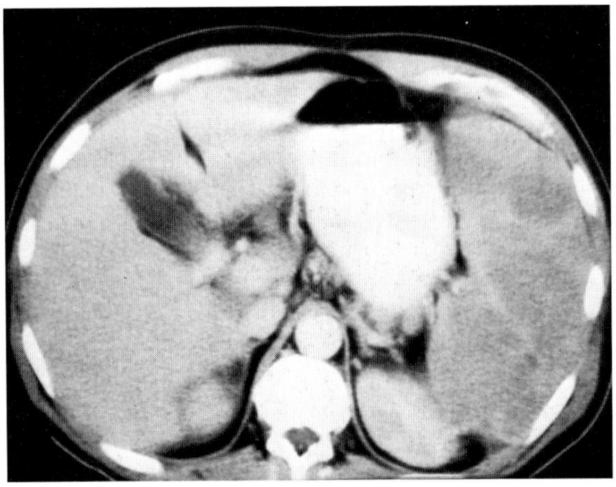

Fig. 8.42. A CT scan of an AIDS patient showing focal low-density lesions due to non-Hodgkin's lymphoma within an enlarged spleen

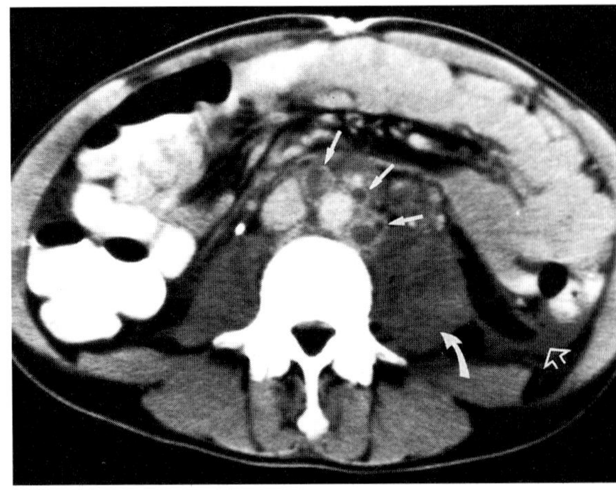

Fig. 8.43. A CT scan of the abdomen of an AIDS patient with the unusual finding of multiple low-density lymph nodes (*arrows*). There is infiltration of the left psoas muscle (*curved arrow*) and ascites (*open arrow*). (Courtesy of Dr. William Brandt)

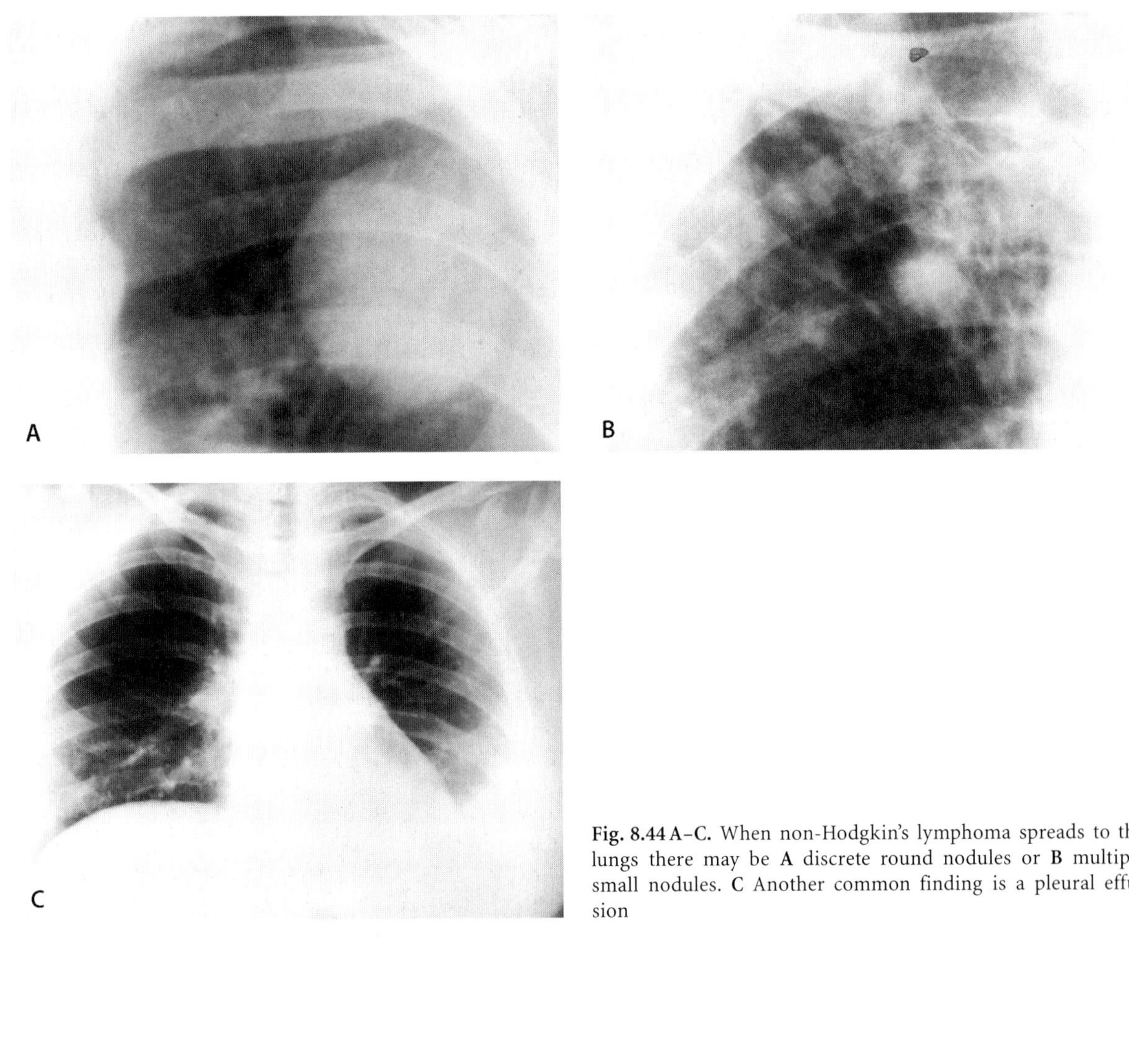

Fig. 8.44 A–C. When non-Hodgkin's lymphoma spreads to the lungs there may be **A** discrete round nodules or **B** multiple small nodules. **C** Another common finding is a pleural effusion

Imaging Findings

The abdomen is the most common site of involvement in AIDS-related lymphoma. Focal masses in the liver occur more often than in normal hosts. Lesions are low density on CT and hypoechoic on ultrasound (Fig. 8.41), although there may be lymphomatous hepatomegaly without focal lesions. Lymphomatous localized splenic lesions are also more common than in the non-AIDS host (Fig. 8.42). Splenomegaly may oocur in the AIDS patient without specific cause, and does not always indicate lymphomatous involvement or other diseases. Renal involvement may produce well-circumscribed or infiltrative masses. Involvement of mesenteric and retroperitoneal lymph nodes is common. Low-density nodal centers are not common in AIDS-related lymphoma, and should suggest mycobacterial disease (Fig. 8.43). Omental infiltration is associated with a poor prognosis. AIDS-related lymphomas involving the gastrointestinal tract produce focal masses, usually accompanied by other manifestations of the disease.

Though far less common than primary involvement of the abdomen, thoracic neoplasms may be primary, presenting with hilar and/or mediastinal lymphadenopathy or confluent masses. More often, thoracic involvement is secondary, with metastatic foci to the lungs: these may present as well-circumscribed parenchymal masses which may show very rapid growth, or as a diffuse reticulonodular pattern (Fig. 8.44). Pleural effusions are the most common thoracic manifestation of AIDS-related lymphoma. Both effusions and parenchymal lung involvement are much more common than in the non-AIDS host. Metastases to bone are rare, but adjacent masses may involve bone directly.

Kaposi's Sarcoma (see also Chap. 42)

Described in 1872, the hemangiosarcoma of Kaposi has been the subject of much misunderstanding. Two variations have been described, depending on the natural history of the tumor. The "classic" version is a peripheral neoplasm, often presenting as pigmented nodules in the lower limbs, which progresses slowly in the majority of patients unless there is a change in the status of the patient's immune system. The other version is described in some texts as the "HIV-related generalized aggressive," but in fact Kaposi described both versions in his two publications in 1872 and 1895, including disseminated generalized spread in a child. A major symposium held in Uganda in 1962 resulted in a monograph describing the collected knowledge of about 1000 cases of Kaposi's sarcoma from all over the world, but predominantly from Central Africa. All the clinical and pathological findings now described in the so-called AIDS-related Kaposi's sarcoma were well documented long before clinical AIDS was known. Similar cases are seen in organ transplant recipients or any other patient who is for any reason immunosuppressed. The slow "classic" variety can be transformed into the "aggressive" version by immunosuppression at any age.

Kaposi's sarcoma does not in itself indicate AIDS. In regions such as sub-Saharan Africa, either can exist separately; therefore, HIV serology must be assessed in every patient with Kaposi's sarcoma at any age.

There are regional differences in distribution and aggression. For example, in the United States, unlike most other AIDS complications, Kaposi's sarcoma is concentrated in certain regions: 30% of California and New York homosexuals with AIDS develop Kaposi's sarcoma, whereas in Kansas only 5% of homosexuals with AIDS develop the tumor. Sexual contacts of male homosexuals experience an increased risk of subsequently developing Kaposi's sarcoma. In HIV-negative individuals, it follows a benign course; this is the pattern for 2% of Kaposi's sarcoma in the homosexual population.

Recently a herpes type virus (HHV-8), also called "Kaposi's sarcoma-associated herpes virus" (Kaposi's sarcoma HV), has been found incorporated into the DNA of Kaposi's sarcoma tumor specimens and is now recognized as the cause. Epidemiologically, spread of Kaposi's sarcoma in the homosexual population has been linked to sexual practices involving fecal contact (raising the possibility of spread by other forms of fecal contact). There is a high prevalence of antibodies to Kaposi's sarcoma HV in HIV-infected American homosexual men, but a low prevalence, similar to that in the population at large, in HIV-positive drug users, hemophiliacs, and women.

In Purvis et al.'s analysis of tumor lesions from 38 Ugandan Kaposi's sarcoma patients, the lesions contained Kaposi's sarcoma HV, and Kaposi's sarcoma HV DNA was also detectable in peripheral blood mononuclear cells. Also noted was the intriguing finding that a high percentage of Kaposi's sarcoma lesions were positive for Epstein-Barr virus sequences. Similar Kaposi's sarcoma HV sequences have been identified in all cases tested of the so-called classic Kaposi's sarcoma, endemic African Kaposi's sarcoma, AIDS-associated epidemic Kaposi's sarcoma, and iatrogenic Kaposi's sarcoma. Examination of serological evidence of antibodies to Kaposi's sarcoma HV has revealed all patients with African endemic Kaposi's sarcoma to be seropositive. Between 2% and 8% of children are positive, confirming the presence of a nonsexual means of spread (conceivably fecal contact due to poor hygiene practices). Kaposi's sarcoma HV may, indeed, be a common childhood febrile infection in ende-

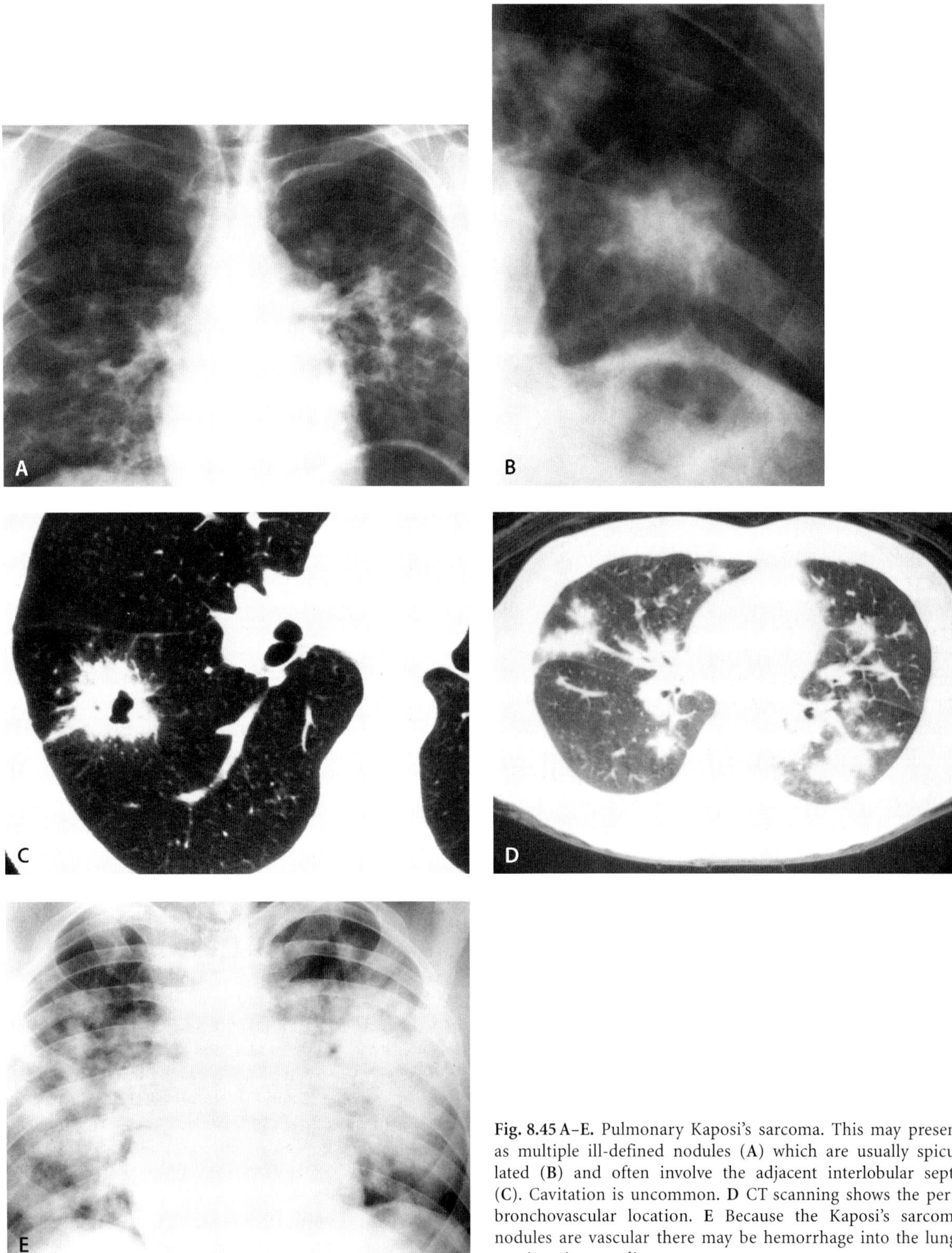

Fig. 8.45 A–E. Pulmonary Kaposi's sarcoma. This may present as multiple ill-defined nodules (**A**) which are usually spiculated (**B**) and often involve the adjacent interlobular septa (**C**). Cavitation is uncommon. **D** CT scanning shows the peribronchovascular location. **E** Because the Kaposi's sarcoma nodules are vascular there may be hemorrhage into the lung, causing airspace disease

mic areas. In Africa and elsewhere young children may develop Kaposi's sarcoma with minimal skin involvement but with lymphadenopathy, extensive internal organ involvement, and a virulent course.

An additional mystifying statistic is that Kaposi's sarcoma is overwhelmingly a male disease even in the almost exclusively heterosexual population of Africa, and there are few concordant couples even in areas of high incidence. Even in pediatric Kaposi's sarcoma and pre-AIDS era Kaposi's sarcoma, a strong male predominance has been noted, except along the eastern seaboard of South Africa.

Kaposi's sarcoma is less common and quite variable in heterosexually transmitted AIDS: it occurs in 8%–18% of heterosexually transmitted AIDS cases in Africa, 30% in Mexico, 6%–9% in the Caribbean, but less than 1% of such cases in USA or India. Patients whose HIV infections is transfusion related rarely develop Kaposi's sarcoma, yet it has developed in patients acquiring HIV via maternal-fetal infection, particularly in the African and Caribbean populations. Kaposi's sarcoma is the most common transplant-associated tumor in Saudi Arabia, but is rare in this setting in Western countries.

It is important to note the clinical variations in Kaposi's sarcoma: although usually characterized by painless deep reddish-purple subcutaneous nodules and similar angiomatous lesions of the mucosae, there may be facial thickening without obvious pigmentation. Kaposi's sarcoma may appear in the gastrointestinal tract or airways without visible skin lesions. Visceral lesions can be solitary or multiple and present as a mass, bleeding, or obstruction. Angiography can demonstrate multiple clinically unsuspected tumors.

It is probable that the development of the aggressive form of Kaposi's sarcoma requires a substantial degree of immunosuppression. In 80% of cases of Kaposi's sarcoma the tumor is the presenting symptom of AIDS. However, particularly in Africa, not every patient with Kaposi's sarcoma has AIDS or is even HIV positive. There is nothing clinically or histologically to distinguish the non-AIDS patient; only serology can do this.

Although chemotherapy shows clinical response in many patients with endemic African Kaposi's sarcoma, epidemic AIDS-related Kaposi's sarcoma does not respond. Lesions will, however, respond well to local palliative radiotherapy.

Imaging Findings

Thoracic manifestations of Kaposi's sarcoma in severely immuno-compromised patients include, most commonly, the development of numerous ill-defined nodules with a basilar predominance which tend to follow the bronchovascular bundles (Fig. 8.45). The nodules may be spiculated in appearance, resulting from tumor involvement of adjacent interlobular septa. Cavitation may rarely occur. As the nodules may be hemorrhagic, they can be surrounded by ill-defined ground-glass densities, which represent bleeding into surrounding lung parenchyma. More severe bleeding may cause frank consolidation. The hemorrhage may clear over time, leading to the false impression that the disease is improving. Pleural effusions are common. There may be lymphadenopathy and this may enhance with contrast injection to some extent in about half of cases, but enhancement is not as dramatic as with bacillary angiomatosis (see above). Nodular lesions in the airways are occasionally visible (Fig. 8.46).

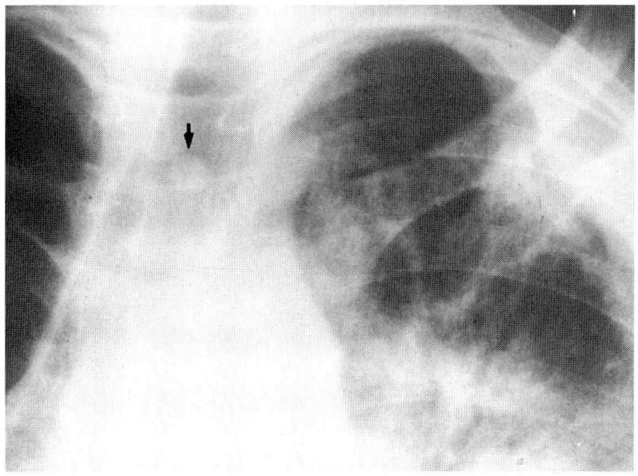

Fig. 8.46. Kaposi's sarcoma may produce nodular lesions in the airways which may occasionally be visualized on chest radiograph, as in this tracheal lesion (*arrow*). Similar nodules may be found in the larynx

When Kaposi's sarcoma involves the internal organs, the most common sites of involvement are the gastrointestinal tract (heavily weighted toward small bowel), lungs, and lymph nodes. Gastrointestinal disease presents as irregular masses in any viscus, which may produce obstruction, deformity, or hemorrhage. The most frequently involved is the duodenum. Air contrast examinations or sonography of the gastrointestinal tract may reveal submucosal nodules, polypoid lesions, or diffuse thickening and distortion. Larger lesions may have central umbilication, producing a target effect. Hepatosplenomegaly may be present. Lymphadenopathy is also seen (Fig. 8.47 A), which may enhance to some extent with contrast injection. Ascites may be present (Fig. 8.47 B).

Bone involvement produces lytic lesions with associated periosteal reaction. Associated marrow involvement may be appreciated on MRI. Kaposi's sarcoma seldom involved the brain (see also Chap. 42).

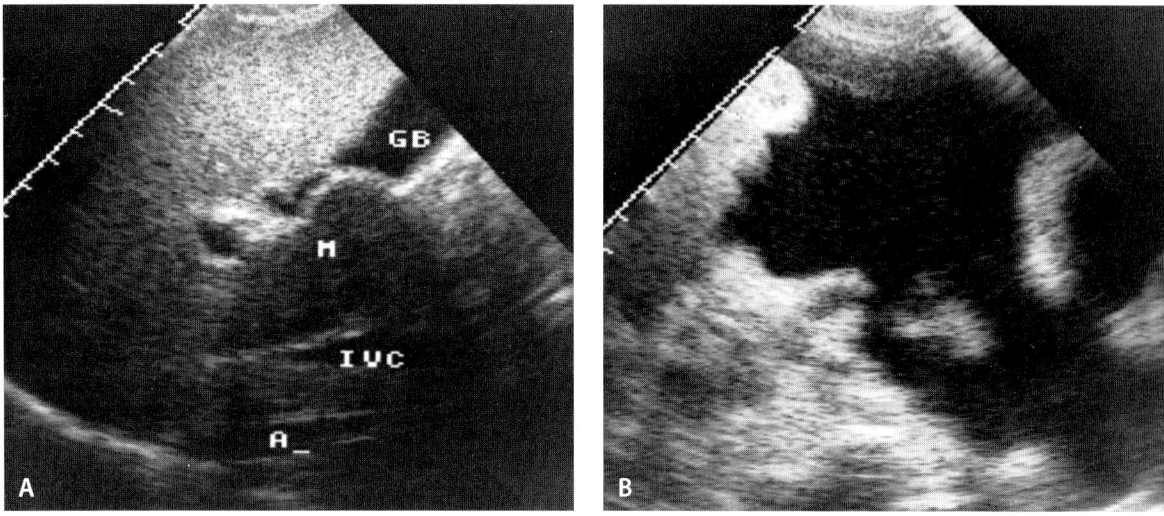

Fig. 8.47 A, B. Kaposi's sarcoma in the abdomen in AIDS. **A** Ultrasonography shows a large periportal nodal mass (*M*) and **B** ascites, which is a frequent finding. *A* Aorta; *GB* gallbladder; *IVC* inferior vena cava. (Courtesy of Dr. William Brandt)

Organisms Likely to Cause AIDS-Related Diarrhea in the Tropics

The most common presentation of AIDS in Africa is "slim disease," a syndrome characterized by chronic diarrhea and weight loss, leading to severe cachexia. This syndrome affects up to 80% of AIDS patients, and as many as 85% of patients have diarrhea (compared with 50% of Western AIDS patients). However, Lucas and colleagues' autopsy study from West Africa indicated that a premortem diagnosis of diarrhea was no more frequent in cachectic patients than in noncachectic patients, and found wasting to be strongly correlated with tuberculosis. Forty-four percent of skeletally wasted cadavers had tuberculosis compared with 39% of moderately wasted and 23% of nonwasted cadavers. This goes against conventional wisdom, that wasting results from an enteropathy such as that caused by cryptosporidiosis or HIV itself. There is speculation that in some patients, a component of wasting may be related to soluble tumor necrosis factor receptor concentrations (reflecting immune activation and high cytokine activity), rather than being entirely attributable to infections.

The coccidian parasites *Cryptosporidium parvum, Isospora belli,* and *Cyclospora*, and the Microsporidia are thought to account for at least half of the cases of persistent AIDS-associated diarrhea in the developing world, with contributions from *Mycobacterium avium* complex, other bacteria, and cytomegalovirus.

Cryptosporidiosis and isosporiasis are protozoan diseases (in the same genus as *Toxoplasma gondii*) which affect the epithelial cells of the gastrointestinal tract. In normal hosts, cryptosporidiosis produces transient episodes of diarrhea. In AIDS patients, the diarrhea is far more severe.

Cryptosporidium was the most common pathogen identified in several AIDS diarrhea studies from Africa and Haiti, and is also common in Central and South America. In a study from Brazil, *Cryptosporidium* and *Isospora* were not found in any of the normal hosts examined, but were present in 19% and 10% of AIDS patients respectively. Examination of the causes of chronic diarrhea in AIDS patients, as compared to the general population in Zambia, showed that *Isospora* occurred in markedly increased numbers in AIDS patients (and was not seen in the general population), and that *Cryptosporidium* was also an important AIDS-related pathogen. *Cryptosporidium* has been documented in 38% of AIDS patients with diarrhea in Mali, and 21% in the Democratic Republic of the Congo. In two Tanzanian studies, cryptosporidiosis and isosporiasis were virtually restricted to HIV-positive individuals with diarrhea. Also in Tanzania, a survey of intestinal parasites showed that the prevalence of *Cryptosporidium parvum, Isospora belli,* and *Strongyloides stercoralis* was higher in HIV-positive than in HIV-negative patients (and higher in AIDS patients than in HIV-positive patients). *Entamoeba histolytica* and *Ascaris lumbricoides* were more frequent in HIV-negative patients. In a study comparing HIV-positive Zambian diarrhea patients with HIV-negative diarrhea patients, only *Isospora belli* and *Cryptosporidium* were seen exclusively in the HIV-positive group, and an increased incidence of *Entamoeba coli* was also seen. Fecal samples from 108 AIDS patients in southern India revealed that a third of patients with diarrhea were positive for *Cryptosporidium* oocytes. In Pape's large Haitian diarrhea study in HIV-positive patients, the most common enteric protozoa included *Cryptosporidium* (30%), *Isospora belli* (12%), *Cyclospora* (11%), *Giardia* (3%), and *Entamoeba histolytica* (1%). Co-infections with *Isospora* and *Cryptosporidium* are seen quite commonly.

Cryptosporidia will involve the biliary tract in 10% of AIDS patients. Multisystemic infections involving the respiratory tract, small intestine, biliary tract, and pancreas have occurred. High death rates are seen in the AIDS population because currently there is no effective treatment, although nitazoxanide has recently been shown to be promising. It also shows activity against *Isospora belli, Entamoeba histolytica, Giardia lamblia, Ascaris lumbricoides, Enterobius vermicularis, Hymenolepis nana,* and *Dicrocoelium dentriticum.*

The ubiquitous Microsporidia species (*Enterocytozoon bieneusi*), a small protozoan parasite, has been described in 33% of Australian AIDS patients with diarrhea. Its contribution to diarrhea in African AIDS patients is probably less significant; it is reported in 2% of patients in Zambia and is not found in patients in Uganda or the Democratic Republic of the Congo.

Cytomegalovirus may produce colitis, with nodular mucosal thickening. Cytomegalovirus infections resulting in diarrhea were identified in only 6% of patients in the Democratic Republic of the Congo and no patients in Uganda and Zambia. Intestinal disease due to atypical mycobacteria is also rare in Africa and has not increased in AIDS patients there.

Although there is no definitive evidence that AIDS increases the likelihood of infection with *Strongyloides* in the tropics, disseminated strongyloidiasis is much more common in HIV-positive patients (and patients placed on steroids). Dissemination may be associated with the adult respiratory distress syndrome, septic shock, and death. Patients with preexisting colonization by *Strongyloides* appear to have increasing intestinal penetration by the larvae, leading to self reinfection with increased burdens of juvenile forms. These pass through the lungs and may produce an acute allergic reaction, clinically manifested by asthma, cough, pulmonary infiltrates, and hypoxia. The organisms and surrounding inflammatory reaction may be visible on plain radiographs as a nodular or reticulonodular pattern or on CT scanning as ill-defined nodular densities, about 2–5 mm in size (Fig. 8.48). The patients often present with a combination of gastrointestinal and respiratory symptomatology. This syndrome is frequently accompanied by gram-negative sepsis. The diagnosis may be made by bronchoalveolar lavage and the presence of *Strongyloides* in the intestine,

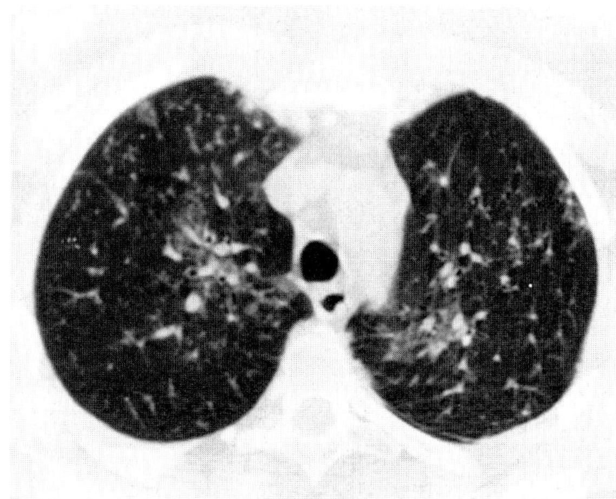

Fig. 8.48. Ill-defined nodules and patchy foci of airspace disease are seen in this patient with asthma: there were *Strongyloides* in both sputum and stool. (Courtesy of Dr. Linda Haramati)

found by examination of the the stool for ova and parasites or by duodenal capsule biopsy. Disseminated strongyloidiasis may involve the CNS (see p. 722, Chap. 13).

Entamoeba histolytica and *Giardia* appear to be more common in patients with AIDS in the United States than in African and other third world nations, probably due to increased male homosexual contact. Although unclean water supplies can transmit these diseases, there appears to be no increased risk in AIDS patients in the developing world. Studies from numerous African countries suggest that there is no significant increase in the incidence of extracellular intestinal parasites, such as *Necator americanus* and *Ascaris,* when AIDS patients are compared with controls.

Reports from areas where typhoid and paratyphoid are endemic show that HIV patients may have a substantial increase over baseline rates of these diseases. This may reflect the decreased activity of the mononuclear cells in AIDS patients against these organisms. Typhoid and paratyphoid in the AIDS patient are characterized by fulminant diarrhea associated with colitis, and often relapse despite adequate treatment.

Nontyphi *Salmonellae* are also a substantial cause of morbidity in HIV in the tropics, and systemic salmonellosis may be an underdiagnosed cause of death. Of 103 patients in Burundi in hospital for *Salmonella* dysentery, 86 were HIV positive (83%).

No etiological agent can be identified in approximately 20%–40% of the patients in Africa, Haiti, and other parts of the developing world who have both AIDS and chronic diarrhea. This may represent the lack of sophisticated laboratories, but it may also indicate a high incidence of AIDS enteropathy: a chronic diarrhea in AIDS patients for which no identifiable pathogen is found and which possibly results from the direct effect of HIV on the mucosa.

Gastrointestinal Symptoms

A reasonable guess as to the possible cause can be made on the basis of gastrointestinal symptoms. Dysphagia or odynophagia suggest *Candida*, cytomegalovirus, or herpes simplex esophagitis. Subacute abdominal pain, vomiting, and weight loss raise the possibility of lymphoma or Kaposi's sarcoma. Severe acute abdominal pain suggests pancreatitis or intestinal perforation due to cytomegalovirus. Right upper quadrant pain suggests hepatic abscess, cholangitis, or cholecystitis. Diarrhea suggests protozoal, parasitic, bacterial, and/or viral disease. Pneumatosis intestinalis should raise the possibility of cryptosporidiosis, rotavirus, cytomegalovirus, *Clostridium difficile*, or *Pseudomonas*.

Many patients with AIDS involving the gastrointestinal tract will have a combination of two or more etiological factors, such as more than one organism or both infection and malignancy. The documentation of one pathogen or a malignancy does not exclude others. All clinical findings should not be attributed to a single primary diagnosis, particularly in the third world, where multiple pathologies are not uncommon even in the absence of AIDS.

Radiographic Manifestations of Gastrointestinal Disease in AIDS: Differential Diagnosis by Anatomical Site

Esophagus and Stomach

Many AIDS patients experience severe dysphagia or odynophagia, which may be due to a variety of etiologies. Air contrast examination of the esophagus and stomach is important to evaluate focal lesions and the condition of the intervening mucosa.

Esophageal disease may be caused by HIV, resulting in multiple discrete, large shallow ulcers. Esophageal herpes simplex virus (HSV) infection produces numerous discrete ulcers which may be surrounded by edema and which are separated by normal mucosa, producing a cobblestone appearance on barium swallow (Fig. 8.49). The rectum and anus may also be involved. Cytomegalovirus is another common cause of esophageal ulceration, characteristically producing large somewhat diamond-shaped ulcers (Fig. 8.50). In the stomach, thickening of mucosal folds and antral stenosis are characteristic findings.

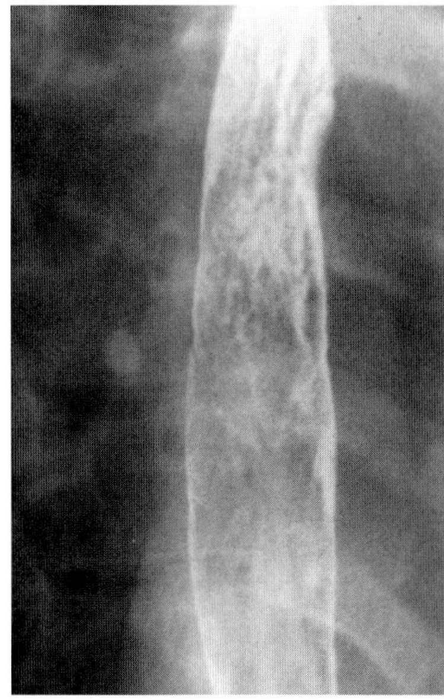

Fig. 8.49. The barium air contrast study of the esophagus of an AIDS patient with herpes simplex esophagitis. There are multiple ulcers separated by areas of normal mucosa

Many of the AIDS patients who complain of dysphagia/odynophagia will have thrush (candidiasis). For example, candidiasis was noted in 21%–40% of AIDS patients in the Democratic Republic of the Congo and in Burundi 31% had this complication. Oral thrush is often found in patients with esophageal candidiasis. A barium swallow early in the course of involvement will show small round plaque-like exophytic lesions on the mucosal surface of the esophagus. In more severe cases, the interstices between plaques, mucosal ulcerations and pseudomembranes produce a "shaggy" appearance (Fig. 8.51; see also p. 626).

Kaposi's sarcoma may involve the esophagus, stomach, small bowel, or large bowel, originating as flat submucosal lesions but enlarging into polypoid masses often demonstrating central umbilication (target lesion). These lesions may be accompanied by enlarged lymph nodes, which may enhance on contrast injection (see Chap. 42).

Small Intestine

In the small bowel, *Isospora belli*, *Cryptosporidium*, and *Microsporidia* all produce a similar hypersecretory state, on barium studies causing dilution and fragmentation as well as fold thickening (Fig. 8.52 A). Isosporiasis may involve the small intestine, the mesenteric and mediastinal lymph nodes, the spleen, and the liver.

Abdominal involvement is common in disseminated histoplasmosis. The gastrointestinal tract will be in-

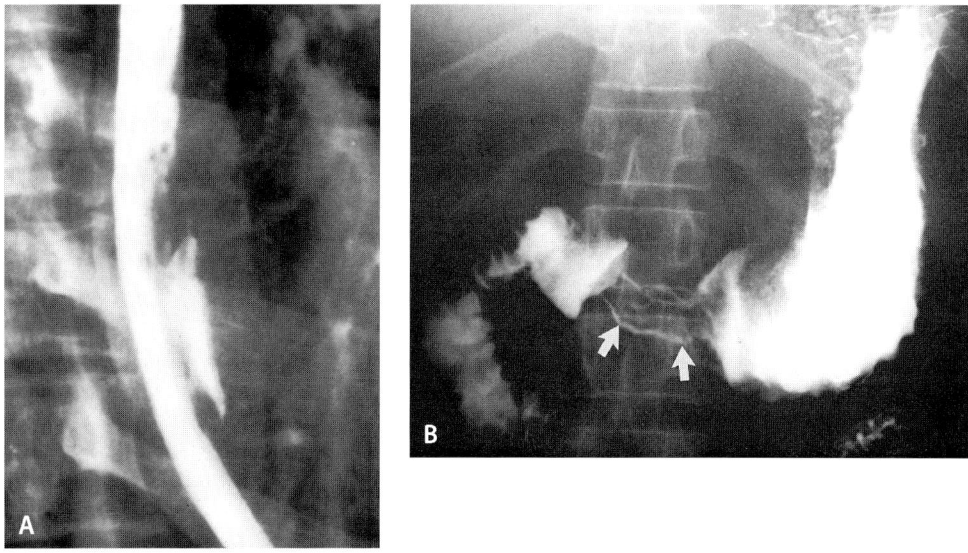

Fig. 8.50 A, B. Cytomegalovirus. **A** A barium swallow shows a large and deep ulcer, which is characteristic of cytomegalic involvement of the esophagus. **B** In the stomach gastritis is often characterized by thickened folds and stenosis of the antral region (*arrows*)

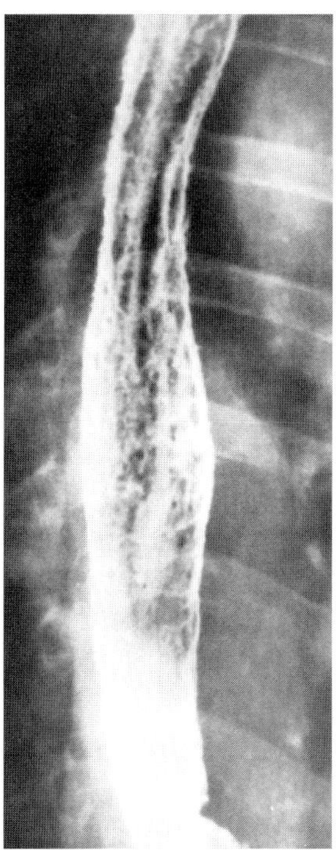

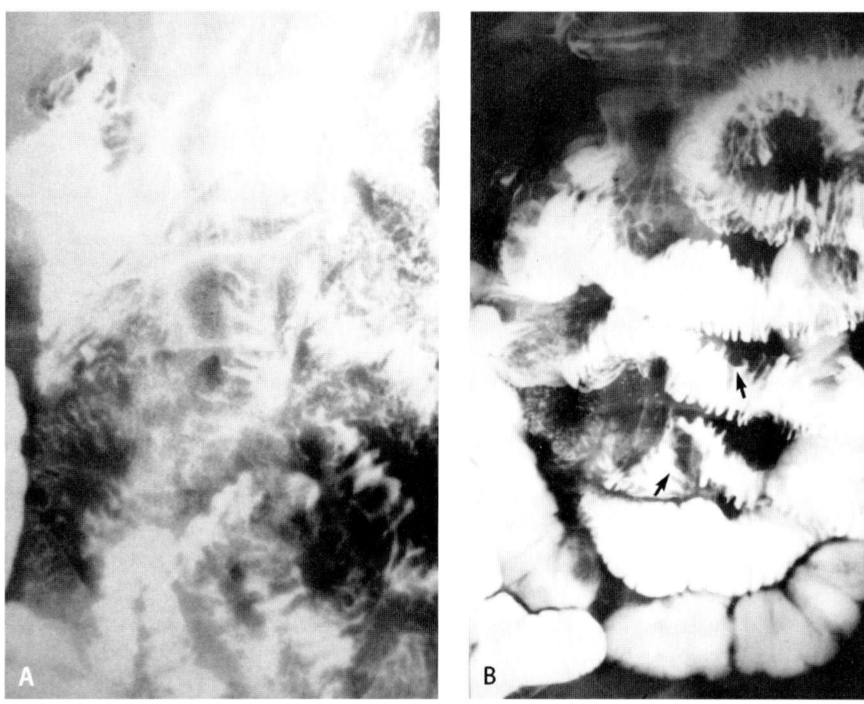

Fig. 8.51 (*left*). The barium swallow of a patient with AIDS and candidiasis shows a "shaggy" appearance of the esophagus because barium is trapped in the interstices between plaque-like lesions

Fig. 8.52 A, B (*middle, right*). The small intestine of AIDS patients is affected by infections and tumors. For example: **A** *Isospora belli* causes thickening of the mucosal folds and dilution of barium. **B** There may be multiple nodules in the small intestine in patients with Kaposi's sarcoma (*arrows*), often associated with thickened mucosal folds. If the nodules ulcerate, they appear as "target" lesions

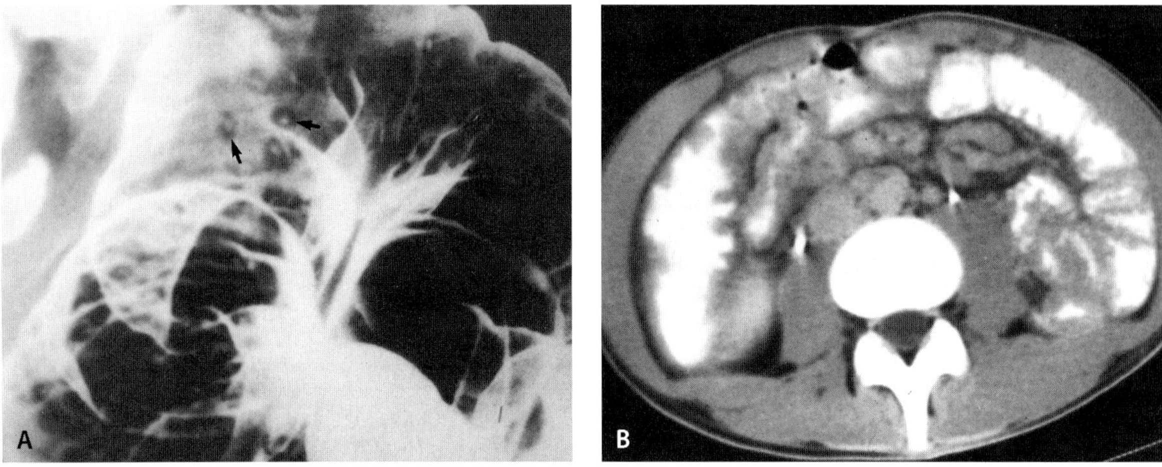

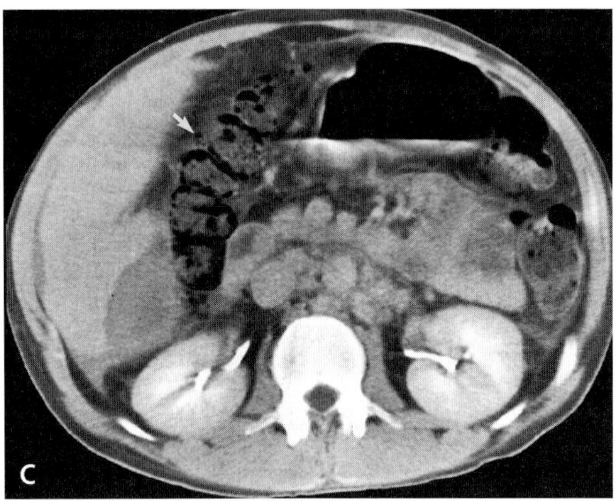

Fig. 8.53 A–C. Cytomegaloviral infection of the colon. **A** Multiple ulcers with surrounding edema (*arrows*), seen in a barium air contrast study, and **B** marked thickening of the bowel wall in a patient with both enteritis and colitis. **C** In another patient there is pneumatosis coli (*arrow*). This is relatively common in AIDS. The differential diagnosis includes cryptosporidiosis, rotavirus, *Clostridium difficile*, and *Pseudomonas* infections. (C courtesy of Dr. William Brandt)

volved 75% of the time; the terminal ileum and ascending colon are particularly often affected. This involvement is manifested by ulcerations, fold thickening, and marked circumferential bowel wall thickening resembling carcinoma (see p. 588).

The bowel may be involved in tuberculosis, particularly the ileocecal region, which is rich in lymphoid tissue. Ulcers, ulcerating masses, fistulae, stenoses, and wall thickening may be seen, producing obstruction, bleeding and perforation. *Mycobacterium avium* complex commonly involves the jejunum as well as the remainder of the small bowel, producing a pattern of irregular thickened folds (see Chap. 5).

Kaposi's sarcoma involving the small bowel may produce nodular fold thickening, often with the characteristic umbilicated lesions (Fig. 8.52 B). The lesions are best demonstrated by compression (see Chap. 42). Cytomegalovirus may also involve the small bowel, particularly the terminal ileum (Fig. 8.53 B).

Colon and Rectum

Cytomegaloviral colitis is common, often involving the cecum and ascending colon. As in the esophagus, multiple deep or shallow ulcers are produced (Fig. 8.53), often associated with a markedly thickened bowel wall and inflammatory changes in the adjacent fat. Pneumatosis coli or perforation may result. Histoplasmosis may produce fold thickening and apple-core lesions in the ileocecal region. Rectal involvement may be seen in herpes simplex virus infections.

Liver and Spleen

Liver CT or ultrasonography is frequently abnormal in AIDS patients with hepatic dysfunction. There is often fatty degeneration and the liver may also be the site of bacterial of fungal abscesses (Fig. 8.54) or focal lesions resulting from disseminated cytomegalovirus infection histoplasmosis, lymphoma, or Kaposi's sarcoma. Focal lesions in the liver or spleen

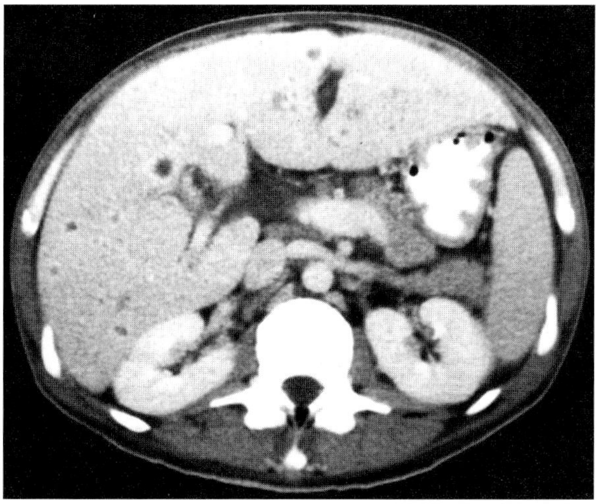

Fig. 8.54. The CT scan of an AIDS patient with multiple cryptococcal abscesses in the liver. There is surrounding enhancement after contrast injection

◄

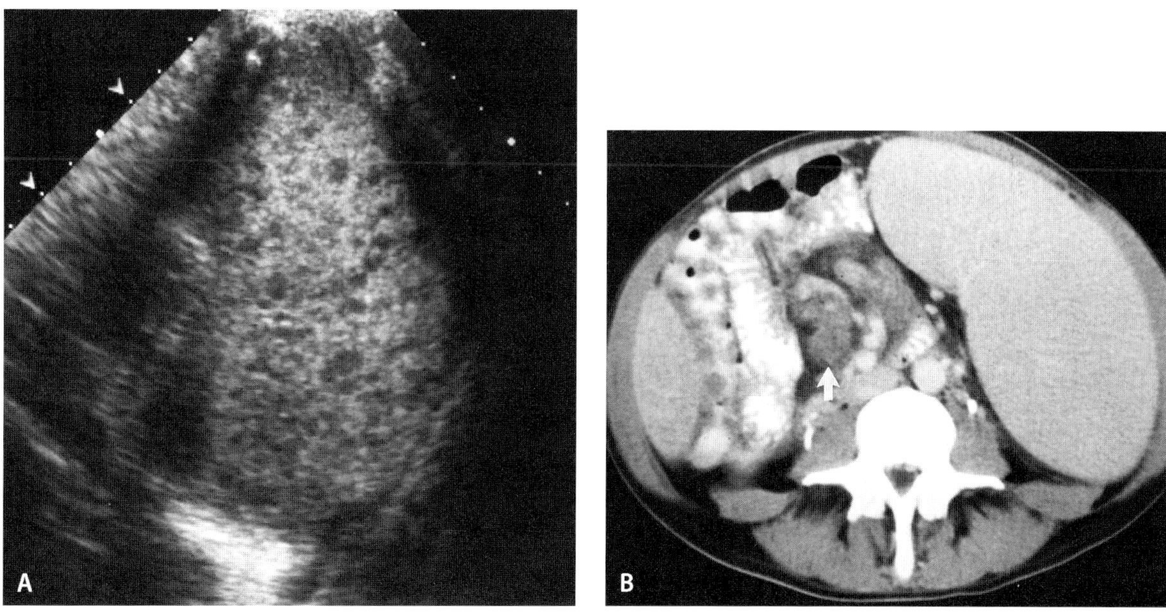

Fig. 8.55 A, B. Mycobacterial infections in AIDS patients. **A** A sonogram shows multiple tuberculous splenic microabscesses. (Courtesy of Dr. William Brandt) **B** A CT scan of another patient shows splenomegaly and lymphadenopathy (*arrow*) due to *Mycobacterium avium* complex

▼

are common in tuberculosis (Fig. 8.55) (see Chap. 5). Bacillary angiomastosis may produce peliosis (multiple blood-filled cystic spaces) of both the liver and spleen (Fig. 8.56). Disseminated histoplasmosis may produce hepatosplenomegaly, foci of splenic hypoattenuation, adrenal masses, and enlarged lymph nodes, with or without low-density centers. *Pneumocystis carinii* may produce focal low-density liver or spleen lesions which may demonstrate rim calcification. Non-Hodgkin's lymphoma may produce multiple focal lesions in the liver which are low attenuation on CT and hypoechoic on ultrasonography. Hepatomegaly and splenomegaly are both common in AIDS patients. The spleen may be enlarged without invoking a secondary process in addition to AIDS, or it may be involved by lymphoma, Kaposi's sarcoma or infection. Nonspecific tropical splenomegaly must be excluded (see Chap. 46).

Biliary System

A wide variety of organisms can cause cholecystitis in AIDS, including *Microsporidia, Enterocytozoon bieneusi, Septata intestinalis,* cytomegalovirus, *Cryptosporidium, Pneumocystis carinii,* and *Isospora belli.* AIDS-related cholangitis may produce an echogenic nodule at the distal end of the common bile duct, thought to represent edema of the ampulla of Vater. AIDS-related cholangiopathy may be due to cryptosporidiosis or cytomegalovirus infection. Patients

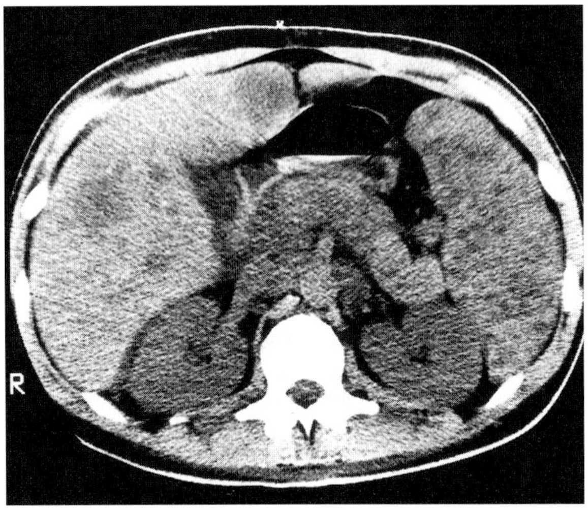

Fig. 8.56. The CT scan of a patient with extensive bacillary angiomatosis, causing peliosis of the liver and spleen. The patient was mistakenly treated for Kaposi's sarcoma, without any benefit, and unfortunately died

Fig. 8.57 A–D. AIDS-related cholangitis causes a variety of changes. **A** Multiple irregular areas of tapered narrowing of the biliary tree tract (cholangiogram). **B** Strictures and areas of dilatation, producing a beaded appearance (cholangiogram). **C** CT scan shows dilatation of portions of the biliary system (*arrows*) but without ductal dilatation in this patient. **D** Ultrasonography shows thickening of the wall of the common bile duct (*arrow*). (Courtesy of Dr. William Brandt)

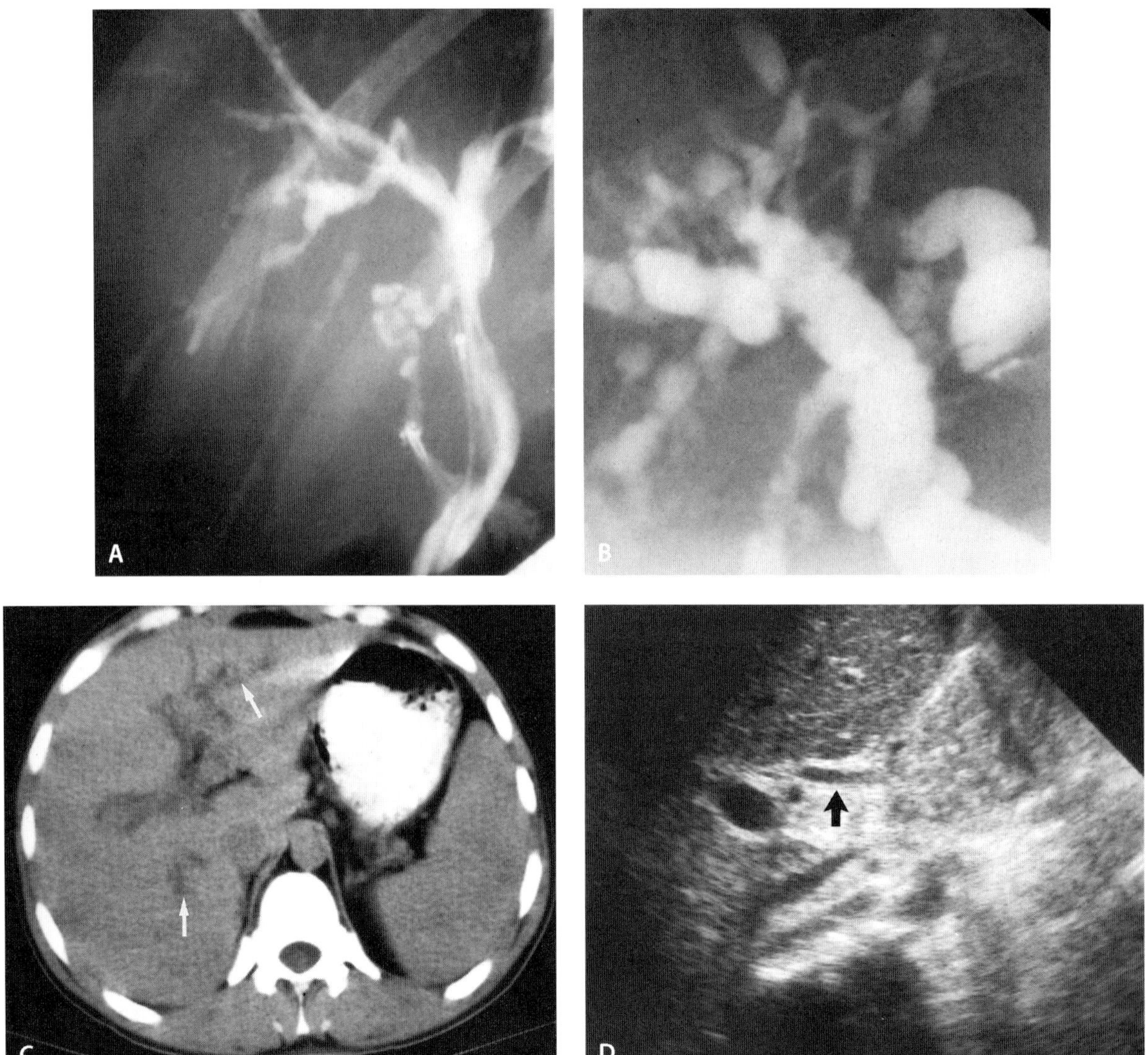

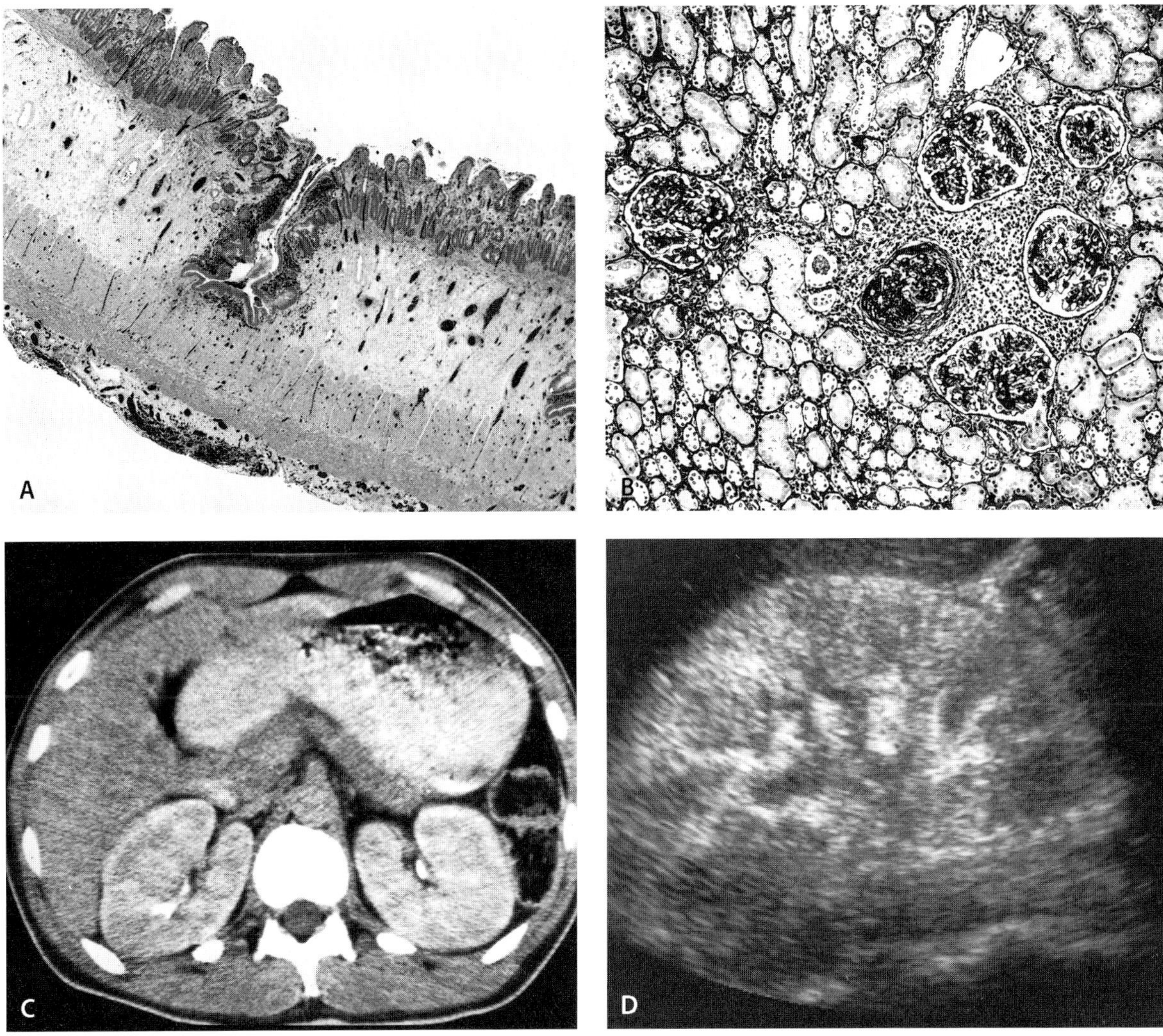

Fig. 8.58 A–D. It is not always possible to identify the cause of the changes in AIDS patients. **A** An ulcer in the small intestine of a child with a history of gastrointestinal bleeding. This might be due to intimal fibrosis, similar to the vasculopathy seen in other groups in children with AIDS, or it might be caused by an unidentified infection. **B** In the kidney there are two patterns. There is an HIV-associated nephropathy which is a focal glomerulosclerosis with interstitial lymphocytic infiltration. This can be one of the presenting clinical symptoms of AIDS in children. In the other group of patients, the changes are nonspecific: there is renal enlargement and the underlying process may be direct HIV in origin. **C** The CT scan of an AIDS patient with diffusely enlarged kidneys due to AIDS nephropathy. **D** Ultrasonography of an enlarged kidney with increased echogenicity, the characteristic finding of AIDS nephropathy. (**A**, **B** from M.A. Greco and D. Zagzag, in D.H. Connor, ed. *The pathology of infectious diseases.* Stamford, Appleton and Lange, 1997, pp 169–181; **C**, **D** courtesy of Dr. William Brandt)

present with right upper quadrant pain, nausea, vomiting, fever, and cholestasis.

On cholangiography, the appearance of AIDS cholangitis is similar to that of sclerosing cholangitis, with diffuse tapered narrowing of the intrahepatic biliary tree (Fig. 8.57 A). There may be focal stricturing or beading of the biliary tree (Fig. 8.57 B), focal areas of intrahepatic ductal dilatation (Fig. 8.57 C), or thickening of the ductal walls or the gallbladder wall. The extrahepatic bile duct may be dilated and thickened but is generally not stenotic (Fig. 8.57 D). Papillary stenosis may, however, be present, with dilatation to the level of the papilla.

Renal Involvement

HIV itself may produce renal disease characterized by progressive renal failure, proteinuria, and diffuse enlargement of the kidneys which are hyperechoic on ultrasonography (Fig. 8.58 B–D). Bacteria, including *Mycobacterium tuberculosis* and fungi may pro-

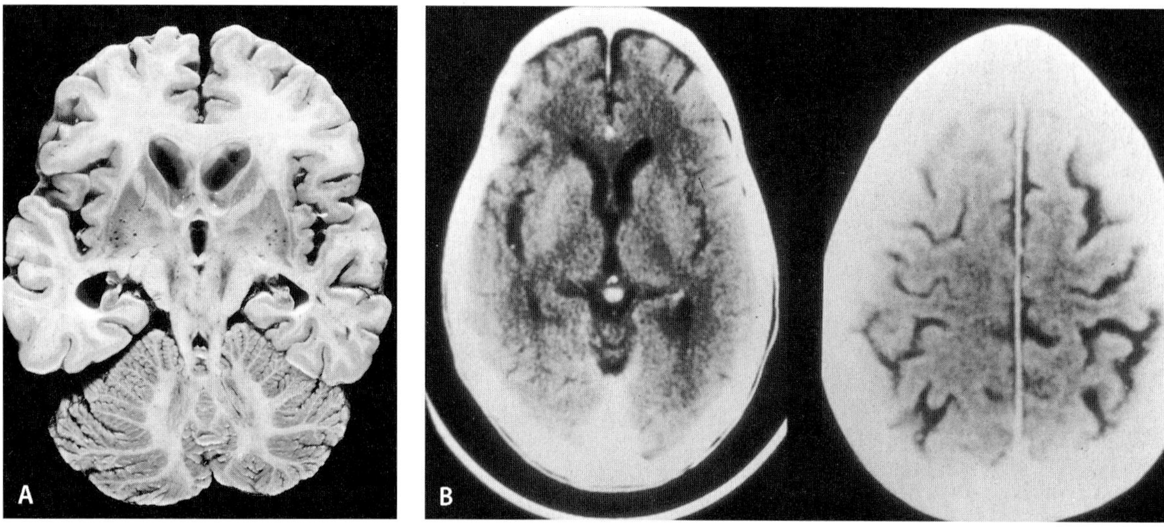

Fig. 8.59 A, B. HIV-1-associated cerebral atrophy. **A** The brain of a very demented adult with HIV encephalitis. The sulci are widened, the ventricles are dilated, and there is loss of cerebral substance. **B** The scans of a 30-year-old AIDS patient showing similar changes with cerebral atrophy, prominent sulci, and dilated ventricles. (**A** from M.K. Rosenblum, in D.H. Connor, ed. *The pathology of infectious diseases*. Stamford, Appleton and Lange, 1997, pp 183–197)

duce renal abscesses. Non-Hodgkin's lymphoma may develop renal involvement, either by direct extension of adjacent adenopathy or by lymphoma intrinsic to the kidneys.

Ascites

The presence of ascites should raise the suspicion of tuberculosis, atypical mycobacteria, Kaposi's sarcoma, bacillary angiomatosis, or lymphoma. Pneumocystis carinii may produce ascites with peritoneal calcification.

Abdominal Lymphadenopathy

As previously noted, the presence of abdominal lymphadenopathy suggests lymphoma or tuberculosis (the latter more likely to be necrotic), atypical mycobacteria (often non-necrotic), Kaposi's sarcoma (mild contrast enhancement), or bacillary angiomatosis (dramatic contrast enhancement).

AIDS and the Cental Nervous System

AIDS produces a variety of neurological symptoms which may result in the patient being referred for imaging. About 30% of patients will have progressive dementia; CNS presentations also include headache, convulsions, meningeal signs, visual impairment, hemiplegia, focal seizures, and peripheral neuropathy. Meningitis, progressive multifocal leukoencephalopathy, cerebral lymphoma, toxoplasmosis, cryptococcosis, and mycobacterial, mycotic, or bacterial cerebral abscesses are common pathological conditions in AIDS.

In Africa, focal neurological findings have been reported in about 10% of HIV-positive adult hospital admissions, and the AIDS dementia complex in 9%–54%. In the HIV-positive autopsies of Lucas and colleagues, 24% died primarily of intracerebral disease, and less than half had normal brains. Cerebral toxoplasmosis was the most common lesion, and this was 12 times more common than primary cerebral lymphoma, with which it can be confused on imaging studies. Tuberculous meningitis was the second most common intracerebral lesion in this study; other causes of CNS pathology included, in descending order, pyogenic meningitis, cryptococcosis, cytomegaloviral encephalitis, and primary CNS lymphoma. In a study of meningitis in AIDS patients from the South African city of Soweto, tuberculosis was also found to be the most common cause of meningitis, followed by bacterial meningitis (most commonly *Streptococcus pneumoniae*), viral meningitis, and cryptococcal meningitis.

Viral Pathogens

HIV itself is the most common organism to affect the brain in the AIDS patient. Direct HIV encephalopathy causes diffuse brain atrophy with enlargement of the fissures, sulci, and ventricles (Fig. 8.59). White matter atrophy predominates, but subcortical gray matter and cortex can also be affected

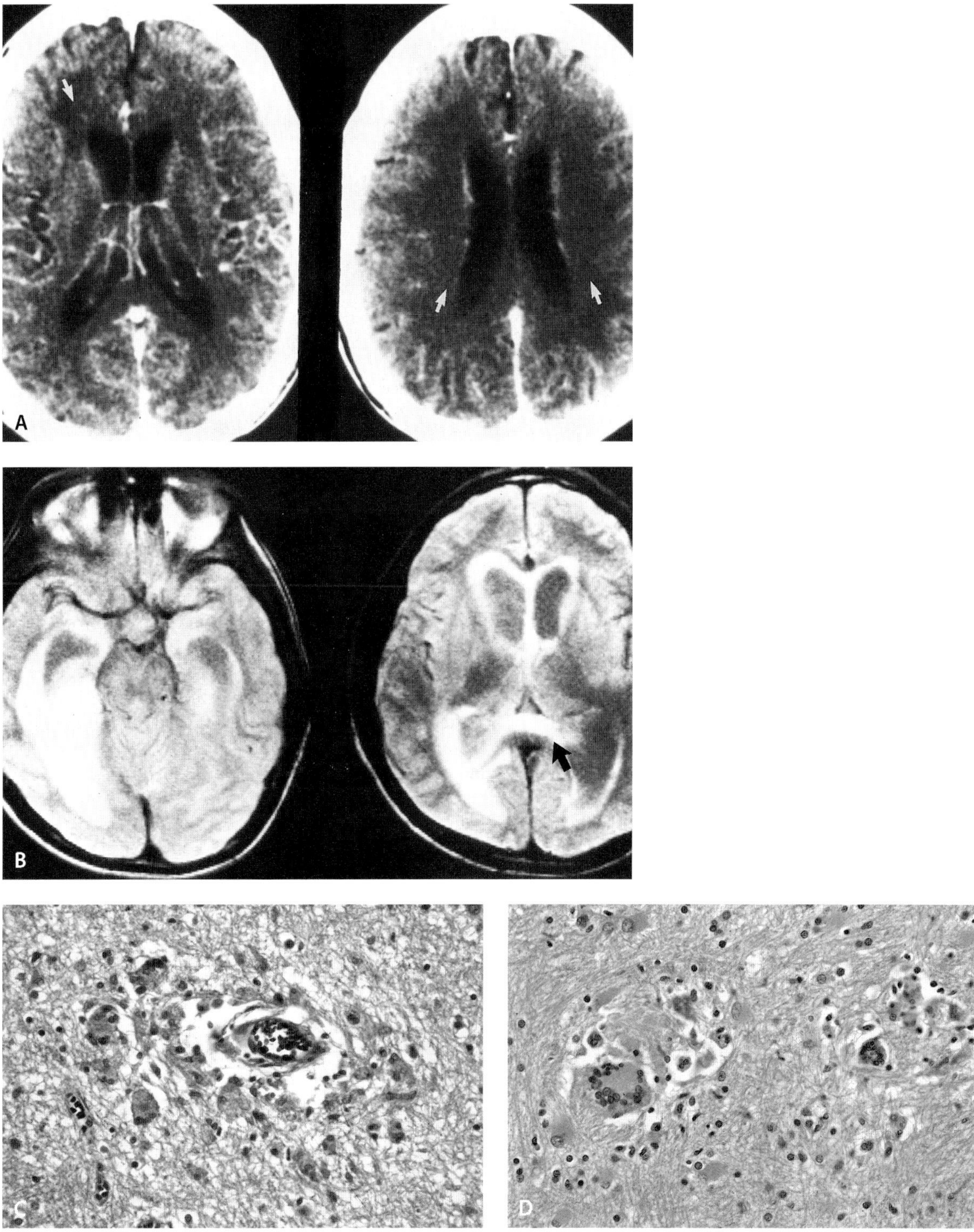

Fig. 8.60 A–D. HIV-associated white matter disease. **A** CT scans show abnormally low-density white matter, best seen in the periventricular regions (*arrows*). (Confirmed at autopsy.) **B** Proton density MR images show hyperintense white matter in the perventricular regions, especially in the splenium of the corpus callosum (*arrow*). This patient had HIV encephalopathy. **C** A section from the deep cerebral white matter of a patient with HIV encephalitis. There is no necrosis and only a moderate perivascular inflammatory reaction, mainly by macrophages, many of which are multinucleated. H & E, ×100. **D** Extensive HIV-1-infected macrophage infiltration of the white matter with marked astrogliosis. There are numerous multinucleated cells. H & E, ×250. (C, D from M.K. Rosenblum, in D.H. Connor, ed. *The pathology of infectious diseases.* Stamford, Appleton and Lange, 1997, pp 183–197)

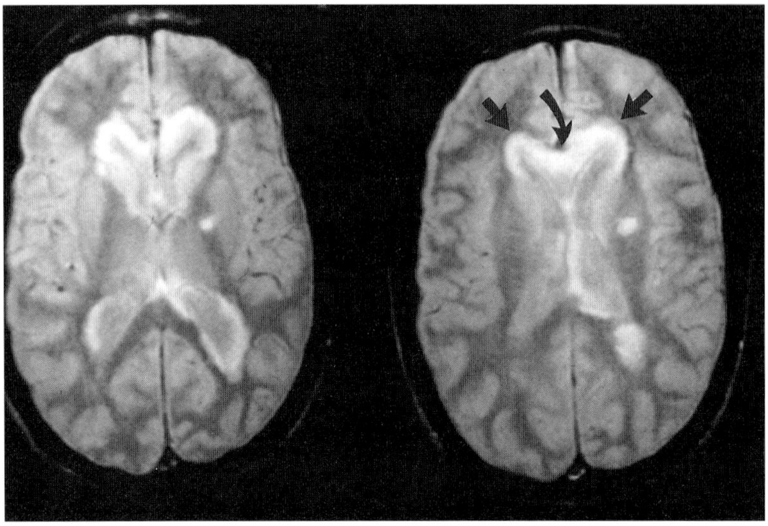

Fig. 8.61. Proton density MR images show marked hyperintensity of the ependyma bifrontally (*arrows*) in this patient with severe cytomegalovirus infection. The genu of the corpus callosum has also been affected (*curved arrow*)

(Fig. 8.60). Magnetic resonance imaging may show hyperintense signals in the white matter of T2-weighted images.

Cytomegalovirus infection may produce ependymitis (Fig. 8.61).

Toxoplasmosis

Toxoplasma gondii, a parasite often found in cats, is the most common focal brain lesion in AIDS. The majority (about two-thirds) of CNS masses in AIDS patients are due to cerebral toxoplasmosis. This condition is common in AIDS in Africa, representing the third most common cause of death in the HIV-positive autopsy study of Lucas and colleagues. It was present in 21% of patients dying with AIDS-defining pathology. CT scanning may aid diagnosis, but even this is not definitive because the appearance of toxoplasmosis and CNS lymphoma may be similar. However, since in the tropics CNS toxoplasmosis is far more common than primary CNS lymphoma, and since the latter is poorly treatable even with sophisticated techniques, focal neurological manifestations should probably be ascribed to toxoplasmosis; antimicrobial therapy may be both diagnostic and therapeutic. Improvement is expected within 2 weeks after initiating treatment.

Imaging Findings

Toxoplasmosis may produce brain abscesses or cysts, most commonly involving the corticomedullary junction, basal ganglia and thalamus (Fig. 8.62 A, B). Lesions are usually multiple, of variable size, and isodense with gray matter; they may be surrounded by edema, and ring enhance with contrast administration. However, lesions may also be solitary. Even with sophisticated MR sequences, toxoplasmosis cannot be reliably distinguished from lymphoma.

Rarely, toxoplasmosis may involve the lungs, presenting with findings resembling pneumocystis carinii pneumonia (Fig. 8.62 C; see also Chap. 45).

Cryptococcosis

The third most common process to involve the CNS in AIDS is cryptococcosis, a relatively frequent opportunistic infection in tropical AIDS, found in 5% of the AIDS deaths in Lucas and colleagues' Ivory Coast autopsy study. CNS disease (meningitis, meningoencephalitis) is most common, followed by lung and skin involvement. Patients with CNS involvement may present with fever, headache, malaise, neck stiffness, nausea, altered mental status, or seizures. Diagnosis is by lumbar puncture with CSF-India ink smears, or, when available, examination for cryptococcal antigen. In a South African study of cryptococcal meningitis, HIV-positive individuals were more likely to suffer neurological complications and/or death than non-HIV patients.

The site of entry of the organism is the lung. A study from India documented that culture of cryptococci from nonneural sites was more frequent in HIV-positive patients than in normal hosts.

Imaging Findings

Although meningitis is the most common manifestation of cryptococcal infection, it is seldom evident on imaging studies. There may be gelatinous pseudocysts, typically within the perivascular spaces sur-

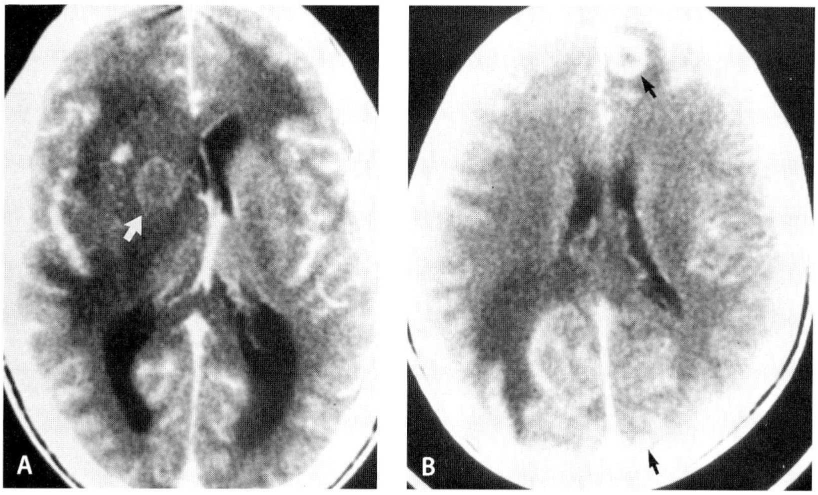

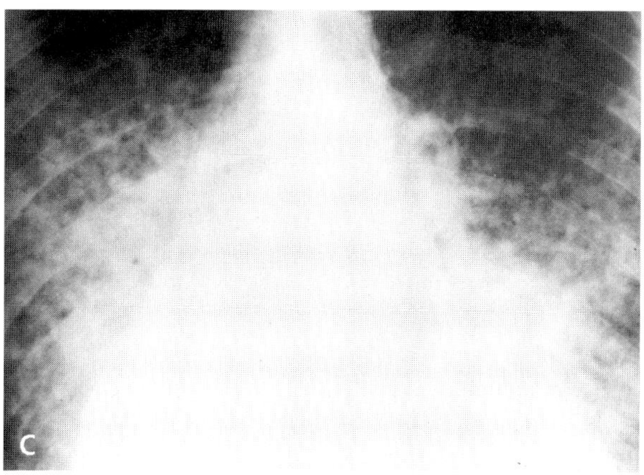

Fig. 8.62 A–C. Cerebral toxoplasmosis. **A** A ring-enhancing lesion centered in the right basal ganglia with surrounding edema (*arrow*): this obstructs the foramina of Monro, with resulting hydrocephalus. There is effacement of the sulci. **B** Multifocal enhancing lesions (*arrows*): this is a frequent finding in toxoplasmosis. **C** Toxoplasmosis may rarely involve the lung, where it produces an appearance similar to *P. carinii* pneumonia

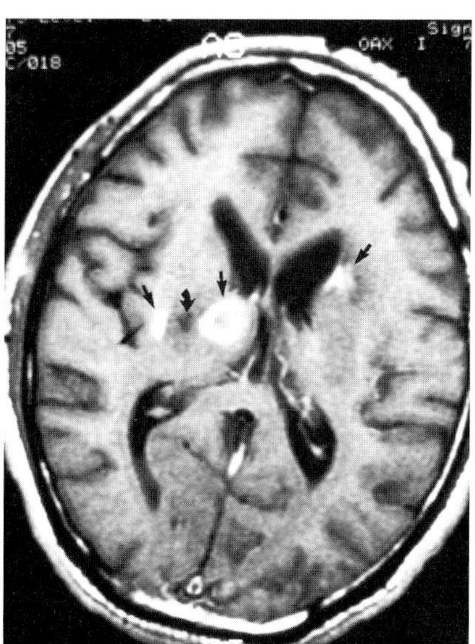

Fig. 8.63. Cryptococosis: There are three enhancing cryptococcomas (*arrows*), and a gelatinous pseudocyst (*curved arrow*) in the region of the basal ganglia

rounding small perforating vessels arising within the basilar cisterns: on CT scanning these cysts produce focal, low-density lesions within the basal ganglia with little surrounding inflammatory reaction. These rarely show contrast enhancement because they remain extraparenchymal, within the perivascular space. MRI, if available, is preferable for identification of pseudocysts, which show increased signal intensity on T2-weighted images. If there are cryptococcomas they may enhance because they are intraparenchymal, therefore violating the blood-brain barrier (Fig. 8.63; see pp. 621–623).

CNS Tuberculosis (see Chap. 5)

Tuberculous involvement of the CNS in the tropics most commonly presents as tuberculous meningitis (Fig. 8.64). This may be manifest on CT as infarctions involving the territories supplied by the lenticulostriate arteries (the basal ganglia or frontal lobes) secondary to arteritis of vessels within the basal subarachnoid space, or by meningeal enhancement in the regions of the basal cisterns. Tuberculo-

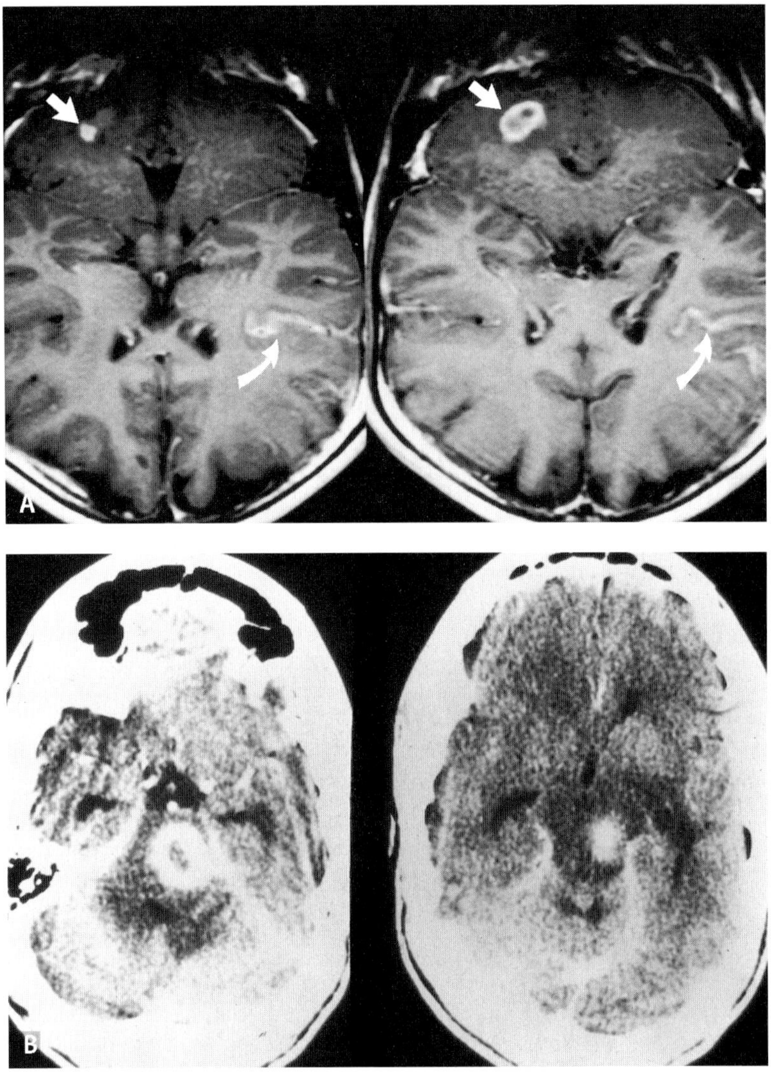

Fig. 8.64 A, B. Cerebral tuberculosis in AIDS patients. **A** Coronal postgadolinium T1-weighted images showing a tuberculoma in the left cerebellar hemisphere (*arrow*) and dense leptomeningeal enhancement in the right sylvian fissure (*curved arrow*) due to tuberculous meningitis. **B** CT images demonstrating a ring-enhancing tuberculoma in the midbrain with surrounding edema

mas are relatively rare, as are tuberculous cerebral abscesses. Tuberculomas appear as focal lesions which may have central necrosis and which may ring enhance or, in the healing phase, calcify. (Fig. 8.64 B). Tuberculous abscesses resemble other pyogenic brain abscesses (see pp. 515–523).

Syphilis (see Chap. 35)

Many HIV-infected individuals also are seropositive for syphilis. Some authors believe that a more severe clinical presentation and faster development of neurosyphilis may occur in the HIV-positive patient. Syphilis should be considered in any AIDS patient exhibiting unexplained skin or CNS findings. Syphilitic arteritis may be the cause of stroke in this group of patients and appears on arteriography as a vasculitis with focal irregularity of the arterial walls. Syphilitic gummas may appear as focal lesions.

Other Intracranial Infections

In addition to tuberculosis and syphilis, intracranial infections in the HIV patient include *Staphylococcus, Streptococcus, Salmonella, Rhodococcus equi, Listeria monocytogenes*, and various fungi (Fig. 8.65). Cerebral involvement by *Nocardia* is most

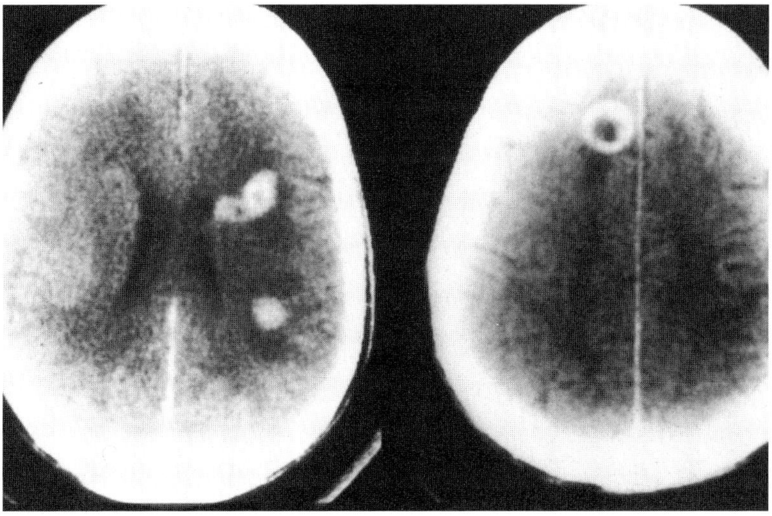

Fig. 8.65 (*left*). The differential diagnosis of cerebral lesions in AIDS patients can be difficult: two scans showing the non-specific appearance of ring-enhancing cerebral abscesses, in this case due to *Candida*

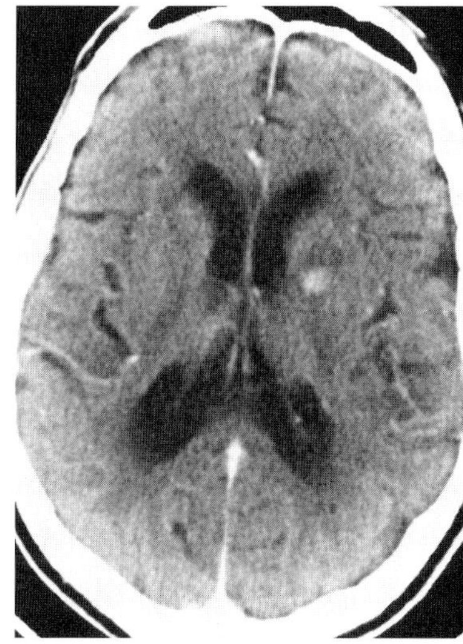

Fig. 8.66 (*right*). The CT scan of an AIDS patient with bacillary angiomatosis, showing good contrast enhancement of a lesion of the left basal ganglia

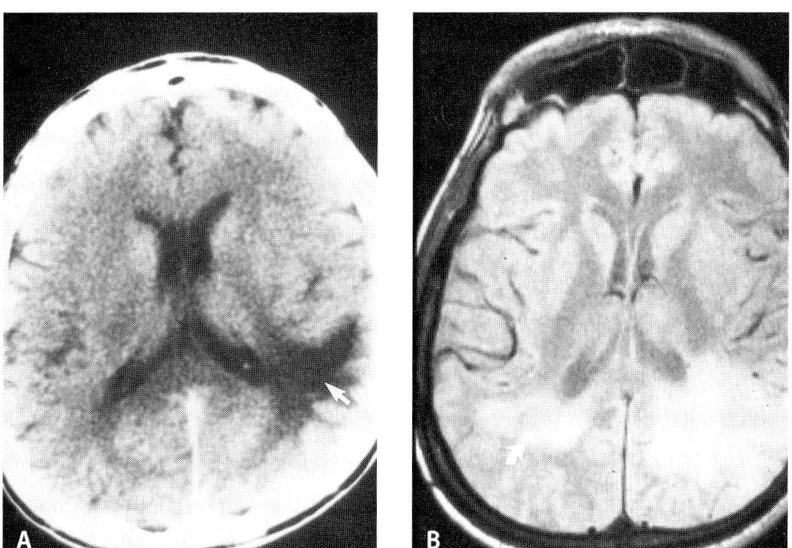

Fig. 8.67 A, B. Leukoencephalopathy. **A** CT of an AIDS patient shows diminished attenuation in the left periatrial white matter (*arrow*) due to progressive multifocal leukoencephalopathy. **B** Similar but more subtle changes on the contralateral side (*curved arrow*) can only be appreciated on a proton density MR image (*right*), demonstrating the superiority of MR for white matter pathology

commonly manifested by ring-enhancing abscesses, single or multiple, frequently associated with subependymal nodules and hydrocephalus. Bacillary angiomastosis may occasionally involve the brain, producing focal, enhancing lesions (Fig. 8.66; see pp. 552–555).

Progressive Multifocal Leukoencephalopathy

Progressive multifocal leukoencephalopathy is a very rare cause of demyelination and white matter necrosis, beginning in the subcortical white matter in the parietal and occipital lobes and progressing to extensive involvement. On CT scanning, there are low-density nonenhancing white matter lesions without a mass effect, while on T2-weighted MR

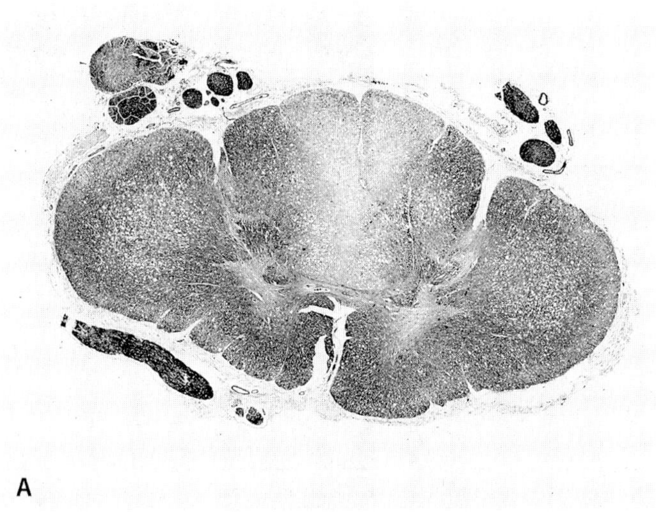

A

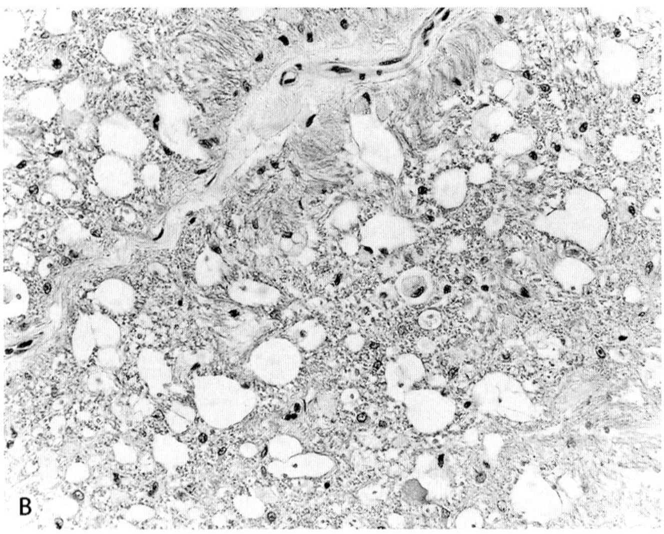

B

Fig. 8.68 A, B. The spinal cord in HIV patients. Selective involvement of the spinal cord is rare; disseminated foci are much more common. However, vacuolar myelopathy is the major cause of spinal cord disorder in AIDS. **A** The lateral and posterior columns are extensively involved with white matter vacuolization. This is the typical distribution in AIDS. There is also degeneration of the gracile tracts shown by the pallor in this section. **B** The lateral column of the same patient showing the vacuolar process, the commonest cause of spinal cord dysfunction. ×250. (From M.K. Rosenblum, in D.H. Connor, ed. *The pathology of infectious diseases*. Stamford, Appleton and Lange, 1997, pp 183–197)

images, affected areas show increased signal (Fig. 8.67). The condition is characterized by progressive motor and visual disturbances and is untreatable and rapidly fatal.

Equally important in AIDS, especially in children, is the neurotropic effect of HIV. The encephalopathy may progress slowly or very rapidly. It usually occurs late in the infection but may be the first evidence of HIV, presenting as progressive weakness, mental deterioration, and occasionally seizures (which may occur when there are no discernible focal lesions). CT or MRI will show cerebral atrophy and hydrocephalus. The basal ganglia and periventricular white matter may be mineralized (siderocalcinosis). Necrotizing myelitis has also been observed in the spinal cord (Fig. 8.68).

CNS Lymphoma

Primary CNS lymphomas were rare before the AIDS era, and even in AIDS patients, lymphomatous involvement of the CNS may be metastatic. CNS lymphoma (usually B-cell, non-Hodgkin's type) is the most common cerebral neoplasm in AIDS, and the second most common mass lesion after toxoplasmo-

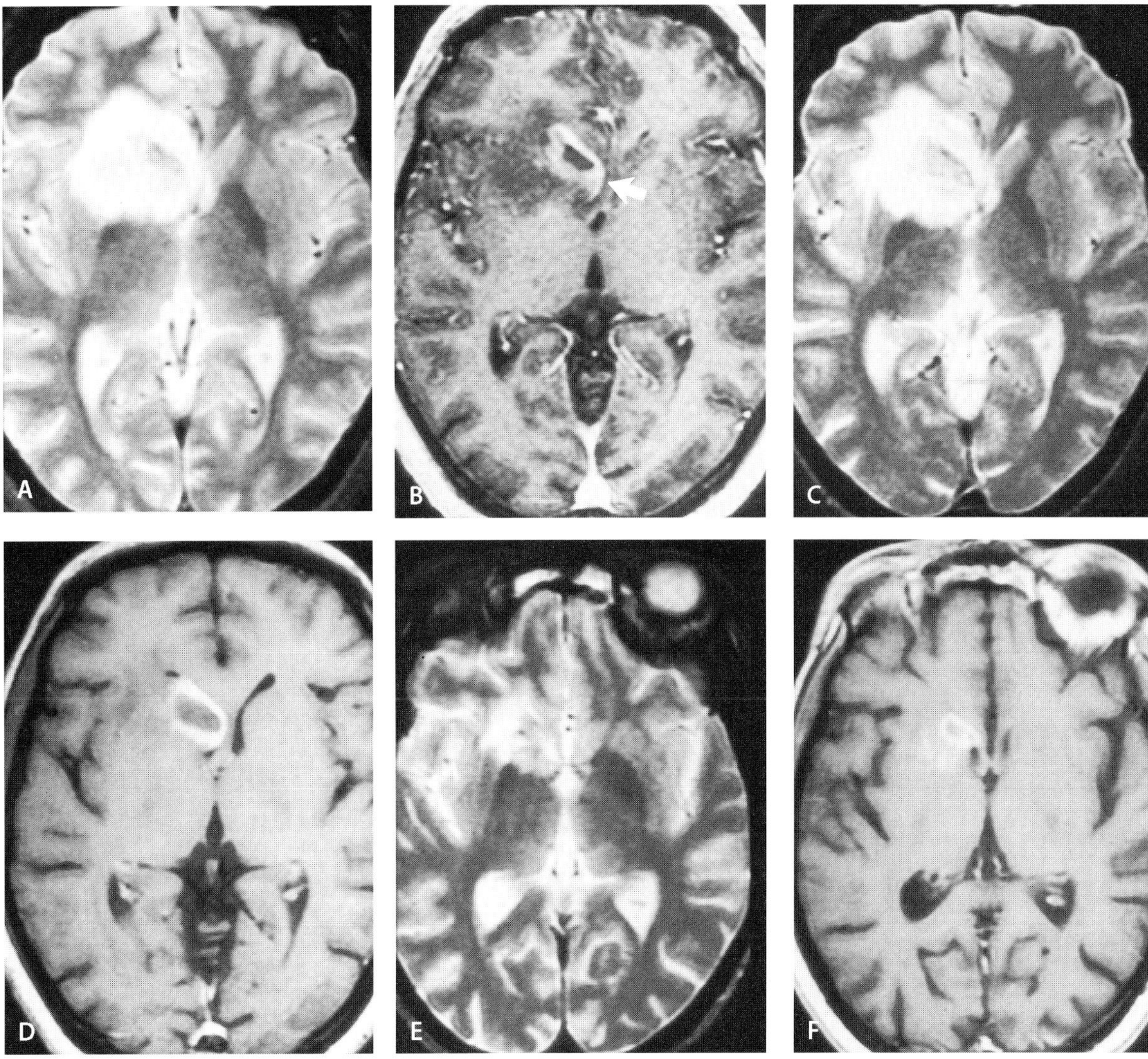

Fig. 8.69 A–F. Serial scans of a young male patient with AIDS suffering from seizures. The initial scans (**A**, **B**) show a hyperintense lesion centered in the right caudate on a T2-weighted image (**A**), with rim enhancement after administratio of gadolinium (**B**). The patient was treated presumptively for toxoplasmosis for 3 weeks and the lesion grew (**C**, **D**) on both T2-weighted (**C**) and enhanced (**D**) images. After these scans and the lack of response to toxoplasmosis therapy, the presumptive diagnosis was changed to lymphoma and radiation therapy was started. Three weeks later (**E**, **F**), the lesion is much smaller on both T2-weighted (**E**) and gadolinium-enhanced (**F**) images. This strategy averted a biopsy. In retrospect, the ependymal involvement seen on **B** (*arrow*) is very suggestive of lymphoma

sis. Lymphoma is more often a solitary lesion than toxoplasmosis, but since toxoplasmosis is far more common, a solitary toxoplasmoma should be in the differential diagnosis when a single lesion is identified. The presence of ependymal spread or major involvement of the corpus callosum favors lymphoma. AIDS lymphomas, unlike CNS lymphomas in the normal host, show ring enhancement rather than homogeneous enhancement on contrast-enhanced CT. This is thought to be due to their rapid growth because they are unchecked by normal immune mechanisms. AIDS lymphomas outgrow their blood supply and become centrally necrotic: hence the ring enhancement, because only the perimeter is viable. On MRI, the lesions are usually hypointense on T1-weighted sequences and iso- or hyperintense on T2-weighted sequences, and they may ring enhance with gadolinium injection (Fig. 8.69). The most common locations are in the periventricular white matter, the corpus callosum, and the basal ganglia. Subependymal spread may be seen when there is contrast enhancement around the ventricle involved. These features may help in the differentiation from toxoplasmosis. However, since CNS lym-

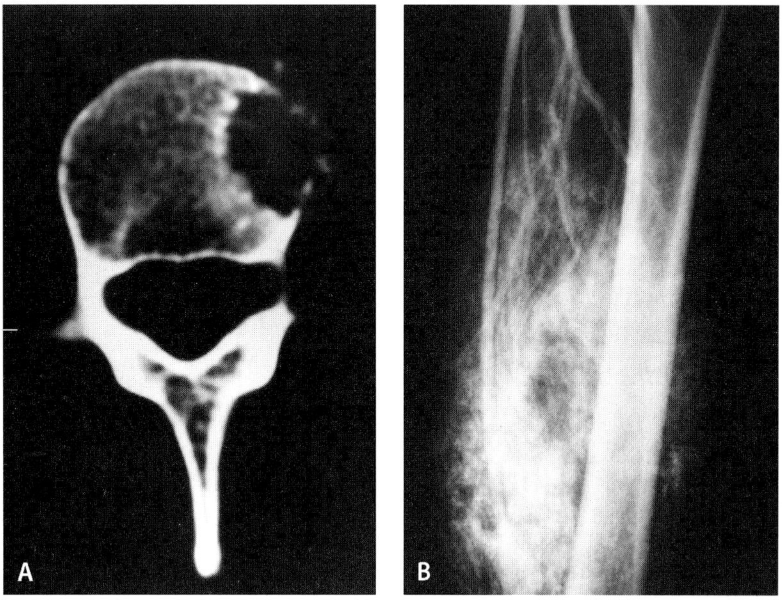

Fig. 8.70 A, B. Skeletal lesions in AIDS. **A** Bacillary angiomatosis causing a well-marginated lytic lesion in a vertebral body. (Courtesy of Dr. B. Herts and *AJR*, 1991) **B** A femoral arteriogram in another patient with marked contrast enhancement of a large mass in leg muscles. This was due to bacillary angiomatosis, confirmed by biopsy

phoma responds poorly to treatment, it is best to give the patient a trial of antibiotic therapy. There should be a recognizable response within 2–3 weeks if the lesion is due to toxoplasmosis.

Bones and Soft Tissues

Patients with AIDS may develop osteomyelitis caused by common organisms such as *Staphylococcus aureus* or *Mycobacterium tuberculosis*, or opportunistic organisms such as *Nocardia, Bartonella henselae*, or fungi: they give rise to soft tissue swelling, and later periostitis and lytic lesions develop in bone. Bacillary angiomatosis is another cause of lytic lesions (Fig. 8.70 A): muscle and soft tissues may also be involved, producing a soft tissue mass which enhances dramatically with contrast (Fig. 8.70 B). Similar lytic lesions of bone, with associated soft tissue abscesses, are also seen in disseminated coccidioidomycosis: in the spine the disc spaces often remain intact (Fig. 8.71). Skeletal tuberculous is a frequent complication (see Chap. 5).

Septic arthritis may be due to common bacteria or opportunistic fungi, but also may be due to the HIV, in which case there is characteristically a brief painful reaction involving primarily the knees and ankles. Patients with AIDS also have an increased incidence of the spondyloarthropathies such as Reiter's disease and psoriatic arthritis.

Pyomyositis, occasionally seen in the normal host in tropical regions, is common in AIDS. It characteristically presents with pain in a group of muscles, fever, and leukocytosis (see Chap. 30). Phlegmonous inflammation progresses to necrosis and abscess formation accompanied by septicemia. *Staphylococcus* is the most common organism (Fig. 8.72), but *Streptococcus, Mycobacteria, Nocardia*, and *Cryptococcus* are additional sources of muscle infections.

Non-Hodgkin's lymphoma may involve bones, particularly in children and often in the leg, causing permeative destruction. Kaposi's sarcoma involves bone less often, but may cause cortical destruction and periosteal reaction (see Chap. 42).

An early soft tissue manifestation of HIV infection, often the presenting symptom, is an AIDS-related parotid cyst (lymphoepithelial cysts). When associated with cervical lymphadenopathy, such cysts are extremely suggestive of HIV infection. They probably result from the systemic lymphoid infiltration which affects many organs and which involves periparotid and intraparotid nodes, resulting in obstruction of intranodal ducts (Fig. 8.74). In children the clinical appearance suggests chronic mumps.

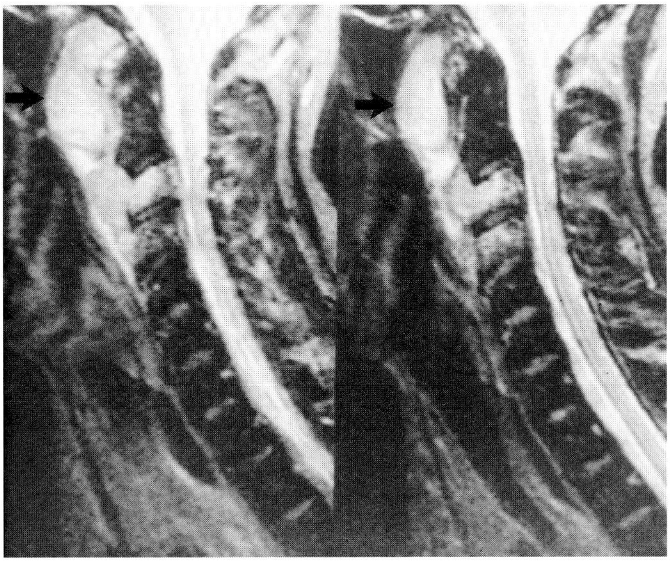

Fig. 8.71. Two scans of the cervical spine showing osteomyelitis of the C3 and C4 vertebral bodies: the disc spaces are spared, which is suggestive of coccidioidomycosis. There is a large prevertebral abscess (*arrow*; see Figs. 6.45, 6.46)

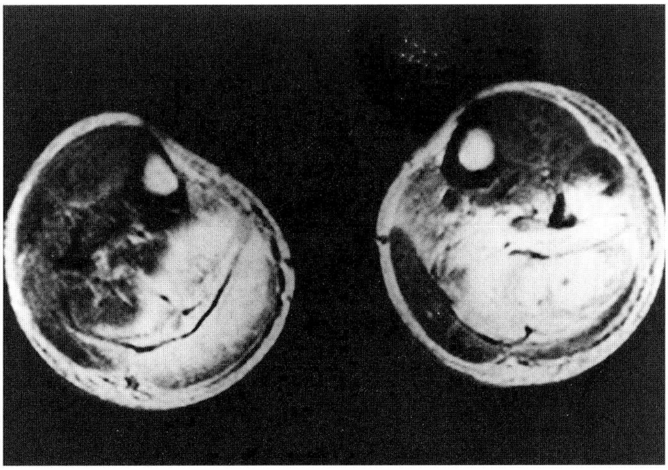

▲

Fig. 8.72. Edema and necrosis of muscle groups in the leg, due to staphylococcal pyomyositis. There is an increased signal on T2-weighted images. (From J. Tehranzadeh, in J.M. Taveras and J.T. Ferrucci, eds. *Musculoskeletal infection in the immunocompromised patients.* Philadelphia, New York, Lippincott-Raven, 1997)

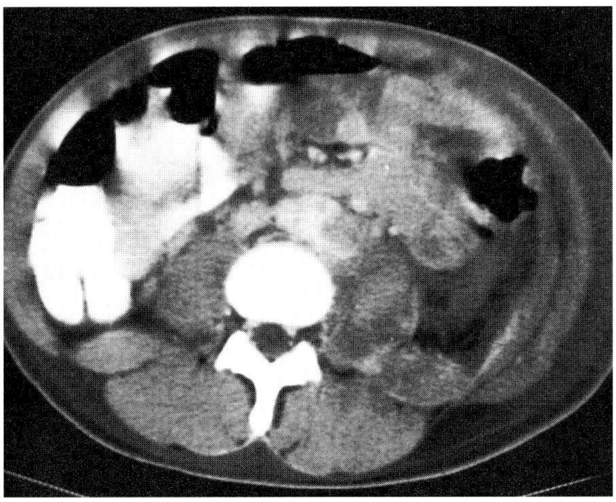

◀

Fig. 8.73. A contrast-enhanced scan. The vascular tumors of Kaposi's sarcoma will enhance after contrast injection, as in this patient with mottled enhancement of periaortic lymph nodes and the involved left psoas muscle

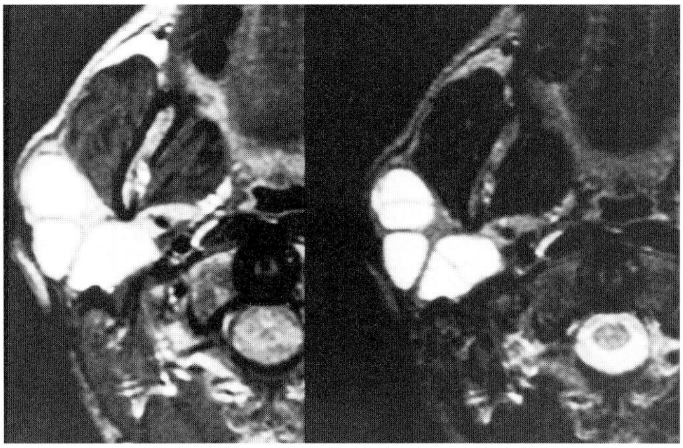

Fig. 8.74. The parotid glands are also affected by the lymphoproliferative process in AIDS, causing chronic swelling: proton density (*left*) and T2-weighted (*right*) axial MR images show multiple parotid cysts in this HIV-positive patient

Antiviral Treatment and Prophylaxis for Opportunistic Infections

The advent of multidrug antiviral therapy, simultaneously attacking different phases of viral replication, has had a profound effect on survival in those able to tolerate the regimen (1998). These drugs remain extremely costly and often cannot be afforded by patients in the developing world. Indeed, because of the assignment of limited available resources to patients with curable diseases, no treatment whatsoever may be offered to those with AIDS.

There has been increasing pressure on pharmaceutical patent holders to lower prices for AIDS drugs sold to the developing world. In March, 1998, Glaxo Wellcome announced a program to offer AZT at substantially reduced cost to pregnant women in developing countries. The proposed abbreviated course is expected to reduce maternal-fetal transmission by half in those receiving the drug, although efficient drug distribution remains a serious problem. More recently, a single maternal and a single newborn oral dose of Nevirapine®, costing very little, has been found to be even more effective. Possible longterm effects have yet to be assessed.

The potential for prophylaxis against opportunistic infections in the developing world faces similar financial limitations and distribution problems. It is interesting to note that the three most common causes of death in the West African autopsy study of HIV-positive patients from Lucas and colleagues were tuberculosis, bacterial sepsis, and cerebral toxoplasmosis. All these conditions can be prevented or treated. Possible prophylactic measures include isoniazid for tuberculosis, trimethoprim-sulfamethoxazole for toxoplasmosis and bacterial infections (and *Pneumocystis carinii*, though uncommon), and 23-valent pneumococcal vaccine for *Streptococcus pneumoniae*. If resources are available, prophylactic measures can be tailored to local risk.

Summary

Because few patients in the tropics with AIDS survive to reach truly profound levels of immunosuppression, the spectrum of opportunistic infections and malignancies varies greatly and differs from that encountered in the developed world. Each geographic location has its own endemic diseases which the patients may already harbor prior to developing AIDS, or may contract after developing AIDS. When assessing imaging findings, geographic, social, and microbiological issues must also be considered in forming an appropriate differential diagnosis. The recent explosion in quality epidemiological and clinical research in the tropics will continue to add key information to this developing field. Whether it will match the huge explosion of HIV and AIDS remains to be seen.

Bibliography

Abouya YL, Beaumel A, Lucas S, et al: *Pneumocystis carinii* pneumonia. *Am Rev Respir Dis* 145:617–620, 1992

Aisu TO, Eriki PP, Morissey AB, et al: Nocardiosis mimicking pulmonary tuberculosis in Ugandan AIDS patients. *Chest* 100:888, 1991

Akhras F, et al: Emerging patterns of heart disease in HIV infected homosexuals: a prospective colour flow Doppler echocardiographic study. *Eur Heart J* 15:68–75, 1994

Allen CM, Craze J, Grundy A: Case report: tuberculous bronchooesophageal fistula in the acquired immunodeficiency syndrome. *Clin Radiol* 43:60–62, 1991

Alteri PI, Clement C, Lazala G, et al: Opportunistic invasion of the heart in Hispanic patients with acquired immunodeficiency syndrome. *Am J Trop Med Hyg* 51:56–59, 1994

Ambrosino MM, Roche KJ, Geiesser NB, et al: Application of thin-section low-dose chest CT (TSCT) in the management of pediatric AIDS. *Pediatr Radiol* 25:393–400, 1995

Amdahl BM, Rubins JB, Daley CL, et al: Impaired natural immunity to pneumolysin during human immunodeficiency virus infection in the United States and Africa. *Am J Respir Crit Care Med* 52:2000–2004, 1995

Amin Z, Miller RF, Shaw PJ: Lobar or segmental consolidation on chest radiographs of patients with HIV infection. *Clin Radiol* 52:541–545, 1997

Ampel NM: Emerging disease issues and fungal pathogens associated with HIV infection. *Emerging Infect Dis* 2:109–116, 1996

Amundson DE, Murray KM, Brodine S, et al: High-dose corticosteroid therapy for *Pneumocystis carinii* pneumonia in patients with aquired immunodeficiency syndrome. *South Med J* 83:711–714, 1989

Ananthasubramanian M, Ananthan S, Vennila R, et al: *Cryptosporidium* in AIDS patients in south India: a laboratory investigation. *J Common Dis* 29:29–33, 1997

Anderson M: Gastroenterological aspects of AIDS in the third world. *Baillieres Clin Gastroenterol* 4:375–383, 1990

Andreula CF, Burdi N, Carell A: CNS cryptococcosis in AIDS: spectrum of MR findings. *J Comput Assist Tomogr* 17:438–441, 1993

Arabi Y, Fairfax MR, Szubi MJ, et al: Adrenal insufficiency, recurrent bacteremia, and disseminated abscesses caused by *Nocardia asteroides* in a patient with acquired immunodeficiency syndrome. *Diagn Microbiol Infect Dis* 24:47–51, 1996

Asiimwe-Okiror G et al: Changes in sexual behaviour and decline in HIV infection among young pregnant women in urban Uganda. *AIDS* 11(14):1757–63, 1997

Atzori C, Bruno A, Chichino G, et al: HIV-1 and parasitic infections in rural Tanzania. *Ann Trop Med Parasitol* 87:585–593, 1993

Balakrishman J, Becker PS, Kumar AJ, et al: Acquired immunodeficiency syndrome: correlation of radiologic and pathologic findings in the brain. *Radiographics* 10:201–215, 1990

Balthazar EJ, Megibow AJ, Barry M, et al: Histoplasmosis of the colon in patients with AIDS: imaging findings in four cases. *AJR* 161:585–587, 1993

Baron A, Steinbach L, LeBoit P, et al: Osteolytic lesions and bacillary angiomatosis in HIV infection: radiologic differentiation from AIDS-related Kaposi's sarcoma. *Radiology* 177:77–81, 1990

Barretto JA, Palaci M, Ferrazoli L, et al: Isolation of *Mycobacterium avium* complex from bone marrow aspirates of AIDS patients in Brazil. *J Infect Dis* 168:777–779, 1993

Barrio JL, Suarez M, Rodriguez JL, et al: *Pneumocystis carinii* pneumonia presenting as cavitating and noncavitating solitary pulmonary nodules in patients with the acquired immunodeficiency syndrome. *Am Rev Respir Dis* 134:1094–1096, 1986

Bartholomew C, Cleghorn F: Retroviruses in the Caribbean. *PAHO Bull* 23:76–80, 1989

Batungwanayo J, Taelman H, Dhote R, et al: Pulmonary tuberculosis in Kigali, Rwanda. *Am Rev Respir Dis* 146:53–56, 1992

Batungwanayo J, Taelman H, Bogaerts J, et al: Pulmonary cryptococcosis associated with HIV-1 infection in Rwanda: a retrospective study of 37 cases. *AIDS* 8:1271–1276, 1994

Batungwanayo J, Taelman H, Lucas S, et al: Pulmonary disease associated with the human immunodeficiency virus in Kigali, Rwanda. A fiberoptic bronchoscopic study of 111 cases of undetermined etiology. *Am J Respir Crit Care Med* 149:1591–1596, 1994

Beach RS, Mantero-Athenza E, Fordyce-Baum, et al: HIV infection in Brazil. *N Engl J Med* 321:830–832, 1989

Beale TJ, Wetton CW, Crofton ME: A sonographic-pathological correlation of liver biopsies in patients with the acquired immune deficiency syndrome (AIDS). *Clin Radiol* 50:761–764, 1995

Bem C: Human immunodeficiency virus-positive tuberculous lymphadenitis in Central Africa: clinical presentation of 157 cases. *Int J Tuberc Lung Dis* 1:215–219, 1997

Benator DA, French AL, Beaudet LM, et al: *Isospora belli* infection associated with acalculous cholecystitis in a patient with AIDS. *Ann Intern Med* 121:663–664, 1994

Benhamou Y, et al: AIDS related cholangiopathy. Critical analysis of a prospective series of 26 patients. *Dig Dis Sci* 38:1113–1118, 1993

Benson ML, Laine FJ: Brain imaging in AIDS. *South Med J* 88:331–337, 1995

Berer M: Reducing perinatal HIV transmission in developing countries. *Bull WHO* 77, 11:871–879, 1999

Bergemann A, Karstaedt AS: The spectrum of meningitis in a population with high prevalence of HIV disease. *Q J Med* 89:499–504, 1996

Berkley S: AIDS in the developing world: an epidemiologic overview. *Clin Infect Dis* 17:s 329–s 336, 1993

Berman A, Espinoza L, Diaz J, et al: Rheumatic manifestations of human immunodeficiency virus infection. *Am J Med* 85:59–64, 1988

Bhoopat L, Thamprasert K, Chaiwun B, et al: Histopathologic spectrum of AIDS-associated lesions in Maharaj Nakorn Chiang Mai Hospital. *Asian Pac J Allergy Immunol* 12:95–104, 1994

Bini EJ, Weinshel EH, et al: Endoscopic evaluation of chronic human immunodeficiency virus-related diarrhea: is colonoscopy superior to flexible sigmoidoscopy? *Am J Gastroenterol* 93:56–60, 1998

Blumberg H, Stephens D: Pyomyositis and human immunodeficiency virus infection. *South Med J* 83:1092–1095, 1990

Bobat R, Moodley D, Coutsoudis A, et al: Breastfeeding by HIV-1-infected women and outcome in their infants: a cohort study from Durban, South Africa. *AIDS* 11:1627–1633, 1997

Borisch-Chappuis B, Nezelof C, Muller H, et al: Rapid communication. Different Epstein-Barr virus expression in lymphomas from immunocompromised and immunocompetent patients. *AJR* 136:751–758, 1990

Borradori L, Schmit JC, Stetzkowski M, et al: *Penicillium marneffei* infection in AIDS. *J Am Acad Dermatol* 31:843–846, 1994

Brancato L, Itescu S, Winchester R: Reiter's syndrome and related rheumatic conditions in HIV infection. *J Musculoskeletal Med* 15:32, 1989

Brody AM, et al: Gastric tuberculosis: a manifestation of acquired immunodeficiency syndrome. *Radiology* 159:347–348, 1986

Bronnimann DA, Adam RD, Galgiani JN, et al: Coccidioidomycosis in the acquired immunodeficiency syndrome. *Ann Intern Med* 106:372–379, 1987

Buckley JA, Padhani AR, Kuhlman JE: CT features of pulmonary nocardiosis. *J Comput Assist Tomogr* 19:726–732, 1995

Buonaguro FM, Tornesello ML, Beth-Giraldo E, et al: Herpesvirus-like DNA sequences detected in endemic, classic, iatrogenic and epidemic Kaposi's sarcoma (KS) biopsies. *Int J Cancer* 65:25–28, 1996

Calabrese L: The rheumatic manifestations of infection with human immunodeficiency virus. *Semin Arthritis Rheum* 18:225–239, 1989

Cantwell MF, Binkin NJ: Tuberculosis in sub-Saharan Africa: a regional assessment of the impact of the human immunodeficiency virus and National Tuberculosis Control Program quality. *Tuber Lung Dis* 77:220–225, 1996

Cantwell MF, Binkin NJ: Impact of HIV on tuberculosis in sub-Saharan Africa: a regional perspective. *Int J Tuber Lung Dis* 1:205–214, 1997

Casado JL, Navas E, Frutos B, et al: *Salmonella* lung involvement in patients with HIV infection. *Chest* 112:1197–1201, 1997

Castro KG, Lieb S, Jaffe HW, et al: Transmission of HIV in Belle Glade, Florida: lessons for other communities in the United States. *Science* 239:193–197, 1988

Cegielski JP, Ramaiya K, Lallinger GJ, et al: Pericardial disease and human immunodeficiency virus in Dar es Salaam, Tanzania. *Lancet* 335:209–212, 1990

Chacin-Bonilla L, Guanipa N, Cano G, et al: Cryptosporidiosis among patients with acquired immunodeficiency syndrome in Zulia State, Venezuela. *Am J Trop Med Hyg* 47:582–586, 1992

Chacko S, John TJ, Babu PG, et al: Clinical profile of AIDS in India: a review of 61 cases, *J Assoc Physicians India* 43:535–538, 1995

Chang L, Miller BL, McBride D, et al: Brain lesions in patients with AIDS: H-1 MR spectroscopy. *Radiology* 197:525–531, 1995

Chang Y, Cesarman EP, Lee F, et al: Identification of herpesvirus-like DNA sequences in AIDS-associated Kaposi's sarcoma. *Science* 266:1865–1869, 1994

Chariyalertsak S, Sirisanthana T, Supparatpinyo K, et al: Seasonal variation of disseminated *Penicillium marneffei* infections in northern Thailand: a clue to the reservoir? *J Infect Dis* 173:1490–1493, 1996

Chattopadhya D, Aggarwal RK, Kumari S: Further evaluation of alternative strategy for HIV testing in India. *J Commun Dis* 28:158–162, 1996

Chechani V, Allam AA, Smith PR, et al: Bronchitis mimicking opportunistic lung infection in patients with human immunodeficiency virus infection/AIDS. *N Y State J Med* 92:297–300, 1992

Chikwem JO, Mohammed I, Okara GC, et al: Prevalence of transmissible blood infections among blood donors at the University of Maiduguri Teaching Hospital, Maiduguri, Nigeria. *East Afr Med J* 74:213–216, 1997

Chinn RJ, Wilkinson ID, Hall-Craggs MA, et al: Toxoplasmosis and primary central nervous system lymphoma in HIV infection: diagnosis with MR spectroscopy. *Radiology* 197:649–654, 1995

Chintu C, Athale UH, Patil PS: Childhood cancers in Zambia before and after the HIV epidemic. *Arch Dis Child* 73:100–105, 1995

Chui DW, Owen RL: AIDS and the gut. *J Gastroenterol Hepatol* 9:291–303, 1994

Clarkston WK, Bonacini M, Peterson I: Colitis due to *Histoplasma capsulatum* in the acquired immune deficiency syndrome. *Am J Gastroenterol* 86:913–916, 1991

Cohen WA: Intracranial bacterial infections in patients with AIDS. *Neuroimaging Clin North Am* 7:223–229, 1997

Colebunders RL, Ryder RW, Nzilambi N, et al: HIV infection in patients with tuberculosis in Kinshasa, Zaire, *Am Rev Respir Dis* 139:1082–1085, 1989

Collins CD, Blanshard C, Gleeson JA, et al: Cytomegalovirus colitis in AIDS: plain abdominal radiograph findings. *Clin Radiol* 48:127–130, 1993

Conces Jr. DJ, Tarver RD: Noninfectious and nonmalignant pulmonary disease in AIDS. *J Thorac Imaging* 6:53–59, 1991

Conlon CP, et al: HIV related enteropathy in Zambia. A clinical microbiological and histological study. *Am J Trop Med Hyg* 42:83–88, 1990

Cooper CR Jr., McGinnis MR: Pathology of *Penicillium marneffei*. An emerging acquired immunodeficiency syndrome-related pathogen. *Arch Pathol Lab Med* 121:798–804, 1997

Coplan NL, Shimony RY, Ioachim HL, et al: Primary pulmonary hypertension associated with human immunodeficiency viral infection. *Am J med* 89:96–99, 1990

Corboy JR, Fink L, Miller WT: Congestive cardiomyopathy in association with AIDS. *Radiology* 165:139–141, 1987

Cortes E, Detels R, Aboulafia D, et al: HIV-1, HIV-2, and HTLV-1 infection in high-risk groups in Brazil. *N Engl J Med* 320:953–958, 1989

Daley CL: Pyogenic bacterial pneumonia in the acquired immunodeficiency syndrome. *J Thorac Imaging* 6:36–42, 1991

Dallabetta G, Mitotti P: Chronic diarrhoea in AIDS patients in the tropics: a review. *Trop Doct* 22:3–9, 1992

Da Silva F, Boudghene F, Lecomte I, et al: Sonography in AIDS-related cholangitis: prevalence and cause of an echogenic nodule in the distal end of the common bile duct. *AJR* 160:1205–1207, 1993

Davachi F, Ngoie K, Ndoko K, et al: Pediatric AIDS and associated cancers in Kinshasa, Zaire. *Antibiot Chemother* 43:140–149, 1991

Davenport C, Dillon WP, Sze G: Neuroradiology of the immunosuppressed state. *Radiol Clin North Am* 30:611–637, 1992

Davies P, Stein M, Latif A, et al: Acute arthritis in Zimbabwean patients: possible relationship to human immunodeficiency virus infection. *J Rheumatol* 16:346–348, 1989

DeCastro S, et al: Heart involvement in AIDS: a prospective study during various stages of the disease. *Eur Heart J* 13:1452–1459, 1992

De Cock KM, Barrere B, Diaby L, et al: AIDS – the leading cause of adult death in the West African city of Abidjan, Ivory Coast. *Science* 249:793–796, 1990

De Cock KM, Selik RM, Soro B: AIDS surveillance in Africa; a reappraisal of case definitions. *BMJ* 303:1185–1188, 1991

De Cock KM, Soro B, Coulibaly IM: Tuberculosis and HIV infection in sub-Saharan Africa. *JAMA* 268:1581–1587, 1992

De Cock KM, Lucas SB, Lucas S, et al: Clinical research, prophylaxis, therapy, and care for HIV disease in Africa. *Am J Public Health* 83:1385–1389, 1993

Defalgue D, et al: Sonographic diagnosis of cholangitis in AIDS patients. *Gastrointest Radiol* 14:143–147, 1989

Dehne KL: Herpes zoster as an indicator of HIV infection in Africa. *Trop Doct* 11:68–74, 1992

De Lorenzo LJ, Huang CT, Maguire GP, et al: Roentgenographic patterns of *pneumocystis carinii* pneumonia in 104 patients with AIDS. *Chest* 91:323–326, 1987

Denning DW, Follansbee SE, Scolaro M, et al: Pulmonary aspergillosis in the acquired immunodeficiency syndrome. *N Engl J Med* 324:654–662, 1991

Desai GA, Mugala DD: Management of empyema thoracis at Lusaka, Zambia. *Br J Surg* 79:537–538, 1992

Deschamps MM, Pape JW, Desvarieux M: A prospective study of HIV-seropositive asymptomatic women of childbearing age in a developing country. *J Acquir Immune Defic Syndr* 6:446–451, 1993

Dina TS: Primary central nervous system lymphoma versus toxoplasmosis in AIDS. *Radiology* 179:823–828, 1991

Donovan B, Bek MD, Pethebridge AM, et al: Heterosexual gonorrhoea in central Sydney: implications for HIV control. *Med J Aust* 154:175–180, 1991

Doumbo O, Rossignol JF, Pichard E, et al: Nitazoxanide in the treatment of cryptosporidial diarrhea and other intestinal parasitic infections associated with acquired immunodeficiency syndrome in tropical Africa. Am J Trop Med Hyg 56:637–639, 1997

Drew WL: Cytomegalovirus infection in patients with AIDS. *J Infect Dis* 158:449–456, 1988

Duong TA: Infection due to *Penicillium marneffei*, an emerging pathogen: review of 155 reported cases. *Clin Infect Dis* 23:125–130, 1996

Eisner MD, Kaplan LD, Herndier B, et al: The pulmonary manifestations of AIDS-related non-Hodgkin's lymphoma. *Chest* 110:729–736, 1996

Elswood BF, Stricker RB: Polio vaccines and the origin of AIDS [see comments]. *Med Hypotheses* 42:347–354, 1994

Elvin KM, Lumbwe CM, Luo NP: *Pneumocystis carinii* is not a major cause of pneumonia in HIV infected patients in Lusaka, Zambia. *Trans R Soc Trop Med Hyg* 83:553–555, 1989

Emmons W, Reichwein B, Winslow DL: *Rhodococcus equi* infection in the patient with AIDS: literature review and report of an unusual case. *Rev Infect Dis* 13:91–96, 1991

Engelbrecht S, Treurnicht FK, Schneider JW, et al: Detection of human herpes virus 8 DNA and sequence polymorphism in classical, epidemic, and iatrogenic Kaposi's sarcoma in South Africa. *J Med Virol* 52:168–172, 1997

Esfandiari A, Jordan WC, Brown CP: Prevalence of enteric parasitic infection among HIV-infected attendees of an inner city AIDS clinic. *Cell Mol Biol* 41:S 19–S 23, 1995

Esfandiari A, Swartz J, Teklehaimanot S: Clustering of giardiosis among AIDS patients in Los Angeles County. *Cell Mol Biol* 43:1077–1083, 1997

Falcone S, Murphy BJ, Weinfeld A: Gastric manifestations of AIDS: radiographic findings on upper gastrointestinal examination. *Gastrointest Radiol* 16:95–98, 1991

Falguera M, Nogues A, Ruiz-Gonzalez A, et al: Transthoracic needle aspiration in the study of pulmonary infections in patients with HIV. *Chest* 106:697–702, 1994

Farthing MJ, Kelly MP, Veitch AM: Recently recognised microbial enteropathies and HIV infection. *J Antimicrob Chemother* 37:61–70, 1996

Field AS, Hing MC, Miliken ST, et al: Microsporidia in the small intestine of HIV-infected patients. *Med J Aust* 158:390–394, 1993

Fink L, Reichek N, St. John Sutton MG: Cardiac abnormalities in acquired immune deficiency syndrome. *Am J Cardiol* 54:1161–1163, 1984

Fish DN, Danziger LH: Neglected pathogens: bacterial infections in persons with human immunodeficiency virus infection. A review of the literature (1). *Pharmacotherapy* 13:415–439, 1993

Fleming AF: Opportunistic infections in AIDS in developed and developing countries. *Trans R Soc Trop Med Hyg* 84:1–6, 1990

Fleming AF: HIV and blood transfusion in sub-Saharan Africa. *Transfus Sci* 18:167–179, 1997

Foltzer MA, Guiney WB, Wager GC, et al: Bronchopulmonary bacillary agiomatosis. *Chest* 104:973–975, 1993

Frager DH, et al: Gastrointestinal complications of AIDS: radiologic features. *Radiology* 158:597–603, 1986

French AL, Beaudet LM, Benator DA, et al: Cholecystectomy in patients with AIDS: clinicopathologic correlations in 107 cases. *Clin Infect Dis* 21:852–858, 1995

Friedman SL: Kaposi's sarcoma and lymphoma of the gut in AIDS. *Baillieres Clin Gastroenterol* 4:455–475, 1990

Friedman EP, Miller RF, Severn A, et al: Cryptococcal pneumonia in patients with the acquired immunodeficiency syndrome. *Clin Radiol* 50:756–760, 1995

Friedman-Kien AE, Saltzman BR: Clinical manifestations of classical, endemic African, and epidemic AIDS-associated Kaposi's sarcoma. *J Am Acad Dermatol* 22:1237–1250, 1990

Gallant JE, Somani J, Chaisson RE, et al: Diagnostic accuracy of three clinical case definitions for advanced HIV disease. *AIDS* 6:295–299, 1992

Gilks CF: What use is a clinical case definition for AIDS in Africa? *BMJ* 303:1189, 1991

Gilks CF: Prophylaxis for HIV-associated infections in the developing world. *J Antimicrob Chemother* 31:119–128, 1993

Gilks CF, Ojoo SA, Ojoo JC, et al: Invasive pneumococcal disease in a cohort of predominantly HIV-1 infected female sex-workers in Nairobi, Kenya [see comments]. *Lancet* 347:718–723, 1996

Giri TK, Pande I, Mishra NM, et al: Spectrum of clinical and laboratory characteristics of HIV infection in northern India. *J Commun Dis*n 27:131–141, 1995

Gnaore E, Sassan-Morokro M, Kassim S, et al: A comparison of clinical features in tuberculosis associated with infection with human immunodeficiency viruses 1 and 2. *Trans R Soc Trop Med Hyg* 87:57–59, 1993

Goldstein JD, Zeifer B, Chao C, et al: CT appearance of primary CNS lymphoma in patients with acquired immunodeficiency syndrome. *J Comput Assist Tomogr* 15:39–44, 1991

Gomez Morales MA, Atzori C, Ludovisi A, et al: Opportunistic and non-opportunistic parasites in HIV-positive and negative patients with diarrhoea in Tanzania. *Trop Med Parasitol* 46:109–114, 1995

Goodman PC: Pulmonary tuberculosis in patients with acquired immunodeficiency syndrome. *J Thorac Imaging* 5:38–45, 1990

Goodman PC: Non-Hodgkin's lymphoma in the acquired immunodeficiency syndrome. *J Thorac Imaging* 6:49–52, 1991

Goodman PC, Schnapp LM: Pulmonary toxoplasmosis in AIDS. *Radiology* 184:791–793, 1992

Gotuzzo E, Frisancho O, Sanchez J, et al: Association between the acquired immunodeficiency syndrome and infection with *Salmonella typhi* or *Salmonella paratyphi* in an endemic typhoid area. *Arch Intern Med* 151:381–382, 1991

Gotuzzo E, Escamilla J, Phillips IA, et al: The impact of human T-lymphotrophic virus type I/II infection on the prognosis of sexually acquired cases of acquired immunodeficiency syndrome. *Arch Intern Med* 152:1429–1432, 1992

Graham BD, McKinsey DS, Driks MR, et al: Colonic histoplasmosis in acquired immunodeficiency syndrome. *Dis Colon Rectum* 34:185–190, 1991

Greco MA, Zagzag D: Human immunodeficiency virus infection lesions in the pediatric AIDS group. In: Connor DH, (ed.) *The pathology of infectious diseases.* Appleton and Lange, Stamford 1997, pp 169–181

Greenberg AE, NSA W, Ryder RW, et al: *Plasmodium falciparum* malaria and perinatally acquired human immunodeficiency virus type 1 infection in Kinshasa, Zaire. *N Engl J Med* 325:105–109, 1991

Greenblatt RM, Lukehart SA, Plummer FA, et al: Genital ulceration as a risk factor for human immunodeficiency virus infection. *AIDS* 2:47–50, 1988

Greyson-Fleg RT: Computed tomography findings in gastrointestinal involvement by opportunistic organisms in acquired immunodeficiency syndrome. *J Comput Assist Tomogr* 10:175–181, 1986

Gupta RK, Jena A, Sharma A, et al: MR imaging of intracranial tuberculomas. *J Comput Assist Tomogr* 12:280–285, 1988

Haller JO, Cohen HL: Gastrointestinal manifestations of AIDS in children (review). *AJR* 162:387–393, 1994

Hansman Whiteman ML, Post MJ, Berger JR, et al: Progressive multifocal leukoencephalopathy in 47 HIV-seropositive patients: neuroimaging with clinical and pathologic correlation. *Radiology* 187:233–240, 1993

Haramati LB, et al: The effect of HIV status on chest radiographic and CT findings in patients with tuberculosis. *Clin Radiol* 52:31–35, 1997

Harries AD: Tuberculosis and human immunodeficiency virus infection in developing countries. *Lancet* 335:387–390, 1990

Hartman TE, Primack SL, Muller NL, et al: Diagnosis of thoracic complications in AIDS: accuracy of CT. *AJR* 162:547–553, 1994

Herskowitz A, et al: Myocarditis and cardiotropic viral infection associated with severe left ventricular dysfunction in late stage infection with human immunodeficiency virus. *J Am Coll Cardiol* 24:1025–1032, 1994

Herts BR, Rafii M, Spiegel G: Soft tissue and osseous lesions caused by bacillary angiomatosis: unusual manifestations of cat-scratch fever in patients with AIDS. *AJR* 157:1249–1251, 1991

Hinnant K, et al: Cytomegaloviral and cryptosporidial cholecystitis in two patients with AIDS. *Am J Surg Pathol* 13:57–60, 1989

Hira SK, Ngandu N, Wadhawan D, et al: Clinical and epidemiological features of HIV infection at a referral clinic in Zambia. *J Acquir Immune Defic Syndr* 3:87–91, 1990

Hopewell PC, Luce JM: Pulmonary involvement in the acquired immunodeficiency syndrome. *Chest* 87:104–112, 1985

Hrdy DB: Cultural practices contributing to the transmission of human immunodeficiency virus in Africa. *Rev Infect Dis* 9:1109–1119, 1987

Hudson CP: *Pneumocystis carinii* pneumonia in Africa [letter; comment]. *Lancet* 347:126, 1996

Hughes A, Corrah T: Human immunodeficiency virus type 2 (HIV2). *Blood Rev* 4:158–164, 1990

Hulnick DH, Megibow AJ, Naidich DP, et al: Abdominal tuberculosis: CT evaluation. *Radiology* 157:199–204, 1985

Hunter G, Bagshawe AF, Baboo KS, et al: Intestinal parasites in Zambian patients with AIDS. *Trans R Soc Trop Med Hyg* 86:543–545, 1992

Hutto C, Parks WP, Lai S: A hospital-based prospective study of perinatal infection with human immunodeficiency virus type 1. *J Pediatr* 118:347–353, 1991

Ioachim HL, Adsay V, Giancotti FR, et al: Kaposi's sarcoma of internal organs. A multiparameter study of 86 cases. *Cancer* 75:1376–1385, 1995

Jablonowski H, Fatkenheuer G, Youle M, et al: Ancillary benefits of *Mycobacterium avium-intracellulare* complex prophylaxis with clarithromycin in HIV-infected patients. *Drugs* 54:16–22; discussion 28–29, 1997

Jacobs P: The malignant lymphomas in Africa. *Hematol Oncol Clin North Am* 5:953–983, 1991

Janeke JB: The ABC (anchored bone conduction) system [letter]. *S Afr Med J* 85:1199–1200, 1995

Jeena PM, Coovadia HM, Chrystal V: *Pneumocystis carinii* and cytomegalovirus infections in severely ill, HIV-infected African infants. *Ann Trop Paediatr* 16:361–368, 1996

Jensen MC, Brant-Zawadzki M: MR imaging of the brain in patients with AIDS. Value of the routine use of iv gadopentetate dimeglumine. *AJR* 160:153–157, 1993

John TJ, Babu PG, Saraswathi NK, et al: The epidemiology of AIDS in the Vellore region, Southern India. *AIDS* 7:421–424, 1993

Kalyesubula I, Musoke-Mudido P, Marum L, et al: Effects of malaria infection in human immunodeficiency virus type 1-infected Ugandan children. *Pediatr Infect Dis J* 16:876–881, 1997

Kanki PJ, Travers KU, Mboup S, et al: Slower heterosexual spread of HIV-2 than HIV-1. *Lancet* 343:943–946, 1994

Kapiga SH, Lwihula GK, Shao JF, et al: Predictors of AIDS knowledge, condom use and high-risk sexual behaviour among women in Dar-es-Salaam, Tanzania. *Int J STD AIDS* 6:175–183, 1995

Kaplan JE, Hu DJ, Holmes KK, et al: Preventing opportunistic infections in human immunodeficiency virus-infected persons: implications for the developing world. *Am J Trop Med Hyg* 55:1–11, 1996

Katz DA, Berger JR, Duncan RC: Neurosyphilis: a comparative study of the effects of infection with human immunodeficiency virus. *Arch Neurol* 50:243–249, 1993

Katzenstein DA, Latif AS, Grace SA, et al: Clinical and laboratory characteristics of HIV-1 infection in Zimbabwe. *J Acquir Immune Defic Syndr* 3:701–707, 1990

Kelly MP: Clinical manifestations of African AIDS. *Br J Hosp Med* 48:734–741, 1992

Kelly PJ, Matthewman LA, Hayter D, et al: *Bartonella (Rochalimaea) henselae* in southern Africa – evidence for infections in domestic cats and implications for veterinarians. *J S Afr Vet Assoc* 67:182–187, 1996

Kelly P, Baboo KS, Wolff M, et al: The prevalence and aetiology of persistent diarrhoea in adults in urban Zambia. *Acta Trop* 61:183–190, 1996

Khalil AM, et al: Magnetic resonance imaging findings in pulmonary Kaposi's sarcoma. A series of ten cases. *Eur Respir J* 7:1285–1289, 1994

Khanna N, Chandramuki A, Desai A, et al: Cryptococcal infections of the central nervous system: an analysis of predisposing factors, laboratory findings and outcome in patients from South India with special reference to HIV infection. *J Med Microbiol* 45:376–379, 1996

Khumalo-Ngwenya B, Luo NP, Chintu C, et al: Gut parasites in HIV-seropositive Zambian adults with diarrhoea. *East Afr Med J* 71:379–383, 1994

Kirchner JT: Opportunistic fungal infections in patients with HIV disease. *Postgrad Med J* 99:209–216, 1996

Kok I, Veenstra J, Rietra PJ, et al: Disseminated *Penicillium marneffei* infection as an imported disease in HIV-1 infected patients. Description of two cases and a review of the literature. *Neth J Med* 44:18–22, 1994

Kool HEJ, et al: HIV seropositivity and tuberculosis in a large general hospital in Malawi. *Trop Geogr Med* 36:128–132, 1990

Kramer MR, Uttanchandani RB: The radiographic appearance of pulmonary nocardiosis associated with AIDS. *Chest* 98:382–385, 1990

Kramer MR, Gregg PA, Goldstein M: Disseminated strongyloidiasis in AIDS and non-AIDS immunocompromised hosts: diagnosis by sputum and bronchoalveolar lavage. *South Med J* 83:1226–1229, 1990

Kreiss JK, Castro KG: Special considerations for managing suspected human immunodeficiency virus infection and AIDS in patients from developing countries. *J Infect Dis* 162:955–960, 1990

Kuhlman JE, Kavuru M, Fishman EK, et al: *Pneumocystis carinii* pneumonia: spectrum of parenchymal CT findings. *Radiology* 175:711–714, 1990

Kumar RM, Uduman SA, Khurranna AK: A prospective study of mother-to-infant HIV transmission in tribal women from India. *J Acquir Immune Defic Syndr Hum Retrovirol* 9:238–242, 1995

Kumar RM, Uduman SA, Khurranna AK: Impact of maternal HIV-1 infection on perinatal outcome. *Int J Gynaecol Obstet* 49:137–143, 1995

Kumar A, Mehra M, Badhan SK, et al: Heterosexual behaviour and condom usage in an urban population of Delhi, India. *AIDS Care* 9:311–318, 1997

Kumar RM, Uduman SA, Khurrana AK: Impact of pregnancy on maternal AIDS. *J Reprod Med* 42:429–434, 1997

Kupfer MC, et al: MRI evaluation of AIDS-related encephalopathy: toxoplasmosis vs. lymphoma. *Magn Reson Imaging* 8:51–57, 1990

Lanjewar DN, Anand BS, Genta R, et al: Major differences in the spectrum of gastrointestinal infections associated with AIDS in India versus the west: an autopsy study. *Clin Infect Dis* 23:482–485, 1996

Lawn SD, et al: Pulmonary tuberculosis: radiological features in West Africans coinfected with HIV. *Br J Radiol* 72:339–344, 1999

LeBlang SD, Whiteman ML, Post MJ, et al: CNS *Nocardia* in AIDS patients: CT and MRI with pathologic correlation. *J Comput Assist Tomogr* 19:15–22, 1995

Leroy V, Whiteman ML, Post MJ, et al: Four years of natural history of HIV-1 infection in African women: a prospective cohort study in Kigali (Rwanda), 1988–1993. *J Acquir Immune Defic Syndr Hum Retrovirol* 9:415–421, 1995

Levy WS, et al: Prevalence of cardiac abnormalities in human immunodeficiency virus infections. *Am J Cardiol* 63:86–89, 1989

Li VC, Clayton S, Cheng-Zhang C, et al: AIDS and sexual practices: knowledge, attitudes, behaviors, and practices of health professionals in the People's Republic of China. *AIDS Educ Prev* 4:1–5, 1992

Liao S, Choi KH, Zhang K, et al: Extremely low awareness of AIDS, sexually transmitted diseases and condoms among Dai ethnic villagers in Yunnan province, China. *AIDS* 11:S27–S34, 1997

Lindan CP, Lieu TX, Giang LT, et al: Rising HIV infection rates in Ho Chi Minh City herald emerging AIDS epidemic in Vietnam. *AIDS* 11:S5–S13, 1997

Logan PM, Finnegan MM: Pulmonary complications in AIDS: CT appearances. *Clin Radiol* 53:567–573, 1998

Long R: The chest roentgenogram in pulmonary tuberculosis patients seropositive for human immunodeficiency virus type 1. *Chest* 99:123–127, 1991

Long PF: A retrospective study of *Nocardia* infections associated with the acquired immune deficiency syndrome (AIDS) [letter]. *Infection* 22:362–364, 1994

Long R, Scalcini M, Manfreda J, et al: Impact of human immunodeficiency virus type 1 on tuberculosis in rural Haiti. *Am Rev Respir Dis* 143:69–73, 1991

Louthrenoo W, Thamprasert K, Sirisanthana T, et al: Osteoarticular penicilliosis marneffei. A report of eight cases and review of the literature. *Br J Rheumatol* 33:1145–1150, 1994

Lubat E, Megibow AJ, Balthazar EJ, et al: Extrapulmonary *Pneumocystis carinii* infection in AIDS: CT findings. *Radiology* 174:157–160, 1990

Lucas SB: Missing infections in AIDS. *Trans R Soc Trop Med Hyg* 84:34–38, 1990

Lucas SB, Diomande M, Hounnou A, et al: HIV-associated lymphoma in Africa: an autopsy study in Cote D'Ivoire. *Int J Cancer* 59:20–24, 1994

Lucas SB, Hounnou A, Peacock C, et al: The mortality and pathology of HIV infection in a west African city [see comments]. *AIDS* 7:1569–1579, 1993

Lucas SB, Hounnou A, Peacock C, et al: Nocardiosis in HIV-positive patients: an autopsy study in West Africa. *Tuber Lung Dis* 75:301–307, 1994

Lucas SB, Peacock CS, Hounnou A, et al: Disease in children infected with HIV in Abidjan, Cote d'Ivoire [see comments]. *BMJ* 312:335–338, 1996

Maher D, Hoffman I: Prevalence of genital infections in medical inpatients in Blantyre, Malawi. *J Infect* 31:77–78, 1995

Major NM, Tehranzadeh J: Musculoskeletal manifestations of AIDS. *Radiol Clin North Am* 35:1167–1189, 1997

Makris AN, Sher S, Bertoli C, et al: Pulmonary strongyloidiasis: an unusual opportunistic pneumonia in a patient with AIDS. *AJR* 161:545–547, 1993

Malin AS, Gwanzura LK, Klein S, et al: *Pneumocystis carinii* pneumonia in Zimbabwe [see comments]. *Lancet* 346:1258–1261, 1995

Mamun KZ, Cheesbrough JS: An assessment of the lower limit of specificity of the clinical definition of AIDS in Africa. *AIDS* 3:323–324, 1989

Manfredi R, Costigliola P, Ricchi E, et al: Sepsis bacteraemia and other infections due to non-opportunistic bacterial pathogens in a consecutive series of 788 patients hospitalized for HIV infection. *Clin Ther* 143:279–290, 1993

Markovitz DM: Infection with the human immunodeficiency virus type 2. *Ann Intern Med* 118:211–218, 1993

Marshall JB: Tuberculosis of the gastrointestinal tract and peritoneum. *Am J Gastroenterol* 88:989–999, 1993

Martin DJ, Schoub BD, Miller GB, et al: AIDS and tuberculosis. *S Afr Med J* 78:533–535, 1990

Martin DJ, Sim JG, Sole GJ, et al: CD4+ lymphocyte count in African patients co-infected with HIV and tuberculosis [see comments]. *J Acquir Immune Defic Syndr Hum Retrovirol* 8:386–391, 1995

Matondo P, Sivapalan S: Sexually transmissible agent and African Kaposi's sarcoma [editorial]. *Int J STD AIDS* 7:4–6, 1996

Matondo P, Zumla A: The spectrum of African Kaposi's sarcoma: is it consequential upon diverse immunological responses? *Scand J Infect Dis* 28:225–230, 1996

Mawar N, Mehendale S, Thilakavathi S, et al: Awareness and knowledge of AIDS and HIV risk among women attending STD clinics in Pune, India. *Indian J Med Res* 106:212–222, 1997

Mbaga JM, Pallangyo KJ, Bakari M, et al: Surgical time of patients with acquired immune deficiency syndrome: experience with 274 patients in Dar-Es-Salaam. *East Afr Med J* 67:95–99, 1990

McGuinness G: Changing trends in the pulmonary manifestations of AIDS. *Radiol Clin North Am* 35:1029–1082, 1997

McGuinness G, Naidich DP, Garay S, et al: AIDS associated bronchiectasis: CT features. *J Comput Assist Tomogr* 17:260–266, 1993

McGuinness G, Scholes JV, Garay SM, et al: Cytomegalovirus pneumonitis: spectrum of parenchymal CT findings with pathologic correlation in 21 AIDS patients. Radiology 192:451–459, 1994

McGuinness G, Gruden JF, Bhalla M, et al: AIDS-related airway disease. *AJR* 168:67–77, 1997

McLeod DT, Neill P, Gwanzura, Latif AS, et al: *Pneumocystis carinii* pneumonia in patients with AIDS in Central Africa. *Respir Med* 84:225–228, 1990

McMillan A, et al: Influence of human immunodeficiency virus infection on treponemal serology in patients who have been treated for syphilis. *J Infect* 21:95–103, 1990

Meeran K: Prevalence of HIV infection among patients with leprosy and tuberculosis in rural Zambia. *Br Med J* 298:364–365, 1989

Mhalu FS, Lyamuya E: Human immunodeficiency virus infection and AIDS in East Africa: challenges and possibilities for prevention and control. *East Afr Med J* 73:13–19, 1996

Michiels JF, Hofman P, Bernard E, et al: Intestinal and extraintestinal *Isospora belli* infection in an AIDS patient. A second case report. *Pathol Res Pract* 190:1089–1094, 1994

Miles PR, Baughman RP, Linnemann CC Jr: Cytomegalovirus in the bronchoalveolar lavage fluid of patients with AIDS. *Chest* 97:1072–1076, 1990

Miller RA: Leprosy and AIDS: a review of the literature and speculations on the impact of CD4+ lymphocyte depletion on immunity to *Mycobacterium leprae*. *Int J Lepr* 59:639–644, 1991

Miller WT Jr, Edelman JM, Miller WT: Cryptococcal pulmonary infection in patients with AIDS: radiographic appearance. *Radiology* 175:725–728, 1990

Miszkiel KA: Spectrum of MRI findings in CNS cryptococcosis in AIDS. *Clin Radiol* 51. 12:842–850, 1996

Modilevsky, T, Sattler FR, Barnes PF: Mycobacterial disease in patients with human immunodeficiency virus infection. *Arch Intern Med* 149:2201–2205, 1989

Molinert HT, Garcia EG, Cruz RR: Prevention of infection with human immunodeficiency virus in Cuba. *PAHO Bull* 23:62–67, 1989

Montano MA, Novitsky VA, Blackard JT, et al: Divergent transcriptional regulation among expanding human immunodeficiency virus type 1 subtypes. *J Virol* 71:8657–8665, 1997

Moore EH, Russell LA, Klein JS, et al: Bacillary angiomatosis in patients with AIDS: multiorgan imaging findings. *Radiology* 197:67–72, 1995

Moosa MY, Coovadia YM: Cryptococcal meningitis in Durban, South Africa: a comparison of clinical features, laboratory findings, and outcome for human immunodeficiency virus (HIV)-positive and HIV-negative patients. *Clin Infect Dis* 24:131–134, 1997

Moreira ED Jr, Silva N, Brites C, et al: Characteristics of the acquired immunodeficiency syndrome in Brazil. *Am J Trop Med Hyg* 48:687–692, 1993

Morgello S, Cho E-S, Nielsen S, et al: Cytomegalovirus encephalitis in patients with acquired immunodeficiency syndrome. *Hum Pathol* 18:289–297, 1987

Morgello S, Soifer FM, Lin CS, et al: Central nervous system *Strongyloides stercoralis* in acquired immunodeficiency syndrome: a report of two cases and review of the literature. *Acta Neuropathol (Berl)* 86:285–288, 1993

Mulder D, Nunn A, Kamali A, et al: Decreasing HIV-1 seroprevalence in young adults in a rural Ugandan cohort [see comments]. *BMJ* 311:833–836, 1995

Murphy D: *The Ukimwi road from Kenya to Zimbabwe*. J. Murray, London, 1983

Murray JF: Tuberculosis and HIV infection: global perspectives. *Respirology* 2:209–213, 1997

Murray JF, Mills J: Pulmonary infectious complications of human immunodeficiency virus infection. *Am Rev Respir Dis* 141:1356–1372, 1990

Naidich DP, Garay SM, Leitman BS, et al: Radiographic manifestations of pulmonary disease in the acquired immunodeficiency syndrome (AIDS). *Semin Roentgenol* 22:14–30, 1987

Narain JP, Hull B, Hospedales CJ, et al: Epidemiology of AIDS and HIV infection in the Caribbean. *PAHO Bull* 23:42–49, 1989

Nathoo KJ, Chigonde S, Nhembe M, et al: Community-acquired bacteremia in human immunodeficiency virus-infected children in Harare, Zimbabwe. *Pediatr Infect Dis J* 15:1092–1097, 1996

Ng'weshemi JZ, Boerma JT, Pool R, et al: Changes in male sexual behaviour in response to the AIDS epidemic: evidence from a cohort study in urban Tanzania. *AIDS* 10:1415–1420, 1996

Nikpoor N, Drum DE, Aliabadi P: Gastric uptake of gallium-67 in AIDS. *J Nucl Med* 33:643–645, 1992

Nunn P, Kibuga D, Elliott A, et al: Impact of human immunodeficiency virus on transmission and severity of tuberculosis. *Trans R Soc Trop Med Hyg* 84:9–13, 1990

Nyberg DA, Federle MP, Jeffrey RB, et al: Abdominal CT findings of disseminated *Mycobacterium avium* in AIDS. *AJR* 145:297–299, 1985

Odehouri K, De Cock KM, Krebs JW, et al: HIV-1 and HIV-2 infection associated with AIDS in Abidjan, Cote d'Ivoire. *AIDS* 3:509–512, 1989

Oksenhendler E, Cadranel J, Sarfati C, et al: *Toxoplasma gondii* pneumonia in patients with the acquired immunodeficiency syndrome. *Am J Med* 88:18N–21N, 1990

Oldham SAA, Castillo M, Jacobson FL, et al: HIV-associated lymphocytic interstitial pneumonia: radiologic manifestations and pathologic correlation. *Radiology* 170:83–87, 1989

Padovani B, et al: Sarcome de Kaposi pulmonaire chez les patients atteints du syndrome d'immunodeficience acquise (SIDA). Apport de al radiographie du thorax et du scanner. *J Radiol* 74:467–472, 1993

Pais P, HIV and India: looking into the abyss. *Trop Med Int Health* 1:295–304, 1996

Pantongrag-Brown T et al: Frequency of abdominal CT findings in AIDS patients with *M. avium* complex bacteraemia. *Clin Radiol* 53:816–819, 1998

Pape JW, Verdier RI, Boncy M, et al: *Cyclospora* infection in adults infected with HIV. Clinical manifestations, treatment, and prophylaxis. *Ann Intern Med* 121:654–657, 1994

Paxton LA: Community based study of treatment seeking among subjects with symptoms of sexually transmitted disease in Uganda. *Br Med J* 317:1630–1631, 1998

Pela AO, Platt JJ: AIDS in Africa: emerging trends. *Soc Sci Med* 28:1–8, 1989

Pfutzner A, Dietrich U, von Eichel U, et al: HIV-1 and HIV-2 infections in a high-risk population in Bombay, India: evidence for the spread of HIV-2 and presence of a divergent HIV-1 subtype. *J Acquir Immune Defic Syndr* 5:972–977, 1992

Pillay T, Pillay DG, Bramdev A: Disseminated histoplasmosis in a human immunodeficiency virus-infected African child. *Pediatr Infect Dis J* 16:417–418, 1997

Pincus PS, Sandler MA, Naude GE, et al: Multiple pulmonary cavities – an unusual complication of *Pneumocystis carinii* pneumonia. *S Afr med J* 72:871–872, 1987

Pitchenik AE: Tuberculosis control and the AIDS epidemic in developing countries. *Ann Intern Med* 113:89–91, 1990

Pitchenik AE, Robinson HA: The radiographic appearance of tuberculosis in patients with the acquired immune deficiency syndrome (AIDS) and pre-AIDS. *Am Rev Respir Dis* 131:393–396, 1985

Pomeroy C, Filice GA: Pulmonary toxoplasmosis: a review. *Clin Infect Dis* 14:863–870, 1992

Poon TP, Tschertkoff V, Pares GF, et al: Spinal cord toxoplasma lesion in AIDS: MR findings. *J Comput Assist Tomogr* 16:817–819, 1992

Popovich MJ, Arthur RH, Helmes E: CT of intracranial cryptococcosis. *AJNR* 11:139–142, 1990

Post MJD, Hensley GT, Moskowitz LB, et al: Cytomegalic inclusion virus encephalitis in patients with AIDS: CT, clinical, and pathologic correlation. *AJNR* 7:275–280, 1986

Post FA, Wood R, Maartens G: CD4 and total lymphocyte counts as predictors of HIV disease progression. *Q J med* 89:505—508, 1996

Prazuck T, Yameogo JM, Heylinck B, et al: Mother-to-child transmission of human immunodeficiency virus type 1 and type 2 and dual infection: a cohort study in Banfora, Burkina Faso. *Pediatr Infect Dis J* 14:940–947, 1995

Prosper M, Omene JA, Ledlie S, et al: Clinical significance of resolution of chest X-ray findings in HIV-infected children with lymphocytic interstitial pneumonitis (LIP). *Pediatr Radiol* 25:S243–S246, 1995

Provenzale JM, Jinkins JR: Brain and spine imaging findings in AIDS patients. *Radiol Clin North Am* 35:1127–1166, 1997

Purvis SF, Katongole-Mbidde E, Johnson JL, et al: High incidence of Kaposi's sarcoma-associated herpesvirus and Epstein-Barr virus in tumor lesions and peripheral blood mononuclear cells from patients with Kaposi's sarcoma in Uganda. *J Infect Dis* 175:947–950, 1997

Quinn TC: The epidemiology of the acquired immunodeficiency syndrome in the 1990s. *Emerg Med Clin North Am* 13:1–25, 1995

Quinn TC, Zacarias RK, St John RK: HIV and HTLV-I infections in the Americas: a regional perspective. *Medicine* 68:189–209, 1989

Radin DR: Disseminated histoplasmosis: abdominal CT findings in 16 patients. *AJR* 157:955–958, 1991

Radin DR: Intraabdominal *Mycobacterium tuberculosis* vs *Mycobacterium avium-intracellulare* infections in patients with AIDS: distinction based on CT findings. *AJR* 156:487–491, 1991

Radin R: HIV infection: analysis in 259 consecutive patients with abnormal abdominal CT findings. *Radiology* 197:712–722, 1995

Radin DR, Baker EL, Klatt EC, et al: Visceral and nodal calcification in patients with AIDS-related *Pneumocystis carinii* infection. *AJR* 154:27–31, 1990

Rankin JA, Collman R, Daniele RP: Acquired immune deficiency syndrome and the lung. *Chest* 94:155–164, 1988

Rao KS, et al: Sexual lifestyle of long distance lorry drivers in India: questionnaire survey. *Br med J* 318:162–163, 1999

Redvanly RD, Silverstein JE: Intra-abdominal manifestations of AIDS. *Radiol Clin North Am* 35:1083–1125, 1997

Richards PJ, et al: Chest imaging in AIDS (review). *Clin Radiol* 53:554–556, 1998

Rigsby MO, Curtis AM: Pulmonary disease from nontuberculous mycobacteria in patients with human immunodeficiency virus. *Chest* 106:913–919, 1994

Rodgers W, Yodlowski M, Mintzer C: Pyomyositis in patients who have the human immunodeficiency virus. *J Bone Joint Surg [Am]* 75:588–592, 1993

Rodrigues LG, Chequer P: AIDS in Brazil, 1982–1988. *PAHO Bull* 23:30–34, 1989

Rodriguez WL, Ramirez-Ronda CH: CNS involvement in AIDS patients as seen with CT and MR: a review. *Assoc Med Puerto Rico* 83:548–551, 1991

Roldan EO, Moskowitz L, Hensley GT: Pathology of the heart in AIDS. *Arch Pathol Lab Med* 111:943–946, 1987

Roles NC: Ritual surgery in East Africa. *East Afr Med J* 43:579–594, 1966

Rosenberg Z, Norman A, Solomon G: Arthritis associated with HIV infection: radiographic manifestations. *Radiology* 173:171–176, 1989

Rosenblum MK: Human immunodeficiency virus infection. Lesions of the central nervous system. In: Connor DH, ed., *The pathology of infectious diseases.* Appleton and Lange, Stamford, 1997, pp 183–197

Rotterdam H: *Microbacterium avium* complex (MAC) infection. In: Connor DH, ed. *The pathology of infectious diseases.* Appleton and Lange, Stamford, 1997, pp 657–669

Rottenberg GT: Fulminant *Toxoplasma gondii* pneumonia in a patient with AIDS. *Clin Radiol* 52:472–473, 1997

Saksena NK, Wang B, Ge YC, et al: Coinfection and genetic recombination between HIV-1 strains: possible biological implications in Australia and South East Africa. *Ann Acad Med Singapore* 26:121–127, 1997

Sandhu JS, Goodman PC: Pulmonary cysts associated with *Pneumocystis carinii* pneumonia in patients with AIDS. *Radiology* 173:33–35, 1989

Saran R, Gupta AK: HIV-2 and HIV-1/2 seropositivity in Bihar. *Indian J Public Health* 39:119–120, 1995

Sauda FC, Zamarioli LA, Ebner Filho W, et al: Prevalence of *Cryptosporidium* sp. *Isospora belli* among AIDS patients attending Santos Reference Center for AIDS, Sao Paulo, Brazil. *J Parasitol* 79:454–456, 1993

Sewankambo N, Mugerwa RD, Goodgame R: Enteropathic AIDS in Uganda. An endoscopic, histological and microbiological study. *AIDS* 1:9–13, 1987

Shah RM, Kaji AV, Ostrum BJ, et al: Interpretation of chest radiographs in AIDS patients: usefulness of CD4 lymphocyte counts. *Radiographics* 17:47–61, 1997

Shanley DJ: Tuberculosis of the spine: imaging features. *AJR* 164:659–664, 1995

Shapiro JM, Romney BM, Weiden MD, et al: *Rhodococcus equi* endobronchial mass with lung abscess in a patient with AIDS. *Thorax* 47:62–63, 1992

Siegel RJ: Human immunodeficiency virus infection lesions in the pediatric AIDS group. In: Connor DH, ed. *The pathology of infectious diseases.* Appleton and Lange, Stamford, pp 161–168, 1997

Simmons JT, Suffredini AF, Lack EE, et al: Nonspecific interstitial pneumonitis in patients with AIDS: radiologic features. *AJR* 149:265–268, 1987

Siraprapasiri T, Thanprasertsuk S, Rodklay A, et al: Risk factors for HIV among prostitutes in Chiangmai, Thailand. *AIDS* 5:579–582, 1991

Sitas F, Taylor L, Madhoo J, et al: Occurrence of human herpes virus 8 in Kaposi's sarcoma and other tumours in South Africa [letter]. *S Afr Med J* 87:1020–1022, 1997

Sitas F, Bezwoda WR, Levin V, et al: Association between human immunodeficiency virus type 1 infection and cancer in the black population of Johannesburg and Soweto, South Africa. *Br J Cancer* 75:1704–1707, 1997

Sor S, Levine MS, Kowalski TE, et al: Giant ulcers of the esophagus in patients with human immunodeficiency virus:

clinical, radiographic, and pathologic findings. *Radiology* 194:447–451, 1995

Srikanth P, John TJ, Jeyakumari H, et al: Epidemiological features of acquired immunodeficiency syndrome in southern India. *Indian J Med Res* 105:191–197, 1997

Stansell JD: Fungal disease in HIV-infected persons: cryptococcosis, histoplasmosis, and coccidioidomycosis. *J Thorac Imaging* 6:28–35, 1991

Staples CA, Kang EY, Wright JL, et al: Invasive pulmonary aspergillosis in AIDS: radiographic, CT, and pathologic findings. *Radiology* 196:409–414, 1995

Steffen HM, et al: Kardiale Beteiligung im Rahmen der HIV-1-Infektion: vorläufige Ergebnisse einer echokardiographischen Untersuchung. *Zet Fur Kardiol* 79:83–88, 1990

Stein N, Spencer D, Kantor A, et al: Radiation therapy in epidemic, AIDS-related Kaposi's sarcoma in southern Africa. *Tumori* 80:216–219, 1994

Stein ME, Lachter J, Spencer D, et al: Chemotherapy for AIDS-related and endemic African Kaposi's sarcoma in southern Africa. *Int J Dermatol* 34:729–732, 1995

Steinbach LS, Tehranzadeh J, Fleckenstein JL, et al: Human immunodeficiency virus infection: musculoskeletal manifestations. *Radiology* 186:833–838, 1993

Styblo K: The impact of HIV infection on the global epidemiology of tuberculosis. *Bull Int Union Tuberc Lung Dis* 66:27–32, 1991

Supparatpinyo K, Khamwan C, Baosoung V, et al: Disseminated *Penicillium marneffei* infection in southeast Asia. *Lancet* 344:110–113, 1994

Suster B, Akerman M, Orenstein M, et al: Pulmonary manifestations of AIDS: review of 106 episodes. *Radiology* 161:87–93, 1996

Sze G, Brant-Zawadzki MN, Norman D, et al: The neuroradiology of AIDS. *Semin Roentgenol* 22:42–53, 1987

Tarimo DS, Kilewo JZ, Minjas JN, et al: Prevalence of intestinal parasites in adult patients with enteropathic AIDS in north-eastern Tanzania. *East Afr Med J* 73:397–399, 1996

Teixidor HS, Godwin TA, Ramirez EA: Cryptosporidiosis of the biliary tract in AIDS. *Radiology* 180:51–56, 1991

Tien RD, Chu PK, Hesselink JR: Intracranial cryptococcosis in immunocompromised patients: CT and MR findings in 29 cases. *AJNR* 12:283–289, 1991

Tien RD, Gean-Marton AD, Mark AS: Neurosyphilis in HIV carriers: MR findings in six patients. *AJR* 158:1325–1328, 1992

Todd J, Balira R, Grosskurth H, et al: HIV-associated adult mortality in a rural Tanzanian population. *AIDS* 11:801–807, 1997

Townsend RR: CT of AIDS-related lymphoma. *AJR* 156:969–974, 1991

Traill ZC, Miller RF, Alin N, et al: *Pseudomonas aeruginosa* bronchopulmonary infection in patients with advanced human immunodeficiency virus disease. *Br J Radiol* 69:1099–1103, 1996

Tshibwabwa-Tumba E, Mwinga A, Pobee JO, et al: Radiological features of pulmonary tuberculosis in 963 HIV-infected adults at three Central African Hospitals. *Clin Radiol* 52:837–841, 1997

Tyndall MW, Ronald AR, Agoki E, et al: Increased risk of infection with human immunodeficiency virus type 1 among uncircumcised men presenting with genital ulcer disease in Kenya. *Clin Infect Dis* 23:449–453, 1996

U.N./W.H.O. AIDS epidemic update – December 1998. Report of the joint U.N. Programme on HIV/AIDS. UNAIDS. Geneva, 1998

Uttamchandani RB, Daikos GL, Reyes RR, et al: Nocardiosis in 30 patients with advanced human immunodeficiency virus infection: clinical features and outcome. *Clin Infect Dis* 18:348–353, 1994

Vanarthos WJ, et al: Diagnostic use of nuclear medicine in AIDS (review). *Radiographics* 12:731–752, 1992

Vetter KM, Djomand G, Zadi F, et al: Clinical spectrum of human immunodeficiency virus disease in children in a west African city. Project RETRO-CI. *Pediatr Infect Dis J* 15:438–442, 1996

von Reyn CF, Waddell RD, Eaton T, et al: Isolation of *Mycobacterium avium* complex from water in the United States, Finland, Zaire, and Kenya. *J Clin Microbiol* 31:3227–3330, 1993

Wall SD, Jones B: Gastrointestinal tract in the immunocompromised host: opportunistic infections and other complications. *Radiology* 185:327–335, 1992

Wall SE, Friedman SL, Margulis AR, et al: Gastrointestinal Kaposi's sarcoma in AIDS: radiographic manifestations. *J Clin Gastroenterol* 6:165–171, 1984

Wasser L, Talavera W: Pulmonary cryptococcosis in AIDS. *Chest* 92:692–695, 1987

Wehn SM, Heinz ER, Burger FC, et al: Dilated Virchow-Robin spaces in cryptococcal meningitis associated with AIDS: CT and MR findings. *J Comput Assist Tomogr* 13:756–762, 1989

Weissman D, Barker TD, Fauci AS: The efficiency of acute infection of CD4+ T cells is markedly enhanced in the setting of antigen-specific immune activation. *J Exp Med* 183:687–692, 1996

Weniger BG, Quinhoes EP, Sereno AB, et al: A simplified surveillance case definition of AIDS derived from empirical clinical data. *J Acquir Immune Defic Syndr* 5:1212–1223, 1992

Wheeler VW, Radcliffe KW: HIV infection in the Caribbean [editorial]. *Int J STD AIDS* 5:79–89, 1994

Whiteman M, Espinoza L, Post MJD, et al: Central nervous system tuberculosis in HIV-infected patients: clinical and radiographic findings. *AJNR* 16:1319–1327, 1995

Wicky S, Cartei F, Mayor B, et al: Radiological findings in nine AIDS patients with *Rhodococcus equi* pneumonia. *Eur Radiol* 6:826–830, 1996

Wolff SD, Kuhlman JE, Fishman EK: Thoracic Kaposi sarcoma in AIDS: CT findings. *J Comput Assist Tomogr* 17:60–63, 1993

World Health Report 1998. *Life in the 21th Century.* World Health Organisation Geneva, 1998

Wyatt SH, Fishman EK: The acute abdomen in individuals with AIDS (review). *Radiol Clin North Am* 32:1023–1043, 1994

Yee J, Wawl S: Gastrointestinal manifestations of AIDS (review). *Gastroenterol Clin North Am* 24:413–434, 1995

Zibrak JD, Silvestri RC, Costello P: Bronchoscopic and radiologic features of Kaposi's sarcoma involving the respiratory system. *Chest* 4:476–479, 1986

Zimmerman PA, Buckler-White A, Alkhatib G, et al: Inherited resistance to HIV-1 conferred by an inactivating mutation in CC chemokine receptor 5: studies in populations with contrasting clinical phenotypes, defined racial background, and quantified risk. *Mol Med* 3:23–36, 1997

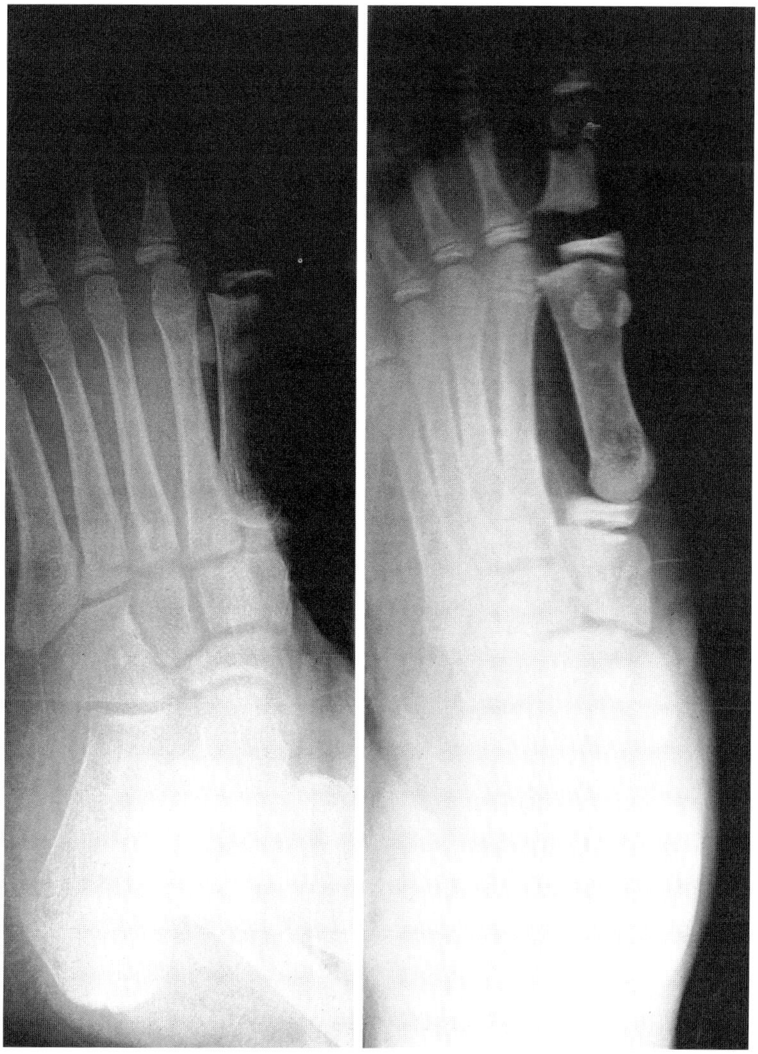

Ex Africa semper aliquid nova.
(Ascribed, perhaps incorrectly, to Pliny)

A young African girl, working in the fields, was bitten in the foot by a snake; she went to the nearest small hospital, where she was treated by Dr. Nutt. When she went home, she was also treated by her traditional practitioner. After a good mixture of Western and African medicine the snake bite was almost forgotten but the whole foot had become infected. An enormous slough developed and discharged pus; she went back to her nearest hospital for daily dressings as ordered by Dr. Nutt and carried out by the African nursing aide. One day, during the dressing, the shaft of the first metatarsal fell out. The nursing aide was rather concerned, looked quickly over his shoulder and replaced the missing bone and bandaged the foot again. Because her progress was not satisfactory, the radiograph was taken to exclude bone infection, which, indeed, it did. (From Palmer, in *"Current status of skeletal roentgenology"*, University of Miami, 1966).

Subject Index*

* (i) pages referring volume 1; (ii) pages referring volume 2.